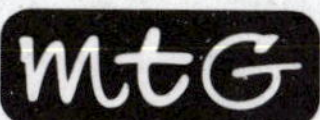

AIIMS EXPLORER

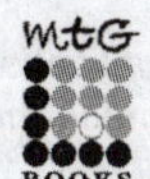

MTG Books

(A unit of MTG Learning Media (P) Ltd.)

New Delhi | Gurgaon

Price : ₹ 375

Revised Edition : August 2014

Published by : **MTG Books**
(A Unit of MTG Learning Media Pvt. Ltd.)

Corporate Office : Plot 99, Sector 44 Institutional Area, Gurgaon, Haryana-122003.
Phone : 0124 - 4951200. Web: mtg.in Email: info@mtg.in

Registered Office : 406, Taj Apt., Ring Road, Near Safdarjung Hospital, New Delhi-110029

Printed at Rajkamal Electric Press, Plot No. 2, Phase-IV, Kundli, Haryana.

Visit **www.mtg.in** for buying books online.

Contents

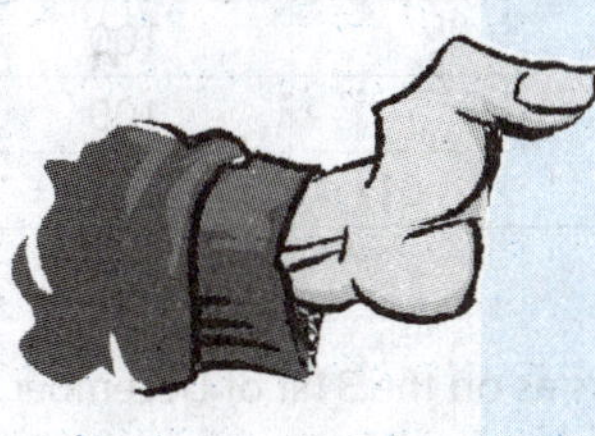

About*

All India Institute of Medical Sciences (AIIMS)

AIIMS, New Delhi conducts MBBS Entrance Test for admission into AIIMS New Delhi and 6 other AIIMS Institutions in India. All India Institute of Medical Sciences (AIIMS) is an autonomous Institution of national importance that awards its own medical degrees and other academic distinctions. The degrees awarded by the Institute are recognised medical qualifications for the purpose of the Indian Medical Council Act and equivalent and treated at par with medical degrees conferred by other Universities.

The Institute (AIIMS, New Delhi) is a residential University in which the faculty members, staff and the students live on campus. There are 8 hostels for undergraduate students (6 for boys and 2 for girls) with a capacity to accommodate 850 students.

Six Other AIIMS

Under the Pradhan Mantri Swasthya Suraksha Yojana six new All India Institutes of Medical Sciences has been established similar to AIIMS New Delhi, there are at Bhopal, Patna, Jodhpur, Rishikesh, Raipur and Bhubaneswar.

Number of Seats and Reservation

S. No.	Location of AIIMS	UR	OBC	SC	ST	OPH	Foreign	Total
1.	New Delhi	37	19	11	05		01	73 (72 Indian)
2.	Bhopal	50	27	15	08			100
3.	Patna	50	27	15	08			100
4.	Jodhpur	50	27	15	08	3% Horizontal		100
5.	Rishikesh	50	27	15	08			100
6.	Raipur	50	27	15	08			100
7.	Bhubaneswar	50	27	15	08			100
Total		337	181	101	53		01	672

Eligibility

Age : He/She should have attained or will attain the age of 17 (seventeen) years as on the 31st of December of the year of admission.

Essential Qualifications: He/She should have passed the 12th Class under the 10+2 Scheme/ Senior School Certificate Examination or Intermediate Science (I.Sc.) or an equivalent examination of a recognised University/Board of any Indian State with ENGLISH, PHYSICS, CHEMISTRY and BIOLOGY.

Minimum Aggregate: He/She should have obtained a minimum of 60% marks in the case of General & OBC and 50% in case of SC/ST candidates in aggregate in ENGLISH, PHYSICS, CHEMISTRY and BIOLOGY.

Course Duration: Minimum 5½ academic years including one year's compulsory internship

Exam Centres: Ahmedabad, Bangaluru, Bhopal, Bhubaneswar, Chandigarh, Chennai, Dehradun, Delhi, Guwahati, Hyderabad, Jammu, Jodhpur, Kochi, Kolkata, Lucknow, Mumbai, Patna and Raipur.

** Subject to change. Please refer latest prospectus.*

Exam Pattern

The competitive entrance examination will be of 3½ hours duration and will have one paper consisting of 200 objective type (multiple choice and assertion-reason type) questions from Physics, Chemistry, Biology and General Knowledge. The distribution of questions is as follows:

Subject	Number of Questions
Total	200
Physics	60
Chemistry	60
Biology(Botany & Zoology)	60
General Knowledge	20

Scheme of Marking

Incorrect responses will be given negative marks. Each correct response will get a score of 1 mark and each incorrect response will get a score of -1/3 (minus-one-third). No credit will be given for the questions not answered. More than one response will be treated as wrong answer and negatively marked.

Standard of Examination

No syllabus for the examination has been prescribed by the Institute. However, the general standard of the competitive entrance examination will be that of 12th class under the 10+2 Scheme/Intermediate Science.

Language of Question Paper

Question paper will be provided either in English or in Hindi according to the choice of candidates. A candidate must select in the space provided in the application form whether he/she prefers to have the question paper in English or Hindi. This choice cannot be changed later at any stage.

Minimum Cut off Marks

Category	Minimum Cut-Off Marks
General including OPH belonging to General category	50%
OBC including OPH belonging to OBC category	45%
SC/ST including OPH belonging to SC/ST category	40%

Declaration of Results

The list of candidates who qualify for admission will be displayed on notice board of Examination Section, AIIMS. The result will also be available on AIIMS website www.aiimsexams.org. The mark of individual candidate will be made available on AIIMS website www.aiimsexams.org on completion of the admission process. Requests of re-evaluation/re-checking of answer sheet will not be entertained under any circumstances. Selected candidates are required to report to the respective AIIMS to undergo medical examination by a Medical Board consisting of Faculty Members set up by the respective Institute. If, in the assessment of the Medical Board, a candidate is found medically unfit to the course, then he/she will be not admitted and the decision of the Medical Board shall be final.

2014 AIIMS

SUCCESS STORY

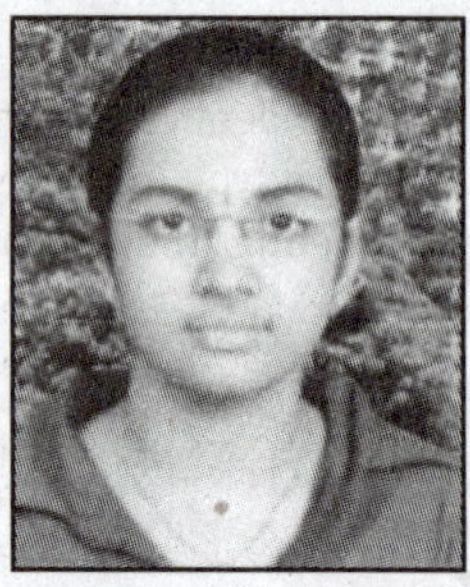

Pattisapu Srividya
1st Rank

- **What is your rank in other medical exams this year?**

I secured 9th rank in JIPMER, 7th in EAMCET, 8th in Manipal Medical Entrance exam and 59th in AIPMT.

- **How did you prepare for AIIMS 2014? How much time did you devote for AIIMS?**

Actually, I haven't particularly prepared for the AIIMS because I was not confident that I could make through it. But I was studying regularly for the other medical exams like JIPMER, EAMCET and AIPMT. I attribute my success to my love towards my studies. I really enjoy my studies but along with that I never compromise on my eight hours of sleep.

- **What is your dream in Medical studies?**

I wish to study more on molecular biology as I am extremely fond of this domain.

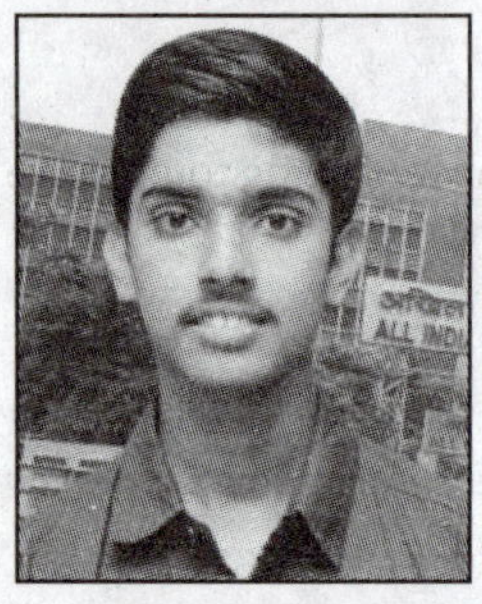

Arvind Subramanian
4th Rank

- **What is your rank in other medical exams this year? Did you target any specific exam to excel among others exams?**

I secured AIR 6, 17, 32 in KEAM, JIPMER, and AIPMT respectively. Yes, I put extra effort to crack Jawaharlal Institute of Postgraduate Medical Education & Research entrance examination. My mind was preoccupied with a desire to achieve good rank in JIPMER this year.

- **Please share your exam preparation strategy. How did you divide your preparation schedule among the three subjects?**

Preparation strategy was to work hard and have clarity on basic concepts of Physics, Chemistry and Biology subjects. I started preparing the various medical competitive examinations simultaneously with my intermediate examinations.

During my Intermediate first year, I invested a lot of time to strengthen Zoology and Botany subjects because these two subjects have vast theory part. Thus, Biology section demanded exam preparation to be started at early.

Then, as I entered Intermediate last year, I also focused on Physics. I made a point to attempt and solve at least 20 numerical a day within a set deadline to boost question-solving speed. This really helped me solve questions in time efficient manner during several entrance examinations.

- **What was your preparation strategy a month before AIIMS 2014 exam?**

A month before the AIIMS 2014 exam, I was busy in revising notes and solving previous years sample papers after 10-15 days. Revision exercise allowed me to analyse my weak area and brought good improvement in my exam preparation.

I also used to take 4-5 mock tests a week, which helped me to improve my question solving speed. And a day before the exam I indulged in activities like listening to music and playing video games to bust exam restlessness.

- **Which subject was the easiest and which was the toughest?**

Chemistry was the easiest section for me. Physics was the toughest as the questions were time consuming in nature.

- **Reasons to pursue MBBS? And your career plan after pursuing the course?**

My elder brother, an MBBS student at JIPMER, was my role model. My brother scored AIR 5 in AIPMT in the year 2011. He inspired me to enter this noble profession. I aspire to become neurologist.

Courtesy : careers360.com

AIIMS TOPPER'S TALK!

- **Why did you choose Medical/Bio stream?**

Ayush : I had passion from childhood to become a Doctor. I am associated with an NGO named Akhil Bharatiya Banvasi Kalyan Ashram, wherein I have supported 10-15 medical camps.

Archana : I appeared for medical entrance exams to enter into good medical college and realise my dream of becoming a good doctor.

Sankalp Dudeja : Basically, I belong to a family of doctors. Both of my parents are doctors. My brother is doing MBBS from M.A.M.C. So, I was naturally inclined towards medical stream.

- **Which exams you appeared for and what is your rank in those exams?**

Ayush : I have appeared in NEET, Manipal, JIPMER and AIIMS. My rank in Manipal is 88, JIPMER – AIR 13 and 5th rank in AIIMS.

Archana : I appeared in AIPMT(Rank 7), AIIMS(Rank1), JIPMER(Rank 1), K-CET(Rank 1), COMED K (Rank 1), Manipal UGET (Rank 1), Kerala PMT (Rank 37). I secured rank 22 in 14th National Science Olympiad (NSO) organised by Science Olympiad Foundation (SOF).

Sankalp : I appeared for the following exams – 1st Rank in AIIMS, DPMT, 3rd Rank in CBSE-PMT, 10th Rank in BHU (Screen.), 12th Rank in MAHE.

- **Any other achievements?**

Ayush : I secured AIR 2 in Kishore Vigyanik Purushkar Competition (KVPY) held in 2012, I cleared all the three olympiads NSEB, NSEP and NSEC and cleared 2nd stage of Chemistry as well as Biology Olympiad and I have attended the orientation-cum-selection camp for the International Biology Olympiad held at HBCSE in Mumbai.

My exact score subjectwise is: Physics-175/180, Chemistry-175/180 and Biology-341/360. My overall score is 691-720.

Archana : I am NTSE and KVPY scholar and secured 97.8 per cent in CBSE XII boards.

Sankalp : I am an NTSE scholar. I secured 2nd rank in 8th National Science Olympiad. I got 95.6% in board exams (12th class).

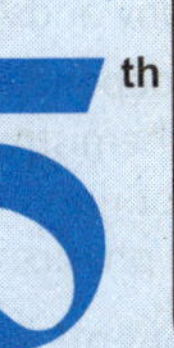

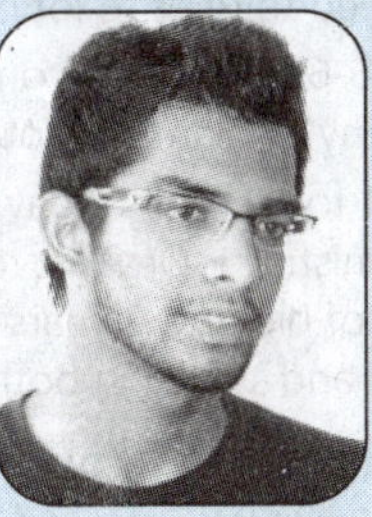

Ayush Goel
1st in NEET (2013)

"Students should do what they love to do, study with interest and passion and take time out for refreshment and should not restrict themselves in timeframes."

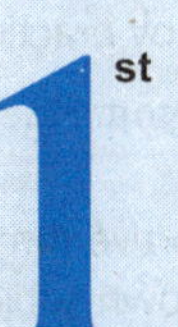

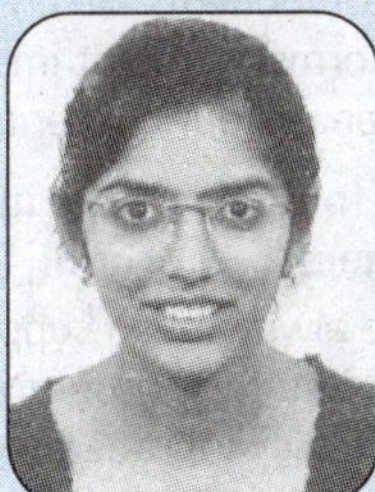

Archana Sasi (2012)
1st in JIPMER, K-CET COMED (K), UGET Manipal
7th in AIPMT
37th in Kerala PMT

"I would advise to readers to make themselves thorough with their concepts and practise objective questions extensively to achieve their goal."

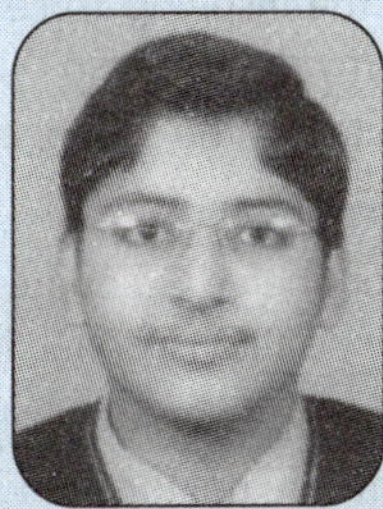

Sankalp Dudeja
1st in DPMT, 3rd in CBSE PMT & 10th in BHU (Screening)

"The stronger your concepts are the better rank you would secure. Be regular and steadfast in your studies. Have faith in God and confidence in yourself."

- **How did you prepare for the examination?**

Ayush : There is no specific topic or chapters to stress upon, however, I would say that less emphasis can be given to Physics and Chemistry because it does not need much revision as compared to Biology. One should spend more time in Biology with special reference to topics like 'Domestication', 'Plants', 'Pollution' etc., because they are data driven topics and we need to refer to lot of data around this subject.

Archana : I studied for 5-6 hours a day on a regular basis. I laid stress on organic Chemistry, mechanics in Physics, morphology and anatomy of plants in Botany and Animal Physiology.

Sankalp : I used to put 1 to 10 hours a day depending on time alloted to school, coaching etc., Physics - Mechanics, Electrostatics; Chemistry - Organic chemistry, Physical chemistry; Biology - Genetics, Taxonomy, Human physiology, Application of biology, 2 years of rigorous preparation is sufficient, I was weak in morphology, families, anatomy etc. in biology and strong in both physics & chemistry.

- **In your words what are the components of an ideal preparation plan?**

Ayush : First of all one should have love for subject he/she is studying, secondly, ample concentration and dedication towards the chosen subject. What you love, you should do that first and it should not be forced on you. Interact more with teachers and friends. Take suitable breaks from study, refresh your mind and come back to study again. Do not restrict yourselves in certain timeframes.

Archana : An ideal preparation plan needs to distribute time evenly subjectwise and topicwise; should be feasible with breaks added suitably and needs to be followed sincerely.

Sankalp : I think the components of an ideal preparation plan are reading understanding application. Of these, 'understanding' forms the most important part (which according to me, is the rank deciding factor). After understanding application of your concepts by practicing the objective questions is also very important.

- **What role did the following play in your success?**
(a) parents (b) teachers (c) school

Ayush : My parents have always been supportive throughout. They never forced me to study against my choice of subject. I was given freedom to choose my own subject. Teachers have been a great inspiration to me throughout my school time. They have encouraged me a lot. I witnessed a dramatic change in my life when I reached to class XIth from class Xth. The teachers' assistance I received during this phase, played an important role in my life and helped me to progress in my studies.

Archana : My parents supported me right throughout , inspiring me to follow my dreams though never putting pressure on me. My teachers made me raise my expectations for myself and were always there to clear my doubts. My school – National Public School, Indiranagar, Bangalore– helped to provide a platform and nurtured my skills. It also exposed me to various competitive exams that helped me find out where I stand.

Sankalp : Parents were the inspiring force behind me. They helped me at each and every step. My brother also helped a lot by clearing my doubts even during the wee hours of the day.

The regular tests conducted at the school also helped in keeping my schedule tight and myself always busy.

- **Your family background?**

Ayush : My father is a Commerce Graduate and is having his own Business. My mother is a housewife and my elder brother is a Doctor in Hindu Rao Hospital, New Delhi.

Archana : My father is the Vice President of Total Gaz India and my mother is an Ophthalmologist.

Sankalp : Both my parents are doctors and are running a private hospital in Sonipat. My elder brother (who got 10th rank in CBSE-PMT last year) is doing MBBS from M.A.M.C.

- **How have our various products like explorers, magazine etc. helped you in your preparation?**

Ayush : The Last Years' Solved Papers of different PMTs in MTG 'Biology Today' Magazine did help me to some extent. It helped me to brush up the topics. The Solved Papers give an idea about the pattern of questions.

Archana : I did not use MTG magazines but found the Objective Books very useful to practise MCQs.

Sankalp : I referred to AIIMS, CBSE-Mains and DPMT explorers for the questions asked in previous years.

- **What mistake you think you shouldn't have made?**

Ayush : I should have focussed more on solving questions rather than reading subjects. In last 2-3 months before the examination, students should focus more on solving questions.

Archana : My mistake was not giving enough focus to NCERT which especially in Biology should be read extensively since questions are often set directly from it.

Sankalp : Thankfully, by the guidance and experience of my parents and elder brother as well as of the teachers, I didn't make any such mistake.

- **What do you think is the secret of your success?**

Ayush : Great confidence on self, interest and passion for the subject. I was very confident on my preparation and was sure of myself to get selected.

Archana : The secret of my success is practising previous years' question papers from different medical entrance exams. The pattern being similar and questions often being repeated, gives a good practice.

Sankalp : There is nothing secret about my success. I worked hard, got proper guidance and took the exams seriously and got this result.

- **Had you not been selected then what would have been your future plan?**

Ayush : I didn't plan that.

Archana : If I was not selected in AIIMS then I would have again attempted entrances next year after a year of intense studying.

Sanklap : I never thought about that.

- **What advice would you like to give our readers who are PMT aspirants?**

Ayush : (a) Trust your teachers. Ultimately, they are the ones who would surely guide you.
(b) Don't study for the sake of studying .
(c) Enjoy and have fun but work hard too.
(d) Never put yourself under too much pressure.
(e) Make friends, interact and study with them.

Archana : I would advise to readers to make themselves thorough with their concepts and practise objective questions extensively to achieve their goal.

Sankalp : I would advise all the PMT aspirants to understand the text rather than cramming. The stronger your concepts are the better rank you would secure. Be regular and steadfast in your studies. Have faith in God and confidence in yourself. ■■■

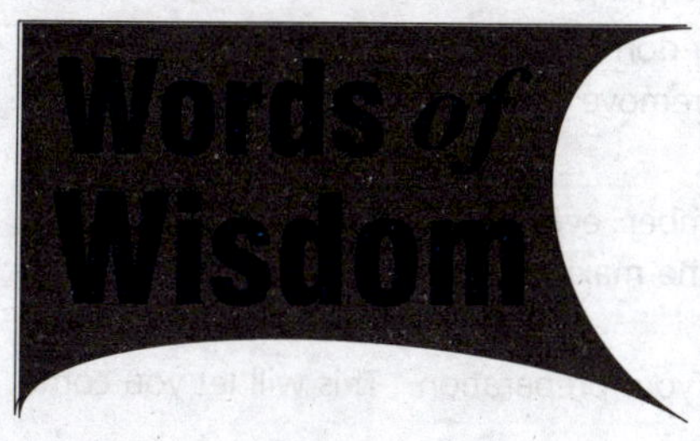

The success mantra is to study NCERT books rather than studying those heavy weight expensive materials. NCERT is the best way to clear your base and concepts in all the three subjects-Physics, Chemistry and Biology. Once your base is clear, scoring in AIPMT is easier for anyone.

Tejaswin Jha, 1st Rank in AIPMT 2014

One should devote two years in thorough and dedicated study during class 11th and 12th to prepare for medical entrance exams. But if somebody starts from class 10 only, then its even better !! Students must take proper guidance from school and coaching and study from good reference books along with NCERT textbooks.

Shreyasi Manish Shah, 4th Rank in AIPMT 2014

How to Prepare For AIIMS

By Sajanjiv S. Nagpal, 2nd Rank in AIIMS 2004

All India Institute of Medical Sciences is the dream destination of all medical aspirants. The exam is quite well known for its different pattern. The charisma attached with the meagre number of seats also makes it a tough deal. About 60,000 candidates appear in the exam out of which only 34 (General Category) make their way through to the institute.

Pattern of the exam

The exam consists of 200 questions out of which 40 are multiple choice questions in the subjects of Physics, Chemistry, Biology each, 20 in G.K. and the rest 60 are Assertion-Reason type questions equally divided between the subjects of Physics, Chemistry and Biology.

AIIMS V/s other PMTs

The paper of AIIMS is quite different from other PMT exams and demands a little care during the preparation for an assured selection. The questions asked are not that straight-forward as they might appear at first sight. It requires concentration, presence of mind and above all confidence that whatever you are marking is true and that you are doing full justice to the question. It is popularly but wrongly believed that graduation level studies are required for AIIMS preparation. It is not. Concentrate on the basics.

Requirements of a good AIIMS preparation plan

- ✓ Don't over-expect. Don't take an extra pressure on your head for AIIMS preparation. The other tensions are already enough.
- ✓ Just keep cool and prepare but keep in mind that for any other PMT and so also AIIMS you should go through the text thoroughly.
- ✓ Don't simply cram facts. Understanding is more important and definitely pays when required.
- ✓ Don't hesitate to clear your doubts. Don't have that feeling that you don't know anything. Everyone has his doubts. After all a rose also has thorns. You are the rose and have to remove your thorns one by one.
- ✓ Start from the important topics so that they are not left out.
- ✓ Try to do the maximum. But remember that you cannot remember everything. Its human to forget. Caution: Don't try to make this tip an excuse. You must remember the maximum as I said, if not everything. After all the competition demands you to be perfect.
- ✓ Share problems with parents. Be it be related to your emotions or to your preparation. This will let you come back on track and concentrate on your studies again.
- ✓ Concentrate on your G.K. You need to keep a track of the events of the past year, besides the basic facts. (HINT: Nobel prizes and other awards are very important)
- ✓ Have a clear concept. This will help you maximum during assertion reason type questions solving.
- ✓ Read quality magazines like Physics for you, Chemistry Today and Biology Today and not just any others of

the plethora available on the book stalls. These magazines present a wider application of the various concepts related to your studies. Such concepts are often asked in the AIIMS paper as assertion reason type or in the conventional MCQ type questions.

- ✓ Read HYFs available in the above mentioned magazines to revise a day before the examination as there is no time to go through the entire books again.

Strategies at the test centre and during the exam

- ✓ Have a light breakfast to avoid tiredness and sleepiness during the exam.
- ✓ Reach the test centre well in time to avoid any anxiety.
- ✓ Don't talk to people. They will always try to push you deep in the sea of pressure in which you are already floating. Try talking to your parents to keep yourself relaxed.
- ✓ Don't unnecessary feel that "I can't believe today is the AIIMS paper"; or "What will I do now, I am not prepared" and other self-demoralizing thoughts like these. Be relaxed, it is just another exam and not an appeal against a death sentence.
- ✓ Read the question carefully. A miss of a word and it could cost you a seat
- ✓ Plan the course of attempting the paper. Gauge its length. Otherwise 3.5 hours are enough I think.
- ✓ Don't go for absolutely wild guesses. Negative marking is stiff.
- ✓ Be careful about the correct marking of answers. Also ensure that the non-writing hand which we generally keep on the answer sheet does not have a pen mark or a stain which may spoil it.
- ✓ After the exam, feel relaxed. You have done what you could. Don't think much about the exam. Your job is over now. Now it is the examiner's turn.

THE BIGGEST MYTH

The biggest myth about the exam is that Assertion Reason type questions are a hurdle which cannot be crossed. For such questions read the text book thoroughly. Read the text book as if trying to find out a reason for every line written. With practice you will develop this habit and subconsciously grasp the chapter as if it written in the form of an Assertion and its Reason. Presence of mind is also required for proper judgement of the correct option especially the choice between a (if both A and R are true and R is the correct explanation of A) and b (if both A and R are true but R is not the correct explanation of A).

Practice such questions from the MTG magazines and MTG's publication, Assertion Reason Type questions for AIIMS.

Follow my suggestions, of course with your own modifications, for success in the exam.

ALL THE BEST!!!

CHAPTERWISE INDEX

PHYSICS

S.No.	Chapter's Name	1994 Ques. No.	Tot.	1995 Ques. No.	Tot.	1996 Ques. No.	Tot.	1997 Ques. No.	Tot.	1998 Ques. No.	Tot.	1999 Ques. No.	Tot.	2000 Ques. No.	Tot.
1	Units and Dimensions	19, 20, 24, 43	4	47, 50	2	42	1	41	1	3	1	40, 41	2	2, 46	2
2	Motion in One Dimension	6	1		0	24, 35	2	23	1		0		0	30	1
3	Motion in Two Dimensions	21	1		0	17, 21, 43	3	9, 11, 53. 56	4	2, 53	2	38, 39	2	53	1
4	Laws of Motion and Friction	12	1	53	1	19, 20, 22	3	10	1	36	1	34, 59	2	1	1
5	Work, Power and Energy	26, 31	2	3, 18, 34	3	16	1	45, 47, 48	3	4, 5, 13, 18	4	36, 47	2	3, 15, 48	3
6	Centre of Mass and Rotational Motion	27	1	15, 20, 36	3	46	1	31, 46, 58	3	1, 21	2	49	1	18, 23, 54	3
7	Gravitation	7, 9, 16, 32, 38, 40	6	6, 16, 31, 59, 60	5	58	1	2, 8, 36, 50, 60	5	28, 41	2	50	1	4, 5	2
8	Properties of Matter	4, 18, 37, 60	4	57	1	15	1	7, 20, 22, 39, 55	5	31, 39, 48	3	37, 44, 56	3		0
9	Oscillation	2	1	21, 32	2		0		0	9, 29, 47	3	35, 43, 45	3	50	1
10	Waves	56, 58	2	40, 48	2	2, 11, 23, 28, 40, 49	6	6, 21, 54	3	14, 24, 26, 30	4	46	1	14, 31	2
11	Heat and Thermo dynamics	1, 3, 8, 11, 15, 17, 35, 47, 49, 55, 59	11	5, 22, 30, 46, 49, 55	6	10, 18, 29, 31, 37, 41, 47, 56, 57	9	13, 24, 28, 30, 40, 49	6	15, 19, 22, 32, 34, 35, 42, 43, 44, 55	10	25, 31, 53	3	12, 13, 44, 45, 49, 58	6
12	Electrostatics	54	1	27, 29, 38	3		0	1, 27	2	12, 49, 50	3	16, 17, 32, 33, 51	5	17, 22, 26, 32, 39, 43	6
13	Current Electricity		0	10, 14, 17, 23, 42, 56, 58	7	3, 60	2	19, 29, 51	3	10	1	10, 52	2	16, 21, 38, 57	4
14	Thermal and chemical effects of current	29	1	26	1	9, 45	2		0	33	1	9	1	20	1
15	Magnetic Effects of Current		0		0		0	15, 27	2		0	3, 30, 57	3	24, 25, 34, 37, 41, 56	6
16	Magnetism		0	2, 25	2	5, 6, 38, 50	4		0	20, 23, 45	3	7, 20, 21, 28, 29, 42	6	35, 36, 60	3
17	Electromagnetic Induction and Alternating Current	10, 45	2	4, 43	2	36	1	12, 17, 26, 37	4	40, 56, 58	3	22, 23, 24	3	11, 33, 42	3
18	Electromagnetic Waves		0		0	33, 34, 59, 53	4	4	1	16, 27, 51	3	8, 19	2	27, 28	2
19	Ray Optics	5, 13, 23, 36, 57	5	28, 35, 44, 51, 52, 54	6	12, 13, 51	3	3, 5, 14, 25, 42, 52	6	6, 7, 37, 38, 46, 54 57, 59, 60	9	18, 27	2	8, 9, 10, 29, 52, 55, 59	7
20	Wave Optics		0		0		0		0			2, 26	2		0
21	Modern Physics	14, 25, 39, 41, 42, 44, 46, 48, 50, 52, 53	11	1, 7, 8, 9, 12, 24, 37, 39, 45	9	1, 4, 7, 8, 14, 25, 27, 30, 32, 39, 44, 48, 52, 54	14	32, 34, 38, 43, 44	5	8, 11, 17, 25, 52	5	1, 13, 14, 54, 55, 58, 60	7	6, 7, 40, 47, 51	5
22	Solids and Semiconductor Devices	22, 28, 30, 33, 34, 51	6	11, 13, 19, 33, 41	5	26, 55	2	16, 18, 33, 35, 59	5		0	4, 5, 6, 11, 12	5	19	1
23	Universe		0		0		0		0		0		0		0
24	Principle of Communication		0		0		0		0		0		0		0

USE THIS INDEX FOR TOPICWISE ANALYSIS OF LAST 14 YEARS AIIMS PAPERS AND REFER TO THESE QUESTIONS WHEN YOU ARE PRACTISING MCQ's CHAPTERWISE

2001		2002		2003		2004		2005		2006		2007	
Ques. No.	Tot.	Ques. No.	Tot.	Ques. No.	Tot.	Ques. No.	Tot.	Ques. No.	Tot.	Ques. No.	Tot.	Ques. No.	Tot.
6, 8, 14, 21, 48	5	1, 2, 50	3	29, 31	1	40	1	15, 39	2		0	9, 37	2
	0	4, 5, 20	3	29, 31	2	19	1		0	2	1	38	1
3, 54	2	3	1		0		0	32	1		0	30	1
51	1	51	0		0	55	1	18, 36, 42	3	20, 48	2	31	1
9, 13, 26, 44	4	21, 57	2	10	1	20	1	20, 21	2	15	1	40	1
2, 41	2	22	1	42	1	2, 15, 45	3	31, 33, 34, 35, 52	5	3, 46. 26	3	17, 18	2
16, 34, 45, 55, 59	5	23, 24, 31, 41, 58	5	1, 11, 47	3		0	22	1	51	1	16, 32, 56	3
33	1	32, 34, 39, 56	4	2, 12, 28, 36	4	5, 14, 52	3	23, 24, 30, 41, 60	5	5, 58	2	15, 33, 39, 55	4
17, 19	2	55, 59	2	14, 57	2	6	1	25	1		0	35	1
28, 50, 58	3	27, 28, 29, 30, 38, 53	6	35, 52	2	1, 23	2		0	4, 30, 36	3	36, 60	2
5, 7, 15, 18, 27, 31, 32, 43, 46,	9	33, 35, 36, 37, 54, 60	6	13, 23, 41, 53, 54, 56	6	12, 28, 39, 43, 53, 58	6	51, 53, 57, 58, 59	5	21, 22, 34, 35, 44, 47, 53, 55, 56	9	22, 34, 54, 57, 58	5
20, 23, 37, 48, 39	5	10, 11, 25	3	6, 19, 20, 24	4	10, 11, 26, 33	4	9, 38,40,	3	6, 12, 13, 24	4	5, 48	2
10, 36, 49, 60	4	40, 45	2	4, 30, 46	3	27	1	28	1		0	43, 50	2
12, 42	2	12	1		0	41	1		0		0	23	1
11	1	14	1	21, 27	2	16, 18, 35, 36	4		0	25	1	6, 7, 49	3
4	1	13, 47	2	22	1	29, 44, 50	3		0	7, 50	2	29, 47	2
29, 40	2	44, 46, 52	3	7, 49	2		0	4, 17, 27, 37	4	31, 59	2	4, 20, 51	3
35	1	15, 17	2	37, 38, 58	3		0	1, 19	2	41	1	13, 45	2
	0	6, 16, 19, 42	4	15, 25, 34, 50, 55	5	17, 22, 30, 42, 49	5	3, 6, 29, 43, 45, 50	6	1, 8, 11, 23, 37	5	1, 2, 21, 41	4
1, 25, 52	3	18, 26, 43, 48	4	16	1	21, 32, 48	3	14, 26, 47.	3	14, 17, 49	3	42	1
22, 24, 30, 47, 53, 57	6	9, 49	2	3, 5, 9, 17, 18, 26, 32, 33, 43, 44, 48, 51, 59, 60	14	3, 4, 7, 8, 9, 24, 25, 31, 34, 47, 51, 54, 56, 59, 60	15	7, 8, 11, 12, 46, 48, 54	7	9, 10, 18, 27, 28, 29, 32, 42, 45, 52, 57	11	8, 14, 24, 25, 26, 44, 52, 59	8
56	1	7, 8	2	8, 40, 45	3	13, 37, 38, 46, 57	5	2, 5, 10, 16, 44, 49, 55, 56	8	16, 19, 33, 38, 39, 43, 54	7	3, 11, 19, 27, 28, 46	6
	0		0		0		0	13	1		0		0
	0		0		0		0		0	40, 60	2	10, 12, 53	3

CHAPTERWISE INDEX

CHEMISTRY

S.No.	Chapter's Name	1994 Ques. No.	Tot.	1995 Ques. No.	Tot.	1996 Ques. No.	Tot.	1997 Ques. No.	Tot.	1998 Ques. No.	Tot.	1999 Ques. No.	Tot.
1	Basic Concepts	82, 85, 102, 105, 107	5	62, 80, 84, 101	4		0	71, 80	2	71, 79, 109	3	61, 71, 72, 73, 76, 82, 92, 98, 107	9
2	Atomic Structure	92, 106, 108	3	85	1	81, 98, 117, 119	4	61, 64, 105, 109, 116, 119	6	63, 82, 92, 111, 113, 110, 119	7	88, 104, 109, 116, 117	5
3	Periodic Properties	88, 91, 93, 95, 111	5	86, 89, 97, 115	4	94, 108	2	108, 117, 120	3	62, 120	2	67	1
4	Chemical Bonding	110, 115	2	108, 114	2	114	1		0		0		0
5	Nuclear Chemistry		0	72	1	80, 102	2	87	1		0	86	1
6	Gaseous and Liquid states	66, 67, 103	3	69, 95, 102	3	73	1	90, 101	2	66, 104, 114	3	62, 80, 97	3
7	Solid state		0		0	111	1		0		0	91	1
8	Mole Concept & Solutions		0	81, 103, 104, 105	4	61, 62, 63, 76, 79, 83, 90, 96	8	66, 76, 97, 102	4	69, 77, 97	3	78, 94, 108	3
9	Colloids, Surface Chemistry & Catalyst	99, 118	2	90	1		0		0	68	1	68	1
10	Equilibrium	68, 97, 104	3	63, 66, 71, 91	4	70, 74, 75, 85, 88, 93, 101, 104, 106	9	65, 68, 92, 106, 112	5	61, 87, 94, 102	4	100	1
11	Kinetics		0	113	1	97,	1	95	1	67, 96	2	84	1
12	Energetics	61, 109	2	96, 118	2	112	1	75, 93, 110, 113	4	74, 100, 106, 112, 115	5	106	1
13	Electrochemistry	63, 89	2	61, 64, 106, 79	4	115, 118	2	84, 99	2	75, 93, 108	3	64, 79, 81, 112, 113, 120	6
14	Redox Reactions		0	98, 109, 117	3	65, 107, 120	3	100	1	64, 84, 99	3	110	1
15	Metallurgy		0	94, 107	2	71, 77, 78, 92	4		0	76	1		0
16	Hydrogen and its Compounds	79, 80	2		0	87	1		0		0		0
17	*s*-block Elements	114	1		0		0		0		0		0
18	*p*-block Elements	65, 78, 81, 83, 96, 100, 113, 116, 120	9	68, 70, 75, 88, 93, 110, 114	7	69, 89, 99, 105, 116	5	63, 72, 78, 94, 111, 114, 118	7	65, 70, 116	3	63, 65, 69, 74, 85, 93, 95, 111, 114	9
19	*d*-and *f*-block Elements	71, 84	2	65, 73, 100	3	72, 82, 100	3	67, 88, 91, 103, 115	5	105	1	75, 102, 115	3
20	Complex compounds		0	67, 83	2		0	69, 77	2	107	1	96	1
21	Purification and Analysis of Compound		0	92	1		0	86	1	83, 101	2	87	1
22	General Organic Chemistry	64, 87	2	78, 111, 112	3	86	1	73, 98	2	72, 73, 89	3	119	1
23	Aliphatic Hydrocarbons	70, 75, 77, 111, 102	5	87, 99	2	68, 103, 110	3	62, 89	2	90	1	103	1
24	Aromatic Hydrocarbons		0		0	113	1	70, 79	2	81, 103, 110	3	70, 90, 99, 105	4
25	Halogen derivatives	72, 94	2	76	1	64	1		0	98	1		0
26	Alcohol, phenols & ethers	74, 98, 117, 119	4	82, 116	2	84, 95	2	83, 85	2	88	1	66	1
27	Aldehyde & Ketone	62, 69, 76, 86	4		0	67, 109	2		0		0	83, 101, 118	3
28	Carboxylic acids & their derivatives	73	1	120	1		0	82, 104, 107	3	78	1	77	1
29	Nitrogen compounds		0	77	1		0	81, 96	2	85, 86, 95	3		0
30	Biochemistry		0		0	91	1		0	91, 117	2	89	1
31	Chemistry in Action	90	1	70	1	66	1	74	1	80	1		0

USE THIS INDEX FOR TOPICWISE ANALYSIS OF LAST 14 YEARS AIIMS PAPERS AND REFER TO THESE QUESTIONS WHEN YOU ARE PRACTISING MCQ's CHAPTERWISE

2000		2001		2002		2003		2004		2005		2006		2007	
Ques. No.	Tot.	Ques. No.	Tot.	Ques. No.	Tot.	Ques. No.	Tot.	Ques. No.	Tot.	Ques. No.	Tot.	Ques. No.	Tot.	Ques. No.	Tot.
99	1		0	113, 114	2	72, 87, 99	3	102, 104	2	75	1		0		0
112	1	65	1	69, 70, 81, 88, 111, 120	6	95	1	90	1	84	1	76	1		0
90, 96, 110	3	68, 76	2		0		0	61	1	70, 110	2	104	1	67, 112	2
	0	69, 77, 89, 106, 116, 119	6	83, 118, 119	3	89	1	74, 119	2		0	70, 72, 102	3	66, 94, 117	3
104, 118	2	117, 118	2		0	104	1	105	1	72, 77	2		0	72, 78, 82, 120	4
79, 91	2		0	68	1		0	120	1	109	1	77	1	73, 75	2
67, 101	2	90, 92	2	86, 87, 94	3		0	94	1	80	1	80, 85, 110	3	62	1
64, 76, 102, 117	4	86, 99, 105	3	66	1	91, 118	2	91	1		0	84, 120	2	68, 98	2
	0	82, 91	2	95, 103, 112	3		0	115	1	78	1	69, 112	2	93	1
73, 78, 86, 98, 114	5	66, 67, 74, 78, 94, 98, 100, 102, 104,111	10	76, 77, 85	3	93, 98, 109	3	64, 72, 93, 95, 96. 101, 117	7	83, 87, 88, 108	4	78, 109	2	64, 77, 110, 119	4
82	1		0	79	1	100	1	99	1	82, 86	2	82, 107	2	116	1
75, 103	2	70, 71	2	84, 101, 115, 116	4	90, 94, 114, 116	4	89, 92, 114	3	81, 85	2	79, 83, 86, 108	4	80, 81, 97, 114	4
	0	88, 93, 97	3	102	1	92, 97	2	97	1	79, 113	2	81, 87, 111	3		0
61, 66	2	115	1	78, 105	2	67	1	66	1	65, 101	2		0		0
109	1	87	1	67	1	73	1		0	71, 114	2		0	70	1
	0		0		0	62, 120	2		0		0		0		0
	0	110	1	93	1	105	1		0	106	1	65	1	92	1
62, 65, 68, 69, 71, 83, 93, 95, 105, 106, 107, 108, 113, 115	14	72, 73, 75, 81, 83, 85, 120	7	80, 91, 107, 108	4	61, 63, 69, 70, 103, 115	6	65, 67, 69, 70, 73, 106	6	61, 67, 68, 74, 102, 103, 104, 107, 111,	9	63, 64, 71, 73, 74, 106	6	65, 79, 83, 87, 104, 105	6
72, 84, 89, 97, 100	5	101	1	89, 92, 117	3	66, 68, 101	3	71, 116	2	66, 105	2	66, 105, 114	3	74, 101, 107	3
63, 77, 92	3	80, 96, 107	3		0	64, 65, 71, 88, 102	5	62, 63, 68, 103	4	62, 63, 64, 73	4	61, 67, 103	3	76, 88, 89, 100, 108	5
87	1	108, 114	2		0		0		0		0		0		0
74, 94, 116, 119	4	62, 63, 95, 103	4	82, 96, 97, 99	4	77, 80, 81, 112, 113	5	78, 79	2	89, 92, 98	3	89, 115, 116	3	99, 118	2
	0		0	74, 75, 100	3		0	77, 112	2	69	1	119	1	84, 103, 113	3
88, 120	2	61, 84	2	98	1	76, 78, 79, 110	4	80, 110	2	115, 120	2	90, 91	2	61, 85, 95	3
80	1		0	65, 90	2	108	1	82, 83	2	90, 91, 93, 112	4	98, 99, 117	3	91, 111	2
81	1	109, 112, 113	3	64, 109, 110	3	86	1	88, 111, 113	3	116	1	92, 100	2	69, 86	2
	0		0	71, 72, 73	3		0	81, 104	2		0		0	109	1
70, 111	2	64	1	104	1	74, 83, 111	3	85	1	94	1	93	1	90, 106	2
85	1		0		0	75, 84, 85	3	75, 76, 86, 87	4	76, 95, 96, 100, 118, 119	6	94	1	63, 71, 96, 102	4
	0		0	62, 106	2	82, 96, 106, 107	4	84, 107, 108	3	97, 99, 117	3	62, 88, 95, 96, 97, 101, 113	7	115	1
	0	79	1	61, 63	2	117, 119	2	98, 100, 118	3		0	68, 75, 118	3		0

CHAPTERWISE INDEX

BIOLOGY

S.No.	Chapter's Name	1994 Ques. No.	Tot.	1995 Ques. No.	Tot.	1996 Ques. No.	Tot.	1997 Ques. No.	Tot.	1998 Ques. No.	Tot.	1999 Ques. No.	Tot.
1	General Biology	148	1	160	1		0	122, 145	2	123	1	140	1
2	Biological Classification	170	1	149, 154, 166	3	138, 142	2	169	1		0		0
3	Kingdom Monera	146, 161	2	152	1		0		0	126	1	142, 144, 147	3
4	Kingdom Fungi						0		0		0		0
5	Plant Kingdom	156, 167, 168, 169	4	150, 165	2	170	1	160	1	139, 122, 130	3	145, 146	2
6	Cell and its Structural Component	142	1	145, 159, 170	3		0		0	147, 179	2	148, 162	2
7	Cell Reproduction	160	1	164	1		0	167	1	177	1	149	1
8	Cell Respiration		0	158, 172	2		0		0	0	0	139	1
9	Enzymes		0	137	1		0		0	0	0	172	1
10	Biomolecules	125	1		0	140, 152	2		0	151	1	161, 178	2
11	Mendelian Genetics	147, 151, 152, 155, 162, 163	6		0		0	126, 148, 164, 168	4	164	1	167	1
12	Hereditary Material	164, 177	2		0	151	1		0	137	1	141	1
13	Anatomy of Flowering Plants		0	147, 153, 155, 178, 179	5	160	1	149, 151, 156	3	153, 154	2	157, 158, 163, 176	4
14	Morphology of Flowering Plants	165, 166	2	148, 151, 156	3	144	1	157	1	135, 138	2	159, 169	2
15	Physiology of Flowering Plants	154, 158, 176, 178	4	157, 162, 163, 180	4	148, 158, 161, 164, 169, 175	6	146, 159, 170, 176, 177	5	121, 127, 149, 178	4	155, 156, 174, 175, 170	5
16	Embryology of Flowering Plants	159	1		0	146, 159	2	166	1	136	1	160, 171	2
17	Growth and Development in Flowering Plants		0		0		0		0		0		0
18	Angiosperm Families		0	167	1		0		0		0		0
19	Ecology and Pollution		0	177	1	150, 153, 154, 155, 162, 167, 168, 179	8	150, 152, 158, 161	4	124, 128, 150, 180	4	165, 166, 173	3
20	Applied Botany		0	146, 161	2	149, 157, 165, 166, 180	5	147, 163	2	148, 152, 156, 161, 176	5	164	1
21	Animal Kingdom	129, 131, 137	3	121, 123, 125, 132, 138, 139, 171, 173, 174	9	121, 122, 123, 125, 128, 129, 136, 137, 131	9	132, 138, 139, 140, 173	5	158, 169, 172	3	122, 123, 135, 152, 153	5
22	Gene and Chromosome	123, 153, 157	3	133	1		0	154	1	165	1		
23	Gene regulation and Applied Genetics	149, 150, 180	3	168, 169, 176	3	171, 177	2	178, 179, 180	3	155	1	143, 168	2
24	Human Genetics & Genetic Disorder	127, 132, 175, 179	4		0		0	131, 134	2		0	125	1
25	Animal Tissue	121, 122, 128, 130, 143	5	122, 124, 127, 135	4		0	136, 137	2		0	133, 179	2

USE THIS INDEX FOR TOPICWISE ANALYSIS OF LAST 14 YEARS AIIMS PAPERS AND REFER TO THESE QUESTIONS WHEN YOU ARE PRACTISING MCQ's CHAPTERWISE

2000		2001		2002		2003		2004		2005		2006		2007	
Ques. No.	Tot.	Ques. No.	Tot.	Ques. No.	Tot.	Ques. No.	Tot.	Ques. No.	Tot.	Ques. No.	Tot.	Ques. No.	Tot.	Ques. No.	Tot.
146	1	146, 164, 166	3	156, 161	2		0	131	1		0		0		0
166	1	150	1	171	1		0				0		0		0
145, 157, 172	3	161, 169	2	173	1	150	1	129	1		0	149, 177	2		0
170	1		0		0		0		0	171	1	141, 145, 150	3	146, 173	2
	0	167	1	142, 143, 150	3		0	153, 158, 176	3		0		0	171, 172	2
168	1	180	1	127, 165, 170, 177	4	157, 171	2	149	1	146, 147, 169	3	135, 153, 180	3	134, 138	2
154	1	122	1	0	0		0		0	143, 145	2		0		0
	0	153	1	130	1		0		0		0		0	141	1
	0	136	1		0	136	1		0	150	1	132	1	140	1
	0		0	160, 179	2		0		0		0	128	1	122, 142	2
122, 123	2	131	1	137, 138	2		0	160	1	141, 154	2	126, 127	2	157, 158	2
	0	177, 178	2		0	135, 143	2		0	170	1	158, 160	2	144	1
142, 178	2	132, 143, 179	3	140, 143, 147, 175	4	151, 158, 175	3	154, 157, 159	4		0	144, 172	2	174	1
	0	142	1		0			178	1	140	1		0	149, 152, 153	3
132, 133, 136, 150, 173	5	141, 155, 156, 163, 171, 174	6	126, 139, 146, 180	4	130, 152, 173, 174	4	173, 174, 175, 179	4	172, 177	2	151, 171, 178, 179	4	143, 147, 148, 150, 151, 176, 178	7
	0	160	1	144, 172, 174	3	154, 160	2	141, 177	2	142	1	154	1	155, 179	2
	0		0		0		0	150, 172	2	158, 160,	2	152	1	175	1
	0	130	1		0		0		0		0	146	1		0
153, 156, 158, 165	4	140, 152	2	148, 149, 162	3	125, 126, 127, 133, 137, 138, 139, 168, 178, 179	10	125, 136, 137, 138	4	128, 131, 137, 148, 149, 156, 163, 164, 173	9	133, 139, 155, 156, 157, 163, 167, 174, 175, 176	10	145, 154, 160, 170, 177	5
126, 139, 160, 163, 167, 174, 176	7	128, 139, 144, 145, 151, 170	6	141	1	153, 159, 162, 166, 172, 177	6	148, 151, 152, 155, 161	5	126, 129, 136, 153, 155	5	143, 147, 148	3	156, 159, 180	3
130, 131, 135, 159, 180	5	134, 135, 148, 157, 158, 176, 162, 172	8	131, 132, 135, 151, 152, 153, 157, 168	8	164, 169	2	122, 164	2	151, 159, 179	3	122, 123, 131	3	124, 166	2
140	1	123, 154	2	129	1	144	1	145, 146	2	139, 144,	2	173	1		0
147	1	129, 168	2	124, 128, 136, 176, 178	5	123, 141	2	121, 140, 142	3	157, 162, 180	3	142, 169	2		0
127	1	175	1		0	155	1	124, 144	2	124, 167	2	130	1	135, 161	2
	0	133	1	164, 167	2	161	1		0		0	136	1		0

CHAPTERWISE INDEX

BIOLOGY

S.No.	Chapter's Name	1994		1995		1996		1997		1998		1999	
		Ques. No.	Tot.	Ques. No.	Tot.	Ques. No.	Tot.	Ques. No.	Tot.	Ques. No.	Tot.	Ques. No.	Tot.
26	Musculo-skeletal system	134	1	128, 130, 144	3	147	1		0		0		0
27	Digestive System and Nutrition	138, 140, 141	3	126	1	124, 127, 132, 133, 139, 145, 163	7		0	141, 174, 175	3	128	1
28	Respiration	139, 144	2	142	1		0	121, 141	2				0
29	Circulatory system and Immunity	145	1		0	126	1	133, 144	2	134, 157	2	121, 126	2
30	Excretion and Osmoregulation		0		0	135, 174	2	123, 175	2	160	1	130, 137	2
31	Reproduction and Embryonic Development		0	131	1		0	135, 172, 174	3	131, 133, 162, 166, 168	5	129, 151	2
32	Nervous system and sense organ	136	1	134, 141, 175	3	173	1	130, 142	2	132, 144, 146, 159, 167, 171	6	131, 177, 180	3
33	Endocrine system	124	1	129	1	130, 134, 176	3	0	0	140, 163	2	127, 132, 134	3
34	Common Human Diseases	133, 171, 172, 173, 174	5	143	1	143	1	125, 129, 143	3	125, 142, 145, 173	4	124, 150, 154	3
35	Growth and Regeneration		0		0		0		0		0	136	1
36	Evolution	126, 135	2	136, 140	2	172	1	153	1	129, 143, 170	3	138	1
37	Drug and Addiction		0		0		0	171	1		0		0
38	Applied Zoology		0		0		0	124, 128, 155, 162	4		0		0
39	Wild Life and Conservation		0		0	156, 178	2	165	1		0		0
40	Human Population & Growth		0		0	141	1	127	1		0		0

USE THIS INDEX FOR TOPICWISE ANALYSIS OF LAST 14 YEARS AIIMS PAPERS AND REFER TO THESE QUESTIONS WHEN YOU ARE PRACTISING MCQ's CHAPTERWISE

2000		2001		2002		2003		2004		2005		2006		2007	
Ques. No.	Tot.	Ques. No.	Tot.	Ques. No.	Tot.	Ques. No.	Tot.	Ques. No.	Tot.	Ques. No.	Tot.	Ques. No.	Tot.	Ques. No.	Tot.
124, 128	2	121	1		0	128	1		0	152	1	129, 164	2	132	1
137, 162	2	173	1	125, 135, 158, 159	4	132, 149	2		0	122	1	124	1	123	1
169	1		0		0	176	1		0		0		0	131	1
134, 155, 179	3	137	1	121, 134	2	122, 124, 163	3	128, 139, 147	3	127, 134, 165, 166	4		0	136, 139, 163, 164, 165	5
129	1		0		0		0		0	138	1		0	168, 169	2
143	1	165	1		0	129, 146, 147, 156, 167	5		0	125, 135, 168	3		0	128, 129	2
141, 161, 164, 171	4	124, 149	2	166	1	140, 145	2	123	1		0	121, 125	2	121, 125, 130, 162	4
125, 151	2		0	0	0	134, 148	2	162	1	123	1	137, 170	2	126, 127	2
121, 144, 148, 175	4	147, 159	2	154, 155, 169	3	131, 165	2	133	1		0	134, 138, 140, 161, 162, 166	6		0
	0		0	163	1	170	1		0	161	1		0		0
128, 152, 177	3	126, 127, 138	3	123	1	180	1	130, 156, 163, 166, 167, 170, 171	7	174, 175, 176	3	165	1	133, 137, 167	3
	0	125	1	122	1	0	0	127, 132, 134, 143, 168	5		0	168	1		0
149	1		0		0	121	1	165, 169, 180	3	132, 133	2		0		0
	0		0		0	142	1	126, 135	2	130,	1	159	1		0
	0		0		0		0		0	178	1		0		0

Model Test Paper–1

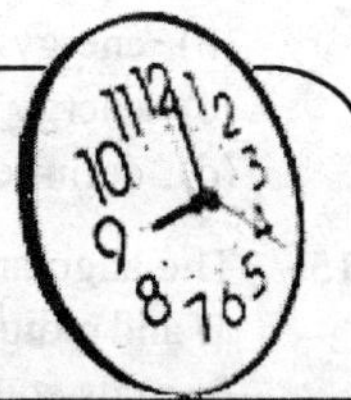

Time : $3\frac{1}{2}$ hours. *Maximum Marks : 200*

PHYSICS

1. What is the dimensional formula for the gravitational constant?
(a) $[M^{-1} L^3 T^{-1}]$ (b) $[M^{-2} L^{-1} T^3]$
(c) $[M^{-1} L^3 T^{-2}]$ (d) $[M^{-2} L^3 T^{-2}]$.

2. An ideal gas is heated from 27°C to 627°C at constant pressure. If initial volume was 4 m^3, then the final volume of the gas will be
(a) 2 m^3 (b) 4 m^3
(c) 6 m^3 (d) 12 m^3.

3. The tension in piano wire is 10 N. What should be the tension in the wire to produce a note of double the frequency?
(a) 5 N (b) 20 N
(c) 40 N (d) 80 N.

4. Which of the following is a dimensionless quantity?
(a) strain (b) stress
(c) specific heat (d) quantity of heat.

5. When we heat a gas-sample from 27°C to 327°C, then the initial average kinetic energy of the molecules was E. What will be the average kinetic energy after heating?
(a) $327E$ (b) $300E$
(c) $2E$ (d) $\sqrt{2}E$.

6. A certain radioactive element has a half-life of 20 years. If we have a block with 10 gm of the element in it, after how many years will there be just 2.5 g of the element in the block?
(a) 40 years (b) 60 years
(c) 80 years (d) 100 years.

7. A ray of light having wavelength 720 nm enters in a glass of refractive index 1.5. The wavelength of the ray within the glass will be
(a) 360 nm (b) 480 nm
(c) 720 nm (d) 1080 nm.

8. The reactance of an inductance of 0.01 Hz to a 50 Hz A.C. is
(a) 6.28 Ω (b) 3.14 Ω
(c) 1.04 Ω (d) 0.59 Ω.

9. Ten identical cells each of potential E and internal resistance r are connected in series to form a closed circuit. An ideal voltmeter connected across three cells, will read
(a) $3E$ (b) $7E$
(c) $10E$ (d) $13E$.

10. Which of the following, when added as impurity into the silicon, produces n-type semiconductor?
(a) P (b) Al
(c) B (d) Mg.

11. A tube closed at one end containing air produces fundamental note of frequency 512 Hz. If the tube is open at both ends, the fundamental frequency will be
(a) 256 Hz (b) 768 Hz
(c) 1024 Hz (d) 1280 Hz.

12. Which of the following is an essential requirement for initiating the fusion reaction?
(a) critical mass (b) thermal neutrons
(c) high temperature (d) critical temperature.

13. If an electron is brought towards another electron, the electric potential energy of the system
(a) increases (b) decreases
(c) becomes zero (d) remains the same.

14. The photoelectrons emitted from a given cathode on the incidence of a given monochromatic beam of light, have a/an
(a) energy spread with a lower limit

(b) energy spread with an upper limit
(c) energy spread with no sharp limits
(d) definite energy only.

15. The angular velocity of rotation of a star (of mass M and radius R) at which the matter starts to escape from its equator, is

(a) $\sqrt{\frac{2GR}{M}}$ (b) $\sqrt{\frac{2GM}{R^3}}$
(c) $\sqrt{\frac{2GM}{R}}$ (d) $\sqrt{\frac{2GM^2}{R}}$

16. Greater accuracy in the determination of the position of a particle with an optical microscope can be had, if the beam of light used
(a) is polarised
(b) has greater intensity
(c) has higher wavelength
(d) has higher frequency.

17. A body of mass 5 kg is raised vertically to a height of 10 m by a force of 170 N. The velocity of the body at this height will be
(a) 37 m/s (b) 22 m/s
(c) 15 m/s (d) 9.8 m/s.

18. An intrinsic semiconductor, at the absolute zero temperature, behaves like a/an
(a) insulator (b) superconductor
(c) *n*-type semiconductor
(d) *p*-type semiconductor.

19. The periodic time of a body executing SHM is 4 sec. After how much interval from time $t = 0$, its displacement will be half of its amplitude?
(a) $\frac{1}{2}$ sec (b) $\frac{1}{3}$ sec
(c) $\frac{1}{4}$ sec (d) $\frac{1}{6}$ sec.

20. Time period of pendulum, on a satellite orbiting the earth is
(a) zero (b) infinity
(c) $1/\pi$ (d) π.

21. For an enclosure maintained at 1000 K, the maximum radiation occurs at wavelenghth λ_m. If the temperature is raised to 2000 K, the peak will be shift to

(a) $\frac{1}{2}\lambda_m$ (b) $\frac{3}{2}\lambda_m$
(c) $\frac{5}{2}\lambda_m$ (d) $\frac{7}{2}\lambda_m$.

22. It is possible to have a positively charged body at
(a) zero potential (b) negative potential
(c) positive potential (d) all of these.

23. If two lenses of power +1.5 D and +1.0 D are placed in contact, then the effective power of combination will be
(a) 2.5 D (b) 4.2 D
(c) 4.5 D (d) 5.4 D.

24. Simple capacitor filters are good for
(a) low voltage supply (b) low current supply
(c) high current supply
(d) low voltage and high current supply.

25. The heat produced by a 100 W heater in 2 minutes is equal to
(a) 16.3 kcal (b) 14.2 kcal
(c) 10.5 kcal (d) 2.8 kcal.

26. Curies temperature of iron is the temperature below which, it is
(a) radioactive (b) superconducting
(c) ferromagnetic (d) diamagnetic.

27. An *X*-ray beam of wavelength 10^{-10} m falls on a crystal of atomic spacing 2×10^{-10} m. The Bragg angle for the second order reflection will be
(a) 15° (b) 30°
(c) 45° (d) 60°.

28. What is the equivalent resistance between *A* and *B* in the given figure?
(a) 10 Ω
(b) 20 Ω
(c) 40 Ω
(d) 50 Ω.

20Ω 20Ω
A 20Ω B
20Ω 20Ω

29. A certain mass of gas at 273 K is expanded to 81 times its volume under adiabatic conditions. If γ= 1.25 for the gas then its final temperature is
(a) 0°C (b) –91°C
(c) –182°C (d) –235°C.

30. In a phase-shift oscillator, the positive feedback is taken from the
(a) anode directly (b) grid and anode
(c) load resistance (d) RC network.

31. The moment of inertia of a disc of mass M and radius R about an axis which is tangential to the circumference of the disc and parallel to its diameter, is

(a) $\frac{3}{2}MR^2$ (b) $\frac{2}{3}MR^2$

(c) $\frac{5}{4}MR^2$ (d) $\frac{4}{5}MR^2$.

32. Crystalline solids are

(a) anisotropic (b) isotopic

(c) amporphus (d) none of these.

33. The motion of a rocket is based on the principle of conservation of

(a) mass (b) kinetic energy

(c) linear momentum (d) angular momentum.

34. Which of the following relation is called as current density?

(a) $\frac{I}{A}$ (b) $\frac{A}{I}$

(c) $\frac{I^2}{A}$ (d) $\frac{I^3}{A^2}$.

35. A body weighed 250 N on the surface assuming the earth to be a sphere of uniform mass density, how much would it weight half way down to the centre of the earth?

(a) 240 N (b) 210 N

(c) 195 N (d) 125 N.

36. Radius of gyration of a body depends upon

(a) axis of rotation (b) translation motion

(c) shape of the body (d) area of the body.

37. Ten identical wires each having a resistance of one ohm are connected in parallel. The combination will have a resistance of

(a) 10 Ω (b) 1 Ω

(c) 0.1 Ω (d) 0.01 Ω.

38. The logic circuit given in the figure performs the logic operation

(a) $\overline{A}BC$

(b) $\overline{A}B\overline{C}$

(c) ABC

(d) $AB\overline{C}$.

A B C Y

39. A nucleus of $_4Be^9$ absorbs an alpha particle and emits a neutron. The resulting nucleus will be

(a) $_6C^{12}$ (b) $_4BE^8$

(c) $_5C^{13}$ (d) $_6C^{13}$.

40. If a *p-n* diode is reverse biased, then the resistance measured by an ohm-meter, will be

(a) zero (b) low

(c) high (d) infinite.

***Directions for Q.41 to 60** : These questions consists of two statements each, printed as **Assertion** and **Reason**. While answering these questions you are required to choose any one of the following four responses.*

(a) If both Assertion and Reason are true and the Reason is a correct explanation of the Assertion.

(b) If both Assertion and Reason are true but Reason is not a correct explanation of the Assertion.

(c) If Assertion is true but the Reason is false.

(d) If both Assertion and Reason are false.

41. *Assertion (A) :* Evaporation has a cooling effect.
Reason (R) : At the surface of the liquid, some of the faster upward-moving molecules have enough kinetic energy to overcome the attractions from other molecules and escape from the liquid. With these faster molecules gone, the average kinetic energy of those left behind is reduced.

42. *Assertion (A) :* Room heaters and refrigerators lose most of their heat by convection.
Reason (R) : A hot surface heats the air next to it. The hot air rises, to be replaced by cooler air which then heats up, and so on.

43. *Assertion (A) :* The diameter of an atom is ~ 10^4 times that of its nucleus.
Reason (R) : The diameter of the nucleus is ~ 10^{-14}m

44. *Assertion (A) :* Many solids have a molar heat capacity close to 25 J mol^{-1} K^{-1}
Reason (R) : The molar heat capacity is the heat capacity per mole.

45. *Assertion (A) :* In conductors the electrons are free to move between atoms.
Reason (R) : In conductors the conduction band is only partly filled. It has unoccupied energy levels.

46. *Assertion :* The relative velocity of two photons travelling in opposite directions is C.
Reason : The rest mass of photon is zero.

47. *Assertion :* Brilliant colours are seen in thin layer of oil on the surface.
Reason : White light is composed of several colours.

48. *Assertion :* Activity of 10^8 undecayed radioactive nuclei of half life 50 days is equal to that of 1.2×10^8 undecayed nuclei of some other material with half life 60 days.
Reason : Activity is proportional to half life.

49. *Assertion :* Any hollow metallic closed container maintained at a uniform temperature can act as a source of black body radiation.
Reason : All metals act as black bodies.

50. *Assertion :* In LCR series circuit. The reasonance occurs at one frequency only.
Reason : At resonance the inductive reactance is equal to the capacitive reactance.

51. *Assertion :* The comets do not obey Kepler's laws of planetary motion.
Reason : The comets do not have elliptical orbit.

52. *Assertion :* Water kept in an open vessel will quickly evaporate on the surface of the moon.
Reason : The temperature at the surface of the moon is much higher than the boiling point of water.

53. *Assertion :* A domestic electrical appliance, working on a three pin, will continue working even if the top pin is removed.
Reason : The third pin is used only as a safety device.

54. *Assertion :* A needle placed carefully on the surface of water may float, whereas a ball of the same material will always sink.
Reason : The bouyancy of an object depends both on the material and shape of the object.

55. *Assertion :* Electric appliances with metallic body, *e.g.* heaters have three-pin connection, whereas an electric bulb has a two pin connection.
Reason : Three pin connection reduces heating of connecting cables.

56. *Assertion :* Machine parts are jammed in winter.
Reason : The viscosity of lubricant used in machine parts increase at low temperatures.

57. *Assertion :* A normal eye can clearly see all the objects beyond a certain minimum distance.
Reason : The human eye has the capacity to suitabily adjust the focal length of its lens to a certain extent.

58. *Assertion :* On a rainy day, it is difficult to drive a car or bus at high speed.
Reason : The value of coefficient of friction is lowered on wetting the surface.

59. *Assertion :* The Sun looks bigger in size at sunrise and sunset than during day.
Reason : The phenomenon of diffraction bends light rays.

60. *Assertion :* The rainbow is seen sometimes in the sky when it is raining. When one sees a rainbow, one's back is towards the Sun.
Reason : Internal reflection from water droplet causes dispersion. The final ray is in the backward direction.

CHEMISTRY

61. The number of unpaired electron in $1s^2\ 2s^2\ 2p^3$ is
(a) 1 (b) 2
(c) 3 (d) 5.

62. The oxidation number of oxygen atom in O_2^{2-} ion is
(a) –1 (b) –2
(c) –3 (d) –5.

63. Maximum covalency of an element of atomic number 7 is
(a) 2 (b) 3
(c) 4 (d) 5.

64. Lithopone, a white pigment, consists of
(a) PbS and MgO (b) $BaSO_4$ and $PbSO_4$
(c) ZnS and $BaSO_4$ (d) Al_2O_3 and $CaCO_3$.

65. The number of electrons required to deposit 1 gm equivalent aluminium (at. wt. = 27) from a solution of aluminium chloride will be
(a) 1 (b) 2
(c) 3 (d) 4.

66. The amount of zinc (at. wt. = 65) necessary to produce 224 ml of H_2 by the reaction with an acid will be
(a) 0.065 gm (b) 0.65 gm
(c) 6.5 gm (d) 7.5 gm.

67. The volume of carbon dioxide gas evolved at S.T.P. by heating 7.3 gm of $Mg(HCO_3)_2$ will be
(a) 1120 ml (b) 2000 ml
(c) 2240 ml (d) 2340 ml.

68. The molarity of pure water is
(a) 1.16 M (b) 5.56 M
(c) 18.36 M (d) 55.56 M.

69. A certain gas diffuses four times as quickly as oxygen. The molecular weight of the gas is
(a) 1 (b) 1.5
(c) 2 (d) 16.

70. The equivalent weight of oxygen, when it is converted to oxide is equal to
(a) molecular weight (b) $\frac{\text{molecular weight}}{2}$
(c) $\frac{\text{molecular weight}}{3}$ (d) $\frac{\text{molecular weight}}{4}$

71. Which of the following is used in photography?
(a) AgCl (b) AgBr
(c) Ag_2S (d) $Ag_2C_2O_4$.

72. In the presence of mercuric ion and concentrated sulphuric acid, the reaction of acetylene with water produces
(a) CH_3-CHO (b) CH_3-COOH
(c) $CH_3-CO-CH_3$
(d) CH_3-CH_2-OH.

73. If an atom is reduced, its oxidation number
(a) increases (b) slightly decreases
(c) does not change (d) sharply decreases.

74. Which of the following has the maximum electronegativity?
(a) F (b) O
(c) C (d) N.

75. The property, which can be classified as an intensive property, is
(a) mass (b) temperature
(c) volume (d) heat capacity.

76. The temperature, at which the density of O_2 at 1 atm. is the same as that of CH_4 at S.T.P. is
(a) 100°C (b) 150°C
(c) 273°C (d) 546°C.

77. The important ore of aluminium is
(a) corundum (b) ruby
(c) kaolin (d) bauxite.

78. Which of the following oxyacids does not exist?
(a) $HBiO_3$ (b) H_3BiO_4
(c) H_3SbO_3 (d) H_3AsO_4.

79. The fractional distillation is used in
(a) crude oil (b) coal tar
(c) petroleum (d) all of these.

80. If *p*H value of a solution is 3 and by adding water, it becomes 6, then the dilution is increased by
(a) 10 times (b) 100 times
(c) 500 times (d) 1000 times.

81. Which of the following kinds of catalysis can be explained by the adsorption theory?
(a) enzyme catalysis (b) acid base catalysis
(c) heterogeneous catalysis
(d) homogeneous catalysis.

82. The element, with atomic number 118, will be
(a) alkali (b) nobel gas
(c) transition element (d) alkaline earth metal.

83. Which of the following molecule has regular geometry?
(a) PF_3 (b) SF_6
(c) H_2O (d) XeF_4.

84. The complete combustion of CH_4 gives
(a) $CO + H_2$ (b) $CO + N_2$
(c) $CO + H_2O$ (d) $CO + N_2O$.

85. Which of the following alkaline earth metal has highest ionic mobility in aqueous solution?
(a) Ca^{2+} (b) Mg^{2+}
(c) Be^{2+} (d) Ba^{2+}.

86. Rutherford's scattering experiment is related to the size of
(a) nucleus (b) proton
(c) electron (d) neutron.

87. Which of the following compounds is not soluble in HNO_3?

(a) CuS (b) CdS
(c) PbS (d) AgCl.

88. Which of the following molecule or ions is a bidentate ligand?
(a) Br_2^+ (b) $CH_3 - C \equiv N$
(c) $C_2O_4^{2-}$ (d) CH_3NH_2.

89. What is the correct bond angle in dimethyl ether?
(a) 109° (b) 110°
(c) 120° (d) 180°.

90. The molality of a solution having 18 gm of glucose (mol. wt. = 180) dissolved in 500 gm of water is
(a) 0.1 M (b) 0.5 M
(c) 0.2 M (d) 2.2 M.

91. Nessler's reagent is used in the test of
(a) NH_3 (b) NH_4^+
(c) NH_4Cl (d) all of these.

92. How many gm of silver will be displaced from a solution of $AgNO_3$ by 4 gm of magnesium?
(a) 4 gm (b) 16 gm
(c) 18 gm (d) 36 gm.

93. The IUPAC name of the compound having the formula CCl_3CH_2CHO is
(a) 1, 1, 1 - trichloropropanal
(b) 1, 2, 1 - dichloromethanal
(c) 2, 2, 2 - trichloropropanal
(d) 3, 3, 3 - trichloropropanal.

94. In the presence of an acid, hydrolysis of methyl cyanide produces
(a) acetic acid (b) methylamine
(c) methyl alcohol (d) formic acid.

95. Chloroform by reacting with concentrated HNO_3 produces
(a) water gas (b) laughing gas
(c) tear gas (d) producer gas.

96. Euchlorine is produced by heating a mixture of
(a) KCl + Conc. HCl (b) $KClO_3$ + Conc. HCl
(c) KCl + Conc. H_2SO_4
(d) K_2ClO_3 + Conc. H_2SO_4.

97. Which of the following is a condensation polymer?
(a) dacron (b) neoprene
(c) teflon (d) polystyrene.

98. Which of the following is the electronic configuration of Cu^{2+} ($Z = 29$)
(a) [Ar] $4s^1 3d^8$ (b) [Ar] $4s^1 3d^{10}$
(c) [Ar] $3d^9$ (d) [Ar] $4s^2 3d^{10} 4p^1$.

99. Atom bomb is based on the principle of
(a) radioactivity (b) nuclear fusion
(c) nuclear fission (d) fusion and fission.

100. In which of the following reaction $K_p > K_c$?
(a) $H_2 + I_2 \rightarrow 2HI$ (b) $N_2 + 3H_2 \rightarrow 2NH_3$
(c) $PCl_3 + Cl_2 \rightarrow PCl_5$ (d) $2SO_3 \rightarrow O_2 + 2SO_2$.

Directions for Q. 101 to 120 : *These questions consists of two statements each, printed as* ***Assertion*** *and* ***Reason****. While answering these questions you a re required to choose any one of the following four responses.*
(a) If both Assertion and Reason are true and the Reason is a correct explanation of the Assertion.
(b) If both Assertion and Reason are true but Reason is not a correct explanations of the Assertion.
(c) If Assertion is true but the Reason is false.
(d) If both Assertion and Reason are false.

101. *Assertion :* Alpha (α)-amino acids exist as internal salt in solution as they have amino and carboxylic acid groups in near vicinity.
Reason : H^+ ion given by carboxylic group (—COOH) is captured by amino group (—NH_2) having lone pair of electrons.

102. *Assertion :* Methanoic acid reduces mercuric chloride to mercurous chloride on heating while ethanoic acid does not.
Reason : Methanoic acid is a stronger acid than ethanoic acid.

103. *Assertion :* Sulphur dioxide and chlorine are both bleaching agents.
Reason : Both are drying agents.

104. *Assertion :* In case the central atom in a molecule is surrounded only by shared pairs of electrons, the molecule has a regular geometry.
Assertion : The shared electron pairs repel each other with equal force so all bonds are equidistant from each other.

105. *Assertion :* Nitrous acid (HNO_2) may act as an oxidising as well as a reducing agent.
Reason : The oxidation number of nitrogen remains same in all the compounds.

106. *Assertion :* The bond order in a molecule can have any value, positive or negative, integral

or fractional or zero.
Reason : The bond order of a molecule depends upon the number of electron in the bonding and antibonding molecular orbitals.

107. *Assertion* : Phenol undergoes Kolbe's reaction whereas ethanol does not.
Reason : Phenoxide ion is more basic than ethoxide ion.

108. *Assertion* : A spectral line will be observed for a $2p_x - 2p_y$ transition.
Reason : The energy is released in the form of wave of light when electron drops from $2p_x$ to $2p_y$ orbital

109. *Assertion* : Aromatic aldehydes and also formaldehyde undergo Cannizzaro reaction with strong alkali.
Reason : Aldehydes which have α-hydrogen atoms undergo cannizzaro reaction.

110. *Assertion* : With halogens and alkali, amides give primary amines having one carbon atom less.
Reason : The reaction of amides with alkali is a qualitative test of amides.

111. *Assertion* : Formic acid reduces mercuric chloride to mercurous chloride on heating, while acetic acid does not.
Reason : Formic acid is a stronger acid than acetic acid.

112. *Assertion (A)* : The graphite is a better lubricant on the moon than on the earth.
Reason (R) : On the moon, there is lack of gravity on the motion of machines.

113. *Assertion* : Enthalpy of graphite is lower than that of diamond.
Reason : Entropy of graphite is greater than that of diamond.

114. *Assertion* : Copper liberates hydrogen from a solution of dilute hydrochloric acid.
Reason : Hydrogen is below copper in the electrochemical series.

115. *Assertion* : Phenol undergoes Kolbe reaction whereas ethanol does not.
Reason : Phenoxide ion is more basic than ethanoxide ion.

116. *Assertion* : Alkali metals impart colour to the flame.
Reason : Their ionisation energies are low.

117. *Assertion* : Bond order in a molecule can assume any value positive or negative; integral or fractional, including zero.
Reason : It depends on the number of electrons in the bonding and antibonding orbitals.

118. *Assertion* : The molecularity of the reaction $H_2 + Br_2 = 2\ HBr$ is two.
Reason : The order of this reaction is 3/2.

119. *Assertion* : Cyclobutane is less stable than cyclopentane.
Reason : Presence of 'blent bonds' causes "loss of orbital overlap".

120. *Assertion* : The Dumans method is more applicable to nitrogen containing organic compounds than the Kjeldahl's method.
Reason : The Kjeldahl's method does not give satisfactory results for compounds in which nitrogen is directly linked to oxygen.

BIOLOGY

121. Single filament of *Nostoc* without mucilage sheath is known as
(a) trichome (b) colony
(c) mycelium (d) hyphae.

122. Which type of cancer is found in lymph nodes and spleen?
(a) leukaemia (b) sarcoma
(c) carcinoma (d) lymphoma.

123. A plant cell has potential to develop into full plant. This property of the plant cell is called
(a) pleuripotency (b) totipotency
(c) tissue culture (d) gene cloning.

124. Phytotron is a device by which
(a) protons are liberated
(b) plants are grown in controlled environment
(c) mutations are produced in plants
(d) leaf fall occurs on abscission layer.

125. When the gametophyte is not formed by spores but by any other part of sporophyte, it is known as
(a) apospory (b) polyspory
(c) multispory (d) germination.

126. Eggs having yolk in their centre and cytoplasm in peripheral layer, are called
(a) centrolecithal (b) microlecithal
(c) isolecithal (d) telolecithal.

127. Passive immunity is defined as immunity
(a) acquired through first exposure to the disease
(b) achieved through vaccination
(c) inherited from the parents
(d) achieved through the sera of other animals enriched in antibodies.

128. Sensation of stomach pain is due to
(a) proprioceptors (b) exteroceptors
(c) interoceptors (d) teloreceptors.

129. Sympathetic nerves in mammals arise from
(a) thoraco-lumbar region
(b) cervical region
(c) sacral region
(d) 3rd, 7th, 9th and 10th cranial nerves.

130. The genes, which are confirmed to differential region of Y-chromosomes only, are called
(a) holandric (b) autosomal
(c) mutant
(d) completely sex-linked.

131. The asexual production of seed is called
(a) fragmentation (b) advention
(c) apomixis (d) self-fertilization.

132. Recent reports of acid rains in big industrial cities are due to the effect of atmospheric pollution by excessive release of
(a) NH_3 by coal gas industries
(b) CO_2 by burning of coal/wood, cutting of forests
(c) NO_2 and SO_2 by burning of fossil fuels.
(d) CO_2 by incomplete combustion of carbon fuel.

133. The C_4 plants differ from C_3 plants with reference to the
(a) substrate that accepts CO_2 in carbon assimilation
(b) number of ATP that are consumed in preparing sugar
(c) type of end product
(d) type of pigment involved in photosynthesis.

134. Perisperm is
(a) peripheral part of endosperm
(b) persistent of *nucellus*
(c) remnant of endosperm
(d) disintegrated secondary nucleus.

135. Translocation of organic materials is best explained by
(a) imbibition theory
(b) transpiration pull
(c) active transport
(d) mass flow hypothesis.

136. How much amount of oxygen is present in one gram of haemoglobin?
(a) 20 ml (b) 13.4 ml
(c) 1.34 ml (d) 40 ml.

137. Which proteolytic enzyme induces lysis of firbin during fibrinolysis?
(a) firbin (b) thrombin
(c) plasmin (d) all of these.

138. Which of the following is an example of sex-linked inheritance?
(a) night-blindness (b) cretinism
(c) anaemia (d) colour-blindness.

139. There is an irregular mating population. If the frequency of an autosomal recessive lethal gene is 0.4, then the frequency of the carriers in a population of 200 individuals is
(a) 96 (b) 72
(c) 36 (d) 104.

140. The compound, which is soluble in water but does not impede the oxygen transportation, is
(a) NO (b) SO_3
(c) SO_2 (d) CO.

141. Major source of sugar in the world is
(a) *Citrulus vulgaris* (b) *Annona squamosa*
(c) *Beta vulgaris*
(d) *Saccharum officinarum*.

142. During photosynthesis oxygen, in glucose comes from
(a) oxygen in air (b) carbon dioxide
(c) water (d) both (a) and (b).

143. Red Data Book deals with
(a) plants on the verge of extinction
(b) plants that are extinct
(c) endemic plant
(d) plant showing photoperiodism.

144. Which of the following correctly represents the flow of genetic information?
(a) DNA → RNA → protein
(b) protein → RNA → DNA
(c) RNA → DNA → protein
(d) RNA → protein → DNA.

145. When ovules at two points are developed, from the inner wall of the unilocular ovary, the placentation is called
(a) marginal (b) basal
(c) parietal (d) superficial.

146. Which of the following is most convincing reasons for increasing population growth in a country?
(a) low population of old people
(b) low mortality rate (c) high birth rate
(d) high population of young children.

147. Which of the following is not applicable to coelenterates?
(a) coelenteron (b) nematoblasts
(c) choanocytes (d) radial symmetry.

148. The horns of Rhinoceros are composed of
(a) chitin (b) cartilage
(c) bone (d) keratin.

149. Chordae tendinae are found in
(a) ventricles of brain (b) atria of heart
(c) joints of legs (d) ventricles of heart.

150. The amphids are cuticular elevations on the ventro-lateral lips of *Ascaris*. These are
(a) tactoreceptors (b) tangoreceptors
(c) chemoreceptors (d) olfactoreceptors.

151. The cell organelle associated with photorespiration is
(a) mesosome (b) lysosome
(c) ribosome (d) glyoxysome.

152. The 3 sub-families of leguminose are distinguished mainly on the basis of
(a) nature and habit of plants
(b) inflorescence and flower characters
(c) nature of gynoecium
(d) nature of fruit and its germination.

153. Which of the following plant yields powerful analgesic?
(a) *Rauwolfia serpentina*
(b) *Ferula asafoetida*
(c) *Carcuma longa*
(d) *Papaver somniferum*.

154. Black wood is obtained from
(a) *Dalbergia* (b) *Acacia*
(c) *Albizzia* (d) *Manihot*.

155. Velamen is found in
(a) *Viscum* (b) *Rosa*
(c) *Vanda* (d) *Santalum*.

156. The shade of a tree is cooler than the shade of a roof due to
(a) transpiration
(b) green leaves
(c) guttation
(d) photosynthesis.

157. Preganglionic sympathetic fibres are
(a) synergic (b) cholinergic
(c) adrenergic (d) hypergonic.

158. Homonids were originated during
(a) miocene (b) palaeocene
(c) pliocene (d) oligocene.

159. Meroblastic cleavage refers to which type of division of eggs?
(a) incomplete (b) spiral
(c) total (d) horizontal.

160. Glycosidic bond is broken during the digestion of
(a) lipid (b) starch
(c) protein (d) all of these.

Directions for Q. 161 to 180 : These questions consist of two statements each, printed as assertion and reason. While answering these questions you are required to choose any one of the following four responses.

(a) If both assertion and reason are true and the reason is a correct explanation of the assertion.
(b) If both assertion and reason are true but the reason in not a correct explanation of the assertion.
(c) If assertion is true but the reason is false
(d) If both assertion and reason are false.

161. *Assertion :* Mitochondria are semi autonomous bodies.

Reason : Mitochondria produce ATP by the breakdown of carbohydrates into CO_2 and H_2O.

162. *Assertion :* Protostele has no pith in centre.
Reason : It is the most primitive stele in plant kingdom.

163. *Assertion :* Some of the monocots show increase in girth
Reason : Vascular cambium is absent in monocot.

164. *Assertion :* Plasma membrane is selectively permeable.
Reason : It allows some solutes to pass through it readily along with solvents.

165. *Assertion :* Plasmolysis occurs due to phenomenon of exosmosis.
Reason : It occurs because of hypertonic solution outside.

166. *Assertion :* Male *Anopheles* does not spread malaria.
Reason : It does not carry *Plasmodium*.

167. *Assertion :* Termites and ants are social insects.
Reason : They make fungus garden in their nests.

168. *Assertion :* In frog cleavage is unequal and holoblastic.
Reason : Their eggs are macrolecithal.

169. *Assertion :* Patella and fabella are sesamoid bones
Reason : They are formed by ossification of tendons.

170. *Assertion :* Deamination occurs by transaminase enzyme in the kidney.
Reason : Removal of an amino group from an amino acid is used in production of Ammonia.

171. *Assertion* : Meiotic division results in the production of four dissimilar cells.
Reason : Synapses occurs during zygotene of meiosis.

172. *Assertion* : Minerals are not part of biologically active substances.
Reason : Some individuals suffer anaemia due to the deficiency of iron.

173. *Assertion* : Submerged plants get CO_2 in the form of carbonates and bicarbonates.
Reason : Stomata are not present in submerged plants.

174. *Assertion* : In alcoholic drink, the alcohol is converted into glucose in the liver.
Reason : Liver cells are able to produce glucose from alcohol by back fermentation.

175. *Assertion* : Generally, a woman does not conceive during the lactation period.
Reason : The hormone 'prolactin' initiates and maintains lactation in a postpartum woman

176. *Assertion* : *Drosophila melanogaster* is widely used in genetic research.
Reason : *Drosophila melanogaster* is a readily available insect.

177. *Assertion* : The 'absorption spectrum' of chlorophyll 'a' shows close correlation with its 'action spectrum'
Reason : Chlorophyll 'a' is present in both the pigment systems I and II.

178. *Assertion* : Ionizing radiations are harmful for the living organism.
Reason : They form toxic photoproducts in the cells.

179. *Assertion* : The development in cockroach is heterometabolous metamorphosis.
Reason : The young ones resemble the adults in all.

180. *Assertion* : The aerobic respiration is bioenergically more efficient than the anaerobic glycolysis.
Reason : The aerobic respiration occurs in the mitochondria, while glycolysis is purely cytosolic.

GENERAL KNOWLEDGE

181. The human skeleton is divided into
(a) two parts (b) three parts
(c) four parts (d) six parts.

182. Who said these words "Play the game in the spirit of the game".
(a) Rajiv Gandhi (b) Indira Gandhi
(c) Chandrashekar (d) Jawahar Lal Nehru.

183. The chief metabolic function of vitamin 'D' is to
(a) afford antiachitic activity
(b) prevent night blindness
(c) prevent blood coagulation
(d) prevent the loss of muscle.

184. The capital of 'Barbados' is
(a) Capetown (b) Bridgetown (c) Belarus (d) Berlin.

185. Mother Teresa won the Nobel Prize for peace in
(a) 1992 (b) 1989
(c) 1984 (d) 1979.

186. First Woman Congress President was
(a) Annie Besant (b) Sarojini Naidu
(c) Indira Gandhi
(d) Vijayalakshmi Pandit.

187. Sri Aurbindo was a great
(a) writer (b) actor
(c) philosopher (d) sport person.

188. "Bharat Bharti" was written by
(a) Amrita Pretam (b) Mulkraj Anand
(c) Suryakant Tripathi
(d) Maithili Saran Gupta.

189. Aravali range is situated in the
(a) north-west region (b) south-west region
(c) north-east region (d) south-east region.

190. 'Prince of Wales Cup' is related with
(a) Golf (b) Hockey
(c) Football (d) Cricket.

191. 'Diesel Engine' was invented by
(a) Carnot (b) H.W. Seeley
(c) Edison (d) Rudolf Diesel.

192. Astrology deals with the study of
(a) space (b) bacteria
(c) plants life
(d) stars and future forecasting.

193. Integrated Rural Development Progress (IRDP) was initiated during
(a) 1975-1976 (b) 1969-1970
(c) 1976-1977 (d) 1980-1981.

194. The natural growth rate of population during any year is the difference between the
(a) birth rate and death rate per 1000
(b) death rate and birth rate per 1000
(c) birth rate and average population
(d) average population and birth rate per 1000.

195. Latitude is the distance in degrees on the earth's surface is measured
(a) north and south poles of the equator
(b) east and west poles of the equator
(c) upper and lower position of the earth
(d) temperature difference between different areas on earth.

196. 'GATT' stands for
(a) general agreement on toures and travels
(b) general agreement on to traffic's and track
(c) general agreement on trade and tourism
(d) general agreement on telephone and telegraph.

197. The attorney general of India is the legal adviser to
(a) Prime Minister on foreign policies
(b) Government of India
(c) President of India
(d) Government on finance policies.

198. First speaker of Lok Sabha was
(a) G.V. Mavalankar
(b) Sardar Hukum Singh
(c) Bali Ram Bhagat
(d) Neelam Sanjiva Reddy.

199. The first chief justice of India was
(a) J.C. Shah (b) S.R. Das
(c) Patanjali Shastri (d) Harilal J. Kania.

200. 'Vande Matram. was first published in
(a) Anand math (b) Vinay patrika
(c) Gitanjali (d) Nandini.

■■■

Model Test Paper–2

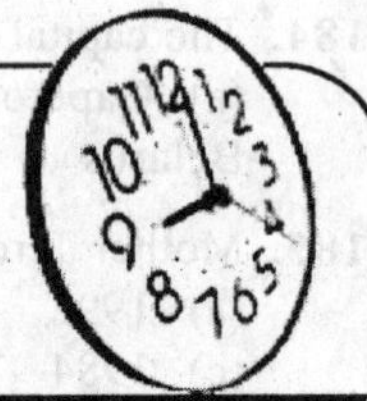

Time : $3\frac{1}{2}$ *hours.* *Maximum Marks* : 200

PHYSICS

1. A person wants to see two pillars distant 11 km as separate and distinct. The distance between the pillars must be approximately
(a) 0.25 m (b) 3 m
(c) 1 m (d) 0.5 m

2. An electromagnetic radiation has an energy 14.4 keV. To which region of electromagnetic spectrum does it belong ?
(a) *X*-rays region (b) Visible region
(c) Infra red region (d) γ-ray region

3. A circuit element *X* when connected to an a.c. supply of peak voltage 200V gives a peak current of 5*A* which is in phase with the voltage. *A* second circuit element *Y*, when connected by itself with the same supply also gives the same value of the peak current, but the current now lags the voltage by 90°. If a series combination of *X* and *Y* is connected to the same supply, what will be the r.m.s. value of the current ?
(a) 5 A (b) $2.5\sqrt{2}$ A
(c) 2.5 A (d) $5\sqrt{2}$ A

4. If applied voltage on a motor is 200 volt and back e.m.f. is 160 volt. The efficiency of the motor is
(a) 50% (b) 80%
(c) 100% (d) 25%

5. The value of relative magnetic permeability (μ_r) for ferromagnetic materials is
(a) $\mu_r = 1$ (b) $\mu_r >> 1$
(c) $\mu_r < 1$ (d) $\mu_r > 1$

6. A circular disc of area $\left(4\hat{i}+5\hat{j}\right) \times 10^{-3}\ m^2$ is placed in a uniform magnetic field of intensity $\left(0.2\hat{i}+0.3\hat{j}\right)$ tesla. The flux crossing the disc will be
(a) 23×10^{-3} weber (b) 23×10^{-2} weber
(c) 23 weber (d) 23×10^{-4} weber

7. The resistance required to be connected in parallel to an ammeter in order to increase its range 10 times, will be
(a) Ten times the resistance of ammeter
(b) Nine times the resistance of ammeter
(c) One tenth of the resistance of ammeter
(d) One ninth of the resistance of ammeter

8. The magnetic flux density applied in a cyclotron is 3.5 tesla. The frequency of the electric field that must be applied between the dees in order to accelerate protons, will be
(a) 5.34×10^7 Hz (b) 3.55×10^7 Hz
(c) 6.53×10^7 Hz (d) None of these

9. The cold junction of a thermocouple is maintained at 10°C. No thermo-e.m.f. is developed when the hot junction is maintined at 530°C. The neutral temperature is
(a) 540°C (b) 520°
(c) 530°C (d) 270°C

10. If two bulbs of wattage 25 and 100 respectively each rated at 220-volt are connected in series with the supply of 440 volt, then which of the bulbs will fuse ?
(a) 100 watt bulb (b) 25 watt bulb
(c) None of these (d) Both (a) and (b)

11. A cell of e.m.f 2 volt and internal resistance 1.5 Ω is connected to the ends of 1 m long wire. The resistance of wire is 0.5 Ω/m. The value of potential gradient on the wire will be
(a) 0.05 V/m (b) 5 V/m
(c) 0.5 V/m (d) 4.005 V/m

12. The resistance of a wire is 10 Ω. Its length is increased by 10% by stretching. The new resistance will now be

(a) 13 Ω (b) 1.2 Ω
(c) 12 Ω (d) 11 Ω

13. The equivalent capacity in the following figure between the points X and Y will be

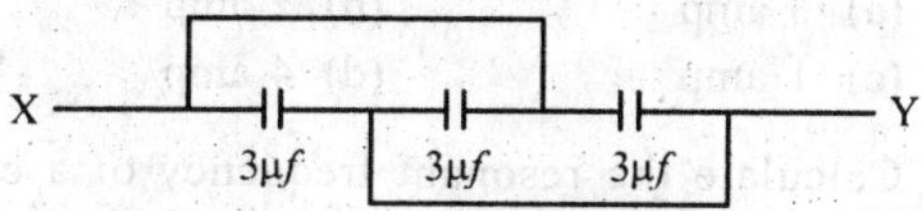

(a) 1 μf (b) 9 μf
(c) 4.5 μf (d) 6 μf

14. Two small spheres each having the charge + Q are suspended by insulating threads of length L from a hook. This arrangement is taken in space where there is no gravitational effect, then the angle between the two suspensions and the tension in each thread will be

(a) $180°, \frac{1}{4\pi\varepsilon_0}\frac{Q^2}{2L^2}$ (b) $90°, \frac{1}{4\pi\varepsilon_0}\frac{Q^2}{L^2}$

(c) $180°, \frac{1}{4\pi\varepsilon_0}\frac{Q^2}{(2L)^2}$ (d) $\frac{1}{180°}, \frac{1}{4\pi\varepsilon_0}\frac{Q^2}{L^2}$

15. The electric flux entering and emanating out of a closed surface is 2×10^3 and 8×10^3 volt-meter respectively. The charge enclosed by the closed surface is

(a) 0.53 μC (b) Zero
(c) 1 coulomb (d) 0.053 μC

16. In Meldis experiment the string vibrates in 7 segments under tension of 9 gm-wt. If the string is to be vibrated in 3 segments, the tension required will be

(a) 61 gm-wt (b) 49 gm-wt
(c) 1.4 gm-wt (d) 13 gm-wt

17. The temperature of the filament of a lamp is 2100 K and its surface area is 4×10^{-4} m². If the emissivity of the filament is 0.453 then the power of lamp is

(a) 400 watt (b) 200 watt
(c) 100 watt (d) 0 watt

18. Equal volumes of monoatomic and diatomic gases of same initial temperature and pressure are mixed. The ratio of the specific heats of the mixture $\left(\frac{C_p}{C_v}\right)$ will be

(a) 1.52 (b) 1.5
(c) 1 (d) 1.53

19. 5 gm air is heated from 4°C to 6°C. If the specific heat of air at constant volume be 0.172 cal/gm-°C, the increase in the internal energy of air will be

(a) 7.2 calorie (b) 17.2 joule
(c) 7.2 erg (d) 1.72 calorie

20. At a certain instant of time the mass of a rocket going up vertically is 100 kg. If it is ejecting 5 kg or gas per second at a speed of 400 m/s, the acceleration of the rocket would be (Taking g = 10 m/s²)

(a) 2 m/s² (b) 10 m/s²
(c) 20 m/s² (d) 1 m/s²

21. If the change in the value of 'g' at a height h above the surface of the earth is the same as at a depth x below its surface then (both x and h being much smaller than the radius of the Earth)

(a) $x = \frac{h}{2}$ (b) $x = 2h$
(c) $x = h$ (d) $x = h^2$

22. A constant torque acting on a circular wheel changes its angular momentum from A_0 to $4A_0$ in 4 second. The magnitude of this torque is

(a) 4 A_0 (b) A_0
(c) $\frac{3A_0}{4}$ (d) 12 A_0

23. A body of 5 kg moves on a frictionless horizontal surface with a speed 3 m/s. It compresses a spring put along its way and stops. What is the compession in spring ? The force constant of spring = 10 kg wt per metre.

(a) 0.2 m (b) 1 m
(c) 0.68 m (d) None of these.

24. A 12 HP motor has to be operated 8 hour/day. How much will it cost at the rate of 1.50 rupees per kilowatt-hour in 10 days ?

(a) Rs. 950 (b) Rs. 1500
(c) Rs. 1000 (d) Rs. 1074.24

25. A man is at rest in the middle of a pond on perfectly smooth ice. He can get himself to the shore by

making use of Newton's
(a) Third law (b) Second law
(c) First law (d) All the laws

26. The mass of a rocket is 10,000 kg. The velocity of the gases escaping from it is 1000 m/s. At what rate should the fuel be burnt so that the rocket may just take off ?
(a) 19.6 kg/minute (b) 19.06 kg/s
(c) 9.8 kg/s (d) 98 kg/s

27. A block of mass 2 kg rests on a rough inclined plane making an angle of 30° with the horizontal. The coefficient of static friction between the block and the plane is 0.7. The frictional force on the block is
(a) $9.8 \times \sqrt{3}\,N$ (b) $0.7 \times 9.8 \times \sqrt{3}\,N$
(c) $9.8\,N$ (d) $0.7 \times 9.8\,N$

28. Which of the following is an example of motion in three dimensions ?
(a) Motion in a vertical circle
(b) Motion of blades of rotating fan
(c) A vertically falling object
(d) Motion of an electron in the atom

29. A pendulum bob of weight $2N$ is pulled to the right by a horizontal force F until the string makes an angle of 30° to the vertical. What is the force and tension in the string needed to sit at 30°?
(a) 3 newton, 3.5 newton
(b) 4 newton, 3 newton
(c) 2 newton, 1 newton
(d) 1.2 newton, 2.3 newton

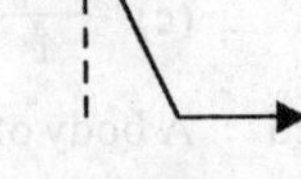

30. Dimensions of permeability of a medium are
(a) $[MLT^{-2}A^{2}]$ (b) $[MLT^{-2}A^{-2}]$
(c) $[ML^{-1}T^{2}A^{-2}]$ (d) $[ML^{-1}T^{-2}A^{-2}]$

31. What is the number of significant figures in 0.002305×10^{-27} kg ?
(a) 4 (b) 6
(c) 7 (d) 3

32. The maximum number of the photoelectrons released in a photocell is independent of
(a) Intensity of radiations incident on cathode surface
(b) Frequency of the incident ray
(c) Nature of the cathode surface
(d) None of the above

33. A transformer has 50 turns in its primary winding and 25 turns in its secondary winding. If the current in the secondary winding is 4 ampere, what is the current in primary winding ?
(a) 3 amp (b) 2 amp
(c) 1 amp (d) 4 amp

34. Calculate the resonant frequency of a circuit consisting of an inductor of 0.2 mH and a capacitor of $2\mu F$ capacitance
(a) 10112 Hz (b) 9000 Hz
(c) 7962 Hz (d) 5550 Hz

35. A circuit having a resistor, an inductor and a capacitor in series is connected to a 150 V A.C. mains. For the circuit $R = 9$ ohm, $X_L = 28$ ohm and $X_c = 16$ ohm. Calculate the current in the circuit
(a) 20 amp (b) 15 amp
(c) 10 amp (d) 7.5 amp

36. The armature current in D.C. motor is maximum when the motor has
(a) Intermediate speed
(b) Just started
(c) Picked up maximum speed
(d) Just been switched off

37. Iron is ferromagnetic
(a) More than 770°C
(b) At normal temperature
(c) At all temperatures
(d) Below 770°C

38. The magnetic moment of a magnet (10 cm × 2 cm × 1 cm) is 1 amp × m². What is the intensity of magnetisation ?
(a) 540 amp/m (b) 4×10^{5} amp/m
(c) 45 amp/m (d) 5×10^{4} amp/m

39. A long straight wire carries a current of 4 amp. A proton travels with a velocity of 4×10^{4} m/s parallel to the wire 0.2 m from it and in a direction opposite to the current. What is the force on which the magnetic field of current exerts on the moving proton ?

(a) 2.56×10^{-20} newton
(b) 5.62×10^{-20} newton
(c) 6.52×10^{-20} newton
(d) 2.56×10^{-20} dyne

40. Which of the following planets is called the goddess of beauty ?
(a) Mars (b) Mercury
(c) Venus (d) Jupiter

Instructions for Q. No. 41 to 60

Directions : Each of the questions given below consists of two statements, an assertions (A) and reason (R). Select the number corresponding to the appropriate response in the answer sheet as follows.

(a) If both assertion and reason are true and the reason is a correct explanation of the assertion
(b) If both assertion and reason are true but the reason is not a correct explanation of the assertion
(c) If the assertion is true, but the reason is false
(d) If both assertion and reason are falses

41. *Assertion (A) :* A pulsar is a source of radiowaves that vary in intensity at regular intervals.
Reason (R) : A pulsar is a rotating neutron star.

42. *Assertion (A):* For a given mass of an ideal gas, at constant temperature the product of the pressure and volume is constant.
Reason (R) : The mean square velocity of the molecules is inversely proportional to their masses at constant temperature.

43. *Assertion (A) :* γ for a diatomic gas is more than for a monoatomic gas.
Reason (R) : The molecules of a monoatomic gas have more degrees of freedom than those of a diatomic gas.

44. *Assertion (A) :* Radio waves can be polarised.
Reason (R) : Sound waves are longitudinal waves.

45. *Assertion (A) :* In series LCR circuit, reasonance occurs when inductive reactance is equal to capacitive reactance.
Reason (R) : At resonance the impedance of the circuit is minimum and is purely resistive.

46. *Assertion (A) :* If a pendulum falls freely, then its time period becomes infinite.
Reason (R) : Free falling body has acceleration equal to g.

47. *Assertion (A) :* Sound waves can not propagate through vaccuum but light waves can.
Reason (R) : Sound waves can not be polarised but light waves can be.

48. *Assertion (A) :* The frequencies of incident, reflected and refracted beam of monochromatic light incident from one medium to another medium are same.
Reason (R) : The incident, reflected and refracted rays are coplanar.

49. *Assertion (A) :* Machine parts are jammed in winter.
Reason (R) : The viscosity of lubricant used in machine parts increases at low temperatures.

50. *Assertion (A) :* The comets do not obey Kepler's laws of planetary motion.
Reason (R) : The comets do not have elliptical orbits.

51. *Assertion (A) :* Lightening conductors are made pointed at the end.
Reason (R) : An oppositely charged electric wind starts from the pointed end.

52. *Assertion (A) :* The internal resistance of a cell depends on the concentration of the electrolyte used in the cell
Reason (R) : Dilution increases the ionisation of the electrolyte.

53. *Assertion (A) :* For a given mass of an ideal gas, the product of the pressure and volume is constant, at constant temperature.
Reason (R) : The root-mean-square speed of the molecules is inversely proportional to the square root of their mass.

54. *Assertion (A) :* The ratio of $C_p/C_{v.}$, for a diatomic gas is more than that for a monoatomic gas.
Reason (R) : The molecules of a monoatomic gas have more degrees of freedom than those of a diatomic gas.

55. *Assertion (A) :* Newton's corpuscular theory of light could not explain refraction of light.

Reason (R) : It predicted that light should travel faster in denser media than in rarer media.

56. *Assertion (A)* : When temperature of a semi-conductor is increased, then its resistance decreases.
Reason (R) : The energy gap between conduction band and valence band is very small.

57. *Assertion (A)* : Electric appliances with metallic body have three connections, whereas an electric bulb has a two pin connection.
Reason (R) : Three pin connections reduce heating of connecting wires.

58. *Assertion (A)* : Environmental damage has increased the amount of ozone in the atmosphere.
Reason (R) : Increase of ozone increases the amount of ultra violet radiation on earth.

59. *Assertion (A)* : The ratio of $\frac{C_p}{C_v}$ is more for helium than for hydrogen gas.
Reason (R) : Atomic mass of helium is more than that of hydrogen.

60. *Assertion (A)* : A number of T.V. programmes can be simultaneously transmitted through water by means of laser.
Reason (R) : Laser beam is not absorbed by water.

CHEMISTRY

61. For a dilute solution, Raoult's law states that
(a) The relative lowering of vapour pressure is proportional to the amount of solute in solution
(b) The relative lowering of vapour pressure is equal to the mole fraction of solute
(c) The lowering of vapour pressure is equal to the mole fraction of the solute
(d) The vapour pressure of the solution is equal to the mole fraction of the solvent

62. The formula of metallic hydroxide (eq. wt = 150) is $M(OH)_2 . xH_2O$. If the atomic wt. of metal is 176 then the value of x will be
(a) 3 (b) 5
(c) 2 (d) 6

63. Why are strong acids generally used as standard solutions in acid-base titrations ?
(a) Strong acids form more stable solutions than weak acids
(b) They can be used to titrate both strong and weak bases
(c) The pH of the equivalence point will always be 7
(d) The salts of the strong acids do not hydrolyse

64. For which of the following reactions $k_p = k_c$?
(a) $H_{2(g)} + Cl_{2(g)} \rightleftharpoons 2HCl_{(g)}$
(b) $N_{2(g)} + 3H_{2(g)} \rightleftharpoons 2NH_{3(g)}$
(c) $2NOCl_{(g)} \rightleftharpoons 2NO_{(g)} + Cl_{2(g)}$
(d) $N_2O_{4(g)} \rightleftharpoons 2NO_{2(g)}$

65. The hydrogen ion concentration in weak acid of dissociation constant k_a and concentration C its nearly equal to
(a) K_aC (b) $\frac{C}{K_a}$
(c) $\sqrt{\frac{K_a}{C}}$ (d) $\sqrt{K_aC}$

66. Diazonium salt decomposes as
$C_6H_5N_2^+Cl^- \rightarrow C_6H_5Cl + N_2$
At 0°C, the evolution of N_2 becomes two times faster when the initial concentration of the salt is doubled. Therefore, it is a
(a) First order reaction with molecularity two
(b) Second order reaction
(c) First order reaction
(d) Second order reaction with molecularity one

67. Milk is an example of
(a) Gel (b) Emulsion
(c) Pure solution (d) Suspension

68. If a chemical change is brought about by one or more methods, in one or more steps, then the amount of heat evolved or absorbed during complete change is the same, whichever method was followed. This rule is known as
(a) Joule Thomson effect
(b) Hess law
(c) Le Chatelier principle
(d) None of these

69. Out of Cu, Ag, Fe and Zn, the metal which can displace all other from their salt solutions is
(a) Zn (b) Cu
(c) Ag (d) Fe

70. Hydrogen oxygen fuel cells are used in space craft to supply
(a) Oxygen
(b) Power for pressure
(c) Power for heat and light
(d) Water

71. Ge(II) compounds are powerful reducing agents, whereas Pb(IV) compounds are strong oxidants. It can be due to
(a) The ionic radii of Pb^{2+} and Pb^{4+} are larger than those of Ge^{2+} and Ge^{4+}
(b) The ionisation potential of lead is less than that of germanium
(c) Lead is moe electropositive than germanium
(d) More pronounced inert pair effect in lead than in germanium

72. Glass reacts with
(a) HNO_3
(b) HF
(c) Olium
(d) $K_2Cr_2O_7$

73. Anhydrous $AlCl_3$ is prepared from
(a) Dry HCl gas + Heated Al metal
(b) Aluminium and Cl_2
(c) Conc. HCl and Al metal
(d) Dil. HCl and aluminium metal

74. In diborane, banana bond is formed between
(a) 2 electrons, 2 atoms
(b) 2 electrons, 1 atom
(c) 2 electrons, 3 atom
(d) 1 electron, 2 atoms

75. Lithopone is a combination of ZnS and
(a) $SrSO_4$ (b) $CaSO_4$
(c) $PbSO_4$ (d) $BaSO_4$

76. Microcosmic salt is
(a) $(NH_4)_2$ $HPO_4.2H_2O$
(b) $Na(NH_4)HPO_4.4H_2O$
(c) $Na_2HPO_4.2H_2O$
(d) None of the above

77. Which of the following statements is false for alkali metals ?
(a) Li^+ ion is exceptionally small
(b) Sodium is amphoteric in nature
(c) Lithium is strongest reducing agent
(d) All alkali metals give blue solution in liquid ammonia

78. Mac Arthur process is used for
(a) Cl (b) Fe
(c) Ag (d) O_2

79. Fenton reagent is
(a) $CuSO_4$ + NaOH (b) $AgNO_3$ + NH_4 OH
(c) $SnCl_2$ + HCl (d) $FeSO_4$ + H_2O_2

80. D_2O is used more in
(a) Pharmaceutical preparations
(b) Nuclear reactor
(c) Chemical industry
(d) Insecticide preparation

81. Arrange the elements in increasing order of atomic radius Na, Rb, K, Mg
(a) Mg, Na, K Rb (b) Na, K, Mg, Rb
(c) Na, K, Mg, Rb (d) Rb, K, Mg, Na

82. Which of the following is paramagnetic ?
(a) Cu^+ (b) Ni^{2+}
(c) Zn^{2+} (d) None of these.

83. Which of the following elements will have the lowest first ionisation energy ?
(a) Li (b) Rb
(c) Mg (d) Ca

84. An element with atomic number 20 will be placed in which period of periodic table ?
(a) 2 (b) 3
(c) 4 (d) 1

85. In modern periodic table, elements are arranged in
(a) Increasing atomic number
(b) Increasing volume
(c) Increasing mass
(d) Alphabetically

86. Anline when treated with HNO_2 and HCl at 0°C gives
(a) A diazo compound
(b) Nitro benzene
(c) Phenol
(d) None of these.

87. Oxalic acid may be distinguished from tartaric acid by
(a) Litmus paper
(b) Ammoniacal silver nitrate solution
(c) Sodium bicarbonate solution
(d) Phenolphthalein

88. The weakest acid among the following is
(a) $CH_2ClCOOH$ (b) CH_3COOH
(c) $CHCl_2COOH$ (d) CCl_3COOH

89. Which compound undergoes aldol condensation?
(a) Ethyl methyl ketone
(b) Phenyl acetaldehyde
(c) Acetaldehyde
(d) All of these

90. Phenol condenses with phthalic anhydride in presence of conc. H_2SO_4 to form
(a) Phenyl red (b) Phenolphthalein
(c) Methyl orange (d) Salicylic acid

91. A gas X at 1 atm is bubbled through a solution containing $1MY^-$ and $1MZ^-$ ions at 25°C. If reduction potential of $Z > Y > X$ then
(a) Y will oxidise both X and Z
(b) Y will oxidise Z and not X
(c) Y will oxidise X and not Z
(d) Y will reduce both X and Z

92. In an electroplating experiment *m* gram of silver is deposited when 4 amp current flows for 2 minutes. The amount (in grams) of silver deposited by 6 amp of current flowing for 40 sec will be
(a) $\frac{m}{4}$ (b) $\frac{m}{2}$
(c) $4m$ (d) $2m$

93. Identify the intensive quantity from the following
(a) Enthalpy and volume
(b) Volume and temperature
(c) Enthalpy and temperature
(d) Temperature and refractive index

94. The extra stability of lyophilic colloid is due to
(a) The smaller size of their particles
(b) A layer of medium of dispersion on their particles
(c) Charge on their particles
(d) The large size of their particles

95. The inversion of cane-sugar is represented by
$C_{12}H_{22}O_{11} + H_2O \rightarrow C_6H_{12}O_6 + C_6H_{12}O_6$
It is a reaction of
(a) Pseudo unimolecular
(b) Unimolecular (c) Second order
(d) None of these

96. The concentration of $[H^+]$ and concentration of $[OH^-]$ of 0.1 M aqueous solution of 2% ionised weak acid is (K_w for water $= 1 \times 10^{-14}$)
(a) 2×10^{-3} M and 5×10^{-12} M
(b) 1×10^{-3} M and 5×10^{-12} M
(c) 0.02×10^{-2} M and 5×10^{-11} M
(d) 3×10^{-12} M and 4×10^{-13} M

97. In which of the following case, does the reaction go farthest to completion ?
(a) $K = 10$ (b) $K = 10^{-2}$
(c) $K = 10^2$ (d) $K = 1$

98. 10 ml of conc. H_2SO_4 (18M) is diluted to one litre. The approx. strength of dilute acid could be
(a) 0.09 N (b) 0.36 N
(c) 0.18 N (d) 18.0 N

99. The hydrogen phosphate of certain metal has formula $MHPO_4$. The formula of metal chloride would be
(a) M_2Cl_2 (b) MCl_2
(c) MCl (d) MCl_3

100. Normality of 2M H_2SO_4 is
(a) $\frac{N}{2}$ (b) 4N
(c) 2N (d) $\frac{N}{4}$

Instructions for Q. No. 101 to 120

Directions : Each of the questions given below consists of two statements, an assertions (A) and reason (R). Select the number corresponding to the appropriate response in the answer sheet as follows.

(a) If both assertion and reason are true and the reason is a correct explanation of the assertion
(b) If both assertion and reason are true but the reason is not a correct explanation of the assertion
(c) If the assertion is true, but the reason is false
(d) If both assertion and reason are falses

101. *Assertion (A) :* Pure water obtained from different sources such as, river, well, spring, sea etc. always contains hydrogen and oxygen combined in the ratio 1 : 8 by mass.
Reason (R) : A chemical compound always contain elements combined together in same proportion

by mass, it was discovered by French chemist, Joseph Proust (1799).

102. *Assertion (A) :* In CO molecule 12 parts by mass of carbon combine with 16 parts by mass of oxygen and in CO_2, 12 parts by mass of carbon combine with 32 parts by mass of oxygen.
Reason (R) : When two elements combine separately with a fixed mass of a third element, then the ratio of their masses in which they do so is either the same or whole number multiple of the ratio in which they combine with each other.

103. *Assertion (A) :* The ratio by volume of gaseous reactants and products is in agreement with their molar ratio.
Reason (R) : Volume of a gas is inversely proportional to the number of moles of a gas.

104. *Assertion (A) :* Enthalpy of graphite is lower than that of diamond.
Reason (R) : Entropy of graphite is greater than that of diamond.

105. *Assertion (A) :* For the combustion reactions, the value of ΔH is always negative.
Reason (R) : the combustion reactions are always endothermic.

106. *Assertion (A) :* The value of enthalpy of neutralisation of weak acid by strong base is numerically less than 57.1 kJ.
Reason (R) : All OH^- ions of strong base are not completely neutralised by H^+ ions obtained from acid.

107. *Assertion (A) :* Copper liberates hydrogen from the solution of dilute hydrochloric acid.
Reason (R) : Hydrogen is below copper in the electrochemical series.

108. *Assertion (A) :* The dehydration of alcohols by conc H_2SO_4 involves the formation of intermediate carbocation.
Reason (R) : The protonated alcohol molecule loses water molecule in the second step.

109. *Assertion (A) :* Acetylene on reacting with sodamide gives sodium acetylide and ammonia.
Reason (R) : Sp hybridised carbon atoms of acetylene are considerably electro-negative.

110. *Assertion (A) :* Chlorine and sulphur dioxide are both bleaching agents.
Reason (R) : Both are reducing agents.

111. *Assertion (A) :* The conjugated dienes are more stable than the corresponding alkenes containing one double bond or even the dienes containing two isolated double bonds.
Reason (R) : Conjugated dienes are regarded as hybrids of several contributing structures.

112. *Assertion (A) :* Alkanes can have an infinite number of conformations.
Reason (R) : In configurational isomerism, the isomers are distinct individual substances.

113. *Assertion (A) :* As a salt such as NaCl dissolves, the Na^+ and Cl^- ions leaving the crystal lattice acquire far greater freedom.
Reason (R) : In thermodynamic terms, the formation of solution occurs with a favourable change in free energy *i.e.* ΔH has a high positive value and $T\Delta S$ a low negative value.

114. *Assertion (A) :* Water is specially effective in screening the electrostatic interactions between the dissolved ions.
Reason (R) : The force of ionic interactions depends upon the dielectric constant (e) of the solvent.

115. *Assertion (A) :* When two uncharged similar atoms are brought very close together, their surrounding electron clouds influence each other, and a force of attraction is built up between them.
Reason (R) : The random variation in the positions of electrons around one nucleus may create a transient electric dipole, which induces a transient opposite electric dipole in the nearby atom.

116. *Assertion (A) :* The equilibrium constant is fixed and a characteristic for any given chemical reaction at a specified temperature.
Reason (R) : The composition of the final equilibrium mixture at a particular temperature depends upon the starting amount of reactants.

117. *Assertion (A) :* The degree of ionization of water is small at 25° C, only about one of every 10^7 molecules in pure water is ionized at any instant.
Reason (R) : In pure water at 25° C, the molar concentration of water is essentially constant.

118. *Assertion (A) :* The p^{ka} of a weak acid becomes equal to pH of the solution at the midpoint of of its titration.
Reason (R) : The molar concentrations of proton acceptor and proton donor become equal at the midpoint of titration of a weak acid.

119. *Assertion (A) :* Maleic and fumeric acids are well defined compounds. These two compound are stereo isomers but not enantiomers.
Reason (R) : Maleic and fumeric acids have same molecular formula but they are not mirror images of each other.

120. *Assertion (A) :* The nearly tetrahedral arrangement of the orbitals about the oxygen atom allows each water molecule to form hydrogen bonds with as many as four neighbouring water molecules.
Reason (R) : In ice each water molecule forms four hydrogen bonds as molecule is fixed in the space.

BIOLOGY

121. Group of related species with the potential, directly or indirectly, of forming fertile hybrids with one another, is called
(a) sibling species (b) subspecies
(c) coenospecies (d) none of these

122. The generalization that the evolution does not proceed back along its own path, or repeat routes is known as
(a) Cope's law (b) Allen's law
(c) Dollo's law (d) Gloger's law

123. Which of these is present only in the inert extracellular stage of the life cycle of virus ?
(a) ribosomes (b) proteins
(c) capsid (d) all of these

124. Erythropoietin hormone that stimulates red blood cell production is
(a) gamma-globulin (b) beta-globulin
(c) alpha-globulin (d) none of these

125. The term infusoria is applied to
(a) bacteria (b) protozoa
(c) rotifers (d) all of these

126. Salmon fish is
(a) anadromous (b) catadromous
(c) both (a) and (b) (d) none of these

127. In obese persons, the adipose (fat) tissues are present beneath the skin in
(a) hypodermis (b) dermis
(c) epidermis (d) all of these

128. Order salientia of phylum amphibia includes
(a) frogs (b) toads
(c) salamanders (d) both (a) and (b)

129. Platelets are derived from
(a) lymphoblast (b) monoblast
(c) myeloblast (d) megakaryoblast

130. ATP synthetase complex is found in inner mitochondrial membrane, and has two major cofactors, these are
(a) F_1 and F_2 (b) T_s and T_n
(c) F_1 and F_0 (d) R_1 and R_2

131. Fine branching protein fibres forming an extracellular network in many vertebrate connective tissues and holding tissues and organs together is called
(a) white elastic fibres
(b) yellow elastic fibres
(c) reticulin fibres (d) none of these

132. Which of the following is cobalt and nucleotide containing vitamin ?
(a) thiamine (b) cyanocobalamine
(c) ascorbic acid (d) none of these

133. Gerdy's fibres are
(a) ligament of neck (b) ligament of ankles
(c) ligament of palm (d) ligament of face

134. Gerlach's valve is present
(a) between right auricle and right ventricle
(b) between aorta and left ventricle
(c) between appendix and caecum
(d) none of these

135. Which of the following is iron storing protein ?
(a) ferritin (b) gamma-globulin
(c) alpha-globulin (d) albumins

136. Which of these first enter lacteals of the villi and then pass into blood vessels in the shoulder area?
(a) glucose (b) vitamin C
(c) amino acids (d) cholesterol

137. Which of the following enzyme is secreted by infants but not by adults ?
(a) rennin (b) pepsinogen
(c) lipase (d) trypsin

138. Which of the following is characterized by an extremely under-weight condition by limiting food consumption ?
(a) amenorrhea (b) bulimina
(c) anorexia nervosa (d) none of these

139. The rare disease progeria is associated with
(a) osteoporosis (b) leukoplakia
(c) premature old age (d) osteoarthritis

140. Synovial fluid is found in
(a) intercellular spaces
(b) around the brain
(c) freely movable joints
(d) internal ear

141. Pashmina wool is obtained from
(a) rabbit (b) goat
(c) sheep (d) deer

142. Desmosomes are related with
(a) cell division (b) cell excretion
(c) cell adherence (d) cytolysis

143. Action potential on outer surface of plasma membrane is
(a) variable (b) neutral
(c) positive (d) negative

144. Which of the following does not produce any digestive enzyme ?
(a) pancreas (b) gastric mucosa
(c) mouth (d) liver

145. Regulator of Basal Metabolic Rate (BMR) is
(a) thyroid hormones
(b) sympathetic nervous system
(c) parasympathetic nervous system
(d) adrenaline

146. Which of the following is a living fossil ?
(a) *Sphenondon* (b) *Latimaria*
(c) *Heloderma* (d) both (a) and (b)

147. Cleistogamy is found in
(a) *Commelina* (b) *Ficus*
(c) *Vallisneria* (d) all of these

148. Restriction enzymes are used in genetic engineering because
(a) they can cut DNA at specific base sequence
(b) they can join different DNA fragments
(c) they are nuclease that cut DNA at variable sites
(d) they are proteolytic enzymes which can degrade harmful proteins

149. Which of the following cell organelles is considered to be rich in hydrolytic enzymes ?
(a) ribosomes (b) ER
(c) lysosomes (d) chloroplast

150. Xanthophyll is chiefly responsible for
(a) yellow colour (b) green colour
(c) red colour (d) no colour

151. The green mould is commonly called
(a) *Penicillium* (b) *Polysiphonia*
(c) *Aspergillus* (d) *Spirogyra*

152. Detritus food chain accounts for more energy flow than grazing food chain because
(a) no organism dies
(b) most organisms die after having been eaten
(c) most organisms die without having been eaten
(d) all of the above are correct

153. The thermal algae can survive in a hot water spring at
(a) 40°C (b) 70°C
(c) 60°C (d) 15°C

154. Endodermal cells can be distinguished by the presence of
(a) elongated cells
(b) barrel shaped cells
(c) thin-walled cells
(d) cambial cells

155. Abscisic acid causes
(a) retardation of growth
(b) faster leaf fall
(c) dormancy of tubers
(d) all of the above

156. The first case of polyembryony was reported in certain
(a) grape seed (b) orange seed
(c) pulse seed (d) mango seed

157. The free energy change ΔG from the conversion of one molecule of glucose to 6 molecules of CO_2 is –686 k cal/mol, yet only about 266 k cal/mol of this is captured within ATP molecules. The rest is

(a) transferred to H_2O molecules
(b) converted to heat
(c) used to form lactate
(d) reutilized in the ATP formation

158. Which of the following plant's roots are medicinal and leaves, flowers and fruits are eaten as vegetables?

(a) *Aleuritis fordii*
(b) *Holostemma adakodien*
(c) *Helianthus annuus*
(d) all of the above

159. Hydrogen cyanide binds to the active site of an enzyme that is part of the pathway that forms ATP in the cells, in this way, it prevents the enzyme activity. Therefore, hydrogen cyanide can best be described as

(a) coenzyme
(b) cofactor
(c) allosteric modulator
(d) competitive inhibitor

160. Which gene sanctuary has been created for an insectivorous plant ?

(a) Kumbhalgarh sanctuary
(b) Bori sanctuary
(b) Nepenthes sanctuary
(c) all of the above

Instructions for Q. No. 161 to 180

Directions : Each of the questions given below consists of two statements, an assertions (A) and reason (R). Select the number corresponding to the appropriate response in the answer sheet as follows.

(a) If both assertion and reason are true and the reason is a correct explanation of the assertion
(b) If both assertion and reason are true but the reason is not a correct explanation of the assertion
(c) If the assertion is true, but the reason is false
(d) If both assertion and reason are falses

161. *Assertion (A) :* Xylem is made of four types of cells.
Reason (R) : This type of composition of the xylem is extremely clear in hydrophytes.

162. *Assertion (A) : Raphanobrassica* is the cross between *Raphanus* and *Brassica*.
Reason (R) : It is allopolyploid.

163. *Assertion (A) :* Auxins were the first growth hormones discovered in plants.
Reason (R) : In most of plants tip movement in seedling stage led to the discovery of auxins.

164. *Assertion (A) :* The frequency of polyploidy is higher in plants than in animals.
Reason (R) : Polyploidy is useful in the natural selection of new species of plants.

165. *Assertion (A) :* Housewives keep cut potatoes pieces submerged in water if not required for immediate use for cooking.
Reason (R) : This helps in softening the potato pieces.

166. *Assertion (A) :* More elastic fibres are found in artery walls than vein walls.
Reason (R) : Elastic fibres are absent from tendons.

167. *Assertion (A) :* The maximum change of potential difference across the membrane during an action potential is 110V approx.
Reason (R) : Action potential is self propagating.

168. *Assertion (A) :* A man's urine turned green when treated with ferric chloride.
Reason (R) : He is suffering from diabetes.

169. *Assertion (A) :* A woman is capable of sueing a man for refusing to own this child whose blood group is O. The blood group of woman is A and man is B.
Reason (R) : Genetically she is right he can be father of the child.

170. *Assertion (A) :* In coronary heart disease, there is impairment of heart muscles.
Reason (R) : Coronary heart disease is due to reduced blood supply.

171. *Assertion (A) : Fasciola hepatica* is hermaphrodite.
Reason (R) : The gonads are well developed

and the male and female genital ducts open into a common chamber, the genital atium.

172. *Assertion (A)* : In mitotic division, most of the ordered sequence of phases takes place during interphase.
Reason (R) : Synthesis of *m* RNA, *t* RNA and ribosomes occurs during G_1-phase and replication of DNA occurs in S-phase.

173. *Assertion (A)* : Role of erythrocytes in CO_2 transport is primary to form HCO_3^- ions for carriage in the plasma and reconvert them back to CO_2.
Reason (R) : About 42% of CO_2 carried in human blood is in the form of erythrocytic carbamino-haemoglobin; which breaks down in the lungs to release oxygen again.

174. *Assertion (A)* : The chewing and lapping mouthparts consist of a long tongue which is formed from the glossae of the labium.
Reason (R) : The galeae are much elongated and coiled, each forming a half tube, which makes complete tube when both are locked together.

175. *Assertion (A)* : When a foreign object, such as a sand grain gets in between the shell and mantle, it results in the formation of a pearl.
Reason (R) : The inner nacreous layer of iridiscent nacre is called the 'mother of pearl' which is formed of many thin and alternating layers of calcium carbonate and concholin.

176. *Assertion (A)* : *Neurospora* is an ideal material for genetical and biochemical studies.
Reason (R) : Because of its suitability in the studies of heredity and genetic material contained within it.

177. *Assertion (A)* : Heterosis is defined as superiority of F_1 hybrid of two genetically dissimilar parents.
Reason (R) : Heterosis can be measured in terms of growth rate, size and yield.

178. *Assertion (A)* : Left-handed DNA is known as B-DNA.
Reason (R) : Right-handed DNA is known as Z-DNA.

179. *Assertion (A)* : Rhizoidal aggregates have been observed at distinct sites on curled root hairs.
Reason (R) : The infection thread is formed by a process of invagination of the hair cell walls in the region of curling.

180. *Assertion (A)* : Mendelian recombinations are due to crossing over.
Reason (R) : Crossing over bring about exchange of genes through chiasmata formation.

GENERAL KNOWLEDGE

181. Which 13th Century Indian poet and discipline of Sufi Saint Hazrat Nizamuddin Aulia is buried next to his mentor in Delhi?
(a) Amir Khusro (b) Salim Shah Chishti
(c) Moin-ud-din chishti
(d) Kublia Khan

182. Men's team final of the NTPC Commonwealth Table Tennis Championship, held during April 2001 in New Delhi, was won by
(a) England (b) Singapore
(c) Nigeria (d) India

183. Which one of the following liquid gases is used as a fuel for a cryogenic engine?
(a) liquid oxygen (b) liquid hydrogen
(c) liquid nitrogen (d) liquid chlorine

184. Who among the following is a Bharatnatyam dancer?
(a) Kaushalya Reddy (b) Navtej Singh Johar
(c) Sunil Mehra (d) Rajeev Lochan

185. Which of the following is not one of the three basic instruments carried by NASA's Mars mission–2001 : *A Space Odyssey*?
(a) MARIE (b) GRS
(c) THEMIS (d) DANICS

186. Osteoporosis is a disease that affects
(a) heart (b) lungs
(c) bones (d) kidneys

187. Which of the following is not a mascot for the 2002 Football World Cup?
(a) Ato (b) Nik
(c) Kaz (d) Mik

188. 'Darshak', which was in the news during April 2001, is a/an
(a) indigenously-built hydrographic survey ship commissioned into the Indian Navy
(b) indigenously-built submarine commissioned into the Indian Navy
(c) indigenously-built missile frigate commissioned into the Indian Navy
(d) none of these

189. Majuli, the world's largest riverine island, is surrounded by waters of the river
(a) Amazon (b) Ganga
(c) Brahmaputra (d) Nile

190. Who among the following is the recipient of Saraswati Samman for the Year 2000 for his novel *Amruta Phala*?
(a) Dr. Indira Parthasarathy
(b) Manoj Das (c) Shri Ramakant Rath
(d) Subir Das

191. Most of the Ajanta paintings were completed during the rule of the
(a) Vardhanas (b) Sakas
(c) Satvahanas (d) Guptas

192. Budhism in Nepal was introduced in the reign of
(a) Samudragupta (b) Ashoka
(c) Chandragupta (d) Harsha

193. Which region of India receives rainfall due to western disturbance in winter?
(a) western region (b) central region
(c) eastern region
(d) north–western region

194. Which bank in India first introduced the Credit Card system?
(a) Andhra Bank (b) Central Bank
(c) Canara Bank (d) State Bank of India

195. The Association of South East Asian Nations (ASEAN) has its headquarters at
(a) Manila (b) Jakarta
(c) Kuala Lumpur (d) Bangkok

196. Certain bacteria living in human digestive system are beneficial because they synthesize vitamin
(a) D (b) B–Complex
(c) K (d) A

197. Who among the following was recently crowned Miss Universe 2001
(a) Miss Greece (b) Miss U.S.A.
(c) Miss Puerto Rico (d) Miss India

198. The Oscar Award for the Best Film for 2001 has been given to
(a) Crouching Tiger, Hidden Dragon
(b) American Beauty
(c) Gladiator
(d) Shakespeare in Love

199. Carnivorous animals are those that live on
(a) gram and grains of different types
(b) grass (c) human flesh
(d) animal flash

200. *Nag* is the name of the indigenously developed
(a) medium range missile
(b) anti–tank missile
(c) torpedo
(d) submarine

■■■

Model Test Paper–3

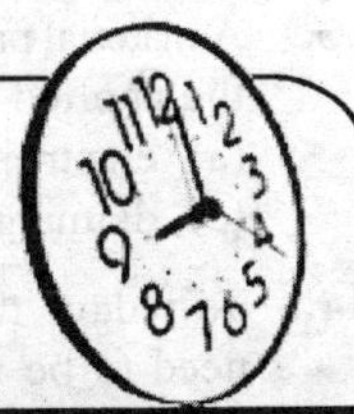

Time : $3\frac{1}{2}$ hours. *Maximum Marks : 200*

PHYSICS

1. There are two combination of n equal resistances. In combination A, all the resistances are in series and in combination B, all the resistances are in parallel. The ratio of the resistances of combination A to that of combination B is
(a) $n^2 : 1$ (b) $n : 1$
(c) $1 : 1/n$ (d) $1 : n^2$

2. If the time period of a magnet is T when $T \alpha \sqrt{x}$, then x represents
(a) length of the magnet
(b) moment of inertia of the magnet
(c) breadth of the magnet
(d) mass of the magnet

3. The electric intensity E, current density J and specific resistance p are related to each other through the relation
(a) $E = p/J$ (b) $E = Jp$
(c) $E = J/p$ (d) $E = JE$

4. The distances of two planets from the Sun are 10^{13} and 10^{12} metres respectively. The ratio of time periods of these two planet is
(a) $10\sqrt{10}$ (b) 100
(c) $1\sqrt{10}$ (d) 10

5. There will be an increase in potential energy of the system, if work is done upon the system by
(a) a conservative force
(b) a non-conservative force
(c) any conservative or nonconservative force
(d) none of the above

6. The amplitude of a particle in SHM decreases from 20 cm to 15 cm in 2 minutes. Its energy decreases by nearly
(a) 22.5% (b) 25%
(c) 50% (d) 12.5%

7. A small masses of rock like material surrounded by vapours of large masses and revolving in highly elliptical orbits are called
(a) meteorites (b) galaxy
(c) comets (d) asteroids

8. In a n - p - n transistor circuit, the collector current is 10 mA. If 90% of the electrons emitted reach the collector, then
(a) the base current will be 2 mA
(b) the emitter current will be 11 mA
(c) the emitter current will be 9 mA
(d) the base current will be 0.1 mA

9. What led to the discovery of proton ?
(a) scattering of α-particles by the heavier nuclei
(b) artificial disintegration of $_7N^{14}$ with α-particles.
(c) artificial disintegration of $_4Be^9$ with α-particles
(d) radioactive decay of certain elements

10. Maxwell's equation involving $d\vec{B}/dt$ is obtained from
(a) Biot-Savart's law (b) Ampere's law
(c) Gauss' law (d) Faraday's law

11. Two coils of self-inductances L_1 and L_2 are placed so close together that effective flux in one coil is completely linked with the other. If M is the mutual inductance between them, then
(a) $M = (L_1L_2)^2$ (b) $M = L_1/L_2$
(c) $M = L_1 L_2$ (d) $M = \sqrt{(L_1L_2)}$

12. The north pole of a bar magnet is rapidly introduced into a solenoid at the end A. Which of the following statements taking place ?
(a) the end A of the solenoid behaves like a north pole
(b) the end A of the solenoid behaves like a south pole
(c) no induced e.m.f. is developed
(d) the end A of the solenoid acquires positive potential

13. A material produces a magnetic field which opposes the applied magnetic field, then it is
(a) electromagnetic (b) paramagnetic
(c) diamagnetic (d) ferromagnetic

14. To reduce the range of voltmeter, its resistance need to be reduced. A voltmeter has resistance R_0 and range V. Which of the following resistances when connected in parallel will convert it into a voltmeter of range V/n ?
(a) $(n-1)R_0$ (b) $(n+1)R_0$
(c) nR_0 (d) none of these

15. What is the magnetic field at the point of intersections of diagonals of a current carrying square loop of each side L while the current through the loop is I ?
(a) $\frac{\mu_0 8\sqrt{2}I}{4\pi L}$ (b) $\frac{\mu_0 4\sqrt{2}I}{4\pi L}$
(c) $\frac{\mu_0\sqrt{2}I}{4\pi L}$ (d) none of these

16. The radius of the trajectory of a charged particle in a uniform magnetic field is proportional to
(a) momentum of the particle
(b) energy of the particle
(c) charge on the particle
(d) magnetic field

17. A wire of resistance 3Ω is cut into three equal pieces, which are joined to form a triangle. The equivalent resistance between any two corners of the triangle is
(a) $\frac{1}{4}\Omega$ (b) $\frac{2}{3}\Omega$
(c) $\frac{3}{2}\Omega$ (d) 4Ω

18. Two capacitors of capacitances 4 μF and 6 μF are connected across a 120 V battery in series with each other. What is the potential difference across the 4 μF capacitor ?
(a) 60 V (b) 48 V
(c) 40 V (d) 72 V

19. The persistence of sound in a hall is called
(a) reverberation (b) acoustics
(c) resonance (d) articulation

20. Which of the following statements is correct about the stationary wave ?
(a) particles at the consecutive anti-nodes are in same phase
(b) particles at the consecutive anti-nodes differ in phase by π
(c) all the particles of the medium vibrate in the same phase
(d) the phase lag between the particles continuously varies with the increase in distance

21. When a tuning fork produces sound waves in air, which one of the following properties of sound is same in the material of tuning fork as well as air?
(a) velocity (b) frequency
(c) wavelength (d) amplitude

22. The relation between velocity amplitude a, the displacement amplitude 'A' and the angular frequency ω of $S.H.M.$ is
(a) $A = \omega a$ (b) $a = \omega A$
(c) $A = \omega\nu$ (d) $a = \omega A^2$

23. Two steam engines X and Y have their source at 1000 K and 1100 K and their sinks are at 500 K and 400 K respectively. If η_x and η_y be their efficiencies, then which of the following statements about their efficiencies is true ?
(a) $\eta_x = \eta_y$ (b) $\eta_x < \eta_y$
(c) $\eta_x > \eta_y$
(d) the data is not sufficient to make the above prediction

24. What are thermal radiations ?
(a) electromagnetic waves
(b) mechanical longitudinal waves
(c) mechanical transverse waves
(d) none of these

25. Cloudy nights are usually warmer, because clouds
(a) have low thermal conductivity
(b) do not radiate heat
(c) do not absorb heat
(d) have high thermal conductivity

26. Let R be the radius of soap bubble and σ be the surface tension of soap solution. If p be the excess of pressure inside the soap bubble, then
(a) $p \propto R\sigma$ (b) $p \propto \frac{R}{\sigma}$
(c) $p \propto \frac{\sigma}{R}$ (d) $p \propto \frac{1}{R_\sigma}$

27. A gale blows over a house. The force due to the gale on the roof is
(a) in the direction of gale
(b) upward (c) downward
(d) in the direction of gale

28. Density of ice is ρ and that of water is σ. What will be the decrease in volume when a mass M of ice melts?
(a) $M\left(\frac{1}{\rho}-\frac{1}{\sigma}\right)$ (b) $\frac{\sigma-\rho}{M}$
(c) $\frac{M}{\sigma-\rho}$ (d) $\frac{1}{M}\left(\frac{1}{\rho}-\frac{1}{\sigma}\right)$

29. A bird is sitting in a wire cage, which is hanging from a spring balance. How will the reading change when the bird flies inside the cage?
(a) it will be more than earlier one
(b) it will be less than earlier one
(c) it will remain unchanged
(d) it cannot be predicted

30. The bulk modulus of rubber is $9 \times 10^8\ Nm^{-2}$. To what depth below the surface of sea should the rubber ball be taken as to decrease its volume by 0.1% ?
(a) 100 m (b) 10 m
(c) 1 m (d) 1 km

31. We have two wires W_1 and W_2. Both are made of same material and have the same length. The radius of cross-section of W_2 wire is twice that of W_1. Same load is suspended from both of them. If the strain in W_1 be 4, then in W_2 it will be
(b) 4 (b) 2
(c) 1 (d) 8

32. Two wires, made of the same material and of same area of cross section, are respectively one metre and two metres long. Force required to change the length of one metre wire by 1 cm is F_1. The force required to change the length of the $2m$ wire by 1 cm will be
(a) F_1 (b) $\frac{F_1}{4}$
(c) $\frac{F_1}{2}$ (d) $2F_1$

33. A planet is revolving around the Sun in an elliptical orbit. Its closest distance from the Sun is r and the farthest distance is R. If the orbital velocity of the planet closest of the Sun be v, then what is the velocity at the farthest point?
(a) $\left(\frac{r}{R}\right)^{1/2}$ (b) $\frac{vR}{r}$
(c) $\frac{vr}{R}$ (d) $v\left(\frac{R}{r}\right)^{1/2}$

34. Which of the following is not true for stationary satellite of the earth ?
(a) it is stationary in space
(b) its angular speed is equal to that of earth about its own axis.
(c) its time period is 24 hours
(d) it revolves from west to east

35. Two identical copper spheres of radius k are in contact with each other. If the gravitational attraction between them is R, then which of the following relations is correct ?
(a) $F \alpha \frac{1}{R^2}$ (b) $F \alpha R^4$
(c) $F \alpha R^2$ (d) $F \alpha \frac{1}{R^4}$

36. If the gravitational mass of a body on the moon be denoted by M_m and that on the earth by M_e, then
(a) $M_m = \sqrt{M_e}$ (b) $M_m = M_e$
(c) $M_m = \frac{1}{6}M_e$ (d) $M_m = 6M_e$

37. If the radius of the circular path of particle going round the circle is double without changing its frequency of rotation, then centripetal force on it will be
(a) doubled (b) unchanged
(c) halved (d) quadrupled

38. It is easier for a swimmer jumping into water from a height to describe a loop in the air by
(a) keeping the arms and legs straight
(b) spreading the arms and legs
(c) pulling the arms and legs closer
(d) none of these

39. Three identical balls each of radius 10 cm and

mass 1 kg each are placed touching one another on a horizontal surface. Where is their centre of mass located ?
(a) at the centre of one ball
(b) at the point of contact of any two spheres
(c) on the horizontal surface
(d) none of these

40. A nucleus of mass number A originally at rest emits α-particle with speed v. What will be the recoil speed of the daughter nucleus ?
(a) $v/(A-4)$ (b) $4v/(A+4)$
(c) $4v(A-4)$ (d) $v/(A+4)$

Instructions for Q. No. 41 to 60

Directions : Each of the questions given below consists of two statements, an assertions (A) and reason (R). Select the number corresponding to the appropriate response in the answer sheet as follows.

(a) If both assertion and reason are true and the reason is a correct explanation of the assertion
(b) If both assertion and reason are true but the reason is not a correct explanation of the assertion
(c) If the assertion is true, but the reason is false
(d) If both assertion and reason are falses

41. *Assertion (A) :* In a radioactive disintegration an electron is emitted by the nucleus.
Reason (R) : Electrons are always present inside the nucleus.

42. *Assertion (A) :* In Rutherford's experiment, α-particles from a radium source were allowed to fall on a 10^{-4} mm thick gold foil. Most of α-particles passed straight through the foil.
Reason (R) : The entire positive charge and nearly whole of the mass of the nucleus is concentrated in the nucleus.

43. *Assertion (A) :* The relative velocity of two photons travelling in opposite direction is C.
Reason (R) : The rest mass of a photon is zero.

44. *Assertion (A) :* Tiny drops of liquid resist deforming forces better than bigger drops.
Reason (R) : Excess pressure inside a drop is directly proportional to the surface tension.

45. *Assertion (A) :* The couple acting on a body is not equal to the rotational K.E. of the body.
Reason (R) : Couple and K.E. have different units

46. *Assertion (A) :* A thin aluminium disc spinning freely about a central pivot is quickly brought to rest when placed between the poles of a strong U-shaped magnet.
Reason (R) : A current induced in a disc rotating in a magnetic field produces a force which tends to oppose the disc's motion.

47. *Assertion (A) :* The period of simple pendulum is independent of the mass of the bob.
Reason (R) : Inertial and gravitational masses are equivalent.

48. *Assertion (A) :* The frequencies of incident, reflected and refracted beam of monochromatic light incident from one medium to another are the same.
Reason (R) : The incident, the reflected and the refracted rays are coplanar.

49. *Assertion (A) :* Radio waves can be polarised.
Reason (R) : Sound waves in air are longitudinal in nature.

50. *Assertion (A) :* A hollow metallic closed container maintained at a uniform temperature can act as a black body for radiations.
Reason (R) : All metals acts as black bodies.

51. *Assertion (A) :* The Sun appears bigger at sunrise and sunset than at mid-day.
Reason (R) : The phenomenon of interference bends light rays.

52. *Assertion (A) :* On a rainyday it is safer to drive a car or a bus at high speed.
Reason (R) : Coefficient of friction is higher on wetting the surface.

53. *Assertion (A) :* Electric appliances with metallic body *e.g.* heaters have two pin connections, whereas an electric bulb has three pin connection.
Reason (R) : Three pin connections reduce heating of connecting wires.

54. *Assertion (A) :* Environmental damage has increased the amount of ozone in the atmosphere.
Reason (R) : Increase of ozone increases the amount of ultraviolet radiation on the earth.

55. *Assertion (A)* : The rainbow is seen sometimes in the sky when it is raining to an observer with his back towards the Sun.
Reason (R) : Total internal reflection from water droplets causes dispersion. The final rays are in the backward direction.

56. *Assertion (A)* : The relative velocity of two photons travelling in opposite directions is C.
Reason (R) : The rest mass of photon is zero.

57. *Assertion (A)* : Brilliant colours are seen in thin layer of oil on the surface.
Reason (R) : White light is composed of several colours.

58. *Assertion (A)* : Activity of 10^8 undecayed radioactive nuclei of half life 50 days is equal to that of 1.2×10^8 undecayed nuclei of some other material with half life 60 days.
Reason (R) : Activity is proportional to half life.

59. *Assertion (A)* : Any hollow metallic closed container maintained at a uniform temperature can act as a source of black body radiation.
Reason (R) : All metals act as black bodies.

60. *Assertion (A)* : In LCR series circuit. The resonance occurs at one frequency only.
Reason (R) : At resonance the inductive reactance is equal to the capacitive reactance.

CHEMISTRY

61. 'Placedo' is often given to patients. It is
(a) a sugar pill
(b) a broad spectrum antibiotic
(c) an anti-depressant
(d) a tonic

62. The presence of a bacterium, virus or foreign protein triggers the production of specialised protein molecules known as antibodies or
(a) immunoglobulin (b) lymphocyte
(c) myoglobin (d) antigen

63. A tyndall effect would most likely be observed in which one of the following ?
(a) sol (b) precipitate
(c) solution (d) solvent

64. Natural rubber is a
(a) polyisoprene (b) polyamide
(c) polyester (d) polysaccharide

65. The radio element has half-life of one day. After three days, the amount of element disintegrated will be
(a) $\frac{1}{16}$ of original amount
(b) $\frac{1}{3}$ of original amount
(c) $\frac{1}{8}$ of original amount
(d) $\frac{7}{8}$ of original amount

66. Which one among the following is not an organometallic compound ?
(a) trimethoxy titanium chloride
(b) trimethyl aluminium
(c) trimethyl boron
(d) tetracarbonyl nickel

67. Which of the following electronic configurations will have the highest magnetic moment ?
(a) d^7 (b) d^4
(c) d^3 (d) d^5

68. Green colour is imparted to the flame by
(a) potassium salt (b) calcium salt
(c) sodium salt (d) barium salt

69. The alkaline earth metals have an outer electronic configuration of
(a) ns^1 (b) ns^2np^6
(c) ns^2 (d) ns^2np^1

70. The energy associated with adenosine triphosphate molecule is stored in
(a) C – O bonds (b) C – N bonds
(c) C – C bonds (d) O – P bonds

71. A peptide bond consists of a
(a) acetal linkage (b) hemiacetal linkage
(c) glycosidic linkage (d) amide linkage

72. In a chemical reaction, negative catalyst will increase the value of
(a) reaction rate
(b) ΔS
(c) ΔH
(d) activation energy

73. Beta rays have greater penetrating power than the alpha rays of similar energy because
(a) α-rays are positively-charged species carrying 2 units of charge
(b) β-rays have negligible mass and consequently very high velocities
(c) β-rays are a steam of electrons with negative charge
(d) α-rays are attracted by the electron while the beta particles are repelled by the cloud

74. I.U.P.A.C. name of complex, $K_3[Al(C_2O_4)_3]$ is
(a) potassium aluminium (III) oxalate
(b) potassium trioxalato-aluminate (III)
(c) potassium alumino oxalate
(d) potassium trioxalato-aluminate

75. From the following oxides of nitrogen which is paramagnetic ?
(a) N_2O_3 (b) N_2O
(c) N_2O_5 (d) NO_2

76. Which will be the major product when an alkyl halide reacts with potassium cyanide ?
(a) nitro compounds (b) isocyanides
(c) nitriles (d) amines

77. Reduction of ethanoic acid with Li AlH_4 produces
(a) ethanoic anhydride (b) ethanal
(c) ethanol (d) lithium ethanoate

78. A tertiary alcohol is obtained
(a) by the reaction of a ketone and a Grignard reaction
(b) when an aldehyde is reduced by $LiAlH_4$
(c) by the reaction is obtained
(d) when a ketone is reduced with $LiAlH_4$

79. •When trichloromethane is slowly oxidised by air in the presence of light the product formed is
(a) phosgene (b) phosphine
(c) carbon-dioxide (d) diethylcarbonate

80. The reaction
N_2O_5 (soln.) $\rightleftharpoons$ $2NO_2$ (soln.) + 1/2 O_2 (g),
is found to be first order with respect to N_2O_5. Given that the first order rate constant is 6.2×10^{-4} S^{-1}, the rate of the reaction when N_2O_5 is 1.25, mol L^{-1} is
(a) 3.10×10^{-5} mol L^{-1} S^{-1}
(b) 7.75×10^{-4} mol L^{-1} S^{-1}
(c) 1.55×10^{-4} mol L^{-1} S^{-1}
(d) 15.50×10^{-4} mol L^{-1} S^{-1}

81. Electrical conductivity is affected by
(a) the viscosity of the solvent (i.e., solute-solvent interaction)
(b) the solvation of ions (i.e., solute-solvent interaction)
(c) the interionic attraction (i.e., solute-solute interaction)
(d) all of these.

82. Of the following combinations, predict the Fe that could lead to a reaction. Use the information provided below : Fe^{3+} (aq) + e^- → Fe^{2+} (aq), E^0 = + 0.77 V
Cl_2 (g) + 2 e^- → Cl^- (aq), E^0 = + 1.36 V
(a) Fe^{2+} (aq) + Cl^- (aq)
(b) Fe^{3+} (aq) + Cl_2 (g)
(c) Fe^{2+} (aq) + Cl_2 (g)
(d) Fe^{3+} (aq) + Cl^- (aq)

83. Bond dissociation energies for H_2(g), Cl_2(g) and HCl(g) are 104, 58 and 103 k cals respectively. The enthalpy of formation of HCl(g) is
(a) 59 k cals (b) –22 k cals
(c) 22 k cals (d) –59 k cals

84. Animal cell swells when placed in
(a) hypotonic solution (b) hypertonic solution
(c) isotonic solution (d) saturated solution

85. Which of the following has 8 : 8 coordination ?
(a) CsCl (b) NaCl
(c) CaF_2 (d) Na_2O

86. For the angular momentum quantum number l = 4, the magnetic quantum number m has a set of
(a) 8 values (b) 5 values
(c) 4 values (d) 9 values

87. The energy of the ground state of the hydrogen atom is -2.17×10^{-18} J per atom. Its value in J mol^{-1} will be
(a) -2.17×10^{-18} J mol^{-1}
(b) -4.34×10^{-18} J mol^{-1}
(c) -2.624×10^{6} J mol^{-1}
(d) -1.312×10^{6} J mol^{-1}

88. Identify the incorrect statement regarding monosaccharides
(a) they also contain either an aldehyde or a keto functional group
(b) all monosaccharides are polyhydroxy com-

pounds containing a number of alcoholic groups

(c) there are about twenty naturally occurring monosaccharides

(d) two important monosaccharides are starch and cellulose

89. The molecular formula of an organic compound with a molecular weight of 78 and empirical formula of CH is

(a) C_4H_4 (b) C_8H_8
(c) C_6H_6 (d) C_3H_3

90. For complete hydrogenation of one mole of propyne, the quantity of hydrogen required is

(a) three moles (b) two moles
(c) one mole (d) less than one mole

91. Treatment of ethyne with ozone followed by treatment with zinc and water, leads to the formation of

(a) formaldehyde (b) an ozonide
(c) a diketone (d) a diol

92. The number of secondary carbons in 2, 2-dimethyl butane is

(a) 1 (b) 0
(c) 4 (d) 2

93. Hard steel can be further hardened by heating it to red hot and then cooling it by plunging it into cold water. This process is called

(a) tempering (b) annealing
(c) quenching (d) smelting

94. Extraction of iron from its ore consists of smelting and refining. Smelting is carried out in a

(a) electric furnace
(b) open health convertor
(c) bessemer convertor
(d) blast furnace

95. The element that does not belong to group 13 of the periodic table is

(a) rubidium (b) aluminium
(c) boron (d) gallium

96. Identify the statement that is not correct as far as structure of diborane is concerned

(a) the hydrogen atoms are not in the same plane in diborane
(b) each boron atom forms four bonds in diborane
(c) there are two bridging hydrogen atoms in diborane
(d) all B-H bonds in diborane are similar

97. Concentrated sulphuric acid has a charring action on carbohydrates because it

(a) has strong acidic properties
(b) has strong affinity towards water
(c) acts as an oxidising agent
(d) is a diprotic acid

98. Which of the following methods is used to remove permanent hardness of water ?

(a) addition of calcium chloride solution to water
(b) addition of sodium carbonate solution to water
(c) addition of magnesium chloride solution to water
(d) boiling water sufficiently

99. The factor that does not affect the rate of a chemical reaction in solution is

(a) the presence of a catalyst
(b) the temperature of the reactions
(c) the concentration of the reactants
(d) a change in pressure

100. Standard electrode potential refers to the electrode potential of

(a) the metal in combination with 1 mol L^{-1} solution of its ions
(b) the metal in combination with its ions of any concentration
(c) the metal alone
(d) the metal in combination with 1 N solution of its ions

Instructions for Q. No. 101 to 120

Directions : Each of the questions given below consists of two statements, an assertions (A) and reason (R). Select the number corresponding to the appropriate response in the answer sheet as follows.

(a) If both assertion and reason are true and the reason is a correct explanation of the assertion
(b) If both assertion and reason are true but the reason is not a correct explanation of the assertion
(c) If the assertion is true, but the reason is false
(d) If both assertion and reason are falses

101. *Assertion (A) :* The lactic acid shows the geometrical isomerism.
Reason (R) : Lactic acid has carbon-carbon double bond.

102. *Assertion (A) :* 2-Hydroxy i.e. butane dioic acid is known as malic acid.
Reason (R) : It is present in unripe apples.

103. *Assertion (A) :* During the fermentation of grape juice, a reddish brown coloured crust is formed.
Reason (R) : Impure potassiam hydrogen tartrate is of reddish brown colour and it is known as argol.

104. *Assertion (A) :* Amines are more basic than ethers and esters.
Reason (R) : Nitrogen is less electronegative than oxygen, it is in better position to accommodate the positive charge of the proton.

105. *Assertion (A) :* An orbital cannot have more than two electrons, moreover, if an orbital has two electrons they must have opposite spins.
Reason (R) : No two electrons in an atom can have same set of all the four quantum numbers

106. *Assertion (A) :* The pairing of electrons in the orbitals of a particular sub-shell does not occur until all the orbitals of the sub-shell are singly occupied.
Reason (R) : Singly occupied orbitals must have the electrons with parallel spins.

107. *Assertion (A) :* Fluorine molecules has bond order one.
Reason (R) : The number of electrons in antibonding molecular orbitals is two less than that in bonding molecular orbitals.

108. *Assertion (A) :* The molality of the solution does not change with change in temperature.
Reason (R) : The molality is expressed in units of moles per 1000 gm of solvent.

109. *Assertion (A) :* The molecularity of the reaction $H_2 + Br_2 \rightarrow 2HBr$ is two.
Reason (R) : The order of this reaction is 3/2.

110. *Assertion (A) :* Sodium ammonium hydrogen phosphate tetrahydrate is used in the bead test.
Reason (R) : The colourless transparent sodium metaphosphate combines with metallic oxides giving coloured orthophosphates.

111. *Assertion (A) :* Alpha (α) - amino acids exist as internal salt in solution as they have amino and carboxylic acid groups in near vicinity.
Reason (R) : H^+ ion given by carboxylic group (-COOH) is captured by amino group ($-NH_2$) having lone pair of electrons.

112. *Assertion (A) :* Methanoic acid reduces mercuric chloride to mercurous chloride on heating while ethanoic acid does not.
Reason (R) : Methanoic acid is a stronger acid than ethanoic acid.

113. *Assertion (A) :* Sulphur dioxide and chlorine are both bleaching agents.
Reason (R) : Both are drying agents.

114. *Assertion (A) :* In case the central atom in a molecule is surrounded only by shared pairs of electrons, the molecule has a regular geometry.
Reason (R) : The shared electron pairs repel each other with equal force so all bonds are equidistant from each other.

115. *Assertion (A) :* Nitrous acid (HNO_2) may act as an oxidising as well as a reducing agent.
Reason (R) : The oxidation number of nitrogen remains same in all the compounds.

116. *Assertion (A) :* The bond order in a molecule can have any value, positive or negative, integral or fractional or zero.
Reason (R) : The bond order in a molecule depends upon the number of electrons in the bonding and antibonding molecular orbitals.

117. *Assertion (A) :* Phenol undergoes Kolbe's reaction whereas ethanol does not.
Reason (R) : Phenoxide ion is more basic than ethoxide ion.

118. *Assertion (A) :* A spectral line will be observed for a $2p_x$-$2p_y$ transition.
Reason (R) : The energy is released in the form of wave of light when electron drops from $2p_x$ to $2p_y$ orbital.

119. *Assertion (A)* : Aromatic aldehydes and also formaldehyde undergo Cannizzaro reaction with strong alkali.
Reason (R) : Aldehydes which have α - hydrogen atoms undergo Cannizzaro reaction.

120. *Assertion (A)* : With halogens and alkali, amides give primary amines having one carbon atom less.
Reason (R) : The reaction of amides with alkali is a qualitative test of amides.

BIOLOGY

121. Where would you find chondrin secreting chondrocytes ?
(a) nerve cells (b) bone
(c) cartilage (d) muscles

122. Dermis in frog's skin comprises
(a) stratum spongiosum and compactum
(b) compactum and malpighian
(c) corneum and malpighian
(d) malpighian and stratum spongiosum

123. Hairs in mammals are developed from
(a) stratum compactum
(b) stratum corneum
(c) stratum germinativum
(d) stratum spongiosum

124. Eutheria are characterised by
(a) skin with glands (b) true- placenta
(c) hair (d) skin with glands

125. In the flying birds, the quill feathers are useful for
(a) giving shape to the bird
(b) gaining external heat
(c) flight in air
(d) preventing loss of heat from the body

126. A four-chambered heart is found in
(a) men
(b) all vertebrates
(c) all animals
(d) some reptiles, birds and mammals

127. Among mammals, placenta is not found in
(a) *Platypus* (b) man
(c) mouse/horse (d) kangaroo

128. Tadpole larva is a connecting link between
(a) reptiles and aves
(b) amphibians and mammals
(c) fishes and amphibians
(d) amphibians and reptiles

129. Ontogenetically, liver is
(a) endodermal (b) mesodermal
(c) ectodermal (d) none of these

130. In frog, micromeres and megameres are formed during
(a) third cleavage (b) second cleavage
(c) first cleavage (d) fourth cleavage

131. Which of the following constitutes symbiosis ?
(a) mutualism and commensalism
(b) commensalism and predation
(c) proto-cooperation and mutualism
(d) commensalism only

132. The type of inter-specific interaction in which one of the species is unaffected, and other is harmed, is called as
(a) predation (b) parasitism
(c) neutralism (d) antibiosis

133. What percentage of Earth surface forms the grassland ?
(a) 48% (b) 10%
(c) 3% (d) 19%

134. Besides leucoplasts, starch grains can be stored in
(a) chromoplasts (b) chloroplast
(c) mitochondria (d) lysosome

135. Fraternal twins are produced when
(a) single ovum is fertilized by two sperms
(b) single fertilized ovum divides into two
(c) two ova are fertilized simultaneously
(d) two ova develop partheno-genetically

136. The genetic constitution of klinefelter's syndrome is
(a) 44 + XY (b) 44 + XO
(c) 44 + XX (d) 44 + XXY

137. Polyploidy brings about
(a) instant speciation (b) gradual speciation
(c) both (a) and (b) (d) none of these

138. The book Voyage of the Beagle has a relationship with which one of the following ?
(a) atavism (b) lamarckism
(c) theory of natural selection
(d) none of these

139. Which of the following statements about photosynthesis is not true ?
(a) photosynthesis is rapid in green light
(b) oxygen is produced during photosynthesis from the breakdown of water
(c) carbon dioxide is absorbed by the leaves in bright light
(d) plants can photosynthesise without an increase in dry weight

140. The products of light reaction in photosynthesis are
(a) ferrodoxin and cytochrome b_6
(b) ATP and NADPH
(c) ADP and glucose
(d) plastoquinone and cytochrome *f*

141. Grana and stroma lamellae are the parts of
(a) chloroplast (b) golgi body
(c) ribosome (d) mitochondria

142. Which of the following plant shows whole plant senescence ?
(a) gram (b) mustard
(c) wheat (d) all of these

143. The pigment phytochrome was discovered by
(a) Borthwick & Hendricks
(b) Skoog (c) Went
(d) Melchers

144. A green scum suddenly appears on the village pond, most likely cause is
(a) increase in O_2 (b) increase in excreta
(c) increase in CO_2
(d) increase in inorganic minerals

145. Which of the following can determine the distribution of a plant of animal species ?
I. rainfall II. temperature
III. sources of fond
IV. sex of the individual
(a) II and IV (b) I and III
(c) I, II and III (d) Only IV

146. Which of the following techniques is an important aspect of *in vitro* culture in the field of experimental embryology ?
(a) aeration (b) aseptic conditions
(c) nutrient medium (d) all of these

147. In a seed, developing from a bitegmic ovule, the testa is the mature
(a) both outer and inner integuments
(b) outer integument (c) inner integument
(d) none of these

148. Which of the following statements is correct
(a) the lateral meristems are present at the tip of the root
(b) the primary permanent tissue can never become meristematic
(c) the secondary meristems are those which develop into permanent tissues
(d) cambium of roots is a primary meristems

149. The example of monocots showing secondary growth in stem is
(a) *Asparagus* (b) *Cocos*
(c) *Lilium* (d) *Yucca*

150. When T.S. of a dicot plant is seen under microscope, the middle region is dark but the outer region is light; the outer region is known as
(a) annual ring (b) sapwood
(c) heartwood (d) growth ring

151. Wounds in plants are healed by the activity of
(a) intercalary meristem
(b) lateral meristem
(c) apical meristem
(d) hemicellulose

152. Wood is a general term for
(a) vessels
(b) secondary xylem
(c) primary xylem
(d) secondary vascular elements

153. The perianth is the term used when
(a) calyx is absent and corolla is similar to calyx
(b) androecium and gynoecium are similar
(c) calyx and corolla are similar
(d) none of these

154. *Utricularia* is a
(a) leafless plant
(b) stemless plant
(c) rootless plant
(d) non-flowering plant

155. Which of the following functions are carried out by the leaf ?
I. photosynthesis II. transpiration
III. respiration IV. translocation
(a) II and III (b) I and II
(c) I and III (d) all of the above

156. Botanical name of pitcher plant is
(a) *Dionoea* (b) *Drosera*
(c) *Nepenthes* (d) *Utricularia*

157. Quinine, important in the treatment of malaria, is extracted from
(a) stem of *Hevea*
(b) bark of *Cinnamon*
(c) bark of *Cinchona*
(d) leaves of *Ocimum*

158. The pulse among following is
(a) *Ocimum sanctum*
(b) *Dalbergia latifolia*
(c) *Coffea arabica* (d) *Cicer arietium*

159. Hemp fibres are obtained from
(a) *Linum* (b) *Cannabis*
(c) *Corchorus* (d) *Hibiscus*

160. Which is a medicinal plant ?
(a) *Aconitum* (b) *Linum*
(c) *Dalbergia* (d) *Tectona*

Instructions for Q. No. 161 to 180

Directions : Each of the questions given below consists of two statements, an assertions (A) and reason (R). Select the number corresponding to the appropriate response in the answer sheet as follows.

(a) If both assertion and reason are true and the reason is a correct explanation of the assertion
(b) If both assertion and reason are true but the reason is not a correct explanation of the assertion
(c) If the assertion is true, but the reason is false
(d) If both assertion and reason are falses

161. *Assertion (A) :* Symbiosis is also furnished by mycorrhiza.
Reason (R) : In this case symbiosis is established between alga and virus.

162. *Assertion (A) :* Starved leaves show protoplasmic respiration.
Reason (R) : They have protein as their respiratory substrates.

163. *Assertion (A) :* R.Q. during anaerobic respiration is always infinity.
Reason (R) : Oxygen is never evolved.

164. *Assertion (A) :* All food chains will come to stand still if bacteria disappear from earth.
Reason (R) : Bacteria are only associated with the soil fertility and hardly have any role for food chains.

165. *Assertion (A) :* Fruits are stored in CO_2 environment.
Reason (R) : With increase in CO_2, the rate of respiration decreases.

166. *Assertion (A) : Monocystis* parasites in one hosts.
Reason (R) : Monocystis is monogenetic.

167. *Assertion (A) :* Chordates have poor regeneration power while non chordates have good regeneration power.
Reason (R) : Non chordates have asexual reproduction so they have good regeneration power.

168. *Assertion (A) :* Earthworms mate in April-June.
Reason (R) : Copulation in earthworm lasts for one month.

169. *Assertion (A) :* Blood takes no part in reproduction in cockroaches.
Reason (R) : Blood in them lacks respiratory pigments.

170. *Assertion (A) :* In a graafian follicle, the primary oocyte and the follicle cells may be considered as sibling cells.
Reason (R) : Both are derived from oogonia.

171. *Assertion (A) :* Glycolysis begins in the cytoplasm and causing split into 2 three-carbon intermediates, then rearranged further to yield two molecules of pyruvate.

Reason (R) : During glycolysis four ATP and two NADPH molecules are produced and net yield is only two ATP molecules.

172. *Assertion (A) :* Translocations involve transfers of genetic material between non-homologous chromosomes.
Reason (R) : Translocation involve shifting, not deleting or adding genetic material which can cause chromosomal defects when gametes are formed.

173. *Assertion (A) :* A tadpole whose thyroid gland has been removed may not metamorphose.
Reason (R) : Calcitonin and thyroxine are produced from thyroid gland. These hormones stimulate protein synthesis which are important for tissue growth and development in amphibian tadpoles.

174. *Assertion (A) :* Gene conversion in eukaryotes occurring mainly at synapsis during meiosis, whereby a donor DNA sequence, a few hundred bases or perhaps a kilobase in length is transferred from one gene to another having substantial sequence homology.
Reason (R) : It may be responsible for much diversity in some mammalian immunoglobulin production.

175. *Assertion (A) :* Cortisol is a protein hormone of mammals which promotes gluconeogenesis and lowers blood pressure.
Reason (R) : Low plasma cortisol level promotes release of corticotropin releasing factor (CRF) from the cortex, causing release in turn of ACTH from the posterior pituitary.

176. *Assertion (A) :* Molecules of 3 phosphoglyceraldehyde get isomerized to produce dihydroxy acetone phosphate.
Reason (R) : The isomerization is catalyzed by the enzyme *phosphate triose isomerase.*

177. *Assertion(A):* Antitranspirants are material applied to plants for retarding transpiration.
Reason (R) : Abscisic acid and phenyl mercuric acetate are not antitranspirants.

178. *Assertion(A):* When the chromosomes are highly coiled and condensed at the time of cell division, it is possible to photograph and count them.
Reason (R) : Each species has a characteristic chromosome number.

179. *Assertion(A):* DNA replicates after mitosis.
Reason (R) : In mitosis the chromosomal number does not stay constant.

180. *Assertion(A):* In collateral vascular bundles phloem is situated towards the inner side.
Reason (R) : In monocot stem the cambium is present.

GENERAL KNOWLEDGE

181. The timc difference between I.S.T. and G.M.T. is
(a) $5\frac{1}{2}$ hrs (b) 9 hrs
(c) $12\frac{1}{2}$ hrs (d) $8\frac{1}{2}$ hrs.

182. 'Pulitzer' prizes are awarded to Americans for excellence in
(a) films (b) social work
(c) journalism (d) meidcine.

183. Doldrum is an area of
(a) low temperature (b) low rainfall
(c) low pressure (d) low humidity.

184. The U.N. Day is observed on
(a) 24th October (b) 24th January
(c) 24th Septemper (d) 24th June.

185. Triputi temple is located in
(a) Karnataka (b) Andhra Pradesh
(c) Tamil Nadu (d) Kerala.

186. Port Blair is situated in
(a) North Andaman (b) South Andaman
(c) Middle Andaman (d) Little Andaman.

187. The first of the GAEL (Global Alliance for the elimination of Leprosy) was held in
(a) New Delhi (b) Bombay
(c) Culcutta (d) Paris.

188. Which of the following are the recipient of Bharat Ratan Award for year 2000.
(a) Lata Mangeshkar
(b) Ustad Bismillah Khan
(c) Asha Bhosle (d) Both (a) and (b).

189. Which mirror is used as a rear view mirror in vehicles?
(a) plain (b) convex
(c) concave (d) spherical.

190. Dronacharya Award is for
(a) best sports persons
(b) best coaches
(c) best persons in archery
(d) best shooters.

191. Tehri Dam is being built on the river
(a) Yamuna (b) Godavari
(c) Kaveri (d) Bhagirathi.

192. The state in South India which generates electricity based on hydel power only is
(a) Karnataka (b) Kerala
(c) Tamil Nadu (d) Andhra Pradesh.

193. The acid present in lemons and oranges is
(a) acetic acid (b) hydrochloric acid
(c) citric acid (d) oxalic acid.

194. Who wrote "Sare Jahanse Achchha Hindustan Hamara"?
(a) Ghalib (b) Iqbal
(c) Nehru (d) Azad.

195. Which country is honoured by having all the three International beauty crowns in the same year
(a) Venezuala (b) Italy
(c) South America (d) India.

196. Who among the following is the author of the book "Bradman's Best"?
(a) Roland Perry
(b) Barry Richards
(c) Richard Mulvaney (d) Jom Brokaw.

197. Which of the following computer viruses is named after a cherry and caffeine soft drink popular with programmes?
(a) Sircam (b) Code Pink
(c) Code Red (d) Malisa.

198. Megger is an instrument to measure
(a) very low resistance
(b) insulation resistance
(c) inductance of a coil
(d) all of the above.

199. A red object, when seen through a thick blue glass, appears
(a) red (b) violet
(c) green (d) black.

200. The most important and the main musical instrument in "Nautanki" from of folk theatre is
(a) nagara (b) tabla
(c) flute (d) mohuri.

■■■

Model Test Paper–4

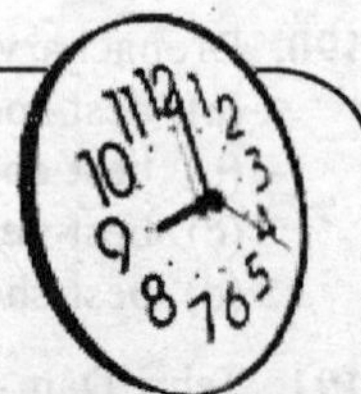

Time : $3\frac{1}{2}$ hours. *Maximum Marks : 200*

PHYSICS

1. In Huygen's wave theory, the focus of all points in the same state of vibration called
(a) wave front (b) a half-period zone
(c) vibrator (d) a ray

2. A spring has been kept fixed with immovable wall and a force of 1 newton has been applied on it. The spring extends upto a length I. Now if 2 newton force is applied on it, it will extend
(a) $2/3\ I$ (b) $3/2\ I$
(c) $2I$ (d) I^2

3. Refractive index is greater for
(a) light of greater wavelength
(b) light of shorter wavelength
(c) light of low frequency
(d) all of these

4. A thin circular copper plate, a sphere and a cube of same mass and material are heated to 100°C temperature. Now if they are allowed to cool, which of the three will cool first ?
(a) sphere (b) copper plate
(c) cube (d) all at same time

5. If we bring N-pole of a magnet towards the coil. The face of the coil acquires
(a) zero-polarity (b) north polarity
(c) south polarity (d) none of these

6. In a closed and organ pipe which of the following notes is not present if fundamental note is 50?
(a) 100 (b) 250
(c) 150 (d) none of these

7. In a semiconductor diode P-side is earthed and N-side is applied a potential of 2 volt, the diode shall
(a) breakdown (b) not conduct
(c) conduct (d) conduct partially

8. The sensitivity of galvanometer depends on
(a) moment of inertia of coil
(b) angle of deflection
(c) earth's magnetic field
(d) none of these

9. If v_e be the escape velocity and v_o be the orbital velocity, then v_e/v_o is equal to
(a) $2\sqrt{2}$ (b) $\sqrt{2}$
(c) $\frac{1}{\sqrt{2}}$ (d) 2

10. A pendulum of time period T is kept suspended in a train accelerating uniformly, then its time period
(a) decreases (b) increases
(c) remains unchanged
(d) none of these

11. The difference in the acceleration due to gravity at the pole and equator is given by
(a) $R\,\omega^2$ (b) $\Omega \cos \theta^2$
(c) $R\omega^2 \cos^2\theta$ (d) $\frac{R\omega^2\theta}{g^2}$

12. If two bulbs one of 60 W and other of 100 W are connected in parallel, then which one of the following will glow more ?
(a) 60 W bulb (b) 100 W bulb
(c) both equally (d) none of these

13. The number of electrons ejected from photoelectric surface depends upon
(a) the wavelength of light
(b) the frequency of light
(c) the intensity of incident light
(d) none of these

14. An n-type semiconductor is formed
(a) only from germanium
(b) when germanium is doped with impurity containing $3d$ valence electrons
(c) when germanium is doped with impurity containing 5-valence electrons
(d) only from pure silicon

15. Which one of the following is essential feature of SHM ?
(a) acceleration is directly proportional to displacement from mean position and is directed towards it
(b) restoring force is inversely proportional to displacement from mean position
(c) acceleration and amplitude
(d) constant amplitude

16. Which of the following wavelengths will suffer maximum deviation while passing through a prism?
(a) orange (b) green
(c) violet (d) red

17. A spectrum which contains all wavelengths without any break is called
(a) continuous emission spectrum
(b) line spectrum
(c) emission spectrum
(d) all of these

18. Seebeck emf depends on
(a) neutral temperature
(b) temperature of cold junction
(c) temperature of hot junction
(d) none of these

19. A hollow cylinder and a solid cylinder having same mass and same diameter are released from rest simultaneously from top of an inclined plane which one will reach bottom first ?
(a) solid (b) hollow
(c) both equally
(d) one with greator density

20. A hollow charged metal sphere has radius r. If the potential difference between its surface and a point at a distance of $3r$ from the centre is V, then electric field intensity at a distance of $3r$ from centre is
(a) $\frac{V}{2}r$ (b) $\frac{V}{4}r$
(c) $-\frac{V}{3r}$ (d) $\frac{V}{6}r$

21. In an A.C. circuit V and I is given by
$V = 100$ sine $(1000\ t)$ volt
$I = 1000 \sin (1000\ t + \pi/3)$ mA The power dissipated in the circuit is
(a) 10 W (b) 25 W
(c) 10^4 W (d) 250 W

22. A series LCR circuit is tuned to resonance. The angular frequency of the applied AC voltage is ω. If resistance of the circuit is R, the impedance of circuit will be
(a) $R^2 + \left(\omega L + \frac{1}{\omega C}\right)^2$ (b) $R + \omega L + \left(\frac{1}{\omega C}\right)$
(c) R (d) $\sqrt{R + \left(\omega L - \frac{1}{\omega C}\right)}$

23. Choose the correct answer
Heat in metals is produced due to
(a) collision of conduction electrons with protons
(b) collision of conduction electrons with atoms
(c) collision of electrons with electrons
(d) in all these ways as mentioned in above options

24. A proton enters a magnetic field parallel to the direction of field, then the path following by it is
(a) straight line (b) hyperbola
(c) circular (d) helical

25. The negative sign in the equation $e = \frac{-d\phi}{dt}$ indicates
(a) induced emf opposes the cause producing it
(b) current density is negative
(c) emf is always taken negative
(d) none of the above

26. Fission reaction was discovered by
(a) Seaborg
(b) Otto Han and Strassman
(c) Einstein (d) S. Hawking

27. If 200 MeV energy is released in a fission of a single nucleus of $_{92}U^{235}$. How many fissions must occur per second to produce a power of kW ?
(a) 3.125×10^{13} (b) 3.12×10^{12}
(c) 0.312×10^{13} (d) none of these

28. Some water drops of radius r each coalesec to form a big drop of radius R. Then rise in temperature is given by
(a) $\left(\frac{3T}{J}\right)\left(\frac{1}{r}-\frac{1}{R}\right)$ (b) $\frac{3T}{J.r}$
(c) $\frac{rT}{J}$ (d) $\frac{3T}{J}\left(\frac{1}{r}+\frac{1}{R}\right)$

29. A long straight conductor is bent into shape as shown. If it carries I ampere

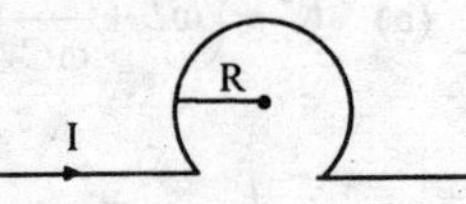

and its radius is R, then magnetic field $(\vec{B})$ at the centre of circular coil is
(a) $\frac{\mu_0 I(\pi+1)}{2\pi R}$ (b) Zero
(c) ∞ (d) $\frac{\mu_0 I(\pi-1)}{2\pi R}$

30. An engineer claims to have made an engine delivering 10 kW power with fuel consumption of 1g sec^{-1}. The calorific value of fuel is 2k cal/gm. His claim is
(a) depends on engine
(b) valid (c) non-valid
(d) depends on load

31. If two drops of same radius are falling through air with a velocity of 5 cm sec^{-1}. If the two drops coalesec to form one drop, the terminal velocity of the drop is
(a) $5\sqrt{2}$ cm/sec (b) 10 cm/sec
(c) 2.5 cm/sec (d) $5 \times 4^{1/3}$ cm/sec

32. The frequency of open organ pipe is f. If half part of the organ pipe is dipped in water, then frequency is
(a) $3f/4$ (b) $f/2$
(c) f (d) zero

33. A particle is acted upon by a force of constant magnitude which is always perpendicular to the velocity of particle. The motion of the particle takes place in a horizontal plane. It follows
(a) it moves in a circular path
(b) velocity is constant
(c) linear momentum is constant
(d) none of these

34. The number of turns in the coil are doubled, the emf will get
(a) quadrupled (b) halved
(c) doubled (d) none of these

35. Nucleus contains
(a) protons, electrons and neutrons
(b) electrons and neutrons
(c) protons and electrons
(d) protons and neutrons

36. Diamond shines due to
(a) total internal reflection
(b) refraction (c) reflection
(d) none of these

37. The frequency of sonometer wire is n. If its tension is increased four times and length is doubled, the new frequency will be
(a) n (b) $2n$
(c) $n/2$ (d) $4n$

38. Which of the following combination would give maximum emf ?
(a) Sb and Bi (b) Fe and Bi
(c) Ni and Cr (d) Cu and Fe

39. According to Bohr's theory, the radius of electron in an orbit described by principal quantum number n and atomic number Z is proportional to
(a) $\frac{n^2}{Z^2}$ (b) $\frac{n^2}{Z}$
(c) Z^2n^2 (d) $\frac{Z^2}{n}$

40. $\frac{kg.m^2}{s^2}$ is the unit of

(a) Momentum (b) Power
(c) Energy (d) Impulse

Instructions for Q. No. 41 to 60

Directions : Each of the questions given below consists of two statements, an assertions (A) and reason (R). Select the number corresponding to the appropriate response in the answer sheet as follows.

(a) If both assertion and reason are true and the reason is a correct explanation of the assertion

(b) If both assertion and reason are true but the reason is not a correct explanation of the assertion

(c) If the assertion is true, but the reason is false

(d) If both assertion and reason are falses

41. *Assertion (A) :* A dip needle becomes vertical at magnetic equator of the earth.
Reason (R) : The magnetic field due to the earth at the magnetic equator is vertical.

42. *Assertion (A) :* When two electrons are brought close to each other, the electrical potential energy increases.
Reason (R) : Work must be done against electrical force of repulsion.

43. *Assertion (A) :* If Young's double slit experiment is performed in water, the fringe with width will decrease
Reason (R) : Wavelength of light in water is smaller than in air.

44. *Assertion (A) :* Interference pattern is obtained on a screen due to two identical coherent sources of monochromatic light. The intensity at the central part of the screen becomes one half if one of the sources is blocked.
Reason (R) : The resultant density is the sum of the densities due to two sources; if one is blocked the intensity obviously reduces to one-half.

45. *Assertion (A) :* Insulators do not allow flow of current through them.
Reason (R) : They have no free charge carriers.

46. *Assertion (A) :* The shape of an automobile is so designed that its front resembles the streamline pattern of the fluid through which it moves.
Reason (R) : the resistance offered by the fluid is maximum.

47. *Assertion (A) :* Two satellites of mass m_1 and m_2 ($m_1 > m_2$) are going around the earth in orbits of radii r_1 and r_2 ($r_1 > r_2$).
Reason (R) : They will have same velocity.

48. *Assertion (A) :* In Thomson's experiment all the positive ions with the same value of specific charge are focussed on the same parabola irrespective of their velocities.
Reason (R) : The ions of same velocities arrive at different points on the same parabola.

49. *Assertion (A) :* In the process of nuclear fission the fragments emit two or three neutrons as soon as they are formed and subsequently emit particles.
Reason (R) : As the fragments contain an excess of neutrons over protons emission of neutrons and particles bring their neutron/proton ratio to stable values.

50. *Assertion (A) :* While passing round the corners of an obstacle the light spreads out to some extent into the region of the geometrical shadow.
Reason (R) : The bending is greater for light of longer wavelengths and less for shorter wavelengths.

51. *Assertion (A) :* An e.m.f. is induced in a circuit whenever there is a change in the magnetic flux linked with the circuit and the magnitude of the induced e.m.f. is equal to the negative rate of change of flux.
Reason (R) : The direction of the induced e.m.f. is such that it opposes the very cause to which it is due.

52. *Assertion (A) :* If a heavy nucleus is split into two medium sized parts, each of the new nuclei will have more binding energy per-nucleon than the original nucleus.
Reason (R) : Combining two light nuclei to form a single relatively heavy nucleus means more binding energy per nucleon in the new nucleus.

53. *Assertion (A) :* When two vibrating tuning forks having frequencies 256Hz and 512Hz are held near each other, beats can not be heard.
Reason (R) : The principle of superposition is valid only if the frequencies of the oscillators are nearly equal.

54. *Assertion (A) :* In the absence of space charge, the potential gradient between cathode and the anode will be uniform.
Reason (R) : The space charge reduces the potential in the cathode and anode region non-uniformly.

55. *Assertion (A) :* A thin aluminium disc, spinning freely about a central pivot, is quickly brought to rest when placed between the poles of strong U-shaped magnet.
Reason (R) : Current induced in the disc rotating in a magnetic field produces a force which opposes the motion of the disc.

56. *Assertion (A) :* When white light is incident on a thin oil film on the surface of water, colours are seen.
Reason (R) : White light is composed of several colours.

57. *Assertion (A) :* The work done in bringing a body from the top to the base along a frictionless inclined plane is the same as the work done in bringing it down along the vertical side.
Reason (R) : The gravitational force on the body along the inclined plane is the same as that along the vertical side.

58. *Assertion (A) :* A vibrating tuning fork sounds louder when its stem is put against a desk top.
Reason (R) : When a wave reaches another denser medium, a part of the wave is reflected.

59. *Assertion (A) :* Isotopes of an element can be separated by using a mass spectrometer.
Reason (R) : Separation of isotopes is possible because of the difference in electron numbers of isotopes.

60. *Assertion (A) :* A large soap bubble expands while a small bubble shrinks, when they are connected to each other by a capillary tube.
Reason (R) : The excess pressure inside bubble (or a drop) is inversely proportional to its radius

CHEMISTRY

61. Consider the following reaction occurring in an automobile
$2C_8H_{18(g)} + 25O_{2(g)} \rightarrow 16CO_{2(g)} + 18H_2O_{(g)}$
The sign ΔH, ΔS and ΔG would be
(a) –, +, + (b) –, +, –
(c) +, –, + (d) +, +, –

62. Equivalent conductance of NaCl, HCl and CH_3COONa at infinite dilution are 126.45, 426.16 and 91 ohm^{-1} cm^2 respectively. The equivalent conductance of CH_3COOH at infinite dilution would be
(a) 390.71 ohm^{-1} cm^2 (b) 253.71 ohm^{-1} cm^2
(c) 101.38 ohm^{-1} cm^2 (d) 678.90 ohm^{-1} cm^2

63. Which does not exist ?
(a) $[CCl_6]^{2-}$ (b) $[GeF_6]^{2-}$
(c) $[SiCl_6]^{2-}$ (d) $[GeF_6]^{2-}$

64. The type of hybridisation of boron in diborane is
(a) sp^3 (b) sp^2
(c) sp^2 (d) sp^3d^2

65. Boron compounds behave as Lewis acids because of their
(a) electron deficient character
(b) covalent nature
(c) acidic nature
(d) ionising property

66. All the following substances react with water. The pair that yields the same gaseous product is
(a) Ca and CaH_2 (b) Na and Na_2O_2
(c) K and KO_2 (d) Ba and BaO_2

67. Epsom salt is
(a) $2CaSO_4.H_2O$ (b) $MgSO_4.2H_2O$
(c) $MgSO_4.7H_2O$ (d) $BaSO_4.2H_2O$

68. Squashes are stored by adding
(a) Na_2SO_3 (b) KCl
(c) Citric acid
(d) Sod. metabisulphite

69. In Goldschmidt aluminothermic process, reducing agent used is
(a) Na (b) Al powder
(c) Coke (d) Al_2O_3

70. Which one of the following pairs of substances on reaction will not evolve H_2 gas ?
(a) iron and H_2SO_4 (aq)
(b) iron and steam
(c) copper and HCl (aq)
(d) sodium and ethanol

71. The oxide that gives hydrogen peroxide on treatment with dil acid is
(a) MnO_2 (b) Na_2O_2
(c) PbO_2 (d) TiO_2

72. The energy required to remove an electron of a gaseous atom from its ground state is called
(a) electrode potential
(b) ionisation energy
(c) potential energy
(d) activation energy

73. Chloride of an element A gives neutral solution in water. In the periodic table, the element A belongs to
(a) fifth group
(b) third group
(c) first group
(d) first transition series

74. If the valency shell electronic configuration of an element is $ns^2 np^5$, this element belongs to the group of
(a) noble gases (b) inert metals
(c) alkali metals (d) halogens

75. Main product of reaction
$CH_3CONH_2 + HNO_2 \rightarrow$? is
(a) CH_3NH_2 (b) $CH_3CH_2NH_2$
(c) CH_3COOH (d) CH_3NO_2

76. Paraldehyde is
(a) a hexamer of formaldehyde
(b) a trimer of acetaldehyde
(c) a trimer of formaldehyde
(d) a hexamer of acetaldehyde

77. An aldehyde when treated with an alkali gives an acid and an alcohol. Such reaction is named as
(a) cannizzaro reaction
(b) hydrolysis reaction
(c) aldol condensation
(d) claisen condensation

78. Reaction $\underbrace{CO + H_2}$ $+ H_2 \xrightarrow[Cr_2O_3\text{-}ZnO]{673\ K,\ 300\ atm.}$ may be used for the manufacture of
(a) HCHO (b) HCOOH
(c) CH_3OH (d) CH_3COOH

79. An organic compound A reacts with sodium metal and forms B. On heating with conc. H_2SO_4, A gives diethyl ether. A and B are respectively
(a) CH_3OH, CH_3ONa
(b) C_3H_7OH, C_3H_7ONa
(c) C_2H_5OH, C_2H_5ONa
(d) C_4H_9OH, C_4H_9ONa

80. Glucose molecule reacts with 'X' number of phenyl hydrazine molecules to yield osazone. The value of 'X' is
(a) 3 (b) 2
(c) 1 (d) 4

81. The sugar present in fruits is
(a) sucrose (b) glucose
(c) fructose (d) galactose

82. To become a carbohydrate a compound must contain at least
(a) 4 carbons (b) 3 carbons
(c) 2 carbons (d) 6 carbons

83. Vitamin D is also known as
(a) reporductive vitamin
(b) ascorbic acid
(c) growth vitamin
(d) sunshine vitamin

84. Zwitter ion is formed by
(a) benzoic acid (b) acetanilide
(c) aniline (d) lysine

85. Aspirin is an acetylation product of
(a) m-hydroxybenzoic acid
(b) o-dihydroxy benzene
(c) o-hydroxybenzoic acid
(d) p-dihydroxy benzene

86. The olefin which on ozonolysis gives CH_3CH_2CHO and CH_3CHO is
(a) 1-pentene (b) 2-butene
(c) 1-butene (d) 2-pentene

87. An isomer of ethanol is
(a) diethyl ether (b) dimethyl ether
(c) methanol (d) ethylene glycol

88. IUPAC name of

$$CH_3-\underset{C_2H_5}{\overset{H}{\underset{|}{\overset{|}{C}}}}-\underset{CH_3}{\overset{C_2H_9}{\underset{|}{\overset{|}{C}}}}-CH_3 \text{ is}$$

(a) 3, 4, 4-trimethyl heptane
(b) 2-ethyl-3, 3-dimethyl heptane
(c) 2-butyl-2-methyl-3 ethyl butane
(d) 3, 4, 4-trimethyl octane

89. The most-suitable method of separation of 1 : 1 mixture of *o*-and *p*-nitrophenols is
(a) crystallisation (b) chromatography
(c) sublimation (d) steam distillation

90. Consider the reaction
$M^{n+}_{(aq)} + ne^- \rightarrow M_{(s)}$
The standard reduction potential values of the metals M_1, M_2 and M_3 are –0.34V, –33.05V and –1.66V respectively. The order of their reducing power will be
(a) $M_1 > M_3 > M_2$ (b) $M_3 > M_2 > M_1$
(c) $M_1 > M_2 > M_3$ (d) $M_2 > M_3 > M_1$

91. Specific conductance of 0.1 N KCl solution at 25°C is 0.012 ohm^{-1} cm^{-1}. The resistance of the cell containing the solution at the same temperature was found to be 55 ohm. The cell constant will be
(a) 0.918 cm^{-1} (b) 0.66 cm^{-1}
(c) 0.142 cm^{-1} (d) 1.12 cm^{-1}

92. $S + \frac{3}{2}O_2 \rightarrow SO_3 + 2x$ k cal

$SO_2 + \frac{1}{2}O_2 \rightarrow SO_3 + y$ k cal

Find out the heat of formation of SO_2
(a) (x + y) (b) (2x + y)
(c) (2x – y) (d) $\frac{2x}{y}$

93. How many layers are adsorbed in chemical adsorption ?
(a) several (b) 2
(c) 1 (d) zero

94. Activation energy of a chemical reaction can be determined by
(a) evaluating rate constants at two different temperatures
(b) evaluating velocities of reaction at two different temperatures
(c) evaluating rate constant at standard temperature
(d) changing concentration of reactants

95. The pH of a solution obtained by mixing 50 ml 0.4N HCl and 50 ml 0.2N NaOH is
(a) 1.0 (b) –log 0.2
(c) –log 2 (d) 2.0

96. In which case K_p is less than K_c ?
(a) $2SO_2 + O_2 \rightleftharpoons 2SO_3$
(b) $H_2 + Cl_2 \rightleftharpoons 2HCl$
(c) $PCl_5 \rightleftharpoons PCl_3 + Cl_2$
(d) $2SO_3 + O_2 \rightleftharpoons 2SO_3$

97. How many grams of dibasic acid (mol. wt. 200) should be present in 100 ml of the aqueous solution to give 0.1N normality ?
(a) 2 g (b) 20 g
(c) 1 g (d) 10 g

98. The ratio between the two mean square speed of H_2 at 50 K and that of O_2 at 800 K is
(a) 1 (b) 2
(c) 4 (d) $\frac{1}{4}$

99. If we mix a pentavalent impurity in a crystal lattice of germanium, what type of semi-conductor formation will occur ?
(a) *p*-type (b) *n*-type
(c) both (a) and (b) (d) none of the two

100. A solid has a structure in which 'W' atoms are located at the corners of a cubic lattice, 'O' atoms at the centre of edges and 'Na' atoms at the centre of the cube. The formula of the compound is
(a) Na_2WO_3 (b) $NaWO_3$
(c) $NaWO_2$ (d) $NaWO_4$

Instructions for Q. No. 101 to 120

Directions : Each of the questions given below consists of two statements, an assertions (A) and reason (R). Select the number corresponding to the appropriate response in the answer sheet as follows.

(a) If both assertion and reason are true and the reason is a correct explanation of the assertion

(b) If both assertion and reason are true but the reason is not a correct explanation of the assertion

(c) If the assertion is true, but the reason is false

(d) If both assertion and reason are falses

101. *Assertion (A)* : Lead is a metal with a high density. It readily dissolves in moderately concentrated nitric acid giving colourless fumes which turn red in contact with air.
Reason (R) : Nitric oxide (NO) is a colourless oxide of nitrogen while NO_2 is a coloured oxide of nitrogen.

102. *Assertion (A)* : The reaction of ammonia solution with calomel is a disproportionation reaction in which mixture of Hg (ii) amido chloride and Hg are formed.
Reason (R) : In a disproportionation reaction species under reaction is neither oxidised nor reduced.

103. *Assertion (A)* : Sodium thiosulphate dissolves the white precipitate of silver chloride.
Reason (R) : The thiosulphate ions act as strong complexing agents.

104. *Assertion (A)* : When $SnCl_2$ solution is added to $HgCl_2$ solution, a milky white precipitate is obtained and on adding excess of $SnCl_2$, a black precipitate is formed.
Reason (R) : The disproportionation of Hg(II) is easier than its reduction only.

105. *Assertion (A)* : The electron affinity of chlorine is greater than that of fluorine.
Reason (R) : Chlorine is more electronegative than fluorine.

106. *Assertion (A)* : The boiling point of *n*-alkanes increases regularly with the increase in the number of carbon atoms.
Reason (R) : The magnitude of van der Waal's forces increases with the increases in molecular mass and molecular size.

107. *Assertion (A)* : *p*-nitroaniline is stronger base than *p*-toluidine.
Reason (R) : The electron with drawing NO_2 group in the *p*-nitroaniline makes it a stronger base.

108. *Assertion (A)* : All the amines, except tertiary amines are capable of forming intermolecular hydrogen bonds.
Reason (R) : Tertiary amines have larger molecules and surface area.

109. *Assertion (A)* : Phenol is strongly acidic than ethanol.
Reason (R) : Phenoxide ion is more stabilized by resonance than ethoxide ion.

110. *Assertion (A)* : The nuclear isomers are the atoms with the same atomic number and same mass number, but with different radioactive properties.
Reason (R) : The nucleus in the excited state will evidently have a different half-life as compared to that in the ground state.

111. *Assertion (A)* : Balloons made of Mylar films are better at containing helium than the conventional rubber balloons
Reason (R) : The root-mean-square speed of helium is very high so helium atoms can effuse rapidly through rubber balloons.

112. *Assertion (A)* : To separate ^{235}U from the more abundant ^{238}U isotope, all the uranium is converted into UF_6.
Reason (R) : UF_6 is one of the few compounds that exists in gaseous state under ordinary conditions.

113. *Assertion (A)* : One mole of helium atoms should occupy 22.4 litre volume at STP.
Reason (R) : Taking 31 pm as radius of helium atom, if we pack together a mole of helium atoms, the mole of atoms should have a volume of 22.4 litre.

114. *Assertion (A) :* A sample of 8.00 moles of chlorine gas in a 4.00 litre tank 27 C leads to a pressure of 49.2 atm according to ideal gas law.
Reason (R) : The actual pressure of the sample of chlorine is nearly 20 atmosphere less than the ideal pressure.

115. *Assertion (A) :* The pressure of a gas is inversely proportional to its volume at constant temperature and *n*.
Reason (R) : The gas volume is directly proportional to *n* at constant temperature and pressure.

116. *Assertion (A) :* Not only is the fraction of oxygen is reduced in diving gases, but nitrogen of normal air is replaced by helium.
Reason (R) : Nitrogen becomes more soluble in the body fluids at high pressure and causes a condition similar to alcohol intoxication.

117. *Assertion (A) :* When one talks after breathing helium, the sound becomes like that of Donald Duck.
Reason (R) : The vocal cords vibrate faster in an atmosphere less dense than air and the pitch of voice is raised.

118. *Assertion (A) :* The reacting gases combine in volumes that are ratios of small whole numbers.
Reason (R) : The partial pressure of a gas in a mixture is given by its mole fraction times the total pressure of the mixture.

119. *Assertion (A) :* The oxidation numbers are artificial, they are useful as a 'book-keeping' device of electrons in reactions.
Reason (R) : The oxidation numbers do not usually represent real charges on atoms, they are simply conventions that indicate what the maximum charge could possibly be on an atom in a molecule.

120. *Assertion (A) :* The structural-pair geometry of Formaldehyde molecule is trigonal planar.
Reason (R) : In H_2CO molecule, the carbon atom is surrounded by 3 sigma bonding electron pairs.

BIOLOGY

121. In which of the following animal, all the three important chordate characters exist throughout life ?
(a) amphibians (b) mammals
(c) *Amphioxus* (d) all of the above

122. Which cranial nerve has the highest number of branches ?
(a) vagus nerve (b) facial nerve
(c) trigeminal (d) all of the above

123. What is common among silver fish, crab, honey bee and prawn ?
(a) metamorphosis (b) compound eye
(c) poison gland (d) all of the above

124. The maximum formation of m-RNA occurs in
(a) ribosome (b) nucleolus
(c) cytoplasm (d) nucleoplasm

125. The most striking example of point mutation is found in a disease, called
(a) down's syndrome (b) night blindness
(c) thalassemia
(d) sickle-cell anaemia

126. At high altitude, the RBCs in the human blood will
(a) increase in number
(b) decrease in size
(c) increase in size (d) decrease in number

127. Typhus disease in humans is caused by
(a) rickettsiae (b) protozoans
(c) virus (d) none of the above

128. Rickettsiae form a group of
(a) bacterium-like prokaryotes
(b) viruses (c) fungi
(d) none of the above

129. In the fertile human female, approximately on which day of the ovulation takes place ?
(a) 14th day (b) 8th day
(c) 1st day (d) 18th day

130. Which of the following is regarded as an unit of nervous tissue?
(a) neuron (b) dendrite
(c) axon (d) myelin sheath

131. Which of the follwing carries absorbed product from digestive tract ?
(a) pulmonary vein
(b) hepatic portal vein
(c) hepatic artery
(d) none of the above

132. Who proposed the 'signal hypothesis' meant for the biosynthesis of secretory type of proteins?
(a) Blobel and Sabatini
(b) Camillo Golgi (c) Baltimore
(c) Sheeler and Bianchi

133. Which of the following carries protein and lipid to other parts of the cell?
(a) rough endoplasmic reticulum
(b) smooth endoplasmic reticulum
(c) both (a) and (b)
(d) none of the above

134. Epidermal layer consisting of dividing cells, is
(a) stratum granulosum
(b) stratum malpighii
(c) stratum lucidum
(d) stratum corneum

135. The tissue having least power of regeneration is
(a) skeletal tissue of long bones
(b) endothelium of blood vessels
(c) epidermis of skin
(d) nervous tissue of brain

136. Which of the following evidences does not favour the Lamarckian concept of inheritance of acquired chracters ?
(a) lack of pigment in cave dwelling animals
(b) presence of webbed toes in aquatic birds
(c) absence of limbs in snakes
(d) melanization in peppered moth

137. A disease caused by eating fish contaminated with mercury, is called
(a) osteosclerosis (b) minimata disease
(c) bright's disease
(d) hashimoto's disease

138. Although much CO_2 is carried in blood, yet blood does not become acidic, because
(a) buffer system of blood plays an important role
(b) CO_2 continuously diffuses through the tissues
(c) CO_2 combines with water to form H_2CO_3, which is neutralized by $NaCO_3$
(d) all of the above

139. The concept that 'population tends to increase geometrically while food supply increases arithmetically' was put forward by
(a) Thomas Malthus (b) Adam Smith
(c) Stuart Mill (d) Charles Darwin

140. The transgenic animals are those which have
(a) foreign DNA is some of its cells
(b) foreign RNA in all its cells
(c) foreign DNA in all of its cells
(d) both (b) and (c)

141. Which of the following metabolic disease occurs only in males ?
(a) Lesch–Nyhan disease
(b) Gaucher's disease
(c) Fabry's disease
(d) Hunter's disease

142. Hurthle cells are present in
(a) spleen (b) liver
(c) thyroid gland (d) lymph

143. Phylogenetic classification is one which is based on
(a) overall similarities
(b) common evolutionary descent
(c) habits
(d) utilitarian system

144. In mitochondira, cristae act as sites for
(a) oxidation-reduction reaction
(b) protein synthesis
(c) breakdown of macromolecules
(d) phosphorylation of flavoporteins

145. A product may bind to the regulatory enzyme's active site, preventing it from binding substrate and temporarity shutting down the metabolic pathway. This is called
(a) allosteric inhibition
(b) competitive inhibition
(c) negative feedback
(d) non-competitive inhibition

146. During the formation of cell wall the secreted outermost layer of cellulose is
(a) primary wall (b) secondary wall
(c) middle lamella (d) both (b) and (c)

147. Segments of DNA which are capable of moving in and out of a chromosome are termed as
(a) transposons (b) recon
(c) muton (d) replicon

148. The transition reactions
(a) connect glycolysis to the Krebs cycle
(b) give off CO_2
(c) utilize NAD^+
(d) include all of the above

149. Who among the following placed gymnosperms between monocots and dicots as third taxon ?
(a) Englar and Prantl
(b) Bentham and Hooker
(c) Hutchinson
(d) all of the above

150. Plasmodesmata are formed around the membranes of
(a) golgi bodies (b) nucleus
(c) chloroplast (d) none of the above

151. Which of the following statements is/are correct?
(a) both plasmids and viruses can serve as vectors
(b) vectors carry only the foreign gene into the host cells
(c) plasmids can carry recombinant DNA but viruses can not
(d) all of the above

152. In hypogynous type of flowers all floral parts arise below the
(a) sepals (b) gynoecium
(c) petals (d) androecium

153. In *Selaginella*, heterosporous spores are
(a) sexual and asexual
(b) large and small
(c) haploid and diploid
(d) all spores are of the same size

154. Which of the following plants contains mercury in their tissues ?
(a) *Fucus* (b) *Laminaria*
(c) both (a) and (b) (d) *Fusarium*

155. Protein 'canaralin' is obtained from
(a) carrots (b) almonds
(c) jack beans (d) grapes

156. Certain pollutants remain unchanged for a long time in the environment. These are not easily degradable and are termed as
(a) persistent (b) non-biodegradable
(c) both (a) and (b) (d) biodergradable

157. When the procedure of bacterial staining is carried out, the negative bacteria stain
(a) purple (b) red
(c) green (d) both (b) and (c)

158. Diatoms are placed under
(a) protozoans (b) fungi
(c) plantae (d) protista

159. A group of isodiametric cells with intercellular spaces must be
(a) prosenchyma (b) collenchyma
(c) sclerenchyma (d) parenchyma

160. Man's utilization of starch as energy source depends on the ability to convert it completely to individual glucose units. This process is initiated by the action of enzymes
(a) *Amylases* (b) *Cellulases*
(c) *Proteases* (d) none of the above

Instructions for Q. No. 161 to 180

Directions : Each of the questions given below consists of two statements, an assertions (A) and reason (R). Select the number corresponding to the appropriate response in the answer sheet as follows.

(a) If both assertion and reason are true and the reason is a correct explanation of the assertion
(b) If both assertion and reason are true but the reason is not a correct explanation of the assertion
(c) If the assertion is true, but the reason is false
(d) If both assertion and reason are falses

161. *Assertion (A) : Gibberella fujikuroi* was first called as *Fusarium moniliforme.*
Reason (R) : Its sexual stage was not discovered.

162. *Assertion (A)* : Tyloses are abundant in duramen.
Reason (R) : They provide rigidity and strength to heartwood.

163. *Assertion (A)* : Gram, pea and mango show epigeal germination.
Reason (R) : In epigeal germination radicle grows after hypocotyl.

164. *Assertion (A)* : Antitranspirants are material applied to plants for retarding transpiration.
Reason (R) : Abscisic acid and phenyl mercuric acetate are not antitranspirants.

165. *Assertion (A)* : The first activity in light reaction of photosynthesis is the photolysis of H_2O.
Reason (R) : PS I is not involved in the photolysis of water.

166. *Assertion (A)* : Olecranon process is present at the distal end of Ulna.
Reason (R) : It articulate with the trochlea.

167. *Assertion (A)* : Mule is an example of heterosis.
Reason (R) : Heterosis is the superiority of offspring to their parents.

168. *Assertion (A)* : Cardiac output is the volume of blood pumped by left or right ventricle in one minute.
Reason (R) : It is calculated by multiplying the heart rate by the stroke volume.

199. *Assertion (A)* : Tea, coffee and alcohols are diuretic.
Reason (R) : They suppress ADH (vasopressin).

170. *Assertion (A)* : Nephritis is the inflammation of kidney.
Reason (R) : It is caused by bacterial infection.

171. *Assertion (A)* : Enzymes are protein that catalyses biochemical reactions.
Reason (R) : The enzyme itself is unchanged in the reaction to take place.

172. *Assertion (A)* : Mimicry is a device adopted by the nature to protect the individuals for their own purposes.
Reason (R) : It helps the animal in self defence and survival.

173. *Assertion (A)* : The sustaining surface for the gliding in certain animals, is a fold or series of folds of the skin known as pataguim.
Reason (R) : The gliding flights are performed by arboreal animals.

174. *Assertion (A)* : Aldosterone is a steroid hormone and is important in the control of sodium and potassium ion concentration in mammals.
Reason (R) : It upgrades sodium ion concentration in the ECF by promoting reabsorption of sodium ions from renal tubules and excretion of potassium ions in urine.

175. *Assertion (A)* : Thyroid stimulating hormone is smallest polypeptide hormone of adenohypophysis of pituitary.
Reason (R) : Its role is to intensify the synthesis of hormones in adrenal cortex under a direct 'feedback' regulation.

176. *Assertion (A)* : There is a gradual decrease in the energy content at successive trophic level from producer to consumer.
Reason (R) : Pyramid of energy shows energy shows energy accumulation pattern at different trophic levels.

177. *Assertion (A)* : Meselson and stahl tested the Watson and Crick theory of DNA replication.
Reason (R) : They confirmed the mechanism of DNA replication by using the isotopic and centrifugation techniques.

178. *Assertion (A)* : Desired improved variety of economically useful crops are obtained by hybridization.
Reason (R) : When an ovary develops into a fruit without fertilization is called hybridization.

179. *Assertion (A)* : Chromosome appears longer during leptotene.
Reason (R) : The term chromosome was coined by Waldeyer.

180. *Assertion (A)* : Chromosome number is halved during Telophase-I.
Reason (R) : Chromosomes whose arms are equal, termed as submetacentric.

GENERAL KNOWLEDGE

181. 'Dazzler' is
(a) virus
(b) mascot for Cricket World Cup 2003
(c) bacteria
(d) none of these

182. Mohemmad Ali is associated with
(a) boxing (b) wrestling
(c) cricket (d) billiards

183. Who won the 2001 Miss World contest at the sun city resort in South Africa
(a) Zerelda Lee (b) Abgani Darego
(c) Diya Mirza (d) Juilet Jane Horne

184. 'Vande Matram' was taken from
(a) raj tarangani
(b) anand math
(c) akbar nama
(d) akbar khosa

185. 'Golden girl' is the biography of
(a) P.T.Usha
(b) Vijaya Lakshmi Pandit
(c) Sarojini Naidu
(d) Indira Gandhi

186. Who is the constitution head of our country?
(a) the President
(b) the Chief Justice
(c) the Attorney General
(d) the Prime Minister

187. When is the World Habitat Day?
(a) october 10 (b) october 8
(c) november 10 (d) october 3

188. Megasthenese visited India during the reign of
(a) Chandragupta II
(b) Chandragupta Maurya
(c) Ashoka
(d) Harsha

189. After returning from South Africa, Gandhiji launched his first successful 'Satyagraha' in
(a) chauri-chaura (b) dandi
(c) bardoli (d) champaran

190. The city which bore the brunt of the recent earthquake in Gujarat on January 26, 2001 is
(a) Ahmedabad (b) Bhuj
(c) Valsad (d) Gandhi Nagar

191. The Raga which is sung early in the morning is
(a) Todi (b) Darbari
(c) Bhopali (d) Bhimpalasi

192. For reproducing sound, CD (company disc) audioplayer uses a
(a) quartz crystal
(b) titanium needle
(c) laser beam
(d) barium titanate ceramic

193. Match List-1 (Books) with List II (Authors) and select the correct answer using the codes given below the Lists :

List I	List II
A. My Music, My Life	1. Laxman Garkward
B. Adha Gaon	2. Rahi Massom Raja
C. Radha	3. Ramakanta Nath
D. The Pilferer	4. Ravi Shankar

(a) A B C D
3 2 4 1
(b) A B C D
4 2 3 1
(c) A B C D
4 1 3 2
(d) A B C D
3 1 4 2

194. Hiroshima day in Japan was remembered on
(a) August 6 (b) August 9
(c) October 7 (d) August 13

195. A test tube baby means fertilisation of the ovum and development taking place in the
(a) test tube
(b) uterus
(c) test tube and uterus respectively
(d) uterus and test tube respectively

196. The Bus started between India and Bangladesh flies from
(a) Delhi (b) Guwahati
(c) Calcutta (d) Asansol

197. Harappas used which type of ancient script?
(a) symbolic (b) hieroglyphic
(c) linear (d) pictographic

198. The fourth Buddist council was held during the reign of
(a) Ashoka
(b) Chandragupta
(c) Kanishka
(d) Chandragupta Vikramaditya

199. Which of the following is not a computer language
(a) BASIC (b) JAVA
(c) SUMATRA (d) FORTRAN

200. Who played the leading role in the founding of the Indian National Congress?
(a) A.O.Hume
(b) Surendranath Banerjee
(c) Gopal Krishna Gokhale
(d) Khan Abdul Ghafer Khan

■■■

Model Test Paper–5

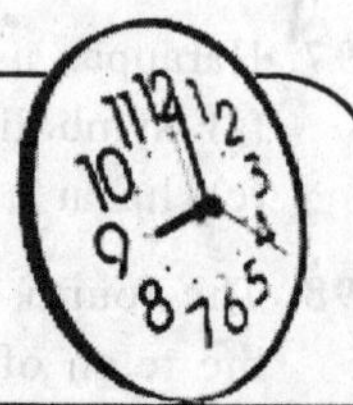

Time : $3\frac{1}{2}$ hours. *Maximum Marks : 200*

PHYSICS

1. Light of wavelength 0.4 μm from a mercury vapour lamp falls on a photocell and causes the emission of photoelectrons for which the stopping potential is 1.5 volt. With light of wavelength 0.6 μm from a sodium lamp, the stopping potential is 0.5. V. The work function of the photoelectric material used in the photocell is
(a) 1.5 eV (b) 2.0 eV
(c) 2.5 eV (d) 3.0 eV.

2. Suppose we convert the masses of a proton and a neutron completely into energies E_p and E_n respectively. Then $(E_p - E_n)$ is
(a) positive (b) zero
(c) negative
(d) positive or negative depending on the proton and the neutron come from the nucleus.

3. The earth's magnetic field acts as if the earth is a bar magnet. Then the equivalent *S*-pole
(a) lies in Australia
(b) is in the northern hemisphere
(c) is located near the equator
(d) coincides with the geographical south pole of the earth.

4. A neutral point is one at which two or more magnetic fields
(a) cancel one another
(b) act in the same direction
(c) combine to give minimum intensity
(d) combine to give maximum intensity.

5. A transparent material has three refractive indices 1.665, 1.650 and 1.68 for yellow, red and blue light respectively. The dispersive power of the substance is
(a) 0.03 (b) 0.018
(c) 2.0 (d) 0.045.

6. A lens of power +4.00 D is kept in contact with another lens. The combination has the focal length of 40 cm. The power of the second lens is
(a) -2.00 D (b) -1.50 D
(c) 2.50 D (d) 3.00 D.

7. The maximum velocity of an electron ejected from a photoelectric emitter when radiation falls on the latter is found to be 2×10^6 ms^{-1}. Assuming the charge to mass ratio of electron (*e/m*) to be 1.8×10^{11} coulomb/kg, the stopping potential is (in volt)
(a) 1.2 (b) 2.1
(c) 11.1 (d) 16.3.

8. Energy is not carried by
(a) longitudinal progressive waves
(b) electromagnetic waves
(c) transverse progressive waves
(d) stationary waves.

9. In nuclear reaction, which is conserved?
(a) charge only (b) momentum only
(c) sum of mass and energy
(d) all of the above.

10. How will the image formed by a convex lens be affected if the upper half of the lens is wrapped in black paper?
(a) the upper half of the image will be absent
(b) size of the image will be reduced to one half
(c) the brightness of image is reduced
(d) there will be no effect.

11. Suppose there are 4 branches of 5 identical cells

connected in series, the internal resistance of each cell being 10 ohm. If the group of cells sends a current of 0.2 ampere through an external resistance of 25 ohm, then the e.m.f of each cell is (in volt)

(a) 1.5 (b) 1.25
(c) 2.5 (d) 1.75.

12. An unknown resistance R_1 is connected in series with a resistance 10 ohm. This combination is connected to one gap of a metre bridge while the other gap is connected to another resistance R_2. The balance point is at 50 cm. Now, when the 10 ohm resistance is removed, the balance point shifts to 40 cm. Then the value of R_1 (in ohm) is

(a) 60 (b) 40
(c) 20 (d) 10.

13. Around a temperature of 25°C, a *p*-type semi-conductor has

(a) neither electrons nor holes
(b) a few free electrons and many holes
(c) a few holes and many free electrons
(d) many holes and many free electrons.

14. Suppose the binding energy per nucleon is plotted as a function of atomic mass number. The curve will have a sharp maximum for helium nucleus. This indicates

(a) helium is radioactive
(b) helium fissions very easily
(c) helium is very stable
(d) the rare occurrence of helium.

15. Two men talk on moon

(a) they hear each other with lower frequency
(b) they hear each other with higher frequency
(c) they can hear each other
(d) they can't hear each other at all.

16. 24 cells, each of internal resistance 0.5 Ω, are to be used to send maximum current through an external resistance of 3 Ω. The cells should be arranged

(a) all in series (b) all in parallel
(c) two rows of 12 cells each
(d) three rows of 8 cells each.

17. A bullet is shot from a gun when the angle of elevation of the gun is 30° and another when the angle of elevation is 60°.
For the two cases, which of the following is true?

(a) horizontal range as well as vertical height attained in both the cases will be same.
(b) horizontal range is same in both the cases but vertical height attained in the second case is three times than in the first case
(c) horizontal range in both the cases will be same but vertical height attained in the second case is two times than in the first case
(d) none of the above.

18. Amount of charge in coulomb required to deposit one gram equivalent in electrolysis is

(a) 96,490 (b) $48.0\sqrt{10^{-10}}$
(c) 6×10^{29} (d) 9608.

19. Given the relativistic mass of a particle

$$m = \frac{m_0}{\left(1-\frac{v^2}{c^2}\right)^{1/2}}$$

where m_0 = rest mass, v = its velocity and c = velocity of light. Which of the following statements is true?

(a) increase in mass is due to its increase in potential energy
(b) increases in mass is equal to the increased in the kinetic energy divided by c^2
(c) there is no increase in mass
(d) mass increases when $v = 0$.

20. A particle is moving eastwards with a velocity of 5 ms^{-1}. In 10 second, the velocity changes to 5 ms^{-1} northwards. The average acceleration in this time is

(a) $\frac{1}{2}$ ms^{-2} towards N
(b) zero
(c) $\frac{1}{\sqrt{2}}$ ms^{-2} towards NE

(d) $\frac{1}{\sqrt{2}}$ ms^{-2} towards NW.

21. The moment of inertia of a thin square plate $ABCD$ of uniform thickness about an axis passing through the centre O and perpendicular to the plane of the plate is

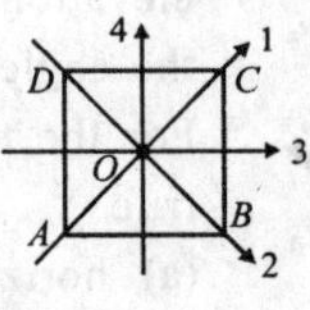

(a) $I_1 + I_2$ (b) $I_3 + I_4$
(c) $I_1 + I_3$ (d) $I_1 + I_2 + I_3 + I_4$.

22. An open and wide glass tube is immersed vertically in mercury in such a way that length 0.05 m extends above mercury level. The open end of the tube is closed and the tube is raised further by 0.43 m. The length of air column above mercury level in tube will be
(a) 0.215 m (b) 0.2 m
(c) 0.1 m (d) 0.4 m.

23. An equiconvex lens is made of material which has a refractive index of 1.6 for blue light and 1.5 for red light. Its focal length for red light is 0.20 m. What is the ratio of focal length for red light to focal length for blue light?
(a) 5/6 (b) 15/16
(c) 1 (d) 6/5.

24. A battery of internal resistance 4 Ω is connected to the network of resistance as shown in the figure. In order that the maximum power can be delivered to the network, the value of R in Ω should be

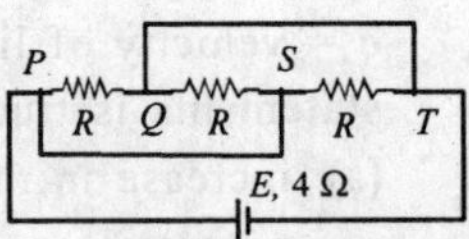

(a) 6 Ω (b) 12 Ω
(c) 8/3 Ω (d) 4/3 Ω.

25. A particle of mass 0.1 kg is projected with a velocity $U = \sqrt{10}$ ms^{-1} making an angle of 30° with the horizontal in x-y plane. The magnitude of the angular momentum of the particle about the point of projection when the particle is at its maximum height (H) is
(a) $\sqrt{\frac{30}{160}}(-\hat{k})$ kg m^2 s^{-1} (b) $\frac{\sqrt{30}}{160}(-\hat{k})$ kg m^2 s^{-1}
(c) zero (d) $\frac{\sqrt{30}}{160}(+\hat{k})$ kg m^2 s^{-1}.

26. An LC circuit has an inductance of 2 H and a capacitance of 2 PF. The capacitor is initially charged with a 10 V battery when the switch S is open. The battery is then removed from the circuit, and the switch is closed so that the capacitor is shorted across the inductor

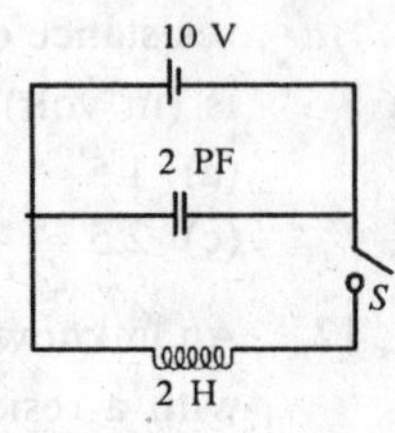

(a) the frequency of oscillation of the circuit is $\frac{10^6}{4\pi}$ Hz
(b) the maximum charge on the capacitor is 2×10^{-11} C
(c) the maximum current in the circuit is 10^{-5} A
(d) the maximum current in the circuit is $\frac{10^{-5}}{\pi}$ A.

27. An incubator made of material of thermal conductivity 2.5×10^{-4} Wm^{-1}K^{-1} has the following dimension $l = 1$ m, $b = 0.5$ m, $h = 0.5$ m and wall thickness $= 1 \times 10^{-2}$ m. The interior of incubator is to be maintained at 40°C by a heater coil placed inside, connected across 100 V supply. If the outside temperature is 20°C, what is the resistance of the heater coil?
(a) 2 kΩ (b) 3 kΩ
(c) 4 kΩ (d) 5 kΩ.

28. The K_α line from molybdenum ($Z = 42$) has a wavelength 0.7078 Å. What will be the wavelength of K_α line of an element whose atomic number is 30?
(a) 1.414 Å (b) 2.12 Å
(c) 2.8 Å (d) 3.5390 Å.

29. An achromatic prism is made by combining two prisms P_1 ($\mu_f = 1.523$, $\mu_c = 1.515$) and P_2 ($\mu_f = 1.666$, $\mu_c = 1.650$). If the angle of prism P_1 is 10° then the angle of the prism P_2 will be
(a) 5° (b) 7.8°
(c) 10.6° (d) 20°.

30. In the circuit shown in figure, the value of the current I is

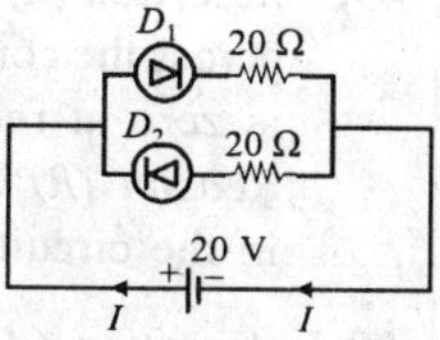

(a) 2 A
(b) 1 A
(c) zero
(d) 0.5 A.

31. Number of condensers, each of capacitance 1 μF and each one which gets punctured if a potential difference just exceeding 500 volt is applied, are provided. Then an arrangement suitable for giving a capacitor 2 μF across which 300 volt may be applied requires atleast

(a) 2 component capacitors
(b) 12 component capacitors
(c) 72 component capacitors
(d) 6 component capacitors.

32. In Young's double slit experiment, the intensity of central maximum is I_0. What will be the intensity at the same site when one slit is closed?

(a) I_0 (b) $I_0/2$
(c) $I_0/4$ (d) $I_0/16$.

33. The total energy of a particle executing simple harmonic motion is proportional to

(a) displacement from equilibrium position
(b) frequency of oscillation
(c) velocity in equilibrium position
(d) square of amplitude of motion.

34. Two racing cars of masses M_1 and M_2 are moving in circles of radii r_1 and r_2 respectively. Their speeds are such that they each move a complete circle in the same time t. The ratio of angular speed of the first to second car is

(a) $M_1 : M_2$ (b) $r_1 : r_2$
(c) 1 : 1 (d) $M_1v_1 : M_2v_2$.

35. If the coefficient of friction of a plane inclined at 45° is 0.5, the acceleration of a body sliding freely on it is

(a) $\frac{9.8}{\sqrt{2}}$ m/s² (b) 9.8 m/s²
(c) 4.9 m/s² (d) $\frac{9.8}{2\sqrt{2}}$ m/s².

36. The moment of inertia of a body (initially at rest) about a given axis is 1.2 kg-m². In order to produce a rotational kinetic energy of 1500 J, an angular acceleration of 25 rad/sec² must be applied about that axis for a period of

(a) 8 sec (b) 2 sec
(c) 1 sec (d) 10 sec.

37. R.M.S. velocity of a particle is V at pressure P. If the pressure increases by two times, then R.M.S. velocity will become

(a) $2V$ (b) V
(c) $0.5V$ (d) $4V$.

38. If the density of oxygen is 16 times that of hydrogen, what will be the corresponding ratio of their velocities of sound waves?

(a) 16 : 1 (b) 4 : 1
(c) 1 : 4 (d) 1 : 16.

39. Hydrogen balloon will carry which of the following body most easily?

(a) 10 kg feather (b) 10 kg iron
(c) 10 kg cotton (d) all of these.

40. Electromotive force is the force, which is able to maintain a constant

(a) resistance
(b) power
(c) current
(d) potential difference.

Instructions for Q. No. 41 to 60

Directions : Each of the questions given below consists of two statements, an assertions (A) and reason (R). Select the number corresponding to the appropriate response in the answer sheet as follows.

(a) If both assertion and reason are true and the reason is a correct explanation of the assertion

(b) If both assertion and reason are true but the reason is not a correct explanation of the assertion

(c) If the assertion is true, but the reason is false

(d) If both assertion and reason are falses

41. *Assertion (A)* : In a nuclear reactor graphite is used as moderator.
Reason (R) : Successive collisions of neutrons with the graphite nuclei result in loss of energy which slows the neutrons down.

42. *Assertion (A)* : White light contains the range of colours in light from violet with a wavelength of 4×10^{-7} m to red light with a wavelength of 7×10^{-7} m.
Reason (R) : When Young's double slit experiment is carried out with white light, multicoloured fringes are formed.

43. *Assertion (A)* : Insulators do not conduct electricity.
Reason (R) : In insulators the forbidden energy gap between the conduction and valence band is wide. On application of electric field the electrons fail to get required energy to cross over to conduction band which, therefore, remains empty.

44. *Assertion (A)* : Soft magnetic materials (*e.g.*, iron) have a high coercivity and do not demagnetise easily.
Reason (R) : Hard magnetic materials (*e.g.*, steel) have a low coercivity and become temporary magnets.

45. *Assertion (A)* : Laser can be used to measure huge distances by the method of pulse reflection.
Reason (R) : Light beam obtained from laser is highly collimative.

46. *Assertion (A)* : The velocity of an electron in an orbit is inversely proportional to the square of the radius of the orbit.
Reason (R) : The angular velocity of the electron is proportional to the radius of the orbit.

47. *Assertion (A)* : The maximum number of electrons in an orbit is $2n^2$ and the maximum number of electrons in a subshell is $2(2l + 1)$
Reason (R) : According to Pauli's exclusion principle no two electrons can have all their quantum numbers identical.

48. *Assertion (A)* : An ammeter is connected in series in an electrical circuit and it should have a low resistance.
Reason (R) : The introduction of the ammeter must not affect the main current.

49. *Assertion (A)* : In series A.C. circuit, the voltage across the combination of capacitor and inductor is zero at resonance.
Reason (R) : At series resonance the current in the circuit is zero.

50. *Assertion (A)* : If two or more different gases are mixed at the same temperature, there will be no exchange of energy among their molecules.
Reason (R) : Different gases at the same temperature have the same average kinetic energy per molecule and this energy is directly proportional to the absolute temperature of the gas.

51. *Assertion (A)* : When energy of hydrogen atom increases from -13.6eV to -1.51eV, its radius increases by 4.24Å.
Reason (R) : The energy of hydrogen atom is given by $E = -\frac{13.6}{n^2}$ eV and the radius is given by $r = 0.53\ n^2$:

52. *Assertion (A)* : The force with which one plate of a parallel plate capacitor is attracted towards the other plate is given by s^2/e_0 per unit area where s is the surface density of charge.
Reason (R) : The electric field due to one charged plate of the capacitor at the location of the other is $E = \sigma/\varepsilon_0$ and the force per unit area is given by $F = \sigma E$.

53. *Assertion (A)* : Air is more elastic than iron.
Reason (R) : Elasticity is directly proportional to compressibility and air is more compressible than iron.

54. *Assertion (A)* : A solid floats in a liquid so that it is just submerged. When the liquid is heated the solid sinks to the bottom.
Reason (R) : Weight of the solid increases with the rise in temperature.

55. *Assertion (A)* : When a man walks on a rough horizontal surface towards east, the frictional force on him is directed towards east.
Reason (R) : Frictional force always opposes the relative motion.

56. *Assertion (A) :* According to special theory of relativity a particle cannot travel with speed of light.
Reason (R) : In that case mass of the particle will be reduced to zero.

57. *Assertion (A) :* Electrons and protons having negligible initial velocity are accelerated through a certain potential difference. Protons will have larger momentum.
Reason (R) : An electron has negative charge while a proton has positive charge.

58. *Assertion (A) :* The velocity of sound in air increases due to the presence of moisture.
Reason (R) : The presence of moisture in air lowers the density of air.

59. *Assertion (A) :* Two systems which are both in thermal equilibrium with a third system are in thermal equilibrium with each other.
Reason (R) : The heat flows spontaneously from a system at a higher temperature to a system at lower temperature.

60. *Assertion (A) :* Tiny drops of liquid resist deforming forces better than bigger drops.
Reason (R) : Excess pressure inside a drop is directly proportional to surface tension.

CHEMISTRY

61. The mass of a neutron is
(a) less than that of a proton
(b) equal to that of an electron
(c) about one quarter of that of a helium atom
(d) much less than that of a hydrogen atom.

62. The difference between heats of reaction at constant pressure and constant volume for the reaction
$2C_6H_6(l) + 15O_2(g) \rightarrow 12\,CO_2(l) + 6H_2O(g)$ at 25° C in kJ is
(a) -7.43 (b) +3.72
(c) -3.72 (d) +7.43.

63. Which one of the following molecules is paramagnetic?
(a) CO (b) N_2O_4
(c) O_3 (d) O_2.

64. One mole of methanol, when burnt in oxygen, gives out 723 kJ mole^{-1} heat. If one mole of oxygen is used, what will be the amount of heat evolved?
(a) 723 kJ (b) 482 kJ
(c) 964 kJ (d) 241 kJ.

65. Chlorine can be liberated from potassium chloride solution by the action of
(a) iodine solution (b) fluorine
(c) sodium chloride (d) potassium iodide.

66. Atomic number of an element is 30. Therefore its possible group in the periodic table is
(a) I *A* (b) II *B*
(c) II *A* (d) I *B*.

67. Oxygen is obtained when one of the following compound is heated.
(a) SiO_2 (b) Fe_2O_3
(c) KNO_2 (d) $KMnO_4$.

68. The electronic configuration $1s^1\ 2s^2\ 2p^5\ 3s^1$ describes which one of the following?
(a) an excited state of fluorine
(b) the ground state of neon atom
(c) an excited state of neon atom
(d) the ground state of fluoride ion.

69. The molecular weight of a gas is 128. The weight of 8.21 litres at 3 atmospheric pressure and 27° C is
(a) 64 g (b) 128 g
(c) 82.1 g (d) 821 g.

70. For the reaction
$$2SO_3(g) \rightleftharpoons 2SO_2(g) + O_2(g)$$
$K_c = 32$. If $[SO_3] = [O_2] = 2$ M, then $[SO_2]$ is
(a) 4 M (b) 8 M
(c) 16 M (d) 0.8 M.

71. 0.2 g of gas *X* occupies a volume of 440 ml and 0.1 g of carbon dioxide occupies 320 ml at the same temperature and pressure. The gas *X* could be
(a) O_2 (b) SO_2
(c) NO (d) C_4H_{10}.

72. Ammonia is considered to be a Lewis base because of
(a) polarity of the molecule
(b) high volatility
(c) presence of lone pair of electrons
(d) the peculiar shape of the molecule.

73. Which of the following oxides of nitrogen is a white solid?
(a) NO (b) NO_2
(c) N_2O_5 (d) N_2O_3.

74. The base catalysed aldol condensation will not occur with
(a) propionaldehyde
(b) benzaldehyde
(c) 2 - methyl propionaldehyde
(d) acetone.

75. When a colourless gas is passed through bromine water only decolourisation takes place. The gas is
(a) SO_2 (b) HCl
(c) HBr (d) H_2S.

76. The mass of a molecule of oxygen in g is
(a) 5.3×10^{23} (b) 1.92×10^{-23}
(c) 10.6×10^{-23} (d) 5.3×10^{-23}.

77. Which of the following statements is correct?
(a) ΔH is positive for exothermic reactions
(b) ΔH is negative for endothermic reactions
(c) enthalpy of fusion is negative
(d) enthalpy of neutralisation of strong acid with a strong base is always the same.

78. An ion, which has 18 electrons in the outermost shell is
(a) Th^{4+} (b) K^+
(c) Cs^+ (d) Cu^+.

79. Hydrogen acts as an oxidising agent in its reaction with
(a) bromine (b) calcium
(c) nitrogen (d) sulphur.

80. pH of 10^{-8} M HCl solution is
(a) 8 (b) 7
(c) 4 (d) between 6 and 7.

81. Which of the following is not an electrophilic substitution ?
(a) $C_6H_6 + CH_3COCl \xrightarrow{AlCl_3} C_6H_5COCH_3 + HCl$
(b) $p\text{-}NO_2C_6H_4Cl + O\bar{H} \longrightarrow p\text{-}NO_2C_6H_4OH + C\bar{l}$
(c) $C_6H_5CH_3 \xrightarrow[\text{conc. } H_2SO_4]{\text{conc. } HNO_3} p\text{-}CH_3C_6H_4NO_2 + H_2O$
(d) $C_6H_6 + C_2H_5Cl \xrightarrow{AlCl_3} C_6H_5C_2H_5 + HCl$.

82. Which of the following is the most reactive towards ring nitration?
(a) benzene (b) toluene
(c) mesitylene (d) m - xylene.

83. Which of the following is the strongest acid?
(a) o - methoxybenzoic acid
(b) salicylic acid
(c) 2, 6 - dihydroxy benzoic acid
(d) benzoic acid.

84. Alkanes and alkenes can be distinguished by their solubility in
(a) alcohol (b) ether
(c) H_2SO_4 (d) water.

85. Which of the following compounds is least soluble in water?
(a) phenol (b) benzene
(c) ethanol (d) benzoic acid.

86. Oils and fats in our food not only provide us energy but also act as carriers of certain vitamins, such as
(a) A and B (b) A and C
(c) B and C (d) A and D.

87. Thermite process is used to extract metals
(a) when their oxides cannot be reduced by carbon

(b) when their carbonates do not yield oxides by thermal decomposition
(c) when their sulphides cannot be converted into oxides by roasting
(d) when their melting points are very high.

88. A sodium salt was mixed with ammonium sulphate and heated. A colourless gas was evolved which was insoluble in hot water. But it dissolved in cold water to give a neutral solution. The sodium salt was
(a) sodium chloride (b) sodium carbonate
(c) sodium nitrate (d) sodium phosphate.

89. A colourless water-soluble organic liquid decomposes sodium carbonate and liberates carbon dioxide. It produces a black precipitate with Tollen's reagent. The liquid is
(a) acetaldehyde (b) acetic acid
(c) formaldehyde (d) formic acid.

90. Among naturally occurring carbohydrates, an instance of a furanose ring is found in
(a) the galactose unit of lactose
(b) the glucose unit of cellulose
(c) the fructose unit of canesugar
(d) the glucose unit of canesugar.

91. If ΔH is the change in enthalpy and ΔE the change in the internal energy accompanying a gaseous reaction,
(a) ΔH is always greater than ΔE
(b) ΔH is always less than ΔE
(c) $\Delta H < \Delta E$ only if the number of moles of the products is greater than the number of moles of the reactants
(d) $\Delta H < \Delta E$ only if the number of moles of the products is less than the number of moles of the reactants.

92. Two useful by-products, obtained in the Solvay process of manufacturing sodium carbonate are
(a) quicklime and carbon dioxide
(b) sodium bicarbonate and ammonium chloride
(c) ammonium chloride solution and quicklime
(d) sodium bicarbonate and carbon dioxide.

93. Two moles of nitrogen and two moles of hydrogen are taken in a closed vessel of five litre capacity and suitable conditions are provided for the reaction. When equilibrium is reached, it is found that half a mole of nitrogen is used up. The equilibrium concentration of ammonia is
(a) 0.4 (b) 0.3
(c) 0.2 (d) 0.1.

94. Which of the following statements does not apply for weak electrolytes?
(a) conductivity of weak electrolytes at moderate concentration is extremely poor
(b) law of chemical equilibrium can be applied to the dissociation of weak electrolytes
(c) dissociation constant for weak electrolyte is very low
(d) degree of dissociation of weak electrolyte is appreciably high at higher concentration.

95. An aqueous solution of colourless metal sulphate M, gives a white precipitate with NH_4OH. This was soluble in excess of NH_4OH. On passing H_2S through this solution a white precipitate is formed. The metal in the metal salt is
(a) aluminium (b) calcium
(c) barium (d) zinc.

96. Formaldehyde and acetaldehyde are manufactured by dehydrogenation of methanol and ethanol respectively. The catalyst used in this reaction is
(a) conc. H_2SO_4 (b) copper
(c) nickel (d) H_3PO_4.

97. Nessler's reagent is
(a) an alkaline solution of $HgCl_2$ and KI
(b) a solution of ammonium hydroxide
(c) a solution of KI and sodium thiosulphate
(d) a solution of I_2.

98. The reaction in which the yield of the product cannot be increased by the application of high pressure is
(a) $PCl_3 (g) + Cl_2 (g) \rightleftharpoons PCl_5 (g)$
(b) $N_2 (g) + O_2 (g) \rightleftharpoons 2NO (g)$
(c) $N_2 (g) + 3H_2 (g) \rightleftharpoons 2NH_3 (g)$
(d) $2SO_2 (g) + O_2 (g) \rightleftharpoons 2SO_3 (g)$

99. The half-life for the reaction $N_2O_5 \rightleftharpoons 2NO_2 + \frac{1}{2}O_2$ is 24 hrs at 30°C. Starting with 10 g of N_2O_5, how many grams of N_2O_5 will remain after a period of 96 hours
(a) 1.25 g (b) 0.63 g
(c) 1.77 g (d) 0.5 g.

100. Aqua regia is a mixture
(a) 1 volume of conc. HCl + 3 volumes of conc. HNO_3
(b) 1 volume of conc. HNO_3 + 3 volumes of conc. HCl
(c) equal volumes of conc. HCl and conc. HNO_3
(d) 1 volume of conc. HCl + 3 volumes of conc. H_2SO_4.

Instructions for Q. No. 101 to 120

Directions : Each of the questions given below consists of two statements, an assertions (A) and reason (R). Select the number corresponding to the appropriate response in the answer sheet as follows.
(a) If both assertion and reason are true and the reason is a correct explanation of the assertion
(b) If both assertion and reason are true but the reason is not a correct explanation of the assertion
(c) If the assertion is true, but the reason is false
(d) If both assertion and reason are falses

101. *Assertion (A) :* To separate from the more abundant isotope, all the uranium is converted into UF_6.
Reason (R) : UF_6 is one of the few compounds that exists of gaseous state under ordinary conditions.

102. *Assertion (A) :* One mole of helium atoms should occupy 22.4 litre volume at STP.
Reason (R) : Taking 31 pm as radius of helium atom, if we pack together a mole of helium atoms, the mole of atoms should have a volume of 22.4 litre.

103. *Assertion (A) :* A sample of 8-00 moles of chlorine gas in a 4-00 litre tank at 27°C leads to a pressure of 49.2 atm according to ideal gas law.
Reason (R) : The actual pressure of the sample of chlorine is nearly 20 atomosphere less than the ideal pressure.

104. *Assertion (A) :* The pressure of a gas is inversely proportional to its volume at constant temperature and *n*.
Reason (R) : The gas volume is directly proportional to *n* at constant temperature and pressure.

105. *Assertion (A) :* Not only is the fraction of oxygen is reducd in diving gases, but nitrogen of normal air is replaced by helium.
Reason (R) : Nitrogen becomes more soluble in the body fluids at high pressure and causes a condition similar to alcohol intoxication.

106. *Assertion (A) :* When one talks after breathing helium, the sound becomes like that of Donald Duck.
Reason (R) : The vocal cords vibrate faster in an atmosphere less dense than air and the pitch of voice is raised.

107. *Assertion (A) :* The reacting gases combine in volumes that are ratios of small whole numbers.
Reason (R) : The partial pressure of a gas in a mixture is given by its mole fraction times the total pressure of the mixture.

108. *Assertion (A) :* The oxidation numbers are artificial, they are useful as a 'book-keeping' device of electron in reactions.
Reason (R) : The oxidation numbers do not usually represent real charges on atoms, they are simply conventions that indicate what the maximum charge could possibly be on an atom in a molecule.

109. *Assertion (A) :* The structural-pair geometry of Formaldehyde molecule is trigonal planar.
Reason (R) : In H_2CO molecule, the carbon atom is surrounded by 3 sigma bonding electron pairs.

110. *Assertion (A) :* The conjugated dienes are more stable than the corresponding alkenes containing one double bond or even the dienes containing two isolated double bonds.
Reason (R) : Conjugated dienes are regarded as hybrids of several contributing structures.

111. *Assertion (A) :* As mole is the basic chemical unit, the concentration of the dissolved solute is usually specified in terms of number of moles of solute.
Reason (R) : The total number of molecules of reactants involved in a balanced chemical equation is known as molecularity of the reaction.

112. *Assertion (A) :* Ionic compounds are made of positive and negative ions arranged in a manner so as to acquire maximum potential energy.
Reason (R) : In order to acquire maximum stability ions in a crystal should be arranged in such a way that the forces cf repulsion should overweight the forces of attraction.

113. *Assertion (A) :* When a trace amount of 'As' is added to extremely pure germanium a *n*-type of semiconductor is obtained.
Reason (R) : Four electrons of impurity are used in forming bonds and fifth electron remains free. This extra electron can serve to conduct electricity.

114. *Assertion (A) :* The half-life time of a first order reaction is always constant and it does not depends upon the initial concentration of reactants.
Reason (R) : For the first order reaction the half-life time is expressed as -

$$t_{1/2} = \frac{2.303}{k}\log 2$$

115. *Assertion (A) :* The kinetics of the reaction-
$mA + nB + pC \rightarrow m'X + n'Y + p'Z$
obeys the rate expression as-

$$\frac{dx}{dt} = k[A]^m[B]^n$$

Reason (R) : The rate of reaction does not depend upon the concentration of C.

116. *Assertion (A) :* The atoms of different elements having same mass number but different atomic number are known as isobars.
Reason (R) : The sum of protons and neutrons, in the isobars is always different.

117. *Assertion (A) :* The nuclear isomers are the atoms with the same atomic number and same mass number, but with different radioactive properties.
Reason (R) : The nucleus in the excited state will evidently have a different half-life as compared to that in the ground state.

118. *Assertion (A) :* In case of isoelectronic ions the ionic size increases with the increase in atomic number.
Reason (R) : The greater the attraction of nucleus, greater is the ionic radius.

119. *Assertion (A) :* Neither pure H_2SO_4 nor pure $HClO_4$ conducts electric current but a mixture of two does.
Reason (R) : Stronger acid $HClO_4$ donates a proton to H_2SO_4 which acts as a base.

120. *Assertion (A) :* The neutrons are better initiators of nuclear reactions than the protons, deutrons or α -particles of the same energy.
Reason (R) : Neutrons are uncharged particles and hence, they are not repelled by positively charged nucleus.

BIOLOGY

121. Which of the following contains hydrolytic enzyme?
(a) mitochondrion (b) lysosome
(c) ribosome (d) peroxisome.

122. Interferon is
(a) anti-viral (b) anti-bacterial
(c) anti-animal cell (d) bacteria.

123. What is the function of centrosome?
(a) cell wall formation (b) cell plate formation
(c) cell differentiation (d) cell division.

124. The vegetation of Rajasthan is
(a) xerophytic (b) deciduous
(c) alpine (d) arctic.

125. Which of the following gas is necessary for germination of pea seeds?
(a) H_2 (b) N_2
(c) O_2 (d) water vapour.

126. If the cell of root in wheat plant has 42 chromosomes, then the number of chromosomes in the synergid cell is

(a) 14 (b) 21
(c) 28 (d) 42.

127. Which of the following represents the correct order in prophase I?
(a) leptotene, zygotene, diplotene, pachytene, diakinesis
(b) leptotene, zygotene, pachytene, diplotene, diakinesis
(c) zygotene, diplotene, pachytene, leptotene, diakinesis
(d) diakinesis, zygotene, diplotene, leptotene, pachytene.

128. Which state in India is the maximum producer of peanut?
(a) Rajasthan (b) Gujarat
(c) Bihar (d) Uttar Pradesh.

129. The genetic preservation of exinct species is done in
(a) gene bank (b) national park
(c) herbarium (d) none of these.

130. Meiosis is best shown in
(a) anther wall (b) pollen grain
(c) gamete (d) microsporangium.

131. If a red eyed wild type *Drosophila* mates with a simple blue eyed (red is dominant while blue is recessive), then the ratio of red and blue eyed is
(a) 3 : 1 (b) 2 : 2
(c) 1 : 2 (d) 1 : 3.

132. Stalk of the ovule is called
(a) hilum (b) tigellum
(c) funicle (d) none of these.

133. Cypsella fruit develops from
(a) superior syncarpous ovary
(b) superior apocarpous ovary
(c) both (a) and (b)
(d) none of these.

134. System of binomial nomenclature in plants was given by
(a) Carolus Linnaeus
(b) Bentham and Hooker
(c) Robert Hooke
(d) Engler and Prantl.

135. The number of ATP formed after combustion of 1 mole of glucose is
(a) 36 (b) 38
(c) 40 (d) 30.

136. Which of the following plant is used in study of the photosynthesis?
(a) *Chlorella* (b) *Asparagus*
(c) *Amaranthus* (d) sunflower.

137. One quantasome contains
(a) 230 chlorophyll molecules
(b) 233 chlorophyll molecules
(c) 330 chlorophyll molecules
(d) some molecules of chlorophyll.

138. The leaf of *Mimosa* on touching becomes flaccid and droops down. This is due to
(a) water goes out of pulvini
(b) water movement
(c) based on water concentration
(d) none of these.

139. The proteins, which regulate life processes, are called
(a) structural protein (b) functional protein
(c) skeletal protein (d) all of these

140. In sex linkage, the speciality is
(a) gene flow
(b) criss-cross inheritance
(c) atavism (d) reversion

141. The modern theory of organic evolution is based on
(a) natural selection (b) genetic variation
(c) isolation (d) all of these

142. Which one of the following pairs is not correctly matched ?
(a) syphilis - *Trichuris trichura*
(b) sleeping sickness - *Trypanosoma gambiense*
(c) dengue fever - *Arbovirus*
(d) plague - *Yersinia pestis*

143. Animals, with radial symmetry in adult and bilateral symmetry in larva, are
(a) coelenterates (b) echinoderms
(c) annelids (d) platyhelminthes

144. In which of the following solution a cell get deplasmolyzed ?
(a) isotonic (b) detonic
(c) hypotonic (d) hypertonic

145. Linolenic acid is unsaturated fatty acid and its content is highest in
(a) sunflower oil (b) coconut oil
(c) cotton oil (d) groundnut oil

146. Common cold is caused by
(a) protozoa (b) unicellular algae
(b) bacteria (d) virus

147. Auxanometer is used to measure
(a) respiration (b) ascent of sap
(c) growth (d) transpiration

148. Stilt roots are present in
(a) *Helianthus* (b) maize
(c) banyan (d) *Tridax*

149. Commissural stigma is present in the family
(a) fabaceae (b) cruciferae
(c) solanaceae (d) liliaceae

150. The geranium oil is obtained from which part of *Pelargonium* ?
(a) roots (b) stem
(c) flower (d) leaves

151. The speed of development and metamorphosis of tadpole into adult frog is controlled by
(a) salinity of water (b) food availability
(c) pH of water (d) thyroid hormone

152. In which of the following, the calcified cartilage is found?
(a) vertebrae of shark
(b) suprascapula of pectoral girdle of frog
(c) scapula of pectoral girdle of man
(d) both 'a' and 'b'

153. Which of the following is a vestigial organ of human ?
(a) wisdom teeth (b) muscle of glottis
(c) hairs (d) intestine

154. A fungal disease of the poultry is
(a) Monoliasis (b) Coccodoisis
(c) Mareks (d) Coryza

155. Which of the following is prototherian ?
(a) *Opposum* (b) kangaroo
(c) *Platypus* (d) all of these

156. *Taenia saginata* differs from *T. solium* in the absence of
(a) hooks upon scolex (b) suckers upon scolex
(c) scolex (d) none of these

157. The term zymase for enzymes, in yeast, was coined by
(a) Louis Pasteur (b) Edward Buchner
(c) Sumner (d) Kuhne

158. Which one of the following is a structural protein?
(a) keratin (b) haemoglobin
(c) amino acid (d) gelatin.

159. Chromosomes start moving towards the pole in .... of mitosis.
(a) anaphase (b) metaphase
(c) prophase (d) telophase.

160. The function of chalaza in hen's egg is to
(a) nourish the embryo
(b) to keep the blastoderm on top
(c) to balance the egg
(d) has no function at all.

Instructions for Q. No. 161 to 180

Directions : Each of the questions given below consists of two statements, an assertions (A) and reason (R). Select the number corresponding to the appropriate response in the answer sheet as follows.

(a) If both assertion and reason are true and the reason is a correct explanation of the assertion
(b) If both assertion and reason are true but the reason is not a correct explanation of the assertion
(c) If the assertion is true, but the reason is false
(d) If both assertion and reason are falses

161. *Assertion (A) :* Bryophytes rarely attains a height of 20 cm.

Reason (R) : Largest bryophyte is *Dawsonia*.

162. *Assertion (A)* : Pyramid of energy is always upright.
Reason (R) : Loss of energy always takes place from one trophic level to another trophic level.

163. *Assertion (A)* : Self pollination takes place in cleistogamous flower.
Reason (R) : Cross pollination is the transfer of pollen grains in two genetically dissimilar flower.

164. *Assertion (A)* : In xerosere lichens are the pioneer.
Reason (R) : No other life form can survive on bare rock substratum.

165. *Assertion (A)* : Mycoplasmas are categorised under kingdom monera.
Reason (R) : They lack rigid cell wall.

166. *Assertion (A)* : PET scanning is more useful than CT scanning.
Reason (R) : PET is a computerised scanning technique.

167. *Assertion (A)* : In zero population growth the size of the population remains same or constant.
Reason (R) : Emigration is equal to immigration.

168. *Assertion (A)* : Bacteria do not have true sexual reproduction.
Reason (R) : Bacteria reproduce only by asexual means.

169. *Assertion (A)* : Karyotyping is done at mitotic metaphase.
Reason (R) : Karyotyping can detect the defect such as monosomy or trisomy.

170. *Assertion (A)* : In insects like bees, ants, & wasps the ploidy level is different in males & females.
Reason (R) : Males show arrhenotoky.

171. *Assertion (A)* : A body of nervous tissue integrating animal sensory and motor functions and providing through conduction pathways to transmit impulses rapidly, along the body.
Reason (R) : In vertebrates it comprises the brain and spinal cord, and in certain invertebrates a pair of solid ventral nerve chains.

172. *Assertion (A)* : The plasmalemmas of animal cells typically have the oligosaccharide chains of their glycolipids and glycopoteins exposed freely on their surfaces.
Reason (R) : These play important roles in immunological responses, in cell-cell adhesion and identification of cell surface changes.

173. *Assertion (A)* : A group of phosphorylated compounds transferring chemical energy required for cell work which depends upon their tendency to donate their phosphate group to water.
Reason (R) : Phosphate bond energy indicates the difference between free energies of reactants and products respectively before and after hydrolysis of a phosphorylated compound.

174. *Assertion (A)* : In placental mammals the placenta is connected to the embryo by the umblical cord and has an essential role in the immunological protection of the embryo.
Reason (R) : In mammals foetal components of the placenta derive initially from the chondroblast connected with embryonic blood stream either through its contact with the yolk sac.

175. *Assertion (A)* : Some bacterial and eukaryotic DNA polymerases can replace a nucleotide and insert incorrectly. DNA ligase then seals the phosphodiester bond. To avoid removing the nucleotide from the wrong strand, cells methylate DNA which has been formed some while; repair enzymes thus distinguish old from new DNA.
Reason (R) : Mutant lacking repair mechanisms are likely to be more susceptible to irradiating sources and express mutations so induced.

176. *Assertion (A)* : The first photochemical reaction in photosynthesis is the evolution of molecular oxygen.
Reason (R) : PS-II consists of the particle coloured dark green and the light gathering pigment complex shown to one side.

177. *Assertion (A)* : Synandrous condition is found in cucurbits.
Reason (R) : The male flower of cucurbits, generally, contains five stamens which are laterally fused (anthers and filaments both).

178. *Assertion (A)* : Hershey and Chase experiment showed that protein is the genetic material of T_2 bacteriophage.
Reason (R) : According to Hershey and Chase, RNA is the genetic material in T_2 bacteriophage.

179. *Assertion (A) :* Many globular proteins also undergo small conformational changes in the course of their biological function.
Reason (R) : These changes are associated with the binding of a ligand.

180. *Assertion (A) :* Elongation and division of cells are promoted by gibberellins.
Reason (R) : Gibberellins increase the formation of hydrolytic enzymes that release energy necessary for growth.

GENERAL KNOWLEDGE

181. The first Indian to receive the Megasaysay award was
(a) Dr. M.C. Modi (b) Vinoba Bhave
(c) Rabindra Nath Tagore
(d) Swami Vivekanand.

182. The first Indian woman to win an Olympic medal is
(a) Karnam Malleswari (b) P.T. Usha
(c) Ashwani Nachppa (d) None of these

183. How many years did Nehru spended in jails ?
(a) fifteen (b) nine
(c) ten (d) five

184. Where is the louvre Museum ?
(a) Paris (b) India
(c) New york (d) China

185. What does a bibliosphilist collect ?
(a) coins (b) stamps
(c) books (d) pens

186. The only category in which either an Indian or a person of Indian origin has not got a nobel prize is
(a) medicine (b) chemistry
(c) physics (d) literature

187. Which of the following is not been crowned as Miss World
(a) Diana Hayden (b) Ashwarya Rai
(c) Yukta Mukhi (d) Sushmita Sen

188. 'Alpha and Omega' means
(a) come and go
(b) the beginning and the end
(c) to win and to loose
(d) none of these

189. Gopichand and Aparna Popat play
(a) tennis (b) badminton
(c) chess (d) Table Tennis

190. The common name of iron oxide is
(a) magnetite (b) haemitite
(c) rust (d) smut

191. One megawatt is equal to
(a) 1,000,000 watts (b) 1000,000 watts
(c) 1,000,000,000 watts (d) 1000 watts

192. The instrument of music in which Ustad Amjad Ali Khan has distinguished himself is
(a) sarod (b) violin
(c) sitar (d) shehnai

193. The longest railway platform in the world is in
(a) India (b) United states
(c) Italy (d) Australia

194. The date which is considered as the date when India became small pox free was
(a) June 5, 1998 (b) July 5, 1995
(c) Dec 1, 1993 (d) Aug 13, 1990

195. The length of the river Indus is the same as
(a) Mahanadi (b) Brahmputra
(c) Kaveri (c) Ganga

196. Which of the following computer viruses is named after cherry and caffein soft drink popular with programmers ?
(a) sircam (b) code pink
(c) code Red (d) malisa

197. 'Rambola' is the original name of poet
(a) Tulsi das (b) Ram das
(c) Soordas (d) Kabir

198. Another name for the inherited blood disease thalassaemia ?
(a) looley's anaemia (b) grave's disease
(c) heamophilia (d) dypnoea

199. The most powerful supercomputer ever made in India is
(a) Param 1000 (b) Java 2000
(c) Arjun 100 (d) Vaibhav 2C.

200. The writer associated with 'Rally for the valley' (Narmada) is
(a) Salman Raished (b) Naipul
(c) Arundhati Roy (d) Isbal Perons

■■■

Model Test Paper–6

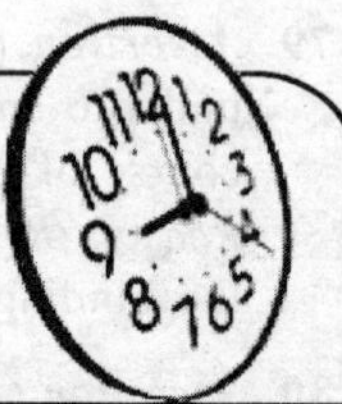

Time : $3\frac{1}{2}$ *hours.* *Maximum Marks* : 200

PHYSICS

1. The temperature of the sink of a Carnot engine is 27ºC. If the efficiency of the engine is 25%, the temperature of the source is

(a) 227ºC (b) 327ºC
(c) 127ºC (d) 27ºC.

2. Which is not a thermodynamical function?

(a) enthalpy (b) workdone
(c) Gibb's energy (d) internal energy.

3. Stream at 100ºC is passing into 1.1 kg of water contained in a calorimeter of water equivalent to 0.02 kg at 15ºC till the temperature of the calorimeter and its contents rises to 80ºC. The mass of the steam condensed in kg is

(a) 0.130 (b) 0.065
(c) 0.260 (d) 0.135.

4. Melting point of ice

(a) increases with increasing pressure
(b) decreases with increasing pressure
(c) is independent of pressure
(d) is proportional to pressure.

5. A fixed amount of nitrogen gas (1 mole) is taken and is subjected to pressure and temperature variation. The experiment is performed at high pressure as well as high temperatures. The results obtained are shown in the fig.

(4) (3) (2) (1)
$\frac{PV}{RT}$ 2 1 0
100 200 300
P (Atoms)

The correct variation of PV/RT with P will be exhibited by

(a) curve (4) (b) curve (3)
(c) curve (2) (d) curve (1).

6. An aluminium rod, Young's Modulus is 7.0×10^9 N/m² has a breaking strain of 0.21. The minimum cross sectional area of the rod in m² in order to support a load of 10^4 N is

(a) 1×10^{-2} (b) 1×10^{-3}
(c) 1.4×10^{-2} (d) 7.1×10^{-4}.

7. In order that a floating object be in a stable equilibrium, its centre of buoyancy should be

(a) vertically above its centre of gravity
(b) vertically below its centre of gravity
(c) horizontally in lines with its centre of gravity
(d) may be anywhere.

8. A crown made of gold and copper weighs 210 gm in air and 198 gm in water. The weight of gold in crown is

(a) 93 gm (b) 100 gm
(c) 150 gm (d) 193 gm.

Density of gold = 19.3 gm/cm³ and
Density of copper = 8.5 gm/cm³.

9. When a 20 gm mass hangs attached to one end of a light spring of length 10 cm, the spring stretches by 2 cm. The mass is pulled down until the total length of the spring is 14 cm. The elastic energy J, stored in the spring is

(a) 2×10^{-3} (b) 4×10^{-2}
(c) 4×10^{-3} (d) 8×10^{-3}.

10. A spring having a spring constant K is loaded with a mass m. The spring is cut into two equal parts and one of these is loaded again with the same mass. The new spring constant is

(a) $K/2$ (b) K
(c) $2K$ (d) K^2.

11. A cord is used to lower vertically a block of mass M at a distance d at a constant downward acceleration of $g/4$. Then the work done by the cord on the block is

(a) $\frac{Mgd}{4}$ (b) $\frac{-Mgd}{4}$
(c) $\frac{3Mgd}{4}$ (d) $\frac{-3Mgd}{4}$.

12. A rifle bullet loses $(1/20)^{th}$ of its speed in passing through a plank. The least number of such planks required to stop the bullet is
(a) 5 (b) 10
(c) 11 (d) 20.

13. Two spheres of masses M and $2M$ are initially at rest at a distance R apart. Due to mutual force of attraction they approach each other. When they are at separation $R/2$, the acceleration of their centre of mass would be
(a) 0 (b) 1 g m/s^2
(c) 3 g m/s^2 (d) 12 g m/s^2.

14. Two masses m and M are connected by a light string that passes through a smooth hole O at the centre of a table. Mass m lies on the table and M hangs vetically. m is moved round in a horizontal circle with O as the centre. If l is the length of the string from O to m then the frequency with which m should revolve so that M remains stationary is
(a) $\frac{1}{2\pi}\sqrt{\frac{Mg}{ml}}$ (b) $\frac{1}{\pi}\sqrt{\frac{Mg}{ml}}$
(c) $\frac{1}{2\pi}\sqrt{\frac{ml}{Mg}}$ (d) $\frac{1}{\pi}\sqrt{\frac{ml}{Mg}}$.

15. A car is moving in a circular track of radius r with a constant speed v. A plumb bob is suspended from the roof of the car by a light spring of length l. The angle made by the string with the vertical is
(a) $\tan^{-1}\left(\frac{v^2}{rg}\right)$ (b) $\tan^{-1}\left(\frac{v^2}{lg}\right)$
(c) $\tan^{-1}\left(\frac{rg}{v^2}\right)$ (d) $\tan^{-1}\left(\frac{lg}{v^2}\right)$.

16. A cord is wound round the circumference of a wheel of radius r. The axis of the wheel is horizontal and its moment of inertia about this axis is I. A weight mg is attached to the end of the cord and is allowed to fall from rest. The angular velocity of the wheel, when the weight has fallen through a distance h, is
(a) $\left[\frac{2gh}{I+mr}\right]^{1/2}$ (b) $\left[\frac{2mgh}{I+mr^2}\right]^{1/2}$
(c) $\left[\frac{2mgh}{I+2mr^2}\right]^{1/2}$ (d) $(2gh)^{1/2}$.

17. At what depth below the surface of the earth is the value of g same as that of a height of 5 km?
(a) 10 km (b) 7.5 km
(c) 5 km (d) 2.5 km.

18. The mass of moon is 1/81 of earth's mass and its radius is 1/4 of that of earth. If the escape velocity from the earth's surface is 11.2 km/s, its value for the moon is
(a) 0.14 km/s (b) 0.5 km/s
(c) 2.5 km/s (d) 5.0 km/s.

19. For a planet moving around the sun in an elliptical orbit of semi-major and semi-minor axes a and b, respectively, and period T,
(a) the torque acting on the planet around the sun is non-zero
(b) the angular momentum of the planet around the sun is constant
(c) the areal velocity is $\frac{\pi ab}{T}$
(d) the planet moves with a constant speed around the sun.

20. A simple pendulum has a time period T. The pendulum is completely immersed in a non-viscous liquid whose density is $1/10^{th}$ of that of the material of the bob. The time period of the pendulum immersed in the liquid is
(a) T (b) $\sqrt{\frac{9}{10}}\,T$
(c) $\sqrt{\frac{10}{9}}\,T$ (d) $\frac{T}{10}$.

21. What is the common base current amplification factor (α) of a transistor, if the common emitter current amplification factor (β) is 200?
(a) 0.895 (b) 0.995
(c) 0.855 (d) 0.915.

22. What isotope will be produced from ${}_{90}Th^{232}$ after 3α decays and two β decays?

(a) ${}_{88}Ra^{218}$ (b) ${}_{86}Rn^{218}$
(c) ${}_{88}Ra^{220}$ (d) ${}_{86}Rn^{220}$.

23. A transformer has a turns ratio of 100. The secondary supplies 16 W of power to a load. Assuming 80% efficiency, find the current in the primary if the input to the primary is 200 V A.C.

(a) 0.3 A (b) 0.2 A
(c) 0.05 A (d) 0.1 A.

24. The load resistance of a single transistor amplifier is 2000 Ω. If the transistor constant $\beta = 100$, what change in base current will produce a change in p.d. of 2 V across the load resistor?

(a) 1 μA (b) 20 μA
(c) 10 μA (d) 15 μA.

25. A convex lens of focal length 10 cm is made of glass of refractive index 1.5. It is immersed in a liquid of refractive index 1.3. What is the new focal length of the lens?

(a) 30.5 cm (b) 32.5 cm
(c) 27.5 cm (d) 33.5 cm.

26. A small source of sound moves along a circle as shown in the figure. The frequencies heard by a stationary listener at *O* when the source is at *A*, *B* and *C* are ν_1, ν_2, and ν_3 respectively. It follows that

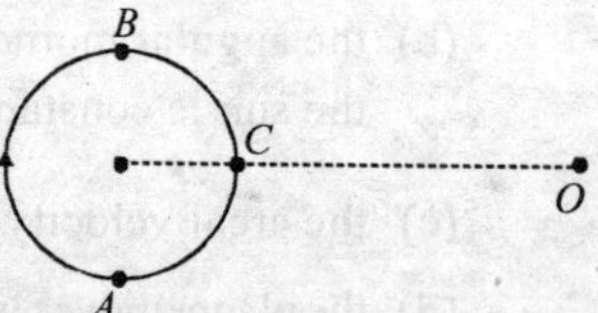

(a) $\nu_1 > \nu_3 > \nu_2$ (b) $\nu_2 > \nu_3 > \nu_1$
(c) $\nu_1 > \nu_2 > \nu_3$ (d) $\nu_3 > \nu_2 > \nu_1$.

27. If more air is pushed into a soap bubble, the pressure in it

(a) remains the same
(b) becomes zero
(c) increases (d) decreases.

28. A particle falls through a vertical distance of 10 m on a fixed smooth plane making an angle α with the horizontal, If its impact with the plane is perfectly elastic, the time interval in seconds between the first and second impacts on the plane is

(a) $\frac{20}{7}\sin\alpha$ (b) $\frac{20}{7}\tan\alpha$
(c) $\frac{20}{7}\cos\alpha$ (d) $\frac{20}{7}$.

29. A small object is projected up along the surface of a rough inclined plane of angle 45°. The object takes η times to descend than to ascend. The coefficient of kinetic friction between the object and plane is

(a) $\left(\frac{\eta-1}{\eta+1}\right)^2$ (b) $\frac{\eta-1}{2\eta^2+1}$
(c) $\frac{\eta-1}{\eta^2+1}$ (d) $\frac{2\eta-1}{\eta^2+1}$.

30. A balloon of mass m descends with a constant acceleration a. To acquire an upward acceleration of the same magnitude, it should reject a mass of

(a) $\frac{m(a+g)}{2g}$ (b) $\frac{2ma}{a+g}$
(c) $\frac{1}{2}\left(\frac{ma}{a+g}\right)$ (d) $\frac{2m}{g}(a+g)$.

31. A ball falls freely under gravity. The distances covered in the first, second and third second of motion are in the ratio

(a) 1 : 2 : 3 (b) 1 : 4 : 9
(c) 1 : 4 : 6 (d) 1 : 3 : 5.

32. A uniform iron chain lies on a horizontal surface. The maximum fraction of the length of the chain that can hang over the edge of the horizontal surface is ......

Given: coefficient of static friction = 0.25.

(a) 10% (b) 15%
(c) 20% (d) 25%.

33. An athlete completes one round of a circular track of radius R in 40 second. The displacement at the end of 2 minute 20 second is

(a) 0 (b) 2R
(c) 2πR (d) 7πR.

34. If $|\vec{\upsilon}_1 + \vec{\upsilon}_2| = |\vec{\upsilon}_1 - \vec{\upsilon}_2|$ and $\vec{\upsilon}_2$ is finite then

(a) $\vec{\upsilon}_1$ is parallel to $\vec{\upsilon}_2$ (b) $\vec{\upsilon}_1 = \vec{\upsilon}_2$

(c) $|\vec{\upsilon}_1| = |\vec{\upsilon}_2|$
(d) $\vec{\upsilon}_1$ and $\vec{\upsilon}_2$ are mutually perpendicular.

35. A car is moving along a straight horizontal road with a speed of 72 km h^{-1}. If the coefficient of static friction between the tyres and the road is 0.5, the shortest distance in which the car be stopped is ...... Given : $g = 10$ m s^{-2}.

(a) 30 m (b) 40 m
(c) 72 m (d) 20 m.

36. To shake off water from a wet cloth, it is common to give it a sudden jerk. In so doing, we are taking advantage of
(a) Newton's first law of motion
(b) Newton's second law of motion
(c) Newton's third law of motion
(d) impulse.

37. A lens of power +2 D and a lens of power –1 D are kept in contact. The combination behaves as:
(a) a lens of power +3 D
(b) a lens of power –3 D
(c) a lens of power +1 D
(d) a lens of power –1 D.

38. Two lenses of power +2 D and –5 D are kept in contact. The focal length of the combination is:
(a) –1/3 m (b) 1/3 m
(c) 3 m (d) –3 m.

39. Two spheres of equal masses but radii R and $2R$ are allowed to fall in a liquid. The ratio of their terminal velocities is:
(a) 1 : 4 (b) 1 : 2
(c) 2 : 1 (d) 1 : 16.

40. The displacement of a body is proportional to the cube of time elapsed. The magnitude of acceleration of the body is:
(a) increasing with time
(b) decreasing with time
(c) constant, but not zero
(d) zero.

Instructions for Q. No. 41 to 60

Directions : Each of the questions given below consists of two statements, an assertions (A) and reason (R). Select the number corresponding to the appropriate response in the answer sheet as follows.

(a) If both assertion and reason are true and the reason is a correct explanation of the assertion
(b) If both assertion and reason are true but the reason is not a correct explanation of the assertion
(c) If the assertion is true, but the reason is false
(d) If both assertion and reason are falses

41. *Assertion (A) :* The internal resistance of a cell depends on the concentration of the electrolyte used in the cell.
Reason (R) : dilution increases the ionisation of the electrolyte.

42. *Assertion (A) :* For a given mass of an ideal gas, the product of the pressure and volume is constant, at constant temperature.
Reason (R) : The root-mean square speed of the molecules is inversely proportional to the square root of their mass.

43. *Assertion (A) :* The ratio of C_p/C_v for a diatomic gas is more than that for a monoatomic gas.
Reason (R) : The molecules of a monoatomic gas have more degrees of freedom than those of a diatomic gas.

44. *Assertion (A) :* Newton's corpuscular theory of light could not explain refraction of light.
Reason (R) : It predicted that light should travel faster in denser media than in rarer media.

45. *Assertion (A) :* When temperature of a semi-conductor is increased, then its resistance decreases.
Reason (R) : The energy gap between conduction band and valence band is very small.

46. *Assertion (A) :* Electric appliances with metallic body have three connections, whereas an electric bulb has a two pin connection.
Reason (R) : Three pin connections reduce heating of connecting wires.

47. *Assertion (A) :* Environmental damage has increased the amount of ozone in the atmosphere.
Reason (R) : Increase of ozone increases the amount of ultraviolet radiation on earth.

48. *Assertion (A)* : The ratio of $\frac{C_p}{C_v}$ is more for helium than for hydrogen gas.
Reason (R) : Atomic mass of helium is more than that of hydrogen.

49. *Assertion (A)* : Machine parts are jammed in winter.
Reason (R) : The viscosity of lubricant used in machine parts increases at low temperatures.

50. *Assertion (A)* : The phenomenon of pair production is not possible unless the energy of gamma ray photon is equal to or greater than 1.20 MeV.
Reason (R) : The rest mass of an electron is 0.51 MeV.

51. *Assertion (A)* : A dip needle becomes vertical at magnetic equator of the earth.
Reason (R) : The magnetic field due to the earth at the magnetic equator is vertical.

52. *Assertion (A)* : When two electrons are brought close to each other, the electrical potential energy increases.
Reason (R) : Work must be done against electrical force of repulsion.

53. *Assertion (A)* : If Young's double slit experiment is performed in water, the fringe width will decrease.
Reason (R) : Wavelength of light in water is smaller than in air.

54. *Assertion (A)* : Interference pattern is obtained on a screen due to two identical coherent sources of monochromatic light. The intensity at the central part of the screen becomes one half if one of the sources is blocked.
Reason (R) : The resultant intensity is the sum of the intensities due to two sources; if one is blocked the intensity obviously reduces to one-half.

55. *Assertion (A)* : If hydrogen and oxygen molecules have the same *rms* speeds, they must be at the same temperature.
Reason (R) : The *rms* speed of a given gas is directly proportional to the square root of its absolute temperature.

56. *Assertion (A)* : Insulators do not allow flow of current through them.
Reason (R) : They have no free charge carriers

57. *Assertion (A)* : The shape of an automobile is so designed that its front resembles the streamline pattern of the fluid through which it moves.
Reason (R) : The resistance offered by the fluid is maximum.

58. *Assertion (A)* : Two satellites of mass m_1 and m_2 ($m_1 > m_2$) are going around the earth in orbits of radii r_1 and r_2 ($r_1 > r_2$).
Reason (R) : They will have same velocity.

59. *Assertion (A)* : It is not possible for a system, unaided by an external agency to transfer heat from a body at a lower temperature to another at a higher temperature.
Reason (R) : It is not possible to avoid the second law of thermodynamics.

60. *Assertion (A)* : In the process of nuclear fission the fragments emit two or three neutrons as soon as they are formed and subsequently particles.
Reason (R) : As the fragments contain an excess of neutrons over proton ratio to stable values.

CHEMISTRY

61. Energy of a electron in H-atom is given by: $E = -13.6/n^2$. Which one of the following statements is true when n is changed from 1 to 4? Energy will:
(a) decrease 4 times (b) increase 16 times
(c) increase 4 times (d) decrease 16 times

62. Of the following a copolymer is:
(a) neoprene (b) nylon
(c) PVC (d) natural rubber

63. Silver acetate when refluxed with Br_2 in CCl_4 gives:
(a) CH_3Br (b) CH_3COBr
(c) C_2H_5Br (d) $BrCH_2COOH$

64. The *p*H of 0.1 M methyl amine ($K_b = 5.0 \times 10^{-4}$) is
(a) 10.38 (b) 9.83
(c) 13.83 (d) 11.83

65. Addition of HOCl to allyl alcohol gives:
(a) 2-chloropropane 1, 3-diol
(b) 2, 3-dichloropane
(c) 3-chloropropane-1, 2-diol
(d) 1, 2, 3-trichloropropane

66. 0.2 g of organic compound on Kjehldahl's analysis gave enough NH_3 to just neutralise 20 cm^3 of 0.1N H_2SO_4. The percentage of nitrogen should be:
(a) 14 (b) 42
(c) 28 (d) 4.2

67. A hydrocarbon with molecular formula C_8H_{18} gives only one monochloro derivative. It should be:
(a) *n*-octane
(b) 2, 2, 4-tri methyl pentane
(c) 2-methyl heptane
(d) 2, 2, 3, 3 tetramethyl butane

68. To make a solution of *p*H 12, the amount of NaOH dissolved in 250 ml of solution should be:
(a) 0.1 (b) 0.3
(c) 0.2 (d) 0.25 g

69. Which of the following is a steroid-hormone?
(a) insulin
(b) adrenaline
(c) testosterone
(d) oxytocin

70. Treatment of propionaldehyde with dilute NaOH causes an aldol condensation to give:
(a) $CH_3CH_2COOCH_2CH_2CH_3$
(b) $CH_3CH_2CH(OH)CH_2CH_2CHO$
(c) $CH_3CH_2CHOHCH(CH_3)CHO$
(d) $CH_3CH_2COOH(CH_3)CHO$

71. If *F* represents 1 faraday & *N* represents avogadro's number then the charge on the electron will be:
(a) *F*/*N* (b) *F*·*N*
(c) *N*/*F* (d) *F*

72. Natural rubber is a polymer of:
(a) 1, 3 butadiene
(b) 1, 2-butadiene
(c) 2-methyl-1, 3 butadiene
(d) 2-chloro-1, 3 butadiens

73. The magnetic moment (in Bm) of a transition metal ion containing three unpaired electron is:
(a) 1.73 (b) 2.45
(c) 3.87 (d) 3.46

74. Which of the following complexes has maximum molar conductivity in the solution:
(a) $CrCl_3$ $6NH_3$ (b) $CrCl_3$ $4NH_3$
(c) $CrCl_3$ $5NH_3$ (d) $CrCl_3$ $3NH_3$

75. Glyptal is polymer of:
(a) ethylene glycol and phthalic acid
(b) phenol and formaldehyde
(c) ethylene glycol and terephthalic acid
(d) melamine and formaldehyde

76. The raw material used for making nylon-6 is:
(a) glycol and phthalic acid
(b) adipic acid and hexamethylene diamine
(c) chloroprene
(d) caprolactum

77. Stephen's reaction is reduction of:
(a) alkyl cyanide with $LiAlH_4$
(b) alkyl isocyanide with Na and C_2H_5OH
(c) alkyl cyanide with $SnCl_2$ and HCl
(d) acylhalide in the presence of Pd/$BaSO_4$

78. Which one of the following legand cannot form chelate?
(a) EDTA (b) 2, 2′, 2″-tripyridine
(c) etheylene diamine (d) pyridine

79. Hydrolysis of an easter gives acid *A* and alcohol *B*. The acid *A* reduces Fehling's solution. Oxidation of alcohol *B* gives acid *A*. The ester is:
(a) methyl formate (b) methyl acetate
(c) ethyl formate (d) ethyl acetate

80. In the laboratory by dehydration of ethyl alcohol ethylene was obtained with 50% yield. The ethylene so obtained reacted with bromine to give ethylene dibromide with 80% yield. If the amount of ethyl alcohol was 0.5 mol then ethylene dibromide produced would be:
(a) 0.1 mol (b) 4.0 mol
(c) 0.2 mol (d) 0.8 mol

81. Lewisite, a poisonous gas used in world war-II, is formed by the action of $AsCl_3$ with:
(a) $CH \equiv CH$ (b) $CH_3 - CH_3$
(c) $CH_2 = CH_2$ (d) C_6H_6

82. Cassiterite is an ore of:
(a) tin (b) lead
(c) mercury (d) iron

83. German silver is an alloy of:
(a) Cu & Zn (b) Ag & Ni
(c) Au. Cu & Zn (d) Cu. Zn & Ni

84. For neutralising 0.183 gms of a monobasic acid dissolved in water, 15 ml of N/10 NaOH were required. The molecular mass of acid is:
(a) 63 (b) 122
(c) 90 (d) 140

85. Anti-Markownikoff's rule involves the formation of an intermediate
(a) carbocations (b) free radicals
(c) carbanions (d) carbenes

86. The rate of a particular reaction quadruples, when the temperature changes from 293 K to 313 K. The activation energy for such reaction would be:
(a) 50.855 KJ mol^{-1} (b) 54.855 KJ mol^{-}
(c) 52.855 KJ mol^{-1} (d) 56.855 KJ mol^{-1}

87. The solubility product of silver carbonate be ksp, its solubility is:
(a) $3\sqrt{\frac{k_{sp}}{8}}$ (b) $3\sqrt{\frac{k_{sp}}{4}}$
(c) $3\sqrt{k_{sp}}$ (d) $3\sqrt{\frac{k_{sp}}{2}}$

88. Two moles of NH_3 gas are introduced into a previously evacuated one litre vessel in which it partially dissociates at high temperature as $2NH_{3\,(g)} \rightleftharpoons N_{2\,(g)} + 3H_{2\,(g)}$. At equilibrium, one mole of $NH_{3\,(g)}$ remains. The value of K_c is:
(a) 3/2 $mol^2\ l^{-1}$ (b) 3/2 mol
(c) 27/16 $mol^2\ l^{-2}$ (d) 27/64 $mol^2 l^{-2}$

89. The heat of combustion of ethane, ethylene and hydrogen are 370.44 k cal, 333.4 kcal and 68.4 kcal respectively. The heat evolved in the formation of ethane ($C_2H_4 + H_2 \rightarrow C_2H_6$) would be:
(a) −31.30 k cal (b) −62.60 k cal
(c) + 31.30 k cal (d) + 62.60 k cal

90. When the pressure is not too high the Van der Waal's equation reduces to:
(a) $PV = RT - \frac{a}{V}$
(b) $PV = RT - \frac{a}{V^2}$
(c) $PV = RT + Rb$
(d) $PV = RT$

91. The enolic form of acetone contains:
(a) 9 sigma bonds, 1 pi bond and two lone pair
(b) 10 sigma bonds, 1 pi bond and 1 lone pair
(c) 8 sigma bonds, 2 pi bonds and 2 lone pair
(d) 9 sigma bonds, 2 pi bonds and 1 lone pair

92. The volume of 0.25 N tribasic acid required to neutralize 0.500 g, of $Ca(OH)_2$ completely is
(a) 45.0 ml (b) 27.0 ml
(c) 54.0 ml (d) .054 ml

93. The number of protons in 1 c.c. of a solution whose $pH = 12$ is:
(a) 6.02×10^{11} (b) 6.02×10^{8}
(c) 6.02×10^{-12} (d) 6.02×10^{23}

94. By increasing the salt concentration ten times in acidic buffer solution, the pH is:
(a) lowered by 1 unit
(b) increased by 2 units
(c) increased by 1 unit
(d) not changed

95. The pH of a solution made by mixing 50 ml of 0.01 M $Ba(OH)_2$ solution with 50 ml of water is:
(a) 8 (b) 12
(c) 10 (d) 7

96. Equal weights of methane and hydrogen are mixed in an empty container at 25°C. The fraction of total pressure exerted by hydrogen is:
(a) 1/2 (b) 1/9
(c) 8/9 (d) 1/4

97. In which of the following compounds iron has lowest oxidation state?

(a) $FeSO_4 \cdot (NH_4)_2 SO_4 \cdot 6H_2O$

(b) $K_4Fe(CN)_5$

(c) $Fe(CO)_5$

(d) K_2FeO_4

98. Potassium permanganate is converted to MnO_2 in a reaction. Equivalent weight of $KMnO_4$ is. Equivalent weight of $KMnO_4$ is:

(a) mol. wt/5 (b) mol. wt/2

(c) mol. wt/3 (d) mol. wt/1

99. A nucleide has half life of 25 min. If 100 gms of the nucleide decays for 100 min, the amount of nucleide left is:

(a) 1.0 gm (b) 4.0 gms

(c) 6.25 gms (d) 12.5 gms

100. Ordinary boron is a mixture of two isotopes B^{11} and B^{10}. If the atomic weight of boron is 10.81, the percentage of B_{11} in the mixture is:

(a) 50% (b) 81%

(c) 19% (d) 60%

Instructions for Q. No. 101 to 120

Directions : Each of the questions given below consists of two statements, an assertions (A) and reason (R). Select the number corresponding to the appropriate response in the answer sheet as follows.

(a) If both assertion and reason are true and the reason is a correct explanation of the assertion

(b) If both assertion and reason are true but the reason is not a correct explanation of the assertion

(c) If the assertion is true, but the reason is false

(d) If both assertion and reason are falses

101. *Assertion (A) :* Alkanes can have an infinite number of conformations.

Reason (R) : In configurational isomerism, the isomers are distinct individual substances.

102. *Assertion (A) :* As a salt such as NaCl dissolves, the Na^+ and Cl^- ions leaving the crystal lattice acquire far greater freedom.

Reason (R) : In thermodynamic terms, the formation of solution occurs with a favourable change in free energy *i.e.,* ΔH has a high positive value and $T \Delta S$ a low negative value.

103. *Assertion (A) :* Water is specially effective in screening the electrostatic interactions between the dissolved ions.

Reason (R) : The force of ionic interactions depends upon the dielectric constant (ε) of the solvent.

104. *Assertion (A) :* When two uncharged similar atoms are brought very close together, their surrounding electron clouds influence each other, and a force of attraction is built up between them.

Reason (R) : The random variation in the positions of electrons around one nucleus may creat a transient electric dipole, which induces a transient opposite electric dipole in the nearby atom.

105. *Assertion (A) :* The equilibrium constant is fixed and a characteristic for any given chemical reaction at a specified temperature.

Reason (R) : The composition of the final equilibrium mixture at a particular temperature depends upon the starting amount of reactants.

106. *Assertion (A) :* The degree of ionization of water is small at 25°C, only about one of every 10^7 molecules in pure water is ionized at any instant.

Reason (R) : In pure water at 25°C the molar concentration of water is essentially constant.

107. *Assertion (A) :* The p^{ka} of a weak acid becomes equal to pH of the solution at the midpoint of its titration.

Reason (R) : The molar concentrations of proton acceptor and proton donor become equal at the midpoint of titration of a weak acid.

108. *Assertion (A) :* Maleic and fumeric acids are well defined compounds. These two compound are stereo isomers but not enantiomers.

Reason (R) : Maleic and fumeric acids have same molecular formula but they are not mirror images of each other.

109. *Assertion (A) :* The nearly tetrahedral arrangement of the orbitals about the oxygen atom allow each water molecule to form hydrogen bonds with as many as four neighbouring water molecules.

Reason (R) : In ice each water molecule forms four hydrogen bonds as each molecules is fixed in the space.

110. *Assertion (A)* : Hydrogen has three isotopes namely protium, deuterium and tritium.

Reason (R) : All the three isotopes of hydrogen have same number of protons in their nuclei.

111. *Assertion (A)* : Sodium ammonium hydrogen phosphate tetrahydrate is used in the bead test.

Reason (R) : The colourless transparent sodium metaphosphate combines with metallic oxides giving coloured orthophosphates.

112. *Assertion (A)* : Lead is a metal with a high density. It readily dissolves in moderately concentrated nitric acid giving colourless fumes which turn red in contact with air.

Reason (R) : Nitric oxide (NO) is a colourless oxide of nitrogen while NO_2 is a coloured oxide of nitrogen.

113. *Assertion (A)* : The reaction of ammonia solution with calomel is a disproportionation reaction in which a mixture of Hg (II) amido chloride and Hg are formed.

Reason (R) : In a disproportionation reaction species under reaction is neither oxidised nor reduced.

114. *Assertion (A)* : Sodium thiosulphate dissolves the white precipitate of silver chloride.

Reason (R) : The thiosulphate ions act as strong complexing agents.

115. *Assertion (A)* : When $SnCl_2$ solution is added to $HgCl_2$ solution, a milky white precipitate is obtained and on adding excess of $SnCl_2$, a black precipitate is formed.

Reason (R) : The disproportionation of Hg(II) is easier than its reduction only.

116. *Assertion (A)* : The electron affinity of chlorine is greater than that of fluorine.

Reason (R) : Chlorine is more electronegative than fluorine.

117. *Assertion (A)* : The boiling point of *n*-alkanes increases regularly with the increase in the number of carbon atoms.

Reason (R) : The magnitude of Van der Waal's forces increases with the increase in molecular mass and molecular size.

118. *Assertion (A)* : *p*-nitroaniline is stronger base than *p*-toluidine.

Reason (R) : The electron withdrawing NO_2 group in the *p*-nitroaniline makes it a stronger base.

119. *Assertion (A)* : All the amines, except tertiary amines are capable of forming intermolecular hydrogen bonds.

Reason (R) : Tertiary amines have larger molecules and surface area.

120. *Assertion (A)* : Phenol is strongly acidic than ethanol.

Reason (R) : Phenoxide ion is more stablized by resonance than ethoxide ion.

BIOLOGY

121. The maximum biomagnification would be in which of the following in case of aquatic ecosystem?

(a) fishes (b) birds
(c) zooplanktons (d) phytoplanktons.

122. In DNA when AGCT occurs, their association is as per which of the following pair?

(a) AG-CT (b) AC-GT
(c) AT-GC (d) all of these.

123. The process of replication in plasmid DNA other than initiation, is controlled by

(a) Plasmid gene (b) bacterial gene
(c) mitochondrial gene
(d) none of these.

124. Cholecystokinin is secreted by

(a) intestine (b) pancreas
(c) adrenal cortex (d) thyroid gland.

125. Koch's postulates are not applicable to

(a) TB (b) leprosy
(c) diphtheria (d) cholera.

126. The problem, due to Rh factor arises when the blood of two (Rh^+ and Rh^-) mix up

(a) in a test tube (b) through transfusion
(c) during pregnancy (d) both 'b' and 'c'.

127. The term 'humulin' is used for
(a) human insulin (b) isoenzyme
(c) hydrolytic enzyme (d) powerful antibiotic.

128. Which one of the following statements about cytochrome P450 is wrong?
(a) it has an important role in metabolism
(b) it contains iron
(c) it is present in coloured cell
(d) it is an enzyme involved in oxidation reactions.

129. Puccinia forms uredia and
(a) pycnia on barberry leaves
(b) aecia on wheat leaves
(c) telia on wheat leaves
(d) aecia on barberry leaves.

130. A few organisms are known to grow and multiply at temperatures of 100-105^0 C.They belong to
(a) thermophilic subaerial fungi
(b) marine archaebacteria
(c) thermophilic sulphur bacteria
(d) hot spring blue-green algae.

131. Botulism caused by *Clostridium botulinum* affects the
(a) spleen
(b) intestine
(c) lymph glands
(d) neuromuscular junction.

132. The functional unit of contractile system in striated muscle is
(a) cross bridges (b) myofibril
(c) sarcomere (d) Z-band.

133. Calcitonin is a thyroid hormone which
(a) elevates potassium level in blood
(b) lowers calcium level in blood
(c) elevates calcium level in blood
(d) has no effect on calcium.

134. Loss of a X-chromosome in a particular cell, during its development, results into
(a) diploid individual
(b) triploid individual
(c) gynandromorphs
(d) both 'a' and 'b'.

135. Which one among the following chemicals is used for causing defoliation of forest trees?
(a) amo-1618 (b) phosphon D
(c) malic hydrazide (d) 2,4-D.

136. Albinism is known to be due to an autosomal recessive mutation. The first child of a couple with normal skin pigmentation was an albino. What is the probability that their second child will also be an albino?
(a) 100% (b) 25%
(c) 50% (d) 75%.

137. Co-factor(prosthetic group) is a part of holoenzyme, it is
(a) loosely attached inorganic part
(b) accessory non-protein substance attached firmly
(c) loosely attached organic part
(d) none of these.

138. A fruit fly is heterozygous for sex-linked genes, when mated with normal female fruit fly, the male specific chromosome will enter egg cell in the proportion
(a) 1 : 1 (b) 2 : 1
(c) 3 : 1 (d) 7 : 1.

139. Which one of the following statements is correct regarding evolution of mankind?
(a) neanderthal man and cro-magnon man were living at the same time
(b) australopithecus was living in Australia
(c) homoerectus is preceded by homohabilis
(d) none of these.

140. The embryonated egg of *Ascaris* represents
(a) an egg with an egg
(b) an egg with gastrula
(c) an egg with blastula
(d) an egg with a juvenile.

141. Elater mechanism for seed dispersal is exhibited by
(a) *Riccia* (b) *Funaria*
(c) *Liverworts* (d) *Marchantia.*

142. The breeding place of *Flamingo* (Hansawar) in India is most likely
(a) Sambhar lake (b) Chilka lake
(c) Rann of Kutch (d) Ghana Vihar.

143. In C_4 plants, CO_2 combines with
(a) phosphoglyceric acid
(b) ribulose diphosphate
(c) phosphoenol pyruvate
(d) phosphoglyceraldehyde.

144. The polygenic genes show
(a) different genotypes
(b) different phenotypes
(c) different karyotypes
(d) none of these.

145. Which of the following statement is without exception for sponges?
(a) they are found only in marine water
(b) they are all radially symmetric
(c) they all have calcareous spicules
(d) they have high regenerative power.

146. What are the most diversed molecules in the cell?
(a) proteins (b) carbohydrates
(c) lipids (d) mineral salts.

147. Which of the following is common among mammals?
(a) they are carnivores
(b) they have ventral nerve cord
(c) they undergo no moulting
(d) they have seven cervical vertebrae.

148. The ornithine cycle removes two waste products from the blood in liver. These products are
(a) CO_2 and urea
(b) ammonia and urea
(c) CO_2 and ammonia
(d) ammonia and uric acid.

149. The black rust of wheat is a fungal disease caused by
(a) *Melampsore lini*
(b) *Claviceps purpurea*
(c) *Albugo candida*
(d) *Puccinia graminis tritici.*

150. The pigment, that absorbs red and far red light in plants is
(a) xanthophyll-II (b) cytochrome
(c) phytochrome (d) carotene.

151. The sympathetic nerves in mammals, arise from
(a) thoraco-lumber nerves
(b) cervical nerves (c) sacral nerves
(d) 3rd,7th,9th and 10th cranial nerves.

152. Identify the correct match between tiger reserve and its state
(a) Bandipur-Tamil Nadu
(b) Palanau-Orissa (c) Manas-Assam
(d) Corbett-Madhya Pradesh.

153. When two genetic loci produce identical phenotypes in *cis* and *trans* position, they are considered to be
(a) pseudoalleles
(b) different genes
(c) multiple alleles
(d) the parts of same gene.

154. Rickettsiae form a group under
(a) fungi
(b) a category between viruses and bacteria
(c) viruses (d) bacteria.

155. Which one of the following statements is correct with reference to a test tube baby?
(a) a prematurely born baby is reared in an incubator
(b) fertilization of the egg and growth of the embryo are effected in a large test tube
(c) fertilization of the egg is effected outside the body, the fertilized egg is then placed in the womb of the mother where the gestation is completed
(d) fertilization of the egg is effected in the female genital tract, it is then taken out and grown in a large test tube.

156. Organisms phenotypically similar but genotypically different are said to be
(a) multizygous (b) heterozygous
(c) homozygous (d) monozygous

157. Which of the following is the most evident source of evolution?
(a) fossils
(b) morphology
(c) embryos
(d) vestigial organs

158. Number of post-zygote nuclear divisions of synkaryon in exconjugant of *Paramecium* is
(a) one (b) five
(c) three (d) eight

159. Gigantism and acromegaly are due to increase of
(a) GH (b) STH
(c) ADH (d) none of these

160. The head of humerus articulated in the pectoral girdle, the joint is
(a) hinge
(b) immovable
(c) pivot joint
(d) ball and socket

Instructions for Q. No. 161 to 180

Directions : Each of the questions given below consists of two statements, an assertions (A) and reason (R). Select the number corresponding to the appropriate response in the answer sheet as follows.

(a) If both assertion and reason are true and the reason is a correct explanation of the assertion
(b) If both assertion and reason are true but the reason is not a correct explanation of the assertion
(c) If the assertion is true, but the reason is false
(d) If both assertion and reason are falses

161. *Assertion (A) :* Some roots perform photosynthesis.
Reason (R) : Trapa & Tinospora have these type of roots.

162. *Assertion (A) :* Water potential is represented by negative sign.
Reason (R) : Pure water has maximum water potential.

163. *Assertion (A) :* Growing plants in soilless culture is called hydroponics.
Reason (R) : This was first developed by Van Helmont.

164. *Assertion (A) :* Molybdenum deficiency causes whiptail disease of cauliflower.
Reason (R) : It is responsible for the synthesis of IAA.

165. *Assertion (A) :* Light is a limiting factor in photosynthesis.
Reason (R) : Pigment other than chlorophyll *a* are called accessory pigments.

166. *Assertion (A) :* Heavy perspiration results in muscular cramps.
Reason (R) : Skin is an accessory excretory organ.

167. *Assertion (A) :* Multiplicative growth takes place in embryos of animals.
Reason (R) : Growth in embryo occurs due to an increase in the number of cells.

168. *Assertion (A) :* Linkage and crossing over are inversely related.
Reason (R) : Crossing over is visible in prophase stage of meiosis-I.

169. *Assertion (A) :* The endocrine part of human pancreas is represented by α and β cells.
Reason (R) : Endocrine gland have ducts.

170. *Assertion (A) :* Inheritance of Kappa particles in *Paramecium* is a type of extra nuclear inheritance.
Reason (R) : Extra nuclear inheritance or cytoplasmic inheritance are inherited through nucleoplasm.

171. *Assertion (A) :* The nucleus is a membrane-bounded body found in cytoplasm of cell and contains DNA in the form of chromosomes.
Reason (R) : The nucleus is therefore the repository of the molecular information that controls the characteristics of cells and their progeny.

172. *Assertion (A) :* Histone proteins are synthesized during the S-phase when DNA synthesis occurs.
Reason (R) : Histone proteins form an association with DNA to form nucleosome.

173. *Assertion (A) :* Annelids, arthropods and molluscs are all protostomial coelomate.

Reason (R) : Adults of all the above have bilateral symmetry, the tube with-in-a-tube body plan and organs derived from three germ layers.

174. *Assertion (A)* : Sponges are primitive multicellular animals, that probably evolved a multicellular structure independently of other multicellular animals.
Reason (R) : Sponges are stationary, remain attached to substratum while water passes over them.

175. *Assertion (A)* : Active transport results in solute movement against a concentration gradient.
Reason (R) : Active transport of Na^+ and K^+ is energized by ATP.

176. *Assertion (A)* : Lichens bear a composite structure consisting of two dissimilar organisms, a fungus and an alga.
Reason (R) : The fungal component of association is either a member of myxophyceae or chlorophyceae.

177. *Assertion (A)* : In C_4 plants, CO_2 fixation occurs at three sites.
Reason (R) : CO_2 fixation occurs in mesophyll cells, bundle sheath cells and vascular cambium.

178. *Assertion (A)* : Reduction division, in *Selaginella*, occurs during microspore formation only.
Reason (R) : It has been proved experimentally by Zacharich in 1963.

179. *Assertion (A)* : In case of *Nepenthes*, lamina is modified to capture insects to get nitrogenous food.
Reason (R) : The plant proteins are broken down to amino acids then absorbed by plants.

180. *Assertion (A)* : Energy can be transformed from one form into another but it can not be created or destroyed.
Reason (R) : When one form of energy is transformed into another form, some useful energy is always lost as heat, hence,energy can not be recycled.

GENERAL KNOWLEDGE

181. What kind of soil is treated with gypsum to make it suitable for cropping ?
(a) alkaline
(b) acidic
(c) water-logged
(d) soil with excessive clay content

182. Where is the world's first Integrated Solar Combined Cycle Power Project proposed to be set up ?
(a) Cuttack (b) Jaipur
(c) Patna (d) Jodhpur

183. Who started the Saka Era which is still used by the Government of India ?
(a) Kanishka (b) Vikramditya
(c) Samudra Gupta (d) Asoka

184. Which of the following districts is on the international border of India ?
(a) Gorakhpur
(b) West Khasi Hills
(c) Kinnaur
(d) Kullu

185. Laterite soil devlop as a result of -
(a) deposits of alluvial
(b) deposition of loess
(c) leaching
(d) continued vegetation cover

186. The variety of coffee largely grown in India is
(a) Old Chicks (b) Coorgs
(c) Aribica (d) Kents

187. Which one of the following is not an example of indirect tax
(a) sales tax
(b) excise duty
(c) custom duty
(d) expenditure tax

188. Structural unemployment arises due to -
(a) deflationary conditions
(b) heavy industry bias
(c) shortage of raw materials
(d) inadequate productive capacity

189. What can be the maximum interval between two sessions of Parliament ?
(a) three months (b) four months
(c) six months (d) nine months

190. Who amongst the following is renowned in Hindustani classical music (vocal) ?
(a) Shovana Narayan
(b) M. S. Subbalakshmi
(c) Pt. Jasraj
(d) M.S.Gopalakrishnan

191. What is the chemical name for 'baking soda' ?
(a) sodium carbonate
(b) sodium bicarbonate
(c) sodium nitrite
(d) sodium nitrate

192. An atomic pile is used for
(a) producing X- rays
(b) conducting nuclear fission
(c) conducting thermonuclear fusion
(d) accelerating atoms

193. Clove the commonly used spice, is obtained from the
(a) root (b) stem
(c) flower bud (d) fruit

194. What is the number of the permanent members of the security council of United Nations Organisation ?
(a) 6 (b) 4
(c) 5 (d) 7

195. Who was honoured with 'Bharat Ratna' on the Republic Day 2000 ?
(a) Pt. Ravi Shankar
(b) K.Kasturirangan
(c) A.P.J. Abdul Kalam
(d) none of these

196. A 'breath test' used by traffic police to check drunken driving uses -
(a) potassium dichormate-sulphuric acid
(b) potassium permanganate sulphuric acid
(c) turmeric on filter paper
(d) silica gel coated with silver nitrate

197. Who is the author of *Business @Speed of Thought?*
(a) Dick Francis (b) john Gray
(c) Bill Gates (d) David Baldacci

198. Anglo-Nubian is a breed of
(a) sheep (b) goat
(c) poultry (d) cattle

199. Who received the Dada Sahib Phalke award 2002 for film excellence ?
(a) Asha Bhosle
(b) Girish Kannad
(c) Dipti Naval
(d) Lata Mangeskar

200. Total no. of moons of planet jupiter is
(a) 18 (b) 16
(c) 17 (d) 30

■■■

Model Test Paper–7

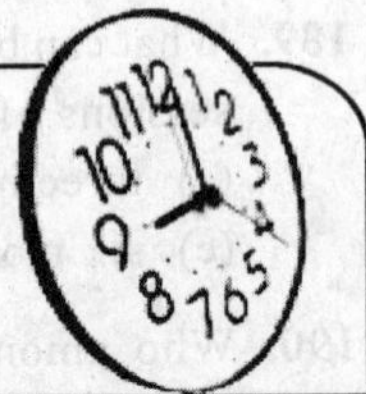

Time : $3\frac{1}{2}$ hours. *Maximum Marks : 200*

PHYSICS

1. If 1000 droplets each of charge q and radius r are mixed to form a big drop, then the potential of big drop, as compared to small droplet, will be
   (a) 10 times (b) 500 times
   (c) 100 times (d) 1000 times

2. In uncontrolled chain reaction, the quantity of energy released, is
   (a) very high (b) normal
   (c) very low (d) first (a) then (b)

3. The angular velocity of the second needle of a watch will be
   (a) π (b) $\frac{60}{\pi}$
   (c) 2π (d) $\frac{\pi}{30}$

4. Which of the following gates can be served as a building block for any digital circuits?
   (a) OR (b) NOT
   (c) AND (d) NAND

5. The energy required to detatch one electron from the Balmer series of hydrogen spectrum will be
   (a) – 13.6 ev (b) – 3.4 eV
   (c) 10.2 eV (d) – 1.5 eV

6. There are five resistance of 1 Ω each. If the first three resistance are joined in parallel and rest two are joined is series, then the final resistance of the combination when joined in series is
   (a) 2/3 Ω (b) 7/3 Ω
   (c) 5/3 Ω (d) 8/3 Ω

7. A train is moving with a constant velocity. If a pendulum is hanging from its roof then its time-period
   (a) remains same (b) increases
   (c) decreases (d) none of these

8. The value of the surface tension of a liquid is 70 dyne/cm. What will be its value in N/m?
   (a) 70 N/m (b) 7×10^2 N/m
   (c) 7×10^{-2} N/m (d) 7×10^3 N/m.

9. In the Young's experiment the distance between two slits is increased by 2 times. What will be fringe width?
   (a) increased by two times
   (b) increased by four times
   (c) decreased by two times
   (d) decreased by four times

10. The force of cohesion is
    (a) maximum in solids
    (b) same in different matters
    (c) maximum in liquids
    (d) maximum in gases

11. The working of a dynamo is based on the principle of
    (a) heating effect of current
    (b) chemical effect of current
    (c) magnetic effect of current
    (d) electromagnetic induction

12. A nucleus emits one α-particle and forms a new nucleus. The mass and charge of the new nucleus is changed in which of the following way?
    (a) mass is reduced by 4 and charge is reduced by 6
    (b) mass is reduced by 2 and charge is reduced by 2
    (c) mass is reduced by 4 and charge is reduced by 2
    (d) mass is reduced by 2 and charge is reduced by 4

13. A boy aims a gun at a bird from a point at a horizontal distance of 100 m. If the gun can impart a velocity of 500 m/s to the bullet, at what height about the board must he aim his gun in order to hit it (Take g = 10 m/s^2)

(a) 20 m (b) 50 m

(c) 40 m (d) 100 m

14. If the momentum of a particle is 2×10^{-23} kg-m/s. then its wavelength will be

(a) 3.3×10^{-11} m (b) 8.2×10^{-5} m

(c) 6.3×10^{-7} m (d) 9×10^{-3} m

15. Atomic number of a nucleus is Z, while its mass number is M. What will be the number of neutrons in its nucleus ?

(a) M (b) $(M - Z)$

(c) Z (d) $(M + Z)$

16. The energy produced in the sun is due to

(a) fission reaction (b) chemical reaction

(c) fusion reaction

(d) motion of electrons and ions

17. In Young's experiment, the distance between slits is 0.28 mm and distance between slits and screen is 1.4 m. Distance between central bright fringe and third bright fringe is 0.9 cm. What is wavelength of used light

(a) 5000 Å (b) 5880 Å

(c) 6000 Å (d) 5800 Å

18. The radius of a planet is 1/4th of Earth's radius and its acceleration due to gravity is double to Earth's acceleration due to gravity. How many times be the value of escape velocity at the planet comparing to its value at the Earth?

(a) $1/\sqrt{2}$ (b) $2\sqrt{2}$

(c) $\sqrt{2}$ (d) 2

19. Initially a tyre at 27°C has 20 atm. pressure. What is the value of temperature when the tyre moves with pressure of 25 atmosphere

(a) 192 K (b) 350 K

(c) 240 K (d) 375 K

20. No. of images formed by an object kept between two plane mirrors at an angle 72° is

(a) 2 (b) 4

(c) 3 (d) 5

21. The half-life of a radioactive substance is 48 hr. How much time it will take to disintegrate to its 1/16th part

(a) 12 hr (b) 48 hr

(c) 16 hr (d) 192 hr

22. According to the Rutherford's atomic model. the electrons inside the atom are

(a) stationary (b) centralized

(c) not stationary (d) none of these

23. The equivalent resistance (R_{AB}) between the points A and B is

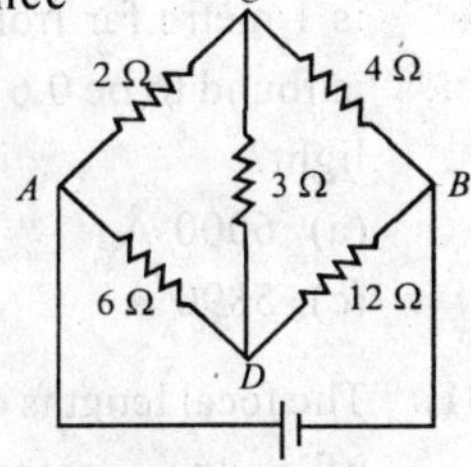

(a) 6 Ω

(b) 7.5 Ω

(c) 4.5 Ω

(d) 8 Ω

24. If a ball is thrown vertically upwards with 40 m/s, its velocity after two sec will be (g = 10ms^{-2})

(a) 10 m/s (b) 30 m/s

(c) 20 m/s (d) 40 m/s

25. A scooter (m = 40 kg) having velocity 4 m/s collides with another scooter (m = 60 kg) having velocity 2 m/s. If the collision is inelastic, then loss in kinetic energy is

(a) 48 J (b) 392 J

(c) 110 J (d) 440 J

26. A sphere of 0.2 m diameter bears 1 microcoulomb charge on it. The maximum electric intensity at a point due to the sphere will be

(a) 9×10^9 N/C (b) 9×10^{-9} N/C

(c) 9×10^5 N/C (d) 9×10^{-5} N/C.

27. A star is receding from earth at a speed 10^5 m/s. The line of wavelength 5700 Å in its spectrum will be shifted by

(a) 1.9 Å (b) 5700 Å

(c) 1.9 metre (d) 1.9 micron.

28. The waves moving from a sitar to a listener in air are
(a) longitudinal progressive
(b) longitudinal stationary
(c) transverse progressive
(d) transverse stationary.

29. Light of wavelength 2×10^{-3} m falls on a slit of width 4×10^{-3} m. The angular dispersion of the central maximum will be
(a) 30° (b) 60°
(c) 90° (d) 180°.

30. The distance between two coherent sources produced by a biprism is 1.0 mm. When the screen is 1 metre far from the sources, the fringe width is found to be 0.6 mm. What is the wavelength of light?
(a) 6000 Å (b) 5896 Å
(c) 5890 Å (d) 7800 Å.

31. The focal lengths of the objective and the eyepiece of an astronomical telescope are 20 cm and 5 cm respectively. If the final image is formed at a distance of 30 cm from the eyepiece, find the magnifying power.
(a) 44.6 (b) 4.68
(c) 64.4 (d) 6.44.

32. The luminous intensity of a 40 watt bulb is 300 candela. Calculate the efficiency of the bulb.
(a) 62.4 lm/watt (b) 42.6 lm/watt
(c) 94.25 lm/watt (d) 25.94 lm/watt.

33. A straight rod partially immersed in water appears to be inclined at 45° with the surface when viewed vertically through air. What is the actual inclination of the rod?
(a) 30° (b) 45°
(c) 53° (d) 60°.

34. Fraunhaufer lines become brighter during solar eclipse because
(a) the sun-rays get diffracted by moon
(b) solar radiations are completely blocked off by the moon and only the photosphere radiations reach the earth
(c) chromosphere radiations are stopped by the moon and only the photosphere radiations reach the earth
(d) photosphere radiations are stopped by the moon, but the chromosphere radiations are able to reach the earth.

35. In a cyclic process the change in internal energy of a system is
(a) minimum but not zero
(b) zero
(c) maximum but not infinite
(d) infinite.

36. The rms speed of the particles of fume of mass 5×10^{-17} kg executing Brownian motion in air at N.T.P. is
(a) 1.5 m/s (b) 3.0 m/s
(c) 1.5 cm/s (d) 3 cm/s.

37. A material breaks under a stress of 10^9 N/m². If the density of the material be 3×10^3 kg/m³, what will be the length of the wire made of that material so that the wire breaks by its own weight when suspended.
(a) 3.4×10^4 m (b) 3.4×10^5 m
(c) 3.4×10^3 m (d) 3.4 m.

38. Which of the following bond is strongest?
(a) ionic (b) covalent
(c) Van der Waals (d) metallic.

39. Surface area of a soap bubble is 1.3×10^{-4} m². The work done to double the surface area will be (surface tension (T) for soap solution $= 3 \times 10^{-3}$ N/m.)
(a) 3.9×10^{-7} joule
(b) 3×10^{-7} joule
(c) 2.6×10^{-4} joule (d) $2.3 \times 10^{+1}$ joule.

40. A spacecraft is launched in a circular orbit very close to earth. What additional velocity should be given to the spacecraft so that it might escape the earth's gravitational pull
(Radius of the earth = 6400 km, $g = 9.8$ m/s²)
(a) 11.2 km/s (b) 3.25 km/s
(c) 8 km/s (d) 20.2 km/s.

Instructions for Q. No. 41 to 60

Directions : Each of the questions given below consists of two statements, an assertions (A) and reason (R). Select the number corresponding to the appropriate response in the answer sheet as follows.

(a) If both assertion and reason are true and the reason is a correct explanation of the assertion

(b) If both assertion and reason are true but the reason is not a correct explanation of the assertion

(c) If the assertion is true, but the reason is false

(d) If both assertion and reason are falses

41. *Assertion (A) :* When light passes from one medium to another of different density the only quantity which is unchanged is its wavelength.
Reason (R) : The wavelength is not related to the refractive index of the medium.

42. *Assertion (A) :* A plane mirror forms a real image when a converging beam of light falls on it.
Reason (R) : When a converging beam is reflected, the angle of reflection is not equal to the angle of incidence.

43. *Assertion (A) :* Light incident normally on the first face of an equilateral glass prism ($\mu = 1.5$) is certain to be totally internally reflected.
Reason (R) : The critical angle for the given glass is less than 60°.

44. *Assertion (A) :* Due to friction kinetic energy of a satellite increases.
Reason (R) : Air friction decreases the total mechanical energy of the system, consequently the planet comes nearer with greater velocity.

45. *Assertion (A) :* Rain drops fall to the earth with uniform velocity.
Reason (R) : All freely falling objects have zero weight.

46. *Assertion (A) :* A stream of water from a tap becomes narrower as it falls.
Reason (R) : The speed of water increases as it falls.

47. *Assertion (A) :* The internal energy of an ideal gas does not change during an isothermal process.
Reason (R) : The decrease in volume of the ideal gas is compensated by a corresponding increase in pressure when its temperature is held constant.

48. *Assertion (A) :* Cathode rays travel with speed of light.
Reason (R) : Cathode rays are electromagnetic in nature.

49. *Assertion (A) :* When a dielectric medium is filled between the plates of a condenser, its capacitance increases.
Reason (R) : The dielectric medium reduces the potential difference between the plates of the condenser.

50. *Assertion (A) :* A thin polythene bag weights the same when empty and when filled with air at atmospheric pressure.
Reason (R) : Air is weightless.

51. *Assertion (A) :* The lightening conductor at the top of high buildings has sharp pointed conductors.
Reason (R) : The surface density of charge at sharp points is very high resulting in setting up of electric wind.

52. *Assertion (A) :* If a convex lens of glass is immersed in water its power decreases.
Reason (R) : In water it behaves as a concave lens.

53. *Assertion (A) :* The power factor in a series of resonant circuit is unity.
Reason (R) : In case of series resonance the inductive and capacitive reactances are equal.

54. *Assertion (A) :* When a current is drawn from a cell, there is a fall in potential difference across its terminals.
Reason (R) : Every cell has internal resistance.

55. *Assertion (A) :* Ammeter is always connected in series with a circuit to measure the current flowing through it.
Reason (R) : Ammeter has very low resistance.

56. *Assertion (A) :* During boiling, if an amount ΔQ of heat is absorbed, $p\Delta V$ is the work done by the system, then $\Delta Q = p\Delta V$

Reason (R) : Boiling is an isothermal process, So Δ U = O in equation $\Delta Q = \Delta U + p\Delta V$, which is based on first law of thermodynamics.

57. *Assertion (A) :* When one mole of an ideal gas expands under adiabatic condition so that its state changes from (P_1, V_1, T_1) to (P_2, V_2, T_2), the work done by the gas is given by $\Delta W = C_v(T_1 - T_2)$.
Reason (R) : During adiabatic expansion $\Delta Q = 0$ and $\Delta U = C_v(T_2 - T_1)$ in the expression $\Delta Q = \Delta U + \Delta W$.

58. *Assertion (A) :* A beam of light which emerges from a convex lens must be convergent.
Reason (R) : A convex lens is a converging lens while a concave lens is diverging lens, whatever may be the medium in which they are placed.

59. *Assertion (A) :* When light passes from one medium to another of different density the only quantity which is unchanged is its wavelength.
Reason (R) : The wavelength of light is not related to the refractive index of the medium.

60. *Assertion (A) :* α - particles produce more intense ionization than β -particles.
Reason (R) : α -particles are positively charged.

CHEMISTRY

61. Which of the following has larger radius?
(a) Ca (b) F
(c) F (d) Na

62. Identify the transition element
(a) $1s^22s^22p^63s^23p^64s^2$
(b) $1s^22s^22p^63s^23p^63d^{10}4s^2\ 4p^1$
(c) $1s^22s^22p^63s^23p^63d^24s^2$
(d) $1s^22s^22p^63s^23p^63d^{10}4s^24p^14d^2$

63. Which of the following is most alkaline?
(a) PH_3 (b) AsH_3
(c) NH_3 (d) SbH_3

64. The oxide that gives hydrogen peroxide (H_2O_2) on the treatment with a dilute acid (H_2SO_4) is
(a) PbO_2 (b) MnO_2
(c) Na_2O_2 (d) TiO_2

65. Catalyst is used to
(a) increase the product
(b) increase the reactants
(c) decrease the product
(d) minimise the time of reaction

66. Chlorobenzene is prepared commercially by
(a) Dow's process
(b) Rasching process
(c) Deacon's process
(d) Etard's process

67. Which of the following is Lewis-acid?
(a) Cl^- (b) S^{--}
(c) Ag^+ (d) C_2H_5OH

68. Which of the following are the constituents of gun metal?
(a) Cu, Sn (b) Cu, Sn, Zn
(c) Cu, Sn, Pb (d) Cu, Zn, Sb, Pb

69. Formaldehyde + ammonia → *Y*, the product *Y* is
(a) methanol
(b) para-formaldehyde
(c) formamide
(d) hexamethylenetetramine

70. Oleic, stearic and palmitic acids are
(a) nucleic acid (b) fatty acids
(c) amino acid (d) nitric acid

71. The most suitable method of the seperation of a mixture of ortho and para-nitrophenol mixed in the ratio of 1 : 1, is
(a) distillation (b) vapourisation
(c) crystallization (d) colour spectrum

72. When primary amine is heated with CS_2 in the presence of excess mercuric chloride it gives isothio cyanate. This reaction is called
(a) Perkin's reaction
(b) Hoffman-bromide reaction
(c) Carbyl-amine reaction
(d) Hoffman mustard oil reaction

73. If N and S both are present in an organic compound, then during Lassaigne's test, both will change into
(a) NaSCN (b) Na_2S and NaCN
(c) Na_2S and NaCNO (d) Na_2SO_3 and NaCN

74. In radioactive decay, the emitted electrons come from
(a) nucleus of the atom
(b) outermost orbit of the atom
(c) inner orbital of the atom
(d) orbit having principal quantum number one

75. $CH_3CONH_2 \xrightarrow{P_2O_5} Z + H_2O$, identify the product Z
(a) CH_3Br (b) CH_3OH
(c) CH_3CN (d) CH_3NH_2

76. Which of the following compound is easily attacked by an electrophile?
(a) 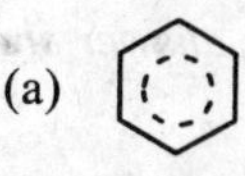 (b) 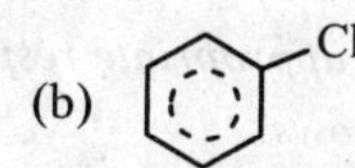

(c) 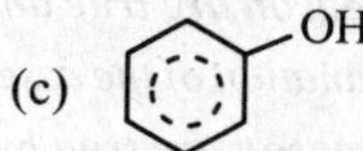

(d) 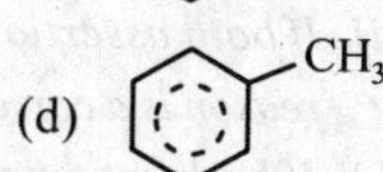

77. Paracetamol is used as a/an
(a) antipyretic (b) antimalarial
(c) antibiotic (d) tranquillizer

78. The number of water molecules in Mohr's salt is
(a) 5 (b) 7
(c) 6 (d) 8

79. A quantum of light energy is called
(a) proton (b) electron
(c) photon (d) neutron

80. Which of the following substance will give amide, when reacted with NH_3 ?
(a) nitrogen
(b) acetyl chloride
(c) hydrogen chloride
(d) potassium chloride

81. The bond order of nitrogen molecule is
(a) 1 (b) 4
(c) 3 (d) 7

82. Half-life of radium is 1580 yrs. Its average life will be
(a) 2.5×10^3 yrs (b) 2.275×10^3 yrs
(c) 1.832×10^3 yrs (d) 8.825×10^2 yrs

83. The reaction between copper and hot concentrated H_2SO_4 produces
(a) SO_3 (b) Cu
(c) H_2 (d) SO_2

84. Electronic configuration $1s^2 2s^2 2p_x^1 2p_y^1 2p_z^1$ represents which of the following elements?
(a) oxygen (b) nitrogen
(c) hydrogen (d) fluorine

85. The pH value of HCl (10^{-12} M) is
(a) −12 (b) −7
(c) 12 (d) 7

86. The function of enzymes in the living system is to
(a) transport oxygen
(b) provide energy
(c) provide immunity
(d) catalyse biochemical reactions

87. Which of the following is used as an anti-knocking material?
(a) T.E.L. (b) glyoxal
(c) freon (d) ethyl alcohol

88. Diazo-coupling is useful to prepare some
(a) dyes (b) pesticides
(c) proteins (d) vitamins

89. Which statement is not correct about alcohol?
(a) alcohol is lighter than water
(b) alcohol of less no. of carbon atoms is less soluble in water than alcohol of more no. of carbon atoms
(c) alcohol evaporates quickly
(d) all of these

90. Arrangement of Na, Rb, K, Mg in the increasing order of atomic radius will be
(a) Mg < Na < K < Rb
(b) Na < Mg < K < Rb

(c) K < Na < Mg < Rb
(d) Rb < K < Mg < Na

91. $C_3H_8 + Cl_2 \xrightarrow{\text{Light}} C_3H_7Cl + HCl$ is an example of which of the following types of reactions?
(a) substitution (b) addition
(c) elimination (d) rearrangement

92. Which of the following possesses highest melting point?
(a) chlorobenzene (b) *m*-dichlorobenzene
(c) *o*-dichlorobenzene (d) *p*-dichlorobenzene

93. Which of the following is not true in case of reaction with heated copper at 300°C?
(a) phenol → benzyl alcohol
(b) secondary alcohol → ketone
(c) primary alcohol → aldehyde
(d) tertiary alcohol → olefin

94. The heat of combusion of methane at 298 K is expressed by $CH_{4\,(g)} + 2O_{2\,(g)} \rightarrow CO_{2\,(g)} + 2H_2O$ and ΔH = 890.2 KJ. Magnitude of Δ E of reaction at this temperature is
(a) infinity (b) equal to ΔH
(c) less than ΔH (d) greater than ΔH

95. Which of the following species participate in sulphonation of benzene ring?
(a) H_2SO_4 (b) SO_3
(c) HSO_3^- (d) SO_2^-

96. IUPAC name of the compound

$$CH_3 - CH = \underset{\displaystyle CH_2 - CH_2 - CH_3}{C} - CH_2 - CH_3$$

(a) 3-ethyl 2-hexene (b) 3 propyl 3-hexene
(c) 3-propyl 2-hexene (d) 4-ethyl 4-hexene

97. pH of a solution can be expressed as
(a) $-\log_e (H^+)$ (b) $\log_e (H^+)$
(c) $-\log_{10} (H^+)$ (d) $\log_{10} (H^+)$

98. The concentration of $[H^+]$ and concentration of $[OH^-]$ of a 0.1 aqueous solution of 2% ionised weak acid is [ionic product of water = 1×10^{-14}]
(a) 0.02×10^{-3}M and 5×10^{-11} M
(b) 2×10^{-3} M and 5×10^{-12}M
(c) 1×10^{-3} M and 3×10^{-11} M
(d) 3×10^{-2} M and 4×10^{-13} M

99. A compound with empirical formula (CH_2O) has a vapour density of 30. Its moleclar formula is
(a) CH_2O (b) $C_3H_6O_3$
(c) $C_2H_4O_2$ (d) $C_6H_{12}O_6$

100. The unit of equivalent conductivity is
(a) S-cm $^{-2}$
(b) ohm – cm^2 (*g*-equivalent)
(c) ohm-cm
(d) ohm $^{-1}$ cm^2 (*g* equivalent) $^{-1}$

Instructions for Q. No. 101 to 120

Directions : Each of the questions given below consists of two statements, an assertions (A) and reason (R). Select the number corresponding to the appropriate response in the answer sheet as follows.

(a) If both assertion and reason are true and the reason is a correct explanation of the assertion
(b) If both assertion and reason are true but the reason is not a correct explanation of the assertion
(c) If the assertion is true, but the reason is false
(d) If both assertion and reason are falses

101. *Assertion (A) :* The number of electron in an neutral atom is always equal to atomic number of that atom.
Reason (R) : The atomic number of the atom is equal to the number of protons in the nucleus of the atom.

102. *Assertion (A) :* The radioactivity of Ra and Ra^{2+} is always same.
Reason (R) : The radioactivity is an extra-nuclear phenomenon.

103. *Assertion (A) :* $_{14}Si^{30}$, $_{15}P^{31}$ and $_{16}S^{32}$ are a group of isotones.
Reason (R) : Isotones are atoms of different elements having different mass numbers of atomic numbers but same number of neutrons in their nuclei.

104. *Assertion (A)* : Nuclear isomers are the atoms with same atomic number, same mass number but with different radioactivity.
Reason (R) : One of the two nuclear isomeric nuclei one may be in the ground state whereas the other in the excited state.

105. *Assertion (A)* : Arenes can be obtained by the reaction of aromatic substrate with an alkylating agent in presence of acidic catalyst.
Reason (R) : This reaction is known as free radical substitution reaction.

106. *Assertion (A)* : Chlorobenzene reacts with potassium cyanide to give benzonitrile,
Reason (R) : Cyanide (CN^-) ion is a strong nucleophile.

107. *Assertion (A)* : Nuclide $_{13}Al^{30}$ is more stable as compared to nuclide $_{20}Ca^{40}$
Reason (R) : Nuclides having an odd number of protons and neutrons are generally less stable.

108. *Assertion (A)* : When butene-1 reacts with bromine (Br_2), two optical isomeres are obtained.
Reason (R) : Product contains one asymmetric carbon atom.

109. *Assertion (A)* : When an atom in group 1A of the periodic table undergoes radioactive decay by emitting a positron, the resulting element belongs to zero group.
Reason (R) : When an atom emits a positron, its atomic number increases by one unit.

110. *Assertion (A)* : A certain element X, forms three binary compounds with chlorine containing 59.68%, 68.95% and 74.75% chlorine respectively. These data illustrate the law of multiple proportions.
Reason (R) : According to law of multiple proportions, the relative amounts of an element combining with some fixed amount of a second element in a series of compounds are the ratios of small whole numbers.

111. *Assertion (A)* : Water has greater dipole-dipole attraction than hydrogen sulphide.
Reason (R) : Oxygen has higher electronegativity than sulphur.

112. *Assertion (A)* : When 20 ml of ethanol is mixed with 20 ml of water, the volume of resulting solution will be less than 40 ml.
Reason (R) : The hydrogen bond between water and alcohol molecules is weaker than hydrogen bond between the like molecules.

113. *Assertion (A)* : Ortho-nitrophenol has much lower boiling point and lower solubility in water than meta and para isomers.
Reason (R) : Ortho-nitrophenol involves intramolecular hydrogen bonding and the possibility of association of the molecules is absent.

114. *Assertion (A)* : All molecules which have polar bonds have net dipole moment.
Reason (R) : Asymmetrical molecules with polar bonds have zero dipole moment.

115. *Assertion (A)* : In the covalent compounds of hydrogen, the hydrogen atom has the electronic configuration analogous to that of hydride ion.
Reason (R) : Hydride ion is formed when hydrogen atom loses an electron.

116. *Assertion (A)* : The bond order of helium is always zero.
Reason (R) : The number of electrons in bonding molecular orbital and antibonding molecular orbital is equal.

117. *Assertion (A)* : The H-N-H bond angle in NH_3 molecule is much greater than H-As-H bond angle in AsH_3.
Reason (R) : Formation of NH_3 molecule involves sp^3 hybridisation, while no hybridisation occurs in AsH_3.

118. *Assertion (A)* : The dipole-moment of CH_3F is greater than that of $CHCl_3$.
Reason (R) : Fluorine has greater electron affinity than that of chlorine.

119. *Assertion (A)* : Stannous chloride ($SnCl_2$) is a non-linear molecule.
Reason (R) : In $SnCl_2$ molecule Sn atom is present in *sp* hybridised state.

120. *Assertion (A)* : The bond angle H-C-H in the methane is the same as the bond angle Cl-C-Cl in the carbon tetrachloride.

Reason (R) : H-C-H bonds in methane are almost non-polar while Cl-C-Cl bonds in carbon tetrachloride are highly polar.

BIOLOGY

121. Transpiration-pull theory operates in
(a) active water absorption
(b) passive water absorption
(c) root pressure
(d) imbibition.

122. Photophosphorylation is a process in which
(a) O_2 comes out of the water by photolysis
(b) phosphoglyceric acid is formed
(c) aspartic acid is formed
(d) light energy is changed and stored into chemical energy in ATP.

123. The primary photochemical reaction in chloroplast occurs in
(a) stroma (b) periplast cavity
(c) quantasome (d) inner membrane.

124. Bacterial photosynthesis occurs in wavelength
(a) ultraviolet (b) blue
(c) red (d) far-red.

125. Which of the following will not be a limiting factor in photosynthesis?
(a) oxygen (b) carbon dioxide
(c) chlorophyll (d) light.

126. In photosynthesis, the special role of light is
(a) activation of chloroplast
(b) photolysis
(b) reduction of carbon dioxide
(d) synthesis of glucose.

127. In C_4-pathway, the first reaction is
(a) addition of CO_2 with PGA
(b) addition of CO_2 with PEPA
(c) addition of CO_2 with RuDP
(d) addition of CO_2 with RMP.

128. Emerson effect has given the view of
(a) two different photochemical reactions in photosynthesis
(b) light and dark reaction in photosynthesis
(c) photophosphorylation
(d) photorespiration.

129. In higher plants, the amount of light utilised in photosynthesis is about
(a) 100 percent (b) 50 percent
(c) 10 percent (d) 1 to 2 percent.

130. The initial enzyme of Calvin cycle is
(a) ribulose diphosphate carboxylase
(b) triose phosphate dehydrogenase
(c) phosphopentokinase
(d) cytochrome oxidase.

131. DCMU, a herbicide, kills plants by
(a) stopping respiration due to inhibition of dehydrogenase enzymes
(b) inhibiting photosystem-II of photosynthesis
(c) inhibiting photosystem-I of photosynthesis
(d) inhibition of photolysis.

132. Transpiration takes place from
(a) leaf
(b) stem
(c) all organs
(d) only aerial parts of land plant.

133. By increasing the CO_2 concentration around leaves in light
(a) stomata open rapidly
(b) stomata close
(c) there is no effect in stomatal movement
(d) stomata open slowly.

134. About what percentage of water absorbed by plants is lost again by transpiration?
(a) 80% (b) 60%
(c) 96% (d) 40%.

135. What happens by spraying of phenyl mercuric acetate (PMA) of abscisic acid (ABA) on leaves?
(a) transpiration rate increases

(b) transpiration rate decreases
(c) water absorption rate increases
(d) guttation rate increases.

136. Which of the following is a bacterial disease?
(a) rabies (b) measles
(c) small pox (d) tuberculosis.

137. For chlorophyll formation in plants, which of the following elements are needed
(a) iron and calcium
(b) calcium and potassium
(c) iron and magnesium
(d) sodium and copper.

138. Viruses are formed of
(a) nucleic acids
(b) DNA and RNA
(c) proteins
(d) proteins and nucleic acids.

139. Formation of fat (lipogenesis) begins in the body when
(a) blood sugar level is high
(b) glucose is converted into glycogen
(c) when liver and muscles cannot store any more glycogen
(d) when glucose combines with glycerol.

140. The reptiles and birds cannot afford to lose water and hence they excrete
(a) ammonia (b) urea
(c) creatinine (d) uric acid.

141. The fertilized secondary nucleus of the ovule, during double fertilization, establishes the
(a) seed coat (b) endosperm
(c) embryo plant (d) pericarp.

142. Kwashiorkor, an African word to signify "rejected ones" affecting children of underdeveloped and developing countries with symptoms of stunted growth, loss of appetite, anaemia, protruding bellies, match-stick legs, resulting in great mortality, is due to the deficiency of
(a) vitamins (b) proteins
(c) fats (d) carbohydrates.

143. Ginger is a stem, not a root because it has
(a) food storage
(b) nodes and internodes
(c) burning taste
(d) flowers.

144. The tusk of the elephant is formed
(a) from incisors
(b) from canines
(c) of prolongation of the skull
(d) by the thickening of the skin of the head.

145. The blood corpuscle which kills bacteria that get into our body is termed
(a) erythrocyte
(b) phagocyte
(c) thrombocyte
(d) eosinophils.

146. Mulberry-growing is associated with the
(a) control of insect pest
(b) silk worm culture (sericulture)
(c) support for the grape vine
(d) fodder for the cattle.

147. Which of the following disease is caused by air pollution?
(a) rheumatism (b) heart failure
(c) bronchitis (d) leukemia.

148. Cataract is caused by
(a) accumulation of dust in the eye
(b) lens getting opaque
(c) nerves supplying the eyes getting weak
(d) conjunction becoming thickened.

149. In fern plant, the ejection of spores with force is achieved by the
(a) sporangiophore (b) annulus
(c) stomium (d) indusium.

150. Which type of soil is best suited for the cultivation of cotton in India?
(a) loamy soil (b) black soil
(c) sandy soil (d) clayey soil.

151. For the first time viruses were crystallised and isolated by

(a) D. Ivanowski (b) F.C. Bawden
(c) K.M. Smith (d) W.M. Stanley.

152. Chlorophyll *a* occurs in
(a) all plants except algae
(b) all green plants except bacteria
(c) fungi only
(d) angiosperms only.

153. K.C. Mehta is famous for his work on
(a) the wheat rust
(b) viral diseases
(c) bacterial diseases
(d) none of the above.

154. Protonema is a stage in the life cycle of
(a) *Selaginella* (b) *Cycas*
(c) *Funaria* (d) *Rhizopus*.

155. Which one of the following is a fossil
(a) *Rhynia* (b) *Equisetum*
(c) *Selaginella* (d) none of the above.

156. Epidermal outgrowths are known as
(a) stem (b) stomata
(c) buds (d) trichomes.

157. Polyadelphous condition refer to
(a) stigma (b) androecium
(c) gynoecium (d) petals.

158. National Botanical Research Institute is situated at
(a) Shimla (b) Cuttack
(c) Delhi (d) Lucknow.

159. Saffron is produced from
(a) stamens of *Hibiscus*
(b) roots of *Rouwalfia*
(c) style and stigma of *Crocus*
(d) petals of *Musa*.

160. Cystolith is
(a) magnesium sulphate crystals
(b) crystals of calcium
(c) calcium carbonate crystals
(d) none of the above.

Instructions for Q. No. 161 to 180

Directions : Each of the questions given below consists of two statements, an assertions (A) and reason (R). Select the number corresponding to the appropriate response in the answer sheet as follows.

(a) If both assertion and reason are true and the reason is a correct explanation of the assertion
(b) If both assertion and reason are true but the reason is not a correct explanation of the assertion
(c) If the assertion is true, but the reason is false
(d) If both assertion and reason are falses

161. *Assertion (A) :* Casparian strips are formed on the inner tangential wall.
Reason (R) : In root, epidermis is not covered by cuticle.

162. *Assertion (A) :* The stem which has undergone secondary growth shows more phloem than xylem.
Reason (R) : Vascular cambium and cork cambium are synonymus.

163. *Assertion (A) :* Double fertilization is occurs in angiosperms only.
Reason (R) : Female gametophyte is not a food supplying structure in them.

164. *Assertion (A) :* Coconut fruit is considered as drupe and tomato a berry.
Reason (R) : Both are simple fleshy fruits.

165. *Assertion (A) :* Green oranges and tomatoes turn orange yellow coloured when sprayed with ABA.
Reason (R) : ABA possess anti-gibberellin property.

166. *Assertion (A) :* Lymph contain more protein than plasma.
Reason (R) : Haemopoietic organs produce lymph.

167. *Assertion (A) :* Patients are given sago starch.
Reason (R) : Sago starch is obtained from palm.

168. *Assertion (A) :* The glomerular filtrate becomes hypotonic in the ascending limb.
Reason (R) : Ascending limb is impermeable to water.

169. *Assertion (A)* : Spermatozoa produced in large number as compared to ova.
Reason (R) : Sperms are smaller than ova.

170. *Assertion (A)* : The coelenteron of *Hydra* is called gastrovascular cavity.
Reason (R) : *Hydra* is a monoblastic animal.

171. *Assertion (A)* : Each liver lobe is a compact network of closely set, branching and anastomosing lobules cemented together by connective tissues containing blood vessels, small blood sinuses and the fine bile canaliculi.
Reason (R) : Each lobule is formed of several large and cuboidal hepatic cells arranged in columns.

172. *Assertion (A)* : Lymphatic interstitium is packed with a gelatinous substance (tissue gel) in which long collagen fibre bundles are suspended to give tensional strength to the tissues. Tissue gel is formed by reticular network of coiled filaments of proteoglycan and a fluid trapped in minute spaces.
Reason (R) : Tissue gel allows transport water molecules, electrolytes, nutrients, O_2, CO_2, cellular waste products and hormones.

173. *Assertion (A)* : Conjunctiva is composed of stratified epithelium and is continuous with the epidermis that lines the eyelids.
Reason (R) : The conjunctiva is thin, little cornified and are not supplied with free nerve endings.

174. *Assertion (A)* : Within a liver cell, sporozoites of malarial parasite actively feed upon its cytoplasm and grow into large and spherical, adult like forms, called cryptozoites.
Reason (R) : Cryptozoites divide into about numerous minute cryptomerozoites by a special multiple fission called schizogony.

175. *Assertion (A)* : The ovarian cycle of follicles is control by gonadotropic hormones, follicles stimulating hormone (FSH) and luteinizing hormone (LH).
Reason (R) : During ovarian cycle follicles undergo maturation, contain a secondary oocyte and produce female sex hormone.

176. *Assertion (A)* : Zygospore fungi produce spores within sporangia.
Reason (R) : During sexual reproduction, a zygospore forms prior to meiosis and production of spores.

177. *Assertion (A)* : Club fungi usually reproduce sexually.
Reason (R) : In club fungi, the dikaryotic stage is prolonged and periodically produces fruiting bodies where spores are produced in basidia.

178. *Assertion (A)* : Rusts and smuts are club fungi that parasitize cereal crops.
Reason (R) : Some smuts enter seeds and exist inside the plant,becoming visible only near maturity.

179. *Assertion (A)* : Bacteria do not move by means of flagella.
Reason (R) : The 360° rotation of the flagellum does not cause the cell to spin and forward movement.

180. *Assertion (A)* : The tropical movements occurring in response to water stimulus are called rheotropic movements.
Reason (R) : Haptotropic movements occur in response to a light.

GENERAL KNOWLEDGE

181. Industrially most advanced state in India is
(a) Gujrat (b) Maharashtra
(c) Punjab (d) Madhya Pradesh

182. Mahabharat consist of
(a) 18 books & 10,000 couplets
(b) 18 books & 5,000 couplets
(c) 15 books & 10,000 couplets
(d) 13 books & 10,000 couplets

183. The maximum percentage of tribal population in India consists of
(a) Bhils (b) Santhals
(c) Nagas (d) Mundas

184. What is the playing time of the shorter version of our National Anthem which is played on ceremonial occassion?

(a) 2 minutes (b) 1 minute
(c) 50 seconds (d) 48 seconds

185. Chaikar koothu is one of the most impressive dance forms of

(a) Kerala (b) Tamil Nadu
(c) Karnataka (d) Goa

186. The autobiography "A Brush with life" has been written by

(a) M.F.Hussain (b) Shobha De
(c) Satish Gujaral (d) Khushwant Singh

187. Of the 109 known elements, how many are occur in nature and how many are produced synthetically in particle accelerators

(a) 79 & 10 (b) 80 & 29
(c) 95 & 14 (d) none of these

188. Asia's oldest and largest Buddhist monastry is situated in

(a) Twang (b) Srilanka
(c) Lhasa (d) Mongolia

189. The Adi granth was compiled by

(a) Guru Ram Das (b) Guru Amar Das
(c) Guru Arjun Dev (d) Guru Teg Bahadur

190. Which of the following is a metal

(a) mercury (b) bromine
(c) chlorine (d) none of these.

191. Which of the following is a cash crop?

(a) gram (b) groundnut
(c) barley (d) jawar

192. Which continent is honoured by having consecutive three term General of U.N.O.

(a) South Africa (b) Australia
(c) South America (d) North America

193. In how many hours a geo stationary satellite completes one round of its orbit?

(a) 1 (b) 6
(c) 8 (d) 24

194. Cattle bone powder is used as fertilizer as it is rich in

(a) N (b) P
(c) Na (d) K

195. Which of the following is considered as the electronic city of India

(a) Hydrabad (b) Bangalore
(c) Calcutta (d) Mumbai

196. The Summer Olympics of 2004 will be organised at which of the following cities?

(a) Rome (b) Athens
(c) Tokyo (d) New Delhi

197. India had not received noble prize in which of the following field?

(a) chemistry (b) physics
(c) medicine (d) literature

198. The well known wonder drug against cancer 'Taxol' is extracted from the tree

(a) neem (b) yew
(c) oak (d) peepal

199. Aluminium in the earth's crust is found as

(a) cryolite (b) bauxite
(c) gypsum (d) none of these

200. Cloves are actually

(a) seeds (b) bark
(c) fruit
(d) unopened floral bud

■■■

Model Test Paper-8

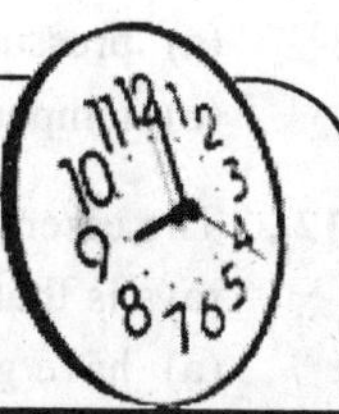

Time : $3\frac{1}{2}$ hours. *Maximum Marks : 200*

PHYSICS

1. The refractive indices of the material of lens for violet, yellow and red colours of light are 1.66, 1.64 and 1.62 respectively, the mean focal length of the lens is 10 cm, then chromatic aberration of the lens between the violet and the red colours is
(a) 0.857 (b) 0.825
(c) 0.625 (d) 1.0

2. Which one of the following nuclear reactions is a source of energy in the sun?
(a) ${}_{56}Ba^{144} + {}_{36}Kr^{92} \rightarrow {}_{92}U^{235} + {}_0n^1$
(b) ${}_2He^3 + {}_2He^3 \rightarrow {}_2He^{14} + {}_0H^1 + {}_1H^1$
(c) ${}_4Be^9 + {}_2He^4 \rightarrow {}_6C^{12} + {}_0n^1$
(d) ${}_{24}Fe^{56} + {}_{43}Ca^{112} \rightarrow 167\ {}_{74}W^{92} + {}_0n^1$

3. If an electron is moving with a speed of 3×10^7 m/s perpendicular to a uniform magnetic field of flux density 0.002 Wb.m^2, then the radius of the path is
(a) 0.084 m (b) 0.064 m
(c) 0.038 m (d) 0.090 m

4. When a sound wave travels from air to water, which of these remains constant?
(a) wavelength (b) frequency
(c) velocity (d) all of these

5. A straight line conductor of length 0.4 m is moved with a speed of 7 m/s perpendicular to a magnetic field of intensity 0.9 Wb/m^2. The induced e.m.f. across the conductor is
(a) 5.04 V (b) 2.52 V
(c) 1.26 V (d) 25.2 V

6. In an intrinsic semiconductor, the fermi level varies linearly with the
(a) thermal conductivity
(b) pressure
(c) temperature
(d) none of these

7. An electron is moving with velocity 10^6 m/s in a circular path of radius 0.0077 m in a magnetic field of 10^{-3} Wb/m^2. The value of *e/m* for the electron is
(a) 1.9×10^{11} C/kg (b) 1.35×10^{11} C/kg
(c) 1.29×10^{11} C/kg (d) 2.6×10^{11}C/kg

8. The coefficient of thermal conductivity of a metal depends upon
(a) thickness of metal plate
(b) temperature difference between two sides
(c) area of plate
(d) all of these

9. A conducting rod is rotated with angular velocity ω in a horizontal plane perpendicular to a uniform magnetic induction *B*. The induced e.m.f. is
(a) ωBI (b) $\frac{\omega BI^2}{2}$
(c) $\frac{BI}{\omega}$ (d) $\frac{\omega^2 BI}{2}$

10. A block of wood is floating in a water tank. The loss of weight of the floating block is equal to
(a) remains same
(b) greater than the weight of block
(c) weight of block
(d) none of these

11. The internal energy of a real gas depends upon

(a) pressure (b) volume
(c) temperature (d) both (b) and (c)

12. The essential distinction between X-rays and γ-rays is that the γ-rays
(a) have greater ionizing power than X-rays
(b) emanate from nucleus, while X-rays emanate from outer part of the atom
(c) have smaller wave-length than X-rays
(d) are more penetrating than X-rays.

13. Which of the following mirror is used by dentist to examine a small cavity?
(a) convex mirror
(b) concave mirror
(c) combination of 'a' and 'b'
(d) none of these

14. The earth E moves in an elliptical orbit with the Sun S at one of the focii as shown in figure. Its speed of motion will be maximum at the point
(a) B
(b) A
(c) C
(d) D

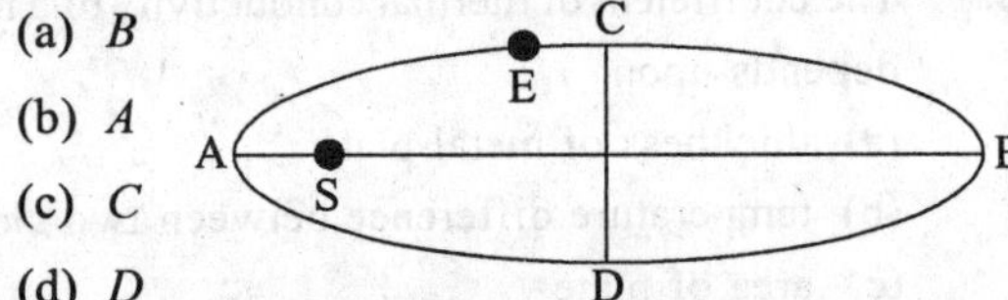

15. A space-station is set-up in space at a distance equal to earth's radius from the surface of earth. Suppose a statellite can be launched from the space station also. If υ_1 and υ_2 be the escape velocities of the satellite on the earth's surface and space station respectively, then
(a) $\upsilon_2 = \upsilon_1$ (b) $\upsilon_2 < \upsilon_1$
(c) $\upsilon_2 > \upsilon_1$ (d) $\upsilon_1^2 = \upsilon_2^2$

16. Current I_0 flows through a solenoid of length L having N number of turns, when it is connected to a DC e.m.f. If charged particle is projected along the axis of solenoid with a speed υ_0, then the force on the charged particle in the solenoid
(a) remains same (b) decreases
(c) increases (d) becomes zero

17. In the arrangement of resistances shown below, the effective resistance between points A and B is

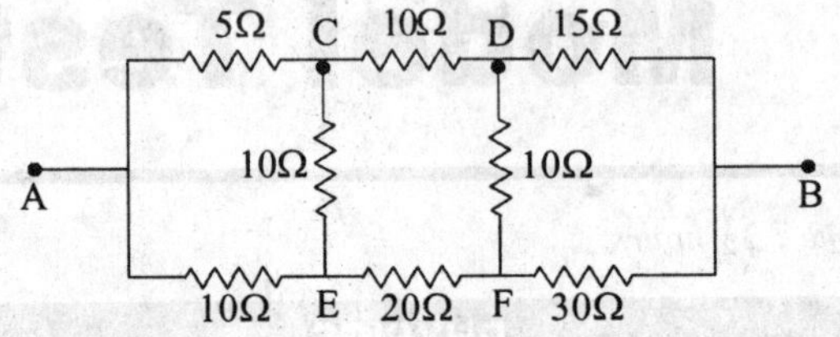

(a) 90 W (b) 30 W
(c) 20 W (d) 110 W

18. Latent heat is defined as the amount of heat absorbed or given out by a body during a change of state, while its
(a) volume remains constant
(b) temperature remains constant
(c) pressure remains constant
(d) none of these

19. A beam of light of wave length λ and illumination L falls on a clean surface of sodium. If n photo electrons are emitted and each has a kinetic energy E, then
(a) $n \propto \lambda$ and $E \propto L$ (b) $n \propto L$ and $E \propto \frac{1}{\lambda}$
(c) $n \propto L$ and $E \propto \lambda$ (d) $n \propto \frac{1}{\lambda}$ and $E \propto \frac{1}{L}$

20. The phenomenon of beats is not observed in the case of visible light waves, because the difference between the two interfering frequencies
(a) has no difference (b) is very high
(c) is very small (d) none of these

21. An aluminium sphere of 10 cm radius is heated from 0°C to 100°C. The change in its volume
(a) 22.6 cm³ (b) 12.3 cm³
(c) 2.0 cm³ (d) 28.9 cm³

22. Two small spheres each carrying a charge q are placed r metre apart. If one of the spheres is taken around the other in a circular path, then work done will be equal to
(a) πρ (b) 2 πρ

(c) $2\pi\rho^2$ (d) zero

23. The electric current, passing through a metallic wire produces heat, because of

(a) the energy released in the ionization of the atoms of the metal

(b) collision of the atoms of the metal with each other

(c) collisions of conduction electrons with each other

(d) collisions of the conduction electrons with the atoms of the metallic wire.

24. Find the ratio of period of rotation of planet (Mars) about the Sun with that of the Earth around it. The mean distance of the Mars from the Sun is 1.42 A.U. and distance of earth from the sun = 1 A.U.

(a) 1.692 : 2 (b) 1 : 1.692

(c) 1.692 : 1 (d) 2 : 1.692

25. Electrical conductivities of Ge and Na are σ_1 and σ_2 respectively. If these substances are heated, then

(a) σ_1 decreases and σ_2 increases

(b) both σ_1 and σ_2 decreases

(c) both σ_1 and σ_2 increase

(d) σ_1 increases and σ_2 decreases

26. If the cross-sectional area of a pipe line increases, the velocity of the flow of liquid

(a) become zero (b) decreases

(c) increases (d) remains same

27. The excess pressure inside a soap bubble of radius (R) and surface tension (T) is

(a) $P = \dfrac{3T}{R}$ (b) $P = \dfrac{4T}{R}$

(c) $P = \dfrac{2T}{R}$ (d) $\dfrac{8T}{R}$

28. A black body radiates heat energy at the rate of 2×10^5 J/s-m² at the temperture of 120°C. Temperature of the black body at which rate of heat radiation is 32×10^5 J/s-m² is

(a) 400 K (b) 600 K

(c) 800 K (d) 200 K

29. Which of the following is not the characteristic of SHM?

(a) displacement time graph is a sine curve

(b) periodic nature

(c) projection of uniform circular motion on any straight line

(d) acceleration zero at the mean position

30. Slope of an adiabatic curve is always

(a) equal to isothermal curve

(b) less than isothermal curve

(c) greater than isothermal curve

(d) either 'b' or 'a'

31. The value of the square of sum of two vectors $\vec{A}$ and $\vec{B}$ with θ as the angle between them is

(a) $\sqrt{A^2 + B^2 - 2AB\sin\theta}$

(b) $\sqrt{A^2 - B^2 + 2AB\cos\theta}$

(c) $\sqrt{A^2 + B^2 + 2AB\cos\theta}$

(d) $\sqrt{A^2 + B^2 + 2AB\sin\theta}$

32. A disc of mass 3 kg is rolling on a horizontal surface with a velocity 0.3 m/s. The total kinetic energy of the disc should be

(a) 0.98J (b) 0.35J

(c) 0.20J (d) 1.26J

33. Myopia is corrected by

(a) bifocal lens (b) concave lens

(c) convex lens (d) cylindrical lens

34. If the plate resistance of a triode valve is $3 \times 10^3\ \Omega$ and amplification factor (μ) is 8, the value of mutual conductance is

(a) $3.6 \times 10^{-4}\Omega^{-1}$ (b) $2.6 \times 10^{-3}\Omega^{-1}$

(c) $1.5 \times 10^{-2}\Omega^{-1}$ (d) $6.3 \times 10^{-3}\Omega^{-1}$

35. When we connected a voltmeter across the terminals of a cell, it measures 6 V. If a resistance of 2 ohms is connected across the terminals of a cell as shown in the figure, then current flowing through this resistance (R) will be

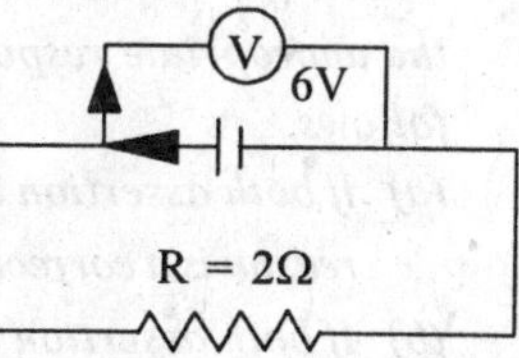

(a) 5A (b) 3A
(c) 2A (d) 7.5A

36. If a man pulls a cart of mass 100 kg with an acceleration of 2 m/sec^2, then force exerted by the man is
(a) 600 N (b) 400 N
(c) 200 N (d) 800 N

37. For steel, the breaking stress is 6×10^6 N/m^2 and the density is 8×10^3 kg/m^3. The maximum length of steel wire, which can be suspended without breaking under its own weight is (g = 10m/s^2)
(a) 140 m (b) 120 m
(c) 75 m (d) 200 m

38. One light-year is approximately equivalent to
(a) 10^{18} m (b) 10^{16} m
(c) 10^{14} m (d) 10^{20} m

39. A 10 A ammeter has a resistance of 0.09 Ω. What resistance of the shunt will enable it read 100 A?
(a) 0.09 Ω (b) 9 Ω
(c) 1 Ω (d) 0.01 Ω

40. A sphere of mass 50 kg is attracted by a second sphere of mass 90 kg with a force equal to a weight of 0.5 mg and their centres are 20 cm apart. The gravitational constant is (weight of sphere = 10^{-6}kg)
(a) 3.3×10^{-11} Nm^2 kg^{-2}
(b) 6.23×10^{-15} Nm^2 kg^{-2}
(c) 4.2×10^{-11} Nm^2 kg^{-2}
(d) 4.36×10^{-11} Nm^2 kg^{-2}

Instructions for Q. No. 41 to 60

Directions : Each of the questions given below consists of two statements, an assertions (A) and reason (R). Select the number corresponding to the appropriate response in the answer sheet as follows.

(a) If both assertion and reason are true and the reason is a correct explanation of the assertion

(b) If both assertion and reason are true but the reason is not a correct explanation of the assertion

(c) If the assertion is true, but the reason is false

(d) If both assertion and reason are falses

41. *Assertion (A)* : A balloon stops rising after attaining a certain maximum height.
Reason (R) : Upthrust due to air decreases with height till it just balances the weight of the balloon.

42. *Assertion (A)* : In series A.C. circuit, the voltage across the combination of capacitor and inductor is zero at resonance.
Reason (R) : At series resonance the current in the circuit is zero.

43. A*Assertion (A)* : It is necessary to use artificial satellite for long distance TV transmission.
Reason (R) : Ionospheric disturbances are minimised by satellite communication.

44. *Assertion (A)* : A table cloth can be pulled from a table without dislodging the dishes.
Reason (R) : To every action there is an equal but opposite reaction.

45. *Assertion (A)* : The dimensions of moment of force are the same as those of work.
Reason (R) : Moment of force is $r \times$ F while works is r.F.

46. *Assertion (A)* : Out of four Indian satellites, Rohini, Aryabhatt, Bhasker and Insat-1B, the time period of Insat-1B is maximum.
Reason (R) : Insat-1B is a communication satellite while others are orbital satellites.

47. *Assertion (A)* : A body is floating completely submerged in a liquid. When it is further pushed inside the liquid it remains in a position in which it is left.
Reason (R) : When a body floats in a liquid completely submerged, there is no net force acting on it.

48. *Assertion (A)* : The fundamental frequency of an open organ pipe increases as the temperature is increased.
Reason (R) : This is because as the temperature increases, the velocity of sound increases more rapidly than length of the pipe.

49. *Assertion (A)* : Alpha particles produce more intense ionisation than beta particles.
Reason (R) : Alpha particles are positively charged.

50. *Assertion (A)* : The lightening conductor at the top of high buildings has sharp pointed ends.
Reason (R) : The surface density of charge at sharp points is very high resulting in setting up of electric wind

51. *Assertion (A)* : In a radioactive disintegration an electron is emitted by the nucleus.
Reason (R) : Electrons are always present inside the nucleus.

52. *Assertion (A)* : In Rutherford's experiment, α - particles from a radium source were allowed to fall on a 10^{-4} mm thick gold foil. Most of α- particles passed straight through the foil.
Reason (R) : The entire positive charge and nearly whole of the mass of the nucleus is concentrated in the nucleus.

53. *Assertion (A)* : The relative velocity of two photons travelling in opposite directions is C.
Reason (R) : The rest mass of a photon is zero.

54. *Assertion (A)* : Tiny drops of liquid resist deforming forces better than bigger drops.
Reason (R) : Excess pressure inside a drop is directly proportional to the surface tension.

55. *Assertion (A)* : The couple acting on a body is not equal to the rotational K.E. of the body.
Reason (R) : Couple and K.E. have different units.

56. *Assertion (A)* : A thin aluminium disc spinning freely about a central pivot is quickly brought to rest when placed between the poles of a strong U-shaped magnet.
Reason (R) : A current induced in a disc rotating in a magnetic field produces a force which tends to oppose the disc's motion.

57. *Assertion (A)* : The period of simple pendulum is independent of the mass of the bob.
Reason (R) : Inertial and gravitational masses are equivalent.

58. *Assertion (A)* : The frequencies of incident, reflected and refracted beam of monochromatic light incident from one medium to another are the same.
Reason (R) : The incident, the reflected and the refracted rays are coplanar.

59. *Assertion (A)* : Radio waves can be polarised.
Reason (R) : Sound waves in air are longitudinal in nature.

60. *Assertion (A)* : A hollow metallic closed container maintained at a uniform temperature can act as a black body for radiations.
Reason (R) : All metals acts as black bodies.

CHEMISTRY

61. An e^- has magnetic quantum number as –3, what is its principal quantum number?
(a) 3 (b) 2
(c) 1 (d) 4.

62. Wavelength associated with electron motion
(a) decreases with increase in speed of e^-
(b) remains same irrespective of speed of electron
(c) increases with increase in speed of electron
(d) is zero.

63. A reaction is $A + B \rightarrow C + D$. Initially, we start with equal concentration of A and B. At equilibrium we find the moles of C is two times of A. What is the equilibrium constant of the reaction ?
(a) 1/4 (b) 2
(c) 4 (d) 1/2.

64. A catalyst in a chemical reaction -
(a) changes the equilibrium constant of a reaction
(b) increases the activation energy of the reaction
(c) does not initiate a reaction
(d) does not change the rate of the reaction.

65. Aromatic compounds undergo-
(a) electrophilic substitution
(b) electrophilic addition
(c) nucleophilic addition reaction
(d) none of these.

66. CH_3COOH is reacted with $CH \equiv CH$ in presence of Hg^{++}, the product is -

(a) $CH_2(OOCCH_3)$ | $CH_2(OOCCH_3)$

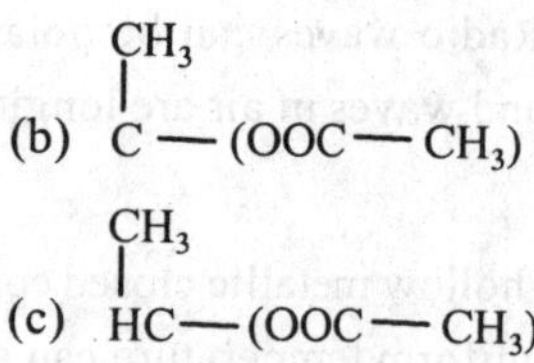

(d) none of these.

67. Which of the following is an electrophile?
(a) $AlCl_3$ (b) NH_3
(C) H_2O (D) $C_2H_5NH_2$.

68. DDT is prepared by reacting chlorobenzene with
(a) $CHCl_3$ (b) $CCl_3 - CHO$
(c) CCl_4 (d) ethane.

69. Which of the following has highest chlorine content?
(a) chloral (b) DDT
(c) pyrene (d) gammexane.

70. Which one of the following is the chiral molecule?
(a) $CHBr_3$ (b) CH_2Cl_2
(c) CH_3Cl (d) CHClBrI.

71. H_2S is passed through an acidified solution of Ag, Cu and Zn. Which forms precipitates ?
(a) Cu (b) Zn
(c) Ag (d) none of these.

72. Which of the following compounds volatilises on heating ?
(a) $ZnCl_2$ (b) $HgCl_2$
(c) $MgCl_2$ (d) none of these.

73. Which of the following oxides reacts with HCl and NaOH ?
(a) N_2O_5 (b) ZnO
(c) CaO (d) CO_2.

74. When acetylene is passed through dil. H_2SO_4 in the presence of $HgSO_4$ the compound formed is
(a) carbide of Hg (b) acetone
(c) C_2H_5OH (d) acetaldehyde.

75. Which metal is protected by a layer of its own oxide ?
(a) Al_2O_3 (b) MgO
(c) Na_2O (d) CaO.

76. The neutralisation of a strong acid by a strong base liberates an amount of energy per mole of H^+ that
(a) depends upon which catalyst is used
(b) depends upon the temperature at which the reaction takes place
(c) depends upon which acid and base are involved
(d) is always the same.

77. Albumin proteins are most abundant in
(A) egg (B) milk
(C) meat (D) soyabean.

78. One of the following is false for Hg
(a) it has high specific heat
(b) it is a metal
(c) it can evolve hydrogen from H_2S
(d) it is less reactive than hydrogen.

79. Equal volumes of methanoic acid and sodium hydroxide are mixed, if x is the heat of formation of water, then heat evolved on neutralisation is
(a) twice of x (b) equal to x
(c) more than x (d) less than x.

80. Which is not a macromolecule?
(a) palmitate (b) starch
(c) DNA (d) insulin.

81. Increase in boiling point of a sucrose solution is 0.1 K, then what is increase in boiling point of the same concentration of NaCl solution ?
(a) 0.4 K (b) 0.2 K
(c) 0.1 K (d) 0.58 K.

82. Specific heat of metal is 0.23 and its chloride contains 87% of chlorine. What is the exact atomic weight of the metal ?
(a) 62 (b) 54
(c) 24 (d) 26.2.

83. 240 g of urea is present in 10 litre solution, the active mass of urea will be
(a) 0.4 mol/lit (b) 0.06 mol/lit
(c) 0.2 mol/lit (d) 0.08 mol/lit.

84. Which of the following is most acidic?
(a) Al_2O_3 (b) MgO
(c) Na_2O (d) CaO.

85. The gas molecules have r.m.s. velocity of its molecules as 1000 m/s. What is its average velocity?
(a) 546 m/s (b) 921.58 m/s
(c) 1012 m/s (d) 960 m/s.

86. The IUPAC name of $C_2H_5CONH_2$ is
(a) propanamide (b) benzamide
(c) methanamide (d) ethanamide

87. The catalyst $SnCl_2$/HCl is used in
(a) Clemmensen reduction reaction
(b) Cannizzaro's reduction reaction
(c) Stephen's reduction reaction
(d) Rosen mund's reduction reaction

88. Which of the following is correct?
(a) german silver-Cu + Zn + C
(b) duralumin-Al + Cu + Mg + Ag
(c) gun metal-Cu + Zn + Sn
(d) solder-Pb + Al

89. The Grignard reagent, on reaction with acetone forms
(a) acetic acid
(b) secondary alcohol
(c) tertiary alcohol
(d) acetaldehyde

90. The order of stability of carbonium ion is
(a) 3° > 1°> 2° > CH_3^+
(b) 3° > 2° > 1° > CH_3^+
(c) CH_3^+ > 1°> 2°> 3°
(d) 2° > 3° > 1° > CH_3^+

91. The bond angle of sp^2-hybrid orbital is
(a) 105° (b) 180°
(c) 120° (d) 109°

92. The positron has mass equal to
(a) deutron (b) proton
(c) electron (d) α-particle

93. The square planar shape is for
(a) $[CrF_6]^{3-}$ (b) $[Cu(NH_3)_4]^{2+}$
(c) BF_4 (d) none of these

94. In which of the following reactions, the hydrogen peroxide is a reducing agent?
(a) $2HI + H_2O_2 \rightarrow 2H_2O + I_2$
(b) $Cl_2 + H_2O_2 \rightarrow 2HCl + O_2$
(c) $2FeCl_2 + 2HCl + H_2O_2 \rightarrow 2FeCl_3 + 2H_2O$
(d) $H_2SO_3 + H_2O_2 \rightarrow H_2SO_4 + H_2O$

95. If $[Zn^{2+}]$ = 0.1 M and E^0 = –0.76 V then half cell potential at 298 K for the reaction $Zn^{2+}(aq) + 2e^- \rightarrow Zn(s)$ is
(a) – 0.698 V (b) –0.789 V
(c) 0.789 V (d) 0.698 V

96. The osmotic pressure of a 5% solution of cane sugar at 15°C is (Mol.wt. of cane sugar = 342)
(a) 3.57 atm (b) 3.45 atm
(c) 2.35 atm (d) 4 atm

97. The pH value of a solution whose hydronium ion concentration 6.2×10^{-9} mol L^{-1} is
(a) 7.75 (b) 7.21
(c) 6.21 (d) 8.21

98. Which of the following metal acts as the most efficient catalyst?
(a) alkaline earth metal
(b) transition metal
(c) alkali metal
(d) coloured metals

99. Silver chloride is soluble in methylamine due to the formation of
(a) $[Ag(CH_3NH_2)_2]Cl$ (b) $Ag(CH_3NH_2)Cl$
(c) AgOH
(d) $Ag + CH_3Cl + NH_4Cl$

100. Which of the following represents noble gas configuration?
(a) $1s^22s^22p^63s^23p^63d^{10}4s^24p^64d^{10}5s^25d^16s^2$
(b) $1s^22s^22p^63s^23p^63d^{10}4s^24f^{14}5s^25p^65p^1$
(c) $1s^22s^22p^63s^23p^63d^{10}4s^24p^64d^{10}5s^25p^6$
(d) $1s^22s^22p^63s^23p^63d^{10}4s^24p^64d^{10}5s^25p^65d^56s^2$

Instructions for Q. No. 101 to 120

Directions : Each of the questions given below consists of two statements, an assertions (A) and reason (R). Select the number corresponding to the appropriate response in the answer sheet as follows.

(a) If both assertion and reason are true and the reason is a correct explanation of the assertion

(b) If both assertion and reason are true but the reason is not a correct explanation of the assertion

(c) If the assertion is true, but the reason is false

(d) If both assertion and reason are falses

101. *Assertion (A) :* The name butanol is not specific, whereas the name butanone represents one specific compound.
Reason (R) : Alcohols show phenomenon of isomerism where as ketones do not show isomerism

102. *Assertion (A) :* Alkenes and cycloalkanes series of hydrocarbons have same general formula.
Reason (R) : Either insertion of a double bond or formation of a ring reduce the number of hydrogen atoms of corresponding alkane by 2.

103. *Assertion (A) :* The carbon atoms of the benzene ring may be numbered for identification of substituent groups, just as a continuous chains of carbon atoms are numbered.
Reason (R) : Smallest set of numbers designating the substituents is the preferred set.

104. *Assertion (A) :* White precipitate of lead chloride ($PbCl_2$) is soluble in concentrated solution of potassium chloride.
Reason (R) : Tetrachloroplumbate (II) ion is formed when chloride ions attacks the Lead (II) chloride.

105. *Assertion (A) :* Mercurous chloride (Hg_2Cl_2) precipitate, on reacting with ammonia solution, gives a mixture of mercury (II) amidochloride and mercury metal.
Reason (R) : The reaction of ammonia and Hg_2Cl_2 involves disproportionation in which simultaneous oxidation and reduction take place.

106. *Assertion (A) :* In a given electrical field beta particles (β) are deflected more than alpha particles (α).
Reason (R) : Beta particles have very low *e* / *m* value as compared to alpha particles.

107. *Assertion (A) :* Neutrons are better projectiles for nuclear reactions than protons or α-particles
Reason (R) : Neutrons are neutral particles and hence, their penetration in nucleus is rather difficult.

108. *Assertion (A) :* The solubility of *n*-alcohols in water decreases with increase in molecular weight.
Reason (R) : The relative proportion of the hydrocarbon part in alcohols increases with the increase in molecular weight which permits enhanced hydrogenbonding with water.

109. *Assertion (A) :* The nitro group, if present in ortho or para positions, would stabilise the phenoxide ion by dispersal of negative charge through mesomeric effect.
Reason (R) : The electron releasing substituents would intensify the negative charge. As a result electron releasing group in phenol should be acid-weakening.

110. *Assertion (A) :* The electronic arrangement with exactly half-filled or completely filled degenerate orbitals would be more stable that any other electronic arrangement.
Reason (R) : The electronic configuration with even or uniform or symmetrical distribution of charge in all directions would evidently be associated with high energy.

111. *Assertion (A) :* The lactic acid shows the geometrical isomerism.
Reason (R) : Lactic acid has carbon-carbon double bond.

112. *Assertion (A) :* 2-hydroxy 1, 4-butane dioic acid is known as malic acid.
Reason (R) : It is present in unripe apples.

113. *Assertion (A) :* During the fermentation of grape juice, a reddish brown coloured crust is formed.
Reason (R) : Impure potassium hydrogen tartrate is of reddish brown colour and it is known as argol.

114. *Assertion (A) :* Amines are more basic than ethers and esters.
Reason (R) : Nitrogen is less electronegative than oxygen, it is in better position to accomodate the positive charge of the proton.

115. *Assertion (A) :* An orbital cannot have more than two electrons, moreover, if an orbital has two electrons they must have opposite spins.
Reason (R) : No two electrons in an atom can have same set of all the four quantum numbers.

116. *Assertion (A) :* The pairing of electrons in the orbitals of a particular sub-shell are singly occupied.
Reason (R) : Singly occupied orbitals must have the electrons with parallel spins.

117. *Assertion (A) :* Fluorine molecule has bond order one.
Reason (R) : The number of electrons in antibonding molecular orbitals is two less than that in bonding molecular orbitals.

118. *Assertion (A) :* Nitrate ion (NO_3^-) is a Bronsted base.
Reason (R) : Bronsted base is a chemical species which can accept H^+ ions.

119. *Assertion (A) :* The molality of the solution does not change with change in temperature.
Reason (R) : The molality is expressed in units of moles per 1000 gm of solvent.

120. *Assertion (A) :* The molecularity of the reaction $H_2 + Br_2 \rightarrow 2HBr$ is two.
Reason (R) : The order of this reaction is 3/2.

BIOLOGY

121. The eukaryotic genome differs from the prokaryotic genome because
(a) the DNA is complexed with histones in prokaryotes
(b) repetitive sequences are present in eukaryotes
(c) the DNA is circular and single stranded in prokaryotes
(d) genes in the former case are organized into operons.

122. In DNA, when AGCT occurs, their association is as per which of the following pair?
(a) AT-GC (b) AG-CT
(c) AC-GT (d) all of these.

123. Edible part in litchi is
(a) endosperm (b) mesocarp
(c) pericarp (d) fleshy aril.

124. Which of the following is the main category of mutation?
(a) somatic mutation
(b) genetic mutation
(c) zygotic mutation
(d) all of these.

125. In soil, water available for plants is
(a) gravitational water
(b) capillary water
(c) chemically bound water
(d) hygroscopic water.

126. Green house effect refers to
(a) production of cereals
(b) cooling of earth
(c) warming of earth
(d) trapping of UV rays.

127. Energy transfer from one trophic level to other in a food chain is
(a) 10% (b) 1%
(c) 20% (d) 2%.

128. Carbon dioxide acceptor in C_3-plants is
(a) PGA (b) PEP
(c) RuDP (d) none of these.

129. In 1984, Bhopal gas tragedy was caused due to leakage of
(a) potassium isocyanate
(b) sodium monoxide
(c) methyl isocyanate
(d) sodium thiocyanate.

130. Land mass occupied by forest is about
(a) 30% (b) 11%
(c) 60% (d) 22%.

131. Which of the following is a secondary pollutant?
(a) PAN (b) CO
(c) aerosol (d) CO_2.

132. Which of the following is related to genetic engineering?
(a) heterosis (b) plastid
(c) mutation (d) plasmid.

133. Which part of the world has a high density of organisms?
(a) deciduous forests (b) grasslands
(c) tropical rain forests (d) savannah.

134. The maximum biomagnification would be in which of the following in case of aquatic ecosystem?
(a) zooplankton (b) fishes
(c) phytoplankton (d) birds.

135. The book '*Genera plantarum*' was written by
(a) Engler & Prantl (b) Bessey
(c) Bentham & Hooker (d) Hutchinson.

136. Columella is a specialized structure found in the sporangium of
(a) *Spirogyra* (b) *Ulothrix*
(c) *Rhizopus* (d) none of these.

137. A system of classification in which a large number of traits are considered is
(a) natural system (b) artificial system
(c) phylogenetic system
(d) synthetic system.

138. Which of the following is true about bryophytes?
(a) they are thalloid
(b) they posses archegonia
(c) they contain chloroplast
(d) all of these.

139. The endosperm of gymnosperm is
(a) diploid (b) triploid
(c) polyploid (d) haploid.

140. In which of the following would you place the plants having vascular tissue lacking seeds?
(a) pteridophytes (b) algae
(c) gymnosperms (d) bryophytes.

141. In prokaryotes, the genetic material is
(a) linear DNA without histones
(b) linear DNA, with histones
(c) circular DNA without histones
(d) circular DNA with histones.

142. Bryophytes have
(a) dominant phase of gametophyte which produces spores
(b) sporophyte is of longer duration
(c) small sporophyte phase and generally parasitic on gametophyte
(d) dominant phase of sporophyte which is parasitic.

143. The antherozoids of *Funaria* are
(a) multiciliated (b) aciliated
(c) monociliated (d) biciliated.

144. DNA is mainly found in
(a) nucleolus (b) nucleus only
(c) cytoplasm only (d) none of these.

145. Which of the following organ has single membrane?
(a) mitochondria (b) nucleus
(c) spherosomes (d) cell wall.

146. An oxidative phosphorylation is the formation of
(a) ATP in respiration
(b) $NADPH_2$ in respiration
(c) ATP in photosynthesis
(d) $NADPH_2$ in photosynthesis.

147. Lactose is a
(a) polysaccharide (b) disaccharide
(c) monosaccharide (d) none of these.

148. The end products of respiration in plants are
(a) sugar and O_2
(b) H_2O and energy
(c) CO_2, H_2O & energy
(d) starch and O_2.

149. The correct sequence in cell cycle is
(a) G_1-S-G_2-M (b) S-G_1-G_2-M
(c) M-G_1-G_2-S (d) S-M-G_1-G_2.

150. The high energy bonds at ATP are between
(a) C-N (b) C-C
(c) P-P (d) C-O.

151. The proper scientific name of cellobiose is
(a) 4N H_2SO_4-β-D-reductase
(b) 4-O-β-glucopyranosyl-D-glucose
(c) 6 NH_3PO_4-α-D-reductase
(d) 8-O-β-D-glucopyranosyl-D-glucose.

152. Feulgen reaction was developed by Feulgen and Rossenbeck to study
(a) protein (b) DNA
(c) lipid (d) RNA.

153. Chromonemata start associating into bivalent chromosomes during
(a) pachytene (b) zygotene
(c) diplotene (d) leptotene.

154. In meiosis, the centromere divides during
(a) anaphase-I (b) prophase I
(c) anaphase II (d) metaphase I.

155. During interphase, RNA and proteins are synthesized in
(a) G_2 phase
(b) S phase
(c) in both G_1 and G_2 phases
(d) G_1 phase.

156. Kreb's cycle takes place in
(a) chloroplast (b) mitochondria
(c) golgi bodies (d) ribosome.

157. Who got the Nobel Prize on working of enzymes in the year 1978?
(a) R. Misra
(b) W. Arber and D. Nathans
(c) G.G. Khorana
(d) Nass and Nass.

158. Plants life originated earlier than animal life because
(a) they can synthesize their food
(b) plants have simple structure
(c) plants are more in number
(d) none of the above.

159. During denaturation of proteins, which of the following bond is broken?
(a) peptide bonds
(b) H-bonds
(c) hydrophobic bonds
(d) electrostatic bonds.

160. End product of respiration is
(a) citric acid (b) malic acid
(c) pyruvic acid (d) none of these.

Instructions for Q. No. 161 to 180

Directions : Each of the questions given below consists of two statements, an assertions (A) and reason (R). Select the number corresponding to the appropriate response in the answer sheet as follows.

(a) If both assertion and reason are true and the reason is a correct explanation of the assertion
(b) If both assertion and reason are true but the reason is not a correct explanation of the assertion
(c) If the assertion is true, but the reason is false
(d) If both assertion and reason are falses

161. *Assertion (A) :* Photosynthesis is an anabolic process.
Reason (R) : Carbohydrate are used up during this process.

162. *Assertion (A) :* C_4 plants are capable of photosynthesizing under very low CO_2 concentration.
Reason (R) : RuBP carboxylase is present in them.

163. *Assertion (A) :* Vitamin deficiency are not seen in plants.
Reason (R) : Vitamins are essential for growth.

164. *Assertion (A) :* Fungi may be heterotrophic or autotrophic.
Reason (R) : Stored food material in fungi is starch.

165. *Assertion (A) :* Peptidoglycan is found in the cell wall of algae.
Reason (R) : Blue green algae are a group of eukaryotes.

16. *Assertion (A) :* Homozygous dominant individual can be used in a test cross to determine the genotype

of an individual showing the recessive phenotype.
Reason (R) : Test cross is a type of back cross.

167. *Assertion (A)* : Fatty liver syndrome is caused due to tobacco addiction.
Reason (R) : Cirrhosis is a disease of kidney.

168. *Assertion (A)* : Aortic semilunar valves become very weak in rheumatic heart disease.
Reason (R) : Rheumatic heart disease includes angina pectoris and coronary thrombosis.

169. *Assertion (A)* : Increase in substrate concentration increases the rate of reaction.
Reason (R) : This is due to occupation of more active sites by substrate molecules.

170. *Assertion (A)* : Stability of a biotic community is governed mainly by its diversity.
Reason (R) : Stability of biotic community is the absence of fluctuations in the population.

171. *Assertion (A)* : If the tadpoles are kept in water containing the element iodine or a weak solution of iodine it undergoes rapid metamorphosis.
Reason (R) : The process of metamorphosis is controlled and regulated by thyroxine hormone, which affects the growth and differentiation of cells.

172. *Assertion (A)* : Fibrinolysis dissolution of fibrin by fibrinolysin caused by the action of proteolytic enzyme system.
Reason (R) : Proteolytic enzyme system is continuously active in the body, but its action is greatly increased by various stress stimuli.

173. *Assertion (A)* : Hydrostatic pressure in blood forces water and low molecular mass solutes of the glomeruli into the Bowman's capsule.
Reason (R) : Kidneys play a major role in regulating the blood pH.

174. *Assertion (A)* : Oynchophora is a small group of animals with molluscan and arthropod affinities.
Reason (R) : It represents an early stage of evolution of annelids.

175. *Assertion (A)* : Emboly involves the invagination and involution through blotting process by the mesentoblast cells.
Reason (R) : Emboly is exhibited by the formation, elongation and ultimate recession of the primitive streak.

176. *Assertion (A)* : The division of extracellular protoplast is called cytokinesis.
Reason (R) : This division is accomplished either through the formation of cell plate in between the newly formed daughter cell or by means of peripheral furrowing.

177. *Assertion (A)* : Plasma membrane is exceedingly thin and not visible as a separate layer.
Reason (R) : It appears merely as a surface layer of cytoplasm.

178. *Assertion (A)* : Ribosomes are not self-replicating particles.
Reason (R) : Lysosomes are membrane bounded vesicles that contain hydrolytic enzymes.

179. *Assertion (A)* : Increase in the quantity of metabolically active protoplasm, accompanied by an increase in cell number and cell size or both called growth.
Reason (R) : Growth, in plants, is not restricted to any specific regions.

180. *Assertion (A)* : The preparation of r-DNA does not require restriction enzymes.
Reason (R) : Because they are not responsible for cleaving plasmid DNA.

GENERAL KNOWLEDGE

181. International Day Against Drug Abuse and Illicit Trafficking is observed on
(a) June 25 (b) July 26
(c) June 26 (d) Aug 26

182. The author of book "What went wrong" is
(a) Atal Bihari Vajpai (b) Kiran Bedi
(c) Sonia Gandhi (d) Seen Smith

183. Which of the following cricket teams set a new record of 12 successive test wins in December 2000.
(a) South Africa (b) Australia
(c) Pakistan (d) India

184. Name of the leader who was regarded by Mahatma Gandhi as his political guru
(a) Gopal Krishan Gokhale
(b) Lord Irwin (c) Leo Jolstoy
(d) Rabindra Nath Tagore

185. Which metal is also known as quick silver
(a) silver (b) mercury
(c) tin (d) zinc

186. Year 2001 is devoted to
(a) physical health (b) mental health
(c) environment (d) none of these

187. Who among the following made a history by becoming the first batsman to complete 10000 runs in one day cricket
(a) Sunil Gawaskar (b) Allen Border
(c) Sachin Tendulkar (d) Saurav Ganguly

188. Whom does the president of India send his resignation if he wants to quit his office
(a) Chief Justice of India
(b) Prime Minister
(c) Vice President of India
(d) Any of these

189. Bombay high is well known in India for
(a) oil exploration (b) hanging garden
(c) fishing in deep sea
(d) atomic reactor.

190. Which of the following is the oldest dynasty of India
(a) Vardhan (b) Kushan
(c) Maurya (d) Gupta

191. The line demarcating the boundary between India and China is called
(a) Radcliffe line (b) 68th parallel
(c) McMohan line (d) Durand line

192. The Jnanpith award for the year 2000-2001 is awarded to
(a) Ms Indira Goswami
(b) Arundhati Roy
(c) Birendra Kumar Bhattacharya
(d) both (a) and (c)

193. Which of the following in news who refused to accept the Arjun award for life time contribution?
(a) Venkatesh Prasad (b) Baljeet Singh Saini
(c) Milkha Singh (d) S. Vijayalakshmi

194. The National Bureau of Plant Genetics Resources (NBPGR) is in
(a) Lucknow (b) Hyderabad
(c) Mumbai (d) New Delhi

195. Who among the following is a famous flute singer
(a) Ravi Shankar (b) Shiv Kumar Sharma
(c) Jakir Hussain
(d) Hariprasad Chaurasia

196. At the equator, the duration of a day is
(a) 10 hrs (b) 12 hrs
(c) 14 hrs (d) 16 hrs

197. RDX is
(a) an instrument to measure blood pressure
(b) a gene
(c) a chemical used in the manufacture of fertilizers
(d) an explosive

198. When the sun reaches its maximum distance from equator, it is known as
(a) solstice (b) eclipse
(c) equinox (d) sidereal day

199. Heavy alcohol consuming people generally die of
(a) blood cancer (b) cirrhosis
(c) liver or stomach cancer
(d) rigor mortis

200. Which country is to host the first Afro Asian Games in 2001.
(a) Japan (b) India
(c) Egypt (d) South Africa

■■■

Model Test Paper–9

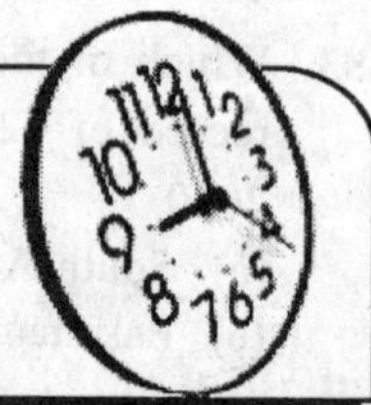

Time : $3\frac{1}{2}$ hours. *Maximum Marks : 200*

PHYSICS

1. The electron in a hydrogen atom makes a transition $n_1 \to n_2$ where n_1 and n_2 are the principal quantum numbers of the two states. Assume the Bohr model to be valid. The time period of the electron in the initial state is eight times that in the final state. What are the possible values of n_1 and n_2 ?
(a) $n_1 = 1, n_2 = 3, n_1 = 2, n_2 = 6$ ...... and so on
(b) $n_1 = 1, n_2 = 2, n_1 = 2, n_2 = 4$ ...... and so on
(c) $n_1 = 2, n_2 = 1, n_1 = 4, n_2 = 2$ ...... and so on
(d) $n_1 = 2, n_2 = 3, n_1 = 3, n_2 = 6$ ...... and so on

2. Two identical bar magnets each of length L and pole strength m are placed at right angles to each other with the north pole of one touching the south pole of the other. Magnetic moment of the system will be
(a) $\frac{mL}{2}$ (b) $\frac{mL}{3}$
(c) $\frac{mL}{\sqrt{2}}$ (d) $(\sqrt{2})\,mL$

3. A concave mirror of focal length 10 cm and a convex mirror of focal length 15 cm are placed facing each other 40 cm apart. A point object is placed between the mirrors, on their common axis and 15 cm from concave mirror. The position of image produced by the successive reflection first on concave mirror then at convex mirror is
(a) 10 cm behind the convex mirror
(b) 6 cm infront of the convex mirror
(c) 6 cm behind the convex mirror
(d) 10 cm infront of the convex mirror

4. A leaky parallel plate capacitor is filled completely with a material having dielectric constant $K = 5$ and electrical conductivity $\sigma = 7.4 \times 10^{-12}\ \Omega^{-1}m^{-1}$. If the charge on the plate at the instant $t = 0$ is $q = 8.85\ \mu C$, then the leakage current at the instant $t = 12$ sec will be
(a) 1.23 μA (b) 0.2μA
(c) 0.1 μA (d) 1.56 μA

5. An AC source of angular frequency ω is fed across a resistor R and a capacitor C in series. The current registered is 1. If now the frequency of the source is changed to $\omega/3$ (but maintaining the same voltage), the current in the circuit is founded to be halved. The ratio of reactance to resistance at the original frequency ω will be
(a) $\sqrt{\frac{5}{7}}$ (b) $\sqrt{\frac{6}{11}}$
(c) $\sqrt{\frac{2}{9}}$ (d) $\sqrt{\frac{3}{5}}$

6. Two guns, situated on the top of a hill of height 10 m, fire one shot each with the same speed $5\sqrt{3}$ m/sec at some interval of time. One gun fired horizontally and other fires upward at an angle of 60° with the horizontal. The shots collide in air at point, the time interval between the firings is
(a) 3 sec (b) 2 sec
(c) 1 sec (d) 4 sec

7. What is increased in a step down transformer?
(a) wattage (b) current
(c) voltage (d) nothing

8. Lines of constant dip are called
(a) isoclinic lines (b) isodynamic lines

(c) isogonic lines (d) isobaric lines

9. An electron and a proton of equal momentum enter a uniform magnetic field normal to the lines of force. If the radii of their paths be r_e and r_p respectively then

(a) $\frac{r_e}{r_p} = \sqrt{\frac{m_p}{m_e}}$ (b) $\frac{r_e}{r_p} = \frac{m_p}{m_e}$

(c) $\frac{r_e}{r_p} = 1$ (d) $\frac{r_e}{r_p}\sqrt{\frac{m_e}{m_p}}$

10. The e.m.f. of a cell is E volt and internal resistance is $r\,\Omega$. The resistance in external circuit is also $r\,\Omega$. The p.d. across the cell will be

(a) $2E$ (b) $\frac{E}{2}$

(c) E (d) $\frac{E}{4}$

11. In an achromatic doublet
(a) convex lens is made of flint glass
(b) concave lens is made of crown glass
(c) convex lens is made of crown glass
(d) both the lenses are made of the same glass

12. The horizontal range of a projectile is $4\sqrt{3}$ times its maximum height. The angle of projector is
(a) 60° (b) 45°
(c) 30° (d) none of these

13. The current gain of a transistor in common base circuit is 0.98. What change in collector current is to be produced in order to produce a change of 5 mA in emitter current ?
(a) 4.9 mA (b) 2.45 mA
(c) 0.196 mA (d) 5.1 mA

14. The binding forces in a metallic crystal are
(a) magnetic forces
(b) Van der Waal forces of attraction
(c) electrostatic forces of attraction
(d) covalent forces

15. The mass of helium nucleus is less than that of its constituent particles by 0.03 amu. The binding energy per nucleon of $_2He^4$ nucleus will be
(a) 3.5 MeV (b) 14 MeV
(c) 7 MeV (d) 21 MeV

16. A radiation worker receives a total dose equivalent of 450 μ S_v during a working week of 30 hour. Calculate the average dose equivalent rate
(a) 15 μ S_v per hour (b) 15 S_v per minute
(c) 45 S_v per second (d) none of these

17. The ratio of the radii of sulphur and helium atoms in the ground state will be
(a) $1 : \sqrt{8}$ (b) 1 : 4
(c) 1 : 8 (d) 1 : 3

18. The energy of a photon is 3×10^{-19} joule. Its momentum is
(a) 10^{-11} kg-m/sec (b) 9×10^{-11} kg-m/sec
(c) 10^{-27} kg-m/sec (d) 3×10^{7} kg-m/sec

19. In Millikan's oil drop experiment, a charged drop of mass 1.8×10^{-14} kg is stationary between the plates. The distance between the plates is 0.90 cm and potential difference between them is 2.0 kV. The number of electrons on the drop is
(a) 5 (b) 50
(c) 500 (d) 0

20. On increasing the length of microscope tube, its magnifying power will
(a) decrease (b) remain unchanged
(c) increase (d) become zero

21. The spectrum of the sun is
(a) line emission and continuous absorption
(b) line emission
(c) line absorption
(d) continuous emission and line absorption

22. A person can not see the objects beyond 50 cm. The power of a lens to correct this vision will be
(a) + 5D (b) – 2D
(c) + 2D (d) 0.5D

23. The frequency from 3×10^9 Hz to 3×10^{10} Hz is
(a) metro high frequency band

(b) super high frequency band
(c) high frequency band
(d) very high frequency band

24. The average power dissipation in a pure capacitor in A.C. circuit is
(a) $2\,CV^2$ (b) zero
(c) $\frac{1}{2}CV^2$ (d) CV^2

25. A metal conductor of length 1m rotates vertically about one of its ends at angular velocity 5 radian per second. If the horizontal component of earth's magnetic field is 0.2×10^{-4} T, the e.m.f. developed between the two ends of the conductor is
(a) 50 mV (b) 5×10^{-4} V
(c) 5 mV (d) 50 μV

26. Research in nuclear and atomic physics caused the invention of
(a) nuclear bombs
(b) generators
(c) motors
(d) hydraulic machines

27. The value of $\frac{d}{dx}(x^2)$ is equal to
(a) $2x$ (b) $\frac{x}{2}$
(c) x (d) x^2

28. The mass and volume of a body are respectively 22.42 g and 4.7 cm³ and the errors in their measurements are 0.01 g and 0.1 cm³. The maximum error in the measurement of density will be
(a) 7% (b) 2.17%
(c) 0.2% (d) 10%

29. A car covers the first half of the distance between two places at a speed of 40 km/h and the other half at 60 km/h. The average speed of the car is
(a) 50 km/h (b) 48 km/h
(c) 40 km/h (d) 60 km/h

30. A helicopter is climbing vertically with a velocity of 15 ms^{-1}, when an object is released from it. If the object hits the ground 4*s* later, the velocity of the object as it hits the ground is
(a) 55 ms^{-1} downwards
(b) 25 ms^{-1} downwards
(c) 0
(d) none of the above

31. The resultant of $\vec{A} \times \vec{0}$ will be equal to
(a) zero vector (b) zero
(c) A (b) unit vector

32. The angle between the two vectors $\vec{A} = 3\hat{i} + 4\hat{j} + 5\hat{k}$ and $\vec{B} = 3\hat{i} + 4\hat{j} - 5\hat{k}$ will be
(a) 90° (b) 45°
(c) zero (d) 180°

33. A rod of mass 5 kilogram is used to push from rest a block of mass 15kg on a frictionless surface. The block moves a distance of 2 metre in 2 second. The net force acting on the stick is
(a) 15 newton
(b) 10 newton
(c) 5 newton
(d) 20 newton

34. When an elevator cabin falls down, the cabin and all the bodies fixed in the cabin are accelerated with respect to
(a) man standing in the cabin
(b) ceiling of the elevator
(c) floor of the elevator
(d) man standing on the earth

35. A particle of mass 4.65×10^{-26} kg moving towards the wall of a vessel with a velocity of 600 m/s. strikes the wall of the vessel at an angle 60° to the normal and rebounds at the same angle at the same speed. Find the impulse of the force received by the wall during the impact
(a) 2.79×10^{-25} newton
(b) 2.79×10^{-23} newton-sec
(c) zero
(d) 4×10^{-20} newton-sec

36. Machine of a constant power makes a body move on a straight path. The distance s travelled in t second is proportional to

(a) $t^{3/2}$ (b) t^3
(c) $t^{1/2}$ (d) t^2

37. The mass of an electron is 9.1×10^{-31} kg. Positron also has the same mass. On meeting they compose a photon by annihilation. What is the energy of photon ? ($c = 3 \times 10^8$ m/s)

(a) 100 eV (b) 10 MeV
(c) 1 keV (d) 1.02 MeV

38. If the value of g at the surface of the earth is 9.8 m/s^2, then the value of g at a place 480 km above the surface of the earth will be (Radius of the earth is 6400 km)

(a) 7.2 m/s^2 (b) 9.8 m/s^2
(c) 8.4 m/s^2 (d) 4.2 m/s^2

39. The intensity of earth's gravitational field at a point situated at a distance of 7400 km from the centre of the earth is 1.5 newton/kg. What is the gravitational potential at the point ?

(a) $+1.11 \times 10^7$ joule kg^{-1}
(b) 5×106 joule kg^{-1}
(c) 10×10^7 joule kg^{-1}
(d) -1.11×10^7 joule kg^{-1}

40. How much of heat is required to heat 2 mole of a monoatomic ideal gas from 0°C to 100°C if no mechanical work is done during heating. The specific heat of gas at constant pressure is 2.5 R, R is the universal gas constant

(a) 378.6 cal (b) 728.2 cal
(c) 592.8 cal (d) 417.1 cal

Instructions for Q. No. 41 to 60

Directions : Each of the questions given below consists of two statements, an assertions (A) and reason (R). Select the number corresponding to the appropriate response in the answer sheet as follows.

(a) If both assertion and reason are true and the reason is a correct explanation of the assertion
(b) If both assertion and reason are true but the reason is not a correct explanation of the assertion
(c) If the assertion is true, but the reason is false
(d) If both assertion and reason are falses

41. *Assertion (A) :* If a convex lens of glass is immersed in water its power decreases.
Reason (R) : In water it behaves as a concave lens.

42. *Assertion (A) :* The power factor in a series resonance circuit is unity.
Reason (R) : In case of series resonance the inductive and capacitive reactances are equal.

43. *Assertion (A) :* When a current is drawn from a cell, there is a fall in potential differences across its terminals.
Reason (R) : Every cell has internal resistance.

44. *Assertion (A) :* Ammeter is always connected in series with a circuit to measure the current flowing through it.
Reason (R) : Ammeter has very low resistance.

45. *Assertion (A) :* During boiling, if an amount dQ of heat is absorbed, pdV is the work done by the system, then $dQ = pdV$
Reason (R) : Boiling is an isothermal process, So $dU = 0$ in equation $dQ = dU + pdV$, which is based on first law of thermodynamics.

46. *Assertion (A) :* When one mole of an ideal gas expands under adiabatic condition so that its state changes from (P_1, V_1, T_1) to (P_2, V_2, T_2), the work done by the gas is given by $\Delta W = C_v (T_1 - T_2)$.
Reason (R) : During adiabatic expansion $\Delta Q = 0$ and $\Delta U = C_v(T_2 - T_1)$ in the expression $\Delta Q = \Delta U + \Delta W$.

47. *Assertion (A) :* A beam of light which emerges from a convex lens must be convergent.
Reason (R) : A convex lens is a converging lens while a concave lens is diverging lens, whatever may be the medium in which they are placed.

48. *Assertion (A) :* When light passes from one medium to another of different density the only quantity which is unchanged is its wavelength.
Reason (R) : The wavelength of light is not related to the refractive index of the medium.

49. *Assertion (A) :* α-particles produce more intense ionization than β-particles.
Reason (R) : α-particles are positively charged.

50. *Assertion (A)* : Lightning conductors protect buildings from damage.
Reason (R) : These send off the charge to earth.

51. *Assertion (A)* : Two bodies of unequal masses dropped from the same height hit the ground with equal kinetic energies.
Reason (R) : The force gravity acting on them are equal.

52. *Assertion (A)* : If the law of gravitation becomes inverse cubelaw even then a line joining the Sun and the planet sweeps equal areas in equal time intervals.
Reason (R) : A planet moves in an elliptical path.

53. *Assertion (A)* : A telescopic objective is rendered achromatic by cementing a convex lens of crown glass and a concave lens of flint glass.
Reason (R) : A convex lens produces greater chromatic aberration than a concave lens.

54. *Assertion (A)* : A solid floats in a liquid so that it is just submerged. When the liquid is heated the solid sinks to the bottom.
Reason (R) : Weight of the solid increases with the rise in temperature.

55. *Assertion (A)* : The resistance of a platinum wire increases as temperature is raised.
Reason (R) : This is because the length of the wire increases as the temperature is raised.

56. *Assertion (A)* : When a dielectric medium is filled between the plates of a condenser, its capacitance increases.
Reason (R) : The dielectric medium reduces the potential difference between the plates of the condenser.

57. *Assertion (A)* : A thin polythene bag weighs the same when empty and when filled with air at atmospheric pressure.
Reason (R) : Air is weightless.

58. *Assertion (A)* : A balloon stops rising after attaining a certain maximum height.
Reason (R) : Upthrust due to air decreases with height till it just balances the weight of the balloon.

59. *Assertion (A)* : In series A.C. circuit, the voltage across the combination of capacitor and inductor is zero at resonance.
Reason (R) : At series resonance the current in the circuit is zero.

60. *Assertion (A)* : It is necessary to use artificial satellite for long distance TV transmission.
Reason (R) : Ionospheric disturbances are minimised by satellite communication.

CHEMISTRY

61. The radius of the nucleus is related to the mass number A by
(a) $R = R_0A^2$ (b) $R = R_0A$
(c) $R = R_0A^{1/2}$ (d) $R = R_0A^{1/3}$
where $R_0 = 10^{-13}$ cm

62. Which of the following species has the highest ionisation energy ?
(a) Al^+ (b) Mg^+
(c) Li^+ (d) Ne

63. As per the modern periodic law the physical and chemical properties of elements are periodic function of their
(a) atomic weight
(b) electronic configuration
(c) atomic volume
(d) atomic size

64. The pH of a solution is increased from 3 to 6. Its H^+ ion concentration will be
(a) reduced by 1000 times
(b) doubled
(c) reduced to half
(d) increased by 1000 times

65. Silver chloride dissolves in excess of NH_4OH. The cation present in this solution is
(a) $[Ag(NH_3)_4]^+$ (b) $[Ag(NH_3)_2]^+$
(c) Ag^+ (d) $[Ag(NH_3)_6]^+$

66. Be^{2+} is isoelectronic with
(a) Li^+ (b) Na^+
(c) Mg^{2+} (d) H^+

67. The cell reaction of a cell is
$Mg_{(s)} + Cu^2{}_{(aq)} \rightarrow Cu_{(s)} + Mg^{2+}{}_{(aq)}$
If the standard reduction potentials of Mg and Cu are – 2.37 and + 0.34 V respectively. The EMF of the cell is
(a) + 2.71 V (b) – 2.03 V
(c) + 2.03 V (d) – 2.71 V

68. 4.5 mole each of H_2 and I_2 are heated in a sealed ten litre vessel. At equilibrium 3 mole of HI were found. The equilibrium constant for

$H_2 + I_2 \rightleftharpoons 2HI$ is

(a) 5 (b) 10
(c) 1 (d) 0.33

69. Mortar is a mixture of
(a) $CaCO_3$ + Silica + H_2O
(b) slaked lime + plaster of paris + H_2O
(c) plaster of paris + silica
(d) slaked lime + silica + H_2O

70. The number of moles of AgCl precipitated when excess of $AgNO_3$ is added to one mole of $[Cr(NH_3)_4Cl_2]Cl$ is
(a) 2.0 (b) 1.0
(c) zero (d) 3.0

71. A mixture contains four solid organic compounds A, B, C and D. On heating only C changes from solid to vapour state. *C* changes from solid to vapour state. C can be separated from rest in the mixture by
(a) fractional distillation
(b) sublimation
(c) distillation (d) crystallisation

72. The homologue of ethyne is
(a) C_3H_8 (b) C_2H_6
(c) C_2H_4 (d) C_3H_6

73. By which of the following reactions can one get N-methyl aniline from aniline ?
(a) benzoylation (b) acetylation
(c) alkylation (d) bromination

74. When an alkyl halides reacts with an alkoxide the product is
(a) ether
(b) unsaturated hydrocarbon
(c) hydrocarbon (d) alcohol

75. Acetaldehyde when treated with dilute NaOH gives
(a) $CH_3CH(OH)—CH_2—CHO$
(b) CH_3COOH
(c) CH_3CH_2OH
(d) $H_3C—CH_3$

76. C_2H_5CHO and $(CH_3)_2CO$ can be distinguished by testing with
(a) fehling solution (b) hydroxylamine
(c) phenyl hydrazine (d) sodium bisulphite

77. Silica is soluble in
(a) H_2SO_4 (b) HNO_3
(c) HCl (d) HF

78. The IUPAC name of

$CH_3—C(Cl)=C(CH_3)—CH(C_2H_5)—CH_2—C\equiv CH$

is
(a) 2-chloro-4-ethyl-3-methyl-hept-2-en-6-yne
(b) 6-chloro-4-ethyl-5-methyl-hept-1-yn-5-ene
(c) 6-chloro-4-ethyl-5-methyl-hept-5en-1-yne
(d) 2-chloro-4-ethyl-3-methyl-hept-6-yn-2-ene

79. Gammexane is
(a) chloral
(b) benzene hexachloride
(c) DDT
(d) hexachloro ethane

80. The ability of an ion to bring about coagulation of a given colloid depends upon
(a) magnitude of its charge
(b) sign of its charge alone
(c) its size
(d) both magnitude and sign of its charge

81. The compound obtained by heating a mixture of a primary amine and chloroform with ethanoic potassium hydroxide (KOH) is
(a) an amide
(b) an alkyl halide
(c) an alkyl isocyanide
(d) an amide and nitro compound

82. The function of enzymes in the living system is to
(a) catalyse biochemical reactions
(b) provide immunity
(c) transport oxygen
(d) provide energy

83. ${}_{92}U^{235} + {}_0n^1 \longrightarrow$ Fission products + Neutron + 3.20×10^{-11} J. The energy released, when 1 gram of ${}_{92}U^{235}$ finally undergoes fission is
(a) 8.21×10^5 kJ (b) 18.60×10^9 kJ
(c) 12.75×10^8 kJ (d) 6.55×10^6 kJ

84. Which one of the following is used to make 'non stick' cookware ?
(a) polyethylene terephthalate
(b) polystyrene
(c) PVC
(d) polytetrafluoroethene

85. Number of water molecules in Mohr's salt is
(a) 5 (b) 6
(c) 7 (d) 8

86. The poisonous gas that comes out with petrol burning in a car is
(a) CO_2 (b) C_2H_6
(c) CH_4 (d) CO

87. Philosopher's wool when heated with BaO at 1100°C gives a compound. Identify the compound
(a) $BaCdO_2$ (b) $Ba + ZnO_2$
(c) $BaZnO_2$ (d) $BaO_2 + Zn$

88. The lanthanide contraction is responsible for the fact that
(a) Zr and Hf have about the same radius
(b) Zr and Nb have similar oxidation state
(c) Zr and Y have about the same radius
(d) Zr and Zn have same oxidation state

89. Which of the following 0.1 m aqueous solutions will have the lowest f.p. ?
(a) KI (b) $C_5H_{10}O_5$
(c) $Al_2(SO_4)_3$ (d) $C_{12}H_{22}O_{11}$

90. Which of the following is redox reaction ?
(a) nitrogen oxides from nitrogen and oxygen by lightning
(b) in atmosphere, O_3 from O_2 by lightning
(c) H_2SO_4 with NaOH
(d) evaporation of water

91. In a reaction

$$CH_2=CH_2 \xrightarrow[\text{acid}]{\text{Hypochlorous}} M \xrightarrow{R} \begin{array}{c} CH_2OH \\ | \\ CH_2OH \end{array}$$

M = Molecule, R = Reagent, M and R are
(a) CH_3CH_2OH and HCl
(b) CH_2Cl-CH_2OH and aq. $NaHCO_3$
(c) CH_3CH_2Cl and NaOH
(d) CH_2-CH_2 (with O bridging, epoxide) and heat

92. Who developed long form of periodic table ?
(a) Mendeleev (b) Niels Bohr
(c) Lothar Mayer (d) Moseley

93. The product D of the reaction

$$CH_3Cl \xrightarrow{KCN} (A) \xrightarrow{H_2O} (B) \xrightarrow{NH_3} (C) \xrightarrow{\Delta} (D) \text{ is}$$

(a) $HCONH_2$ (b) CH_3CN
(c) $CH_3CH_2NH_2$ (d) CH_3CONH_2

94. The IUPAC name of $K_3[Fe(CN)_6]$
(a) potassium ferrohexacyanate (II)
(b) potassium hexaferrocyanate (III)
(c) potassium ferrocyanide (II)
(d) potassium hexacyanoferrate (III)

95. Among the following compound which have more than one type of hybridisation for carbon atom?
(i) $CH_3-CH_2-CH_2-CH_3$
(ii) $H_3C-CH=CH-CH_3$
(iii) $H_2C=CH-C\equiv CH$
(iv) $H-C\equiv C-H$
(a) (iii) and (iv) (b) (i)
(c) (ii) and (iii) (d) (iv)

96. If the equilibrium constant for the reaction

$2AB \rightleftharpoons A_2 + B_2$ is 49.

What is the value of equilibrium constant for

$$AB \rightleftharpoons \frac{1}{2}A_2 + \frac{1}{2}B_2 \text{ ?}$$

(a) 7 (b) 2401
(c) 49 (d) 0.02

97. The reagent used for converting ethanoic acid to ethanol is
(a) PCl_3 (b) BH_3
(c) $LiAlH_4$ (d) $K_2Cr_2O_7/H^+$

98. Compound A reacts with PCl_5 to get B which on treatment with KCN followed by hydrolysis gave propionic acid. What are A and B respectively?
(a) C_2H_5Cl and $C_2H_5Cl_2$
(b) C_2H_6 and C_2H_5Cl

(c) C_3H_8 and C_3H_7Cl
(d) C_2H_5OH and C_2H_5Cl

99. In Wurtz reaction the reagent used is
(a) Na/dry ether (b) Na/liq. NH_3
(c) Na (d) Na/dry alcohol

100. Which one of the following reactions is an example for calcination process ?
(a) $2ZnS + 3O_2 \rightarrow 2ZnO + 2SO_2$
(b) $2Zn + O_2 \rightarrow 2ZnO$
(c) $2Ag + 2HCl + (O) \rightarrow 2AgCl + H_2O$
(d) $MgCO_3 \rightarrow MgO + CO_2$

Instructions for Q. No. 101 to 120

Directions : Each of the questions given below consists of two statements, an assertions (A) and reason (R). Select the number corresponding to the appropriate response in the answer sheet as follows.

(a) If both assertion and reason are true and the reason is a correct explanation of the assertion
(b) If both assertion and reason are true but the reason is not a correct explanation of the assertion
(c) If the assertion is true, but the reason is false
(d) If both assertion and reason are falses

101. *Assertion (A) :* In case of degenerate orbitals if two electrons with opposite spins are placed in the same orbital, a state of high stability will be obtained.
Reason (R) : The most stable electronic arrangement is one in which there is maximum number of paired electrons in the degenerate set of oi bitals.

102. *Assertion (A) :* In transition elements *ns* orbital is filled up first and $(n-1)d$ afterwards, during ionization *ns* electrons are lost prior to $(n-1)$ d electrons.
Reason (R) : The effective nuclear charge felt by $(n-1)d$ electrons is higher as compared to that by *ns* electrons.

103. *Assertion (A) :* The carbonic acid is stronger acid than phenol.
Reason (R) : The hybrid of bicarbonate ion has two equivalent contributing structures, while hybrid of phenoxide ion does not contain such equivalent contributing structures.

104. *Assertion (A) :* Water has greater dipole-dipole attraction than hydrogen sulphide.
Reason (R) : Oxygen has higher electronegativity than sulphur.

105. *Assertion (A) :* When 20 ml of ethanol is mixed with 20 ml of water, the volume of resulting solution will be less that 40 ml.
Reason (R) : They hydrogen bond between water and alcohol molecules is weaker than hydrogen bond between the like molecules.

106. *Assertion (A) :* Ortho-nitrophenol has much lower boiling point and lower solubility in water than meta and para isomers.
Reason (R) : Ortho-nitrophenol involves intramolecular hydrogen bonding and the possibility of association of the molecules is absent.

107. *Assertion (A) :* All molecules which have polar bonds have zero dipole moment.
Reason (R) : Asymmetrical molecules with polar bonds have zero dipole moment.

108. *Assertion (A) :* In the covalent compounds of hydrogen, the hydrogen atom has the electronic configuration analogous to that of hydride ion.
Reason (R) : Hydride ion is formed when hydrogen atom loses an electron.

109. *Assertion (A) :* The bond order of helium is always zero.
Reason (R) : The number of electrons in bonding molecular orbital and antibonding molecular orbital is equal

110. *Assertion (A) :* The H—N—H bond angle in NH_3 molecule is much greater than the H—As—H bond angle in AsH_3.
Reason (R) : Formation of NH_3 molecule involves sp^3 hybridisation, while no hybridisation occurs in AsH_3.

111. *Assertion (A) :* Cyclobutane is less stable than cyclopentane.
Reason (R) : The presence of bent bonds causes loss of orbital overlap.

112. *Assertion (A) :* A spectral line will be seen for the transition *2px* to *2py*.
Reason (R) : Energy is released in the form of

wave of light when the electron drops from *2px* to *2py* orbital.

113. *Assertion (A) :* Sodium ions are discharged in preference of hydrogen ions at mercury cathode.
Reason (R) : The nature of the cathode affects the order of discharge of ions.

114. *Assertion (A) :* Among halogens fluorine can oxidise an element to its highest oxidation state.
Reason (R) : Due to small size of fluoride ion it is difficult to oxidise fluoride ion to fluorine. Hence reverse reaction takes place more easily.

115. *Assertion (A) :* A triester of glycerol and palmitic acid on boiling with aqueous sodium hydroxide gives a solid cake having soapy touch.
Reason (R) : Free glycerol is liberated which is a greasy solid.

116. *Assertion (A) :* When an atom in group 1A of the periodic table undergoes radioactive decay by emitting a positron, the resulting element belongs to zero group.
Reason (R) : When an atom emits a positron, its atomic number increases by one unit.

117. *Assertion (A) :* A certain element X, forms three binary compounds with chlorine containing 59.68%, 68.95% and 74.75% chlorine respectively. These data illustrate the law of multiple proportions.
Reason (R) : According to law of multiple proportions, the relative amounts of an element combining with some fixed amount of a second element in a series of compounds are the ratios of small whole numbers.

118. *Assertion (A) :* The name butanol is not specific, whereas the name butanone represents one specific compound.
Reason (R) : Alcohols show phenomenon of isomerism where as ketones do not show isomerism.

119. *Assertion (A) :* Alkenes and cycloalkanes series of hydrocarbons have same general formula.
Reason (R) : Either insertion of a double bond or formation of a ring reduce the number of hydrogen atoms of corresponding alkane by 2.

120. *Assertion (A) :* The carbon atoms of the benzene ring may be numbered for identification of substituent groups, just as a continuous chains of carbon atoms are numbered.
Reason (R) : Smallest set of numbers designating the substituents is the preferred set.

BIOLOGY

121. Pollination by snail and slug is known as
(a) ornithophilous (b) chiropterophilous
(c) entomophilous (d) malacophilous

122. Single filament of *Nostoc* without mucilage sheath is known as
(a) mycelium (b) colony
(c) trichome (d) hyphae

123. Which of the following is dissolved in water for making Bordeaux mixture?
(a) calcium chloride (b) copper sulphate
(c) sodium chloride (d) none of these

124. Phytotron is a device by which
(a) mutations are produced in plants
(b) plants are grown in controlled environment
(c) protons are liberated
(d) leaf fall occurs on abscission layer

125. Middle piece of a mammalian sperm contains
(a) nucleus (b) centriole
(c) mitochondria (d) vacuole

126. Antiserum contain
(a) antigens (b) leucocytes
(c) antibodies (d) none of these

127. Mechanism of uric acid excretion, in a nephron, is
(a) osmosis (b) diffusion
(c) secretion (d) ultrafiltration

128. Secretion of which of the following is under neurosecretory nerve axons ?
(a) pineal
(b) adrenal cortex
(c) anterior pituitary (d) posterior pituitary.

129. Galapagos islands are associated with the name of
(a) Wallace (b) Malthus
(c) Darwin (d) Lamarck

130. Malathion, parathion belong to group of
(a) triazines
(b) carbamates
(c) pyrethenoids
(d) organophosphates

131. In sweet peas, genes C and P are necessary for colour in flowers. The flowers are white in the absence of either or both the genes. What will be the percentage of coloured flowers in the offspring of the cross Ccpp × ccPp?
(a) 25% (b) 50%
(c) 75% (d) 100%

132. The plants in desert, in order to tolerate water stress, have
(a) no stomata
(b) long root system to reach the water level
(c) stipular spines
(d) stems which are converted into leaf type

133. Positive pollution of soil is due to
(a) reduction in soil productivity
(b) addition of wastes on soil
(c) excessive use of fertilizers
(d) all of these

134. The lining of bone marrow cavity is called
(a) endosteum (b) endomyosium
(c) endoneurium (d) endothelium

135. Which of the following is an example of sex-linked inheritance ?
(a) anaemia (b) cretinism
(c) night-blindness (d) colour-blindness

136. If the rate of addition of new members increases with respect to the individual host of the same population, then the graph obtained has
(a) declined growth
(b) exponential growth
(c) zero population growth
(d) none of these

137. Plants which can withstand wide range of temperature tolerance are called
(a) stenothermic
(b) eurythermic
(c) monothermic
(d) mesothermic

138. Starch and cellulose are the compounds of many units of
(a) glycerol (b) fatty acids
(c) amino acids (d) simple sugars

139. Which of the following is most convincing reasons for increasing population growth in a country?
(a) high birth rate (b) low mortality rate
(c) low population of old people
(d) high population of young children

140. Where does the conversion of harmful prussic acid into potassium sulphocyanide takes place?
(a) spleen (b) liver
(c) bone marrow (d) lymph glands

141. Knock-knee disease is due to
(a) hormonal imbalance
(b) genetical abnormality in males
(c) deficiency in tyrosine amino acid
(d) excess fluoride concentration in water body

142. In mammals, the digestion of starch starts from
(a) mouth (b) stomach
(c) oesophagus (d) duodenum

143. The major constituent of vertebrate bone is
(a) sodium chloride
(b) calcium phosphate
(c) potassium hydroxide
(d) calcium carbonate

144. The amphids are cuticular elevations on the ventro-lateral lips of *Ascaris*. These are
(a) chemoreceptors
(b) tangoreceptors
(c) tactoreceptors
(d) olfactoreceptors

145. Polyploidy leads to rapid formation of new species, because of
(a) genetic recombination
(b) mutation therapy
(c) isolation behaviour
(d) development of multiple sets of chromosomes

146. During interphase, RNAs and proteins are synthesized in
(a) G_1-phase (b) S-phase
(c) G_2-phase (d) all of these

147. Photosynthetic pigments in chloroplast are embedded in the membrane of
(a) matrix (b) photoglobin
(c) thylakoids (d) chloroplast envelope

148. Bulliform cells are present in
(a) mesophyll (b) epidermis
(c) bundle sheath (d) vascular bundles

149. Preganglionic sympathetic fibres are
(a) adrenergic (b) cholinergic
(c) synergic (d) hypergognic

150. Enzymes with two sites are called
(a) apoenzyme (b) holoenzyme
(c) allosteric enzyme (d) conjugate enzyme

151. Meroblastic cleavage refers to which type of division of eggs ?
(a) total (b) spiral
(c) incomplete (d) horizontal

152. Glycosidic bond is broken during the digestion of
(a) protein (b) starch
(c) lipid (d) all of these

153. The presence of continuous phenotypic variation in an F_1-generation suggests that a character is inherited by
(a) epistasis
(b) recombination
(c) gene linkage
(d) polygenic inheritance

154. 'Genera Plantarum' was written by
(a) Bessey
(b) Linnaeus
(c) Hutchinson
(d) Bentham and Hooker

155. Zonula adherens is a kind of
(a) desmosome (b) mesosome
(c) filament (d) membrane

156. Schuffner's dots are seen in red blood corpuscles of man due to which of the following disease ?
(a) kala-azar (b) filaria
(c) malaria (d) diabetes

157. In *Selaginella*, reduction division occurs during the formation of
(a) sperms (b) microspores only
(c) megaspores only (d) both (b) and (c).

158. The process of the escape of liquid from the tip of uninjured leaf is called
(a) guttation (b) transpiration
(c) evaporation (d) evapo-transpiration.

159. Diabetes insipidus occurs due to hyposecretion of
(a) oxytocin (b) vasopressin
(c) thymosine (d) insulin

160. Which of the following RNAs picks up specific amino acid from amino acid pool in the cytoplasm to ribosome during protein synthesis ?
(a) *t*-RNA (b) *m*-RNA
(c) *r*-RNA (d) all of these

Instructions for Q. No. 161 to 180

Directions : Each of the questions given below consists of two statements, an assertions (A) and reason (R). Select the number corresponding to the appropriate response in the answer sheet as follows.

(a) If both assertion and reason are true and the reason is a correct explanation of the assertion
(b) If both assertion and reason are true but the reason is not a correct explanation of the assertion
(c) If the assertion is true, but the reason is false
(d) If both assertion and reason are falses

161. *Assertion (A) :* Smoke reduces photosynthesis.
Reason (R) : Smoke contains SO_2 and oxides of nitrogen and hydrocarbons.

162. *Assertion (A) :* Putrefying bacteria decompose proteins of dead plants and animals to ammonia.
Reason (R) : Nitrosomonas and *Nitrobacter* perform the process of ammonification.

163. *Assertion (A) :* A tree growing near Bombay does not show prominent annual rings.
Reason (R) : Annual rings are not seen in dicot root though secondary growth occur in them.

164. *Assertion (A) :* Long day plants and short day plants are misnomers.
Reason (R) : Short day plant and long day plant growing in same location could not flower on the same day.

165. *Assertion (A) :* Blue and red both the lights are used directly for light reactions of photosynthesis.
Reason (R) : The absorption spectrum represents the graph plotted between the amount of CO_2 consumed and different wavelength of light absorbed by the same pigment.

166. *Assertion (A) :* Carbohydrates are more suitable to provide energy in the body than fat and proteins.
Reason (R) : Wheat and rice are the source of carbohydrates.

167. *Assertion (A) :* Oxygen enters the blood from alveolar air while carbon dioxide leaves the blood to enter the alveolar air.
Reason (R) : This is due to difference in the partial pressure of the gases.

168. *Assertion (A) :* Pulse can be feel on veins in each heart beat.
Reason (R) : Veins are deeply seated in the body.

169. *Assertion (A) :* Insulin is an anabolic hormone.
Reason (R) : It affects antagonistic to glucagon.

170. *Assertion (A) :* A man is unable to pass on a sex linked gene to his son.
Reason (R) : Sex linked genes are present on X-chromosome only.

171. *Assertion (A) :* Coenzyme is a non-protein group without which certain enzymes are inactive or incomplete.
Reason (R) : Coenzymes not only provide a point of attachment for the chemical group being transformed but also influence the properties of the group.

172. *Assertion (A) :* Transmission of the nerve impulse across a synapse is accomplished by neurotransmitters.
Reason (R) : Transmission across a synapse usually requires neurotransmitters because there is small space, the synaptic cleft, that separates one neuron from another.

173. *Assertion (A) :* It is the brain, not the sense organs, that interprets the stimulus.
Reason (R) : Sense organs are transducers; they transform the energy of a stimulus to the energy of nerve impulses.

174. *Assertion (A) :* Cartilage (protein matrix) and bone (calcium matrix) are rigid connective tissues.
Reason (R) : Blood is connective tissue in which plasma is the matrix.

175. *Assertion (A) :* Hair cells on the basilar membrane (the organ of Corti) are responsible for hearing.
Reason (R) : Pressure waves, which begin at the oval window, cause the basilar membrane to vibrate so that the cilia of the hair cells touch the tectorial membrane. This causes the hair cells to initiate nerve impulses, which are carried by the auditory nerve to the brain.

176. *Assertion (A) :* The gramineous type of stomata are commonly found in graminae and cyperaceae.
Reason (R) : The gramineous stomata possess guard cells of which the middle portions are much narrower than the ends so that cells appear in surface view like dumpbells.

177. *Assertion (A) :* The innermost distinct layer of the cortex is known as endodermis.
Reason (R) : The cells of endodermis are non-living and characterised by the presence of casparian strips.

178. *Assertion (A) :* Adenine can not pair with cytosine.
Reason (R) : Because there would be two hydrogen atoms near one of the bonding positions and none at the other.

179. *Assertion (A) :* Either megasporophyllous or microsporophyllous leaves occur in gymnosperms.
Reason (R) : The megasporophyllous leaves are small and less developed whereas microsporophyllous leaves are large, scaly and well developed.

180. *Assertion (A) :* Flagella found in green algae are of whiplash type.
Reason (R) : The flagella found in green algae have a smooth surface and are called tinsel or acronematic.

GENERAL KNOWLEDGE

181. Who gave the slogan 'Inquilab Zindabad'
(a) Mahatma Gandhi
(b) S.C.Bose
(c) Shaheed Bhagat Singh
(d) Lok Manya Tilak

182. Name the website which broke the cricket match fixing story earlier this year?
(a) bazee.com (b) tehelka.com
(c) tazaakhabar.com (d) goforcricket.com

183. 'Sati' was abolished by
(a) Lord William Bentinck
(b) Lord Cavin
(c) Lord Mountbatten
(d) none of these

184. The Kaziranga Wild Life Sanctuary is reserved for which animal
(a) great Indian bustard
(b) rhinoceros
(c) white elephants
(d) white tiger

185. The first feature film (talkie) to be produced in India was
(a) Hatimtai (b) Alam Ara
(c) Pundalik (d) Harish Chandra

186. The first writer to use Urdu as the medium of poetic expression was
(a) Amir Khusru (b) Mirza Ghalib
(c) Faiz (d) Bahadur Shah Zafar

187. Name the director of Indian origin who has become a celebrity after his film. The 'Sixth Sense' became a hit?
(a) Mira Nair (b) Shabana Azmi
(c) Girish Karnad (d) Manoj Shyamalan

188. The Alamatti dam is on the river
(a) godavari (b) krishna
(c) mahanadi (d) cauvery

189. Which one of the following dances involves solo performance
(a) bharatnatyam (b) kuchipudi
(c) mohiniattam (d) odissi

190. Tricolour was adopted as the National Flag in the
(a) Lahore congress
(b) Belgaum congress
(c) Allahabad congress
(d) Haripura congress

191. Which two states has a common High Court?
(a) Himachal Pradesh and Uttar Pradesh
(b) Haryana and Punjab
(c) Gujarat and Maharashtra
(d) Kerala and Tamil Nadu

192. Who is called the father of white revolution?
(a) Dr. Kurien Verghese
(b) Manjunda Swamy
(c) M.S.Swaminathan
(d) U.K.Rao

193. Which state has the highest number of illiterates in India?
(a) Bihar (b) Andhra Pradesh
(c) Orissa (d) Uttar Pradesh

194. The soil group which covers the largest area in India is the
(a) alluvial soil (b) black soil
(c) red soil (d) laterite soil

195. Teacher's day is celebrated in memory of
(a) Nehru (b) Rajaji
(c) Dr. Radhakrishnan (d) Kamaraj

196. The incidence of collapse of World Trade Tower took place on
(a) 11 September (b) 11 October
(c) 13 May (d) 13 September

197. The head of all the three defence field is
(a) Admiral (b) Air Chief Marshell
(c) General (d) President

198. The variety of coffee largely grown in India is
(a) old chicks (b) coorgs
(c) Arabica (d) kents

199. An atomic pile is used for
(a) producing X-rays
(b) conducting nuclear fission
(c) conducting thermonuclear fusion
(d) accelerating atoms

200. Who amongst the following won the Nobel Prize at least twice
(a) Winston Churchill (b) Octavio Paz
(c) Madame Curie (d) George Choupak

■■■

Model Test Paper–10

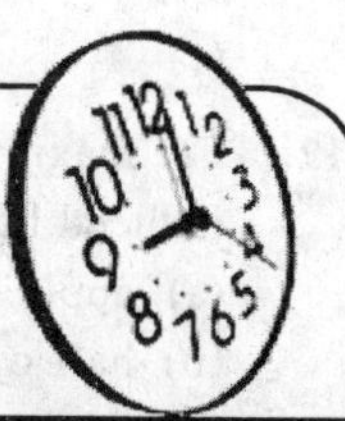

Time : $3\frac{1}{2}$ hours. *Maximum Marks : 200*

PHYSICS

1. Density of nuclear matter varies with A as
(a) $d \propto A^3$ (b) $d \propto A$
(c) $d \propto A^2$ (d) $d \propto A^0$

2. The unit of luminous intensity is
(a) watt (b) candle power
(c) photon (d) candela

3. For a transistor, the current amplification factor is 0.8. The transistor is connected in C.E. configuration. The change in the collector current when the base current changes by 6 mA is
(a) 4.8 m A (b) 2.8 m A
(c) 6.8 m A (d) 5.8 m A

4. If I_1 and I_2 be the currents in a diode under space charge limited conditions for the plate voltages of 400 volt and 200 volt respectively, then the ratio $\frac{I_1}{I_2}$ will be equal to
(a) $2\sqrt{2}$ (b) $\sqrt{2}$
(c) 2 (d) $\frac{1}{2}$

5. A double convex lens of focal length 20 cm is made of glass of refractive index $\frac{2}{3}$. When placed completely in water $\left({}_a\mu_w, \frac{4}{3}\right)$, its focal length will be
(a) 80 cm (b) 17.7 cm
(c) 15 cm (d) 22.5 cm

6. The K.E. of the electron is E when the incident wavelength is λ. To increase the K.E. of the electron to 2 E, the incident wavelength must be
(a) $\frac{h\lambda}{E\lambda - hc}$ (b) $\frac{h\lambda}{E\lambda + hc}$
(c) $\frac{hc\lambda}{E\lambda + hc}$ (d) $\frac{hc\lambda}{E\lambda - hc}$

7. The focal lengths of objective and the eye-piece of a compound microscope are f_o and f_e respectively. Then
(a) $f_o > f_e$ (b) $f_o = f_e$
(c) $f_o < f_e$ (d) None

8. A plane mirror is approaching you at 10 cm per second. You can see your image in it. At what speed will your image approach you
(a) 10 cm/sec (b) 20 cm/sec
(c) 5 cm/sec (d) 15 cm/sec

9. In Millikan's oil drop experiment an oil drop of radius r and charge q is held in equilibrium when the applied potential is V. If the radius of the drop is 2 r for the same charge then the potential required to keep it in equilibrium will be
(a) V (b) $4V$
(c) $2V$ (d) $8V$

10. When two tuning forks A and B are sounded together x beats/s are heard. Frequency of A is n. Now when one prong of fork B is loaded with a little wax, the number of beats/s decrease. The frequency of fork B is:
(a) $n + x$ (b) $n - x^2$
(c) $n - x$ (d) $n - 2x$

11. A resistor R, an inductor L, a capacitor C and ammeters A_1, A_2, A_3 and A_4 are connected to an oscillator in the circuit shown in the figure. When the frequency of the oscillator is increased, that at resonant frequency, the reading of ammeter A_4 is same as that of

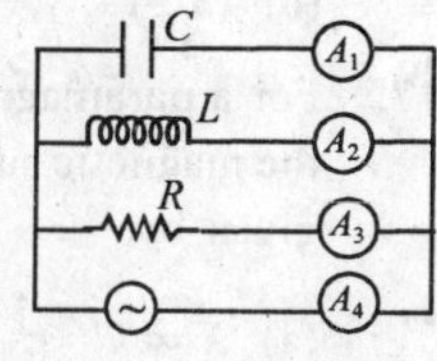

(a) A_1 (b) A_3

(c) A_2 (d) A_1, A_2 and A_3

12. For maximum output power in D.C. motor, the induced back e.m.f. (E) should be
(a) applied voltage
(b) half of applied voltage
(c) double of applied voltage
(d) one third of applied voltage

13. A cylinder of radius R made of a material of thermal conductivity K_1 is surrounded by a cylindrical shell of inner radius R and outer radius $2R$ made of a material of thermal conductivity K_2. The two ends of the combined system are maintained at two different temperatures. There is no loss of heat across the cylindrical surface and the system is in steady state. The effective thermal conductivity of the system is:
(a) $K_1 + K_2$ (b) $\frac{K_1K_2}{K_1+K_2}$
(c) $\frac{K_1+3K_2}{4}$ (d) $\frac{3K_1+K_2}{4}$

14. A step up transformer operates on a 230 volt line and supplies to a load 2 amp. The ratio of primary to secondary windings is 1 : 25. Determine the primary current.
(a) 12.5 amp (b) 8.8 amp
(c) 50 amp (d) 25 amp

15. Susceptibility has the unit of
(a) tesla (b) am^{-2}
(c) am^2 (d) no units

16. When an ideal diatomic gas is heated at constant pressure, the fraction of the heat energy supplied which increases the internal energy of the gas is:
(a) (2/5) (b) (3/7)
(c) (3/5) (d) (5/7)

17. For a paramagnetic material, the dependence of the magnetic susceptibility X on the absolute T is given by
(a) $X \propto T$ (b) $X \propto \frac{1}{T}$
(c) $X \propto$ constant × T (d) X = constant

18. The magnetic induction at the centre of a current carrying loop of radius R is proportional to
(a) R (b) R^2
(c) $\frac{1}{R}$ (d) $\frac{1}{R^2}$

19. The door of a working refrigerator inside a room is left open. The correct statement out of the following one is
(a) the room will be cooled slightly
(b) the room will be cooled to the temperature inside the refrigerator
(c) the room will be warmed up gradually
(d) the temperature of the room will remain unaffected

20. A circular coil of wire carries a current. PQ is a part of very long wire carrying a current and passing close to the circular coil. If the directions of currents are those shown in figure. What is the direction of the force acting on PQ?

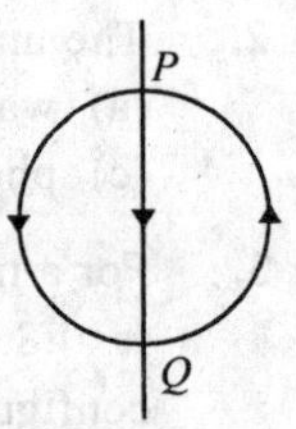

(a) parallel to PQ, towards P.
(b) at right angles to PQ, to the right.
(c) parallel to PQ, towards Q.
(d) at right angles to PQ, to the left.

21. There are n cells each of emf E and internal resistance R connected as shown in figure. A resistance r divided these cells into x and $(n-x)$ cells. The value of current through each cell and through the resistor r is

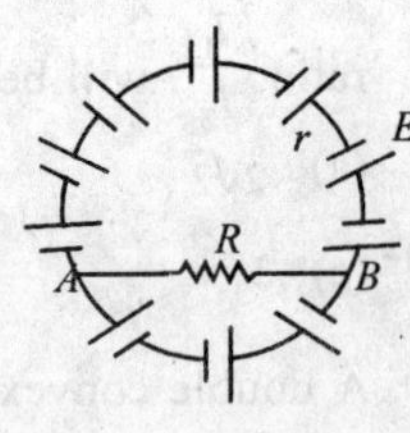

(a) 0, 0 (b) $\frac{E}{R}, \frac{E}{r}$
(c) $\frac{E}{r}, \frac{E}{R}$ (d) $\frac{E}{R}, 0$

22. For an adiabatic expansion of a prefect gas the value of $\Delta P/P$ is equal to:
(a) $\frac{\Delta V}{V}$ (b) $-\gamma\frac{\Delta V}{V}$
(c) $\gamma\frac{\Delta V}{V}$ (d) $-\gamma^2\frac{\Delta V}{V}$

23. An ammeter has a resistance G ohm and a range i ampere. The value of resistance used in parallel, to convert it into an ammeter of range nI ampere is

(a) nG (b) $(n-1)G$

(c) $\frac{G}{n}$ (d) $\frac{G}{n-1}$

24. A wire of resistance R is stretched so that its length increases by 10%. The resistance of the wire increases by

(a) 11% (b) 21%

(c) 15% (d) 28%

25. The freezing point on a thermometer is marked as 20° and the boiling point as 150°. A temperature of 60°C will be ready on this thermometer will be read as:

(a) 40° (b) 65°

(c) 98° (d) 110°

26. You are travelling in a car during a thunder storm. In order to protect yourself from lightning, you would prefer to

(a) remain in the car

(b) get out and lie flat on the ground

(c) take shelter under a tree

(d) touch the nearest electrical pole.

27. The capacitance between the points A, B in the circuit shown is

(a) 20 μ F

(b) 16 μ F

(c) 4 μ F

(d) 18 μ F

(Circuit: 4 μF, 10 μF, 4 μF in series between A and B; 4 μF across upper; 4 μF across lower)

28. Which of the following expression does not represent SHM?

(a) $A \cos \omega t$ (b) $A \sin \omega t + B \cos \omega t$

(c) $A \sin 2\omega t$ (d) $A \sin^2 \omega t$

29. In the given figure, the equivalent resistance between A and B is

(a) 29 Ω

(b) $\frac{17}{24}$ Ω

(c) $\frac{4}{3}$ Ω

(d) $\frac{24}{17}$ Ω

(Circuit: 3 Ω, 4 Ω, 2 Ω, 6 Ω, 8 Ω, 6 Ω between A and B)

30. Two charges 1 μ C each of opposite polarity are separated by 0.2 m. The force acting on another 1 μ C charge placed at the midpoint on the line joining the two charges will be

(a) zero (b) 1.8 N

(c) 0.9 N (d) 2.7 N

31. Which of the following figures represents the motion of a body moving in straight line under constant acceleration:

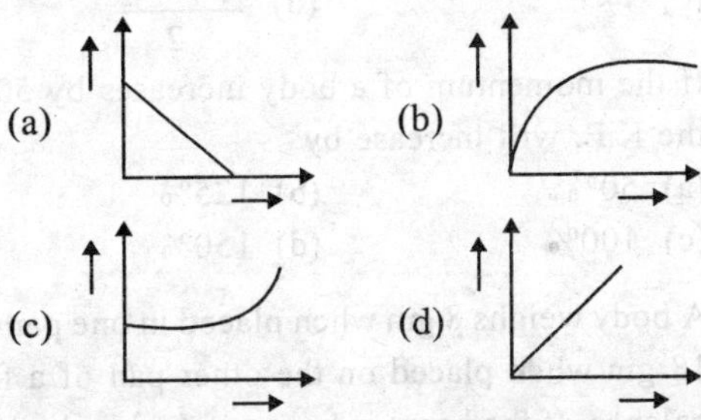

32. A shell is fired from a cannon with a velocity v m/sec at an angle θ with the horizontal direction. At the highest point in its path, it explodes into two pieces of equal masses. One of the pieces retraces its path to the cannon and the speed in m/sec of the other piece immediately after the explosion is

(a) $\frac{\sqrt{3}}{2} v \cos \theta$ (b) $2v \cos \theta$

(c) $3v \cos \theta$ (d) $\frac{3}{2} v \cos \theta$

33. If the density of the earth becomes one half but the radius remains the same, then the value of g on its surface will be

(a) $2g$ (b) $\frac{3g}{2}$

(c) $\frac{g}{2}$ (d) $\frac{g}{4}$

34. The earth's radius is R and acceleration due to gravity at its surface is g. If a body of mass m is sent to a height of $R/5$ from the earth's surface, the PE increases by:

(a) mgh (b) $\frac{5}{6} mgh$

(c) $\frac{4}{5} mgh$ (d) $\frac{6}{7}$ mgh

35. A ladder placed on a smooth floor slips. If at a given instant the velocity with which the ladder is slipping is v_1 and the velocity of that part of ladder which touching the wall is v_2, then the velocity of the centre of the ladder at the instant is

(a) v_1 (b) $\frac{(v_1+v_2)}{2}$

(c) v_2 (d) $\frac{\sqrt{v_1^2+v_2^2}}{2}$

36. If the momentum of a body increases by 50%, the K.E. will increase by

(a) 50% (b) 125%

(c) 100% (d) 150%

37. A body weighs 8 gm when placed in one pan and 18 gm when placed on the other pan of a false balance. If the beam is horizontal when both the pans are empty, the true weight of the body is

(a) 13 gm (b) 15.5 gm

(c) 12 gm (d) 15 gm

38. A stone is thrown at an angle θ with the horizontal such that the horizontal range is equal to the maximum height. The value of tan θ will be

(a) 1 (b) 3

(c) 2 (d) 4

39. The displacement of particle as a function of time is shown in figure. The figure indicates

(a) the particle starts with a certain velocity, but the motion is retarded and finally the particle stops.

(b) the acceleration of the particle is constant throughout

(c) the velocity of particle is constant throughout

(d) the particle starts with constant velocity, the motion is accelerated and finally the particle moves with constant velocity.

40. A block A of mass 2 kg rests on another block B of mass 8 kg which rests on a horizontal floor. The coefficient of friction between A and B is 0.2 while that between B and floor is 0.5. When a horizontal force of 25 N is applied on the block B, the force of friction between A and B is:

(a) Zero (b) 5.0 N

(c) 3.9 N (d) 49 N

Instructions for Q. No. 41 to 60

Each of the questions given below consists of two statements, an assertion (A) and reason (R). Encircle the number corresponding to the appropriate response in the answer sheet as follows.

(a) *If both assertion and reason are true and the reason is a correct explanation of the assertion.*

(b) *If both assertion and reason are true but the reason is not a correct explanation of the assertion.*

(c) *If the assertion is true, but the reason is false.*

(d) *If both assertion and reason are false.*

41. *Assertion :* Germanium is a very good conductor of electricity.

Reason : The number density of free electrons for germanium is 8×10^{28} m^{-3}

42. *Assertion :* Semiconductors devices are easily damaged if they start to overheat.

Reason : At around 100 – 150° C breakdown in semiconductors occurs; there is a sudden fall in resistance, and a huge increase in current.

43. *Assertion :* A metal has resistance.

Reason : When free electrons drift through a metal, they make occasional collisions with the lattice. These collisions are inelastic and transfer energy to the lattice as internal energy.

44. *Assertion :* The conduction properties of a semiconductor can be kept unchanged by doping it with tiny amount of impurities.

Reason : A diode can be made by doping a piece of silicon so that a current in one direction increases its resistance while a current in the opposite direction decreases it.

45. *Assertion :* Heating engineers use *u*-values, rather than *k*-values when calculating heat losses through walls, windows and roofs.

Reason : The *u*-value of a single brick wall is 1.7 Wm^{-2} K^{-1}

46. *Assertion :* Reciprocal of resistivity is called the specific conductance.
Reason : Reciprocal of resistance is called the thermal conductivity.

47. *Assertion :* When some metals are cooled towards absolute zero, a transition temperature is reached at which the resistance suddenly falls to zero.
Reason : Some specially developed metal compounds have transition temperatures above 100 K.

48. *Assertion :* Total current out of a junction is equal to the total current into the junction.
Reason : In a complete circuit, charge is never gained or lost.

49. *Assertion :* Many solids have a molar heat capacity close to 25 J $mol^{-1} K^{-1}$
Reason (: The molar heat capacity is the heat capacity per mole.

50. *Assertion :* Energy levels must have negative values.
Reason : When detached from atom, an electron is at an energy level of zero. When attached, energy is given off and so the energy of electron is below zero and is, therefore, negative.

51. *Assertion :* A body can have acceleration even if its velocity is zero at a given instant of time
Reason : A body is momentarily at rest when it reverses its direction of motion

52. *Assertion :* Frequency of a simple pendulum when taken to moon will be reduced to 1/6 of its value on earth
Reason : The value of g on the moon is 1/6 that on the earth

53. *Assertion :* The dimensions of angular momentum are ML^2T^{-1}
Reason : Angular momentum is equal to the product of moment of inertia and angular velocity

54. *Assertion :* The accumulation of electrons between the anode and the cathode is called the space charge. In the absence of space charge, the potential gradient between cathode and the anode will be uniform
Reason : The space charge, reduces the potential in the cathode and anode region non-uniformly

55. *Assertion :* In electrolysis, the quantity of electricity needed for depositing 1 mole of silver is different from that required for 1 mole of copper
Reason : The molecular weight of silver and copper are different.

56. *Assertion :* An electron and a photon both travelling with same speed enter in a region containing a uniform magnetic field. They trace circles of equal radii but in opposite directions.
Reason : The radii of the circular path traced by a charged particle is independent of the mass of the particle and depends only on the charge and the velocity of the particle.

57. *Assertion :* The phenomenon of pair production is not possible unless the energy of gamma ray photon is equal to or greater than 1.02 MeV.
Reason : The rest mass of an electron is 0.51 MeV.

58. *Assertion :* When light passes from one medium to another of different density the only quantity which is unchanged is its wavelength.
Reason : The wavelength is not related to the refractive index of the medium.

59. *Assertion :* A plane mirror forms a real image when a converging beam of light falls on it.
Reason : When a converging beam is reflected, the angle of reflection is not equal to the angle of incidence.

60. *Assertion :* Light incident normally on the first face of an equilateral glass prism ($\mu = 1.5$) is certain to be totally internally reflected.
Reason : The critical angle for the given glass is less than 60°.

CHEMISTRY

61. What is not true about B_2H_6?
(a) there are two types of H-atoms in the molecule
(b) it has different conformations like C_2H_6
(c) the molecule is electron deficient
(d) both the boron (B) atoms lie in one plane

62. A certain unsaturated hydrocarbon on reductive ozonolysis produces glyoxal and formaldehyde. The hydrocarbon can be

(a) 1, 3-butadiene
(b) mixture of ethyne and ethane
(c) 2-butene (d) ethyne

63. If the solubility product of MOH is 1×10^{-10} mol^2 dm^{-6}, then pH of its aqueous solution will be
(a) 12 (b) 6
(c) 9 (d) 3

64. Which of the following will produce toluene with Zn dust?
(a) picric acid (b) *p*-cresol
(c) benzaldehyde
(d) benzene carbaldehyde

65. Which of the following statement about H_2O_2 is false?
(a) it can act as oxidant as well as reductant
(b) it is a pale blue liquid
(c) the two hydroxyl groups in H_2O_2 lie in same plane
(d) H_2O_2 can be oxidised by ozone

66. Cryoscopic constant is a characteristic feature of
(a) solvent (b) solution
(c) solute (d) none of these

67. The number of π bonds present in acrylonitrile is
(a) 2 (b) 3
(c) 1 (d) 4

68. A substance on treatment with dilute H_2SO_4 gives out a colourless gas which produces turbidity with lime water and also turns potassium dichromate green. The anion present in the substance is
(a) CO_3^{2-} (b) SO_3^{2-}
(c) NO_2^- (d) S^{2-}

69. $CH_3CONH_2 + P_2O_5 \longrightarrow \ldots\ldots$
The organic compound formed in the above reaction is
(a) CH_3COOH (b) CH_3CN
(c) CH_3CHO (d) CH_3NC

70. 4.12 mg of a certain monohydric alcohol produces 1.12 cm^3 of methane at STP on treatment with Grignard's reagent. The molecular mass of the alcohol is
(a) 32 (b) 16
(c) 82.4 (d) 46

71. The reagent used for protection of amino group during the nitration of aniline is
(a) acetic acid (b) PCl_5
(c) acetic anhydride (d) $SOCl_2$/pyridine

72. An organic halide is shaken with aqueous NaOH followed by the addition of dil. HNO_3 and silver nitrate solution gave white ppt. The substance can be
(a) C_6H_5Cl (b) $C_6H_5CH_2Cl$
(c) $C_6H_4(CH_3)Br$ (d) p-$C_6H_4Cl_2$

73. $X \xrightarrow{-\alpha} Y \xrightarrow{-\beta} Z \xrightarrow{-\beta} W$
In the above sequence of reaction, the elements which are isotopes of each other are
(a) X and Z (b) Y and Z
(c) X and W (d) Z and W

74. The compound iso-octane has the formula
(a) C_8H_{16}
(b) $CH_3{\cdot}C(CH_3)_2{\cdot}(CH_2)_3{\cdot}CH_3$
(c) $(CH_3)_2CH{\cdot}(CH_2)C(CH_3)_3$
(d) $C_6H_5(CH_3)_2$

75. Streptomycin is effective in the treatment of
(a) tuberculosis (b) typhoid
(c) malaria (d) cholera

76. The radius of nth orbit for hydrogen is given by the expression
(a) $0.529 \times n$ Å (b) $5.29 \times n^2$ Å
(c) $52.9 \times n^2$ Å (d) $0.529 \times n^2$ Å

77. Ra-226 belongs to distintegration series
(a) $4n$ (b) $4n + 2$
(c) $4n + 1$ (d) $4n + 3$

78. According to VSEPR theory
(a) electron pairs around the central atom in a molecule must remain as far apart as possible
(b) a non-bonding pair of electrons takes up more room on the surface of the atom than a bonding pair
(c) both (a) and (b) are correct
(d) none of these

79. Which of the following is antiseptic dye?
(a) indigo (b) alizarin
(c) gentian violet (d) none of these

80. The difference between 5.0 g and 5.00 g is that
(a) 5.0 has one significant figure while 5.00 has three significant figures
(b) both represent the same quantity
(c) 5.0 has two significant figures while 5.00 has three significant figures
(d) none of these

81. Which one of the following does not contain oxygen?
(a) bauxite (b) dolomite
(c) cryolite (d) zincite

82. Which of the following is the main product of reaction between $RCONH_2$ and Br_2/KOH?
(a) RCH_2NH_2 (b) RCOOH
(c) $R-N=C=O$ (d) RNH_2

83. The name *Aquadag* is associated with
(a) some kind of polymer
(b) colloidal sol of graphite in oil
(c) colloidal sol of graphite in water
(d) none of these

84. Which of the following is expected to be optically active?
(a) $CH_3CH = CH{\cdot}CH_3$
(b) $C_2H_5CH(CH_3)C_3H_7$
(c) $(CH_3)_4C$
(d) $(C_2H_5)_2CH{\cdot}CH_3$

85. Consider the reactions
$C_{(s)} + 2H_{2\,(g)} \rightarrow CH_{4\,(g)}, \quad \Delta H = -x$ kcal
$C_{(g)} + 4H_{(g)} \rightarrow CH_{4\,(g)}, \quad \Delta H = -x_1$ kcal
$CH_{4\,(g)} \rightarrow CH_{3\,(g)} + H_{(g)}, \quad \Delta H = +y$ kcal
The bond energy of C – H bond is
(a) $x/4$ kcal mol^{-1}
(b) $x_1/4$ kcal mol
(c) y kcal mol^{-1}
(d) x_1 kcal mol

86. For which of the following reactions is the equilibrium constant independent of temperature
(a) $N_{2\,(g)} + O_{2\,(g)} \rightleftharpoons 2NO_{(g)}$
(b) $2NO_{2\,(g)} \rightleftharpoons N_2O_{4\,(g)}$
(c) $SO_{2\,(g)} + \frac{1}{2}O_{2\,(g)} \rightleftharpoons SO_{3\,(g)}$
(d) equilibrium constant is never independent of temperature

87. The second ionisation potential of an element M is the energy required to
(a) remove 2 moles of electron from one mole of gaseous atoms
(b) remove one mole of electrons from one mole of any gaseous cation of the element
(c) remove one mole of electron from one mole of gaseous anion
(d) remove one mole of electrons from one mole of unipositive gaseous ion of the element

88. The co-ordination and oxidation number of *X* in the compound $[X(SO_4)(NH_3)_5]Cl$ will be
(a) 10 and 3 (b) 6 and 3
(c) 2 and 6 (d) 6 and 4

89. If bond energies $N\equiv N$, $H-H$ and $N-H$ bonds are 945, 437 and 389 kJ respectively, ΔH for the following gaseous reaction is
$N_2 + 3H_2 \rightarrow 2NH_3$
(a) +1478 kJ (b) –156 kJ
(c) –1478 kJ (d) –78 kJ

90. Which of the following gaseous atoms has highest value of IE_1?
(a) Al (b) Mg
(c) Si (d) P

91. Which of the following is weakest base?
(a) NH_3 (b) $C_6H_5NH_2$
(c) $C_2H_5NH_2$ (d) $(C_2H_5)_2NH$

92. Isopropyl alcohol on oxidation gives
(a) acetone (b) propanoic acid
(c) propene (d) propane

93. Which of the following acids will be able to give silver mirror test?
(a) acetic acid (b) carboxylic acids
(c) butyric acid (d) formic acid

94. Identify the product *B* in the reaction
$CH_3CHO \xrightarrow{CH_3MgI} A \xrightarrow{\text{Hydrolysis}} B$
(a) CH_3OH (b) $(CH_3)_2CHOH$
(c) CH_3CH_2OH (d) $(CH_3)_3COH$

95. The conductivity of an aqueous solution of strong electrolyte
(a) bears no relationship with concentration
(b) remains constant at all concentration

(c) decreases with increases dilution
(d) increases slightly with dilution

96. Which of the following has the highest protective power on lyophobic colloids?
(a) gum arabic (b) albumin
(c) starch (d) gelatin

97. Out of the following hydrogen halides, which one has the highest boiling point?
(a) HI (b) HCl
(c) HBr (d) HF

98. When formaldehyde is heated with ammonia, the compound formed is
(a) methylamine
(b) hexamethylenetetramine
(c) amino formaldehyde
(d) formalin

99. For the transformation $^{14}_{7}N + ? \rightarrow ^{14}_{6}C + ^{1}_{1}H$ bombarding particle is
(a) proton (b) deutron
(c) neutron (d) electron

100. The hybrid state of positively charged carbon in vinyl ($CH_2 = CH^+$) cation is
(a) sp^2 (b) sp^3
(c) sp (d) unpredictable

Instructions for Q. No. 101 to 120

Each of the questions given below consists of two statements, an assertion (A) and reason (R). Encircle the number corresponding to the appropriate response in the answer sheet as follows.
(a) *If both assertion and reason are true and the reason is a correct explanation of the assertion.*
(b) *If both assertion and reason are true but the reason is not a correct explanation of the assertion.*
(c) *If the assertion is true, but the reason is false.*
(d) *If both assertion and reason are false.*

101. *Assertion* : The dipolemoment of CH_3F is greater than that of $CHCl_3$.
Reason : Fluorine has greater electron affinity than that of chlorine.

102. *Assertion* : Stanous chloride ($SnCl_2$) is a non-linear molecule.
Reason : In $SnCl_2$ molecule Sn atom is present in *sp* hybridised state.

103. *Assertion* : The bond angle H—C—H in the methane is the same as the bond angle Cl—C—Cl in the carbon tetrachloride.
Reason : H—C—H bonds in methane are almost non-polar while Cl—C—Cl bonds in carbon tetrachloride are highly polar.

104. *Assertion* : Xenon difluoride is a linear molecule having F—Xe—F bond angle of 180°.
Reason : Formation of XeF_2 molecule takes place by sp^3d hybridization of Xe orbitals.

105. *Assertion* : Molecule which gives rise to fluorescence is referred to as a fluorophore.
Reason : Aromatic amino acids, flavins and vitamin-A are important fluorophores.

106. *Assertion* : When two or more empty orbitals of equal energy are available, one electron must be placed in each until they are all half filled.
Reason : The pairing of electrons is an unfavourable phenomenon.

107. *Assertion* : The combining of atomic orbitals from two atoms is termed as hybridisation.
Reason : The process of hybridisation involves the combination of orbitals of different energies.

108. *Assertion* : The elements belonging to alkali metal group are most electropositive in their respective periods of periodic table.
Reason : The positive charge density on their positive ions is highest in the respective periods.

109. *Assertion* : The atomic mass actually is expressed in terms of atomic mass unit (amu).
Reason : The actual mass of an atom in gms is very small

110. *Assertion* : The atomic mass of carbon atom is expressed as 12.011 amu.
Reason : All carbon atoms have six protons and six neutrons in their nuclei.

111. *Assertion* : The enthalpy of formation of gaseous oxygen molecules at 298 K and under a pressure of one atmosphere is zero.

Reason : The entropy of formation of gaseous oxygen molecules under the same conditions is zero.

112. *Assertion* : A tri-ester of glycerol and palmitic acid on boiling with aqueous NaOH gives a solid cake having soapy touch
Reason : Free glycerol is liberated, which is a greasy solid.

113. *Assertion* : Amongst the halogens, fluorine can oxidise the elements to highest oxidation states
Reason : Due to small size of fluoride ion, it is difficult to oxidise fluoride ion to fluorine. Hence, reverse reaction takes place more easily.

114. *Assertion* : Nitrogen is unreactive at room temperature but becomes reactive at elevated temperatures (on heating) in presence of catalysts
Reason : In nitrogen molecules, there is extensive delocalization of electrons.

115. *Assertion* : Fluorescein is an adsorption indicator
Reason : The indicator fluorescein is a dye

116. *Assertion* : White precipitate of lead chloride ($PbCl_2$) is soluble in concentrated solution of potassium chloride.
Reason : Tetrachloroplumbate (II) ion is formed when chloride ions attacks the lead (II) chloride.

117. *Assertion* : In a given electrical field β-particles are deflected more than α-particles
Reason : β-particles have very low *e/m* value as compared to α-particles.

118. *Assertion* : Neutrons are better projectiles for nuclear reactions than protons or α-particles.
Reason : Neutrons are neutral particles and hence, their penetration in nucleus is rather difficult.

119. *Assertion* : The solubility of n-alcohols in water decreases with increase in molecular weight.
Reason : The relative proportion of the hydrocarbon part in alcohols increases with the increase in molecular weight which permits enhanced hydrogen bonding with water.

120. *Assertion* : The nitro group, if present in ortho or para positions, would stabilise the phenoxide ion by dispersal of negative charge through mesomeric effect.
Reason : The electron releasing substituents would intensity the negative charge. As a result electron releasing groups in phenol should be acid-weakening.

BIOLOGY

121. The umbilical cord in the mammals contain
(a) placenta (b) allantoic artery
(c) umbilicus (d) both (b) and (c)

122. Fraternal twins are
(a) monozygotic (b) siamese
(c) dizygotic (d) both (b) and (c)

123. Which of the following technique is used to measure cerebral blood volume?
(a) PET-scanning (b) ECG
(c) CT-scanning (d) EEG

124. Mark the incorrect statement about immunisation schedule:
(a) one booster dose of tetanus toxoid is given preferably 4 weeks before the expected date of delivery to the female who is immunised previously
(b) two doses of tetanus toxoid, the first dose between 16 and 24 weeks and the second dose between 24 and 32 to non-immunised females.
(c) one dose of tetanus toxoid is given 6 weeks before pregnancy to non immunised females
(d) first DPT dose is given between age of 3-12 months.

125. Following autosomal dominant disease is characterised by very long extremeties, spider like fingers and dislocation of eye lens
(a) Von willebrand's disease
(b) Huntington chorea
(c) Marfan syndrome
(d) Cat-cry syndrome

126. Match the commercial names of following:
(a) propoxur as furadan, carbofuran as temik and aldicarb as baygon
(b) propoxur as baygon, carbofuran as furadan and aldicarb as temik
(c) propoxur as temik, carbofuran as furadan and aldicarb as baygon

(d) propoxur is simazine, carbofuran as furadan and aldicarb as baygon

127. Monoclonal antibodies are effective as
(a) immuno suppressants in renal grafting
(b) immuno repressants in renal grafting
(c) immuno suppressants in cornea transplantation
(d) both (a) and (c)

128. The proper formation of collagen in a healing wound requires
(a) high levels of adrenocortical hormones
(b) cholesterol (c) vitamin C
(d) vitamin D.

129. Diversification of placental mammals took place in:
(a) paleocene (b) eocene
(c) miocene (d) pleistocene

130. Marine life can be classified into three main categories:
(a) plankton, nekton, benthonic
(b) phytoplankton. zooplankton and benthonic
(c) phytoplankton zooplankton and benthonic
(d) plankton, nektons and phytoplankton

131. Amensalism is
(a) an interaction between two living individuals of same species in which one organism does not allow other organism to grow or live near it.
(b) an interaction between two living individuals of different species which allow the growth of both organisms simultaneously.
(c) an interaction between two living individuals of different species in which one organism does not allow other organism to grow or live near it.
(d) it is the relationship between two living individuals of different species in which one is benefitted while the other is neither harmed nor benefitted except to a negligible extent.

132. International Union of Conservation of Nature and Natural Resources (IUCN) describes endangered species as:-
(a) the species which are in danger of extinction and whose survival is unlikely if the causal factors continue to be operating
(b) which are vulnerable and rare
(c) the species with very small populations in the world
(d) all of these

133. Which human chromosome contains the HLA complex?
(a) chromosome 11 (b) chromosome 23
(c) chromosome 48 (d) chromosome 6

134. Tobacco smoke contains radioactive
(a) polonium-210 (b) cesium-138
(c) polonium-220 (d) carbon-14

135. *Neopilina* a living fossil was
(a) discovered in 1952, a connecting link between annelida and mollusc
(b) discovered in 1957, a connecting link between annelida and arthropoda
(c) discovered in 1954, a connecting link between annelida and mollusc
(d) none of these

136. Which of the following is correct about cockroach?
(a) nocturnal, omnivorous, fussorial, protandrous
(b) fossorial, carnivorous, protandrous hermaphrodite
(c) diurnal, omnivorous, fussorial, protandrous
(d) monoecious, omnivorous, diurnal, formation ootheca

137. Amphetamines have been used to treat all of the following disorders except
(a) attention-deficit hyperactivity disorder
(b) mild depression
(c) anorexia nervosa (d) obesity.

138. Which is true about gemmule formation?
(a) it is shown by fresh water sponges under favourable conditions
(b) it is shown by marine and fresh water sponges under favourable conditions
(c) it is shown by marine sponges under unfavourable conditions
(d) it is a feature of fresh water and marine sponges under unfavourable conditions

139. Myocardial infarction is
(a) inadequate flow of blood to a part of the heart caused by obstruction to its blood supply.

(b) death of a part of heart muscle following cessation of blood supply to it.
(c) heart pain of short duration usualy located in front of the chest
(d) hardening of blood vessels.

140. Vitamin B_{12} (cyanocobalamine) deficiency may be produced by
(1) pernicious anemia (2) Crohn's disease
(3) ileal resection (4) chronic pancreatitis
(a) 1 and 2 (b) 2 and 4
(c) 1, 2, 3, 4 (d) none of these.

141. The free part of the soft palate which hangs down freely as a small flap is called
(a) rugae (b) uvula
(c) frenulum (d) sulcus terminalis

142. Stroke volume is increased by
(a) sympathetic stimulation
(b) decreased systematic blood pressure
(c) increased preload
(d) increased heart rate.

143. Mark the correct statement:
(a) *Petromyzon* is marine, unisexual with 8 pairs of cranial nerves
(b) *Petromyzon* is marine and fresh water form unisexual with 12 pairs of cranial nerves
(c) *Myxine* is marine, unisexual
(d) *Petromyzon* is marine and fresh water form, unisexual with 10 pairs of cranial nerves

144. Negative symptoms of Schizophrenia include
(a) hallucination
(b) cognitive deficits
(c) loose associations
(d) strong behaviour.

145. First instar larva of house fly is:
(a) limbless and has one pair of posterior abdominal spiracles
(b) limbless and has one pair of anterior prothoracic and one pair of posterior abdominal spiracles
(c) limbless and has one pair of anterior prothoracic spiracles
(d) having 3 pairs of legs and one pair of posterior abdominal spiracles

146. DNA banking is particularly useful when
(a) a specific disease mutation is known to exist within a family
(b) a child has been shown to have a genetic disease due to a new dominant mutation
(c) the gene for a particular disease in a family has not yet been identified, but its pattern of inheritancen is clear
(d) a family is known to be segregating a balanced robertsonian translocation.

147. Gynandromorphs develop in *Drosophila* when the two cells in the two-celled proembryo will have one of the following chromosomal sets
(a) 2A + XX in one cell and 2A + X in the other
(b) 2A + XXX in both the cells
(c) 2A + X in both the cells
(d) all of these

148. The organism used for alcohol fermentation is
(a) *Pseudomonas* (b) *Aspergillus*
(c) *Penicillium* (d) *Saccharomyces*

149. The twining of tendrils around a support is a good example of
(a) nastic movements (b) phototropism
(c) thigmotropism (d) chemotropism

150. The sexual reproduction is absent in
(a) *Ulothrix* (b) *Spirogyra*
(c) *Volvox* (d) *Nostoc*

151. Which of the following has a cup shaped chloroplast?
(a) *Chlamydomonas* (b) *Spirogyra*
(c) *Pinus* (d) *Funaria*

152. Clinostat is used in studies on
(a) growth movements
(b) respiration
(c) osmosis
(d) photosynthesis

153. The female gametophyte of a typical dicot at the time of fertilization is
(a) 6-celled (b) 7-celled
(c) 8-celled (d) 4-celled

154. Haploid plants (or cells in culture) derived from microspore culture are preferred over diploids for mutation studies, because in haploids
(a) haploid cells can be easily cultured
(b) dominant mutations express immediately
(c) recessive mutations express immediately
(d) mutations are readily induced

155. Mendel studied inheritance for seven pairs of characters in pea. For a study of independent assortment seven characters can be arranged in 21 possible pairs. If you are told that in one of these 21 pairs, independent assortment was not observed in repeated later studies, what would be your reaction?
(a) all the later workers must have committed mistakes
(b) it is impossible
(c) Mendel's principle of independent assortment is not universal
(d) Mendel might not have studies all the 21 combinations

156. When the hilum, chalaza and micropyle of the ovule lie in the same longitudinal axis, it is known as
(a) orthotropous ovule
(b) amphitropous ovule
(c) anatropous ovule
(d) camphylotropous ovule

157. The maximum formation of *m*-RNA occurs in
(a) cytoplasm (b) ribosome
(c) nucleolus (d) nucleoplasm

158. Pyrenoids are the centre of the formation of
(a) starch (b) enzyme
(c) protein (d) fat

159. Haploid plants can be obtained by culturing
(a) young leaves (b) pollen grains
(c) endosperm (d) root lips

160. The floral formula ⊕ ⚥ K_{2+2} C_{x4}, A_{2+4}, $G_{(2)}$ is representative of
(a) *Brassica nigra* (b) *Solanum nigrum*
(c) *Allium cepa* (d) *Helianthus annuus*

Instructions for Q.No. 161 to 180

Each of the questions given below consists of two statements, an assertions (A) and reason (R). Encircle the number corresponding to the appropriate response in the answer sheet as follows.
(a) *If both assertion and reason are true and the reason is a correct explanation of the assertion*
(b) *If both assertion and reason are true but the reason is not a correct explanation of the assertion*
(c) *If the assertion is true, but the reason is false*
(d) *If both assertion and reason are false*

161. *Assertion* : Prophase I is the longest phase in meiosis.
Reason : It is divisible into five sub phases.

162. *Assertion* : Ribosomes occur in both eukaryotes and prokaryotes.
Reason : Organelle ribosomes do not occur in prokaryotes.

163. *Assertion* : Herkogamy promotes self pollination.
Reason : Prepotency is a self sterility technique.

164. *Assertion* : Root cap has no role in water absorption.
Reason : It has no direct relation with vascular system.

165. *Assertion* : Pollination in *Pinus* is anemophilous.
Reason : The pollen grains germinates *in situ.*

166. *Assertion* : DDT is found to be in body water.
Reason : DDT is soluble in water.

167. *Assertion* : The bones of middle ear are primarily responsible for locating the source.
Reason : Middle ear bones are two in number.

168. *Assertion* : Arboviruses are transmitted by animals.
Reason : They have single stranded DNA genome.

169. *Assertion* : Glucose has the lowest renal clearance.
Reason : It is completely reabsorbed.

170. *Assertion* : Notochord is present in protochordate vertebrates.
Reason : Notochord is always formed of bones.

171. *Assertion* : Phaeochromocytoma is a tumour of adernal cortex
Reason : Phaeochromocytoma leads to secondary hypertension

172. *Assertion* : Unit membrane of Robertson's model has a thickness of 75 Å
Reason : Membrane thickness could be 50-100 Å.

173. *Assertion* : Boring of pinna and nose of Indian women is inherited to next generation
Reason : When an individual acquires characters in its life time, they are transmitted to next generation

174. *Assertion* : *Pila* is asymmetrical
Reason : *Pila* shows torsion

175. *Assertion* : Rupture of a cerebral blood vessel may lead to sudden interruption of a blood flow to a portion of brain. This is called cerebrovascular accident.
Reason : Hypertension may cause vasodilation of cerebral blood vessels

176. *Assertion* : Cells of quiscent centre have low DNA, RNA & protein
Reason : It could be the site of hormone synthesis.

177. *Assertion* : Maximum evolution of oxygen of *Spirogyra* is observed in red & blue region
Reason : Blue & red region shows minimum photosynthetic activity

178. *Assertion* : Bacteriochlorophyll-*b* is found in *Rhodopseudomonas*
Reason : It's structure is not yet known.

179. *Assertion* : The bark is economically useful
Reason : The bark of Juglans is used for cleaning and shining teeth

180. *Assertion* : The first link in any food chain is a green plant
Reason : Because they alone have the capacity to fix the CO_2 in presence of sun light.

GENERAL KNOWLEDGE

181. The guardian of the constitution of India is
(a) Indian Parliament
(b) Supreme Court of India
(c) Prime Minister of India
(d) High Court of India.

182. Who is the new Director-General of UNESCO?
(a) Koichiro Matsuura
(b) Fiederico Mayor Zaragoza
(c) Ms. Gro Harlem Brundtland
(d) Thabo Mbeki.

183. With which of the following countries has India recently signed an extradition treaty?
(a) Israel (b) Russia
(c) France (d) UAE.

184. Nasir Hussain is cricket captain of which country?
(a) Bangladesh (b) Kenya
(c) England (d) Scotland.

185. The amount of money (in rupees) allegedly paid as kickbacks in the Bofors case in
(a) Rs. 102 crore (b) Rs. 56 crore
(c) Rs. 64 crore (d) Rs. 75 crore.

186. *Mr. Editor, How Close are You to the PM* is a book authored by
(a) Vinod Mehta (b) N. Ram
(c) Dileep Padgaonkar (d) Prabhu Chawla.

187. According to the Reserve Bank of India's New Credit Policy for the second half of 1999-2000, the Cash Reserve Ratio (CRR) has been reduced from 10 per cent to
(a) 9 per cent (b) 8 per cent
(c) 7 per cent (d) 6 per cent.

188. Name the country where people have voted against a republican form of Government
(a) Britain (b) Australia
(c) Jordan (d) Thailand.

189. WHO's Vision 2020 visualises to eliminate
(a) AIDS (b) hepatitis-C
(c) avoidable blindness
(d) none of these.

190. In which of the following places a baby boy was born as the world's six billionth inhabitant?
(a) Kosovo (b) Vienna
(c) Tokyo (d) Islamabad.

191. Which of the following is/are the Sydney 2000 Olympic mascot(s)?
(a) Millie (the *Echidna*)

(b) Olly (the *Kookaburra*)
(c) Syd (the *Platypus*) (d) all of these.

192. Who among the following is currently the Chairperson of the National Commission for Women?
(a) Hema Malini (b) Vibha Parthasarthy
(c) Abha Sharma (d) Mohini Giri.

193. Which one of the following films was named as the Best feature Film for the 47th National Film Awards announced on July 6, 2000?
(a) Vaanaprastham (Malayalam)
(b) Uttara (Bengali)
(c) Hey Ram (Hindi)
(d) Shaheed Udham Singh (Punjabi).

194. Who among the following won the Wimbledon 2000 Women's Singles title held in July
(a) Serena Williams (b) Venus Williams
(c) Lindsay Davenport (d) Martina Hingis.

195. National Waterway Number 1 will be linking which of the following two cities?
(a) Allahabad - Haldia
(b) Agra - Patna
(c) Cochin - Salem
(d) Dibrugarh - Haldia.

196. Who among the following is the President of International Court of Justice?
(a) Al-Khasawnch (b) Syed Pirzaba
(c) Gilbert Guillaume (d) Don Mckinnon.

197. Who among the following becomes the first and the only star from the Indian Cinema to be waxed at the famous Madame Tussaud's Wax Museum in London?
(a) Dilip Kumar
(b) Shatrughan Sinha
(c) Amitabh Bachchan
(d) Shah Rukh Khan.

198. Who among the following heads the reserach team on the Human Genome Project in Britain?
(a) Dr. Michael Dexter (b) Dr. John Sulston
(c) Dr. Andrew Hynes (d) Dr. John Dexter.

199. Sonal Mansingh is the exponent of which of the following dance forms?
(a) odissi (b) yakshagana
(c) manipuri (d) kuchipudi.

200. The booker prize winner for 2000 Margret Atwood has written which of the following book?
(a) The blind assassin (b) Survival
(c) Life before man (d) all of these.

■■■

ANSWERS

MODEL TEST PAPER - 1

1. (c) 2. (d) 3. (c) 4. (a)
5. (c) 6. (a) 7. (b) 8. (b)
9. (a) 10. (a) 11. (c) 12. (c)
13. (a) 14. (b) 15. (b) 16. (d)
17. (b) 18. (a) 19. (b) 20. (b)
21. (a) 22. (d) 23. (a) 24. (b)
25. (d) 26. (c) 27. (b) 28. (b)
29. (c) 30. (d) 31. (c) 32. (a)
33. (c) 34. (a) 35. (d) 36. (a)
37. (c) 38. (d) 39. (a) 40. (c)
41. (a) 42. (a) 43. (b) 44. (b)
45. (a) 46. (b) 47. (b) 48. (c)
49. (c) 50. (a) 51. (b) 52. (c)
53. (a) 54. (c) 55. (c) 56. (a)
57. (b) 58. (a) 59. (b) 60. (a)
61. (a) 62. (b) 63. (c) 64. (c)
65. (a) 66. (b) 67. (a) 68. (d)
69. (c) 70. (d) 71. (b) 72. (a)
73. (a) 74. (a) 75. (b) 76. (c)
77. (d) 78. (b) 79. (d) 80. (d)
81. (c) 82. (b) 83. (b) 84. (c)
85. (d) 86. (a) 87. (d) 88. (c)
89. (b) 90. (c) 91. (d) 92. (d)
93. (d) 94. (b) 95. (c) 96. (b)
97. (a) 98. (c) 99. (c) 100. (d)
101. (a) 102. (b) 103. (c) 104. (a)
105. (c) 106. (a) 107. (c) 108. (d)
109. (c) 110. (b) 111. (b) 112. (a)
113. (b) 114. (d) 115. (c) 116. (a)
117. (a) 118. (b) 119. (a) 120. (b)
121. (a) 122. (b) 123. (b) 124. (b)
125. (a) 126. (a) 127. (d) 128. (c)
129. (a) 130. (a) 131. (c) 132. (c)
133. (a) 134. (b) 135. (d) 136. (c)
137. (c) 138. (d) 139. (b) 140. (c)
141. (d) 142. (c) 143. (a) 144. (a)
145. (c) 146. (d) 147. (a) 148. (d)
149. (d) 150. (c) 151. (d) 152. (b)
153. (d) 154. (a) 155. (c) 156. (a)
157. (b) 158. (c) 159. (a) 160. (b)
161. (a) 162. (b) 163. (d) 164. (a)
165. (a) 166. (a) 167. (b) 168. (c)
169. (a) 170. (d) 171. (a) 172. (d)
173. (a) 174. (d) 175. (b) 176. (a)
177. (a) 178. (c) 179. (c) 180. (b)
181. (a) 182. (d) 183. (a) 184. (b)
185. (d) 186. (a) 187. (c) 188. (d)
189. (a) 190. (a) 191. (d) 192. (d)
193. (c) 194. (a) 195. (a) 196. (b)
197. (b) 198. (a) 199. (d) 200. (a)

MODEL TEST PAPER - 2

1. (b) 2. (a) 3. (c) 4. (b)
5. (b) 6. (d) 7. (d) 8. (a)
9. (d) 10. (b) 11. (c) 12. (c)
13. (b) 14. (c) 15. (d) 16. (b)
17. (b) 18. (b) 19. (d) 20. (b)
21. (b) 22. (c) 23. (c) 24. (d)
25. (a) 26. (d) 27. (b) 28. (d)
29. (d) 30. (b) 31. (a) 32. (b)
33. (b) 34. (c) 35. (c) 36. (b)
37. (d) 38. (d) 39. (a) 40. (c)
41. (a) 42. (b) 43. (d) 44. (b)
45. (a) 46. (a) 47. (b) 48. (b)
49. (a) 50. (a) 51. (a) 52. (a)
53. (b) 54. (d) 55. (a) 56. (a)
57. (c) 58. (d) 59. (b) 60. (a)
61. (b) 62. (b) 63. (b) 64. (a)
65. (d) 66. (c) 67. (a) 68. (b)
69. (a) 70. (c) 71. (d) 72. (b)
73. (a) 74. (c) 75. (d) 76. (b)
77. (b) 78. (c) 79. (d) 80. (b)
81. (a) 82. (b) 83. (b) 84. (c)
85. (a) 86. (a) 87. (b) 88. (b)
89. (d) 90. (b) 91. (c) 92. (b)
93. (d) 94. (b) 95. (a) 96. (a)
97. (c) 98. (b) 99. (b) 100. (b)
101. (a) 102. (b) 103. (c) 104. (b)
105. (c) 106. (c) 107. (d) 108. (a)
109. (a) 110. (c) 111. (a) 112. (b)
113. (c) 114. (a) 115. (a) 116. (c)
117. (b) 118. (a) 119. (a) 120. (a)
121. (c) 122. (c) 123. (c) 124. (c)
125. (d) 126. (a) 127. (a) 128. (d)
129. (d) 130. (c) 131. (c) 132. (b)
133. (c) 134. (c) 135. (a) 136. (d)
137. (a) 138. (c) 139. (c) 140. (c)
141. (b) 142. (c) 143. (d) 144. (d)
145. (a) 146. (a) 147. (a) 148. (a)
149. (c) 150. (a) 151. (a) 152. (c)
153. (b) 154. (b) 155. (d) 156. (b)
157. (b) 158. (b) 159. (d) 160. (c)
161. (c) 162. (a) 163. (b) 164. (c)
165. (b) 166. (b) 167. (b) 168. (c)
169. (a) 170. (a) 171. (a) 172. (a)
173. (c) 174. (c) 175. (a) 176. (a)
177. (b) 178. (d) 179. (a) 180. (a)

181. (a) 182. (c) 183. (b) 184. (b)
185. (d) 186. (c) 187. (d) 188. (a)
189. (c) 190. (b) 191. (d) 192. (b)
193. (c) 194. (c) 195. (b) 196. (c)
197. (c) 198. (c) 199. (a) 200. (b)

MODEL TEST PAPER - 3

1. (c) 2. (c) 3. (b) 4. (b)
5. (b) 6. (c) 7. (c) 8. (b)
9. (b) 10. (c) 11. (d) 12. (a)
13. (c) 14. (d) 15. (a) 16. (a)
17. (b) 18. (d) 19. (a) 20. (b)
21. (b) 22. (b) 23. (b) 24. (a)
25. (a) 26. (c) 27. (b) 28. (a)
29. (b) 30. (a) 31. (c) 32. (b)
33. (c) 34. (a) 35. (b) 36. (b)
37. (a) 38. (c) 39. (d) 40. (c)
41. (c) 42. (b) 43. (b) 44. (b)
45. (c) 46. (a) 47. (b) 48. (b)
49. (b) 50. (c) 51. (c) 52. (d)
53. (d) 54. (d) 55. (a) 56. (b)
57. (b) 58. (c) 59. (c) 60. (a)
61. (a) 62. (a) 63. (a) 64. (a)
65. (d) 66. (a) 67. (d) 68. (d)
69. (c) 70. (d) 71. (d) 72. (d)
73. (b) 74. (b) 75. (d) 76. (c)
77. (c) 78. (a) 79. (a) 80. (b)
81. (d) 82. (c) 83. (b) 84. (a)
85. (a) 86. (d) 87. (d) 88. (d)
89. (c) 90. (b) 91. (c) 92. (a)
93. (c) 94. (d) 95. (a) 96. (d)
97. (b) 98. (b) 99. (d) 100. (a)
101. (d) 102. (a) 103. (a) 104. (a)
105. (a) 106. (b) 107. (a) 108. (a)
109. (c) 110. (a) 111. (a) 112. (b)
113. (c) 114. (a) 115. (c) 116. (a)
117. (c) 118. (d) 119. (c) 120. (b)
121. (c) 122. (a) 123. (c) 124. (b)
125. (c) 126. (d) 127. (a) 128. (a)
129. (a) 130. (a) 131. (a) 132. (d)
133. (d) 134. (b) 135. (d) 136. (d)
137. (d) 138. (a) 139. (a) 140. (b)
141. (a) 142. (d) 143. (a) 144. (d)
145. (a) 146. (d) 147. (b) 148. (c)
149. (d) 150. (b) 151. (a) 152. (b)
153. (c) 154. (a) 155. (d) 156. (c)
157. (c) 158. (d) 159. (b) 160. (a)
161. (c) 162. (a) 163. (a) 164. (c)
165. (a) 166. (a) 167. (c) 168. (d)
169. (a) 170. (b) 171. (b) 172. (d)
173. (a) 174. (a) 175. (d) 176. (a)
177. (c) 178. (d) 179. (d) 180. (d)
181. (a) 182. (c) 183. (c) 184. (a)
185. (b) 186. (b) 187. (a) 188. (d)
189. (b) 190. (b) 191. (d) 192. (b)
193. (c) 194. (b) 195. (d) 196. (a)
197. (c) 198. (b) 199. (d) 200. (a)

MODEL TEST PAPER - 4

1. (a) 2. (c) 3. (b) 4. (b)
5. (b) 6. (a) 7. (d) 8. (d)
9. (b) 10. (a) 11. (a) 12. (b)
13. (c) 14. (c) 15. (a) 16. (c)
17. (a) 18. (d) 19. (a) 20. (c)
21. (b) 22. (c) 23. (b) 24. (a)
25. (a) 26. (b) 27. (a) 28. (a)
29. (d) 30. (c) 31. (d) 32. (c)
33. (a) 34. (c) 35. (d) 36. (a)
37. (a) 38. (a) 39. (b) 40. (c)
41. (d) 42. (a) 43. (a) 44. (d)
45. (a) 46. (c) 47. (c) 48. (c)
49. (a) 50. (b) 51. (b) 52. (b)
53. (c) 54. (a) 55. (a) 56. (b)
57. (c) 58. (b) 59. (c) 60. (a)
61. (b) 62. (a) 63. (a) 64. (a)
65. (a) 66. (a) 67. (c) 68. (d)
69. (b) 70. (c) 71. (b) 72. (b)
73. (c) 74. (d) 75. (c) 76. (b)
77. (a) 78. (c) 79. (c) 80. (a)
81. (c) 82. (b) 83. (d) 84. (d)
85. (c) 86. (d) 87. (b) 88. (d)
89. (d) 90. (d) 91. (b) 92. (c)
93. (c) 94. (a) 95. (a) 96. (a)
97. (c) 98. (a) 99. (b) 100. (b)
101. (a) 102. (c) 103. (a) 104. (c)
105. (c) 106. (a) 107. (d) 108. (c)
109. (a) 110. (a) 111. (a) 112. (b)
113. (c) 114. (b) 115. (b) 116. (a)
117. (a) 118. (b) 119. (a) 120. (a)
121. (c) 122. (a) 123. (b) 124. (b)
125. (d) 126. (a) 127. (a) 128. (a)
129. (a) 130. (a) 131. (b) 132. (a)
133. (b) 134. (b) 135. (d) 136. (d)
137. (b) 138. (a) 139. (a) 140. (c)
141. (a) 142. (c) 143. (b) 144. (a)
145. (b) 146. (a) 147. (a) 148. (d)
149. (b) 150. (d) 151. (a) 152. (b)
153. (b) 154. (c) 155. (c) 156. (c)
157. (b) 158. (d) 159. (d) 160. (a)
161. (a) 162. (b) 163. (d) 164. (c)
165. (d) 166. (b) 167. (a) 168. (b)
169. (a) 170. (b) 171. (b) 172. (a)
173. (c) 174. (a) 175. (d) 176. (d)
177. (a) 178. (c) 179. (b) 180. (d)
181. (b) 182. (a) 183. (b) 184. (b)
185. (a) 186. (a) 187. (d) 188. (b)

189. (d) 190. (b) 191. (a) 192. (c)
193. (b) 194. (a) 195. (c) 196. (c)
197. (d) 198. (c) 199. (c) 200. (a)

MODEL TEST PAPER - 5

1. (a) 2. (c) 3. (b) 4. (a)
5. (d) 6. (b) 7. (c) 8. (d)
9. (d) 10. (c) 11. (a) 12. (c)
13. (b) 14. (c) 15. (d) 16. (c)
17. (b) 18. (a) 19. (b) 20. (d)
21. (a, b, c) 22. (c) 23. (d) 24. (b)
25. (b) 26. (a, b, c) 27. (c) 28. (a)
29. (a) 30. (b) 31. (c) 32. (c)
33. (d) 34. (c) 35. (d) 36. (b)
37. (b) 38. (b) 39. (b) 40. (d)
41. (b) 42. (a) 43. (a) 44. (d)
45. (a) 46. (d) 47. (a) 48. (a)
49. (c) 50. (a) 51. (a) 52. (d)
53. (d) 54. (c) 55. (b) 56. (c)
57. (b) 58. (a) 59. (a) 60. (b)
61. (c) 62. (a) 63. (b) 64. (b)
65. (b) 66. (b) 67. (d) 68. (a)
69. (b) 70. (b) 71. (b) 72. (c)
73. (c) 74. (b) 75. (a) 76. (d)
77. (d) 78. (d) 79. (b) 80. (d)
81. (b) 82. (c) 83. (b) 84. (c)
85. (b) 86. (d) 87. (a) 88. (c)
89. (d) 90. (c) 91. (d) 92. (c)
93. (c) 94. (d) 95. (d) 96. (a)
97. (a) 98. (b) 99. (b) 100. (b)
101. (b) 102. (c) 103. (b) 104. (b)
105. (a) 106. (a) 107. (b) 108. (a)
109. (a) 110. (a) 111. (b) 112. (d)
113. (a) 114. (a) 115. (a) 116. (c)
117. (a) 118. (d) 119. (a) 120. (a)
121. (b) 122. (a) 123. (b) 124. (a)
125. (c) 126. (b) 127. (b) 128. (b)
129. (a) 130. (d) 131. (a) 132. (c)
133. (a) 134. (a) 135. (c) 136. (a)
137. (a) 138. (a) 139. (b) 140. (b)
141. (d) 142. (a) 143. (b) 144. (c)
145. (a) 146. (d) 147. (c) 148. (b)
149. (b) 150. (d) 151. (d) 152. (d)
153. (a) 154. (a) 155. (c) 156. (a)
157. (b) 158. (a) 159. (a) 160. (c)
161. (b) 162. (a) 163. (b) 164. (b)
165. (b) 166. (b) 167. (a) 168. (c)
169. (b) 170. (a) 171. (b) 172. (a)
173. (a) 174. (c) 175. (b) 176. (a)
177. (a) 178. (d) 179. (a) 180. (a)
181. (b) 182. (a) 183. (c) 184. (a)
185. (c) 186. (b) 187. (d) 188. (b)
189. (b) 190. (c) 191. (a) 192. (a)
193. (a) 194. (b) 195. (b) 196. (c)
197. (a) 198. (a) 199. (a) 200. (c)

MODEL TEST PAPER - 6

1. (c) 2. (b) 3. (a) 4. (b)
5. (d) 6. (d) 7. (a) 8. (d)
9. (d) 10. (c) 11. (d) 12. (c)
13. (a) 14. (a) 15. (a) 16. (b)
17. (a) 18. (c) 19. (b, c) 20. (c)
21. (b) 22. (d) 23. (d) 24. (c)
25. (b) 26. (b) 27. (d) 28. (d)
29. (c) 30. (b) 31. (d) 32. (c)
33. (b) 34. (d) 35. (b) 36. (a)
37. (c) 38. (a) 39. (c) 40. (a)
41. (a) 42. (b) 43. (d) 44. (a)
45. (a) 46. (c) 47. (d) 48. (b)
49. (a) 50. (a) 51. (d) 52. (a)
53. (a) 54. (d) 55. (e) 56. (a)
57. (c) 58. (c) 59. (a) 60. (a)
61. (b) 62. (b) 63. (a) 64. (d)
65. (a) 66. (a) 67. (d) 68. (a)
69. (c) 70. (c) 71. (a) 72. (c)
73. (c) 74. (a) 75. (a) 76. (d)
77. (c) 78. (d) 79. (a) 80. (c)
81. (a) 82. (a) 83. (d) 84. (b)
85. (b) 86. (c) 87. (b) 88. (c)
89. (a) 90. (a) 91. (a) 92. (c)
93. (b) 94. (c) 95. (b) 96. (c)
97. (c) 98. (c) 99. (c) 100. (b)
101. (b) 102. (c) 103. (a) 104. (a)
105. (c) 106. (b) 107. (a) 108. (a)
109. (a) 110. (b) 111. (a) 112. (a)
113. (c) 114. (a) 115. (c) 116. (c)
117. (a) 118. (d) 119. (c) 120. (a)
121. (d) 122. (c) 123. (b) 124. (a)
125. (b) 126. (d) 127. (a) 128. (c)
129. (c) 130. (b) 131. (d) 132. (c)
133. (b) 134. (c) 135. (d) 136. (b)
137. (b) 138. (a) 139. (c) 140. (d)
141. (d) 142. (b) 143. (c) 144. (b)
145. (c) 146. (a) 147. (d) 148. (c)
149. (d) 150. (c) 151. (a) 152. (b)
153. (a) 154. (b) 155. (c) 156. (b)
157. (a) 158. (c) 159. (b) 160. (d)
161. (b) 162. (a) 163. (c) 164. (c)
165. (b) 166. (b) 167. (b) 168. (b)
169. (b) 170. (d) 171. (a) 172. (b)
173. (a) 174. (b) 175. (b) 176. (a)
177. (d) 178. (d) 179. (d) 180. (a)
181. (a) 182. (d) 183. (a) 184. (c)
185. (c) 186. (c) 187. (d) 188. (b)
189. (c) 190. (b) 191. (b) 192. (b)
193. (c) 194. (c) 195. (d) 196. (a)
197. (c) 198. (b) 199. (a) 200. (c)

MODEL TEST PAPER - 7

1. (c) 2. (a) 3. (d) 4. (d)
5. (b) 6. (b) 7. (a) 8. (c)
9. (c) 10. (a) 11. (d) 12. (c)
13. (a) 14. (a) 15. (b) 16. (c)
17. (c) 18. (a) 19. (d) 20. (b)
21. (d) 22. (c) 23. (c) 24. (c)
25. (a) 26. (c) 27. (a) 28. (a)
29. (a) 30. (a) 31. (b) 32. (c)
33. (c) 34. (d) 35. (b) 36. (c)
37. (a) 38. (b) 39. (a) 40. (b)
41. (d) 42. (c) 43. (a) 44. (a)
45. (b) 46. (a) 47. (c) 48. (d)
49. (a) 50. (c) 51. (a) 52. (c)
53. (a) 54. (a) 55. (a) 56. (d)
57. (a) 58. (d) 59. (d) 60. (b)
61. (b) 62. (c) 63. (c) 64. (c)
65. (d) 66. (c) 67. (c) 68. (b)
69. (d) 70. (b) 71. (a) 72. (d)
73. (b) 74. (a) 75. (c) 76. (b)
77. (a) 78. (c) 79. (c) 80. (b)
81. (c) 82. (b) 83. (d) 84. (b)
85. (d) 86. (d) 87. (a) 88. (a)
89. (b) 90. (a) 91. (a) 92. (d)
93. (a) 94. (d) 95. (b) 96. (a)
97. (c) 98. (b) 99. (c) 100. (d)
101. (a) 102. (c) 103. (a) 104. (a)
105. (c) 106. (a) 107. (b) 108. (a)
109. (c) 110. (a) 111. (a) 112. (c)
113. (a) 114. (d) 115. (c) 116. (a)
117. (a) 118. (d) 119. (c) 120. (b)
121. (b) 122. (d) 123. (c) 124. (d)
125. (a) 126. (b) 127. (b) 128. (a)
129. (d) 130. (a) 131. (b) 132. (d)
133. (b) 134. (c) 135. (b) 136. (d)
137. (c) 138. (d) 139. (c) 140. (d)
141. (b) 142. (b) 143. (b) 144. (a)
145. (b) 146. (b) 147. (c) 148. (b)
149. (b) 150. (b) 151. (d) 152. (a)
153. (a) 154. (c) 155. (a) 156. (d)
157. (b) 158. (d) 159. (c) 160. (c)
161. (a) 162. (d) 163. (a) 164. (b)
165. (b) 166. (d) 167. (b) 168. (a)
169. (b) 170. (c) 171. (b) 172. (b)
173. (c) 174. (a) 175. (a) 176. (a)
177. (a) 178. (b) 179. (d) 180. (c)
181. (b) 182. (a) 183. (b) 184. (c)
185. (a) 186. (c) 187. (c) 188. (a)
189. (c) 190. (a) 191. (b) 192. (a)
193. (d) 194. (b) 195. (b) 196. (b)
197. (a) 198. (b) 199. (b) 200. (d)

MODEL TEST PAPER - 8

1. (c) 2. (b) 3. (a) 4. (b)
5. (b) 6. (c) 7. (c) 8. (d)
9. (b) 10. (c) 11. (d) 12. (c)
13. (b) 14. (b) 15. (b) 16. (d)
17. (c) 18. (b) 19. (b) 20. (b)
21. (a) 22. (d) 23. (c) 24. (c)
25. (d) 26. (b) 27. (b) 28. (c)
29. (c) 30. (c) 31. (c) 32. (c)
33. (b) 34. (b) 35. (b) 36. (c)
37. (c) 38. (b) 39. (d) 40. (d)
41. (a) 42. (c) 43. (b) 44. (b)
45. (a) 46. (a) 47. (a) 48. (a)
49. (a) 50. (a) 51. (c) 52. (b)
53. (b) 54. (b) 55. (c) 56. (a)
57. (b) 58. (b) 59. (b) 60. (c)
61. (d) 62. (a) 63. (c) 64. (c)
65. (a) 66. (c) 67. (a) 68. (b)
69. (c) 70. (d) 71. (a) 72. (b)
73. (b) 74. (d) 75. (c) 76. (d)
77. (a) 78. (c) 79. (d) 80. (a)
81. (b) 82. (d) 83. (a) 84. (a)
85. (b) 86. (a) 87. (c) 88. (c)
89. (c) 90. (b) 91. (c) 92. (c)
93. (b) 94. (b) 95. (b) 96. (b)
97. (d) 98. (b) 99. (a) 100. (c)
101. (c) 102. (a) 103. (b) 104. (a)
105. (a) 106. (c) 107. (c) 108. (c)
109. (b) 110. (c) 111. (d) 112. (a)
113. (a) 114. (a) 115. (a) 116. (b)
117. (a) 118. (a) 119. (a) 120. (c)
121. (b) 122. (a) 123. (d) 124. (c)
125. (b) 126. (c) 127. (a) 128. (d)
129. (c) 130. (a) 131. (a) 132. (d)
133. (c) 134. (b) 135. (c) 136. (d)
137. (a) 138. (c) 139. (d) 140. (a)
141. (c) 142. (c) 143. (d) 144. (b)
145. (c) 146. (b) 147. (c) 148. (a)
149. (c) 150. (b) 151. (b) 152. (b)
153. (c) 154. (c) 155. (b) 156. (b)
157. (a) 158. (b) 159. (c) 160. (c)
161. (c) 162. (c) 163. (b) 164. (d)
165. (d) 166. (c) 167. (d) 168. (c)
169. (a) 170. (b) 171. (a) 172. (b)
173. (b) 174. (d) 175. (a) 176. (a)
177. (a) 178. (b) 179. (c) 180. (d)
181. (c) 182. (b) 183. (b) 184. (a)
185. (b) 186. (b) 187. (c) 188. (c)
189. (a) 190. (c) 191. (c) 192. (a)
193. (c) 194. (d) 195. (b) 196. (b)
197. (d) 198. (a) 199. (c) 200. (b)

MODEL TEST PAPER - 9

1.	(c)	2.	(d)	3.	(c)	4.	(b)
5.	(d)	6.	(c)	7.	(b)	8.	(a)
9.	(c)	10.	(b)	11.	(c)	12.	(c)
13.	(a)	14.	(c)	15.	(c)	16.	(a)
17.	(c)	18.	(c)	19.	(a)	20.	(a)
21.	(d)	22.	(b)	23.	(b)	24.	(b)
25.	(d)	26.	(a)	27.	(a)	28.	(b)
29.	(b)	30.	(b)	31.	(a)	32.	(a)
33.	(c)	34.	(d)	35.	(b)	36.	(a)
37.	(d)	38.	(c)	39.	(d)	40.	(c)
41.	(c)	42.	(a)	43.	(a)	44.	(a)
45.	(d)	46.	(a)	47.	(d)	48.	(d)
49.	(b)	50.	(a)	51.	(d)	52.	(b)
53.	(c)	54.	(c)	55.	(c)	56.	(a)
57.	(c)	58.	(a)	59.	(c)	60.	(b)
61.	(d)	62.	(c)	63.	(b)	64.	(a)
65.	(b)	66.	(a)	67.	(a)	68.	(c)
69.	(d)	70.	(b)	71.	(b)	72.	(d)
73.	(c)	74.	(a)	75.	(a)	76.	(a)
77.	(d)	78.	(a)	79.	(b)	80.	(d)
81.	(c)	82.	(a)	83.	(a)	84.	(d)
85.	(b)	86.	(d)	87.	(c)	88.	(a)
89.	(c)	90.	(a)	91.	(b)	92.	(b)
93.	(d)	94.	(d)	95.	(c)	96.	(a)
97.	(c)	98.	(d)	99.	(a)	100.	(d)
101.	(d)	102.	(a)	103.	(a)	104.	(a)
105.	(c)	106.	(a)	107.	(d)	108.	(c)
109.	(a)	110.	(a)	111.	(c)	112.	(d)
113.	(a)	114.	(b)	115.	(c)	116.	(c)
117.	(a)	118.	(c)	119.	(a)	120.	(b)
121.	(d)	122.	(c)	123.	(b)	124.	(b)
125.	(c)	126.	(c)	127.	(c)	128.	(d)
129.	(c)	130.	(d)	131.	(a)	132.	(d)
133.	(d)	134.	(a)	135.	(d)	136.	(b)
137.	(b)	138.	(d)	139.	(d)	140.	(b)
141.	(d)	142.	(d)	143.	(b)	144.	(a)
145.	(d)	146.	(a)	147.	(c)	148.	(b)
149.	(b)	150.	(c)	151.	(c)	152.	(b)
153.	(d)	154.	(d)	155.	(a)	156.	(c)
157.	(d)	158.	(a)	159.	(b)	160.	(a)
161.	(b)	162.	(c)	163.	(b)	164.	(c)
165.	(c)	166.	(c)	167.	(a)	168.	(d)
169.	(b)	170.	(a)	171.	(a)	172.	(a)
173.	(a)	174.	(b)	175.	(a)	176.	(a)
177.	(c)	178.	(a)	179.	(d)	180.	(c)
181.	(c)	182.	(b)	183.	(a)	184.	(b)
185.	(b)	186.	(a)	187.	(d)	188.	(b)
189.	(c)	190.	(a)	191.	(b)	192.	(a)
193.	(a)	194.	(b)	195.	(c)	196.	(a)
197.	(d)	198.	(c)	199.	(b)	200.	(c)

MODEL TEST PAPER - 10

1.	(d)	2.	(d)	3.	(a)	4.	(a)
5.	(c)	6.	(c)	7.	(c)	8.	(b)
9.	(d)	10.	(a)	11.	(b)	12.	(b)
13.	(c)	14.	(c)	15.	(d)	16.	(d)
17.	(b)	18.	(c)	19.	(c)	20.	(d)
21.	(d)	22.	(b)	23.	(d)	24.	(b)
25.	(c)	26.	(a)	27.	(c)	28.	(d)
29.	(c)	30.	(b)	31.	(d)	32.	(c)
33.	(c)	34.	(b)	35.	(d)	36.	(b)
37.	(c)	38.	(d)	39.	(a)	40.	(a)
41.	(d)	42.	(a)	43.	(a)	44.	(c)
45.	(c)	46.	(b)	47.	(a)	48.	(b)
49.	(a)	50.	(a)	51.	(b)	52.	(c)
53.	(a)	54.	(a)	55.	(b)	56.	(d)
57.	(a)	58.	(d)	59.	(c)	60.	(a)
61.	(b)	62.	(a)	63.	(c)	64.	(b)
65.	(c)	66.	(a)	67.	(b)	68.	(b)
69.	(b)	70.	(c)	71.	(c)	72.	(b)
73.	(c)	74.	(c)	75.	(a)	76.	(d)
77.	(b)	78.	(c)	79.	(c)	80.	(c)
81.	(c)	82.	(d)	83.	(c)	84.	(b)
85.	(b)	86.	(d)	87.	(d)	88.	(b)
89.	(d)	90.	(d)	91.	(b)	92.	(a)
93.	(d)	94.	(b)	95.	(d)	96.	(d)
97.	(c)	98.	(d)	99.	(c)	100.	(c)
101.	(d)	102.	(c)	103.	(b)	104.	(b)
105.	(b)	106.	(a)	107.	(d)	108.	(c)
109.	(a)	110.	(b)	111.	(a)	112.	(d)
113.	(b)	114.	(b)	115.	(d)	116.	(a)
117.	(c)	118.	(c)	119.	(c)	120.	(b)
121.	(b)	122.	(c)	123.	(a)	124.	(c)
125.	(c)	126.	(b)	127.	(a)	128.	(c)
129.	(b)	130.	(a)	131.	(c)	132.	(a)
133.	(d)	134.	(a)	135.	(a)	136.	(a)
137.	(c)	138.	(d)	139.	(b)	140.	(c)
141.	(b)	142.	(a, b, c)	143.	(d)	144.	(b)
145.	(a)	146.	(c)	147.	(c)	148.	(d)
149.	(c)	150.	(d)	151.	(a)	152.	(a)
153.	(b)	154.	(c)	155.	(c)	156.	(a)
157.	(d)	158.	(a)	159.	(b)	160.	(a)
161.	(a)	162.	(b)	163.	(b)	164.	(c)
165.	(b)	166.	(d)	167.	(d)	168.	(d)
169.	(a)	170.	(c)	171.	(d)	172.	(c)
173.	(d)	174.	(c)	175.	(c)	176.	(b)
177.	(c)	178.	(b)	179.	(b)	180.	(a)
181.	(b)	182.	(a)	183.	(d)	184.	(c)
185.	(c)	186.	(a)	187.	(a)	188.	(b)
189.	(c)	190.	(a)	191.	(d)	192.	(b)
193.	(a)	194.	(b)	195.	(a)	196.	(c)
197.	(c)	198.	(b)	199.	(a)	200.	(d)

■■■

SOLVED PAPER

AIIMS - 1994

Time : 3½ Hours

Max. Marks : 200

PHYSICS

1. For Boyle's law to hold good, the gas should be
   (a) perfect and at constant temperature but variable mass
   (b) perfect and of constant mass and temperature
   (c) real and at constant temperature but variable mass
   (d) real and of constant mass and temperature.

2. The composition of two simple harmonic motions of equal periods at right angles to each other and with a phase difference of π, results in the displacement of the particle along a
   (a) straight line (b) circle
   (c) hexagon (d) ellipse.

3. The bulb of one thermometer is spherical, while that of other is cylindrical. If both of them have equal amounts of mercury, which one will respond quickly to the temperature ?
   (a) elliptical (b) spherical
   (c) cylindrical (d) both (b) and (c).

4. The surface tension of a liquid decreases with a rise in
   (a) diameter of container
   (b) temperature of the liquid
   (c) thickness of container
   (d) viscosity of the liquid.

5. The angle of a prism is 6° and its refractive index for green light is 1.5. If a green ray passes through it, the deviation will be
   (a) 3° (b) 30°
   (c) 0° (d) 15°.

6. A body 'A' is dropped vertically from the top of a tower. If another identical body 'B' is projected thrown from the same point at the same instant, then
   (a) both 'A' and 'B' will reach the ground simultaneously
   (b) 'A' will reach the ground earlier than 'B'
   (c) 'B' will reach the ground earlier than 'A'
   (d) either 'A' or 'B'.

7. Two satellites of mass m_1 and m_2 ($m_1 > m_2$) are going around the earth in orbits of radius r_1 and r_2 ($r_1 > r_2$). Which statement about their velocities is correct?
   (a) $v_1 < v_2$ (b) $v_1 > v_2$
   (c) $v_1/r_1 = v_2/r_2$ (d) $v_1 = v_2$.

8. If C_P and C_V are the specific heats for a gas at constant pressure and at constant volume respectively, then the relation $C_P - C_V = R$ is exact for
   (a) ideal gas and nearly true for real gases at high pressure
   (b) ideal and real gases at all pressures
   (c) ideal gas and nearly true for real gases at moderate pressure
   (d) ideal gas at all pressure and real gas at moderate pressure.

9. In what manner does the escape velocity of a particle depend upon its mass?
   (a) m^0 (b) m^2
   (c) m^{-1} (d) m.

10. A small piece of metal wire is dragged across the gap between the pole pieces of a magnet in 0.4 sec. If magnetic flux between the pole pieces is known to be 8×10^{-4} Wb, then induced emf in the wire, is
    (a) 4×10^{-3} V (b) 8×10^{-3} V
    (c) 2×10^{-3} V (d) 6×10^{-3} V.

11. The frequency of a tuning fork is 256. It will not resonate with a fork of frequency
    (a) 738 (b) 256
    (c) 768 (d) 512.

12. If the normal force is doubled, the coefficient of friction, is
    (a) doubled (b) halved
    (c) not changed (d) tripled.

13. At what angle of incidence will the light reflected from glass ($m = 1 \cdot 5$) be completely polarized ?
(a) $56 \cdot 3^o$ (b) $40 \cdot 3^o$
(c) $72 \cdot 8^o$ (d) $51 \cdot 6^o$.

14. Which of the following is not true for the given statement: Photoelectric effect supports the quantum nature of light?
(a) if metal surface is faintly illuminated, then photoelectrons leave the surface
(b) there is a minimum frequency of light below which no photoelectrons are emitted
(c) electric charge of the photoelectrons is quantized
(d) None of these

15. In a vessel, the gas is at a pressure P. If the mass of all the molecules is halved and their speed is doubled, then the resultant pressure will be
(a) P (b) $4P$
(c) $P/2$ (d) $2P$.

16. If the radius of earth shrinks by one percent and its mass remaining the same, then acceleration due to gravity on the earth's surface will
(a) remain constant (b) decrease
(c) increase (d) either (b) or (c).

17. A gas behaves as an ideal gas at
(a) high pressure and low temperature
(b) low pressure and high temperature
(c) high pressure and high temperature
(d) low pressure and low temperature.

18. The radius of a soap bubble is r and the surface tension of soap solution is T. Keeping the temperature constant, the extra energy needed to double the radius of the soap bubble by blowing, is
(a) $16\ \pi r^2 T$ (b) $32\ \pi r^2 T$
(c) $8\ \pi r^2 T$ (d) $24\ \pi r^2 T$.

19. The dimension of the modulus of rigidity, is
(a) $[ML^{-2}T^{-2}]$ (b) $[MLT^{-2}]$
(c) $[ML^{-1}T^{-1}]$ (d) $[ML^{-1}T^{-2}]$.

20. One nanometre is equal to
(a) 10^{-7} cm (b) 10^9 mm
(c) 10^{-9} m (d) 10^{-6} cm.

21. A particle revolves round a circular path. The acceleration of the particle is inversely proportional to
(a) mass of particle (b) radius
(c) velocity (d) both (a) and (b).

22. A certain logic circuit has A and B as the two inputs and Y as the output. What is the logic gate in the circuit, if the truth table of the circuit is as shown

	A	B	Y
(a) XOR	0	0	0
(b) OR	0	1	1
(c) NOR	1	0	1
(d) NAND	1	1	0

23. Two lenses of power + 12 D and - 2 D are combined together. What is their equivalent focal length ?
(a) $16 \cdot 6$ cm (b) 10 cm
(c) $8 \cdot 33$ cm (d) $12 \cdot 5$ cm.

24. How many wavelengths of Kr_{86} are there in one metre?
(a) $2348123 \cdot 73$ (b) $1553164 \cdot 13$
(c) $652189 \cdot 63$ (d) $1650763 \cdot 73$.

25. A metal plate gets heated, when cathode rays strike against it, due to
(a) linear velocity of cathode rays
(b) kinetic energy of cathode rays
(c) angular velocity of cathode rays
(d) potential energy of cathode rays.

26. A missile is launched with a velocity less than the escape velocity. The sum of its kinetic and potential energies, is
(a) positive (b) zero
(c) negative (d) first (b) then (c).

27. If the earth is treated as a sphere of radius R and mass M, its angular momentum about the axis of its rotation with period T, is
(a) $\frac{MR^2T}{2\pi}$ (b) $\frac{4\pi MR^2}{5T}$
(c) $\frac{\pi MR^3}{T}$ (d) $\frac{2\pi MR^2}{T}$

28. A pure semiconductor has a/an
(a) finite resistance which decreases with temperature
(b) infinite resistance at 0°C
(c) finite resistance which increases with temperature
(d) finite resistance which does not depend upon temperature.

29. Antimony and Bismuth are usually used in thermocouple, because

(a) a constant thermo e.m.f. is produced
(b) higher thermo e.m.f. is produced
(c) a negative thermo e.m.f. is produced
(d) lower thermo e.m.f. is produced.

30. With an increase in temperature, the electrical conductivity of intrinsic semiconductor
(a) remains unchanged (b) increases
(c) decreases (d) first (b) then (c).

31. Kinetic energy, with any reference, must be
(a) negative (b) zero
(c) positive (d) both (b) and (c).

32. All the known planets move in
(a) elliptical path (b) straight path
(c) hyperbolic path (d) circular path.

33. The dual nature of light is exhibited by
(a) photoelectric effect
(b) diffraction and reflection
(c) diffraction and photoelectric effect
(d) refraction and interference.

34. The neutron was discovered by
(a) Rutherford (b) Marie Curie
(c) James Chadwick (d) Pierre Curie.

35. Approximately, the temperature corresponding to 1 eV energy, is
(a) 7.6×10^2 K (b) 7.7×10^3 K
(c) 7.1×10^{-2} K (d) 7.2×10^3 K.

36. One cannot see through fog, because
(a) refractive index of the fog is infinity
(b) fog absorbs the light
(c) light is scattered by the droplets
(d) light suffers total reflection at droplets.

37. The potential energy possessed by a soap bubble, having surface tension equal to 0.04 N/m of diameter 1 cm, is
(a) $6\pi \times 10^{-6}$ J (b) $2\pi \times 10^{-6}$ J
(c) $8\pi \times 10^{-6}$ J (d) $4\pi \times 10^{-6}$ J.

38. There is no atmosphere on the moon, because
(a) escape velocity of gas molecules is less than their root mean square velocity
(b) it is closer to the earth and also it has the inactive inert gases in it
(c) escape velocity of gas molecules is greater than their root mean square velocity
(d) it is too far from the sun and has very low pressure in its outer surface.

39. In nuclear reactors, the controlling rods are made of
(a) stainless steel (b) cadmium
(c) plutonium (d) graphite.

40. The orbital speed of jupiter, is
(a) equal to the orbital speed of earth
(b) greater than the orbital speed of earth
(c) proportional to the distance from the earth
(d) less than the orbital speed of earth.

41. In Bohr model of hydrogen atom, which of the following is quantised ?
(a) linear momentum of electron
(b) linear velocity of electron
(c) angular momentum of electron
(d) angular velocity of electron.

42. In a boiling water reactor, the boiling water is used as a
(a) moderator (b) fuel
(c) controller (d) coolant.

43. Which of the following physical quantity has the dimensions of $[ML^2T^{-3}]$?
(a) pressure (b) work
(c) impulse (d) power.

44. What is missing in the following nuclear reaction
${}_1H^2 + {}_1H^2 \rightarrow {}_2He^3 + ?$
(a) positron (b) meson
(c) neutron (d) electron.

45. The concept of rotating magnetic field, which is the basis of practically all alternating current machinery, was conceived by
(a) Plank (b) Tesla
(c) Franck and Hertz (d) Young.

46. A strong argument for the particle nature of cathode rays is that they
(a) travel through vacuum
(b) cast shadow
(c) get deflected by electric and magnetic field
(d) produce fluorescence.

47. A bulb contains one mole of hydrogen mixed with one mole of oxygen at temperature *T*. The ratio of r.m.s. values of velocity of hydrogen molecules to that of oxygen molecules, is
(a) 4 : 1 (b) 1 : 16
(c) 1 : 4 (d) 16 : 1.

48. The shortest wavelength of X-rays, emitted from a X-ray tube, depends upon

(a) nature of glass material in the tube
(b) current in the tube
(c) atomic number of the target material
(d) voltage applied to the tube.

49. A constant pressure air thermometer gave a reading of 47.5 units of volume when immersed in ice-cold water, and 67 units in a boiling liquid. The boiling point of the liquid, is
(a) 125°C (b) 100°C
(c) 135°C (d) 112°C.

50. β-rays, emitted from a radioactive material, are known as
(a) charged particles emitted by nucleus
(b) neutral particles
(c) electrons orbiting around the nucleus
(d) electromagnetic radiations.

Directions: *These questions consist of two statements each, printed as Assertion and Reason. While answering these questions you are required to choose any one of the following four responses.*
(a) If both Assertion and Reason are true and the Reason is a correct explanation of the Assertion.
(b) If both Assertion and Reason are true but Reason is not a correct explanation of the Assertion.
(c) If Assertion is true but the Reason is false.
(d) If both Assertion and Reason are false.

51. *Assertion*: The energy gap between the valence band and conduction band is greater in silicon than in germanium.
Reason: Thermal energy produces fewer minority carriers in silicon than in germanium.

52. *Assertion*: In the process of nuclear fission, the fragments emit two or three neutrons as soon as they are formed and subsequently emit particles.
Reason: As the fragments contain an excess of neutrons over protons, emission of neutrons and particles bring their neutron/proton ratio to stable values.

53. *Assertion*: If a heavy nucleus is split into two medium sized parts, each of the new nuclei will have more binding energy per nucleon than the original nucleus.
Reason: Joining two light nuclei together to give a single nucleus of medium size means more binding energy per nucleon in the new nucleus.

54. *Assertion*: In the absence of an externally applied electric field, the displacement per unit volume of a polar dielectric material is always zero.
Reason: In polar dielectrics, each molecule has a permanent dipole moment but these are randomly oriented in the absence of an externally applied electric field.

55. *Assertion*: It is not possible for a system, unaided by an external agency to transfer heat from a body at a lower temperature to another at a higher temperature.
Reason: It is not possible to violate the Second Law of Thermodynamics.

56. *Assertion*: When two vibrating tuning forks having frequencies 256 Hz and 512 Hz are held near each other, beats cannot be heared.
Reason: The principle of superposition is valid only if the frequencies of the oscillators are nearly equal.

57. *Assertion*: A single lens produces a coloured image of an object illuminated by white light.
Reason: The refractive index of the material of lens is different for different wavelengths of light.

58. *Assertion*: Resonance is a special case of forced vibration in which the natural frequency of vibration of the body is the same as the impressed frequency and the amplitude of forced vibration, is maximum.
Reason: The amplitude of forced vibrations of a body increases with an increase in the frequency of the externally impressed periodic force.

59. *Assertion*: At room temperature water does not sublimate from ice to steam.
Reason: The critical point of water is much above the room temperature.

60. *Assertion*: The shape of an automobile is so designed that its front resembles the streamline pattern of the fluid through which it moves.
Reason: The resistance offered by the fluid is maximum.

CHEMISTRY

61. The heat liberated when 1.89 g of benzoic acid is burnt in a bomb calorimeter at 25°C increases the temperature of 18.94 kg of water by 0.632°C. If the specific heat of water at 25°C is 0.998 cal/g-deg, the value of the heat combustion of benzoic acid is
(a) 881.1 kcal (b) 771.4 kcal
(c) 981.1 kcal (d) 871.2 kcal.

62. When ethanal is treated with fehling's solution, it gives a precipitate of
(a) Cu_2O (b) Cu
(c) Cu_3O (d) CuO.

63. Which of the following is not true about e.m.f. of a cell?
(a) work calculated from it is not the maximum work obtainable from the cell
(b) it is maximum voltage obtainable from the cell
(c) it is the potential difference between two electrodes when no current is flowing in circuit
(d) it is responsible for the flow of steady current in the cell.

64. Which of the following compounds will be most easily attacked by an electrophile ?
(a) [benzene] (b) [chlorobenzene, Cl]
(c) [phenol, OH] (d) [toluene, CH_3]

65. Which of the following shows bond in silicone?
(a) Si-C-Si-C-Si (b) Si-Si-Si-Si
(c) -Si-O-Si-O-Si- (d) Si-C-Si-O-Si.

66. If the density ratio of O_2 and H_2 is 16 : 1, then ratio of their V_{rms} will be
(a) 1 : 1 (b) 1 : 4
(c) 16 : 1 (d) 1 : 16.

67. Which of the following gases will have the highest rate of diffusion ?
(a) CO_2 (b) N_2
(c) NH_3 (d) O_2.

68. Which one is the strongest of the following acids?
(a) CCl_3COOH (b) HCOOH
(c) $CH_2ClCOOH$ (d) CH_3COOH.

69. In Wolf-Kishner reduction, the carbonyl group of aldehydes and ketones is converted into
(a) $-CH_2OH$ (b) $-CH_2-$
(c) $-CH_3$ (d) -CHOH-.

70. When propyne is treated with aqueous H_2SO_4, in the presence of $HgSO_4$, the product formed is
(a) acetone (b) ether
(c) aldehyde (d) propanal.

71. Which metal is present in brass, bronze and german-silver ?
(a) Mg (b) Al
(c) Zn (d) Cu.

72. When alkyl halides are heated, with dry Ag_2O, they give
(a) diethyl ether (b) ester
(c) benzene (d) ketone.

73. Which of the following is called an ethanoic acid?
(a) CH_3CH_2COOH
(b) HCOOH
(c) $CH_3CH_2CH_2COOH$
(d) CH_3COOH.

74. Ethyl alcohol exhibits acidic character on reacting with
(a) hydrogen iodide (b) acetic acid
(c) sodium metal (d) all of these.

75. The type of isomerism not exhibited by alkenes is
(a) chain isomerism (b) metamerism
(c) position isomerism (d) stereoisomerism.

76. Which of the following compound gives Cannizzaro's reaction ?
(a) CH_3CH_2CHO (b) HCHO
(c) $(CH_3)_2CHCHO$ (d) CH_3CHO.

77. The formation of 2-butene as a major product by dehydration of 2-butanol is in accordance with
(a) Blanc rule (b) Huckel rule
(c) Markiownikoff's rule
(d) Saytzeff's rule.

78. $MgCl_2 \cdot 6\,H_2O$ when heated gives
(a) magnesium dichloride
(b) magnesium oxide
(c) magnesium oxychloride
(d) magnesium chloride.

79. Permanent hardness of water can be removed by adding
(a) Na_2CO_3 (b) K
(c) $Ca(OCl)Cl$ (d) Cl_2.

80. Which of the following metal reacts with water ?
(a) copper (b) nickel
(c) sodium (d) silver.

81. Which of the following is an alum ?
(a) $FeSO_4(NH_4)_2SO_4 \cdot 6H_2O$
(b) $NaAlO_2$
(c) $Na_2SO_4 \cdot Al_2(SO_4)_3 \cdot 24\,H_2O$
(d) $KCl \cdot MgCl_2 \cdot 6H_2O$.

82. The number of electrons in $[_{19}K^{40}]^{-1}$ is
(a) 28 (b) 19
(c) 40 (d) 20.

83. Which of the following glasses is the most heat resistant ?
(a) bottle glass (b) flint glass
(c) water glass (d) pyrex glass.

84. Number of water molecules in Mohr's salt is
(a) 7 (b) 5
(c) 8 (d) 6.

85. The molecular mass of a volatile substance may be measured by
(a) Liebig's method
(b) Hofmann's method
(c) Victor Meyer's method
(d) none of these.

86. Which of the following will not undergo aldol condensation ?
(a) propionaldehyde (b) acetone
(c) formaldehyde (d) acetaldehyde.

87. Heterolytic fission of an organic covalent bond gives only
(a) anion (b) free radicals
(c) cation (d) both (a) and (c).

88. Which of the following elements will have the highest electron affinity ?
(a) chlorine (b) nitrogen
(c) phosphorus (d) flourine.

89. In which cell the free energy of a chemical reaction is directly converted into electricity ?
(a) concentration cell (b) fuel cell
(c) lead storage battery
(d) lechlanche cell.

90. Aspirin is an acetylation product of
(a) m-hydroxybenzoic acid
(b) o-hydroxybenzoic acid
(c) p-dihydroxybenzene
(d) o-dihydroxybenzene.

91. Which of the following is a strong reducing agent?
(a) Cr (b) Cl
(c) Na (d) Ca.

92. The number of electrons and neutrons of an element is 18 and 20 respectively. Its mass number is
(a) 37 (b) 17
(c) 38 (d) 22.

93. Which is an oxidising substance amongest the following?
(a) SO_2 (b) CO_2
(c) SO_3 (d) NO_2.

94. When chloroform is exposed to air and sunlight, it gives
(a) mustard gas
(b) phosgene
(c) carbon tetrachloride
(d) lewisite.

95. The long form of Periodic Table is based on
(a) mass of the atom (b) atomic number
(c) shapes of the atom (d) electronegativity.

96. Which of the following gas is produced in the reaction: $KO_2 + CO_2$?
(a) O_2 (b) H_2
(c) CO (d) N_2.

97. Which of the following is a Lewis-acid ?
(a) Br^- (b) Cl^-
(c) S^- (d) Ag^+.

98. Which one of the following can differentiate between C_2H_5OH and CH_3OH ?
(a) H_2O (b) HCl
(c) $I_2 + KOH$ (d) NH_3.

99. A catalyst is used to
(a) minimise the time of rate of reaction
(b) increases the product
(c) decrease the product
(d) none of these.

100. The number of water molecules in gypsum and plaster of paris is respectively
(a) 5 and 2 (b) 2 and 1/2
(c) 7 and 2 (d) 2 and 1.

101. Which of the following is called Baeyer's reagent?
(a) alkaline $KMnO_4$ solution
(b) saturated $KMnO_4$ solution
(c) acidic $KMnO_4$ solution
(d) neutral $KMnO_4$ solution.

102. The weight of a metal of equivalent weight 12, which will give 0.475 g of its chloride, is
(a) 0.18 g (b) 0.12 g
(c) 0.24 g (d) 0.16 g.

103. A mixture of 40 g of oxygen and 40 g of helium has a total pressure of 0.9 atm. The partial pressure of oxygen is
(a) 0.5 atm (b) 0.1 atm

(c) 0.9 atm (d) 0.2 atm.

104. The law of equilibrium was first given by
(a) Boyle (b) Goldberg
(c) Waage (d) both (b) and (c).

105. A bivalent metal has the equivalent weight of 12. The molecular weight of its oxide will be
(a) 36 (b) 24
(c) 40 (d) 32.

106. The position of both an electron and helium atom is known within 1.0 nm. The momentum of the electron is known within 5.0×10^{-26} kg ms^{-1}. The minimum uncertainty in the measurement of the momentum of the helium atom is
(a) 7.0×10^{-26} kg ms^{-1} (b) 5.0×10^{-26} kg ms^{-1}
(c) 8.0×10^{-26} kg ms^{-1} (d) 6.0×10^{-26} kg ms^{-1}.

107. According to Dalton's atom theory, the smallest particle in which matter can exist, is called
(a) an electron (b) an atom
(c) a molecule (d) an ion.

108. Which of the following expression gives the de Broglie relationship?
(a) $\lambda = \frac{h}{mp}$ (b) $\frac{h}{mv} = p$
(c) $\lambda m = \frac{v}{p}$ (d) $\lambda = \frac{h}{mv}$.

109. Which of the following statement regarding entropy is correct ?
(a) at absolute zero temperature, the entropy of all crystalline substances is taken to be zero
(b) at 0°C, the entropy of all crystalline substances is taken to be zero
(c) at absolute zero temperature,entropy of a perfect crystalline substance is taken to be zero
(d) at 0°C, the entropy of a perfect crystalline substance is taken to be zero.

110. The compound containing co-ordinate bond is
(a) SO_3 (b) O_3
(c) H_2SO_4 (d) all of these.

Directions: *These questions consist of two statements each, printed as Assertion and Reason. While answering these questions you are required to choose any one of the following four responses.*
(a) If both Assertion and Reason are true and the Reason is a correct explanation of the Assertion.
(b) If both Assertion and Reason are true but Reason is not a correct explanation of the Assertion.
(c) If Assertion is true but the Reason is false.
(d) If both Assertion and Reason are false.

111. *Assertion*: The first ionization energy of aluminium is lower than that of magnesium
Reason: The ionic radius of aluminium is smaller than that of magnesium.

112. *Assertion*: Alkanes having more than three carbon atoms exhibit chain isomerism
Reason: All carbon atoms in alkanes are *sp*-hybridized.

113. *Assertion*: A solution of $KMnO_4$ is decolourized by SO_2.
Reason: SO_2 is acidic in character.

114. *Assertion*: Helium and berylium having similar outer electronic configuration of type ns^2.
Reason: Both are chemically inert.

115. *Assertion*: Ionic compounds tend to be non-volatile.
Reason: The inter-molecular forces in these compounds are weak.

116. *Assertion*: Reaction of conc. H_2SO_4 on NaBr & NaI does not give HBr and HI.
Reaction: Both HBr and HI are oxidized by conc. H_2SO_4 to Br_2 and I_2.

117. *Assertion*: Ethers behave as bases in the presence of mineral acids.
Reason: Due to the presence of lone pair of electrons on the oxygen.

118. *Assertion*: Physical adsorption of molecules on surface requires activation energy.
Reason: Because the bonds of the adsorbed molecules are broken.

119. *Assertion*: The boiling point of ethanol is much higher than that of diethyl ether.
Reason: In ethanol, the molecules are associated by the formation of intermolecular hydrogen bonding, whereas in diethyl ether it is not possible.

120. *Assertion*: Halogens do not occur in free state.
Reason: Halogens are highly reactive.

BIOLOGY

121. Cartilage is formed by
(a) chondrocytes (b) osteoblasts
(c) osteoclasts (d) fibroblasts.

122. Achondroplasia is a disease related with the defect in the formation of
(a) membrane (b) cartilage
(c) bone (d) mucosa.

123. Philadelphia chromosome is found in the patient suffering from
(a) albinism
(b) insomia
(c) myelocytic leukaemia
(d) hepatitis.

124. Diabetes insipidus occurs due to the hyposecretion of
(a) thymosine (b) oxytocin
(c) insulin (d) vasopressin.

125. Steroid hormones are almost similar in structure to
(a) triglyceride (b) tyrosine
(c) coenzyme-A (d) cholesterol.

126. The golden age of reptiles was
(a) mesozoic era (b) palaeozoic era
(c) proterozoic era (d) coenozoic era.

127. Colour blindness, in which all colours are perceived as gray, is termed as
(a) monochromasia (b) chromasia
(c) dichromasia (d) all of these.

128. Which of the following layer of epidermis in man provides the main protection of body against water loss and the entry of disease causing organisms ?
(a) stratum lucidium (b) stratum spirosum
(c) stratum germinativum
(d) stratum corneum.

129. Which of the following cell type is capable of giving rise to other cell types in sponges ?
(a) archaeocytes (b) pinacocytes
(c) collencytes (d) thesocytes.

130. Outer covering of cartilage is known as
(a) endosteum (b) perichondrium
(c) peritonium (d) periosteum.

131. Which of the following is made up of a single bone in mammals ?
(a) lower jaw (b) hyoid
(c) zygomatic arch (d) upper jaw.

132. The daughters born to haemophilic father and normal mother could be
(a) haemophilic (b) normal
(c) carrier (d) all of these.

133. Schuffner's dots are seen in red blood corpuscles of man due to which of the following disease?
(a) malaria (b) kala-azar
(c) diabetes (d) filaria.

134. The contractile element present in a striated muscle fibril, between two successive Z-lines, is called
(a) sarcomere (b) sarcoplasm
(c) sarcosomes (d) all of these.

135. Which of the following is a vestigial structure in python ?
(a) hind limbs (b) teeth
(c) poison glands (d) scales.

136. Which of the following cranial nerve of man is both sensory and motor ?
(a) olfactory (b) optic
(c) trigeminal (d) vagus.

137. Which of the following is respiratory organ of scorpion ?
(a) gills (b) lungs
(c) ctenidia (d) book lungs.

138. Which of the following is an essential fatty acid in mammals ?
(a) palmitic acid (b) stearic acid
(c) gama-linolenic acid (d) acetic acid.

139. The state, during which the respiratory centre is inhibited, is termed as
(a) anoxia (b) asphyxia
(c) suffocation (d) choking.

140. Glissonian cirrhosis is a disease related with
(a) liver (b) lung
(c) pancreas (d) spleen.

141. Which of the following does not produce any digestive enzyme ?
(a) pancreas (b) mouth
(c) gastric mucosa (d) liver.

142. Zonula adherens is a kind of
(a) filament (b) desmosome
(c) membrane (d) mesosome.

143. Lymphoid tissue is found in
(a) lymph nodes (b) thymus
(c) tonsils (d) all of these.

144. Hamburger's phenomenon is also known as
(a) chloride shift mechanism

(b) sodium-potassium pump
(c) carbonic acid shift mechanism
(d) hydrogen shift mechanism.

145. Which of the following carries blood rich in food materials, such as glucose and amino acids, from intestine to liver ?
(a) renal portal vein
(b) dorsal aorta
(c) hepatic portal vein
(d) mesenteric artery.

146. Bacteria with flagella all over its body, is called
(a) monotrichous (b) amphitrichous
(c) lophotrichous (d) peritrichous.

147. Which of the following terms represents a pair of contrasting character ?
(a) homozygous (b) allele
(c) heterozygous (d) phenotypes.

148. 'Genera Plantarum' was written by
(a) Hutchinson (b) Bessey
(c) Bentham and Hooker
(d) Linnaeus.

149. A set of bacterial clones, each containing a plasmid or phage, is called
(a) gene library (b) gene pool
(c) genophore (d) genome.

150. The transfer of genetic material of one bacterium to another by virus is called
(a) transcription (b) translation
(c) replication (d) transduction.

151. Maize has ten pairs of chromosomes. How many linkage groups will be present, if all the genes are mapped?
(a) 20 (b) 5
(c) 40 (d) 10.

152. The complete set of chromosome, inherited as a single unit, from one parent, is known as
(a) genome (b) linkage
(c) gene pool (d) genotype.

153. Which of the following are initiator codons ?
(a) UGA and UAG (b) UUU and UUC
(c) AUG and GUG (d) UAA and UAG.

154. A pigment, which absorbs red and far red light, is
(a) cytochrome (b) phytochrome
(c) xanthophyll (d) carotene.

155. The epistatic effect, in which the dihybrid cross 9 : 3 : 3 : 1 between Aa Bb' Aa bb is modified as
(a) dominance of one allele on another allele of both loci
(b) interaction between two alleles of different loci
(c) dominance of one allele on another allele of same loci
(d) interaction between two alleles of same loci.

156. Which of the following is known as 'resurrection plant'?
(a) *Rafflesia* (b) *Selaginella*
(c) *Chlorella* (d) *Welwitschia.*

157. The jumping genes are called
(a) cistrons (b) mutons
(c) transposons (d) recons.

158. The leaves of *Mimosa pudica* droop down, when touched due to
(a) seismonasty (b) photonasty
(c) epinasty (d) nyctinasty.

159. When pollen grains are not transferred from anthers to stigma in a flower, due to the barrier, it is called
(a) cleistogamy (b) herkogamy
(c) dichogamy (d) heterogamy.

160. The pairing of homologous chromosomes in meiosis is known as
(a) bivalent (b) synapsis
(c) disjunction (d) synergids.

161. Nodules with nitrogen fixing bacteria are present in
(a) wheat (b) cotton
(c) mustard (d) gram.

162. Which of the following explains, how progeny can possess the combinations of traits that none of the parent possessed ?
(a) law of segregation
(b) chromosome theory
(c) law of independent assortment
(d) polygenic inheritance.

163. The presence of continuous phenotypic variation in an F_1-generation suggests that a character is inherited by
(a) gene linkage
(b) epistasis
(c) polygenic inheritance
(d) recombination.

164. The new strand synthesised, in small pieces and then joined together during DNA replication, is called
(a) dead strand (b) lagging strand
(c) leading stand (d) all of these.

165. *Parkinsonia* is a good example of
(a) winged fruit
(b) phyllode
(c) parachute mechanism
(d) phylloclade.

166. Inflorescence, which begins as a dichasial cyme and ends in a monochasial cyme, is called
(a) cyathium (b) biparous
(c) verticillaster (d) thyrsus.

167. Cyanobacteria is a new name for
(a) mycoplasma (b) *Nostoc*
(c) myxophyceae (d) myxomycetes.

168. The thallus of *Volvox* is called
(a) coenocyte (b) filament
(c) heterotrichous (d) coenobium.

169. The similarity between bacterium and cyanobacterium is in the presence of
(a) chloroplast (b) flagella
(c) 80 S ribosomes (d) nucleoid.

170. The five-kingdom classification was suggested by
(a) Engler and Prantl (b) Eichler
(c) Bentham and Hooker
(d) Whittaker.

Directions: *These questions consist of two statements each, printed as Assertion and Reason. While answering these questions you are required to choose any one of the following four responses.*
(a) If both Assertion and Reason are true and the Reason is a correct explanation of the Assertion.
(b) If both Assertion and Reason are true but Reason is not a correct explanation of the Assertion.
(c) If Assertion is true but the Reason is false.
(d) If both Assertion and Reason are false.

171. *Assertion*: A cholera patient is given glucose, electrolytes and water.
Reason: These plasmolyse the disease causing germs.

172. *Assertion*: It is considered advantageous to give the polio vaccine orally.
Reason: It prevents reinfection by causing intestinal immunity.

173. *Assertion*: Calamine lotion is recommended for applying on chickenpox rashes.
Reason: It gives relief by attenuating the chickenpox virus.

174. *Assertion*: Typhoid carriers may be cured by surgical removal of their spleen.
Reason: The disease germs remain concentrated in it.

175. *Assertion*: A father may be a haemophilic only if his mother is carrier.
Reason: The father cannot pass on a sex-linked gene to his son.

176. *Assertion*: Plants possessing C_4-pathway of carbon fixation have a higher net primary productivity than the C_3-pathway possessing plants.
Reason: For each unit weight of fixed carbon, C_4-pathway possessing plants require less water than the C_3-pathway possessing plants.

177. *Assertion*: A single strand of *m*-RNA is capable of forming a number of different polypeptide chains.
Reason: Termination codons occur in *m*-RNA.

178. *Assertion*: Action spectrum of photosynthesis compares well with the absorption spectrum of chlorophyll.
Reason: Chlorophyll is the only pigment which can absorb and convert light energy into chemical energy.

179. *Assertion*: The non-allelic genes for red hair and freckles are usually inherited together.
Reason: The genes for red hair and freckles are located on same chromosome in close association

180. *Assertion*: Chromosomal aberrations are caused by a break in the chromosome or its chromatid.
Reason: Duplication, deficiency, transversion and translocations are the result of chromosomal aberrations.

GENERAL KNOWLEDGE

181. The world's biggest airport is situated in
(a) USA (b) India
(c) Britain (d) France.

182. 'OSI' is stands for
(a) open system information
(b) open system interface

(c) out dated system insertion
(d) open system interconnection.

183. Which of the following official document is related with India?
(a) green paper
(b) white paper (c) yellow book
(d) blue book.

184. A chest disease, whose attack causes difficult breathing and suffocation, is known as
(a) blood-pressure (b) arthritis
(c) cancer (d) asthma.

185. 'Panchayat' is the parliament of
(a) Nepal (b) Spain
(c) Iran (d) Bangladesh.

186. Which of the following are the vital organs?
(a) eyes (b) nostrils
(c) heart (d) ears.

187. Which of the following city has the largest statue in India ?
(a) Madras (b) Delhi
(c) Hyderabad (d) Bombay.

188. 'Skylab' is a
(a) a series of U.S. space probes to explore the solar system
(b) re-usable manned space craft
(c) USA's space station in which astronauts lived and worked in space
(d) a large space craft equipped for manned mission of long duration.

189. The first European invader of Indian soil was
(a) Macmillan
(b) Marco polo
(c) Alexander the great
(d) Fahien.

190. 'Adi Granth' was written by
(a) Guru Gobind Singh
(b) Guru Arjun Dev
(c) Guru Teg Bahadur
(d) Guru Nanak Dev.

191. The height of 'Kanchanjunga peak' in Himalayas, is
(a) 8535 m (b) 8848 m
(c) 8470 m (d) 8611 m.

192. 'Damodar River' is the sorrow of
(a) Maharashtra (b) Bengal
(c) Nagaland (d) Assam.

193. The longest railway tunnel in the world is, located at
(a) South Africa (b) America
(c) Japan (d) China.

194. 'Dhariwal' is known for the production of
(a) Fertilisers (b) soaps
(c) woolen goods (d) sport goods.

195. 'Kozhikode' is the new name of which of the following city?
(a) Paradeep (b) Cochin
(c) Calicut (d) Khandala.

196. Rubber plants are mostly located in
(a) West Bengal and Bihar
(b) Andhra Pradesh and Tamil Nadu
(c) Maharashtra and Himachal Pradesh
(d) Karnataka and Kerla.

197. The capital of Lakshadweep, is
(a) Kavaratti (b) Port Blair
(c) Kohima (d) Silvasa.

198. Which of the following state is most adversely affected by trophical cyclones?
(a) Gujrat (b) Assam
(c) Kerala (d) Orissa.

199. Which of the following is not a Rabi crop?
(a) groundnut (b) wheat
(c) oil seeds (d) gram.

200. The place, which experiences minimum temperature in winter is
(a) Shimla (b) Srinagar
(c) Manali (d) Leh.

❖ ❖ ❖

SOLUTIONS

PHYSICS

1. (b) : According to Boyle's law, the volume (V) of a given mass of a perfect gas at constant temperature is inversely proportional to its pressure (P). Mathematically, $V \propto (1/P)$ or $PV = K$.

2. (a)

3. (c) : The surface area of the cylindrical bulb will be larger than that of the spherical bulb. Hence heat will be quickly transmitted to mercury through the cylindrical bulb. Therefore thermometer with cylindrical bulb will respond quickly to the temperature.

4. (b) : The surface tension of a liquid decreases with a rise in temperature except the molten cadmium and copper. For small range of temperatures, the variation of surface tension is given by the formula $S_t = S_0(1 - at)$, where S_0 and S_t are the surface tensions of liquid at 0°C and t°C respectively and a is the coefficient of surface tension with temperature.

5. (a) : Given: Angle of prism (A) = 6°. We know that deviation $(d) = (m-1)A = (1\cdot5-1)6 = 0\cdot5\times6 = 3°$.

6. (a) : As the body 'A' is dropped from rest $\therefore h = \frac{1}{2}gt_A^2 \Rightarrow t_A = \sqrt{\frac{2h}{g}}$

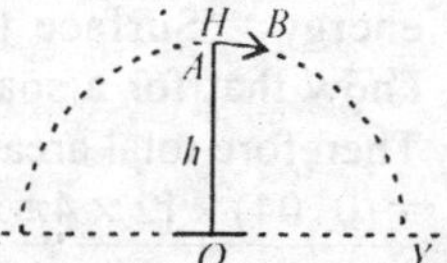

As the body B is given a horizontal velocity at the time of release, it is going to follow the same trajectory as a body on a projectile motion, projected with a velocity having the same horizontal component as the horizontal velocity of B given at H. So the time taken by B from H to Y is same as that from X to H.

Now let the vertical component of velocity at X be v then at H

$$0 = v^2 - 2gh \qquad [\because \text{ at } H, v = 0]$$

$$\Rightarrow v^2 = 2gh \Rightarrow v = \sqrt{2gh}$$

and $0 = v - gt$

$$\Rightarrow t = \frac{v}{g} = \frac{\sqrt{2gh}}{g} = \frac{\sqrt{2h}}{g}$$

$$\therefore t_B = t = \frac{\sqrt{2h}}{g} = t_A$$

7. (a) : We know that for a satellite of mass m moving in an orbit of radius r, $\frac{GM_e m}{r^2} = \frac{mv^2}{r}$ or

$$v = \sqrt{\frac{GM_e}{r}} \propto \sqrt{\frac{1}{r}} \text{ or } \frac{v_1}{v_2} = \sqrt{\frac{r_2}{r_1}}.$$

Since $r_1 > r_2$, therefore $v_1 < v_2$.

8. (c)

9. (a) : Escape velocity $(v_e) = \sqrt{2gR_e}$. Therefore it is independent of the mass of the particle or it will depend on m^0.

10. (c) : Given: Time (t) = 0·4 sec and magnetic flux (ϕ) = 8×10^{-4} Wb. We know from the Faraday's law of electromagnetic induction that the induced e.m.f. in the wire $(\varepsilon) = \frac{d\phi}{dt} = \frac{8\times10^{-4}}{0\cdot4} = 2\times10^{-3}$ V.

11. (a) : Given: Frequency of the tuning fork (f) = 256. We know that fork of the frequency 256 will resonate only with those forks, whose frequency is an integral multiple of 256 (*i.e.* 512 and 768). Since the frequency 738 is not an integral multiple of 256, therefore it will not resonate with the fork having frequency 256.

12. (c)

13. (a) : Given: Refractive index of glass (m) = 1.5. We know from the Brewster's law, $\tan i_p = m = 1.5$. Therefore $i_p = \tan^{-1} 1\cdot5 = 56\cdot3°$ ...(where i_p is the angle of reflected light).

14. (c)

15. (d) : Given: Initial pressure of the gas (P_1) = P; Initial mass of the gas molecules (m_1) = m; Final mass of gas molecules (m_2) = $0\cdot5\,m$; Initial speed of molecules (v_1) = v and final speed of the molecules (v_2) = $2v$. We know that pressure of the gas $(P) = \frac{1}{3}\times\frac{mn}{V}\times v^2 \propto mv^2$

$$\text{or } \frac{P_1}{P_2} = \frac{m_1}{m_2}\times\left(\frac{v_1}{v_2}\right)^2 = \frac{1}{0\cdot5}\times\left(\frac{1}{2}\right)^2 = \frac{1}{2} \text{ or } P_2 = 2P_1.$$

...(where P_2 is the resultant pressure).

16. (c) : Acceleration due to gravity on the earth's surface is given by $g = \frac{GM_e}{R_e^2}$

Now, R_e shrinks by 1%, so the new value for radius of the earth is 0.09 R_e.

$$\therefore\ g' = \frac{GM_e}{(0.09)^2 R_e^2} = \frac{g}{0.0081} > g$$

17. **(b) :** At low pressure and high temperature, the effect of molecular attraction becomes negligible and the behaviour of a gas tends to that of an ideal gas.

18. **(d) :** Given: Initial radius of soap bubble = r; Surface tension of soap solution = T and final radius of soap bubble = $2r$. We know that energy to blow the soap bubble of radius r, $(E_1) = 2 \times 4\pi r^2 \times T = 8\pi r^2 T$ and energy to blow a soap bubble of radius $2r$, $(E_2) = 2 \times 4\pi(2r)^2 T = 32\pi r^2 T$. Therefore extra energy needed $= E_2 - E_1 = 32\pi r^2 T - 8\pi r^2 T = 24\pi r^2 T$.

19. **(d) :** The modulus of rigidity

$$(\eta) = \frac{\text{Shearing stress}}{\text{Shearing strain}} = \frac{F/A}{\phi} = \frac{[MLT^{-2}]}{[L^2]} = [ML^{-1}T^{-2}].$$

20. **(c)**

21. **(b) :** The centripetal acceleration $(a) = \frac{mv^2}{r} \propto \frac{1}{r}$. Therefore acceleration of the particle is inverely proportional to radius.

22. **(a) :** XOR gate gives the output for dissimilar values of inputs. The Boolean expression for XOR gate is $Y = A \cdot \overline{B} + \overline{A} \cdot B$. It is read as "$Y$ equals A and B negated OR A negated AND B".

23. **(b) :** Given: Power of first lens $(P_1) = +12$ D and power of second lens $(P_2) = -2$ D. We know that power of the combination $(P) = P_1 + P_2 = 12 + (-2) = +10$ D.

$\therefore$ Equivalent focal length $(F) = \frac{1}{P} = \frac{1}{10}$ m = 10 cm.

24. **(d)**

25. **(b) :** When cathode rays strike a metal plate, their kinetic energy is transformed into heat energy, which increases the temperature of the plate.

26. **(c) :** When the missile is launched with a velocity less than the escape velocity, it will be influenced by our gravitation and so it will constitute a bound system for which the total energy will be negative.

27. **(b) :** Given: Radius of sphere = R and mass of sphere = M. We know that angular momentum $(I\omega) = \frac{2}{5}MR^2 \times \frac{2\pi}{T} = \frac{4\pi\ MR^2}{5T}$.

28. **(a) :** Since a semiconductor has a negative temperature coefficient of resistance, its resistance decreases with temperature.

29. **(b) :** Antimony and bismuth are the pair of metals producing a higher thermo e.m.f. in comparison with other pairs of metals. Therefore this pair is usually used in thermocouple.

30. **(b)**

31. **(c) :** Kinetic energy is equal to $\frac{1}{2} \times mv^2$, where v is velocity and its square is always positive. Therefore kinetic energy is always positive.

32. **(a)**

33. **(c) :** Diffraction exhibits wave nature of light and photoelectric effect exhibits quantum nature of light. Therefore diffraction and photoelectric effect exhibit the dual nature of light.

34. **(c)**

35. **(b) :** Given: Energy $(E) = 1$ eV $= 1.6 \times 10^{-19}$ J. Average kinetic energy per molecule $(E) = 1.6 \times 10^{-19}$ J

$$= \frac{3}{2}kT \text{ or } T = \frac{2 \times (1.6 \times 10^{-19})}{3k} = \frac{2 \times (1.6 \times 10^{-19})}{3 \times (1.38 \times 10^{-23})}$$
$$= 7.7 \times 10^3 \text{ K.}$$

...(where k is Boltzman constant $= 1.38 \times 10^{-23}$).

36. **(c)**

37. **(c) :** Given: Surface tension in soap bubble $(T) = 0.04$ N/m and diameter of soap bubble $(d) = 1$ cm $= 0.01$ m or radius $(r) = 0.005$ m. We know that potential energy = Surface tension × Surface area. We also know that for a soap bubble, there are two surfaces. Therefore total area $= 2 \times 4\pi r^2$. Thus potential energy $= (0.04) \times [2 \times 4\pi \times (0.005)^2] = 8\pi \times 10^{-6}$ J.

38. **(a)**

39. **(b) :** Cadmium is a good absorber of neutrons and it effectively controls the rate of fission. Therefore in nuclear reactors, the controlling rods are made of cadmium.

40. **(d) :** Orbital velocity $(v_o) = \sqrt{\frac{GM}{r}} \propto \frac{1}{r}$ (where r is the distance from sun). Since the distance of jupiter from the sun is greater than the distance between the sun and the earth, therefore orbital speed of jupiter is less than the orbital speed of earth.

41. **(c) :** As per Bohr's model of hydrogen atom, the angular momentum of an electron around the nucleus, is an integral multiple of $\frac{h}{2\pi}$. Thus angular momentum $= mvr = \frac{nh}{2\pi}$ where n is an integer. Therefore the angular momentum can have only discrete values. *i.e.* it is quantised.

42. (d)

43. (d) : Dimension of work (W) = force × distance $= [MLT^{-2}][L] = [ML^2T^{-2}]$, power $(P) = \frac{\text{work}}{\text{time}} = \frac{[ML^2T^{-2}]}{[T]} = [ML^2T^{-3}]$; pressure $(p) = \frac{\text{force}}{\text{area}} = \frac{[ML^2T^{-2}]}{[L^2]} = [ML^{-1}T^{-2}]$ and impulse = force × time $= [MLT^{-2}][T] = [MLT^{-1}]$. Therefore power has the same dimension as given in the question.

44. (c) : Given: Nuclear reaction: ${}_1H^2 + {}_1H^2 \rightarrow {}_2He^3$ + ?. We know that the balanced equation of the nuclear reaction is ${}_1H^2 + {}_1H^2 \rightarrow {}_2He^3 + {}_0n^1$. Where ${}_0n^1$ is the symbol of neutron. Therefore neutron will be added in the given equation to complete it.

45. (b) **46. (c)**

47. (a) : Given: One mole of hydrogen mixed with one mole of oxygen. We know that r.m.s. velocity $(v_{rms}) = \sqrt{\frac{3RT}{M}} \propto \sqrt{\frac{1}{M}}$ or $\frac{(v_{rms})_H}{(v_{rms})_O} = \sqrt{\frac{M_O}{M_H}} = \sqrt{\frac{32}{2}} = \frac{4}{1}$.
or $(v_{rms})_H : (v_{rms})_O = 4 : 1$.

48. (d)

49. (d) : Given: Initial volume $(V_1) = 47.5$ units; Temperature of ice-cold water $(T_1) = 0°C = 273$ K and final volume $(V_2) = 67$ units. We know from the Charles law, $\frac{V_1}{T_1} = \frac{V_2}{T_2}$ or $T_2 = \frac{V_2}{V_1} \times T_1 = \frac{67}{47.5} \times 273 = 385$ K = 112°C. T_2 is the boiling point of the liquid.

50. (a)

51. (a) : Mathematically, the number of e–h pairs in the intrinsic semiconductor is given by

$$n \propto T^{\frac{3}{2}} e^{-\frac{\Delta \acute{c}}{8\&}} \text{ which gives}$$

$$\Delta E \propto kT\left[\frac{3}{2}\ln T - \ln n\right]$$

Now since in silicon the number of e–h pairs is less than that in Germanium, the energy gap ΔE in silicon is more than that in Ge. [Note that for intrinsic semiconductor, the number of e–h pairs is same as the number of minority or majority carriers].

52 (a)

53. (b) : In the case of fission of a heavy nucleus, it gets broken up into small nuclei which are stable. These small nuclei are stable because their N/Z ratios are small compared to their parent nucleus. Their stability comes from the fact that they are having more binding energy per nucleon.

54. (a) : The displacement vector is given by
$\vec{D} = \varepsilon_0 \vec{E} + \vec{P}$ where
$\vec{E}$ = applied electric field and
$\vec{P}$ = polarisation or dipole moment per unit volume
$= n\vec{p} \times 2$ [$\vec{p}$ is the component of dipole moment of each molecule in direction $\vec{E}$ and n is the no. of molecules per unit volume]
Now in the absence of an electric field ($\vec{E} = 0$) the polarisation vector $\vec{P}$ vanishes (because $\vec{p}$ is there if $\vec{E}$ is there). Therefore displacement $\vec{D} = 0$

55. (a) : The statement given in the Assession is itself a form of the second law of thermodynamics which cannot be violated.

56. (c) : The principle of superposition does not state that the frequencies of the oscillation should be nearly equal. And for beats to be heard the condition is that the difference in frequencies of the two oscillations be not more than 16 times per sec for a normal human ear to recognise it. Hence we cannot hear beats in the case of two tuning forks vibrating at frequencies 256 Hz and 512 Hz respectively.

57. (a) : Due to the variation of the retractive index of the material of the lens, the focal length also varies accordingly. Now as white light is composed of different colours of light, each colour will produce its own image based on the focal length for that colour. This particular phenomenon for a single lens is known as chromatic aberration.

58. (c) : Resonance occurs when the frequency of the applied force becomes nearly equal to the natural frequency of vibration of the body. During resonance the amplitude of the forced vibration reaches its maximum value.

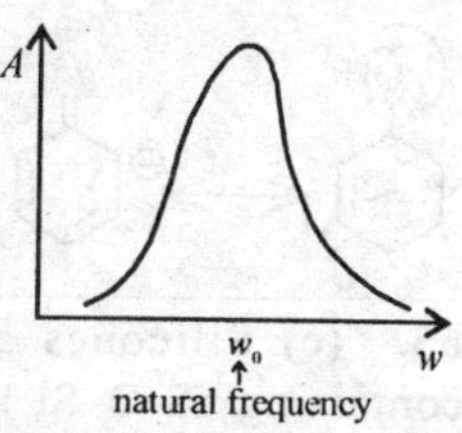

So, if we increase the frequency of the externally impressed periodic force, the amplitude of the forced vibration does not increase but it decreases. So the given reason is false.

59. (c) : We cannot get steam directly from ice. There is one intermediate state called water whose temperature has to be raised to 100°C before we can get steam. Critical point is that temperature at which a gas can be liquefied by applying pressure. So, water cannot have a critical point.

60. (c) : The resistance offered by the fluid should be minimum with that shape.

CHEMISTRY

61. (b) : Given: Weight of benzoic acid = 1.89 g; Temperature of bomb calorimeter = 25°C = 298 K; Mass of water (m) = 18.94 kg = 18940 g; Increase in temperature (t) = 0.632°C and specific heat of water (s) = 0.998 cal/g-deg. We know that heat gained by water or heat liberated by benzoic acid (Q) = $m\,s\,t$ = $18940 \times 0.998 \times 0.632 = 11946.14$ cal. Since 1.89 g of acid liberates 11946.14 cal of heat, therefore heat liberated by 122 g of acid $= \dfrac{11946.14 \times 122}{1.89}$

= 771126.5 cal = 771.12 kcal.

...(where 122 g is the molecular weight of benzoic acid)

62. (a) : $CH_3CHO + 2CuO \rightarrow CH_3COOH + Cu_2O\downarrow$.
(Blue) (Red ppt)

Thus in this reaction, precipitate of copper oxide (Cu_2O) is formed.
Fehling solution is an alkaline solution of cupric ion complexed with sodium potassium tartrate.

63. (a) : E.M.F. is defined as the potential difference between two electrodes when current is flowing in circuit. It is the maximum work obtainable from the cell.

64. (c) : –OH group in phenol can release electrons to the ring better than $-CH_3$ gp in toluene. Cl atom has electron withdrawing effect which inhibits electrophile attack.

(Resonance structures of phenol: $\ddot{O}H$ on ring $\longleftrightarrow$ $\overset{\oplus}{O}H$ with $\ominus$ at ortho $\longleftrightarrow$ $\overset{\oplus}{O}H$ with $\ominus$ at para $\longleftrightarrow$ $\overset{\oplus}{O}H$ with $\ominus$ at ortho)

65. (c) Silicones are organic silicon polymers containing Si–O–Si linkages.

```
     R       R       R
     |       |       |
 -O-Si-O-Si-O-Si-O-
     |       |       |
     O       O       O
     |       |       |
 -O-Si-O-Si-O-Si-O-   (cross linked silicon)
     |       |       |
     R       R       R
```

66. (b) : $\dfrac{\rho O_2}{\rho H_2} = \dfrac{16}{1} \Rightarrow \dfrac{mO_2}{mH_2} = \dfrac{16}{1}$

$V_{rms} \propto \left(\dfrac{1}{m}\right)^{1/2} \Rightarrow \dfrac{V_{rms}(O_2)}{V_{rms}(H_2)} = \left(\dfrac{mH_2}{mO_2}\right)^{1/2} = \left(\dfrac{1}{16}\right)^{1/2} = \dfrac{1}{4}$

67. (c) Rate of diffusion $\propto (1/M)$
M = molecular mass
$M(CO_2) = 44$ $M(N_2) = 28$
$M(NH_3) = 17$ $M(O_2) = 32$
Therefore, rate of NH_3 diffusion is greater than other.

68. (a) : More is the no. of Cl atoms attached to α – carbon of COOH group, greater is the acidity due to high electronegativity of Cl – atoms (it pulls electrons towards it).

69. (b) : Wolf – Kishner reduction :
Aldehyde and Ketones are reduced to hydrocarbons in the presence of excess of hydrazine and strong base on heating.

$$\underset{\substack{|\\H}}{R-C}=O + H_2N\,NH_2 \xrightarrow[200^\circ C]{KOH} \underset{\substack{|\\H}}{R-CH_2} + N_2 + H_2O$$

70. (a) : Ketones are formed on hydration of alkynes (other than acetylene) by following Markownikoff's rule.

$$CH_3C\equiv CH + H\text{–}OH \xrightarrow[H_2O,\ 60^\circ C]{HgSO_4} CH_3\text{–}\overset{\substack{OH\\|}}{C}=CH_2 \xrightarrow{\text{tautomerism}} CH_3\text{–}\overset{\substack{O\\||}}{C}\text{–}CH_3$$

71. (d) : Bronze is an alloy of Cu and Sn.
Brass is an alloy of Cu and Zn.
German-silver is an alloy of Cu, Zn and Ni.

72. (a) : $R-X \xrightarrow[\Delta]{\text{Dry } Ag_2O} \underset{\text{Diethyl ether}}{R-O-R}$

73. (d) : Ethanoic Acid – CH_3COOH
[Ethane → 2 C–atom]

74. (c) : $2CH_3CH_2OH + \underset{\text{metal}}{Na} \longrightarrow 2CH_3CH_2O^-Na^+ + H_2$

Formation of alkoxide indicates the acidic nature of alcohols as alkoxides are electrovalent compounds and are written as RO^-M^+.

75. (b) : Metamerism is due to presence of different alkyl groups attached to the same polyvalent functional group or atom.
∴ This kind of isomerism is not possible in case of alkenes.

76. (b) : Only HCHO does not have α – hydrogens which is the requirement of cannizarro reaction.

$$2HCHO \xrightarrow{NaOH} CH_3OH + HCOONa$$

77. (d) : According to Saytzeff's rule, in the dehydration of secondary and tertiary alcohols, when there is a possibility of formation of two isomers, the hydrogen atom is preferentially eliminated from the adjacent carbon atom with the fewer number of hydrogen atoms.

$$CH_3-CH_2-\underset{OH}{\underset{|}{CH}}-CH_3 \xrightarrow[-H_2O]{H^+} CH_3-CH_2-\overset{\oplus}{CH}-CH_3 \xrightarrow{-H^+} \underset{2-\text{butene}}{CH_3-CH=CH-CH_3}$$

78. **(b) :** $MgCl_2 \cdot 6H_2O \xrightarrow{\text{Heat}} MgCl_2 . 2H_2O \xrightarrow{\Delta}$.

$\underset{\text{Oxychloride}}{Mg_2OCl_2} \xrightarrow[\text{air}]{\text{Heat}} MgO$

79. **(a) :** When hard water is treated with a certain amount of washing powder (Na_2CO_3) the chlorides and sulphates of calcium and magnesium are converted into their respective carbonates, which get precipitated. As a result of this, the hardness of water can be removed.

$CaSO_4 + Na_2CO_3 \longrightarrow CaCO_3 \downarrow + Na_2SO_4$.

80. **(c) :** Sodium reacts with water yielding NaOH and H_2 gas.

$2H_2O + 2Na \rightarrow 2\ NaOH + H_2$

81. **(d) :** The term alum is used for all the double sulphates having the composition, $M_2SO_4.M'_2(SO_4)_3.24H_2O$, where M stands for monovalent basic radicals such Na^+, K^+ etc. and M' for trivalent basic radicals such as Al^{3+}, Cr^{3+} etc.

82. **(d) :** Atomic No. = 19

e^- present originally = 19

total no. of e^- = 19+1 (from –ve charge) = 20

83. **(d) :** Boron sesquioxide B_2O_3 is used in making borosilicates, heat resistant pyrex glass. Pyrex glass contains 14% B_2O_3.

84. **(d) :** Mohr salt is $Fe(SO_4) \cdot (NH_4)_2SO_4 \cdot 6H_2O$.

85. **(b), (c) :** According to Avogadro hypothesis, the mass of 22.4 L of the vapour of any volatile substance at NTP is equal to the molecular mass of the substance.

86. **(c) :** Formaldehyde does not contain α-hydrogen so will not undergo Aldol condensation.

87. **(d) :** Heterolytic fission : unequal distribution of bonded pair of e^- after cleavage.

$$A-B \longrightarrow \underset{\text{Anion}}{A^{\ominus}} + \underset{\text{Cation}}{B^{\oplus}}$$

88. **(a) :** In general, electron affinity decreases down the group. But due to inter-electronic repulsions in small sized F-atom, chlorine has got larger E.A. than that of F.

89. **(b) :** Fuel cell *e.g.*

$H_2(g) + O_2(g) \longrightarrow 2H_2O(l)$

90. **(b) :** Aspirin (Acetyl salicylic acid) is obtained by heating salicylic acid (o-hydroxy benzoic acid) with acetyl chloride and glacial acetic acid.

$$\underset{\text{Salicylic acid}}{C_6H_4(OH)COOH} + CH_3COCl \xrightarrow[CH_3COOH]{\text{Pyridine}} \underset{\text{Aspirin}}{C_6H_4(OCOCH_3)COOH}$$

91. **(c) :** Ionisation energy for Na is very low as compared to other alkaline earth metal or transition elements. So it acts as a good reducing agent.

92. **(c) :** Mass no. = No. of protons + No. of neturons

No. of protons = No. of electrons

$\Rightarrow$ No. of protons = 18

$\Rightarrow$ Mass No. = 20 + 18 = 38

93. **(c) :** SO_3 acts as strong oxidising agent. *e.g.*

$2SO_3 + S \xrightarrow{100°C} 3SO_2$

$5SO_3 + 2P \longrightarrow 5SO_2 + P_2O_5$

$SO_3 + HBr \longrightarrow SO_2 + Br_2 + H_2O$

94. **(b) :** When $CHCl_3$ is exposed to sunlight and air, it slowly decomposes into phosgene and hydrogen chloride.

$$Cl-\overset{Cl}{\overset{|}{\underset{Cl}{\underset{|}{C}}}}-H + [O] \xrightarrow[\text{air}]{\text{light}} Cl-\overset{Cl}{\overset{|}{\underset{Cl}{\underset{|}{C}}}}-OH \longrightarrow HCl + \underset{\text{(Phosgene gas)}}{Cl_2C=O}$$

95. **(b) :** Modern periodic table (*i.e.* long form of table) is based on the periodic law which says that physical and chemical properties of the elements are periodic function of their atomic numbers.

96. **(a) :** $2\ KO_2 + CO_2 \rightarrow K_2CO_3 + \frac{3}{2}O_2$.

97. **(d) :** Ag^+ can accept electron pair so it acts as lewis acid.

98. **(c) :** Iodoform test is positive for ethanol (not for methanol)

$$CH_3CH_2OH \xrightarrow[KOH]{I_2} \underset{\text{Iodoform}}{CHI_3} + HCOO^-K^+$$

99. **(a) :** A catalyst speeds up the reaction both in forward and backward direction, maintaining the equilibrium constant same.

100. (b) : Gypsum : $CaSO_4 \cdot 2H_2O$

Plaster of paris : $CaSO_4 \cdot \frac{1}{2} H_2O$.

$$CaSO_4 \cdot 2H_2O \xrightarrow{120°C} CaSO_4 \cdot \frac{1}{2} H_2O + \frac{3}{2} H_2O$$

101. (a) : Alkaline $KMnO_4$ solution is called Baeyer's reagent and is used for characterisation of olefinic bond in the compound. Purple colour of $KMnO_4$ disappears and brown ppt. due to MnO_2 appears.

$$>C=C< + \underset{\text{(Purple)}}{MnO_4^-} \longrightarrow -\overset{|}{\underset{|}{C}}-\overset{|}{\underset{|}{C}}- + \underset{\text{(Brown ppt)}}{MnO_2}$$

102. (b) : $\frac{\text{Equivalent weight of metal}}{\text{Equivalent weight of compound}} = \frac{\text{Weight of metal}}{\text{Weight of compound}}$

$$\Rightarrow \frac{12}{12+35.5} = \frac{\text{Weight of metal}}{0.475}$$

$\Rightarrow$ Weight of metal = 0.12 g

103. (b) : No. of mole of $O_2 = \frac{\text{Mass}}{\text{Mol. mass}} = \frac{40}{32}$
$= 1.25$ mol

No. of mole of He $= \frac{40}{4} = 10$ mol

mole fraction of $O_2 = \frac{1.25}{1.25+10} = \frac{1.25}{11.25} = \frac{1}{9}$

Partial Pressure of Oxygen $= \frac{1}{9} \times 0.9$ atm.
$= 0.1$ atm.

104. (d) : According to Goldberg and wage, and rate at which substance reacts is directly proportional to its active mass (*i.e.* molar concentration);
$aA + bB = xX + yY$

$K_c = \frac{[X]^x [Y]^y}{[A]^a [B]^b}$ K_c = equilibrium constant

105. (c) : Atomic wt. of metal $= 2 \times 12$
$= 24$

$\therefore$ mol. wt. of its oxide $= 24 + 16$
$= 40$

106. (b) : The Heisenberg uncertainty principle, $\Delta x \times \Delta p \le \frac{h}{4\pi}$, where Δx = Uncertainty in position, Δp = Uncertainty in momentum and $\frac{h}{4\pi}$ = constant.

As Δx is same for electron and helium and $\frac{h}{4\pi}$ is a constant, therefore minimum uncertainty in the measurement of the momentum of the helium atom will be same as that of an electron which is 5.0×10^{-26} kg/ms^{-1}.

107. (b) : Dalton's theory say that an atom is the smallest and indivisible component of all materials.

108. (d) : de Broglie relation is $(\lambda) = \frac{h}{mv} = \frac{h}{p}$, where m = mass, v = velocity, p = momentum, λ = wavelength.

109. (c) : This is the statement of third law of thermodynamics. In a perfect crystal, at absolute zero temperature, each constituent of lattice must have the lowest energy, so it leads to perfect order, therefore zero entropy.

110. (d) : HO–S(→O)(↓O)–OH   O←S(=O)(–O–)... (O=O with coordinate bond to S, ↓O)

All of them therefore contain co-ordinate bonding.

111. (a) The elements of group III have $ns^2\ np^1$, configuration. Since *p*–electrons are held less tightly than *s*–electrons. The first IE of each element is low as compared to the first IE of alkaline earth metal.

112. (c) : Chain isomerism occurs due to difference in the arrangement of C–atoms in the chain. Simplest compound exhibiting chain Isomerism is butane. e.g.

$CH_3CH_2CH_2CH_3$ $CH_3-\overset{\overset{CH_3}{|}}{CH}-CH_3$

n – butane   *Iso* butane

All carbon atoms in all alkanes are sp^3 hybridised.

113. (a) : Acidified $KMnO_4$ is reduced by acidic SO_2.

$[SO_2 + 2H_2O \rightarrow H_2SO_4 + 2H]\ 5$

$[2H + O \rightarrow H_2O] \times 5$

$2KMnO_4 + 3H_2SO_4 \rightarrow K_2SO_4 + 2MnSO_4 + 3H_2O + 5[O]$

$2KMnO_4 + 5SO_2 + 2H_2O \rightarrow K_2SO_4 + 2MnSO_4 + 2H_2SO_4$

114. (c) : Helium : Z = 2; $1s^2$
Berylium : Z = 4; $1s^2, 2s^2$

Helium is an inert gas while beryllium is reactive due to unfilled 2*p* valence shells.

115. (a) Intermolecular force of attraction involves dipole-dipole and weak van der waal's forces in the Ionic compounds.

116. (a) : H_2SO_4 when react with NaBr and NaI, give out Br_2 and I_2 as concentrated H_2SO_4 is a strong oxidising agent.

117. (a) : Due to the presence of lone pair of electrons on oxygen atoms, ether behave as base and form stable oxonium salts with mineral acids.

$$C_2H_5OC_2H_5 + HCl \longrightarrow C_2H_5\overset{\oplus}{\underset{H}{O}}C_2H_5Cl^-$$

Diethyl oxonium chloride

118. (a) : Adsorption is an exothermic process, the heat of adsorption is taken up by the surface of the catalyst which is utilised in enhancing the chemical activity of the reacting molecule.

119. (a)

120. (a) : Due to their high reactivity, halogens are not found in free state.

BIOLOGY

121. (a) : At the time of cartilage formation, chondrification starts in mesenchymal cells and chondroblast cells are formed at the centre of chondrification. Then chondroblasts become entrapped in the extracellular matrix that they secrete, they are now known as chondrocytes. With this entrapment cartilage begins to form.

Mesenchymal cells → chondroblasts → chondrocytes → cartilage

122. (b) : Achondroplasia is a defect in the formation of cartilage at the epiphyses of long bones, producing a form of dwarfism.

123. (c) : Philadelphia chromosome is an abnormal chromosome-21 that has lost part of its long arm. It is found in leukocyte culture of many patients with chronic myelocytic leukaemia.

124. (d) : Diabetes insipidus is the inability of the kidneys to respond to vasopressin. Vasopressin is released in response to a fall in the water content of blood plasma and leads to an increase in the permeability to water of the distal and collecting tubules of the nephron in the kidney. As a result of which the reabsorption of water from the glomerular filtrate is increased. Diabetes insipidus is characterized by micturating dilute urine several times a day.

125. (d) : Cholesterol is the precursor of steroid hormones possessing a complex basic structure.

Structure of cholesterol

126. (a) : Mesozoic era is the middle era in the geological time scale, dating from about 230-270 million years ago. It is known as the 'Age of Reptiles'. It is divided into three main periods, *i.e.* Triassic, Jurassic and Cretaceous.

127. (a) : Colour blindness, in which all colours are perceived as grey, is termed monochromasia. The person suffering from this disease is completely colour blind.

128. (d) : Stratum corneum is the outermost layer of epidermis of man. Its cells are dead, flattened and dry, containing a high proportion of the protein. It provides the main protection of the body against water loss and the entry of disease causing organisms.

129. (a) : Archaeocytes of sponges are short and blunt, with lobose pseudopodia, a large nucleus and a large quantity of RNA. These are considered to be the undifferentiated 'totipotent' cells, which may transform into all other types of cells including sex cells.

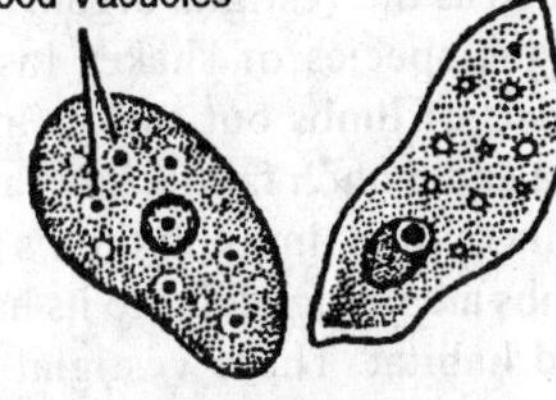

Archaeocytes

130. (b) : The surface of cartilage is surrounded by irregular connective tissue forming the perichondrium.

131. (a) : Each ramus of lower jaw or mandible is formed of a single large membrane bone (dentary), which is broad and flat in the back but narrow and conical in front. The front ends of both dentaries medially join by a symphysis.

132. (c) : Haemophilia is recessive character and is therefore masked in heterozygous condition.

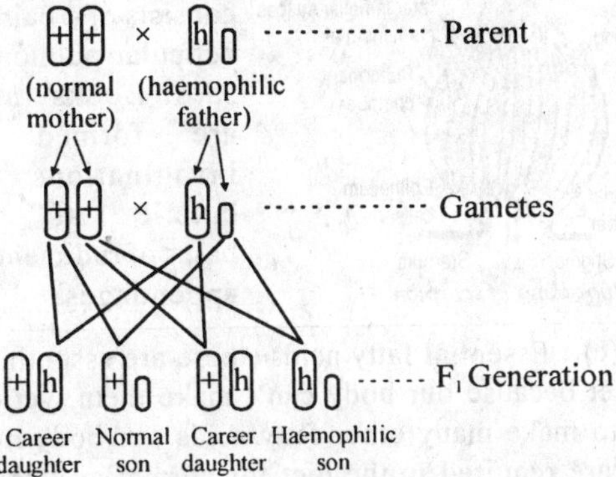

Thus the daughters born to heamophilic father and normal mother would be career but phenotypically normal.

133. (a) : During malaria, RBCs of man gets somewhat enlarged and irregular in shape. A number of orange or yellow eosinophilic granules of unknown nature, called Schuffner's dots appear in its cytoplasm.

134. (a) : Sarcomere is a contractile element in a striated muscle fibril (myofibril). Each sarcomere is joined to the next one by Krause's membrane (Z-line).

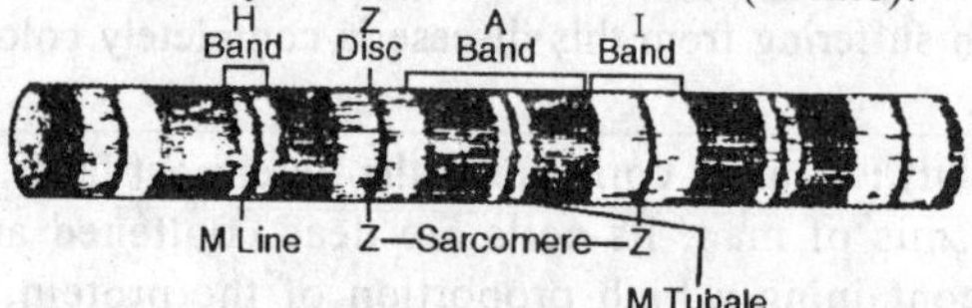

Striated muscle fibril

135. (a) : Python have hind limbs as the vestigial organ. Most of the species of shakes lost all traces of limbs but snakes in the boa and python family have a tiny pairs of hind limbs. Python's hind limbs are vestigial due to its habits and habitat. These vestigial legs can actually be seen as a pair of spur's that sticks out where the body ends and tail begins. These legs rarely do any harm.

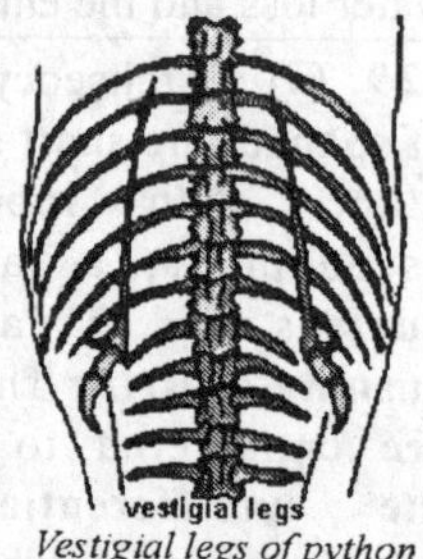

Vestigial legs of python

136. (c) : Trigeminal nerve (cranial nerve V) is one of the pairs of nerves that arise from the anterior end of the vertebrate hindbrain to supply impulses to the mouth and the jaws. It carries sensory nerve fibres from the head surface and mouth cavity and motor nerve fibres serving the jaw muscles.

137. (d) : The respiratory organ of scorpion is book lung. It consists of 4 pairs of cuticular pulmonary sacs. Books lungs are formed by invaginations of cuticle at the bases of rudimentary appendages.

Blood
Pulmonary vein
Lamellae containing blood
Inter lamellar spaces containing air
Pulmonary chamber
Atrial chamber
Epithelium cells
Stigma
Air
Sternum

Book lungs of scorpion

138. (c) : Essential fatty acids (these are essential in our diet because our body can't make them, yet use them to make many other fatty acids our body must have) are required in the diet for normal growth. In mammals, the deficiency of linoleic and gamma-linolenic acid causes poor growth, scaly skin, hair loss and eventually death.

139. (a) : Anoxia is a deficiency in oxygen reaching the tissues that is severe enough to damage the brain permanently.

140. (a) Glissonian cirrhosis is inflammation of peritoneal coat of the liver.

141. (d) : Liver does not produce any digestive enzyme though it helps in digestion by formation of bile, helping in fat metabolism, by storing and releasing carbohydrate etc.

142. (b) : Zonula adherens is a kind of desmosome, which comprises of band of contractile actin filaments near the apical end of each epithelial cell, just under the cell membrane.

143. (d) : Lymphoid tissue (lymphatic tissue) is found in the lymph nodes, tonsils, thymus and spleen. It produces lymphocytes, which have a life span of only a few days and must be constantly replaced.

144. (a) : During transport, most of CO_2 is passed into erythrocytes. A major part (nearly 70%) forms carbonic acid and then bicarbonate.

$$CO_2 + H_2O \rightleftharpoons H_2CO_3 \rightleftharpoons H^+ + HCO_3^- \quad (\leftrightarrow Cl^-)$$

$$\downarrow$$

$$HHb \rightleftharpoons H^+ + Hb^-$$

A seizable portion of bicarbonate passes out into the plasma in return from chloride (Cl^-). It is called chloride shift or Hamburger's phenomenon.

145. (c) : Venous pathway comprising the hepatic portal vein, carries blood rich in absorbed food materials, such as glucose and amino acids, from intestine to the liver. These materials may be stored, converted or released to the general circulation via the hepatic vein.

146. (d) : *Peritrichous* bacterial cell bears a large number of flagella which are distributed evenly all over the cell surface. *Proteus vulagaris* and *Bacillus typhosus* are the common examples.

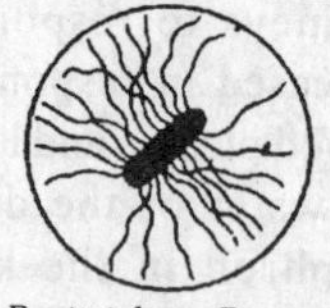

Peritrichous Bacteria

147. (b) : "Allele" is a term which indicates alternative forms of the same gene. For example "D" and "d" are two *allelomorphs* of the gene for plant height. In pure tall or pure dwarf plants, same allele is duplicated (DD or dd), while in hybrid tall both the alleles will be present (Dd). An individual is having only one allele or in other words two identical alleles, is known as *homozygous* (DD or dd). Similarly, an individual, having two different alleles will be called *heterozygous* or hybrid (Dd). Phenotype is observable or measurable distinctive structural or functional characteristic of an individual with regard to one or more characters which is a result of gene products brought to expression in a given enviroment.

148. (c) : Bentham and Hooker's system of classification first appeared in a three - volume book in Latin, named *Genera Plantarum*. The system is based on groups of plant characters which are correlated with each other.

149. (a) : The aggregate of all the genes and their alleles present in an interbreeding population is known as gene pool. Genome is a complete set of chromosomes where every gene / chromosome is represented singly as in a gamete. In bacteria the heredity material is mainly made of spherical or cylindrical structure called nucleoid (genophore).

150. (d) : Transcription is synthesis of RNA, made up of a partricular sequence of nucleotides, by matching with DNA, made up of a corresponding sequence of nucleotides. Translation is synthesis of a polypeptide made up of a particular sequence of amino acids by matching with an RNA made up of a corresponding sequence of nucleotides. Replication is production by duplication of exact copies of complex molecules, such as must occur during the growth and reproduction of any living thing. The only biological molecule in which the original molecules serve as a direct method for the construction of the new DNA. Transduction is the process in which usually a bacteriophage picks up DNA from one bacteria cell and incorporated into another host genome.

151. (d) : The number of linkage groups present in an individual corresponds to number of chromosomes in its one genome (all the chromosomes if haploid or homologous pairs if diploid). It is known as principle of limitation of linkage groups. Maize has 10 linkage groups, as it has 10 pairs of chromosomes.

152. (a) : Genome is the complete but single set of chromosomes as found in gametes or gametophytic cells where each chromosome is represented single. Linkage is the phenomenon of certain genes staying together during inheritance through generations without any change or separation due to their being present on the same chromosome. Gene pool is the aggregate of all the genes and their alleles present in an interbreeding population. Genotype is the gene complement or genetic constitution of an individual with regard to one or more characters irrespective of whether the genes are expressed or not.

153. (c) : In most cases the initiating codon is AUG, which otherwise codes for methionine. The corresponding codon on *m*RNA is usually AUG, but rarely it could be GUG also. When GUG is used as the initiating codon, it does not code valine, but initiating methionine molecule should be found in the formylated methionine.

154. (b) : The phytochrome is a pigment involved in the perception of photoperiodic stimuli controlling flowering, lettuce seed germination and other morphogenetic phenomena. Phytochrome is a protein with a chromophore prosthetic group that resembles, in basic structure, the open - chain tetrapyrrole chromophore of the algal pigment 6 - phycocyanin.

155. (d) : In the phenomenon of epistasis, two independent non-allelic genes affect the same trait of individual in such a way that one overmasks the expression of other. Epistasis can be of the following types - (i) due to recessive allele : *a* masks the effect of *B*, due to a dominant allele : *A* masks the effect of *B*.

156. (b) : A small group of xerophytic species,e.g., *Selaginella lepidophylla* and *S.pilifera*, are cespitose in habit and when dry they coil closely together their rosette like shoots, by a cohesion mechanism, to form a ball-like structure and quickly unroll into a graceful green plant when moisture is readily available. Such plants are sold as curiosities under the name of "resurrection plants".

157. (c) : Transposons are movable genetic elements, which are somewhat similar to a jumping gene. Actually, they are not exactly jumping genes (discovered by Barbara Mc Clintok in maize). They are found in bacteria. Unlike jumping genes, they leave a copy of themselves in the original position when they move to a new site. This phenomenon is significant in antibiotic resistance.

158. (a) : Seismonasty is a nastic movement. When any organ of *Mimosa pudica* is touched, the stimulus reaches the base of the leaf. Owing to this stimulus, the turgor of lower half of pulvinus is lost and the leaf droops down.

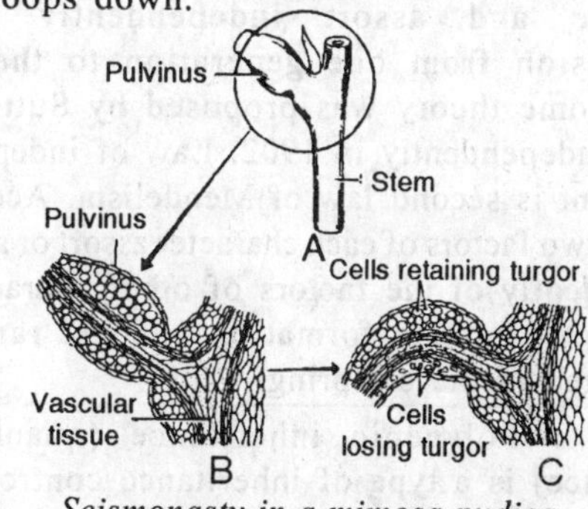

Seismonasty in a mimosa pudica

159. (b) : In some flowers, there is a group of plants which set seeds without exposing their sex organs. Such flowers are called cleistogamous and the phenomenon cleistogamy. Dichogamy refers to maturation of male and female sex organs at different times. Heterogamy term is used for cross - pollination.

160. (b) : Zygotene stage of meiosis is characterised by pairing of homologous chromosomes (synapsis). This pairing is brought about in a zipperlike fashion and may start at centromere, at chromosome ends or at any other position. Two homologous chromosomes are called bivalent while they are pairing during meiosis. The homologous chromosomes break their connection and separate out during Anaphase 1 of meiosis. The process of separation is named as disjunction. Synergids are elongated cells present at the micropylar end of the embryo sac.

161. (d) : Gram is *Cicer arietinum* of leguminosae family. *Rhizobium* forms nodules on the roots of legume plants. They develop the ability to fix nitrogen only when they are present inside the root nodules.

162. (b) : A polygene is defined as a gene where a dominant allele controls only a unit or partial quantitative expression of a trait. In polygenic inheritance, a cross between two pure breeding parents does not produce dominant trait of one parent but instead an intermediate trait is exhibited. The Law of segregation is the first law of Mendelism. According to it, the two factors of a character which remain together in an individual do not get mixed up but keep their identity distinct, separate at the time of gametogenesis or sporogensis, get randomly distributed to different gametes and then get paired again in different offspring as per the principle of probability. Chromosomal theory of inheritance believes that chromosomes are vehicles of hereditary information, possess Mendelism factors or genes, segregate and assort independently during transmission from one generation to the next. chromosome theory was proposed by Sutton and Boveri independently in 1902. Law of independent assortment is second law of Mendelism. According to it, the two factors of each character assort or separate independently of the factors of other characters at the time of gamete formation and get randomly re-arranged in the offspring.

163. (c) : Polygenic inheritance (quantitative inheritance) is a type of inheritance controlled by one or more genes in which the dominant alleles have cumulative effect with each dominant alleles expressing a part or unit of the trait, the full trait being shown only when all the dominant alleles are present. The genes involved in quantitative inheritance are called polygenes. Polygenic inheritance is further characterised by the occurrence of inheritance forms (continuous variations) between the parental types.Linkage is the phenomenon of certain genes staying together during inheritance through generations without any change or separation due to their being present on the same chromosome. Epistasis is the phenomenon by which a gene suppresses the phenotypic expression of a nonallelic gene. Recombination is the new combination of genes which is possible only due to exchange of genetic material between homologous chromosome.

164. (b) : When the double helix of DNA unwinds, DNA replication on one of the two strands (3' to 5' strand) can easily proceeds continuously in 5' to 3' direction. This is the leading strand. On the other strand (5' - 3') if the synthesis has to take place in 5' to 3' direction, it has to be synthesized in a direction opposite to that on the leading strands. This strand is the lagging strand and on this strand synthesis takes place in segments discontinuously and these segments are then fused to create an intact lagging strand. This behaviour where the leading strand is synthesized continuously and the lagging strand is synthesized discontinuously is calld semi - discontinuous replication.

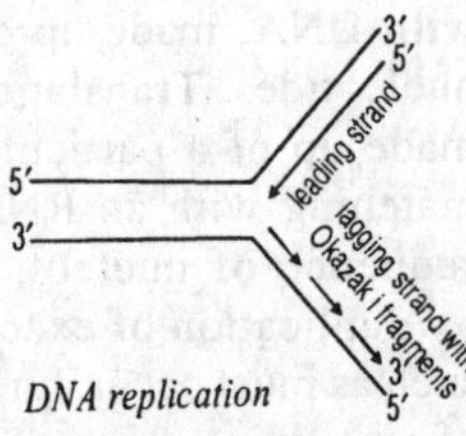

DNA replication

165. (b) : *Parkinsonia aculeata* is a xerophyte. In *Parkinsonia aculeata,* the rachis ends in a spine. Rachis branches are elongated, flattened and green to function as *phyllodes*. They bear small leaflets which fall off very early. Winged fruit has special flat ourgrowths or wings, shows dispersal by wind. In *Cypsela*, the hairy pappus functions as umbrella of parachute. Phylloclades are flattened green stems of unlimited growth which have taken over the function of photosynthesis.

166. (c) : In Biparous or Dichasial Cyme, a terminal flower is subtended by two lateral branches which also end in flowers. The process is repeated. Cyathium has a small conical

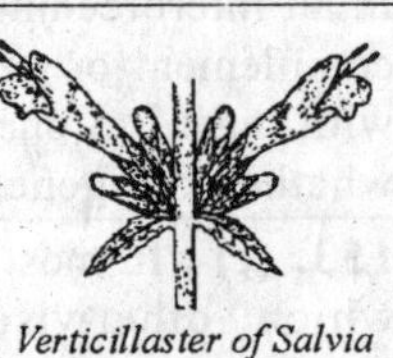
Verticillaster of Salvia

receptacle surrounded by an involucre of generally five green or coloured bracts having nectariferous glands. Internally, the inflorescence contains pedicellate achlamydeous and unisexual flowers of both the types, male and female. Verticillaster is an inflorescence which has two clusters, each having 3 - 9 flowers, develop on a node in the axils of opposite leaves. Each cluster consists of a dichasial cyme with monochasial branches. Thyrsus is cymose clusters borne acropetally on an axis.

167. (c) : Myxophyceae is the older name of cyanophyceae or blue-green algae (according to Fritsch's classification).

168. (d) : The term 'coenobium' means united life. All the cells of *Volvox* act in union particularly in movement.

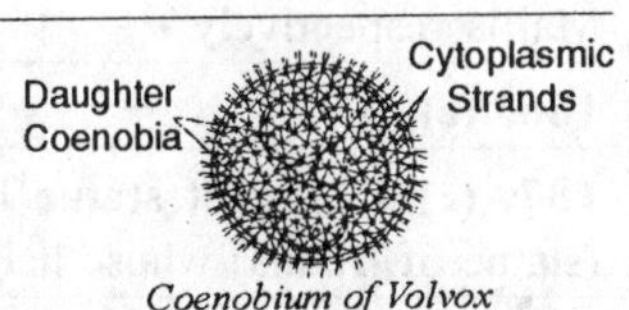

Coenobium of Volvox

169. (d) : Nucleoid consists of a single circular strand of DNA duplex which is repeatedly folded with the help of RNA to form a nearly compact oval or spherical structure. DNA is naked,i.e., it is not associated with histone proteins. There is no organised membrane through mesosome.

170. (d) : The five kingdom classification of whittaker has the following characteristics.
As the viruses are on the border line of living and nonliving matter, they have been left out.
Monera was the kingdom of prokarytes,
Protista - kingdom of unicellular eukaryotes,
Fungi - kingdom of multicellular decomposers,
Plantae - kingdom of multicellular producers or Metaphyta and
Animalia is the kingdom of multicellular consumers or Metazoa.

171. (c) : Cholera is an acute infections disease which is caused by *Vibrio cholerae*. The stools and the vomit of a cholera patient are full of cholera germs and these may get into a healthy person when contaminated food or drink is taken by mouth. Since a large quantity of fluid and salts are rapidly lost through stools and vomit, therefore, the most important treatment is to replace the lost fluid and salts equally rapidly.

172. (a) : The first polio vaccine was prepared by Jones Salk (1953) at university of Pitsburg by killing polio virus with formaldehyde. The killed virus is called "salk vaccine" and injected to develop immunity. Sabin *et al* prepared an oral vaccine known as OPV (oral polio vaccine).

173. (c) **174. (a)**

175. (a) : Haemophilia is a X - linked disease. As a person receives X chromosome from mother and Y from father, therefore the person may be a haemophilic if his mother is carrier of the disease. The person will be certainly haemophilic if his mother is haemophilic.

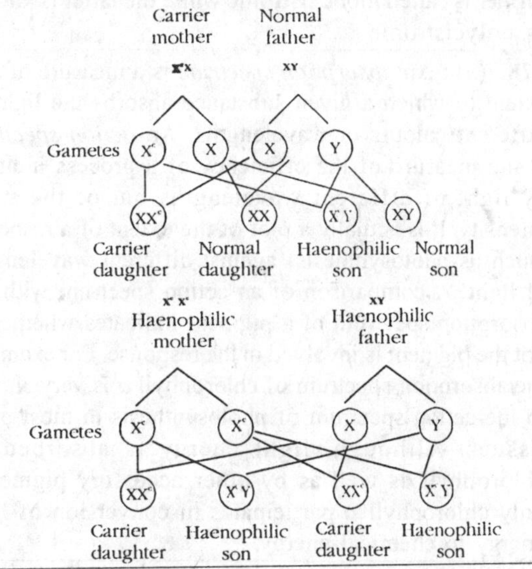

176. (c) : C_3 plants exclusively fix CO_2 *via* the Calvin-Benson pathway. The leaf cells of C_4 plants possess two types of chloroplast, bundle sheath cells and mesophyll cells. The mesophyll cells of C_4 plants exhibit high activity of phosphoenolpyruvate (PEP) carboxylase, which catalyses the fixation of CO_2 with PEP to form oxaloacetic acid. The bundle sheath cells exhibit high RuBP carboxylase and the other enzymes of the Calvin-Benson cycle. C_4 plants are highly productive photosynthetically in view of the low affinity of RuBP carboxylase for its substrate. But CO_2 is concentrated as C_4 acids due to the activity of the PEP carboxylase, which in effect maintains high pool levels of CO_2. C_4 plants is related to very high light-harvesting saturation points. C_4 plants exhibit low rates of photorespiration only in bundle sheath cells. C_4 plants are adapted to high temperature. C_4 plants show better utilization of available water but it cannot be the cause of its higher productivity.

177. (b) : *m*RNA brings instructions from the DNA for the formation of particular type of polypeptide. The instructions are present in the base sequence of its nucleotides. *m*RNAhas methylated region at the 5′ terminus. It functions as a cap for attachment with ribosome. Cap is followed by an initiation codon (AUG) either immediately or after a small non-coding region. Then there is coding region followed by termination codon (UAA, UAG or UGA). An *m*RNA may specify only a single polypeptide or a number of them. The former is called monocistronic while the latter is known as polycistronic.

178. (a) : An *absorption spectrum* is a measure of the extent to which a given substance absorbs the light of different colours or wavelengths. An *action spectrum* is the measure of the efficiency of a process induced by light of different wavelengths but of the same intensity. It is actually a plot of the extent of a response (such as photosynthesis) against different wavelengths of light. A comparison of an action spectrum with the absorption spectrum of a pigment indicates whether or not the pigment is involved in the response. For example, the absorption spectrum of chlorophyll *a* is very similar to the action spectrum of photosynthesis in most plant tissues. Although, light energy is absorbed by chlorophyll as well as by other accessory pigments, only chlorophyll *a* participates in conversion of light energy to chemical energy.

179. (a) : Linkage is association of two or more non-allelomorphic genes, so that they tend to be passed from generation to generation as an inseparable unit and fail to show independent assortment due to their being in same chromosome. Separation of such genes into different chromosomes occurs from time to time as a result of crossing-over. The nearer such genes are to each other on a chromosome the less often closely linked they are said to be. Red hair and freckles are examples of linkage.

180. (b) : Variations in the structure and number of chromosomes are called chromosomal aberrations. Strucural changes can be of following types : (i) *deficiency*, which involves loss of a part of chromosome, (ii) *duplication*, which involves addition of a part chromosome, (iii) *inversion* which involves a reverse order of the genes in a part of chromosome and (iv) translocation, which involves exchange of segments between non - homologous chromosomes.

GENERAL KNOWLEDGE

181. (a) : The world biggest airport at Dallas (Taxas) is situated in U.S.A. and it covers over 7000 hectares.

182. (d)

183. (b) : White paper is the policy statement published by the governments on the subjects of great public importance.

184. (d)

185. (a) : The parliaments of Spain, Bangladesh, Nepal and Iran are Crotes, Jatiya Sansad, Panchayat and Majlis respectively.

186. (c)

187. (c) : Largest statue is situated in Hyderabad (statue of Budha) whose height is 17·3 metres.

188. (c)

189. (c) : Marco polo, Fahein, Macmillan and Alexander the great are the first European to visit China, first chinese pilgrim who came to India, first British Prime Minister to visit India and first European invander of Indian soil respectively.

190. (b)

191. (a) : The heights of Everest, Godwin austen, Kanchanjunga and Mukahi are 8848 m, 8611 m, 8535 m and 8470 m respectively.

192. (b):

193. (c) : The longest railway tunnel is situated in Japan. The length of the tunnel is 21kilometres.

194. (c)

195. (c) : 'Calicut' which is situated about 65 kilometres from tellicherry, is re-named as Kozhikode.

196. (d)

197. (c) : Portblair, Silvasa, Kavaratti and Kohima are the capitals of Andman and Nicobar, Dadar and Nagar Haveli, Lakshadweep and Nagaland respectively.

198. (d)

199. (a) : Wheat, gram, oil seeds etc. ar ethe rabi crops but groundnut is the jayad crop.

200. (d)

SOLVED PAPER
AIIMS - 1995

Time : 3½ Hours Max. Marks : 200

PHYSICS

1. The velocity of photons is proportional to (where υ = frequency)
(a) $1/\sqrt{\upsilon}$ (b) υ
(c) υ^2 (d) $\sqrt{\upsilon}$.

2. Susçeptibility is positive for
(a) non-magnetic substances
(b) paramagnetic substances
(c) diamagnetic substances
(d) ferromagnetic substances.

3. Two particles are seen to collide and move jointly together after the collision. During such a collision, for the total system,
(a) both the mechanical energy and the linear momentum are conserved
(b) linear momentum is conserved but not the mechanical energy
(c) neither the mechanical energy nor the linear momentum is conserved
(d) mechanical energy is conserved but not the linear momentum.

4. The power factor varies between
(a) 0 to 1 (b) 2 and 2.5
(c) 1 to 2 (d) 3.5 to 5.

5. A metal rod at a temperature of 150°C, radiates energy at a rate of 20 W. If its temperature is increased to 300°C, then it will radiate at the rate of
(a) 40.8 W (b) 17.5 W
(c) 68.3 W (d) 37.2 W.

6. The radius vector, drawn from the Sun to a planet sweeps out equal areas in equal lines. This is the statement of
(a) Kepler's third law
(b) Kepler's first law
(c) Newton's third law
(d) Kepler's second law.

7. A tin nucleus has charge +50*e*. If the proton is at 10^{-12} m, from the nucleus, then the potential at this position, is (charge on proton is 1.6×10^{-19} C)
(a) 7.2×10^8 V (b) 14.4×10^4 V
(c) 14.4×10^8 V (d) 7.2×10^4 V.

8. According to Bohr's principle, the relation between principal quantum number (*n*) and radius of orbit, is
(a) $r \propto \frac{1}{n}$ (b) $r \propto n$
(c) $r \propto \frac{1}{n^2}$ (d) $r \propto n^2$.

9. The α-rays are
(a) electromagnetic radiation
(b) stream of electrons
(c) stream of uncharged particles
(d) stream of positively charged particles.

10. The internal resistance of a cell of e.m.f. 2 volts is 0.1 Ω. It is connected to a resistance of 3.9 Ω. The voltage across the cell will be (in volts)
(a) 1.95 V (b) 0.5 V
(c) 2 V (d) 1.9 V.

11. If a p-n diode is reverse biased, then the resistance measured by an ohm-meter, will be
(a) high (b) zero
(c) infinite (d) low.

12. A nucleus of $_4Be^9$ absorbs an alpha particle and emits a neutron. The resulting nucleus will be
(a) $_5C^{13}$ (b) $_6C^{12}$
(c) $_6C^{13}$ (d) $_4BE^8$.

13. The logic circuit given in the figure performs the logic operation

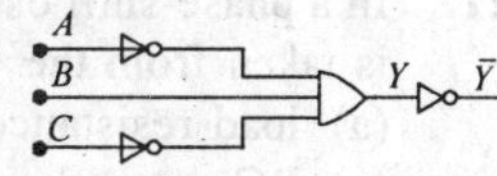

(a) ABC (b) $AB\overline{C}$

(c) $A\bar{B}C$ (d) $\bar{A}B\bar{C}$.

14. Ten identical wires each having a resistance of one ohm are connected in parallel. The combination will have a resistance of

(a) $0.1\ \Omega$ (b) $10\ \Omega$

(c) $0.01\ \Omega$ (d) $1\ \Omega$.

15. Radius of gyration of a body depends upon

(a) shape of the body (b) axis of rotation

(c) area of the body (d) translation motion.

16. A body weighed 250 N on the surface assuming the earth to be a sphere of uniform mass density, how much would it weigh half way down to the centre of the earth?

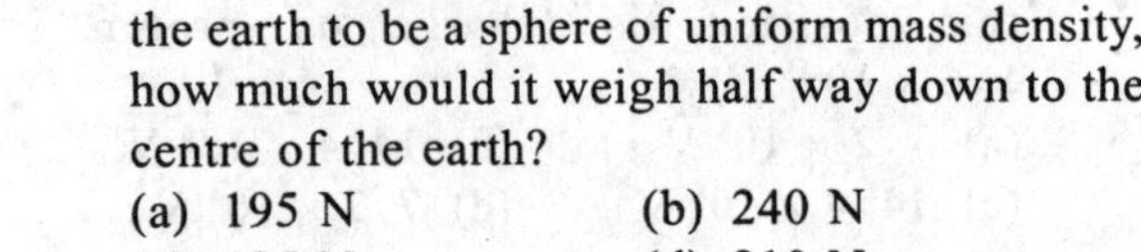

(a) 195 N (b) 240 N

(c) 125 N (d) 210 N.

17. Which of the following relation is called as current density ?

(a) $\frac{I^2}{A}$ (b) $\frac{A}{I}$

(c) $\frac{I^3}{A^2}$ (d) $\frac{I}{A}$.

18. The motion of a rocket is based on the principle of conservation of

(a) linear momentum

(b) mass

(c) angular momentum

(d) kinetic energy.

19. Crystalline solids are

(a) amporphus (b) anistropic

(c) isotropic (d) none of these.

20. The moment of inertia of a disc of mass M and radius R about an axis which is tangential to the circumference of the disc and parallel to its diameter, is

(a) $\frac{5}{4}MR^2$ (b) $\frac{3}{2}MR^2$

(c) $\frac{4}{5}MR^2$ (d) $\frac{2}{3}MR^2$.

21. In a phase-shift oscillator, the positive feedback is taken from the

(a) load resistance (b) anode directly

(c) RC networks (d) grid and anode.

22. A certain mass of gas at 273 K is expanded to 81 times its volume under adiabatic conditions. If $\gamma = 1.25$ for the gas then its final temperature is

(a) -182°C (b) 0°C

(c) -235°C (d) -91°C.

23. What is the equivalent resistance between A and B in the given figure

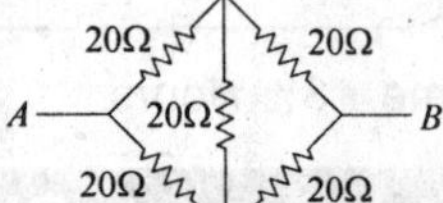

(a) $40\ \Omega$

(b) $10\ \Omega$

(c) $50\ \Omega$

(d) $20\ \Omega$.

24. An X-ray beam of wavelength 10^{-10} m falls on a crystal of atomic spacing 2×10^{-10} m. The Bragg angle for the second order reflection will be

(a) 45° (b) 15°

(c) 60° (d) 30°.

25. Curie temperature of iron is the temperature below which, it is

(a) ferromagnetic (b) radioactive

(c) dimagnetic (d) superconducting.

26. The heat produced by a 100 W heater in 2 min. is equal to

(a) 10.5 kcal (b) 16.3 kcal

(c) 2.8 kcal (d) 14.2 kcal.

27. Simple capacitor filters are good for

(a) high current supply

(b) low voltage supply

(c) low voltage and high current supply

(d) low current supply.

28. If two lenses of power + 1.5 D and + 1.0 D are placed in contact, then the effective power of combination will be

(a) 4.5 D (b) 2.5 D

(c) 5.4 D (d) 4.2 D.

29. It is possible to have a positively charged body at

(a) positive potential (b) zero potential

(c) negative potential (d) all of these.

30. For an enclosure maintained at 1000 K, the maximum radiation occurs at wavelength λ_m. If the temperature is raised to 2000 K, the peak will shift to

(a) $\frac{5}{2}\lambda_m$ (b) $\frac{1}{2}\lambda_m$

(c) $\frac{7}{2}\lambda_m$ (d) $\frac{3}{2}\lambda_m$.

31. Time period of pendulum, on a satellite orbiting the earth, is
(a) $1/\pi$ (b) zero
(c) π (d) infinity.

32. The periodic time of a body executing SHM is 4 sec. After how much interval from time $t = 0$, its displacement will be half of its amplitude ?
(a) $\frac{1}{4}$ sec (b) $\frac{1}{2}$ sec
(c) $\frac{1}{6}$ sec (d) $\frac{1}{3}$ sec .

33. An intrinsic semiconductor, at the absolute zero temperature, behaves like a/an
(a) n-type semiconductor
(b) insulator
(c) p-type semiconductor
(d) superconductor.

34. A body of mass 5 kg is raised vertically to a height of 10 m by a force of 170 N. The velocity of the body at this height will be
(a) 15 m/s (b) 37 m/s
(c) 9.8 m/s (d) 22 m/s.

35. Greater accuracy in the determination of the position of a particle with an optical microscope can be had, if the beam of light used
(a) has higher wavelength
(b) is polarised
(c) has higher frequency
(d) has greater intensity.

36. The angular velocity of rotation of a star (of mass M and radius R) at which the matter starts to escape from its equator, is
(a) $\sqrt{\frac{2GM}{R}}$ (b) $\sqrt{\frac{2GR}{M}}$
(c) $\sqrt{\frac{2GM^2}{R}}$ (d) $\sqrt{\frac{2GM}{R^3}}$.

37. The photoelectrons emitted from a given cathode on the incidence of a given monochromatic beam of light, have a/an
(a) energy spread with no sharp limits
(b) energy spread with a lower limit
(c) definite energy only
(d) energy spread with an upper limit.

38. If an electron is brought toward another electron, the electric potential energy of the system
(a) becomes zero (b) increases
(c) remains the same (d) decreases.

39. Which of the following is an essential requirement for initiating the fusion reaction ?
(a) high temperature
(b) critical mass
(c) critical temperature
(d) thermal neutrons.

40. A tube closed at one end containing air produces fundamental note of frequency 512 Hz. If the tube is open at both the ends, the fundamental frequency will be
(a) 1024 Hz (b) 256 Hz
(c) 1280 Hz (d) 768 Hz.

41. Which of the following, when added as impurity into the silicon, produces n-type semi-conductor ?
(a) B (b) P
(c) Mg (d) Al

42. Ten identical cells each of potential E and internal resistance r are connected in series to form a closed circuit. An ideal voltmeter connected across three cells, will read
(a) $10E$ (b) $3E$
(c) $13E$ (d) $7E$.

43. The reactance of an inductance of 0.01 H to a 50 Hz A.C. is
(a) 1.04 Ω (b) 6.28 Ω
(c) 0.59 Ω (d) 3.14 Ω.

44. A ray of light having wavelength 720 nm enters in a glass of refractive index 1.5. The wavelength of the ray within the glass will be
(a) 720 nm (b) 360 nm
(c) 1080 nm (d) 480 nm.

45. A certain radioactive element has a half-life of 20 years. If we have a block with 10 g of the element in it, after how many years will there be just 2.5 g of the element in the block ?
(a) 80 years (b) 40 years
(c) 100 years (d) 60 years.

46. When we heat a gas-sample from 27°C to 327°C, then the initial average kinetic energy, of the molecules was E. What will be the average kinetic energy after heating ?
(a) $2E$ (b) $327E$
(c) $\sqrt{2}\,E$ (d) $300E$.

47. Which of the following is a dimensionless quantity?
(a) specific heat (b) strain
(c) quantity of heat (d) stress.

48. The tension in piano wire is 10 N.What should be the tension in the wire to produce a note of double the frequency ?
(a) 40 N (b) 5 N
(c) 80 N (d) 20 N.

49. An ideal gas is heated from 27°C to 627°C at constant pressure. If initial volume was 4 m^3, then the final volume of the gas will be
(a) 6 m^3 (b) 2 m^3
(c) 12 m^3 (d) 4 m^3.

50. What is the dimensional formula for the gravitational constant ?
(a) $[M^{-1}L^3T^{-2}]$ (b) $[M^{-1}L^3T^{-1}]$
(c) $[M^{-2}L^3T^{-2}]$ (d) $[M^{-2}L^{-1}T^3]$.

Directions: *These questions consist of two statements each, printed as Assertion and Reason. While answering these questions you are required to choose any one of the following four responses.*
(a) If both Assertion and Reason are true and the Reason is a correct explanation of the Assertion.
(b) If both Assertion and Reason are true but Reason is not a correct explanation of the Assertion.
(c) If Assertion is true but the Reason is false.
(d) If both Assertion and Reason are false.

51. *Assertion*: The rainbow is seen sometimes in the sky when it is raining. When one sees a rainbow, one's back is towards the Sun.
Reason: Internal reflection from water droplet causes dispersion. The final ray is in the backward direction.

52. *Assertion*: The sun looks bigger in size at sunrise and sunset than during day.
Reason: The phenomenon of diffraction bends light rays.

53. *Assertion*: On a rainy day, it is difficult to drive a car or bus at high speed.
Reason: The value of coefficient of friction is lowered on wetting the surface.

54. *Assertion*: A normal human eye can clearly see all the objects beyond a certain minimum distance.
Reason: The human eye has the capacity to suitably adjust the focal length of its lens to a certain extent.

55. *Assertion*: Machine parts are jammed in winter.
Reason: The viscosity of lubricant used in machine parts increase at low temperatures.

56. *Assertion*: Electric appliances with metallic body, *e.g.*, heaters have three-pin connection, whereas an electric bulb has a two pin connection.
Reason: Three pin connection reduces heating of connecting cables.

57. *Assertion*: A needle placed carefully on the surface of water may float, whereas a ball of the same material will always sink.
Reason: The buoyancy of an object depends both on the material and shape of the object.

58. *Assertion*: A domestic electrical appliance, working on a three pin, will continue working even if the top pin is removed.
Reason: The third pin is used only as a safety device.

59. *Assertion*: Water kept in an open vessel will quickly evaporate on the surface of the moon.
Reason: The temperature at the surface of the moon is much higher than the boiling point of water.

60. *Assertion*: The comets do not obey Kepler's laws of planetary motion.
Reason: The comets do not have elliptical orbits.

CHEMISTRY

61. How many electrons are delivered at the cathode during electrolysis by a current of 1 A in 60 seconds
(a) $3 \cdot 74 \times 10^{20}$ (b) $6 \cdot 0 \times 10^{23}$
(c) 7.48×10^{21} (d) $6 \cdot 0 \times 10^{20}$.

62. Which of the following compound turns black on the addition of ammonium hydroxide ?
(a) $CuCl_2$ (b) $PbCl_2$
(c) AgCl (d) Hg_2Cl_2.

63. A buffer solution contains 0 · 1 M of acetic acid and 0 · 1 M of sodium acetate. What will be its pH ? (p^{k_a} of acetic acid is 4 · 75)
(a) 5 · 00 (b) 4 · 00
(c) 5 · 25 (d) 4 · 75.

64. By the electrolysis of aqueous solution of $CuSO_4$, the products obtained at both the electrodes are
(a) O_2 at anode and H_2 at cathode
(b) H_2 at anode and Cu at cathode
(c) O_2 at anode and Cu at cathode
(d) $H_2S_2O_8$ at anode and O_2 at cathode.

65. In order to protect, iron from corrosion, the iron is coated with
(a) zinc (b) nickel
(c) tin (d) copper.

66. In $N_2 + 3H_2 \rightarrow 2NH_3$ reversible reaction, increase in pressure will favour
(a) reversible reaction (b) forward direction
(c) irreversible reaction
(d) backward direction.

67. Which of the following complex has square planar structure ?
(a) $[Ni(CN)_4]^{2-}$ (b) $Ni(CO)_4$
(c) $[Zn(NH_3)_4]^{2+}$ (d) $[NiCl_4]^{2-}$.

68. Which of the following is the least stable and its existence is doubtful ?
(a) SnI_4 (b) CI_4
(c) PbI_4 (d) GeI_4.

69. Two different gases enclosed in different flasks A and B at same temperature and pressure were found to contain same number of molecules. The ratio of volumes of the flasks A and B must be
(a) 1 : 3 (b) 1 : 1
(c) 1 : 4 (d) 1 : 2.

70. The oxidation number of phosphorus and basicity of acid in pyrophosphoric acid respectively are
(a) + four and three (b) + one and four
(c) + five and four (d) + three and one.

71. In which of the following reaction $K_p > K_c$?
(a) $PCl_3 + Cl_2 \rightarrow PCl_5$ (b) $H_2 + I_2 \rightarrow 2HI$
(c) $2SO_3 \rightarrow O_2 + 2SO_2$
(d) $N_2 + 3H_2 \rightarrow 2NH_3$.

72. Atom bomb is based on the principle of
(a) nuclear fission (b) radioactivity
(c) fusion and fission
(d) nuclear fusion.

73. Which of the following is the electronic configuration of Cu^{2+} (Z=29)
(a) $[Ar]3d^9$ (b) $[Ar]4s^1 3d^8$
(c) $[Ar]4s^2 3d^{10} 4p^1$ (d) $[Ar]4s^1 3d^{10}$.

74. Which of the following is a condensation polymer?
(a) teflon (b) dacron
(c) polystyrene (d) neoprene.

75. Euchlorine is produced by heating a mixture of
(a) KCl + conc. H_2SO_4 (b) KCl + conc. HCl
(c) K_2ClO_3 + conc. H_2SO_4
(d) $KClO_3$ + conc. HCl

76. Chloroform by reacting with conc. HNO_3 produces
(a) tear gas (b) water gas
(c) producer gas (d) laughing gas.

77. In the presence of an acid, hydrolysis of methyl cyanide produces
(a) methyl alcohol (b) acetic acid
(c) formic acid (d) methylamine.

78. The IUPAC name of the compound having the formula CCl_3CH_2CHO is
(a) 2, 2, 2-trichloropropanal
(b) 1, 1, 1-trichloropropanal
(c) 3, 3, 3-trichloropropanal
(d) 1, 2, 1-dichloromethanal.

79. How many gm of silver will be displaced from a solution of $AgNO_3$ by 4 gm of magnesium ?
(a) 18 gm (b) 4 gm
(c) 36 gm (d) 16 gm.

80. Nessler's reagent is used in the test of
(a) NH_4Cl (b) NH_3
(c) NH_4^+ (d) all of these.

81. The molality of a solution having 18 gm of glucose (mol. wt = 180) dissolved in 500 gm of water is
(a) 0·2 M (b) 0·1 M
(c) 2·2 M (d) 0·5 M.

82. What is the correct bond angle in dimethyl ether ?
(a) 120° (b) 109°
(c) 180° (d) 110°.

83. Which of the following molecule or ions is a bidentate ligand ?
(a) $C_2O_4^{2-}$ (b) Br_2^+
(c) CH_3NH_2 (d) $CH_3\text{-}C \equiv N$.

84. Which of the following compounds is not soluble in HNO_3 ?
(a) PbS (b) CuS
(c) AgCl (d) CdS.

85. Rutherford's scattering experiment is related to the size of
(a) electron (b) nucleus
(c) neutron (d) proton.

86. Which of the following alkaline earth metal has highest ionic mobility in aqueous solution ?
(a) Be^{2+} (b) Ca^{2+}
(c) Ba^{2+} (d) Mg^{2+}.

87. The complete combustion of CH_4 gives
(a) $CO + H_2O$ (b) $CO + H_2$
(c) $CO + N_2O$ (d) $CO + N_2$.

88. Which of the following molecule has regular geometry ?
(a) H_2O (b) PF_3
(c) XeF_4 (d) SF_6.

89. The element, with atomic number 118, will be
(a) transition element (b) alkali
(c) alkaline earth metal
(d) noble gas.

90. Which of the following kinds of catalysis can be explained by the adsorption theory ?
(a) heterogeneous catalysis
(b) enzyme catalysis
(c) homogeneous catalysis
(d) acid base catalysis.

91. If pH value of a solution is 3 and by adding water, it becomes 6, then the dilution is increased by
(a) 500 times (b) 10 times
(c) 1000 times (d) 100 times.

92. The fractional distillation is used in
(a) petroleum (b) crude oil
(c) coal tar (d) all of these.

93. Which of the following oxyacids does not exist ?
(a) H_3SbO_3 (b) $HBiO_3$
(c) H_3AsO_4 (d) H_3BiO_4.

94. The important ore of aluminium is
(a) kaolin (b) corundum
(c) bauxite (d) ruby.

95. The temperature, at which the density of O_2 at 1 atm, is the same as that of CH_4 at S.T.P., is
(a) 273°C (b) 100°C
(c) 546°C (d) 150°C.

96. The property, which can be classified as an intensive property, is
(a) volume (b) mass
(c) heat capacity (d) temperature.

97. Which of the following has the maximum electronegativity ?
(a) C (b) F
(c) N (d) O.

98. If an atom is reduced, its oxidation number
(a) does not change (b) increases
(c) sharply decreases (d) slightly decreases.

99. In the presence of mercuric ion and conc. sulphuric acid, the reaction of acetylene with water produces
(a) $CH_3\text{-}CO\text{-}CH_3$ (b) $CH_3\text{-}CHO$
(c) $CH_3\text{-}CH_2\text{-}OH$ (d) $CH_3\text{-}COOH$.

100. Which of the following is used in photography?
(a) Ag_2S (b) $AgCl$
(c) $Ag_2C_2O_4$ (d) $AgBr$.

101. The equivalent weight of oxygen, when it is converted to oxide is equal to
(a) $\frac{\text{molecular weight}}{3}$ (b) molecular weight
(c) $\frac{\text{molecular weight}}{4}$ (d) $\frac{\text{molecular weight}}{2}$.

102. A certain gas diffuses four times as quickly as oxygen. The molecular weight of the gas is
(a) 2 (b) 1
(c) 16 (d) 1.5.

103. The molarity of pure water is
(a) 18.36 M (b) 1.16 M
(c) 55.56 M (d) 5.56 M.

104. The volume of carbon dioxide gas evolved at S.T.P. by heating 7.3 gm of $Mg(HCO_3)_2$ will be
(a) 2240 ml (b) 1120 ml
(c) 2340 ml (d) 2000 ml.

105. The amount of zinc (at. wt. = 65) necessary to produce 224 ml of H_2 by the reaction with an acid will be
(a) 6.5 gm (b) 0.065 gm
(c) 7.5 gm (d) 0.65 gm.

106. The number of electrons required to deposit 1 gm equivalent aluminium (at. wt. = 27) from a solution of aluminium chloride will be
(a) 3 (b) 1
(c) 4 (d) 2.

107. Lithopone, a white pigment, consists of
(a) ZnS and $BaSO_4$ (b) PbS and MgO
(c) Al_2O_3 and $CaCO_3$ (d) $BaSO_4$ and $PbSO_4$.

108. Maximum covalency of an element of atomic number 7 is
(a) 4 (b) 2
(c) 5 (d) 3.

109. The oxidation number of oxygen atom in O_2^{2-} ion is

(a) - 3 (b) - 1
(c) - 5 (d) - 2.

110. The number of unpaired electrons in $1s^2 2s^2 2p^3$ is
(a) 3 (b) 1
(c) 5 (d) 2.

Directions: *These questions consist of two statements each, printed as Assertion and Reason. While answering these questions you are required to choose any one of the following four responses.*
(a) If both Assertion and Reason are true and the Reason is a correct explanation of the Assertion.
(b) If both Assertion and Reason are true but Reason is not a correct explanation of the Assertion.
(c) If Assertion is true but the Reason is false.
(d) If both Assertion and Reason are false.

111. *Assertion*: The duma's method is more applicable to nitrogen containing organic compounds than the kjeldahl's method.
Reason: The kjeldahl's method does not give satisfactory results for compounds in which nitrogen is directly linked to oxygen.

112. *Assertion*: Cyclobutane is less stable than cyclopentane.
Reason: Presence of 'bent bonds' causes "loss of orbital overlap".

113. *Assertion*: The molecularity of the reaction $H_2 + Br_2 = 2HBr$ is two.
Reason: The order of this reaction is 3/2.

114. *Assertion*: Bond order in a molecule can assume any value positive or negative; integral or fractional, including zero.
Reason: It depends on the number of electrons in the bonding and antibonding orbitals.

115. *Assertion*: Alkali metals impart colour to the flame.
Reason: Their ionisation energies are low.

116. *Assertion*: Phenol undergoes Kolbe reaction whereas ethanol does not.
Reason: Phenoxide ion is more basic than ethoxide ion.

117. *Assertion*: Copper liberates hydrogen from a solution of dilute hydrochloric acid.
Reason: Hydrogen is below copper in the electrochemical series.

118. *Assertion*: Enthalpy of graphite is lower than that of diamond.
Reason: Entropy of graphite is greater than that of diamond.

119. *Assertion*: Sulphur dioxide and chlorine are both bleaching agents.
Reason: Both are reducing agents.

120. *Assertion*: Formic acid reduces mercuric chloride to mercurous chloride on heating, while acetic acid does not.
Reason: Formic acid is a stronger acid than acetic acid.

BIOLOGY

121. Stomach in vertebrates is the chief site for digestion of
(a) carbohydrates (b) fats
(c) proteins (d) all of these.

122. Diapedesis is
(a) formation of WBC (b) formation of pus
(c) passage of WBC (d) bursting of WBC.

123. In *Leucosolenia,* food is stored in
(a) archaeocytes (b) choanocytes
(c) amoebocytes (d) porocytes.

124. Inheritance of ABO blood groups illustrates
(a) euploidy (b) polyploidy
(c) incomplete dominance
(d) multiple allelism.

125. Which of the following animals has a tetramorphic colony ?
(a) *Porpita* (b) *Obelia*
(c) *Velella* (d) *Physalia.*

126. Glycosidic bond is broken during the digestion of
(a) lipid (b) protein
(c) starch (d) all of these.

127. Intervertebral disc is made up of
(a) calcified cartilage (b) elastic cartilage
(c) hyaline cartilage (d) fibrous cartilage.

128. During muscle contraction actin and myosin form
(a) actomyosin (b) actoplasm
(c) plastosine (d) myoplasm.

129. Stenson's duct is associated with
(a) cardiac gland (b) parotid gland
(c) thyroid gland (d) paratoid gland.

130. The protoplasmic segment of a striated muscle

fibre is termed as
(a) sacroplasm (b) metamere
(c) sarcomere (d) neuromere.

131. Meroblastic cleavage refers to which type of division of eggs ?
(a) incomplete (b) total
(c) horizontal (d) spiral.

132. Which of the following monkey has prehensile tail?
(a) spider monkey (b) loris
(c) rhesus monkey (b) tarsiers

133. Cis-trans test is related with
(a) crossing over (b) mutation
(c) genetic map (d) heredity.

134. Schneiderian membrane is found in
(a) loop of henle (b) trachea
(c) Bowman's capsule (d) nasal mucosa.

135. Lining of intestine of man is
(a) brush border (b) ciliated
(c) non-keratinized (d) keratinized.

136. Homonids were originated during
(a) miocene (b) pliocene
(c) oligocene (d) palaeocene.

137. Enzymes with two sites are called
(a) allosteric enzyme (b) apoenzyme
(c) conjugate enzyme (d) holoenzyme.

138. Camouflage of *Chameleon* is associated with
(a) chromoplast (b) chromosome
(c) chromatophore (d) chromomere.

139. A vertebrate bone, which directly develops from mesenchyme, is called
(a) endochondrial bone
(b) dermal bone
(c) replacing bone (d) all of these.

140. Earliest fossil form in phylogeny of horse is
(a) *Merychippus* (b) *Equus*
(c) *Mesohippus* (d) *Eohippus*.

141. Preganglionic sympathetic fibres are
(a) synergic (b) adrenergic
(c) hypergonic (d) cholinergic.

142. Bohr effect is related with
(a) reduced carbon level in lymph
(b) reduced oxygen level in haemoglobin
(c) oxidised phosphorus level in blood
(d) reduced carbon dioxide level in blood.

143. In gout patients, high level of which of the following is found in blood ?
(a) cholesterol (b) urea
(c) amino acid (d) uric acid.

144. During muscle contraction, energy is provided by
(a) acetyl-CoA (b) phosphagen
(c) AMP (d) Glucose.

145. Desmosomes are found in
(a) epithelial tissue (b) muscular tissue
(c) nervous tissue (d) all of these.

146. The shade of a tree is cooler than the shade of a roof due to
(a) transpiration (b) guttation
(c) photosynthesis (d) green leaves.

147. Raphides are the crystals of
(a) calcium oxalate (b) calcium
(c) calcium phosphate (d) calcium carbonate.

148. When micropyle, chalaza and funicle are in a straight line, the ovule is called
(a) orthotropous (b) anatropous
(c) amphitropous (d) campylotropous.

149. In phylogenetic classification, the groups are arranged
(a) following the evolutionary trends
(b) according to floral similarities
(c) according to their morphological characters
(d) according to their complexities.

150. Triphasic life cycle is found in
(a) *Chondrus* (b) *Laminaria*
(c) *Polysiphonia* (d) *Macrocystis*.

151. Velamen is found in
(a) *Viscum* (b) *Vanda*
(c) *Santalum* (d) *Rosa*.

152. Which of the following is a cyanophage ?
(a) S-13 (b) $\phi \times 174$
(c) SV-40 (d) LPP-1.

153. In which of the following, reticulate chloroplast is found ?
(a) *Oedogonium* (b) *Spirogyra*
(c) *Ectocarpus* (d) *Ulothrix*.

154. Hornworts are represented by
(a) hepaticopsida (b) bryopsida
(c) anthoceratopsida (d) psilopsida.

155. Bulliform cells are present in
(a) bundle sheath (b) mesophyll
(c) vascular bundles (d) epidermis.

156. Black wood is obtained from
(a) *Dalbergia* (b) *Albizzia*
(c) *Manihot* (d) *Acacia*.

157. The growth hormones, responsible for 'bolting', are
(a) coumarins (b) auxins
(c) gibberellins (d) kinetins.

158. Aerobic respiration produces more usable chemical energy than fermentation, because fermentation involves
(a) formation of lactic acid
(b) complete oxidation of food
(c) partial oxidation of food
(d) evolution of CO_2 and alcohol.

159. Photosynthetic pigments in chloroplast are embedded in the membrane of
(a) thylakoids
(b) matrix
(c) chloroplast envelope
(d) photoglobin.

160. Which of the following are famous for chromosome heredity ?
(a) Morgan & Sutton
(b) Beadle & Tatum
(c) Bridges & Morgan
(d) Sutton & Boveri.

161. Which of the following plant yields powerful analgesic ?
(a) *Rauwolfia serpentina*
(b) *Carcuma longa*
(c) *Papaver somniferum*
(d) *Ferula asafoetida*.

162. Decapitation of plant leads to the activation of axillary buds due to
(a) increase in cytokinins
(b) more light availability
(c) auxin translocation
(d) all of these.

163. How many quanta of light are required to evolve one oxygen molecule in photosynthesis ?
(a) three (b) eight
(c) four (d) two.

164. During interphase, RNAs and proteins are synthesized in
(a) G_2-phase (b) G_1-phase
(c) S-phase (d) all of these.

165. Antherozoids of *Dryopteris* are
(a) sickle-shaped and multiflagellate
(b) coiled and multiflagellate
(c) sickle shaped and biflagellate
(d) coiled and biflagellate.

166. The 3 sub-families of leguminosae are distinguished mainly on the basis of
(a) nature and habit of the plants
(b) nature of gynoecium
(c) nature of fruit and its germination
(d) inflorescence and flower characters.

167. Pollinium is found in family
(a) asclepidaceae (b) rubiaceae
(c) solanaceae (d) myrtaceae.

168. Polyploidy leads to rapid formation of new species, because of
(a) isolation behaviour
(b) genetic recombination
(c) development of multiple sets of chromosomes
(d) mutation therapy.

169. Teminism is same as
(a) transcription
(b) translation
(c) reverse transcription
(d) DNA synthesis.

170. The cell organelle associated with photorespiration is
(a) mesosome (b) ribosome
(c) peroxisome (d) lysosome.

Directions: *These questions consist of two statements each, printed as Assertion and Reason. While answering these questions you are required to choose any one of the following four responses.*
(a) If both Assertion and Reason are true and the Reason is a correct explanation of the Assertion.
(b) If both Assertion and Reason are true but Reason is not a correct explanation of the Assertion.
(c) If Assertion is true but the Reason is false.
(d) If both Assertion and Reason are false.

171. *Assertion*: The third cleavage in frog is latitudinal.
Reason: The mitotic spindle orients parallel to the polar axis.

172. *Assertion*: The aerobic respiration is bioenergetically more efficient than the anaerobic glycolysis.
Reason: The aerobic respiration occurs in the mitochondria, while glycolysis is purely cytosolic.

173. *Assertion*: In mammals, a secondary plate is developed.
Reason: The development of secondary plate is mainly in response to the shifting of internal areas.

174. *Assertion*: The development in cockroach is heterometabolous metamorphosis.
Reason: The young ones resemble the adults in all.

175. *Assertion*: In cells engaged in active secretion, as in pancreas, the rough endoplasmic reticulum is well developed.
Reason: Ribosomes attached to endoplasmic reticulum are actively engaged in protein synthesis.

176. *Assertion*: 'Lac Operon Model' is applicable only to *E.coli*.
Reason: *E.coli.* lacks a definite nucleus.

177. *Assertion*: Ionizing radiations are harmful for the living organism.
Reason: They form toxic photoproducts in the cells.

178. *Assertion*: In woody stems, the amount of heart wood continues to increase year after year.
Reason: The activity of the cambial ring continues uninterrupted.

179. *Assertion*: The 'absorption spectrum' of chlorophyll '*a*' shows close correlation with its 'action spectrum'.
Reason: Chlorophyll '*a*' is present in both the pigment systems I and II.

180. *Assertion*: C_4-plants photosynthesize more efficiently than C_3-plants.
Reason: C_4-plants have a shorter carbon dioxide fixation cycle.

GENERAL KNOWLEDGE

181. 'Vande Matram' was first published in
(a) Gitanjali (b) Anand math
(c) Nandini (d) Vinay patrika.

182. The first chief justice of India, was
(a) Patanjali Shastri (b) J.C. Shah
(c) Harilal J. Kania (d) S.R. Das.

183. First speaker of Lok Sabha, was
(a) Bali Ram Bhagat (b) G.V. Mavalankar
(c) Neelam Sanjiva Reddy
(d) Sardar Hukum Singh.

184. The attorney general of India is the legal adviser to
(a) president of India
(b) prime minister of foreign policies
(c) government of finance policies
(d) government of India.

185. 'GATT' stands for
(a) general agreement on trade and tourism
(b) general agreement on toures and travels
(c) general agreement on telephone and telegraph
(d) general agreement on to traffics and track

186. Latitude is the distance in degrees on the earth's surface measured
(a) upper and lower position of the earth
(b) north and south poles of the equator
(c) temperature difference between different areas on earth
(d) east and west poles of the equator.

187. The natural growth rate of population during any year is the difference between the
(a) birth rate and average population
(b) birth rate and death rate per 1000
(c) average population and birth rate per 1000
(d) death rate and birth rate per 1000.

188. Intergrated Rural Development Progress (IRDP) was initiated during
(a) 1976-77 (b) 1975-1976
(c) 1980-1981 (d) 1969-1970.

189. Astrology deals with the study of
(a) plants life
(b) space
(c) stars and future forecasting
(d) bacteria.

190. 'Diesel Engine' was invented by
(a) Edison (b) Carnot
(c) Rudolf Dieself (d) H.W. Seeley.

191. 'Prince of Wales cup' is related with
(a) Football (b) Golf
(c) Cricket (d) Hockey.

192. Aravali range is situated in the
(a) north-east region (b) north-west region
(c) south-east region (d) south-west region.

193. 'Bharat Bharti' was written by
(a) Suryakant Tripathi
(b) Amrita Preetam
(c) Maithili Saran Gupta
(d) Mulkraj Anand.

194. Sri Aurbindo was a great
(a) philosopher (b) writer
(c) sport person (d) actor.

195. First Woman Congress President, was
(a) Indira Gandhi
(b) Annie Besant
(c) Vijayalakshmi Pandit
(d) Sarojini Naidu.

196. Mother Teresa won the Nobel Prize for peace in
(a) 1984 (b) 1992
(c) 1979 (d) 1989.

197. The capital of 'Barbados' is
(a) Belarus (b) Capetown
(c) Berlin (d) Bridgetown.

198. The chief metabolic function of vitamin 'D' is to
(a) prevent blood coagultaion
(b) afford antiachitic activity
(c) prevent the loss of muscle
(d) prevent night blindness.

199. Who said these words 'Play the game in the spirit of the game'
(a) Chandrasekhar (b) Rajiv Gandhi
(c) Jawahar Lal Nehru (d) Indira Gandhi.

200. The human skeleton is divided into
(a) four parts (b) two parts
(c) six parts (d) three parts.

SOLUTIONS

PHYSICS

1. **(b) :** Velocity of photons $(c) = \upsilon\lambda \propto \upsilon$. Therefore velocity (c) is proportional to frequency (υ).

2. **(b)**

3. **(b) :** In an inelastic collision, the kinetic energy is not conserved but linear momentum is conserved. In this sort of a collision there is loss in K.E. of the system.

4. **(a)**

5. **(c) :** Given: Initial temperature of metal rod (T_1) = 150°C = 423 K; Rate of radiated energy (E) = 20 W and final temperature (T_2) = 300°C = 573 K. We know from the Stefan's law $E \propto T^4$ or $\frac{E_1}{E_2} = \left(\frac{T_1}{T_2}\right)^4 = \left(\frac{423}{573}\right)^4$ = 0.293. Therefore final radiated energy

$$(E_2) = \frac{E_1}{0 \cdot 293} = \frac{20}{0 \cdot 293} = 68 \cdot 3 \text{ W}.$$

6. **(d)**

7. **(d) :** Given: Charge $(Q) = 50e = 50 \times (1 \cdot 6 \times 10^{-19})$ C; Distance of proton from nucleus $(r) = 10^{-12}$ m and charge on proton $(e) = 1 \cdot 6 \times 10^{-19}$ C. We know that potential

$$(V) = \frac{1}{4\pi\,\varepsilon_0} \times \left(\frac{Q}{r}\right) = 9 \times 10^9 \times \frac{50 \times 1 \cdot 6 \times 10^{-19}}{10^{-12}}$$
$$= 7 \cdot 2 \times 10^4 \text{ V}.$$

8. **(d) :** According to Bohr's principle, the radius of orbit

$$(r) = \frac{\varepsilon_0\, n^2 h^2}{\pi\; mZe^2} \propto n^2$$

where n = principal quantum number.

9. **(d)**

10. **(a) :** Given: Internal resistance of the cell (r) = $0 \cdot 1\ \Omega$; E.M.F. of the cell (E) = 2 V and external resistance $(R) = 3 \cdot 9\ \Omega$. We know that voltage $(V) = E - Ir$

$$= E - \frac{E}{R+r} \cdot r = 2 - \frac{2}{3 \cdot 9 + 0 \cdot 1} \times 0 \cdot 1 = 1 \cdot 95 \text{ V}.$$

11. **(a)**

12. **(b) :** When one α-particle is absorbed and one neutron is emitted then the balance equation shows that resulting nucleus will be carbon. The balance equation is

$${}_4Be^9 \;+\; {}_2He^4 \;\rightarrow\; {}_0n^1 \;+\; {}_6C^{12}$$
(α-particle) (neutron)

From this equation, we find that atomic weight is 12 and atomic mass number is 6. Since both these values are meant for carbon (C), therefore resulting nucleus will be, ${}_6C^{12}$.

13. **(c) :** The output of the given logic circuit is

$$Y = \overline{\overline{A} + B + \overline{C}}$$
$$\Rightarrow \overline{Y} = \overline{A} + B + \overline{C}$$

So, applying De Morgan's theorem,

$$\overline{\overline{Y}} = \overline{\overline{A}} \,.\, \overline{B} \,.\, \overline{\overline{C}}$$
$$\Rightarrow \text{Y} = A\,\overline{B}\,C$$

∴ The given circuit will perform the logic operation $A\,\overline{B}\,C$.

14. **(a) :** Given: No. of wires = 10 and resistance of each wire = 1 Ω. We know that relation for equivalent resistance of wires connected in parallel

$$\frac{1}{R_{eq}} = \underbrace{\frac{1}{1} + \frac{1}{1} + \frac{1}{1} + \ldots\ldots + \frac{1}{1}}_{\text{10 terms}}$$

$$\therefore R_{eq} = \frac{1}{10} = 0 \cdot 1\ \Omega.$$

15. **(b)**

16. **(c) :** Given: Weight of the body on the earth's surface (W) = 50 N and depth $(d) = \frac{R}{2}$. We know that weight of the body at a distance (d) from the surface of the earth $= W\left(1 - \frac{d}{R}\right) = 250 \times \left(1 - \frac{R/2}{R}\right) = 250 \times \frac{1}{2}$ = 125 N.

Aliter : Given: Weight of the body on the surface of the earth

mg = 250 N

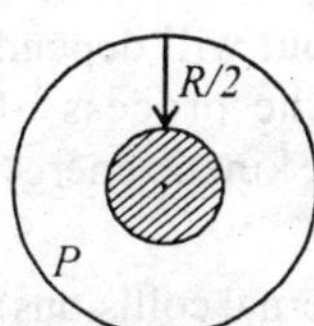

When we move down a distance $R/2$ towards the earth's centre, the value of acceleration due to gravity decreases. First let's calculate the value of acceleration due to gratvity at a depth $R/2$ below the surface. What we have to remember here is that the whole mass of the earth is not going to be effective at a depth of $R/2$. Let, ρ be the uniform mass density of the earth. Then the effective mass of earth at a depth $R/2$ below is

$$M' = \frac{4}{3}\pi\left(\frac{R}{2}\right)^3 \times \rho = \frac{4}{3}\pi R^3\rho \times \frac{1}{8} = \frac{M}{8}$$

Where M = mass of earth on the surface

Now $g' = \frac{GM'}{\left(\frac{R}{2}\right)^2} = 4\frac{GM'}{R^2} = 4\times\frac{GM}{8R^2} = \frac{g}{2}$

$$\Rightarrow mg' = \frac{mg}{2} = \frac{250}{2} = 125 \text{ N}$$

17. (d) : If a current I in a conductor is uniformely distributed over the area of cross-section (A) of the conductor, then the ratio I/A is called the current density at any point on the area. It is represented by joule. Its unit is amp/m^2 and it is a vector quantity.

18. (a)

19. (b) : Crystalline solids have regular periodic arrangements of particles. They are anisotropic and have different properites in different directions.

20. (a) : Given: Mass of the disc = M and radius = R. We know that moment of inertia of a disc about diameter = $\frac{1}{4}MR^2$. And from the theorem of parallel axes, the required moment of inertia = $\frac{1}{4}MR^2 + MR^2$

$$= \frac{5}{4}MR^2.$$

21. (c)

22. (a) : Given: Initial temperature (T_1) = 273 K; Initial volume (V_1) = V; Final volume (V_2) = 81 V and γ = 1.25. We know that under adiabatic condition $T_1V_1^{\gamma-1}$ $= T_2V_2^{\gamma-1}$ or $\frac{273}{T_2} = \left(\frac{V_2}{V_1}\right)^{\gamma-1} = \left(\frac{81V}{V}\right)^{1.25-1} = (81)^{0.25} = 3$ or

$T_2 = \frac{273}{3} = 91$ K = – 182°C (where T_2 is the final temperature of the gas).

23. (d) : This is a case of balanced wheatstone bridge. Since the resistances in upper and lower arms are in series, therefore equivalent resistance in upper arm $(R) = R_1 + R_2 = 20 + 20 = 40\ \Omega$ and equivalent resistant of lower arm $R' = R_3 + R_4 = 20 + 20 = 40\ \Omega$. Now the equivalent resistances R and R' are in parallel. Therefore their resultant resistance

$$R'' = \frac{40\times40}{40+40} = \frac{1600}{80} = 20\ \Omega.$$

24. (d) : Given: Wavelength (λ) = 10^{-10} m and atomic spacing (d) = 2×10^{-10} m. We know from the Bragg's law, $2d\sin\theta = 2\lambda$ or $\sin\theta = \frac{\lambda}{d} = \frac{10^{-10}}{2\times10^{-10}} = 0.5$.

Therefore $\theta = \sin^{-1} 0.5 = 30°$.

25. (a)

26. (c) : Given: Power of heater (P) = 100 W and time (t) = 2 min = 120 sec. We know that work done to produce heat (W) = $P\times t$ = 100 × 120 = 12000 J

$$= \frac{12000}{4.2\times1000} = 2.8 \text{ kcal.}$$

27. (d)

28. (b) : Given: Power of first lens (P_1) = + 1.5 D and power of second lens (P_2) = + 1.0 D. We know that power of the combination (P) = $P_1 + P_2$ = 1.5 + 1.0 = 2.5 D.

29. (d)

30. (b) : Given: Temperature (T_1) = 1000 K; Wavelength at maximum radiation $\lambda = \lambda_m$ and final temperature (T_2) = 2000 K. We know from the Wein's displacement law $\lambda_m \times T$ = constant. Therefore when the temperature is doubled, the peak will shift to half the original value.

31. (d) : On an artificial satellite orbiting the earth the acceleration is given by $\frac{GM}{R^2}$ towards the centre of the earth. Now for a body of mass m on the satellite the graviational force due to earth is $\frac{GMm}{R^2}$ towards the centre of the earth. Let the reaction force on the surface of the satellite be N, then

$$\frac{GMm}{R^2} - N = m\left(\frac{GM}{R^2}\right)$$

$$\Rightarrow N = 0$$

That is on the satellite there is a state of weightlessness or $g = 0$

∴ The time period of the simple pendulum,

$$T = 2\pi\sqrt{\frac{l}{g}} = \infty$$

32. **(d) :** Given: Time period $(T) = 4$ sec and displacement $(y) = \frac{a}{2}$ or $\frac{y}{a} = \frac{1}{2}$. We know that displacement equation $(y) = a \sin \frac{2\pi}{T} t$ or $\frac{y}{a} = \sin \frac{2\pi}{T} t$ or $\frac{1}{2} = \sin \frac{2\pi}{T} t$ or $\frac{2\pi}{T} t = \sin^{-1} \frac{1}{2} = \frac{\pi}{6}$ or $t = \frac{T}{12} = \frac{4}{12} = \frac{1}{3}$ sec

(where t is the interval of time).

33. **(b)**

34. **(d) :** Given: Mass of body $(m) = 5$ kg; Height of the body $(h) = 10$ m and force $(F) = 170$ N. We know that work done by the force $= F \times h = 170 \times 10 = 1700$ J and potential energy $= mgh = 5 \times 10 \times 10 = 500$ J. Now kinetic energy of the body (K.E.) $= 1700 - 500 = 1200$ J. Therefore if the velocity of the body is v, then kinetic energy $1200 = \frac{1}{2} mv^2 = \frac{1}{2} \times 5 \times v^2$ or $v^2 = \frac{1200 \times 2}{5} = 480$ or $v = \sqrt{480} \cong 22$ m/s.

35. **(c) :** We know that the resolving power of a microscope is given by

$R = \frac{2\mu \sin\theta}{\lambda}$ Where μ = the refractive index of the medium between the object and the objective

θ = angle subtended by the radius of the objective on any one object

λ = wavelength of light used

$\therefore$ for greater accuracy, wavelength of light used should be smaller, or conversely, the frequency of the light should be higher.

36. **(d) :** Given: Mass of star $= M$ and radius of the star $= R$. We know that escape angular velocity of the star

$$(\omega_e) = \frac{v_e}{R} = \frac{1}{R}\sqrt{\frac{2GM}{R}} = \sqrt{\frac{2GM}{R^3}}.$$

$$\left(\text{where escape velocity } (v_e) = \sqrt{\frac{2GM}{R}}\right).$$

37. **(d) :** When light of suffciently high energy (greater than the work function) falls an a metal, there is a chance that photoelectric effect takes place, *i.e.*, an electron might come out of the metarial surface. Now the energy of the electron that comes out will depend upon how much energy it loses in the process of collision inside the metarial surface. The kinetic energy of the electron is given by

$K.E. = h\upsilon - h\upsilon_0 -$ (Energy loss due to internal collisions)

Now in the most ideal case, if the energy loss is 0 then $K.E.$ is $K.E._{max}$ *i.e.*

$K.E._{max} = h\upsilon - h\upsilon_0$

And in the worst case, Energy loss $= hv - hv_0$, then $K.E. = 0$

Hence, the photo electrons coming out of the cathode have an energy spread with an upper limit.

38. **(b) :** If two charges are of the same sign, they repel each other. Thus if two electrons are brought closer, some work is done against the force of repulsion. Therefore the electric potential energy of the system increases.

Aliter : e ●——r——● e

Mathematically, the potential due to one electron at the position of the other electron is $\frac{-Ke}{r}$ and hence the potential of the other electron $= -\frac{Ke(-e)}{r} = \frac{Ke^2}{r}$, where r is the distance between the two electrons. Now if r decreases, $P.E.$ increases.

39. **(a)**

40. **(a) :** Given: Frequency of fundamental note when tube is closed $(n_1) = 512$ Hz. We know that frequency of fundamental note for closed organ pipe $(n_2) = \frac{v}{2l}$ and for open pipe $(n_1) = \frac{v}{4l}$ or $n_2 = 2n_1 = 2 \times 512 = 1024$ Hz.

41. **(b) :** Phosphorous is pentavalent and silicon is tetravalent. Therefore when it is doped with pentavalent impurity, it forms a n-type semiconductor.

42. **(b) :** Given: Initial number of cells $(n_1) = 10$; Potential of each cell $= E$; Internal resistance of each cell $= r$ and final number of cells $(n_2) = 3$. We know from the Ohm's law, total voltage of ten cells $= 10 \times E = 10E$ and total resistance in ten cells $= 10 \times r = 10r$. Therefore current in the circuit $(I) = \frac{10E}{10r} = \frac{E}{r}$ or potential difference across three cells $= I \times 3r = \frac{E}{r} \times 3r = 3E$.

(Since the voltmeter is ideal, therefore it will read $3E$).

43. (d) : Given: Inductance (L) = 0·01 H and frequency (n) = 50 Hz. We know that the reactance (X_L) = ωL = $2\pi n \times L = 2 \times \pi \times 50 \times 0{\cdot}01 = 3{\cdot}14\ \Omega$.

44. (d) : Given: Wavelength (λ_0) = 720 nm and refractive index (μ) = 1·5. Since the velocity of light in a medium is given by $C = n\lambda$ and n remaining same for different media we have,

$$n = \frac{c}{\lambda} = \frac{c'}{\lambda'}$$

$$\therefore \lambda' = \frac{c'\lambda}{c}$$

$$\text{Again } c' = \frac{c}{\mu}$$

$$\text{Hence } \lambda' = \frac{\lambda}{\mu}$$

c = speed is vacuum
c' = speed in medium
μ = refractive index of the medium

Therefore, wavelength of the ray in glass $(\lambda) = \frac{\lambda_0}{\mu} = \frac{720}{1{\cdot}5} = 480$ nm.

45. (b) : Given: Half-life $(T)_{1/2}$ = 20 years; Initial mass of element (N_0) = 10 g and final mass of element (N) = 2·5 g. Let the number of half-lives needed for the material to bring it down to 2 g from 10 g be n. We know that the final mass of element is given by

$$N = N_0\left(\frac{1}{2}\right)^n$$

$$\Rightarrow \frac{N}{N_0} = \left(\frac{1}{2}\right)^n \Rightarrow \frac{2{\cdot}5}{10} = \left(\frac{1}{2}\right)^n$$

$$\Rightarrow \left(\frac{1}{2}\right)^2 = \left(\frac{1}{2}\right)^n \Rightarrow n = 2$$

Therefore time taken to disintegrate the element from the block (t) = $(T)_{1/2} \times n = 20 \times 2 = 40$ years.

46. (a) : Given: Initial temperature (T_1) = 27°C = 300 K; Final temperature (T_2) = 327°C = 600 K and initial average kinetic energy (E_1) = E. We know that average kinetic energy (E) = $\frac{3}{2}kT \propto T$. Therefore $\frac{E_1}{E_2} = \frac{T_1}{T_2}$. $= \frac{300}{600} = \frac{1}{2}$ or $E_2 = 2E_1 = 2E$ (where E_2 is final kinetic energy).

47. (b) : Strain = $\frac{\text{Extension in length}}{\text{Original length}} = \frac{[L]}{[L]} = [L^0]$. Therefore strain is a dimensionless quantity.

48. (a) : Given: Initial tension in the piano wire (T_1) = 10 N; Initial frequency of note (n_1) = n and final frequency of the note (n_2) = $2n$. We know that frequency (n) = $\frac{1}{2\pi}\sqrt{\frac{T}{m}} \propto \sqrt{T}$. Therefore $\frac{n_1}{n_2} = \sqrt{\frac{T_1}{T_2}}$ or $\left(\frac{n}{2n}\right)^2 = \frac{10}{T_2}$. Therefore final tension $\frac{1}{4} = \frac{10}{T_2}$ or T_2 = $10 \times 4 = 40$ N.

49. (c) : Given : Initial temperature (T_1) = 27°C = 300 K; Final temperature (T_2) = 627°C = 900 K and initial volume (V_1) = 4 m³. We know from the Charle's law $\frac{V_1}{T_1} = \frac{V_2}{T_2}$ or $V_2 = V_1 \times \frac{T_2}{T_1} = 4 \times \frac{900}{300} = 12\ \text{m}^3$.

50. (a) : Gravitationalconstant(G)

$$= \frac{(\text{Force})(\text{Distance})^2}{(\text{Mass})^2} = \frac{[MLT^{-2}][L^2]}{[M]^2}\ [M^{-1}L^3T^{-2}].$$

51. (a) : The rainbow is seen during or after raining as there are lot of water droplets suspended in the air at that time. As the rainbow is caused by the total internal reflection of the sunlight from the droplets, the final ray is in the backward direction and so one always sees a rainbow in a direction opposite to the sun.

sun ray

52. (b) : During sunrise and sunset, the ray of light from the sun has to travel a longer distance to reach the eyes. As only longer wavelengths can reach the eyes, the angle subtended by the rays of light on the retina is greater than that during the day. That's why the sun looks bigger during sunrise and sunset.

53. (a)

54. (b) : The human eye has the capacity to suitably adjust the focal length of the eye and is done with the help of the cilliary muscles. These muscles get relaxed when we see an object at a distance. And they get strained when we view close by. But these muscles cannot get strained more than a certain limit and that's why we cannot see an object clearer if it is closer than a certain minimum distance from the eye known as the 'least distance for clear vision'.

55. (a)

56. (c) : In case the circuit inside becomes faulty, an electric appliance might end with some charge. Because of which on touching the appliance, the user might get a shock. The third pin provided is for grounding purpose so that all accumulated charges might get discharged to the ground and the appliance remains safe. Now appliances like heater, where there can be more charge accumulation than the electric bulb, grounding is a must. That's why, electric appliances with metallic body, such as heaters have three pin connections.

57. (c) : The buoyancy of an object is the resultant of all the contact forces that are present at the points of contact of the body and the fluid and is perpedicular to the surface at that point. Hence the force of buoyancy depends upon the area of contact of the body with the fluid. The force of buoyancy is more in case of the needle than in the case of the ball. Now it might so happen that the force of buoyancy (B) is greater than the weight (mg) of the needle, in which case the needle might float. But in the case of the ball, $B < mg$, and so the ball sinks.

58. (a) : The third pin is used for grounding purposes so that it leaves the user safe while handling the appliance by making the extra charge on it get discharged.

59. (c) : Since the escape velocity on the surface of the moon is much less than that on earth, so the water molecules get evaporated faster.

60. (b)

CHEMISTRY

61. (a) : Charge = Current × time = 1 × 60 = 60 coulombs

Charge carried by one electron = 1.6×10^{-19}C

No. of electrons = $\dfrac{60}{1.6\times10^{-19}} = 3.74 \times 10^{20}$

62. (d) : The black substance obtained is a mixture of mercury and mercuric aminochloride.

$$Hg_2Cl_2 + 2NH_4OH \longrightarrow \underbrace{Hg\begin{matrix}NH_2\\Cl\end{matrix} + Hg}_{\text{Black}} + NH_4Cl + H_2O$$

63. (d) : Applying the equation :

$$pH = \log\frac{[Salt]}{[Acid]} + pK_a$$

⇒ Here, $pH = pk_a + \log 1$, $pH = 4.75$

64. (c) : Oxygen is oxidised at anode while Cu^{2+} is reduced at cathode. Therefore copper deposits on cathode and oxygen is evolved at anode.

65. (a) : Corrosion or rusting is a surface phenomenon and thus Iron is protected by coating it with a thin film of Zn which is inert to moisture and air by a process called Electroplating.

66. (b) : According to Le-Chateliar Principle increase in pressure will favour the direction where there are lesser no. of species.

67. (a) : $Ni^{2+}(d^8)$:

	3d	4s	4p
Ni^{2+}	⇅ ⇅ ⇅ ↑ ↑	□	□ □ □
$[Ni(CN)_4]^{2-}$:	⇅ ⇅ ⇅ ⇅ xx	xx	xx xx □

∴ dsp^2 hybridisation and square planer structure.

68. (c) : Non-existence of PbI_4 can be explained on the basis of strong oxidising nature of Pb^{4+}. The I^- ions are reducing agents, i.e., in presence of this ion, Pb^{4+} ion is reduced to Pb^{2+} ion.

$$Pb^{4+} + 2I^- \rightarrow Pb^{2+} + I_2.$$

69. (b) : The Avogadro's law states that same volume of all gases at the same temperature and pressure, contain equal number of molecules. Hence ratio of volumes must be 1 : 1.

70. (c) : Pyrophosphoric acid : $H_4P_2O_7$

Let Oxidation state of P be x

$\Rightarrow 4 \times (+1) + 2x + 7 \times (-2) = 0$

$\Rightarrow 4 + 2x - 14 = 0$

$\Rightarrow x = +5$

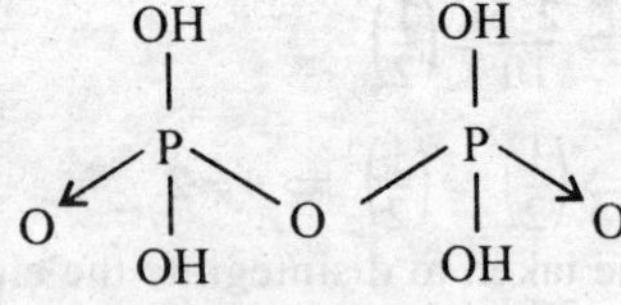

basicity of acid is four.

71. (c) : As $K_p = K_c(RT)^{\Delta n}$

So if Δn = +ve then only, $K_p > K_c$

Where Δn is the difference in number of moles of gaseous products of gaseous reactants.

72. (a) : Nuclear fission is the break up of large unstable nuclei to give smaller more stable nuclei with the release of large amount of energy.

73. (a) : Cu (Z = 29) : $[Ar]4s^1 3d^{10}$

Cu^{2+} : $[Ar]3d^9$.

74. (b) : Dacron is formed by condensation of ethylene glycol and dimethyl terephthalate with the elimination of CH_3OH molecules.

$HOCH_2CH_2OH + CH_3OOC-\langle\bigcirc\rangle-COOCH_3 \xrightarrow{Heat}$

$(CH_2CH_2-OOC-\langle\bigcirc\rangle-COO)_n + CH_3OH$

Dacron

75. (d) : When $KClO_3$ is heated with conc. HCl, a mixture of chlorine and chlorine dioxide is obtained [called Euchlorine]

$[KClO_3 + HCl \rightarrow KCl + HClO_3] \times 2$

$2HClO_3 + 2HCl \rightarrow 2ClO_2 + Cl_2 + 2H_2O$

$2KClO_3 + 4HCl \rightarrow 2KCl + 2ClO_2 + Cl_2 + 2H_2O$

76. (a) : $CHCl_3 + HNO_3 \rightarrow CCl_3NO_2$
Cloropicrin
(Tear gas)

77. (b) : $CH_3CN \xrightarrow[H_2O]{H^+} CH_3-CO-NH_2 \xrightarrow[H_2O]{H^+} CH_3COOH + NH_3$.
(Acetic acid)

78. (c) : $\overset{3}{(Cl_3C} - \overset{2}{CH_2} - \overset{1}{CHO})$

IUPAC name is :

3, 3, 3 – trichloropropanal

79. (c) : Given: Weight of magnesium = 4 gm, We know that $\frac{\text{Weight of silver displaced } (M)}{\text{Weight of magnesium}}$

$= \frac{\text{Equivalent weight of silver}}{\text{Equivalent weight of magnesium}}$ or $\frac{M}{4} = \frac{108}{12}$

or $M = \frac{108 \times 4}{12} = 36$ gm.

80. (d) : $NH_4^+ + OH^- \rightarrow NH_3 + H_2O$

To the aqueous solution of ammonium salt when Nessler's reagent is added, brown coloured precipitate is formed.

$K_2HgI_4 + NH_4Cl + 4KOH \longrightarrow$ (Hg–NH₂, Hg–I bridged by O) + $KI + KCl + H_2O$

(Nessler's reagent) (Brown ppt.)

81. (a) : Moles of glucose $= \frac{\text{mass}}{\text{Molecular mass}} = \frac{18}{180}$

$\Rightarrow$ Molality $= \frac{0.1}{500} \times 1000 = 0.2M$

82. (d) : The oxygen atom in ethers is sp^3 hybridized. Two of the hybrid orbitals overlap with hybrid orbitals of two carbon atoms to form sigma bonds and the bond angle is R–O–R, 110°

83. (a) : A molecule or an ion, which can attach itself to a metal ion from two different positions, is known as bidentate ligand or ion.

$C_2O_4^{2-}$: $O=C-O^{\ominus}$ / $O=C-O^{\ominus}$

It contains two donation sites so it is a bidentate ligand.

84. (c) : $PbS + 2HNO_3 \rightarrow Pb(NO_3)_2 + H_2S$

$CuS + 2HNO_3 \rightarrow Cu(NO_3)_2 + H_2S$

$CdS + 2HNO_3 \rightarrow Cd(NO_3)_2 + H_2S$

85. (b) : In this experiment, when a thin foil of gold was bombarded by α–particles but most of the α–particles went straight and very few got large deflections. Conclusion was drawn that nucleus is very small and very compact.

86. (c) : Due to the high heat of hydration of small cations, ionic mobility for the small cations is low. Order of Ionic mobility is :

$Be^{2+} < Mg^{2+} < Ca^{2+} < Ba^{2+}$.

87. (a) : $CH_4 + O \rightarrow CO + H_2O$

88. (d) : S : [⇅] [⇅|↑|↑] ground state

S : [↑] [↑|↑|↑] [↑|↑| | |] excited state

Six unpaired electrons, form bonds with six fluorine atoms. It has regular octahedral shape.

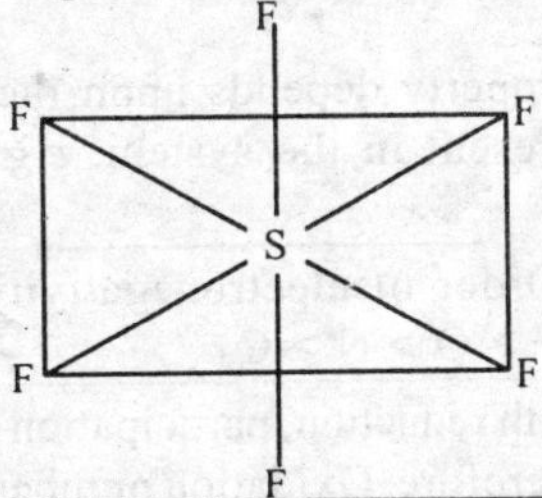

89. (d) : Electronic configuration of element with atomic number 118 will be $[Rn]5f^{14} 6s^2 6p^6$. Since its electronic configuration in the outermost orbit (ns^2np^6) resembles with that of inert or noble gases, therefore it will be a noble gas element.

90. (a) : Adsorption of reactants on the solid surface of the catalysts affect the rate of reaction between the reactants. Reaction proceeds more rapidly after adsorption *e.g.* contact process. So heterogenous catalysis can be best understood in the light of adsorption phenomenon.

91. (c) : Given: Initial pH = 3 and final pH = 6. We know that pH $\propto$ Dilution. Therefore initially $[H^+] = 10^{-3}$ and after dilution $[H^+] = 10^{-6}$. Thus increase in dilution

$= \dfrac{\text{Original } H^+ \text{ concentration}}{\text{Concentration of } H+ \text{ after dilution}} = \dfrac{10^{-3}}{10^{-6}} = 10^3$

= 1000 times.

92. (d) : Fractional distillation : In this process the distillate is collected in fractions under different temperature. *e.g.* It is used these days for distillation of coal tar, petroleum, and crude oil etc.

93. (d) : Arsenic forms two oxyacids H_3AsO_3 and H_3AsO_4. Antimony forms only one oxyacid H_3SbO_3 and bismuth forms only one oxyacid $HBiO_3$. Therefore H_3BiO_4 does not exist.

94. (c) : Bauxite is $Al_2O_3.2H_2O$

95. (a) : The density of O_2 at S.T.P. $(d_1) = \dfrac{32}{22\cdot4}$ gm/litres and that of CH_4 at S.T.P. $(d_2) = \dfrac{16}{22\cdot4}$ gm/litres.

We know that $d_1T_1 = d_2T_2$ or $T_2 = \dfrac{d_1T_1}{d_2}$

$= \dfrac{32}{22\cdot4} \times \dfrac{273}{1} \times \dfrac{22\cdot4}{16} = 546 \text{ K} = 273^\circ\text{C}.$

(where T_1 at STP is 273 K).

96. (d) : Intensive property is that which is independent of the amount of the substance present in the system *e.g.* density, temperature, concentration etc.

Extensive property depends upon the amount of the substance present in the system. *e.g.* volume, mass etc.

97. (b) : Order of electronegativity is

$F > O > N > C$

98. (c) : With reduction, participation of atom electron decreases, therefore, Oxidation number also decreases.

99. (b) : $CH \equiv CH \xrightarrow[H_2O]{H_2SO_4/HgSO_4} CH_3CHO$

Here, addition of water is according to Markownikoff's rule.

100. (d) : As AgBr is sensitive to light, it is used for making photographic films.

Solution of sodium thiosulphate is used as fixer. It forms a soluble complex with silver halides.

$AgBr + 2Na_2S_2O_3 \longrightarrow Na_3[Ag.(S_2O_3)_2] + NaBr$

101. (c) : $O_2 + 4e^- \longrightarrow 2O^{2-}$

$\therefore$ Equivalent weight of oxygen $= \dfrac{\text{molecular weight}}{4}$

102. (a) : rate of diffusion $\propto \dfrac{1}{\sqrt{M}}$

M = Molecular mass

$\Rightarrow \dfrac{r_x}{r_{o_2}} = 4 = \sqrt{\dfrac{M_{O_2}}{M_x}}$

r_x = rate of diffusion of x (gas)

M_x = Molecular mass of x

$\Rightarrow \dfrac{r_x}{r_{o_2}} = 4 = \sqrt{\dfrac{MO_2}{M_x}}$

$\Rightarrow 16 = \dfrac{32}{M_x} \Rightarrow M_x = 2$

103. (c) : Density of water = 1 g/cm³ and its molecular weight = 18. Therefore 1000 cm³ of water will weigh 1000 g of water. We also know that molarity

$= \dfrac{\text{Mass of water}}{\text{Molecular weight}} = \dfrac{1000}{18} = 55\cdot56 \text{ M}.$

104. (b) : $Mg(HCO_3)_2 \rightarrow MgO + 2CO_2 + H_2O$

146 g give 22.4 Litre of CO_2

$\Rightarrow$ 7.3 g will give $= \dfrac{22.4}{146} \times 7.3$

$\Rightarrow$ = 1.12 litre of CO_2

= 1120 ml of CO_2

105. (d) : $Zn + H_2SO_4 \rightarrow ZnSO_4 + H_2$

65 g Zn will give 22.4 litre of H_2 at STP

$\Rightarrow$ 224 ml of H_2 corresponds to $\dfrac{65}{22400} \times 224$

= 0.65 g Zn

106. (a) : $Al^{3+} + 3e^- \rightarrow Al$

Therefore, 3 moles of electron is required to deposite 1 mole of Al.

107. (a) : Lithopone is $(ZnS + BaSO_4)$. It is used as a filler in rubber and paper industry.

108. (a) : The electronic configuration, of an element of atomic number 7, is $1s^2\ 2s^2\ 2p_x^{\ 1}, 2p_y^{\ 1}\ 2p_z^{\ 1}$. Thus the valency shell is second principal shell which has only four orbitals. Therefore the element can form maximum of four covalent bonds. Thus the covalency is 4.

109. (d) : Oxygen atom is monoatomic and oxidation number of an element in a monoatomic ion, is equal to the charge on the ion. *i.e.* -2.

110. (a) : There are three unpaired electrons.

1s	2s	2p		
⇅	⇅	1	1	1

111. (b) : Duma's method can be applied in case of all nitrogenous compounds. But Kjeldahl's method cannot be used in case of nitro, azo and azoxy compounds.

112. (a) : In cyclobutane, there is angle strain as bond angle (C–C–C) is close to 90°. Due to this kind of angle effecting overlapping of orbitals cannot take place.

113. (b) : Molecularity of reaction is the no. of molecules acting in the rate determing step while order of reaction is the sum total of all powers to which concentration are raised in the rate law expression. So both may or may not be same.

114. (a) : Bond order is the half of the difference between bonding and antibonding electrons i.e.,

$$\text{B.O.} = \frac{1}{2}\left[\begin{pmatrix}\text{No. of e}^-\text{s in}\\ \text{bonding M.O.}\end{pmatrix} - \begin{pmatrix}\text{No. of e}^-\text{s in}\\ \text{antibonding M.O.}\end{pmatrix}\right]$$

Greater the bond order, greater is the stability in the molecule.

115. (a) : Alkali metals have very low value of ionisation energy as compared to other metals. So Alkali metals easily get excited and impact to flame.

116. (c) :

Phenol is acidic in nature due to the acidity of phenolic proton (due to reasonance stabilisation) but there is no such stabilisation in ethane.

117. (d) : Cu cannot liberate H_2 from a solution of dilute HCl as hydrogen is above copper in the electrochemical series.

$$E^\circ_{H^+/½H_2} = \pm 0.00$$
$$E^\circ_{Cu^{2+}/Cu} = +0.34$$

118. (b) : Greater entropy of graphite is related to its structure as graphite is less compact and rigid than diamond. ΔH°_f for graphite is zero, but the ΔH°_f for diamond is 2 kJ/mol. That is because graphite is the standard state for carbon, not diamond.

119. (c) : SO_2 in presence of moisture acts as a bleaching agent. This is due to the reducing nature of SO_2. But bleaching action is only temporary.

$$SO_2 + 2H_2O \longrightarrow H_2SO_4 + 2[H]$$

Similarity, Cl_2 in pressure of moisture give out nascent oxygen (oxidation) and cause bleaching.

$$Cl_2 + H_2O \longrightarrow 2HCl + [O]$$

Here, bleaching action is permanent.

120. (b) : $HCOOH + 2HgCl_2 \xrightarrow{\Delta} Hg_2Cl_2 + CO_2 + 2HCl$

Reducing property of formic acid is due to – CHO group.

BIOLOGY

121. (c) : Stomach in vertebrates is the chief site for digestion of proteins. Because HCl is secreted here which alters the pH suitable for protein digestion. At the same time gastric pepsin is secreted by the stomach which digests protein. On the other hand carbohydrate digestion in the stomach depends on the action of salivary amylase and fat digestion is minimal in stomach due to the restriction of gastric lipase activity there.

122. (c) : Diapedesis is passage of blood cells, especially leucocytes, by amoeboid movements through the unruptured wall of a capillary vessel.

123. (c) : In *Leucosolenia,* food is stored in amoebocytes. Amoebocytes receive the partly digested food particles from choanocytes, complete its digestion and distribute the digested material throughout the body. Rest is stored in them.

124. (d) : Inheritance of ABO blood groups illustrates multiple allelism. Here, a single gene codes for an enzyme that is responsible for the addition of sugar residues to a specific glycoprotein on the membrane of red blood cells. Three different alleles of this gene are known. All three alleles have arisen by mutation from a single ancestor.

125. (d) : *Physalia* is tetramorphic in nature. It consists of

(i) a gastrozooid with mouth but no tentacle,

(ii) a small dactylozooid with a long slender tentacle,

(iii) a large dactylozooid with an enormous nematocyst bearing fishing tentacle and

(iv) a branched gonozooid which bears both male and female gonophores.

126. (c) : Starch is a complex polysaccharide carbohydrate, formed by polymerization (condensation) of several hundred glucose subunits by glycosidic bonds. Starch is easily broken down by amylase during digestion.

127. (d) : Intervertebral disc is made up of fibrous cartilage. The intervertebral discs are somatic derivatives. The spaces between developing vertebral bodies firstly become mesenchymal cells, these cells subsequently form the fibrocartilage of the annulus fibrous of the intervertebral discs.

128. (a) : Actomyosin is a protein complex found in

muscles. It is formed between molecules of actin and myosin present in adjacent thick and thin muscle filaments. These actomyosin complexes are involved in the process of muscle contraction.

129. (b) : Parotid glands are yellowish, flattened and the largest salivary glands located in the cheeks near the ears. The single, long, thick Stenson's duct from each gland opens in the vestibule in buccal cavity opposite to the second molar of its side. In man, inflammation and enlargement of these glands due to virus infection is a condition known as mumps.

130. (a) : Sarcoplasm is the protoplasm of the fibres of striated muscle, excluding the myofibrils.

131. (a) : Meroblastic cleavage refers to incomplete type of division of eggs. This occurs in macrolecithal and centrolecithal eggs. In such a cleavage, the furrows divide the small amount of active cytoplasm of animal pole or periphery of egg and most of the yolky portion of vegetal pole or central area of egg remains undivided.

132. (a) : Spider monkey (*Ateles paniscus*) has prehensile tail and belongs to new world monkeys. They are mostly found in tropical forests from Mexico to Brazil.

133. (b) : *Cis-trans* test is a test that determines whether two mutations that have the same effect occur in the same gene or in different genes. The mutation may be in either the *cis*-position (*i.e.*, on the same chromosome) or the *trans*-position (one on each homologue).

134. (d) : Schneiderian membrane is found in nasal mucosa. The olfactory organs of vertebrates have a lining of olfactory mucous membrane or schneiderian membrane. It is made up of basal cells, supporting cells and elongated neurosensory cells.

135. (a) : Brush border is the outer surface of columnar epithelial cells lining the intestine, kidney of man. With a light microscope, it appears as a narrow layer with vertical striations. But the electron microscope shows it to be made of fine hairline processes called microvilli. These greatly increase the surface area of the cell for absorption of dissolved substances.

136. (b) : Pliocene was the epoch of the tertiary, which followed the miocene. In the pliocene, the homonids such as *Australopithecus* and *Homo erectus*, which eventually led to man, became clearly distinguishable from the apes.

137. (a) : Allosteric site is a part of an enzyme to which a specific effector or modulator can be attached. This attachment is reversible. Allosteric enzymes possess an allosteric site in addition to their active site. This site is as specific in its relationship to modulators as active sites are to substrates.

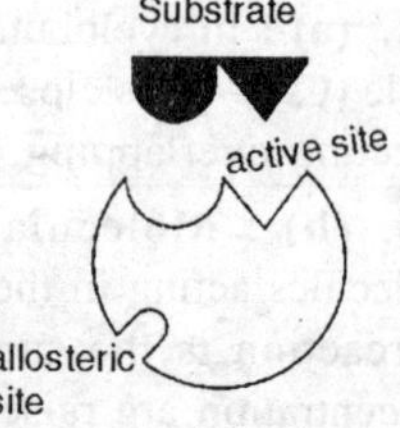

An allosteric enzyme having allosteric site and active site

138. (c) : Chromatophores lie in the skin of certain animals with permanent radiating processes containing pigment that can be concentrated or dispersed within the cell under nervous and/or hormonal stimulation, effecting colour changes. They often result in camouflage in *Chameleon.*

139. (b) : Dermal bone (membrane bone) is a vertebrate bone developing directly from mesenchyme rather than from pre-existing cartilage (cartilage bone). It is largely restricted to bones of cranium, jaws and pectoral girdle.

140. (d) : According to fossils, the evolution of modern horse began in the eocene epoch in North America with a fox-sized species originally named *Eohippus*. But later on, it was renamed *Hyracotherium.* After its origin, *Hyracotherium* spread throughout Europe and Asia.

141. (d) : Cholinergic nerve fibre releases acetylcholine from its end when stimulated by a nerve impulse. In vertebrates, motor fibres to striped muscle, parasympathetic fibres to smooth muscle, and preganglionic sympathetic fibres are all cholinergic.

142. (b) : Bohr effect is the phenomenon whereby the affinity of the respiratory pigment of the blood for oxygen is reduced, and the level of carbon dioxide is increased. This facilitates gaseous exchange, because more oxygen is released in the tissues where the amount of carbon dioxide is rising due to metabolic activity. At the same time, more oxygen is taken up at the lungs where the amount of carbon dioxide is low.

143. (d) : Gout is hereditary metabolic disease in the form of acute arthritis. It is marked by inflammation of the joints. In gout patients, excessive uric acid in blood and iron urates of sodium in and around of joints are present.

144. (b) : In the resting muscle, creatine is combined with phosphoric acid to form phosphagen (creatine phosphate). When the muscle contracts, creatine phosphate (phosphagen) is split back into creatine and phosphoric acid, with the release of energy. This energy is responsible for the actual muscle contraction through the medium of ATP.

145. (a) : Desmosomes are junctional complexes in which adjacent membranes possess disc - shaped

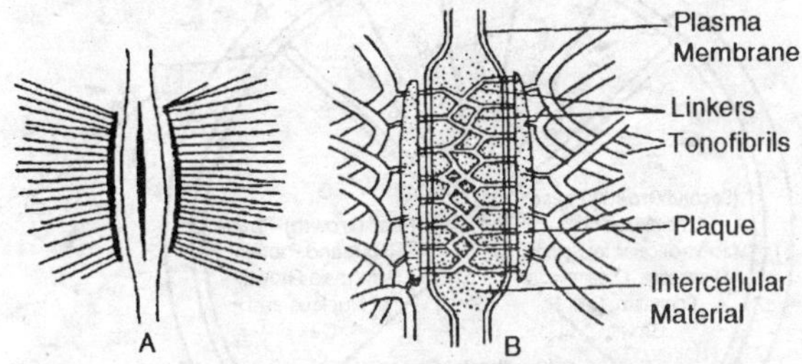

Structure of desmosome. A, in section. B, detailed reconstruction

thickenings of about 0.5 μm diameter, a number of tonofibrils and *trans*-membrane linkers embedded in dense intercellular material. Desmosomes function as spot welds and are hence called spot desmosomes. They occur in epithelia.

146. (a) : Large amount of absorbed water are translocated to the leaves and are lost to the surrounding atmosphere. Transpiration has cooling effect on the plant as well as on the surrounding atmosphere. A roof causes shade, but due to lack of any transpiration like system, it fails to give the same cooling effect as given by a plant.

147. (a) : Calcium oxalate crystals are present in raphides of almost all the plants organs and are particularly common in storage organs, pith and cortical tissues. The shape of the crystal is variable. Needle like or acicular crystal called raphides are found in aroids (*e.g. Colocasia, Amorphophallus, Impatiens*) and many aquatic plants (*e.g., Pistia, Eichornia* etc.).

148. (a) : The ovule where micropyle comes to lie close to the funiculus due to unilateral growth of the ovule are called anatropous. This is the most common

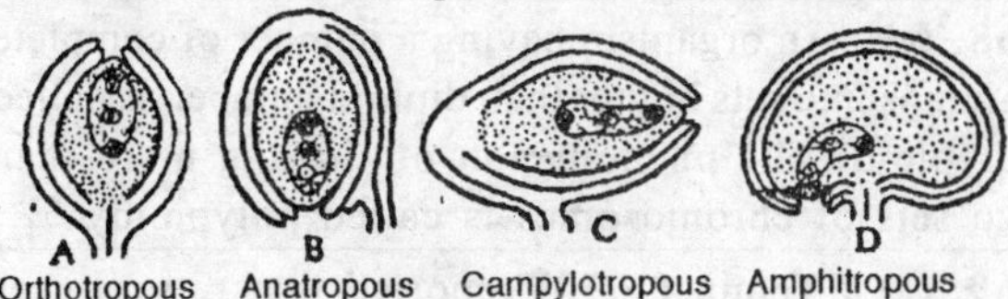

Types of ovule

type of ovule in the angiosperms. Where the curvature of the ovule also affects the nucellus so that the latter becomes horse - shoe - shaped. The ovuale is called amphitropous. In campylotropous ovule, the curvature is less than that in the anatropous ovules.

149. (a) : Darwin proposed the theory of evolution, in which he brought forward the fact that the present - day plants originated from some ancestral ones after undergoing periodical modifications due to environmental changes, therefore, all living plants today are related to each other in one way or the other. Thus later classification is also called vertical classification as it mainly depends upon evolutionary relationship or presumed ancestry.

150. (c) : In *Polysiphonia,* a multicellular gametophytic phase alternate with two sporophytic phases (*viz.* a *carposporophyte* which is attached to gametophyte and a tetrasporophyte. It is independent of gametophyte).

151. (b) : The cells of velamen are dead and empty. The water absorbed by them is later taken by the living cells of the root.

152. (d) : LPP-1 was the first cyanophage to be discovered by Safferman and Morris. It was so named because in can infect three different blue green algae which are *Lyngbya, Phormidium* and *Plectonema.*

153. (a) : In *Oedogonium,* the longitudinal bands of chloroplast get interconnected showing reticulations. The pyrenoids are located on every point of cross connection of the bands of chloroplast.

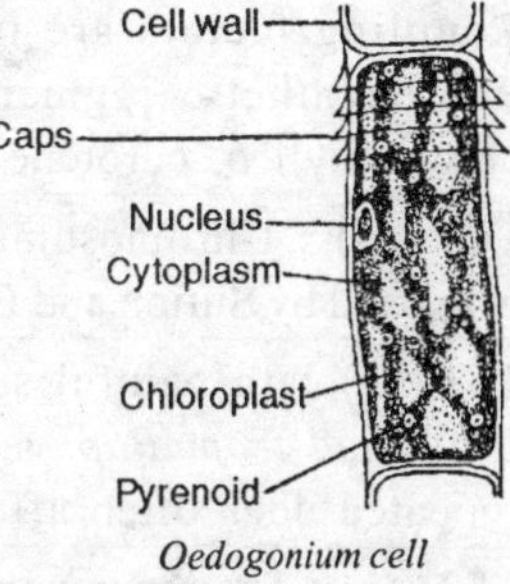

Oedogonium cell

154. (c) : The hornworts are so called because their capsule resembles the horn of animals. *Anthoceros* of this class is considered as a link between the bryophytes and pteridophytes as it is believed to have given rise to *Rhynia* (a fossil pteridophytes).

155. (d) : Bulliform cells are present in epidermis. These epidermal cells are found in the upper leaf epidermis of poaceae and other monocotyledons. Turgor changes in bulliform cells are responsible for the inrolling and unrolling of leaves. *e.g.* maiza, psamma grasses.

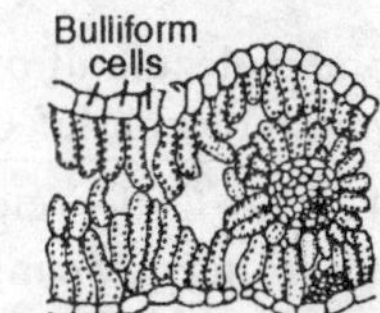

Bulliform cell in leaf epidermis

Therefore they are also called motor cells. They are highly vacuolate and can store water.

156. (a) : *Dalbergia latifolia* is also called Kali Shisham.The sapwood is narrow and pale yellowish white in colour, often with a purple tinge. The heartwood ranges in colour from golden brown through shades of light rose, purple with darker streaks, to deep purple with rather distant, nearly black lines, darkening with age.

157. (c) : Gibberellins play an important role in controlling a balance between internode growth and leaf development. In rosette forming plants (*e.g.*, cabbage) internode growth is poor but leaves are large. So the leaves appear to arise in tufts. This internode suddenly elongates and the stem becomes normal just before flowering.This is called bolting.

158. (c) : During aerobic respiration complete oxidation of food takes place. Thus during it a glucose molecule produce 38 ATP while during fermentation the food is oxidise partially and instead of $CO_2 + H_2O$ formation it results in formation of ethyl alcohol and water with net production of 2ATP.

159. (a) : Thylakoid membrances possess photosynthetic pigments and coupling factors. Coupling factors are involved in ATP synthesis. Photosynthetic pigments include chlorophyll *a*, chlorophyll *b*, carotene and xanthophylls.

160. (d) : Chromosome theory of inheritance was proposed by Sutton and Boveri independently in 1902.

161. (c) : In painful spasmodic affections, opium (*obtained from Papaver somniferum*) is large and repeated does often affords immediate relief.

162. (c) : The auxin content is maximum in stem tip. It is responsible for apical dominance (suppression of lateral buds). Decapitation results in translocation of auxins towards lower side. Hence lateral buds (axillary buds) get activated.

163. (b) : Number of oxygen molecules released per photon or quantum of light is known as quantum yield. Its value is $\frac{1}{8}$ to $\frac{1}{10}$. In other words evolution of one molecule of oxygen or consumption / fixation of one molecule of CO_2 requires 8 - 10 quanta.

164. (d) : Cell cycle consists of two stages, a long nondividing growing I (Interphase) - phase and a short dividing M (Metaphase) - phase. Both have substages. I - phase represents interphase. Interphase is a series of chages that take place in a newly formed cell and its nucleus before it becomes capable of division again. It is divisible into three stages G_1, S and G_2.

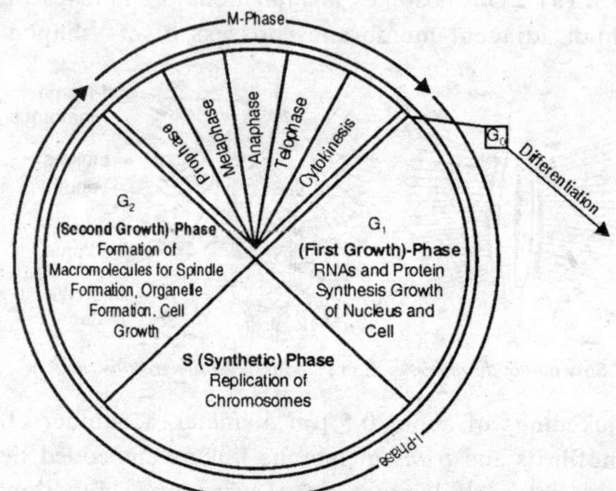

165. (b) : The mature antheridium of *Dryopteris* consists of a jacket layer composed of two ring - shaped cells and either one or two cap cells (cover cells). Inside the jacket layer there are 20 to 50 large spirally coiled atherozoids contained within their mother cells. The antherozoids are motile and multiciliate.

166. (d) : A large taxon, mostly treated as distinct order comprising 3 families : papilionaceae (Fabaceae), caesalpiniaceae and mimosaceae. Of all these families papilionaceae is predominantly herbaceous with a few shurbs and trees, but both the caesalpiniaceae and mimosaceae are chiefly arborescent. The flowers in racemose inflorescence, bisexual, actino or zygomorphic are usually highly ornamental. Stamens few to numerous, basifixed, mostly dehisce longitudinally. Ovary monocarpellary, superior, unilocular, placentation marginal.

167. (a) : The presence of pollinium is the characteristic feature of family asclepiadaceae. *e.g.*madar.

168. (c) : An organism having a number of complete chromosome sets higher than diploid number is called polyploid. The phenomenon of having more than two sets of chromosomes is called polyploidy.

169. (c) : Temin (1970) reported that retroviruses operate a central dogma reverse (inverse flow of information) or teminism inside host cells. Genomic RNA of these viruses first synthesizes DNA through reverse transcription. DNA then transfers information to messenger RNA which takes part in translation of the coded information to form polypeptide.

170. (c) : Plant peroxisomes found in photosynthetic cells perform photorespiration. For this, they are associated with chloroplast. Mesosomes are plasmalemma infoldings found in bacteria. Ribosomes are popularly known as protein factories due to their involvement in protein synthesis. Lysosomes take part in intracellular digestion of various types of materials and autolysis of cell.

171. (b) : Third eleavage of frog is latitudinal. Here, the unequally distributed yolk makes its influence felt. The mitotic spindles orient parallel to the polar axis and displaced as they are toward animal pole. The four blastomeres not only cleave latitudinally, but unequally.

172. (b) : The reaction of glycolysis occurs in the cytoplasm and do not require the presence of oxygen. The conversion of one molecule of glucose to two molecules of pyruvate results in a net gain of two ATP and two NADH molecules. 2 NADH produces 6 ATP (3 ATP per NADH molecule). Thus, glycolysis yields total 8 ATP. The kerbs cycle is far more efficient in the release of energy than are either glycolysis or fermenfation. The reactions of the krebs cycle require the presence of oxygen and are confined to the mitochondria. Total ATP produced during krebs cycle is 24.

173. (a) : In mammals, secondary plate is developed when the response comes for shifting the internal areas of body organs.

174. (c) : The development of cockroach is heterometabolous metamarophosis. It is gradual or incomplete metamorphosis. They have terrestrial youngs called nymphs. Nymphs look similar to adults but they lack the wings that gradually develop during several moults. The stages are –

egg → *nymph* (several instars) → *adult*

175. (a)

176. (b) : In *E. coli*, synthesis of β galactosidase, an enzyme meant for hydrolysis of lactose into glucose and galactose, has been studied in considerable detail.

$$\text{Lactose} \xrightarrow{\beta \text{ galactosidase}} \text{glucose} + \text{galactose}$$

If β galactosides (e.g. lactose) are not supplied to *E. coli* cells, the presence of β galactosidase is hardly detectable, but as soon as lactose is added, production of enzyme β galactosidase increases as much as 10,000 times. The enzyme quantity again fall down as quickly as the substance (i.e. lactose) is removed. Such enzymes, whose synthesis can be induced by adding substrate are known as "inducible enzymes". F. Jacob and J. Monod in 1961, on the basis of their study on the inducible system for the synthesis of β - galactosidase enzyme in *E. coli*, proposed a model in order to explain the induction or repression of enzyme synthesis. The model is popularly known as "operon model",

E. coli like other bacteria has incipient nucleus, i.e. nucleoid.

177. (c) : The ionizing radiations can have direct effect on chromosomes. They may directly break chromosomes or alter one of the DNA bases or indirectly may initiate a chain of chemical reactions. The biological effect also depends on the kind of cell and stage of nuclear cycle.

178. (a) : As a result of continued secondary growth for several years, the older parts of the stem and its old branches have a part of its secondary xylem renderd non - functional. Such a modified and non - functional secondary xylem is called the heart wood or *duramen*, the functional outer younger rings of secondary xylem constitute the sap wood or *alburnum*. With the passage of time and addition of new outer rings of secondary xylem more rings of the sap wood are changed into heart wood. This leads to the increase in the thickness of heart wood, whereas the sap wood remains of about the same thickness.

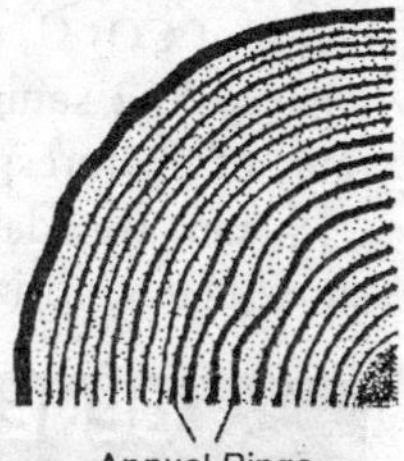

179. (a) : An *absorption spectrum* is a measure of the extent to which a given substance absorbs the light of different colours or wavelengths. An *action spectrum* is the measure of the efficiency of a process induced by light of different wavelengths but of the same intensity. It is actually a plot of the extent of a response (such as photosynthesis) against different wavelengths of light. A comparison of an action spectrum with the absorption spectrum of a pigment indicates whether or not the pigment is involved in the response. For example, the absorption spectrum of chlorophyll *a* is very similar to the action spectrum of photosynthesis in most plant tissues. Although, light energy is absorbed by chlorophylls as well as by other accessory pigments, only chlorophyll *a* is involved in photosystem I and II.

180. (b) : The initial work of Kortschak, Hartt and Barr, which demonstrated that rapidly photo-synthesizing sugarcane plants fix CO_2 into aspartic and malic acids, was confirmed by Hatch and Slack. Hatch and Slack proposed this pathway as Hatch and Slack pathway and named such plant as C_4 plants (as the products are four carbon compounds).

C_4 plants possess two types of chloroplasts bundle sheath cells and mesophyll cells. The mesophyll cells of C_4 plants exhibit high activity of phosphoenolpyruvate (PEP) carboxylase, which catalyzes the fixation of CO_2 with PEP to form oxaloacetic acid. The bundle sheath cells exhibit high RuBP carboxylase and the other enzymes of the Calvin - Benson cycle. C_4 plants are highly productive photosynthetically in view of the low affinity of the RuBP carboxylase for its substrate. But CO_2 is concentrated as C_4 acids due to the activity of the PEP carboxylase, which in effect maintains high pool levels of CO_2 C_4 plants are related to very high light - harvesting saturation points. C_4 plants exibit low rates of photorespiration only in bundle sheath cells. C_4 plants are adapted to high temperature. C_4 plants show better utilization of available water.

GENERAL KNOWLEDGE

181. (b)

182. (c) : First chief justice of India was Shri Harilal J. Kania in the duration between 1950-51.

183. (b)

184. (d) : The attorney general of India is the legal adviser to the government of India. He is appointed by the president of India on the advice of the Prime Minister.

185. (d)

186. (b) : The equator, which divides the earth into the northern and southern and southern hemispheres is designated as latitude.

187. (b)

188. (a) : IRDP programme with some modifications was taken up in 2300 blocks of different cities to provide full employment in these blocks within 5 years. This was initiated during the year of 1976-77.

189. (c)

190. (c) : Rudolf Dieself invented the diesel engine in 1895. He was a German scientist.

191. (b)

192. (b) : Aravali range is one of the oldest mountain in the world, which is situated in north-western India.

193. (c)

194. (a) : Aurbindo was a great philospher. He set up an ashram in Pondichery in 1910.

195. (b)

196. (c) : Mother Teresa came to India, when she was 18 years old and took up teaching as a profession. She established a 'Missionaries of charity'.

197. (d)

198. (b) : Vitamin 'D' regulates the absorption of calcium and phosphorus from the intestinal track and affords antiachitic activity.

199. (c)

200. (b) : The human skeleton is divided into two parts. *i.e.*, the axial skeleton and appendicular skeleton. The axial skeleton consists of the head, neck and trunk while the appendicular skeleton is made up of arms and legs.

❖ ❖ ❖

SOLVED PAPER
AIIMS - 1996

Time : 3½ Hours Max. Marks : 200

PHYSICS

1. A nucleus emits one α-particle and forms a new nucleus. The mass and charge of the new nucleus is changed in one of the following way
   (a) mass is reduced by 2 and charge is reduced by 2
   (b) mass is reduced by 4 and charge is reduced by 6
   (c) mass is reduced by 2 and charge is reduced by 4
   (d) mass is reduced by 4 and atomic no. is reduced by 2.

2. If at same temperature and pressure, the densities for two diatomic gases are d_1 and d_2 respectively, then the ratio of velocities of sound in these gases will be
   (a) $\sqrt{\frac{d_2}{2d_1}}$ (b) $\sqrt{\frac{d_2}{d_1}}$
   (c) $\sqrt{\frac{2d_1}{d_2}}$ (d) $\sqrt{\frac{d_1}{d_2}}$

3. The equivalent resistance between A and C of the given circuit, is 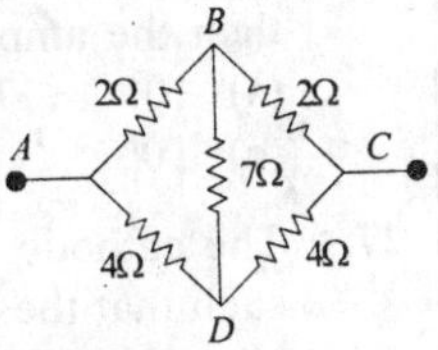
   (a) 8 Ω
   (b) $\frac{32}{12}\Omega$
   (c) $\frac{1}{3}\Omega$ (d) $\frac{8}{3}\Omega$.

4. Which of the following will deflect in electric field?
   (a) cathode-ray (b) X-rays
   (c) ultra-violet rays (d) γ-rays.

5. The working of a dynamo is based on the principle of
   (a) chemical effect of current
   (b) heating effect of current
   (c) electromagnetic induction
   (d) magnetic effect of current.

6. A galvanometer can be changed into ammeter by providing
   (a) high resistance in series
   (b) low resistance in series
   (c) high resistance in parallel
   (d) low resistance in parallel.

7. The energy produced in the sun is due to
   (a) chemical reaction (b) fission reaction
   (c) fusion reaction (d) all of these.

8. Plate current will be maximum, when
   (a) grid is negative while anode is positive
   (b) both the grid and anode are positive
   (c) grid is positive while anode is negative
   (d) both the grid and anode are negative.

9. Thermocouple thermometer is based on
   (a) Peltier effect (b) Seebeck effect
   (c) photoelectric effect
   (d) Compton effect.

10. On increasing the temperature of a substance gradually, its colour becomes
    (a) yellow (b) red
    (c) white (d) green.

11. A source of frequency 240 Hz is moving towards an observer with a velocity of 20 m/s. The observer is now moving away the source with a velocity of 20 m/s. Apparent frequency heard by observer, if velocity of sound is 340 m/s, is
    (a) 268 Hz (b) 270 Hz
    (c) 360 Hz (d) 240 Hz.

12. When light rays enter in a glass slab, their wavelength
    (a) remains unchanged
    (b) decreases
    (c) increases
    (d) either (a) or (b).

13. A convex lens of focal length 40 cm is in contact with a concave lens of focal length 25 cm. The power of the combination, is
(a) + 6.67 D (b) - 6.5 D
(c) - 1.5 D (d) + 6.5 D.

14. Photoelectric effect of light is due to
(a) photons (b) protons
(c) electric effect (d) quanta.

15. Extra pressure inside a soap bubble of radius (r) is proportional to
(a) r^2 (b) r
(c) $1/r^2$ (d) $1/r$.

16. If a spring of mass 30 kg has spring constant of 15 N/m, then its time period, is
(a) 2π sec (b) $2\sqrt{2\pi}$ sec
(c) $2\sqrt{2}$ sec (d) $2\pi\sqrt{2}$ sec.

17. If the radii of circular paths of two particles of same masses are in the ratio 1 : 2, then to have a constant centripetal force, their velocities should be in a ratio of
(a) 4 : 1 (b) $1 : \sqrt{2}$
(c) 1 : 4 (d) $\sqrt{2} : 1$.

18. Ratio of the amount of heat radiation, transmitted through the body to the amount of heat radiation incident on it, is known as
(a) transmittance (b) conductance
(c) absorbance (d) inductance.

19. A body of mass m is placed on a rough surface with coefficient of friction (μ) inclined at θ. If the mass is in equilibrium, then
(a) $\theta = \tan^{-1}\left(\frac{m}{\mu}\right)$ (b) $\theta = \tan^{-1}(\mu)$
(c) $\theta = \tan^{-1}\left(\frac{\mu}{m}\right)$ (d) $\theta = \tan^{-1}(1/\mu)$.

20. The forces, which meet at one point but their lines of action do not lie in one plane, are called
(a) non-coplanar concurrent forces
(b) coplanar concurrent forces
(c) non-coplanar non-concurrent forces
(d) coplanar non-concurrent forces.

21. Which of the following is constant in a projectile motion?
(a) velocity of projection
(b) horizontal component of the velocity
(c) vertical component of the velocity
(d) all of these.

22. Which of the following is a non-conservative force?
(a) electrostatic force (b) viscous force
(c) interatomic force (d) gravitational force.

23. The equation of a wave is given by: $y = 10\sin\left(\frac{2\pi t}{30} + \alpha\right)$. If the displacement is 5 cm at $t = 0$, then the total phase at $t = 7.5$ sec will be
(a) $\frac{2\pi}{3}$ rad (b) $\frac{\pi}{3}$ rad
(c) $\frac{\pi}{2}$ rad (d) $\frac{2\pi}{5}$ rad.

24. The displacement of a body is given to be proportional to the cube of time elapsed. The magnitude of the acceleration of the body, is
(a) constant but not zero
(b) increasing with time
(c) zero
(d) decreasing with time.

25. If ${}_{92}U^{238}$ undergoes successively 8 α-decays and 6 β-decays, then the resulting nucleus is
(a) ${}_{82}U^{210}$ (b) ${}_{82}U^{208}$
(c) ${}_{82}U^{214}$ (d) ${}_{82}U^{206}$.

26. If the plate resistance of a triode is 3.3×10^{-3} Ω and its mutual conductance is 3×10^3 mhos, then the amplification factor is nearly equal to
(a) 10^3 (b) 10^{-2}
(c) 10^6 (d) 10^1.

27. The cathode of a photoelectric cell is charged, such that the work function changes from W_1 to W_2 (where $W_2 < W_1$). If the currents, before and after the changes are I_1 and I_2 respectively and all other conditions remaining unchanged, then
(a) $I_1 = I_2$ (b) $I_1 < I_2$
(c) $I_1 > 2I_2$ (d) $I_1 > I_2$.

28. A lightly damped oscillator with a frequency (ω) is set in motion by harmonic driving force of frequency (n). When $n < \omega$, then response of the oscillator is controlled by
(a) oscillator frequency
(b) spring constant

(c) damping coefficient
(d) inertia of the mass.

29. The temperature of a gas is held constant, while its volume is decreased. The pressure exerted by the gas on the walls of the container increases, because its molecules
(a) strike the walls more frequently
(b) strike the walls with higher velocities
(c) are in contact with the walls for a shorter time
(d) strike the walls with larger force.

30. Threshold frequency for a metal is 10^{15} Hz. If the light of wavelength 4000 Å falls on its surface, then which of the following statement is correct?
(a) photoelectrons come out with a velocity of 100 m/sec
(b) no photoelectric emission takes place
(c) photoelectrons come out with a velocity of 124 m/sec
(d) photoelectrons come out with a velocity of 9.8 m/sec.

31. The volume of a gas expands by 0.25 m^3 at a constant pressure of 10^3 N/m. The work done is equal to
(a) 250 watt (b) 2·5 erg
(c) 250 newton (d) 250 joule.

32. If voltage across an X-ray tube is doubled, then energy of X-rays emitted by this tube would
(a) become half (b) be doubled
(c) remain the same (d) be quardrupled.

33. The velocity of electromagnetic waves in free space is 3×10^8 m/sec. The frequency of a radio wave of wave length 150 m, is
(a) 20 kHz (b) 45 MHz
(c) 2 kHz (d) 2 MHz.

34. In general, the wavelength of microwaves, is
(a) more than that of infrared waves
(b) more than that of radiowaves
(c) less than that of infrared waves
(d) less than that of ultraviolet waves.

35. A boy of mass 40 kg is standing in a lift, which is moving downwards with an acceleration 9·8 m/s^2. The apparent weight of the boy is (Take g = 9·8 m/s^2)
(a) 40 × 9·8 N (b) 0 N
(c) 40/9·8 N (d) 40 N.

36. The magnetic flux linked with a coil, in webers, is given by the equation: $\phi = 5t^2 + 3t + 16$. The induced e.m.f. in the coil in the fourth second will be
(a) 145 V (b) 10 V
(c) 210 V (d) 108 V.

37. Critical temperature can be defined as the temperature
(a) at which the volume of a gas becomes zero
(b) at which there is no motion between the molecules
(c) above which a gas cannot be liquified, no matter however high the pressure may be
(d) at which a gas is converted into its liquid state.

38. A tape-recorder records sound in the form of
(a) magnetic energy
(b) electrical energy
(c) variable resistance on the tape
(d) magnetic field on the tape.

39. The H_α line of hydrogen
(a) has a wavelength smaller than that of the H_β line
(b) has a wavelength 4860 Å
(c) is emitted in the transition from the second excited state to the first excited state
(d) has a wavelength 6060 Å.

40. An observer standing by the side of a road hears the siren of an ambulance, which is moving away from him. If the actual frequency of the siren is 2,000 Hz, then the frequency heard by the observer will be
(a) 2000 Hz (b) 1990 Hz
(c) 4000 Hz (d) 2100 Hz.

41. Calorimeters are made of which of the following?
(a) wood (b) glass
(c) metal (d) either (a) or (b).

42. Light year is the unit of
(a) velocity (b) time
(c) intensity of light (d) distance.

43. Angle between two vectors of magnitudes 12 and 18 units, when their resultant is 24 units is
(a) 82°31′ (b) 63°51′
(c) 89°16′ (d) 75°52′.

44. Emission of β-rays in radioactive decay results in the change of
(a) both mass and charge
(b) mass but not in charge

(c) either mass and charge
(d) charge but not in mass.

45. If a steady current of 4 A maintained for 40 minutes, deposits 4.5 g of zinc at the cathode end, then its chemical equivalent, is
(a) 47×10^{-5} g/C (b) 26×10^{-6} g/C
(c) 51×10^{-7} g/C (d) 36×10^{-6} g/C.

46. When the axis of rotation passes through its centre of gravity, then the moment of inertia of a rigid body is
(a) reduced to its minimum value
(b) zero
(c) increased to its maximum value
(d) infinity.

47. A perfect gas is contained in a cylinder kept in vacuum. If the cylinder suddenly bursts, then the temperature of the gas
(a) is increased
(b) becomes zero K
(c) remains unchanged
(d) is decreased.

48. The hydrogen atom can give spectral lines in the Lyman, Balmer Paschen series. Which of the following statement is correct?
(a) Paschen series is in the visible region
(b) Lyman series is in the infra-red region
(c) Balmer series is (solely) in ultra violet-region
(d) Balmer series is in the visible region (partly).

49. A closed organ pipe and an open organ pipe of the same length produce four beats, when sounded together. If the length of the closed organ pipe is increased, then the number of beats will
(a) remains the same (b) increase
(c) decrease (d) first (d) then (a).

50. A permanent magnet attracts
(a) some substances and repels others
(b) all substances
(c) ferromagnetic substances and repels all other
(d) only ferromagnetic substances.

Directions: *These questions consist of two statements each, printed as Assertion and Reason. While answering these questions you are required to choose any one of the following four responses.*
(a) If both Assertion and Reason are true and the Reason is a correct explanation of the Assertion.
(b) If both Assertion and Reason are true but Reason is not a correct explanation of the Assertion.
(c) If Assertion is true but the Reason is false.
(d) If both Assertion and Reason are false.

51. *Assertion*: The frequencies of incident, reflected and refracted beam of monochromatic light incident from one medium to another are same.
Reason: The incident, reflected and refracted rays are coplanar.

52. *Assertion*: A laser beam of 0.2 W power can drill holes through a metal sheet, whereas a 1000 W torch-light cannot.
Reason: The frequency of laser light is much higher than that of torch light.

53. *Assertion*: A pulsar is a source of radio waves that varies in intensity at regular intervals.
Reason: A pulsar is a rorating neutron star.

54. *Assertion*: The relative velocity of two photons travelling in opposite direction is the velocity of light.
Reason: The rest mass of a photon is zero.

55. *Assertion*: The temperature coefficient of resistance is positive for metals and negative p-type semiconductors.
Reason: The effective charge carriers in metals are negatively charged whereas in p-type semiconductors they are positively charged.

56. *Assertion*: The ratio C_p/C_v is more for helium gas than for hydrogen gas.
Reason: All metals acts as black bodies.

57. *Assertion*: A hollow metallic closed container maintained at a uniform temperature can act as a source of black body radiation.
Reason: All metals act as black bodies.

58. *Assertion*: The square of the period of revolution of a planet is proportional to the cube of the semi-major axis of the ellipse
Reason: Sun's gravitational field is inversely proportional to the square of its distance from the planet.

59. *Assertion*: Environmental damage has increased the amount of ozone in the atmosphere.
Reason: Increase of ozone increases the amount of ultraviolet radiation on earth.

60. *Assertion*: Electric appliances with metallic body. *e.g.*, heaters, presses etc., have three pin

connections, whereas an electric bulb has a two pin connection.
Reason: Three pin connections reduce heating of connecting cables.

CHEMISTRY

61. The percentage of oxygen in NaOH is
(a) 16% (b) 4%
(c) 40% (d) 8%.

62. Which of the following is the correct representation of relative lowering of vapour pressure ?
(a) $\frac{P^0}{\Delta P} = \frac{P^0 - P}{P^0}$ (b) $\frac{P^0 - P}{P^0}$
(c) $\frac{P^0}{P^0 - P}$ (d) $\frac{\Delta P}{P^0} = \frac{P^0 - P}{P^0}$

63. The number of moles of water present in 180 gm of water is
(a) 18 (b) 5
(c) 100 (d) 10.

64. What happens when chloroform is left open in air in the presence of sunlight ?
(a) polymerisation takes place
(b) explosion takes place
(c) no reaction takes place
(d) phosgene, a poisonous gas is formed.

65. Which of the following metal does not liberate H_2 from dilute H_2SO_4 ?
(a) Zn (b) Al
(c) Cu (d) Mg.

66. Glycerol is not used in
(a) explosive (b) cosmetics
(c) soaps (d) matches.

67. Which of the following is formed, when benzaldehyde reacts with alcoholic KCN ?
(a) benzoin (b) benzyl alcohol
(c) benzoin acid (d) ethyl benzoate.

68. Ozonolysis of acetylene gives
(a) HCHO (b) CH_3CHO
(c) CHO-CHO (d) none of these.

69. Chlorine oxidises sodium thiosulphate to form
(a) Na_2SO_3 (b) Na_2O
(c) Na_2SO_4 (d) Na_2CO_3.

70. Which of the following is a characteristic of a reversible reaction ?
(a) it never proceeds to completion
(b) it can be influenced by a catalyst
(c) it proceeds only in forward direction
(d) number of moles of reactants and products are equal.

71. Bauxite, an ore of aluminium is purified by
(a) Hall's process (b) Serpek's process
(c) Bayer's process (d) all of these.

72. Blister copper is
(a) alloy of copper (b) pure copper
(c) copper containing 1% impurity
(d) ore of copper.

73. Which of the following gas molecules have equal total kinetic energy and translational kinetic energy ?
(a) O_2 (b) He
(c) CH_4 (d) N_2.

74. The pH of 0.001 (N) acetic acid solution, which is 10% dissociated, is
(a) 3 (b) 1
(c) 4 (d) 2.

75. The strongest bronsted base among the following anions is
(a) ClO_3^- (b) ClO^-
(c) ClO_4^- (d) ClO_2^-.

76. The boiling point of a compound is raised by
(a) intermolecular hydrogen bonding
(b) volatility of compound
(c) intramolecular hydrogen bonding
(d) non-polarity in the molecules.

77. Thermite is a mixture of
(a) Zn + Mg (b) Fe + Al
(c) Fe_2O_3 + Al (d) Cu + Mg.

78. Silicon is an important constituent of
(a) alloys (b) rocks
(c) vegetables (d) animals.

79. How many litres of ammonia gas at S.T.P. would be needed to prepare 100 ml of 2·5 M ammonium hydroxide solution ?
(a) 5·6 lit (b) 0·056 lit
(c) 11·2 lit (d) 0·56 lit.

80. A radioactive nuclide decays at such a rate that after 96 min, only 1/8th of the original amount remains. The value of half-life of the nuclide is
(a) 32 min (b) 12 min
(c) 48 min (d) 24 min.

81. The maximum number of electrons, present in an orbit that is represented by azimuthal quantum number (l) = 3, will be
(a) 8 (b) 2
(c) 14 (d) 6.

82. Which of the following compounds is known as white vitriol ?
(a) $ZnSO_4 \cdot 7H_2O$ (b) $CaCO_4 \cdot 2H_2O$
(c) $Na_2SO_4 \cdot 7H_2O$ (d) $MgSO_4 \cdot 7H_2O$.

83. Avogadro's number of oxygen atom weighs
(a) 32 g (b) 8 g
(c) 56 g (d) 16 g.

84. In the reaction sequence: $CaC_2 \xrightarrow{H_2O} A \xrightarrow[HgSO_4]{\text{dil } HgSO_4} B \xrightarrow{H_2/Ni} C$, the term 'C' is
(a) CH_3CHO (b) HCHO
(c) C_2H_5OH (d) CH_3OH.

85. The equilibrium constant of a reaction is 300. If the volume of a reaction flask is trippled, the equilibrium constant will be
(a) 300 (b) 100
(c) 600 (d) 150.

86. Which of the following carbonium ion will be most stable ?
(a) $(CH_3)_2CH^+$ (b) CH_3^+
(c) $CH_3CH_2^+$ (d) $(CH_3)_3C^+$.

87. The volume of 3.0 N-H_2O_2 strength is
(a) 16.8 litres (b) 4.2 litres
(c) 33.6 litres (d) 8.4 litres.

88. Which of the following is the strongest base ?
(a) H_2^+ (b) H
(c) HCO_3^- (d) H^-.

89. Bismuth chloride ($BiCl_3$), on hydrolysis, yields a white precipitate of
(a) bismuth hydroxide (b) bismuth oxyacid
(c) bismuth oxychloride
(d) none of these.

90. Ostwald's dilution law is applicable to only
(a) strong electrolytes (b) solute
(c) weak electrolytes (d) solvent.

91. Which of the following contains cobalt ?
(a) vitamin B_{12} (b) haemoglobin
(c) chlorophyll (d) vitamin D.

92. Which of the following is a sulphide ore ?
(a) carnallite (b) magnetite
(c) copper pyrites (d) malachite.

93. The pH value of human blood is about
(a) 4.5 to 5.6 (b) 2.3 to 3.4
(c) 7.3 to 7.5 (d) 3.5 to 4.3.

94. In the P^{3-}, S^{2-} and Cl^- ions, the increasing order of size is
(a) $S^{2-} < Cl^- < P^{3-}$ (b) $Cl^- < S^2 < P^{3-}$
(c) $S^{2-} < P^{3-} < Cl^-$ (d) $P^{3-} < S^{2-} < Cl^-$.

95. Absolute ether is diethyl ether, which
(a) is obtained from williamson's synthesis
(b) is mixed with absolute alcohol
(c) is totally free from moisture and peroxides
(d) contains trace of peroxide.

96. The number of molecules in 4.25 g of ammonia is approximately
(a) 3.5×10^{23} (b) 0.5×10^{23}
(c) 2.5×10^{23} (d) 1.5×10^{23}.

97. The rate, at which a substance reacts, depends upon its
(a) equivalent mass (b) molecular mass
(c) active mass (d) atomic mass.

98. The maximum energy is possessed by an electron, when it is present
(a) in first excited state
(b) in nucleus
(c) at infinite distance from the nucleus
(d) in ground energy state.

99. Which of the following compounds will undergo hydrolysis ?
(a) $NaNO_3$ (b) KCl
(c) NH_4Cl (d) NaCl.

100. Which of the following is the correct sequence of atomic weights of the given elements ?
(a) Ni > Co > Fe (b) Fe > Co > Ni
(c) Co > Fe > Ni (d) Co > Ni > Fe.

101. Which of the following indicator is known as metal indicator ?
(a) phenolphthalein (b) phenol red
(c) eriochrome-Black-T
(d) methyl orange.

102. Which of the following species is isotonic with $_{37}Rb^{86}$?
(a) $_{38}Sr^{87}$ (b) $_{36}Kr^{84}$
(c) $_{39}Y^{89}$ (d) $_{37}Mg^{85}$.

103. Hydrolysis of beryllium carbide produces
(a) acetylene (b) methane
(c) ethene (d) none of these.

104. If active mass of a 6% solution of a compound is 2, its molecular weight will be
(a) 30 (b) 15
(c) 60 (d) 22.

105. Which of the following molecules is paramagnetic?
(a) P_2O_5 (b) NO_2
(c) $H_2S_2O_7$ (d) N_2O_5.

106. The aqueous solution of which of the following salt will have the lowest pH ?
(a) $NaClO_3$ (b) $NaClO$
(c) $NaClO_4$ (d) $NaClO_2$.

107. In the reaction: $2P_2O_5 + 2HNO_3 \rightarrow P_4O_{10} + x$, the term x is
(a) N_2O_4 (b) H_2O only
(c) N_2O_5 (d) PNO_3.

108. If a neutral atoms is converted into a cation, then its
(a) atomic weight increases
(b) size increases
(c) atomic weight decreases
(d) size decreases.

109. Which of the following is urotropine ?
(a) hexamethylene tetramine
(b) hexamethyl-diamine
(c) heximethylene triamine
(d) none of these.

110. Which of the following alkanes is optically active?
(a) 3-methyl hexane (b) propane
(c) 2, 3, 4-trimethyl pentane
(d) 2-methyl butane.

Directions: *These questions consist of two statements each, printed as Assertion and Reason. While answering these questions you are required to choose any one of the following four responses.*
(a) If both Assertion and Reason are true and the Reason is a correct explanation of the Assertion.
(b) If both Assertion and Reason are true but Reason is not a correct explanation of the Assertion.
(c) If Assertion is true but the Reason is false.
(d) If both Assertion and Reason are false.

111. *Assertion*: In crystal lattice, size of the cation is larger in a tetrahedral hole than in an octahedral hole.
Reason: The cations occupy more space than anions in crystal packing.

112. *Assertion*: The enthalpy of formation of gaseous oxygen molecules at 298 K under a pressure of one atm is zero.
Reason: The entropy of formation of gaseous oxygen molecules under the same conditions is zero.

113. *Assertion*: Aniline hydrogen sulphate, on heating, forms a mixture of ortho and para amino benzene sulphonic acids.
Reason: The sulphonic acid group is electron withdrawing.

114. *Assertion*: The atoms in a covalent molecule are said to share electrons, yet some covalent molecules are polar.
Reason: In a polar covalent molecule, the shared electrons spend more time than the average near one of the atoms.

115. *Assertion*: In electrolysis, the quantity of electricity needed for depositing. 1 mole of silver is different from that required for 1 mole of copper.
Reason: The molecular weights of silver and copper are different.

116. *Assertion*: Nitrogen is unreactive at room temperature but becomes reactive at elevated temperatures (on heating) or in the presence of catalysts.
Reason: In nitrogen molecules, there is extensive delocalization of electrons.

117. *Assertion*: Electrons are ejected from a certain metal when either blue or violet light strikes the metal surface. However, only violet light causes electron ejection from a second metal.
Reason: The electrons in the first metal require less energy for ejection.

118. *Assertion*: Sodium ions are discharged in preference to hydrogen ions at a mercury cathode.
Reason: The nature of cathode can affect the order of discharge of cations.

119. *Assertion*: A special line will be seen for a $2p_x \rightarrow 2p_y$ transition.
Reason: Energy is released in the form of waves of light when the electron drops from $2p_x$ to $2p_y$ orbital.

120. *Assertion*: Amongst the halogens, fluorine can oxidise the elements to the highest oxidation state.
Reason: Due to small size of fluoride ions, it is difficult to oxidise fluoride ions to fluorine. Hence reverse reaction takes place more easily.

BIOLOGY

121. The amphids are cuticular elevations on the ventro-lateral lips of *Ascaris*. These are
(a) tactoreceptors (b) chemoreceptors
(c) olfactoreceptors (d) tangoreceptors.

122. *Hydra* recognises its prey by
(a) chemical stimulus of prey
(b) nematocyst
(c) mechanical stimulus of prey
(d) some special organs.

123. The major constituent of vertebrate bone is
(a) potassium hydroxide
(b) sodium chloride
(c) calcium carbonate
(d) calcium phosphate.

124. The function of ductus choledochus is to carry
(a) urine (b) ova
(c) sperms (d) bile.

125. Which of the following gland controls egg production and moulting in insects ?
(a) corpus callosum (b) corpora allata
(c) corpora cardiaca (d) all of these.

126. Chordae tendinae are found in
(a) ventricles of brain (b) joints of legs
(c) ventricles of heart (d) atria of heart.

127. In mammals, the digestion of starch starts from
(a) oesophagus (b) mouth
(c) duodenum (d) stomach.

128. Which of the following is flightless bird ?
(a) ostrich (b) emu
(c) kiwi (d) all of these.

129. The camel's hump is composed of a tissue, which provides water when oxidised is, called
(a) areolar (b) skeletal
(c) adipose (d) muscular.

130. Wharton's duct is the duct of
(a) submandibular salivary gland
(b) parotid gland
(c) submaxillary gland
(d) all of these.

131. The horns of *Rhinoceros* are composed of
(a) chitin (b) bone
(c) keratin (d) cartilage.

132. Sharpey's perforating fibres are related with
(a) muscle contraction
(b) fixing of teeth
(c) heart contraction
(d) all of these.

133. Knock knee disease is due to
(a) deficiency in tyrosine amino acid
(b) hormonal imbalance
(c) excess fluoride concentration in water body
(d) genetical abnormality in males.

134. Sweat glands, in human skin, are located in the
(a) malpighian layer of epidermis
(b) dermis of skin
(c) subdermal layer of fat cells
(d) glandular layer of epidermis.

135. Where the conversion of harmful prussic acid into potassium sulphocyanide takes place ?
(a) bone marrow (b) spleen
(c) lymph glands (d) liver.

136. Which of the following is not applicable to coelenterates ?
(a) choanocytes (b) coelenteron
(c) radial symmetry (d) nematoblasts.

137. Function of contractile vacuole in protozoa is
(a) osmoregulation (b) locomotion
(c) respiration (d) digestion of food.

138. Animals belonging to order rodentia have
(a) long canines (b) long incisors
(c) long molars (d) short incisors.

139. How many teeth grow only once in the life of a man?
(a) 20 (b) 8
(c) 32 (d) 12.

140. Glycosidic link is broken in digestion of
(a) starch (b) protein
(c) lipid (d) all of these.

141. Which of the following is most convincing reasons for increasing population growth in a country ?
(a) low population of old people
(b) high birth rate
(c) high population of young children
(d) low mortality rate.

142. Radial symmetry is usually exhibited in animals, which
(a) are aquatic
(b) have ciliary mode of feeding
(c) are attached to some substratum (sedentary).
(d) none of these.

143. Which of the following has been declared a killer disease under Factory Act ?
(a) tuberculosis (b) asbestosis
(c) shigellosis (d) silicosis.

144. In *Gloriosa*, the tendrillar part is formed by
(a) leaf petiole (b) stipule
(c) axillary bud (d) leaf apex.

145. If PH of stomach is 1 · 6, then which enzyme will digest protein ?
(a) amylase (b) trypsin
(c) erypsin (d) pepsin.

146. When ovules at two points are developed, from the inner wall of the unilocular ovary, the placentation is called
(a) marginal (b) parietal
(c) superficial (d) basal.

147. Yellow bone marrow is found especially in the medullary cavity of
(a) short bones (b) spongy bones
(c) long bones (d) all of these.

148. Carbon dioxide is necessary for photosynthesis. The chemical used to remove this gas most effectively from entering a control apparatus is
(a) calcium oxide (b) distilled water
(c) potassium hydroxide solution
(d) sodium carbonate.

149. `Sudan Black B' stain is used to stain
(a) nucleic acid (b) protein
(c) polysaccharide (d) lipid.

150. Life in biosphere is abundant between
(a) 200 m below sea level to 6000 m above sea level
(b) 6000 m below sea level to 6000 m above sea level
(c) 11000 m below sea level to 9000 m above sea level
(d) 6000 m below sea level to 2000 m above sea level.

151. Which of the following correctly represents the flow of genetic information ?
(a) DNA → RNA →protein
(b) RNA → DNA →protein
(c) RNA → protein → DNA
(d) protein → RNA → DNA.

152. Starch and cellulose are the compounds of many units of
(a) amino acids (b) glycerol
(c) simple sugars (d) fatty acids.

153. An ecological pyramid of biomass is the representation of the ecosystem's
(a) energy flow through each trophic level
(b) population in each food web
(c) tissue organisation at each trophic level.
(d) all of these.

154. Which part of the world has a high density of organisms ?
(a) deciduous forests
(b) grasslands
(c) tropical rain forests
(d) savannahs.

155. In a lake, the upper warmer oxygen rich circulating water layer zone is referred to
(a) limnetic zone (b) epilimnion
(c) profundal zone (d) hypolimnion.

156. Red Data Book deals with
(a) plants on the verge of extinction
(b) endemic plant
(c) plants showing photoperiodism
(d) plants that are extinct.

157. Which of the following is not a correct match ?
(a) Aflatoxin - *Aspergillus parasiticus*
(b) Bengal famine-*Helminthosporium*
(c) Redrust of tea-*Melampsora*
(d) Tikka disease of groundnut-*Cercospora*.

158. How many cytochromes are involved in the electron transport chain ?
(a) five (b) two
(c) six (d) four.

159. In gymosperm, the endosperm is a formed by
(a) fusion of two polar nuclei
(b) fertilised egg
(c) fusion of one polar nucleus
(d) germination of one megaspore.

160. Krantz anatomy is seen in
(a) *Euphorbia hirta*
(b) *Citrus indica*

(c) *Mangifera indica*
(d) *Zea mays.*

161. During photosynthesis, oxygen in glucose comes from
(a) oxygen in air (b) water
(c) carbon dioxide (d) both (b) and (c).

162. The niche of a population is the
(a) set of conditions that it interacts
(b) place where it lives
(c) set of conditions and resources it uses
(d) geographical area that it covers.

163. The best source of vitamin C is
(a) *Citrus indica* (b) *Glycine max*
(c) *Emblica officinalis*
(d) *Arachis hypogea.*

164. The molar ratio of chlorophyll and xanthophyll is
(a) 4 : 1 (b) 3 : 1
(c) 1 : 1 (d) 2 : 1.

165. Shifting cultivation requires
(a) alternate crop pattern on a particular area
(b) huge amount of commercial fertiliser
(c) excessive soil erosion for crop production
(d) long time for the regeneration of soil.

166. Major source of sugar in the world is
(a) *Citrullus vulgaris* (b) *Beta vulgaris*
(c) *Saccharum officinarum*
(d) *Annona squamosa.*

167. *Penicillium* does not allow the growth of bacterium *Staphylococcus*. This sort of relationship is called
(a) commensalism (b) antagonism
(c) ammensalism (d) mutualism.

168. The reflectivity percentage of incident light on the earth is meteorologically called as
(a) reradiation (b) tornado
(c) irrefraction (d) albedo.

169. Plants which can withstand wide range of temperature tolerance are called
(a) monothermic (b) stenothermic
(c) mesothermic (d) eurythermic.

170. Which of the following is not a correct match?
(a) chord moss-*Funaria*
(b) maiden hair fern-*Ginkgo*
(c) walking fern-*Camptosorus*
d) bog moss-*Sphagnum*.

Directions: *These questions consist of two statements each, printed as Assertion and Reason. While answering these questions you are required to choose any one of the following four responses.*
(a) If both Assertion and Reason are true and the Reason is a correct explanation of the Assertion.
(b) If both Assertion and Reason are true but Reason is not a correct explanation of the Assertion.
(c) If Assertion is true but the Reason is false.
(d) If both Assertion and Reason are false.

171. *Assertion*: *Drosophila melanogaster* is widely used in genetic research.
Reason: Drosophila melanogaster is readily available insect.

172. *Assertion*: Genetic drift accentuates speciation.
Reason: Hardy-Weinberg equilibrium seems to retard speciation.

173. *Assertion*: Acetylcholine participates in the nerve impulse transmission across a synapse.
Reason: Acetylcholine is secreted by adrenergic fibres.

174. *Assertion*: The final reabsorption of water from urine into blood occurs through the collecting duct of a mammalian nephron, resulting in the production of hyperosmotic urine.
Reason: The loop of Henley is responsible for the formation of a sodium gradient across the depth of the cortical intersitium of a mammalian kidney.

175. *Assertion*: A correct concentration of auxin and cytokinin is required for the development of root and shoot in a callus.
Reason: When the ratio of kinetin to auxin is high, then only shoots develop. But when the ratio is low then only roots develop.

176. *Assertion*: Generally, a woman does not conceive during the lactation period.
Reason: The hormone 'prolactin' initiates and maintains lactation in a postpartum woman.

177. *Assertion*: Virus-free plants can be produced from virus infected plants by means of meristems tissue culture.
Reason: The virus fails to grow during the growth of host tissue in the artificial medium.

178. *Assertion*: Indiscriminate exploitation of economically important wild plants may lead to their extinction.

Reason: Non-conservation of their germplasm is responsible for this.

179. *Assertion*: Alpine forests consist of dwarf shrubs mainly of junipers, silver firs and rhododendrons.
Reason: Alpine forests occur in the Himalayas above the altitude of 3500 metres.

180. *Assertion*: *Azolla pinnata* is used as a biofertilizer in rice cultivation.
Reason: *Azolla* performs dinitrogen fixation with the help of symbiotic bacterium *Bacillus sp.*

GENERAL KNOWLEDGE

181. Which of the following state has the largest land area?
(a) Andhra Pradesh (b) Uttar Pradesh
(c) Madhya Pradesh (d) Maharashtra.

182. The Muslim league demanded a separate state for the Muslims in the year
(a) 1940 (b) 1920
(c) 1946 (d) 1930.

183. The term 'Carat' is used to express
(a) shape of gold (b) weight of gold
(c) purity of gold (d) type of gold.

184. The Mughal emperor who wrote his autobiography, was
(a) Humayun (b) Akbar
(c) Babar (d) Shahjahan.

185. The national award instituted for sport's coaches, is
(a) Dronachrya award (b) Arjun award
(c) Maulana Abul Kalam award
(d) Nehru award.

186. The Hall of Nation's, is located at
(a) Calcutta (b) Mumbai
(c) New Delhi (d) Madras.

187. The first sultan of Lodhi dynasty, was
(a) Bahlol Lodhi (b) Sikandar Lodhi
(c) Afzal Lodhi (d) Ibrahim Lodhi.

188. Sudden breaking of rock layers below the earth, results
(a) valconoes (b) floods
(c) earthquakes (d) cyclones.

189. Finance-commission is constituted after every
(a) four years (b) two years
(c) five years (d) three years.

190. 'Duck' is associated in which of the following sports?
(a) Cricket (b) Hockey
(c) Basket ball (d) Golf.

191. 'Tides' are caused by
(a) violent activity under the sea
(b) seismic vibrations under earth
(c) gravitational pull of the Sun and moon
(d) low pressure formed on the sea.

192. 'Lunar space craft' is used for
(a) study of the energy, liberated by Sun
(b) study of moon
(c) study of the earth from satellite
(d) transmission of radio signals.

193. Which of the following country, is the largest producer of copper?
(a) India (b) USA
(c) Russia (d) Japan.

194. Which of the following is the deepest lake in the world?
(a) Dal lake (b) Baikal lake
(c) Naini lake (d) Vooler lake.

195. In which of the following movement, Mahatma Gandhi gave the slogan 'Do or Die'?
(a) Quit India movement
(b) Dandi march
(c) non-coorperation movement
(d) Khilafat movement.

196. Which of the following is the capital of Denmark?
(a) Tokyo (b) Ottawa
(c) Copenhagen (d) Rome.

197. At which place did Mahavira got enligenment?
(a) Sarnath (b) Gaya
(c) Vaishali (d) Lumbani.

198. Battle of Haldighati was fought in
(a) 1756 A.D. (b) 1576 A.D.
(c) 1756 B.C. (d) 1576 B.C.

199. How many members in Rajya Sabha are nominated by the President of India?
(a) 12 (b) 10
(c) 13 (d) 11.

200. Who decides the question of disqualification of a Member of Parliament?
(a) supreme court (b) speaker
(c) election commission
(d) president.

❖❖❖

SOLUTIONS

PHYSICS

1. (d) : When one α-particle is emitted, the mass (A) is reduced by 4 and atomic no. (Z) is reduced by 2. Therefore for new nucleus, mass no. is ($A - 4$) and atomic no. is ($Z - 2$).

2. (b) : The velocity of sound in a gas is given by

$$v = \sqrt{\frac{\gamma p}{d}} \quad \text{where } \gamma = \frac{C_p}{C_V}$$

p = pressure d = density

∴ For two gases at constant pressure,

$$\frac{v_1}{v_2} = \sqrt{\frac{d_2\gamma_1}{d_1\gamma_2}}$$

For a diatomic gas $\gamma_1 = \gamma_2 = \frac{7}{5}$

$$\therefore \frac{v_1}{v_2} = \sqrt{\frac{d_2}{d_1}}$$

3. (b) and (d) : From the given circuit, we find that R_{BD} is ineffective as it is a balanced wheatstone bridge. Since both the upper resistances are in a series combination, therefore their equivalent resistance (R_U) = 2 + 2 = 4 Ω. Similarly both the lower resistances are in a series combination, therefore their equivalent resistance (R_L) = 4 + 4 = 8 Ω. Now we see that both the resistance R_U & R_L are in a parallel combination. Therefore equivalent resistance between

$$A \text{ and } C = \frac{R_U \times R_L}{R_U + R_L} = \frac{4\times 8}{4+8} = \frac{32}{12}\ \Omega = \frac{8}{3}\ \Omega.$$

4. (a)

5. (c) : Dynamo operates on the principle of the production of dynamically induced e.m.f. Therefore whenever flux is cut by the conductor, some e.m.f. is produced in it according to the law of electromagnetic induction.

6. (d)

7. (c) : Fusion of hydrogen nuclei into helium nuclei is continuously taking place in the sun, with the continuous liberation of energy. Thus energy produced in the sun is due to fusion reaction.

8. (b) : When both the grid and anode are positive, the maximum electrons will reach the plate. Thus the current will be maximum when both grid and anode are positive.

9. (b) : Seebeck discovered that on heating one of the junctions of a thermocouple, when keeping the other cold, a current is produced in the circuit. This effect is known as Seebeck effect. Therefore thermocouple thermometer is based on Seebeck effect.

10. (a) : The Wein's law states that the temperature $(T) \propto \frac{1}{\lambda_m}$. Therefore on increasing the temperature, the wavelength will decrease. Since the yellow colour is of lower minimum wavelength, therefore colour of substance becomes yellow.

11. (d) : The frequency of the source v_0 = 240 Hz

The velocity of the source u_s = +20 m/s

(as it moves towards the observer)

The velocity of the observer u_0 = – 20 m/s

(as it moves away from the source)

Applying Doppler's effect

$$v = v_0\left[\frac{v+u_0}{v-u_s}\right]$$

$$= 240 \times \left[\frac{340+(-20)}{340-20}\right] = 240 \text{ Hz}$$

12. (b) : Wave speed (v) = $n\lambda \propto \lambda$. When light rays enter in a glass slab (*i.e.* relative denser medium), their velocity is decreased. Thus their wavelength also decreases.

13. (c) : Given: Focal length of a convex lens (f_1) = 40 cm = 0.4 m and focal length of a concave lens (f_2) = – 25 cm = – 0.25 m (minus sign due to concave lens). We know that relation for the focal length of the combination of lenses $\frac{1}{f} = \frac{1}{f_1} + \frac{1}{f_2}$

$$= \frac{1}{0\cdot 4} + \frac{1}{-0\cdot 25}$$

$$= 2.5 - 4 = -1.5 \text{ D or power } (P) = \frac{1}{f} = -1.5 \text{ D}.$$

14. **(a) :** Phenomenon of emission of electrons from a metallic surface, when light of suitable wavelength falls on it, is called photoelectric effect. And the incident light is in the form of small packets of light or bundle of particles known as photons. Therefore photoelectric effect of light is due to photons.

15. **(d) :** Extra pressure inside a soap bubble $(P) = \frac{4T}{r} \propto \frac{1}{r}$.

We know that the extra pressure inside a concave surface over the outside is given by $\frac{2T}{r}$. But since in the case of soap bubble, there are two surfaces (one inside and the other outside), therefore the total extra pressure in a soap bubble is $\frac{2T}{r} + \frac{2T}{r} = \frac{4T}{r}$.

16. **(d) :** Given: Mass $(m) = 30$ kg and spring constant $(k) = 15$ N/m. We know that in simple harmonic motion, time period $(T) = 2\pi\sqrt{\frac{m}{k}} = 2\pi\sqrt{\frac{30}{15}} = 2\pi\sqrt{2}$ sec.

17. **(b) :** Given: Radius of first particle $(r_1) = r$ and radius of second particle $(r_2) = 2r$. We know that when a particle is moving in a circular path, then the centripetal force

$(F) = \frac{mv^2}{r}$ or $F \cdot r \propto v^2$ or $r \propto v^2$. Therefore,

$\frac{r_1}{r_2} = \left(\frac{v_1}{v_2}\right)^2$ or $\frac{v_1}{v_2} = \sqrt{\frac{r_1}{r_2}} = \sqrt{\frac{1}{2}}$ or $v_1 : v_2 = 1 : \sqrt{2}$.

18. **(a)**

19. **(b) :** The situation of the body is shown in the figure. We know that the maximum force of friction is given by $F_{max} = \mu N = \mu mg\cos\theta$

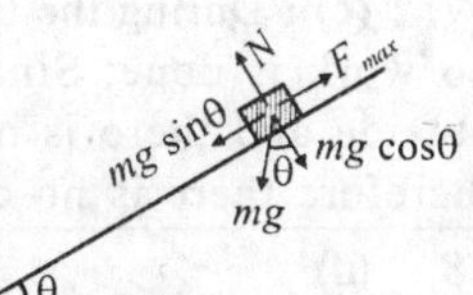

Since the body is in equilibrium,

$$F_{max} = mg\sin\theta$$
$$\Rightarrow \mu\, mg\cos\theta = mg\sin\theta$$
$$\Rightarrow \tan\theta = \mu \Rightarrow \theta \Rightarrow \tan^{-1}(\mu)$$

20. **(a)**

21. **(b) :** If a body is in the projectile motion, then its velocity can be resolved into horizontal and vertical components. And the body is subjected to the acceleration due to gravity (g), which is vertically downwards. Therefore horizontal component remains constant, while vertical component first decreases, becomes zero and then increases in the magnitude.

22. **(b)**

23. **(a) :** Given: Equation of wave $y = 10\sin\left(\frac{2\pi t}{30} + \alpha\right)$; Displacement $(y) = 5$ cm; Initial time $(t_1) = 0$ and final time $(t_2) = 7.5$ sec. We know that displacement of the wave at $t = 0$,

$y = a\sin\alpha = 10\sin\alpha$ or $\sin\alpha = \frac{1}{2}$ or $\alpha = \frac{\pi}{6}$. Therefore

total phase at $t = 7.5$, $\phi = \frac{2\pi \times 7.5}{30} + \frac{\pi}{6} = \frac{\pi}{2} + \frac{\pi}{6} = \frac{2\pi}{3}$.

24. **(b) :** Given that displacement of the body,

$$y \propto t^3$$

or $y = kt^3$

$$\therefore\ v = \frac{dy}{dt} = 3kt^2$$

or $a = \frac{dv}{dt} = 6kt \propto t$

$\therefore$ The magnitude of the acceleration of the body increases with time.

25. **(d) :** Due to 8 α-decays, the atomic mass decreases by 32 and atomic number will reduce by 16. And due to 6 β-decays, the atomic number increases by 6. Therefore resulting nucleus is $_{82}U^{206}$.

26. **(d) :** Given: Plate resistance of a triode $(r_p) = 3.3 \times 10^3\ \Omega$ and mutual conductance $(g_m) = 3 \times 10^3$ mhos. We know that amplification factor $(m) = g_m \times r_p = (3 \times 10^{-3}) \times (3.3 \times 10^3) = 10^1$.

27. **(a) :** The current depends on the intensity of the incident radiation. Therefore if the energy of radiation is more than work function (W), then the current will remain the same.

28. **(b) :** Given: Frequency of damped oscillator $= \omega$; Frequency of harmonic driving force $= n$ and $n < \omega$. We know that if $n < \omega$, then vibrations are nearly in phase with the impressed force or the response of the oscillator is controlled by spring constant.

29. **(a)**

30. **(b) :** Given: Threshold frequency $(f_0) = 10^{15}$ Hz and wavelength of light $(\lambda) = 4000$ Å. We know that threshold wavelength $(\lambda_0) = \frac{c}{f_0} = \frac{3 \times 10^8}{10^{15}} = 3 \times 10^{-7}$ m $= 3000$ Å. Since $\lambda > \lambda_0$, therefore no photoemission will take place.

31. **(d) :** Given: Change in volume of a gas $(dV) = 0.25\ m^3$ and constant pressure $(P) = 10^3\ N/m^2$. We know that work done $(W) = P \cdot dV = 10^3 \times 0.25 = 250$ joule.

32. (c) : The energy of X-rays depends upon the characteristic of the target material. Therefore energy of the X-rays remains the same.

33. (d) : Given: Velocity of electromagnetic waves in free space $(v) = 3 \times 10^8$ m/sec and wavelength (λ) = 150 m. We know that frequency $(f) = \frac{v}{\lambda} = \frac{3 \times 10^8}{150} = 2 \times 10^6$ Hz = 2 MHz.

34. (a) : The wavelength of microwave ranges from 1 mm (where it merges into infra-red) to 120 mm (where it merges into the radio waves). Therefore their wavelength is more than that of infra-red waves.

35. (b) : Given: Mass of boy $(m) = 40$ kg; Acceleration $(a) = 9.8$ m/s^2 and acceleration due to gravity $(g) = 9.8$ m/s^2. We know that apparent weight of the boy $= m(g - a) = 40(9.8 - 9.8) = 0$.

36. (b) : Given: Magnetic flux $(\phi) = 5t^2 + 3t + 16$. We know that the induced e.m.f. (E)

$$= \frac{d\phi}{dt} = \frac{d}{dt}(5t^2 + 3t + 16) = 10t + 3.$$ Therefore induced e.m.f., when $t = 3$, $(E_3) = (10 \times 3) + 3 = 33$ V and induced e.m.f. when $t = 4$, $(E_4) = (10 \times 4) + 3 = 43$ V. Therefore e.m.f. induced in the fourth sec $= E_4 - E_3 = 43 - 33 = 10$ V.

37. (c)

38. (d) : A tape is coated with tiny magnet particles. These particles get magnetized, when electric signal passes through them. Thus, a tape recorder records sound in the form of magnetic field on the tape.

39. (c) : H_α line is emitted, when the electron jumps from the $n = 3$ orbit (second excited state) to the $n = 2$ orbit (first excited state). And H_β line is also emitted, when the electron jumps from the $n = 4$ orbit to the $n = 2$ orbit.

40. (b) : When the source is moving away from the observer, then the frequency of sound heard by him, must be less than the actual frequency (i.e. 1990 Hz).

41. (c) : From the principle of calorimetry, the heat lost by a hot body is equal to heat gained by the cold body. Therefore during this process, heat exchange must be quick, otherwise some heat is lost due to radiations. As the metals are good conductors, therefore heat exchange will be quicker.

42. (d)

43. (d) : Given: Magnitude of first vector $(\vec{A}) = 12$; Magnitude of second vector $(\vec{B}) = 18$ and resultant of the given vectors $(\vec{R}) = 24$. We know that resultant vector $|\vec{R}| = 24 = \sqrt{A^2 + B^2 + 2AB \cos\theta}$

$$= \sqrt{(12)^2 + (18)^2 + 2 \times 12 \times 18 \cos\theta}$$ or

$(24)^2 = 144 + 324 + 432 \cos\theta$ or $432 \cos\theta = 108$ or $\cos\theta = \frac{108}{432} = 0.25$ or $\theta = \cos^{-1} 0.25 = 75°52'$.

44. (d) : β–decay is a process in which a neutron is converted into a proton and an electron or a proton into a neutron and a positron :

$$n \to p + e^- + \bar{\nu}$$
$$p \to n + e^+ + \bar{\nu}$$

Now as the process of β–decay is associated with the increase of atomic number of the parent nucleus, so the charge of the nucleus changes by keeping the mass number constant as we lose a neutron and gain a proton.

45. (a) : Given: Current $(I) = 4$ A; Time $(t) = 40$ min = 2400 sec and weight deposited on cathode $(m) = 4.5$ g. We know from the Faraday's law of electrolysis that the weight deposited $(m) = 4.5 = z \times I \times t$ or

$$z = \frac{4.5}{I \times t} = \frac{4.5}{4 \times 2400} = 47 \times 10^{-5} \text{ g/c.}$$

(where z is the electrochemical equivalent of zinc)

46. (a)

47. (c) : During the free expansion of a perfect gas, no work is done. Since no heat is supplied from outside and there is no change in internal energy, therefore there is no change in temperature.

48. (d)

49. (b) : The fundamental frequency of the closed organ pipe is given by

$$\nu_{open} = \frac{v}{2L}$$

The beat frequency is $\nu_{open} - \nu_{close} = 4$

Now if we increase the length of the closed pipe then the frequency ν_{close} is going to decrease.

∴ The beat frequency $\nu_{open} - \nu_{close}$ is going to increase.

50. (d) : A permanent magnet induces magnetic field only in ferromagnetic substances and visibly attracts them.

51. (b) : Because of the change of the refractive

index of the medium, the wavelength of light changes in different media. But as we know $c = \upsilon\lambda$

$\Rightarrow \upsilon = \frac{c}{\lambda} = \frac{c'}{\lambda'}$

Hence the frequency υ remains constant.

52. **(c) :** A laser is a highly monochromatic and near-perfect parallel beam of light, due to which the beam can be focussed by a converging lens to a very small spot. As the intensity of the beam is too high, it can drill holes through a metal sheet even if the power is 0.2 W. But even a torch-light of 1000 W power cannot drill holes in such a metal sheet, because the light is less intense and the beam is not parallel.

53. **(a) :** A neutron star is composed of neutrons which behave as a degenerate fermi gas. Because of the action of the magnetic field inside a neutron star the ionized gas radiates light, radio waves and X-rays.

54. **(b) :** As the rest mass of a photon is zero, it always moves with the speed of light. And as we know that no material body can ever travel with a speed more than the speed of light in vacuum. Now as the two photons move with speed c of light opposite to each other, their relative velocity is also c.

55. **(b) :** In case of metals when we increase the temperature, the relative movement of the atoms as well the free electrons increase. Becasue of which there is more collisions and more loss of energy. Due to which the resistance increases and it gives a positive temperature coefficient of resistance for metals.

But in the case of a semiconductor (p-type or n-type) the charge carriers are electrons and holes. So the conductivity will depend upon the number of such electron-hole pairs. At any time this number of electron-hole pairs is proportional to $T^{3/2} e^{-\Delta E/2KT}$, where ΔE is the band gap. Now with increase of temperature, the concentration of the electron-hole pairs increases which leads to an increase of conductivity or conversely a decrease of resistivity. So, a p-type semiconductor has a negative temperature coefficient of resistance.

56. **(d) :** We know that $\gamma = \frac{C_p}{C_v}$ for a gas is given by $\gamma = 1 + \frac{2}{n}$ where n is the degrees of freedom. Now for a monatomic gas like hydrogen, $n = 3$

$\therefore \gamma = 1 + \frac{2}{3} = 1.67$

And for a diatomic gas, $n = 5$

$\therefore \gamma = 1 + \frac{2}{5} = 1.4$

$\therefore \gamma_{He} < \gamma_H$

57. **(c) :** All metals have got different physical characteristics, due to which they will be having different emissive and abosorptive powers, so all metals cannot act as black bodies. But a hollow metallic closed container can act as a blackbody. If a small hole is made on the surface of the hollow container whose inner surface is painted black and the shape is as shown in the figure, then any radiation that enters the hole has a good chance of being absorbed after multiple reflections taking place on the inner surface of the container. And thus it can act as a blackbody.

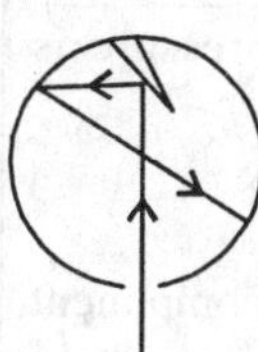

58. **(b) :** To make our calculations easy, let's that the semi major axis of the ellipse be equal to the average distance of the sun from the planet. By applying Newton's law,

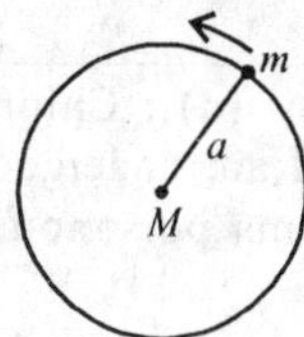

$$\frac{GMm}{a^2} = m(\omega^2 a)$$

ω = angular velocity of the planet

$= \frac{2\pi}{T}$ (T = time period of the planet)

$$\therefore \quad \frac{GMm}{a^2} = m\frac{(2\pi)^2}{T^2}a$$

$$\Rightarrow \quad T^2 = \left(\frac{4\pi^2}{GM}\right)a^3$$

$$\Rightarrow \quad T^2 \propto a^3$$

59. **(d) :** Environmental damage has actually decreased the amount of ozone by making holes in the ozone layer because of which more UV radiation from sun enters our atmosphere.

60. **(c) :** The buoyancy of an object is the resultant of all the contact forces that are present at the points of contact of the body and hence the force of buoyancy depends upon the area of contact of the body with the fluid. The force of buoyancy is more in case of the needle than in the case of the ball. Now it might so happen that the force of buoyancy (B) is greater than the weight (mg) of the needle, in which case the needle might float. But in the case of the ball, $B < mg$, and so the ball sinks.

CHEMISTRY

61. (c) : Molecular weight of NaOH is 40

Atomic weight of oxygen is 16

$\Rightarrow$ Percentage of oxygen $= \frac{16}{40} \times 100 = 40\%$

62. (d) : Relative lowering of vapour pressure is written as :

$$\frac{\Delta P}{P^0} = \frac{P^0 - P}{P^0}$$

P^0 = Vapour pressure of pure component

P = Vapour pressure of component in solution

63. (d) : Molecular weight of water = 18

$\therefore$ No. of moles of water $= \frac{\text{Mass}}{\text{Molecular mass}}$

$= \frac{180}{18} = 10$ moles

64. (d) : Chloroform in the presence of sun light and air, undergoes reaction with oxygen (in air) and forms poisonous phosgene gas.

$$\text{Cl}-\overset{\text{H}}{\underset{\text{Cl}}{\text{C}}}-\text{Cl} + [\text{O}] \xrightarrow{\text{sun light}} \text{Cl}_2\text{C}=\text{O} + \text{HCl}$$

65. (c) : Cu is below hydrogen in the electro-chemical series, so cannot liberate H_2 from dilute H_2SO_4.

$E^\circ(Cu^{2+}/Cu) = +0.34$

66. (d) : Glycerol : CH_2OH | CH–OH | CH_2OH

Its, derivatives like trinitroglycerol are used as explosive.

67. (a) : $2C_6H_5CHO \xrightarrow{\text{alc. KCN}} C_6H_5CH(OH)COC_6H_5$.

Benzaldehyde Benzoin

Thus in this reaction benzoin is formed. The reaction is known as benzoin condensation.

68. (b) : $CH \equiv CH \xrightarrow{O_3}$ CH–CH (ozonide, with O bridge and O–O) $\longrightarrow$ CHO–CHO glyoxal

69. (c) : $Cl_2 + 2Na_2S_2O_3 \rightarrow Na_2SO_4 + 2NaCl + SO_2$

70. (b) : Reversible reactions are those reactions in which there is equilibrium established at every infinitesimal step. But the rate of forward and backward reactions can be speed up by the influence of a catalyst.

71. (d) : Hall's and Bayer's processes are used if aluminium ore contains iron oxide as impurity, while Serpek's process is used when SiO_2 is present as an impurity.

72. (c) : 'Blister copper' is impure copper (98–99% Cu) obtained after treatment of sulphide ore.

73. (b) : The total kinetic energy of a molecule is the sum of its translational, vibrational and rotational kinetic energies. The monoatomic molecules do not possess vibrational and rotational kinetic energies. Hence noble gases (like He, Ar etc) fulfill the criteria.

74. (c) : Concentration of acetic acid = 0.001N for 10% dissociation, the effective concentration of H^+ is one-tenth of total concentration.

Therefore effective concentration $= \frac{1}{10} \times 0.001$ N

$= 0.0001$ N

$\Rightarrow pH = -\log[H^+] = 4$

75. (b) : Strongest acid among $HClO_4$, $HClO_3$, $HClO_2$ and HClO is $HClO_4$ (due to greater no. of attached O-atoms) and weakest is HClO. But the corresponding conjugate base of HClO *i.e.* ClO^- is the strongest Bronsted base.

76. (a) : Intermolecular H–bonding raise the boilding point of a compound as more energy is required to break the Hydrogen bonding between the molecules.

77. (c) : Thermite is a mixture of Fe_2O_3 and Al in the ratio 3 : 1. Thermite reaction involves the displacement of a metal from its oxide by more electropositive metal releasing large amount of energy.

$Fe_2O_3 + Al \rightarrow 2Fe + Al_2O_3$

78. (b) : Silicon is present in soil, rocks etc. in the form of silica (SiO_2) or silicates or aluminosilicates.

79. (a) : Given: Volume of hydroxide solution = 100 ml . We know that molecular weight of ammonia (NH_3) = 17 and molecular weight of 2.5 M-NH_4OH = 42.5 g NH_3 in 1000 ml solution. Since 1000 ml contains 42 . 5 g of NH_3, therefore 100 ml will contain = 4.25 gm NH_3.

Thus number of moles $= \frac{4 \cdot 25}{17} = \frac{1}{4}$. Therefore volume of NH_3 at STP $= \frac{22 \cdot 4 \times 1}{4} = 5 \cdot 6$ litres.

80. (a) : $N = \left(\frac{1}{2}\right)^n N_0$.

N_0 = Initial amount, N = Amount at 't' time

n = no. of half lives.

Given, $\frac{N}{N_0} = \frac{1}{8}$

$\Rightarrow \left(\frac{1}{2}\right)^n = \frac{1}{8} = \left(\frac{1}{2}\right)^3$

$\Rightarrow n = 3$

As by definition, $n = \frac{\text{total time}}{\text{half life time}}$

$\Rightarrow$ half life time $= \frac{96}{3} = 32$ minutes.

81. **(c) :** $l = 3$ corresponds to f–orbitals. Since there are seven f–orbitals and each orbital accomodates 2 electrons, so maximum no. of electrons is 14.

82. **(a) :** White vitriol : $ZnSO_4.7H_2O$

It is prepared by reacting zinc with dilute sulphuric acid.

$Zn + H_2SO_4 \rightarrow ZnSO_4 + H_2$

83. **(d) :** Weight of $6 \cdot 023 \times 10^{23}$ molecules of oxygen $(O_2) = 32$ g. Since the oxygen is diatomic, therefore weight of Avogadro's number of oxygen atom $= \frac{32}{2}$ $= 16$ g.

84. **(c) :** Reaction sequence is;

$$\underset{\text{Acetylene}}{\underset{(A)}{CaC_2 \xrightarrow[2CaO]{H_2O} C_2H_2}} \xrightarrow[HgSO_4]{\text{dil. } H_2SO_4} \underset{\text{Acetaldehyde}}{\underset{(B)}{CH_3\text{–}CHO}} \xrightarrow{H_2/Ni}$$

$$\underset{\text{Ethanol (C)}}{CH_3CH_2OH}$$

85. **(a) :** Equilibrium constant of reaction is independent of volume change.

86. **(d) :** Tertiary Carbocation is most stable as more electron releasing effect by methyl group to the carbocation.

$$\overset{\oplus}{C}H_3 : \quad CH_3 \rightarrow \overset{\oplus}{C}H_2 ; \quad CH_3 \rightarrow \underset{\oplus}{\overset{CH_3 \downarrow}{CH}} \; ; \quad CH_3 \rightarrow \overset{CH_3 \downarrow}{\underset{\downarrow CH_3}{C^{\oplus}}}$$

87. **(a) :** $2H_2O_2 \rightarrow 2H_2O + O_2$

g/L strengh of $H_2O_2 = \frac{68}{22.4} \times V$

$\Rightarrow N = \frac{\text{Strength}}{\text{Equivalent mass}} = \frac{68}{22.4} \times \frac{V}{17} \Rightarrow$

$V = 5.6 \times$ Normality
$= 5.6 \times 3 = 16.8$ litres

88. **(d)** **:** Hydride ion is a strong base, stronger than OH^-, OMe^- etc.

89. **(c) :** Except NF_3 and BF_3, all other trihalides of this group are hydrolysed by water.

$$BiCl_3 + H_2O \rightarrow \underset{\text{oxychloride}}{BiOCl} + 2HCl.$$

90. **(c) :** According to ostwald's dilution law, the degree of dissociation of a weak electrolyte is proportional to the square root of dilution.

$\alpha = \sqrt{\frac{K}{C}}$

α = degree of dissociation, C=concentration
K = Equilibrium constant (dissociation)

91. **(a) :** Vitamin B_{12} contains Cobalt, while Hemoglobin contains Iron and Chlorophyll contains Magnesium.

92. **(c) :** Chemical formula for magnetite is Fe_3O_4, malachite is $CuCO_3.Cu(OH)_2$, carnallite is $KCl \cdot MgCl_2 \cdot 6H_2O$ and copper pyrites is $CuFeS_2$. Therefore copper pyrites is a sulphide ore.

93. **(c) :** Human blood is slightly alkaline *i.e.* pH of 7.3 to 7.5 (pH=7 is neutral).

94. **(b) :** In isoelectronic species, the size of ions decreases as nuclear charge or atomic weight increases. (Atomic weight of P = 30, S = 32 and Cl = 35). Therefore $Cl^- < S^{2} < P^{3-}$.

95. **(c) :** Absolute ether is 100% pure diethyl ether, totally free from any impurities.

96. **(d) :** Given: Weight of ammonia = 4.25 g. We know that 17 g of ammonia (NH_3) contains $6 \cdot 02 \times 10^{23}$ molecules. Therefore number of molecules in 4.25 of

$NH_3 = \frac{6 \cdot 02 \times 10^{23} \times 4 \cdot 25}{17} = 1 \cdot 50 \times 10^{23}$.

97. **(c) :** According to law of mass action, rate depends on active mass or simply concentration.

98. **(c) :** As the electron goes away from nucleus its energy increases sharply.

99. **(c) :** $NH_4Cl + H_2O \rightarrow NH_3 + H_2O + HCl$

100. **(d) :** Fe (Z = 26); Co (Z = 27); Ni (Z = 28)

Fe (Z = 26); Atomic wt. = 55.85
Co (Z = 27); Atomic wt. = 58.93
Ni (Z = 28); Atomic wt. = 58.69

101. **(c) :** Eriochrome black - T :

(structure: HO_3S–naphthalene(OH, NO_2)–N=N–naphthalene(OH))

(unionised form)

102. (a) : Isotonic species are those which have identical numbers of neutrons.

${}_{37}Rb^{86}$; $n = 86 - 37 = 49$
${}_{38}Sr^{87}$; $n = 87 - 38 = 49$
${}_{36}Kr^{84}$; $n = 84 - 36 = 48$
${}_{39}Y^{89}$; $n = 89 - 39 = 50$
${}_{37}Mg^{85}$; $n = 85 - 37 = 48$

103. (b) : Berylium carbide (Be_2C), on hydrolysis evolves methane.

$$Be_2C + 4H_2O \rightarrow 2Be(OH)_2 + CH_4$$

104. (a) : Given: Percentage of solution = 6 and active mass of the compound = 2 = 2M solution or 2 moles/litre. Since 100 ml solution contains 6 g, therefore 1000 ml solution contains $= \frac{6 \times 1000}{100} = 60$ g, therefore molecular weight of the compound $= \frac{60}{2} = 30$.

105. (b) : NO_2 contains an unpaired electron so exhibit paramagnetism.

$$O{=}\dot{\underset{\cdot\cdot}{N}}\rightarrow O$$

106. (c) : $NaClO_4$, on hydrolysis, gives strongest acid $HClO_4$ as compared to other salts. This is strongly ionized and gives highest concentration of H^+. Therefore aqueous solution of $NaClO_4$ will have lowest pH value.

107. (c) : $2P_2O_5 + 2HNO_3 \rightarrow P_4O_{10} + N_2O_5 + H_2O$.

108. (d) : After the removal of electron, to form cation, there is more effective nuclear charge on remaining electrons in the cation. So size decreases.

109. (a) : When formaldehyde reacts with ammonia, it forms hexamethylene tetramine, which is known as urotropine

$$\underset{\text{Formaldehyde}}{6\,HCHO} + 4\,NH_3 \rightarrow \underset{\text{Urotropine}}{(CH_2)_6N_4} + 6\,H_2O.$$

110. (a) : 3 – methyl Hexane is

$$CH_3-CH_2-CH_2-\overset{\overset{CH_3}{|}}{\underset{*}{C}H}-CH_2CH_3$$

C* = Chiral carbon atom (due to which it is optically active)

111. (d) : In crystal lattice tetrahedral void is smaller than the octahedral void due to the concerned geometry. Anions are larger in size than cations so anions occupy more space.

112. (c) : The heat of formation of all the elements in their standard states are arbitrarily assumed to be zero.

113 (d)

$$\underset{\text{Aniline}}{C_6H_5NH_2} + H_2SO_4 \rightarrow C_6H_5\overset{+}{N}H_3H\overset{-}{S}O_4 \xrightarrow{200^\circ C} C_6H_5NHSO_3H \xrightarrow{\text{rearrangement}} \underset{\text{(Para)}}{p\text{-}NH_2C_6H_4SO_3H}$$

114. (a) : In covalent bonding, there is sharing of electrons between two atoms but this sharing may or may not be due to the differences in the electro negativities of two concerned atoms.

115. (b) : $Ag^+ + e^- \rightarrow Ag$
$Cu^{2+} + 2e^- \rightarrow Cu$

For deposition of Ag, 1 mole of electrons is required while for Cu, 2 moles of electrons are required. So quantity of electricity needed for depositing is different.

116. (c) : At elevated temperature or in the presence of catalyst, strong bonds between two N-atom rupture, and make N_2 molecule to active.

117. (a) : Ionisation of first electron requires lesser energy as compared to the second electron ionisation.

118. (a) : Hydrogen ions are discharged in preference to sodium normally but at mercury electrode, sodium ion are discharged first due to the formation of amalgam (Na / Hg).

119. (d) : No transition can take place between $2p_x \rightarrow 2p_y$ as $2p_x$ and $2p_y$ are degenerate orbitals.

120. (b) : Due to high electronegativity and high heat of dissociation fluorine oxidise the elements to their highest oxidation state.

BIOLOGY

121. (b) : The amphids of *Ascaris* are chemoreceptors, while the other sensory papillae are tangoreceptors. Amphid is opening of an amphidial gland.

122. (b) : Nematocysts are stinging cells of (*Hydra*) coelenterates. The poison present in its hollow thread is helpful in capturing the prey.

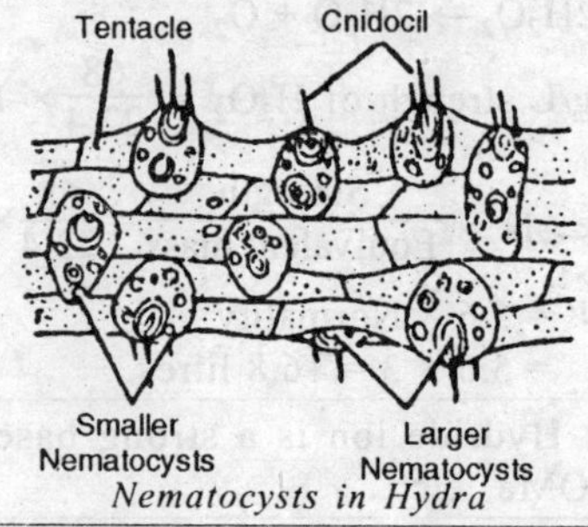

Nematocysts in Hydra

123. (d) : Bone is a hard connective tissue that makes up most of the skeleton of vertebrates. It consists of fine-branched cells (osteoblasts) embedded in a matrix, which they have secreted. The matrix is made up of 30% protein (collagen) and 70% inorganic matter, mainly calcium phosphate.

124. (d) : The right and the left hepatic ducts join to form a common hepatic duct which again joins to the duct of gall bladder (Cystic duct) forming a common bile or ductus choledocus.

125. (b) : Corpora allata and corpora cardiaca glands are found in insects. They produce hormones that control factors like gamete production, metamorphosis, growth and moulting. General body growth is controlled by the corpora cardiaca and moulting and egg production by the corpora allata.

126. (c) : Chordae tendinae (tendinous cords) are tough strands of connective tissue that run from the underside of the bicuspid and tricuspid valves to muscles in the walls of the left ventricles of the heart respectively.

127. (b) : Saliva comes in mouth and is secreted by the salivary gland, which has ptyalin enzyme that is a starch splitting enzyme. Thus salivary secretion stands digestion of starch in mouth.

128. (d) : Ostrich, Emu, Kiwi all are flightless birds. They all are under subclass Neornithes. Tail is short and usually ended in a pygostyle. The retrices are arranged in a semicircle around the pygostyle.

129. (c) : Adipose tissue are modified areolar tissue. The type of tissues present in hump of camel is unilocular adipocytes, These are fatty tissues and can transform fat cells to water through oxidation whenever body needs it.

130. (a) : Wharton's duct is the duct of submandibular salivary gland, opening into the mouth at the side of the frenum linguae.

131. (c) : The horns of *Rhinoceros* are composed of keratin. It is generally known as keratin fibre horn. It has no skeletal element and made by keratinized cells of epidermis and consists of matted keratin fibres bound together. It is a permanent epidermal structure and if broken it grows again.

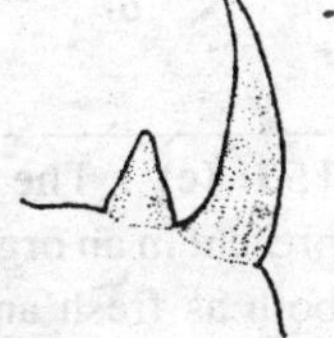

Fibre horn (Rhinoceros)

132. (b) : Sharpey's perforating fibres are collagenous fibres, which pass from the peridontal membrane into the cementum and jaw bones. It fixes the teeth firmly in the sockets.

133. (c) : Fluoride exposure disrupts the synthesis of collagen and leads to the breakdown of collagen in bone, tendon, muscle. Knock knee is a condition where the legs are bowed inwards in the standing position. The bowing usually occurs at or around the knee, so that on standing with the knees together, the feet are far apart.

134. (b) : Sweat glands are epidermal glands embedded in the dermis of the skin of mammals. It secretes a

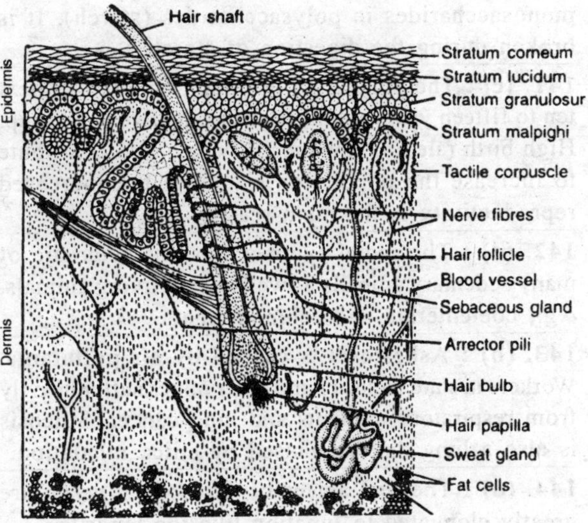

T.S. of skin showing sweat gland

hypertonic solution of salts and other small molecules present in blood. It is a long coiled tubular gland.

135. (d) : Prussic acid is a toxic substance. Non-lethal amounts of prussic acid are rapidly detoxified in liver by reaction with sulphide and sulphocyanate is formed and is readily excreted in urine.

136. (a) : Choanocytes are also called collar cells, which are found in sponges. The flagellated collar cells in sponges, maintain the flow of food bearing water.

137. (a) : The function of contractile vacuole in protozoa is hydrostatic or osmoregulatory. The mechanism which is assumed to effect water regulation is the contractile vacuole. The vacuole periodically increases in volume (diastole) to get filled with water and contracts (systole) to discharge its water content to the surrounding environment and this is the basic mechanism of osmoregulation, *e.g. Amoeba*.

138. (b) : Order rodentia includes rat and squirrel. It also includes gnawing mammals, with a pair of large countinually growing chiesel like incisors, in upper and lower jaws.

139. (d) : The number of milk teeth which are replacable for the 2nd time is 20. In adult human, total number of teeth is 32. Therefore, the teeth that grow only once in the life of a man is 32 – 20 or 12.

140. (a) : The glycosidic link is a link joining monosaccharides in polysaccharides (starch). It is broken during the digestion of starch.

141. (c) : The population of young children in next ten to fifteen years attains the reproductive age group. High birth rate and low mortality rate also contribute to increase the population size. But the increased reproductivity is the main reason.

142. (d) : The radial symmetry is characteristic of many sedentary animals as well as free living animals. *e.g.*, coelenterata and echinodermata.

143. (b) : Asbestosis is caused by air pollutants. Workers in slate factories and other mines suffer heavily from respiratory ailments and lung cancer. Silicosis is also a lung disease caused by silica inhalation.

144. (d) : The leaf apices of *Gloriosa superba* are greatly elongated to function like the tendrils.

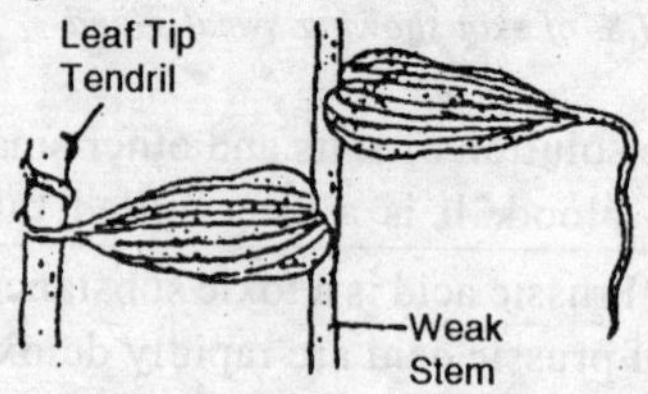

Leaf apices of Gloriosa superba

145. (d) : Pepsin is an enzyme that catalyses the partial hydrolysis of proteins to polypeptides. It is secreted by gastric gland.

146. (b) : In parietal placentation, two or more longitudinal placentae develop along the wall of a syncarpous or compound pistil. The ovary is usually unilocular. In marginal placentation, a single longitudinal placenta having one or two alternate rows of ovules occur along the wall of the ovary, called central suture. In superficial placentation, the ovules develop on the whole inner surface of the ovary including the septa, if present. In basal placentation, the pistil can be monocarpellary or syncarpous. The ovary is unilocular. It bears a single placenta at the base with generally a single ovule.

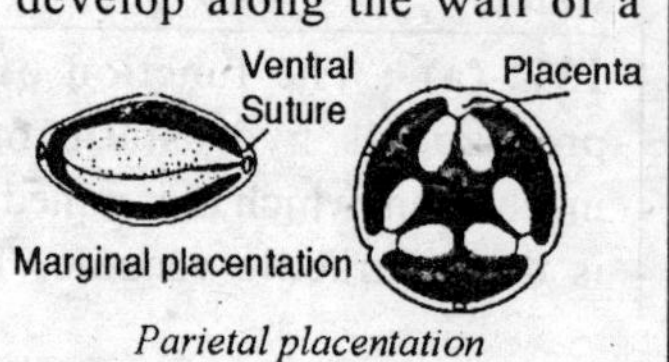

Parietal placentation

147. (c) : Bone marrow is of two types; red and yellow. The yellow marrow is found especially in medullary cavity of long bones, while red in spongy bones.

148. (c) : Like other alkali metals, potassium hydroxide combines with CO_2 as such :-

$$2KOH + CO_2 \rightarrow K_2CO_3 + H_2O$$

149. (d) : Lipid is stained with 'Sudan Black B' protein with bromophenol blue. And for nucleic acid Feulgen stain is used.

150. (a) : Biosphere is stretched above 9000 m above sea level to 11000 m below. But life is abundant in between 6000 m above sea level to 200 m below the sea level.

151. (a) : The flow of intrinsic information from DNA to *m*RNA and then to polypeptide is called central dogma of molecular biology.

$$\text{DNA} \xrightarrow{\text{transcription}} \text{RNA} \xrightarrow{\text{translation}} \text{Polypeptide}$$

152. (c) : Starch consists of two components amylose and amylopectin. Both amylose and amylopectin are formed by the condensation of α - D - glucose. A chain of cellulose molecule contains 6000 or more glucose residues. The successive glucose residues are joined together by 1 - 4 β.- linkages.

α-1 : 6 Linkage

α-1 : 4 Linkage

Structure of starch

153. (c) : The amount of living or organic matter present in an organism is called biomass. It is measured both as fresh and dry weight. Pyramid of biomass is a graphic representation of biomass present sequence wise per unit area of different trophic levels with producers at the base and top carnivores kept at the tip. Maximum biomass occurs in producers. There is a progressive reduction of biomass found in herbivores, primary carnivores, secondary carnivores.

154. (c) : Tropical rain forests are mainly found in central America, along Amazon and Orinoco rivers, South America, Congo river basin of Africa, Malagasy Republic and South east Asia including India. Diversity of life is so high that a hectare of the forest may have as many as 200 species of trees, 70% - 80% of all insects and 80 - 85% of all brids are known from tropical forests.

155. (b) : Distinct zonation and stratification are characteristic features of lakes and large ponds. The warmer upper part of the lake or epilimnion becomes temporarily isolated from the colder lower part or hypolimnion, by a thermocline zone that acts as a barrier to exchange of materials. Consequently, the supply of the oxygen in the hypolimnion and nutrients in the epilimnion may run short.

156. (a) : Red Data book is maintained by IUCN.

157. (c) : Red rust of tea is caused by an alga *Cephaleuros*, a green alage. It is parasitic on a number of higher plants. *Melampsora lini* causes rust of linseed. *Helminthosporium oryzae* causes leaf spot disease of rice commonly called sesame or brown leaf sopt of rice. It causes Bengal famine in 1942 - 43. Circular necrotic dark brown or blackish leaf spot develop in groundnut due to *Cercospora* called as Tikka disease.

158. (d) : The electron transport system is a chain of carriers consisting of nicotinamide adenine dinucleotide (NAD), flavin nucleotides (FAD, sometimes FMN), coenzyme Q (CoQ) and the cytochromes (cyt b,c,a,a_3). Nonheme iron proteins also seem to be involved but their role is not known exactly.

159. (d) The ovule of gymnosperms consists of a parenchymatous mass of cells called the nucellus or the megasporangium. The nucellus encloses a single diploid megaspore mother cell that undergoes meiosis to form a linear tetrad of 4 haploid megaspores, out of which only one remains functional, whereas the rest degenerate. The functional megaspore form female gametophyte. As the female gametophyte is formed prior to fertilization, therefore, endosperm is haploid in case of gymnosperm.

160. (d) : The leaves of C_4 plants are characterized by a sheath of parenchyma cells that are radially arranged around each vascular bundle. The vascular

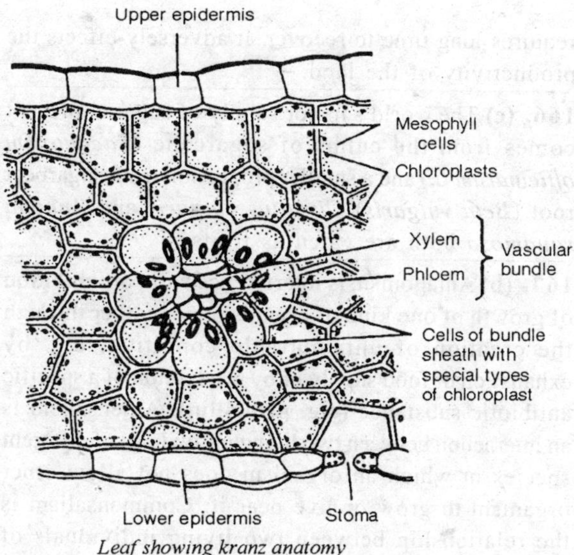

Leaf showing kranz anatomy

bundle in turn is enclosed by loosely packed,"spongy" mesophyll cells. This is known as kranz anatomy and is characteristic of C_4 plants such as sugarcane, sorghum, maize, various grasses originating in the tropics and indeed, many other species of plants.

161. (b) : Ruben and Kamen (1941) and Ruben *et al* (1941) suspended *Chlorella* in water having nonradioactive heavy isotope of oxygen, ^{18}O, instead of natural oxygen ^{16}O. The suspension was illuminated. Oxygen evolved was tested by means of mass spectrometer. It was found to be heavy isotope, ^{18}O.This is possible only if oxygen evolved during photosynthesis comes from splitting of water.

$$6CO_2 + 12H_2{}^{18}O \xrightarrow[\text{chlorophyll,enzymes}]{\text{light}}$$

$$C_6H_{12}O_6 + 6H_2O + 6^{18}O_2 \uparrow$$

162. (c) : The habitat of an organism is the place where it lives. The ecological niche, however includes not only the physical space occupied by an organism but also its functional role in the community and its position in environmental gradients of temeprature, moisture, pH, soil and other conditions of existence.

163. (c) : *Emblica officinalis* (amla) is the best source of vitamin C, though the citrus fruits also contain considerable amounts of the vitamin C.

164. (d)

165. (d) : One of the major consequences of shifting cultivation is that the top soil burnt during practice requires long time to recover. It adversely effects the productivity of the land.

166. (c) The world's major supply of sugar at present comes from the culms of sugarcane (*Saccharum officinarum L.*) and a smaller proportion from sugarbeet root (*Beta vulgaris*) *Citrullus vulgaris* and *Annona squamosa* both are eaten as fruits.

167. (b) Antagonism is interference with, or inhibition of growth of one kind of organism by another through the creation of unfavourable condition, e.g. by exhaustion of food supply or by production of a specific antibiotic substance (e.g. penicillin). Amensalism is an interaction between two living individuals of different species in which an organism does not allow other organism to grow or live near it. Commensalism is the relationship between two living individuals of different species in which one is benefitted while the other is neither harmed nor benefitted except to a negligible extent.

168. (d) : The term albedo refers the reflected light from the earth surface into 100/incident light. Snow has high albedo whereas sea has less.

169. (d) For the relative degree of tolerance a series of terms have come into general use in ecology that use the prefixes steno -, meaning "narrow", and eury-, meaning "wide".

170. (c) *Adiantum* is a walking fern.

171. (a) : *Drosophila* may be the readily available insect but its main importance is the presence of a number of behavioural genes (mutants described as sluggish, non-climbing, flightless, easily shocked etc.) and marked sexual behaviour. The chromosomes present in it can be easily studied. In 1910, Morgan started his work on fruit fly.

172. (d) : Random fluctuation in allele frequencies is called genetic drift. The effect of genetic drift is negligible in large population but in small breeding population fixation or homozygosity would have occured. So there is no question for speciation. On the other hand, according to Hardy Weinberg law at equilibrium, *both gene frequencies and genotype frequencies will remain constant from generation to generation in an infinitely large interbreeding population in which mating is at random and no selection, migration or mutation occur.*

173. (c) : Acetylcholine is secreted by cholinergic neurons. Acetylcholine made by these neurons taken up into synaptic vesicles by a vesicular transporter. It must be rapidly removed from the synapse if repolarization is to occur. The removal occurs by way of hydrolysis of acetylcholine to choline and acetate, a reaction catalysed by acetylcholinesterase.

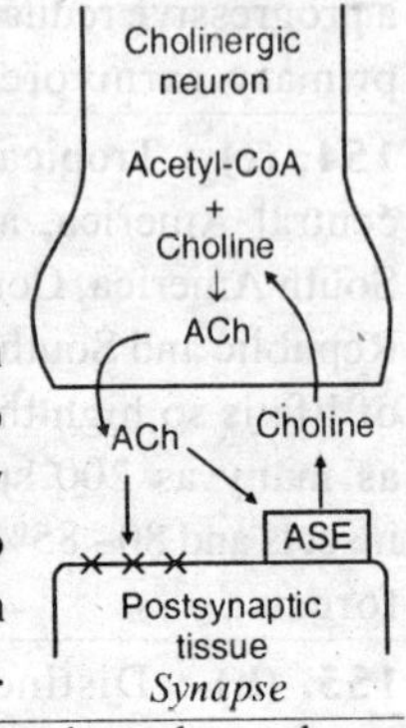

Synapse

174. (b) : The effect of collecting duct depends on the presence of vasopressin over there. This hormone increases the permeability of the collecting duct to water. Gradually the rate of reabsorption from the filtrate increases and it becomes hyperosmotic.
There is graded increase in the osmolality of the interstitium of the pyramids. Na^+, K^+ and Cl^- are transported out of the thick segment of the ascending limb. The Na^+ is actively transported out of the cells into the interstitium by Na^+K^+ ATPase.

175. (a) : The relative ratio of cytokinin (Kinetin) to auxin (IAA) was considered important in determining the nature of organogensis in tobacco pith tissue. It was shown that high level of kinetin caused bud initiation, while high concentration of auxin favoured rooting.

176. (b) : Generally, a woman does not conceive during the lactation period. Lactation stimulates prolactin secretion and there is evidence that prolactin inhibits GnRH secretion, and antagonizes the action of ganadotropins on the ovaries. Ovulation is inhibited, and the ovaries are inactive, so estrogen and progesterone output falls to low levels. Thus during lactation a woman does not conceive. Only 5–10% chances are there during lactation period. This can also be interpreted as mechanism devised by nature so that mother can look after the new born child by providing it with milk.

177. (a) Pathogen free clones of plants can be obtained through shoot - tip culture because shoot apical meristem is usually free of the pathogens. The shoot tips are virus - free also and as shoot tips are grown in artificial medium, virus cannot grow there. Virus can grow in host cells only.

178. (a) In modern era a high yielding variety developed at one place is immediately distributed to all parts of the globe. Naturally the low yielding wild varieties are discarded. The discarded wild varieties automatically disappear. They and their genes cannot be regained.

179. (b) Alpine tundra is the highest altitudinal biome which occurs near the top of very high mountains having permanent snow.i.e. at the height to approximate 3500 metres, i.g. in Himalayas "alpine tundra" vegetation is found. It is a treeless region and lies above the timber - line. Trees of lower region becomes tiny shrubs in this area (e.g. *Rhododendron, Jumiperus, Abies*). Other constituents of alpine tundra are lichens, mosses, grasses, herbs and small shrubs like *Artemesia, Arenaria, Primula* and *Anemone*.

180. (c) Nitrogen fixing cyanobacteria (blue - green alage) form symbiotic association with several plants,e.g. cycad roots, lichens, liverworts, *Azolla*. Out of these, *Azolla - Anabaena* association is of great importance to agriculture. *Azolla pinnata* is a free floating fresh water form which multiplies rapidly, doubling every 5 - 7 days. *Anabaena azolla* resides in the leaf cavities of the fern. It fixes nitrogen. A part of the fixed nitrogen is excreted in the cavities and becomes available to the fern. The decaying fern plants release the same for utilization of the rice plants. When field is dried at the time of harvesting,the fern functions as the green manure, decomposing and enriching the field for the next crop.

GENERAL KNOWLEDGE

181. (c)

182. (a) : In 1940, the Muslim league led by Jinnah, passed a resolution demanding partition of the country and the creation of a new state called Pakistan after independence.

183. (c)

184. (c) : The Babar was a great scholar. His autobiography 'Tuzuk-i-Babri' is a classic of world literature.

185. (a)

186. (c) : The Hall of Nation's is located in Pragati Maidan in the capital of India *i.e.* New Delhi.

187. (a)

188. (c) : Earthquake is shaking of earth's crust sometimes accompained by elevation or depression. But often no lasting effect is visible on the surface, except the damage done by shaking.

189. (c)

190. (a) : In cricket, when the batsman is out without scoring any run, it is called 'duck'.

191. (c)

192. (b) : A series of Russian moon probes luna-2 was the frist probe to hit the moon on 3rd Sept. 1959. Luna-2 was the first to soft land on the moon in 1966.

193. (b)

194. (b) : Baikal lake is the deepest lake in the world, located in Siberia. It's average depth is 700 metres.

195. (a)

196. (c) : Ottawa, Rome, Tokyo and Copenhagen as the capitals of Canada, Italy, Japan and Denmark respectively.

197. (c)

198. (b) : Rana Pratap, the ruler of Mewar was defeated by the Mughal forces led by Mansingh and Asaf Khan.

199. (a)

200. (c) : The election commission recommends the disqualification of a member of parliament, while orders are issued by the president.

SOLVED PAPER
AIIMS - 1997

Time : 3½ Hours Max. Marks : 200

PHYSICS

1. A charged hollow sphere does not produce an electric field at any
(a) inner point (b) outer point
(c) beyond 2 metres (d) beyond 10 metres

2. Time-period of a pendulum on a satellite, orbiting around the earth, is
(a) 0 (b) ∞
(c) $1/\pi$ (d) π

3. Chromatic aberration of lens can be corrected by
(a) providing different suitable curvature to its two surfaces
(b) proper polishing of its two surfaces
(c) suitably combining it with another lens
(d) reducing its aperture

4. Which of the following is the infrared wavelength?
(a) 10^{-4} cm (b) 10^{-5} cm
(c) 10^{-6} cm (d) 10^{-7} cm

5. A beam of light in air enters into the water. Which of the following characteristics of light will not change?
(a) colour (b) velocity
(c) amplitude (d) frequency

6. Whenever stationary waves are set up, in any medium, then
(a) condensations occur at nodes
(b) refractions occur at antinodes
(c) maximum strain is experienced at the nodes
(d) no strain is experienced at the antinodes

7. When there are no external forces, the shape of a small liquid drop is determined by
(a) surface tension of the liquid
(b) density of the liquid
(c) viscosity of air
(d) temperature of air

8. At sea level, the value of g is minimum at
(a) the poles (b) the equator
(c) 45° south latitude (d) 45° north longitude

9. What happens, when we multiply a vector by −2 ?
(a) direction reverses and unit changes
(b) direction reverses and magnitude is doubled
(c) direction remains unchanged but unit changes
(d) neither direction reverses nor unit changes but the magnitude is doubled

10. Conservation of linear momentum is equivalent to
(a) Newton's law of gravity
(b) Newton's first law of motion
(c) Newton's second law of motion
(d) Newton's third law of motion

11. What can be the angle between $\vec{P}+\vec{Q}$ and $\vec{P}-\vec{Q}$?
(a) 0° (b) 90°
(c) 180° (d) between 0° and 180°

12. In Lenz's law, there is a conversion of
(a) charge (b) energy
(c) current (d) momentum

13. The temperature of the sun is measured with
(a) pyrometer
(b) gas thermometer
(c) platinum resistance thermometer
(d) vapour pressure thermometer

14. The objectives with large apertures are used in telescopes for
(a) greater magnification
(b) greater resolution
(c) reducing lens aberrations
(d) ease of manufacture

15. If the magnetic field is parallel to a surface, then magnetic flux at right angle to the surface, is
(a) zero (b) infinite

(c) small but not zero (d) large but not infinite

16. In some substances, charge can flow at ordinary temperature, but not at very low temperatures. These substances are called
(a) conductors (b) insulators
(c) dielectrics (d) semiconductors

17. A choke coil should have
(a) high resistance and low inductance
(b) high resistance and high inductance
(c) low resistance and high inductance
(d) low resistance and low inductance

18. In a pure semiconductor crystal, if current flows due to breakage of crystal bonds, then the semi-conductor, is called
(a) donor (b) acceptor
(c) intrinsic semi-conductor
(d) extrinsic semi-conductor

19. A battery of emf 10 V and internal resistance 3 Ω is connected to a resistor. If the current in the circuit is 0.5 A, what is the resistance of the resistor?

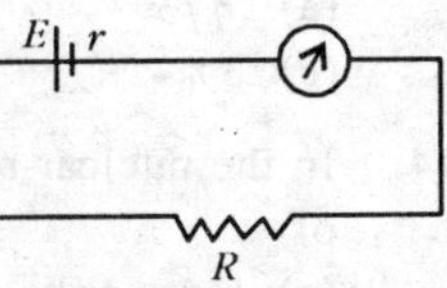

(a) 13 Ω (b) 15 Ω
(c) 17 Ω (d) 19 Ω

20. When a large bubble rises from the bottom of a lake to the surface, its radius is doubled. The atmospheric pressure is equal to that of a column of water of height H. The depth of the lake is
(a) $8H$ (b) $7H$
(c) $2H$ (d) H

21. If a star is moving towards the earth, then the spectrum lines are shifted towards
(a) red (b) infrared
(c) blue (d) green

22. Viscous force exerted by the liquid flowing between two plates in a streamline flow depends upon the
(a) area of the plates
(b) pressure of the liquid
(c) temperature of the liquid
(d) level of the liquid surface

23. The ratio of magnitudes of average velocity to average speed, is
(a) always less than one
(b) always equal to one
(c) always more than one
(d) equal to or more than one

24. During melting process, the heat given to a body is utilised in
(a) increasing the temperature
(b) increasing the density of the material
(c) increasing the average distance between the molecules
(d) decreasing the mass of the body

25. If two mirrors are kept at 60° to each other and a body is placed at the middle, then total number of images formed, is
(a) six (b) five
(c) four (d) three

26. In an A.C.circuit containing only capacitance, the current
(a) leads the voltage by 180°
(b) lags the voltage by 90°
(c) leads the voltage by 90°
(d) remains in phase with the voltage

27. Two charged spheres separated by a distance 'd' exert some force on each other. If they are immersed in a liquid of dielectric constant 2, then what is the force exerted, if all other conditions are same?
(a) $F/2$ (b) F
(c) $2F$ (d) $4F$

28. Which of the following instrument is used to measure temperature of the source from its thermal radiations?
(a) thermometer (b) thermopile
(c) pyrometer (d) barometer

29. A wire of radius r has resistance R. If it is stretched to a radius of $r/2$, its resistance becomes
(a) 0.5 R (b) 2 R
(c) 4 R (d) 16 R

30. If thermal conductivity of rod is 4, then its thermal resistivity will be
(a) 0.25 (b) 1.0
(c) 4.0 (d) 16.0

31. The mass moment of inertia, of a body depends upon
(a) angular velocity of the body
(b) angular acceleration of the body

(c) mass of the body
(d) distribution of mass and axis of rotation

32. During the production of X–rays, if voltage is increased then the
(a) wavelength decreases
(b) minimum wavelength increases
(c) intensity decreases
(d) intensity increases

33. In a diode, when there is a saturation current, the plate resistance (r_p), is
(a) zero (b) infinite quantity
(c) data insufficient (d) some finite quantity

34. The binding energy per nucleon of deuteron ($_1H^2$) and helium atom ($_2He^4$) is 1.1 MeV and 7 MeV respectively. If two deuteron atoms react to form a single helium atom, the released energy, is
(a) 13.9 MeV (b) 26.9 MeV
(c) 23.6 MeV (d) 19.2 MeV

35. In p–type semiconductor, major current carriers are
(a) electrons (b) negative ions
(c) mobile holes (d) both 'a' and 'b'

36. If the mass of a body on the earth surface is M, then its mass on the moon surface, is
(a) 6 M (b) 2 M
(c) M (d) $M/6$

37. In a coil of self-inductance 5 henry, the rate of change of current is 2 ampere per second. The e.m.f. induced in the coil, is
(a) 10 V (b) – 10 V
(c) 5 V (d) – 5 V

38. Electron-volt (eV) is the unit of
(a) energy (b) charge
(c) current (d) potential

39. If 'S' is stress and 'Y' is Young's modulus of a wire material, then energy stored in the wire per unit volume, is
(a) $\dfrac{S^2}{2Y}$ (b) $\dfrac{2Y}{S^2}$
(c) $\dfrac{S}{2Y}$ (d) $2S^2Y$

40. We plot a graph having temperature in °C along X–axis and in °F along Y–axis. If the graph is a straight line, then it
(a) intercepts the positive X–axis
(b) intercepts the positive Y–axis
(c) passes through the origin
(d) intercepts negative axis of both X and Y

41. The dimension of Plank's constant is
(a) $[ML^2T^{-1}]$ (b) $[ML^3T^{-1}]$
(c) $[ML^{-2}T^{-1}]$ (d) $[M^0L^{-1}T^{-3}]$

42. A convex lens is placed in a medium in which it behaves like a glass plate. The refractive index of the medium, will be
(a) equal to refractive index of air
(b) more than the refractive index of glass
(c) equal to the refractive index of glass
(d) less than the refractive index of glass

43. In Bohr's model, the atomic radius of the first orbit is r_0. The radius of the third orbit, is
(a) $r_0/3$ (b) r_0
(c) $3\,r_0$ (d) $9\,r_0$

44. In the nuclear reactions, there is a conservation of
(a) mass only (b) energy only
(c) momentum only (d) all of these

45. A molecule of mass m of an ideal gas collides with the wall of a vessel with a velocity v and returns back with the same velocity. The change in the linear momentum of the molecule is
(a) 2 mv (b) 4 mv
(c) 5 mv (d) 10 mv

46. If there is a change of angular momentum from J to 4J in 4 sec, then the torque, is
(a) 0.75 J (b) 3/4 J
(c) 5/4 J (d) 4/3 J

47. If a point charge moves round in a circle about a charge q, then work done by the charge, is
(a) zero (b) $\dfrac{1}{4\pi\varepsilon_0}\times\dfrac{q}{r}$
(c) $\dfrac{1}{4\pi\varepsilon_0}\times\dfrac{q^2}{r}$ (d) $\dfrac{1}{4\pi\varepsilon_0}\times\dfrac{q^2}{r^2}$

48. If a spring extends by x on loading, then energy stored by the spring is (if T is the tension in the spring and k is the spring constant)
(a) $\dfrac{T^2}{2x}$ (b) $\dfrac{T^2}{2k}$

(c) $\frac{2k}{T^2}$ (d) $\frac{2T^2}{k}$

49. If the temperature of a black body increases from 7°C to 287°C, then rate of energy radiation is

(a) 16 times (b) 8 times
(c) 4 times (d) 2 times

50. The value of acceleration due to gravity 'g', at earth's surface is 10 m/s^2. Its value at the centre of the earth which is assumed to be sphere of radius 'R' and uniform mass density, is

(a) 2.5 R m/s^2 (b) 5 R m/s^2
(c) 10 R m/s^2 (d) 0

Directions: *These questions consist of two statements each, printed as Assertion and Reason. While answering these questions you are required to choose any one of the following four responses.*

(a) If both Assertion and Reason are true and the Reason is a correct explanation of the Assertion.
(b) If both Assertion and Reason are true but Reason is not a correct explanation of the Assertion.
(c) If Assertion is true but the Reason is false.
(d) If both Assertion and Reason are false.

51. *Assertion*: Insulators do not allow flow of current through themselves.
Reason: They have no free charge carriers.

52. *Assertion*: For the sensitivity of a camera, its aperture should be reduced.
Reason: Smaller the aperture, larger is its power.

53. *Assertion*: When a body is projected at an angle 45°, its range is maximum.
Reason: For maximum of range, the value of sin 2θ should be equal to one.

54. *Assertion*: Sound waves cannot propagate through vacuum but light waves can.
Reason: Sound waves cannot be polarised but light waves can be.

55. *Assertion*: Lead is more elastic than rubber.
Reason: If the same load is attached to lead and rubber wires of the same cross-sectional area, the strain of lead is very much less than that of rubber.

56. *Assertion*: A cyclist leans inwards while taking a turn, while a man sitting in a car leans outwards on a curve.
Reason: Centripetal acceleration is acting towards the centre of the curve.

57. *Assertion*: If an electron and proton enter an electric field with equal energy, then path of electron is more curved than that of proton.
Reason: Electron has a tendency to form curve.

58. *Assertion*: If ice cap of the pole melts, the day length will shorten.
Reason: Ice will flow towards the equator and decrease the moment of inertia of the earth. This increases the frequency of rotation of the earth.

59. *Assertion*: When the temperature of a semiconductor is increased, then its resistance decreases.
Reason: The energy gap between conduction band and valence band is very small.

60. *Assertion*: If a pendulum falls freely, then its time period becomes infinite.
Reason: Free falling body has acceleration, equal to g

CHEMISTRY

61. "It is impossible to determine simultaneously the position and velocity of small particles such as electron". It is a statement of

(a) Hund's rule
(b) Aufbau's principle
(c) Pauli's rule
(d) Heisenberg's uncertainty principle

62. In which of the following methane is formed?

(a) $CH_3COOH \xrightarrow{[H]}$
(b) $CH_3COOH \xrightarrow{NaOH/CaO}$
(c) $CH_3COOH \xrightarrow{[O]}$
(d) $CH_3CH_2COOH \xrightarrow{NaOH/CaO}$

63. Which of the following is an alloy of aluminium?

(a) magnalium (b) duralumin
(c) brass (d) both 'a' and 'b'

64. The total number of orbitals in a shell can be given in the form of n. The principal quantum number is

(a) $2n$ (b) n^2
(c) $2n^2$ (d) $(n+1)$

65. A solution wiht pH = 2 is more acidic than one with a pH = 6, by a factor

(a) 4000 (b) 5000
(c) 8000 (d) 10 000

66. Vapour pressure of benzene at 30°C is 121.8 mm. when 15 g of a non-volatile solute is dissolved in 250 g of benzene, its vapour prssure is decreased to 120.2 mm. The molecular weight of the solute is
(a) 35.67 g (b) 356.7 g
(c) 432.8 g (d) 502.7 g

67. Which of the following compound, on reaction with NaOH and Na_2O_2, gives yellow colour?
(a) $Zn(OH)_2$ (b) $Al(OH)_3$
(c) $Cr(OH)_3$ (d) $CaCO_3$

68. A base, as defined by Bronsted theory, is a substance which can
(a) accept protons
(b) donate protons
(c) lose a pair of electrons
(d) gain a pair of electrons

69. In the compound Lithium tetra-hydroaluminate, the ligand is
(a) H (b) H^+
(c) H^- (d) F^-

70. Reduction of benzoyl chloride with $Pd/BaSO_4$ produces
(a) benzene (b) benzaldehyde
(c) benzoic acid (d) benzoyl cyanide

71. Which of the following, on reaction with H_2S, does not produce metallic sulphide?
(a) $CdCl_2$ (b) $ZnCl_2$
(c) $COCl_2$ (d) $CuCl_2$

72. The BCl_3 is a planar molecule where as NCl_3 is pyramidal, because
(a) B–Cl bond is more polar than N–Cl bond
(b) N–Cl bond is more covalent than B–Cl bond
(c) nitrogen atom is smaller than boron atoms
(d) BCl_3 has no lone pair but NCl_3 has a lone pair of electrons

73. The isomers, which can be converted into another form by rotation of the molecules around single bond, are
(a) conformers (b) enantiomers
(c) diastereomers (d) geometrical isomers

74. Nylon–66 is made by using
(a) succinic acid (b) benzylchloride
(c) benzaldehyde (d) adipic acid

75. For the reaction $H_2\ (g) + I_2\ (g) \rightarrow 2\ HI\ (g)$ the change in enthalpy (ΔH) will be
(a) $= \Delta E$ (b) $> \Delta E$
(c) $< \Delta E$ (d) either 'b' or 'c'

76. How many atoms of carbon are present in a diamond weighing 0.5 carat? (one carat weighs 200 mg and assume the diamond to be pure carbon)
(a) 5×10^{21} (b) 6×10^{22}
(c) 7×10^{19} (d) 8×10^{12}

77. Which of the following compound is not coloured?
(a) $Na_2[CuCl_4]$ (b) $Na_2[CdCl_4]$
(c) $K_4[Fe(CN)_6]$ (d) $K_3[Fe(CN)_6]$

78. Potash alum is used as
(a) catalyst (b) disinfectant
(c) mordant (d) coolant

79. Which of the following is not an aromatic compound?
(a) benzene (b) cyclohexane
(c) ortho xylene (d) picric acid

80. If 0.189 g of a chlorine containing organic compound gave 0.287 g of silver chloride, then the percentage of chlorine in the organic compound is
(a) 35.47 (b) 35.57
(c) 37.57 (d) 45.37

81. The main product (70% to 80%) of the reaction between m–dinitrobenzene with NH_4HS is

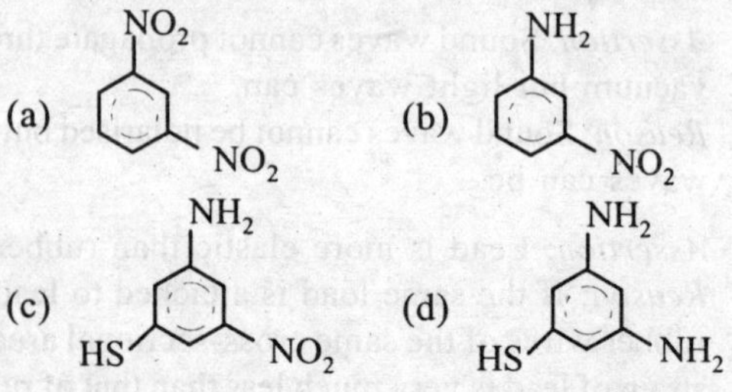

82. $R - CH_2 - CH_2OH$ can be converted into RCH_2CH_2COOH. The correct sequence of the reagents is
(a) KCN and H^+ (b) PBr, KCN and H_2
(c) PBr_3, KCN and H^+ (d) HCN, PBr_3 and H^+

83. Which of the following compound is glycerine?
(a) one primary – OH group is present
(b) two primary – OH groups are present
(c) one secondary – OH group is present
(d) two secondary – OH groups are present

84. How many electrons flow when a current of 5 amperes is passed through a conductor for 200 seconds?
(a) 6.241×10^{21} (b) 6.0241×10^{21}
(c) 6.241×10^{22} (d) 6.0241×10^{22}

85. Which of the following statements is not true about alcohols?
(a) lower alochols have fiery taste and strong smell
(b) as molecular mass increases the boiling point increases
(c) lower alcohols are water insoluble and their solubility increases with molecular weight
(d) lower alcohols are water soluble and their solubility decreases with molecular weight

86. The most suitable method of the separation of a 1 : 1 mixture of ortho – and para – nitrophenols is
(a) filtration (b) sublimation
(c) crystallisation (d) steam distillation

87. Which of the following is not emitted by radioactive substance?
(a) proton (b) positron
(c) α – rays (d) β – rays

88. Brass is an alloy of copper (Cu) and
(a) Al (b) Sn
(c) Zn (d) Ag

89. Formation of polyethylene, from calcium carbide, takes place as follows:
$CaC_2 + 2H_2O \longrightarrow Ca(OH)_2 + C_2H_2$;
$C_2H_2 + H_2 \longrightarrow C_2H_4$;
$n\,(C_2H_4) \longrightarrow (-CH_2-CH_2-)n$. The amount of polyethylene obtained from 64.1 kg of CaC_2 is
(a) 7 kg (b) 14 kg
(c) 21 kg (d) 28 kg

90. If a gas occupies a volume of 300 cc at 27°C and 620 mm pressure, then the volume of the gas at 47°C and 640 mm pressure, is
(a) 310 cc (b) 410 cc
(c) 500 cc (d) 600 cc

91. Which of the following can give iodometric titration?
(a) Fe^{+3} (b) Cu^{+2}
(c) Pb^{+2} (d) Ag^{+2}

92. In the reaction : $I_2 + I^- \rightarrow I_3^-$, the Lewis base is
(a) I^- (b) I_2
(c) I_3^- (d) none of these

93. The enthalphy change of a reaction does not depend upon
(a) state of reactants and products
(b) nature of reactants and products
(c) different intermediate reaction
(d) initial and final enthalpy change of a reaction

94. Ammonia, on reaction with excess of chlorine, gives
(a) NCl_3 and HCl (b) N_4 and NH_4Cl
(c) NCl_3 and NH_4Cl (d) N_2 and HCl

95. The extra amount of energy, which the molecules of the reactants have to absorb, so that their energy becomes equal to the threshold energy, is called
(a) kinetic energy (b) potential energy
(c) chemical energy (d) activation energy

96. Reaction of nitrous acid with aliphatic primary amine will give
(a) dye (b) alcohol
(c) nitrite (d) diazonium salt

97. The maximum amount of $BaSO_4$ precipitated on mixing $BaCl_2$ (0.5 M) with H_2SO_4 (1 M) will corrrespond to
(a) 0.5 M (b) 1.0 M
(c) 1.5 M (d) 2.0 M

98. If 1, 3 – dibromopropane reacts with Zinc and NaI, the product obtained is
(a) propene (b) propane
(c) cyclopropane (d) hexane

99. A current of 9.95 amperes flowing for 10 minutes, deposits 3 gm of a metal. Equivalent weight of the metal is
(a) 12.5 (b) 18.5
(c) 21.5 (d) 48.5

100. The oxidatioin state of chromium in potassium dichromate is
(a) + 2 (b) – 2
(c) – 5 (d) + 6

101. The compressibility factor of an ideal gas is
(a) 1 (b) 2
(c) 4 (d) 6

102. Which of the following is not affected by the temperature ?
(a) molarity (b) molality
(c) normality (d) formality

103. Which of the following does not react with AgCl?
(a) $NaNO_3$ (b) NH_4OH
(c) Na_2CO_3 (d) $Na_2S_2O_3$

104. In a reaction of C_6H_5Y, the major product (> 60%) is m–isomer. The group Y is
(a) – Cl (b) – OH
(c) – NH_2 (d) – COOH

105. Particle nature of the electron was experimentally demonstrated by
(a) de Broglie (b) Schrodinger
(c) Max Bon (d) J.J. Thomson

106. In the gas phase reaction $C_2H_2 + H_2 \rightleftharpoons C_2H_6$, the equilibrium constant can be expressed in
(a) mole litre^{-1} (b) mole litre^{-2}
(c) mole^{-1} litre^{-1} (d) litre mole^{-1}

107. 1 – butyne reacts with cold alkaline $KMnO_4$ to produce
(a) CH_3CH_2COOH
(b) $CH_3CH_2CH_2COOH$
(c) $CH_3CH_2COOH + CO_2$
(d) $CH_3 - CH_2 - COOH + HCOOH$

108. The electronic configuration $1s^2\ 2s^2\ 2p^5\ 3s^1$ shows
(a) ground state of fluorine atom
(b) excited state of fluorine atom
(c) excited state of neon atom
(d) excited state of ion O_2^-

109. Generally, the limit of visible spectrum is
(a) 1000 to 3000 Å (b) 4000 to 7000 Å
(c) 8000 to 10000 Å (d) 12000 to 15000Å

110. In the reaction : $S + 3/2\ O_2 \longrightarrow SO_3 + 2x$ kcal and $SO_2 + 1/2\ O_2 \longrightarrow SO_3 + y$ kcal, heat of formation of SO_2 is
(a) $(x + y)$ (b) $(x - y)$
(c) $(2x + y)$ (d) $(2x - y)$

Directions: *These questions consist of two statements each, printed as Assertion and Reason. While answering these questions you are required to choose any one of the following four responses.*

(a) If both Assertion and Reason are true and the Reason is a correct explanation of the Assertion.
(b) If both Assertion and Reason are true but Reason is not a correct explanation of the Assertion.
(c) If Assertion is true but the Reason is false.
(d) If both Assertion and Reason are false.

111. *Assertion*: The bond angle of PBr_3 is greater than PH_3 but the bond angle of NBr_3 is less than NH_3.
Reason: Size of Br is less than hydrogen.

112. *Assertion*: Heat of neutralization for both HNO_3 and HCl with NaOH is 53 . 7 kJ/mole.
Reason: NaOH is a strong electrolyte/base.

113. *Assertion*: Decrease in free energy causes spontaneous reaction.
Reason: Spontaneous reactions are invariably exothermic reactions.

114. *Assertion*: Liquid ammonia is used for refrigeration.
Reason: It vapourises quickly.

115. *Assertion*: Tungsten has very high melting point.
Reason: Tungten is a covalent compound.

116. *Assertion*: Hydrogen has only one electron in its orbit. But it produces several spectral lines.
Reason: There are many excited energy levels available.

117. *Assertion*: Ionisation potential of Be (atomic no.4) is less than B (atomic no. 5).
Reason: The first electron released from Be is of *p*-orbital but that from B is of *s*-orbital.

118. *Assertion*: NO_3^- is planar while NH_3 is pyramidal.
Reason: N in NO_3^- is sp^2 and in NH_3 is sp^3 hybridized.

119. *Assertion*: N_2 and NO^+ both are diamagnetic substance.
Reason: NO^+ is isoelectronic with N_2.

120. *Assertion*: Na_2SO_4 is soluble in water while $BaSO_4$ is not.
Reason: Lattice energy of $BaSO_4$ exceeds its hydration energy.

BIOLOGY

121. The compound, which is soluble in water but does not impede the oxygen transportation, is
(a) NO (b) SO_2
(c) CO (d) SO_3.

122. The branch of biology dealing with the process of improvement of human race by selective breeding is called
(a) euphenics (b) euthenics
(c) obstetrics (d) eugenics.

123. Waste product of adenine and guanine metabolism are excreted by man as
(a) uric acid (b) urea
(c) allantoin (d) ammonia.

124. Scientists pin-pointed the location of colour-processing perception centres in human visual cortex by a method named
(a) CT scanning
(b) PET scanning
(c) ultra-sound imaging
(d) NMR imaging.

125. The disorders such as alkaptonuria and phenylketonuria are refered to as
(a) infectious disease
(b) acquired disease
(c) congenital disease (d) all of these.

126. There is an irregular mating population. If the frequency of an autosomal recessive lethal gene is 0.4, then the frequency of the carriers in a population of 200 individuals is
(a) 96 (b) 36
(c) 104 (d) 72.

127. If the rate of addition of new members increases with respect to the individual host of the same population, then the graph obtained has
(a) zero population growth
(b) declined growth
(c) exponential growth
(d) none of these.

128. To yield milk, cow is given
(a) stilbesterol (b) sorbitol
(c) gonadotropin (d) prolactin.

129. The disease, in which thick cough, stops the passage of throat and form a layer of mucous membrane, is called
(a) tuberculosis (b) tetanus
(c) diphtheria (d) pertussis.

130. Ora serrata is
(a) gland present in oral cavity of frog
(b) a part of third wall of retina of eye
(c) present in utriculus of ear
(d) oral cavity of protochordates

131. Which of the following is an example of sex-linked inheritance?
(a) night-blindness (b) anaemia
(c) colour-blindness (d) cretinism.

132. Chloragogen cells of earthworm are similar to the vertebrate organ
(a) kidney (b) liver
(c) spleen (d) lung.

133. The type of immunoglobulin present in the colostrum secreted from mammary gland is
(a) IgD (b) IgC
(c) IgM (d) IgE.

134. A pregnant woman, who has done amniocentesis test, finds an extra barr body in her embryo. The syndrome which is likely to be associated with embryo is
(a) Edward's syndrome
(b) Down's syndrome
(c) Klinfelter's syndrome
(d) Patau's syndrome.

135. The preparation of sperm before penetration of ovum is called
(a) insemination (b) coition
(c) spermiation (d) capacitation.

136. Which proteolytic enzyme induces lysis of fibrin during fibrinolysis?
(a) fibrin (b) plasmin
(c) thrombin (d) all of these.

137. The lining of bone marrow cavity is called
(a) endoneurium (b) endosteum
(c) endothelium (d) endomyosium.

138. The endocrine gland of insects, which secretes the juvenile hormone, is
(a) corpora albicans (b) corpora allata
(c) corpora myecaena (d) all of these.

139. Quill feathers at the base of quill wings are called
(a) coverts (b) remiges
(c) down feathers (d) barbules.

140. Structure which remains unchanged during metamorphosis of frog's tadpole is
(a) intestine (b) lung
(c) nervous system (d) heart.

141. How much amount of oxygen is present in one gram of haemoglobin?
(a) 20 ml (b) 1.34 ml
(c) 40 ml (d) 13.4 ml.

142. Otoconium is found in
(a) synovial fluid (b) perilymph
(c) otolithic membrane (d) haemolymph.

143. Exaggerated dread is a death disease which is known as
(a) haemotophobia (b) algophobia
(c) pathophobia (d) myophobia.

144. Antiserum contains
(a) leucocytes (b) antigens
(c) antibodies (d) all of these.

145. The branch, which is associated with diagnosis, prevention and cure of mental disorders is called
(a) neurology (b) psychiatry
(c) neuropsychiatry (d) psychology.

146. Translocation of organic materials is best explained by
(a) imbibition theory
(b) active transport
(c) mass flow hypothesis
(d) transpiration pull.

147. Which of the following is the largest and edible bud?
(a) cabbage (b) onion
(c) cauliflower (d) *Agave*.

148. When a tall and red flowered individual is crossed with a dwarf and white flowered individual, phenotype in the progeny is dwarf and white. What will be the genotype of tall and red flowered individual ?
(a) TtRr (b) TTRR
(c) TTRr (d) TtRR.

149. An insectivorous plant having glandular structures on its leaf secreting sticky fluid is
(a) sundew plant (b) aldrovanda
(c) venus fly trap (d) all of these.

150. Positive pollution of soil is due to
(a) excessive use of fertilizers
(b) reduction in soil productivity
(c) addition of wastes on soil
(d) all of these.

151. Perisperm is
(a) peripheral part of endosperm
(b) remnant of endosperm
(c) disintegrated secondary nucleus
(d) persistant of nucellus.

152. The biome, which is characterised by broad-leaved vegetation, life-resistant resinous plants and drought-evading plants, is known as
(a) steppes (b) chapparal
(c) deciduous forest (d) savannah.

153. Which of the following compound has very important role in prebiotic evolution?
(a) CH_4 (b) SO_2
(c) SO_3 (d) NO.

154. Genes present on Y-chromosome are called
(a) polygenic gene (b) basic gene
(c) pleiotropic gene (d) holandric gene.

155. The carnivorous fish, *Gambusia*, which is introduced in the lakes and ponds to control a deadly disease in India, feeds on the larva of
(a) dragon fly (b) *Nepenthes*
(c) *Anopheles* (d) all of these.

156. The C_4-plants differ from C_3-plants with reference to the
(a) substrate that accepts CO_2 in carbon assimilation
(b) type of end product
(c) type of pigment involved in photosynthesis
(d) number of ATP that are consumed in preparing sugar.

157. The plants in desert, in order to tolerate water stress, have
(a) stipular spines
(b) no stomata
(c) stems which are converted into leaf type
(d) long root system reach the water level.

158. The sphere of living matter together with water, air and soil on the surface of earth is called
(a) lithosphere (b) atmosphere
(c) biosphere (d) hydrosphere.

159. Which of the following prevents the photo-oxidation and destruction of pigments ?

(a) phycoerythrin (b) phytochrome
(c) phytohormone (d) phycocyanin.

160. Meiosis in *Dryopteris* takes place during
(a) gamete formation
(b) spore formation
(c) sex organ formation
(d) spore germination.

161. Recent reports of acid rains in big industrial cities are due to the effect of atmospheric pollution by excessive release of
(a) NH_3 by coal gas industries
(b) NO_2 and SO_2 by burning of fossil fuels
(c) CO_2 by incomplete combustion of carbon fuel
(d) CO_2 by burning of coal/wood, cutting of forests.

162. The process in which the amount of DNA, RNA and protein can be known at a time is called
(a) cellular fractioning
(b) autoradiography
(c) phase-contrast microscopy
(d) tissue culture.

163. The hexaploid wheat is obtained by
(a) chromosomes map (b) hybridomas
(c) hybridisation (d) both (b) and (c).

164. In sweet peas, genes C and P are necessary for colour in flowers. The flowers are white in the absence of either or both the genes. What will be the percentage of coloured flowers in the offspring of the cross Ccpp × ccPp?
(a) 75% (b) 25%
(c) 100% (d) 50%

165. Which plant species is on the verge of extinction due to over-exploitation?
(a) *Gloriosa* (b) *Podophyllum*
(c) *Ceritella* (d) all of these.

166. The asexual production of seed is called
(a) fragmentation (b) apomixis
(c) self-fertilization (d) both (a) & (b).

167. If mitotic division is restricted in G_1-phase of a cell cycle, then the condition is known as
(a) S-phase (b) G_2-phase
(c) M-phase (d) G_0-phase.

168. Epistatic effect, in which the dihybrid cross 9 : 3 : 3 : 1 between AaBb × AaBb is modified as
(a) interaction between two alleles of the same loci
(b) dominance of one allele on another allele of the same loci
(c) interaction between two alleles of different loci
(d) dominance of one allele on another allele of both loci.

169. Potato is included in solanaceae family because
(a) it is epipetallous
(b) it is pentamerous
(c) ovary is slightly diverted from its position
(d) all the above.

170. The chemical compounds which are produced by host plants due to infection as a defence reaction to pathogen, are called
(a) phytotron (b) phytotoxin
(c) phytoalexins (d) phytol.

Directions: *These questions consist of two statements each, printed as Assertion and Reason. While answering these questions you are required to choose any one of the following four responses.*
(a) If both Assertion and Reason are true and the Reason is a correct explanation of the Assertion.
(b) If both Assertion and Reason are true but Reason is not a correct explanation of the Assertion.
(c) If Assertion is true but the Reason is false.
(d) If both Assertion and Reason are false.

171. *Assertion*: In alcoholic drink, the alcohol is converted into glucose in the liver.
Reason: Liver cells are able to produce glucose from alcohol by back fermentation.

172. *Assertion*: After ovariectomy, menstrual cycle in woman may be stopped
Reason: Ovarian hormones induce menstrual cycle.

173. *Assertion*: Cold-blooded animals have no fat layer.
Reason: Cold-blooded animals use their fat for metabolic process during hibernation.

174. *Assertion*: In morula stage, the cells divide without any increase in size.
Reason: Zona pellucida remains undivided till cleavage is complete.

175. *Assertion*: In the descending limb of loops of Henle, the urine is hypertonic, while in ascending limb of loops of Henle, the urine is hypotonic.
Reason: Descending limb is impermeable to Na^+, while ascending limb is impermeable to H_2O.

176. *Assertion*: Submerged plants get CO_2 in the form of carbonates and bicarbonates.

Reason: Stomata are not present in submerged plants.

177. *Assertion*: Thick cuticle is mostly present in disease resistance plants.
Reason: Disease causing agents cannot grow on cuticle and cannot invade the cuticle.

178. *Assertion*: Amber codon is a termination codon.
Reason: If in *m*-RNA, a termination codon is present, the protein synthesis stops abruptly whether the protein synthesis is completed or not.

179. *Assertion*: Plasmids are single-stranded extra-chromosomal DNA.
Reason: Plasmids are possessed by eucaryotic cells.

180. *Assertion*: In apomixis, the plants of new genetic sequence are produced.
Reason: In apomixis, two individuals of same genetic sequence meet.

GENERAL KNOWLEDGE

181. The largest continent is the world,.is
(a) North America (b) Asia
(c) South America (d) Europe.

182. The tomb of Quatab Shahi is situated, in
(a) Allahabad (b) Hyderbad
(c) Agra (d) Aligarh.

183. Hiroshima day is observed on
(a) August 1 (b) July 17
(c) August 6 (d) July 27.

184. Doctors before starting their service take oath in the name of a scientist to work honestly. The name of this scientist, is
(a) Hippocrates (b) Darwin
(c) Plato (d) Socrates.

185. The 'AIDS DAY' is observed on
(a) 1st Dec (b) 20th Dec.
(c) 1st June (d) 1st May.

186. The Halley's comet will be seen next in
(a) 2066 (b) 2058
(c) 2068 (d) 2062.

187. One who obtained the Nobel prize of 1993 for peace along with Nelson Mandela, was
(a) Yasser Arafat (b) F.W. deKlark
(c) Gorbachov (d) Desmond Tutu.

188. Deep Blue is a
(a) computer which plays chess
(b) blue whale
(c) computer which gives weather report
(d) computer operating system.

189. 'Confucianism' is famous in
(a) China (b) Malaysia
(c) Myanmar (d) Japan.

190. 'Dachigam Wild life Sanctuary' in Kashmir is associated with which of the following animal?
(a) Panther (b) Sagul
(c) Horned toed deer (d) Hangul.

191. The name of the sheep, which was cloned for the first time, is
(a) Molly (b) Dolly
(c) Holly (d) Polly.

192. The male cricketer, who scored maximum runs, in a one day cricket match is
(a) Saeed Anwar (b) Kapil Dev
(c) Azharuddin (d) Vivian Richards.

193. Issac Asimov is associated with
(a) movies awards (b) football
(c) writing of science novels
(d) antibiotics.

194. When the Olympic Games were not played?
(a) 1920 (b) 1912
(c) 1924 (d) 1916.

195. Which of the following state has the highest number of illiterates?
(a) Uttar Pradesh (b) Bihar
(c) Andhra Pradesh (d) Orissa.

196. Asian Games were held in India in
(a) 1956 and 1986 (b) 1951 and 1982
(c) 1962 and 1986 (d) 1962 and 1984.

197. The 'Royal Flying Doctor Service' is in
(a) Germany (b) Japan
(c) Australia (d) Canada.

198. The 'Principality of Liechtenstein' is situated in between Switzerland and
(a) Germany (b) Italy
(c) France (d) none of these.

199. The 'Statue of Liberty' was gifted to USA by
(a) Germany (b) Canada
(c) Greece (d) France.

200. Writer of 'Future Shock' is
(a) Bernard Shaw (b) Sewitzer
(c) Bertrond Russell
(d) Alwyn Toffler

❖❖❖

SOLUTIONS

PHYSICS

1. (a) : Let us consider a charged hollow sphere with charge q. The charge q is on the surface of the sphere. We have to calculate the electric field at an interior point P distance r from the centre. If we imagine a Gaussian spherical surface through the point P and concentric with the given shell, we can use the Gauss theorem,

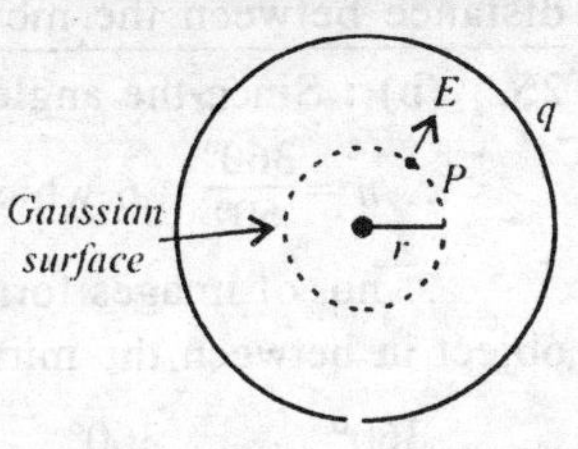

$E \times 4\pi r^2 = \frac{q'}{E_0}$ where q' is the charge enclosed by this Gaussian surface = 0

$\therefore E = 0$

2. (b) : On an artificial satellite orbiting the earth the acceleration is given by $\frac{GM}{R^2}$ towards the centre of the earth. Now for a body of mass m on the satellite the gravitational force due to earth is $\frac{GMm}{R^2}$ towards the centre of the earth. Let the reaction force on the surface of the satellite be N, then

$$\frac{GMm}{R^2} - N = m\left(\frac{GM}{R^2}\right)$$

$\Rightarrow N = 0$

That is on the satellite there is a state of weightlessness or $g = 0$

$\therefore$ The time period of the simple pendulum,

$$T = 2\pi\sqrt{\frac{l}{g}} = \infty$$

3. (c) : The chromatic aberration formed by a convex lens is considered positive and that by a concave lens is considered negative, as they have got exactly oposite characteristics. So the chromatic aberration formed by one lens can be nullified by the suitable use of the second lens.

4. (a) 5. (d) 6. (d)

7. (a) : For very small drops, the potential energy due to gravity is insignificant as compared to that due to surface tension. Therefore the shape of the liquid drop is determined by the surface tension.

8. (b) : Due to the rotation of the earth, the acceleration due to gravity for earth changes and at the equator, its value is given by $g' = g - w^2R$

And at poles, $g' = g$

$\therefore$ The value of acceleration due to gravity is minimum at the equator.

9. (b) : Negative sign reverses the direction. Since magnitude of the number is 2, therefore magnitude of the vector is doubled.

10. (b) : The law of conservation of linear momentum states that in absence of an external force, the linear momentum of a body remains constant. And Newton's first law states that until and unless an external force is applied a body in a state of rest will tend to be in a state of rest and body in motion will tend to keep on moving without a charge of speed and direction. In other words if a body is in a state of rest then its momentum is zero and the first law tells that the body tries to preserve its zero momentum. And when in motion (momentum 'mv'), the body tries to preserve its momentum mv again. Which is the law of conservation of momentum.

11. (d) : $\vec{P}+\vec{Q}$ and $\vec{P}-\vec{Q}$ are diagonals of a parallelogram whose sides are $\vec{P}$ and $\vec{Q}$. Thus the angle between them may be between 0° and 180°.

12. (b)

13. (a) : Pyrometer can measure temperature from 800°C to 6000°C. Therefore temperature of the sun is measured by pyrometer.

14. (b) : Objective of large aperture is used in a telescope, so that it may collect sufficient light and form a bright image.

15. (a) : The magnetic flux through a surface is given by

$$\phi = \vec{B}.\vec{A} = BA\cos\theta$$

Now since the magnetic field $\vec{B}$ is parallel to the surface, so the magnetic flux in a direction perpendicular to the surface will be $\phi = BA\cos 90° = 0$

16. (d) : The electrical resistance of a semiconductor decreases with the rise in temperature. Therefore at absolute zero temperature, a semiconductor becomes an insulator.

17. (c) : In a choke coil, we use a low resistance and a high inductance to reduce the current in an a.c. circuit. We use a high inductance in place of a high resistance because the inductance does not consume power, so we don't lose any energy in the form of heat.

18. (c) : In the case of an intrinsic semiconductor (say Si) where each Si is having 4 outermost electrons, its crystal structure consists of making 4 covalent bonds with 4 negihbouring Si atoms. Each bond consists of two eletrons.

```
     Si    Si
     ||    ||
Si══Si═══Si══Si
     ||  ↑  ||
     Si  |  Si
     (broken)
```

Now if one of the bonds get broken due to some reason (collisions or high temperature) then one electron gets freed and it will be having sufficient energy to cross the band gap and be ready for conduction. So in intrinsic semiconductors, current flows due to breakage of crystal bonds.

19. (c) : Given : E.M.F. of the battery (E) = 10 volts; Internal resistance (r) = 3 Ω and current (I) = 0.5 A.

We know that current (I) $= \frac{E}{R+r}$ or $0.5 = \frac{10}{R+3}$ or

$0.5R + 1.5 = 10$ or $0.5R = 8.5$ or $R = \frac{8.5}{0.5} = 17\ \Omega$

20. (b) : Given : Initial radius of the bubble = r; Final radius of the bubble = $2r$ and initial pressure at the surface (P_1) = column of water height H. When radius of a bubble becomes double, its volume (V_2) becomes 8 times. Also from the Boyle's law, $P_1V_1 = P_2V_2$ or $P_2 = \frac{P_1V_1}{V_2} = \frac{H \times 8V}{V} = 8H$. Therefore depth of the lake $= 8H - H = 7H$.

21. (c) : If a star is moving towards the earth (*i.e.* observer), the frequency of its radiation will increase or the wavelength will decrease. Therefore the spectrum lines will shift towards blue end of the spectrum.

22. (a) : Viscous force $(F) = \eta A \times \frac{dv}{dx} \propto A$ (where A is the area of the plates).

23. (a)

24. (c) : The heat given to the melting solid is used in displacing the molecules from their original position and making their order irregular. It increases the average distance between the molecules.

25. (b) : Since the angle of inclination $\theta = 60°$

$\therefore n = \frac{360°}{60°} = 6$ which is even

$\therefore$ no. of images formed for any position of the object in between the mirrors = 6 − 1 = 5

$(n) = \frac{360°}{\theta} - 1 \Rightarrow \frac{360°}{60} - 1 \Rightarrow 6 - 1 \Rightarrow 5$

26. (c) : In a purely capacitive circuit, where there is no resistance, the current i flowing through it deposits a charge dq on the capacitor in time that is

$dq = idt$

$\Rightarrow i = \frac{dq}{dt}$

$E = E_0 \sin\omega t$

Now using Kirchoff's law, if total charge deposited on the capacitor is q then

$\frac{q}{C} = E_0 \sin\omega t$

$\Rightarrow q = CE_0 \sin\omega t$

$\Rightarrow i = \frac{dq}{dt} = CE_0\omega \cos\omega t = i_0 \cos\omega t$ where

$i_0 = \frac{E_0}{\left(\frac{1}{C\omega}\right)}$ = peak current

$\therefore i = i_0 \cos\omega t = i_0 \sin\left(\omega + \frac{\pi}{2}\right)t$

and $E = E_0 \sin\omega t$

Hence current is leading the voltage in phase by $\frac{\pi}{2}$

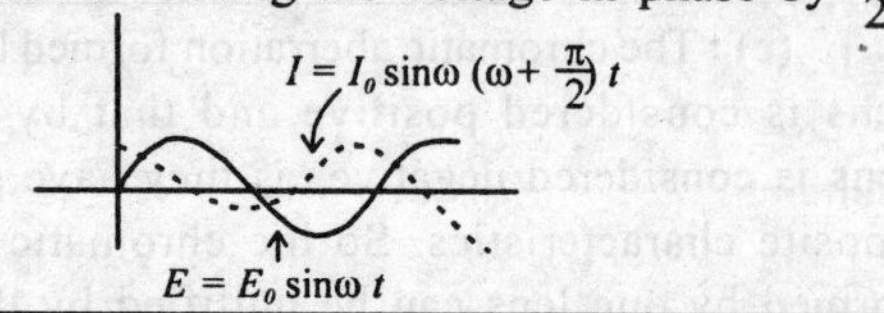

27. (a) : Given : Distance between two charges = d and dielectric constant (k) = 2. Force between two charged spheres $(F) = \frac{1}{4\pi\varepsilon_0} \times \frac{q_1q_2}{r_2}$, where ε_0 is permitivity of free space. and force for a medium with dielectric constant k,

$$F' = \frac{1}{k} \times \frac{1}{4\pi\varepsilon_0} \times \frac{q_1 q_2}{r_2} = \frac{F}{k} = \frac{F}{2}.$$

28. **(c)**

29. **(d)** : Given : Initial radius of wire $(r_1) = r$; Initial resistance $= R$ and final radius of wire (r_2) = 0.5 r. Let L_1 and A_1 be the length and cross-sectional area of original wire and L_2, A_2 be the values for the stretched wire.

Therefore, $L_1 \times \pi r_1^2 = L_2 \times \pi r_2^2$ or

$L_1 r = L_2 \times (0.5r)^2$ or $\frac{L_1}{L_2} = \frac{1}{4}$ and $\frac{A_1}{A_2} = \frac{\pi (r)^2}{\pi (0.5r)^2} = 4.$

Resistance $(R) = \rho \frac{L}{A} \propto \frac{L}{A}$ or

$\frac{R_1}{R_2} = \frac{L_1}{L_2} \times \frac{A_2}{A_1} = \frac{1}{4} \times \frac{1}{4} = \frac{1}{16}$ or $R_2 = 16\ R_1$

30. **(a)** : Thermal resistivity =

$$\frac{1}{\text{Thermal conductivity}} = \frac{1}{4} = 0.25$$

31. **(d)**

32. **(a)** : Wavelength $(\lambda) = \frac{hc}{eV} \propto \frac{1}{V}$. Therefore if voltage is increased then wavelength is decreased.

33. **(b)** : Plate resistance $(r_p) = \frac{\delta V}{\delta I}$ (where δV is the change in voltage and δI is the change in current. At saturation, current $\delta I = 0$. Therefore at saturation $(r_p) = \frac{\delta V}{0} = \infty.$

34. **(c)** : Given : binding energy per nucleon of deuteron $({}_1H^2)$ = 1.1 MeV and binding energy per nucleon of helium ${}_2He^4$ = 7 MeV. Total binding energy of two deuteron atoms $({}_1H^2)$ $(1p + 1n)$ = 2 (2 × 1.1) = 4.4 MeV and total binding energy of helium atom $({}_2H^4)$ $(2p + 2n)$ = 4 × 7 = 28 MeV. Therefore energy released on forming helium nucleus from two deuterons = 28 – 4.4 = 23.6 MeV. The reaction taking place is schematically represented as

$({}_1H^2 + 2 \times 1.1 \text{ MeV}) + ({}_1H^2 + 2 \times 1.1 \text{ MeV}) \longrightarrow ({}_2He^4 + 4 \times 7 \text{ MeV})$

35. **(c)**

36. **(c)** : Mass is the matter contained in a body. It remains constant irrespective of the place where the body is taken. Therefore mass of the body on the moon surface is M.

37. **(b)** : Given : Inductance of the coil (L) = 5 H and rate of change of current $\left(\frac{dI}{dt}\right) = 2$ A/sec. The induced e.m.f. $= -L\left(\frac{dI}{dt}\right) = -5 \times 2 = -10$V.

38. **(a)**

39. **(a)** : Given : Stress on the wire = S and Young's modulus of the material = Y. Energy stored per unit volume $= \frac{1}{2} \times$ Stress × Strain

$$= \frac{1}{2} \times S \times \frac{\text{Stress}}{Y} = \frac{1}{2} \times S \times \frac{S}{Y} = \frac{S^2}{2Y}$$

40. **(b)** : We know that

$$\frac{C}{100} = \frac{F - 32}{180}$$

$\Rightarrow F = \frac{9}{5}C + 160$, which gives us a straight line with positive intercept on the Y axis :

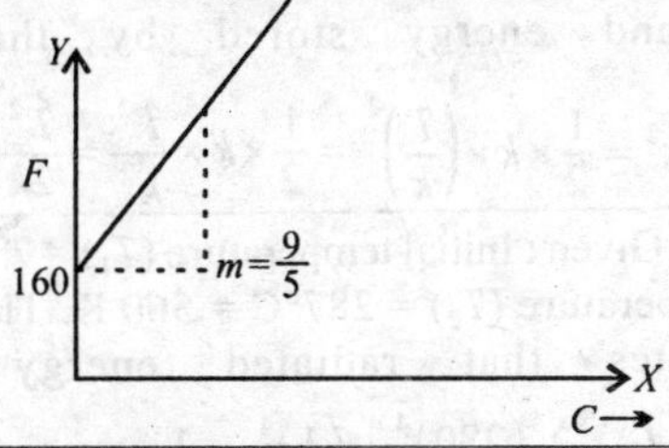

41. **(a)** : Planck's constant (h) =

$$\frac{\text{Energy in each photon}}{\text{Frequency of radiation}} = \frac{[E]}{[\nu]} = \frac{[ML^2T^{-2}]}{[T^{-1}]} = [ML^2T^{-1}].$$

42. **(c)** : We know from the lens maker's formula the focal length,

$$\frac{1}{f} = \left(\frac{\mu_2 - \mu_1}{\mu_1}\right)\left(\frac{1}{R_1} - \frac{1}{R_2}\right)$$

Now for the lens to behave like a glass plate its focal length will be infinity ($f = \infty$)

$\therefore\ \mu_2 - \mu_1 = 0 \Rightarrow \mu_2 = \mu_1$

That is, the refractive index of the medium should be equal to the refractive index of glass.

43. **(d)** : Given : Radius of the first orbit $(r_1) = r_0$.

Radius of nth orbit (r_n) $= \frac{\varepsilon_0 h^2}{\pi m Z e^2} \times n^2 \propto n^2$ or

$\frac{r_0}{r_3} = \left(\frac{n_1}{n_3}\right)^2 = \left(\frac{1}{3}\right)^2 = \frac{1}{9}$ or $r_3 = 9r_0$. ...(where r_3 = radius of the third orbit)

44. (d)

45. (a) : Given : Mass of the molecule = m; Initial velocity of the molecule = v. Initial momentum = mv and final momentum = $-mv$ (minus sign due to motion in the opposite direction). Therefore change in linear momentum of the molecule = Final momentum – Initial momentum = $-mv - mv = -2mv$

$\therefore$ The magnitude of change of linear momentum $= 2mv$

46. (b) : Given Initial angular momentum $(J_1) = J$; final angular momentum $(J_2) = 4J$ and time $(t) = 4$ sec. Torque = Rate of change of angular momentum

$$= \frac{J_2 - J_1}{t} = \frac{4J - J}{4} = \frac{3}{4}J.$$

47. (a) : Since the charge is moving in a circle or along an equipotential surface, therefore work done will be zero.

48. (b) : Extension of spring = x, tension on spring = T and spring constant = k. Now extension of spring $x = \frac{T}{k}$ and energy stored by the spring

$$E = \frac{1}{2} \times kx^2 = \frac{1}{2} \times k \times \left(\frac{T}{k}\right)^2 = \frac{1}{2} \times k \times \frac{T^2}{k^2} = \frac{T^2}{2k}.$$

49. (a) : Given : Initial temperature $(T_1) = 7°C = 280K$; Final temperature $(T_2) = 287°C = 560$ K. The Stefan's law states that radiated energy $E \propto T^4$

or $\frac{E_1}{E_2} = \left(\frac{T_1}{T_2}\right)^4 = \left(\frac{280}{560}\right)^4 = \left(\frac{1}{2}\right)^4 = \frac{1}{16}$

or $E_2 = 16\,E_1$.

50. (d) : Acceleration due to gravity at a depth h from the earth's surface

$$g' = g\left(1 - \frac{h}{R}\right) = g\left(1 - \frac{R}{R}\right) = g(1-1) = 0.$$

51. (a) : In an insulator, the valance band is completely filled and the conduction band is completely empty. There is no charge carriers at all in the conduction band. Moreover as the energy gap $Eg >> KT$, where T is the room temperature, so no electron can jump from the valance band to the conduction band at low temperatures and even at higher temperatures.

conduction band

$Eg >> KT$

valance band

52. (c)

53. (a) :

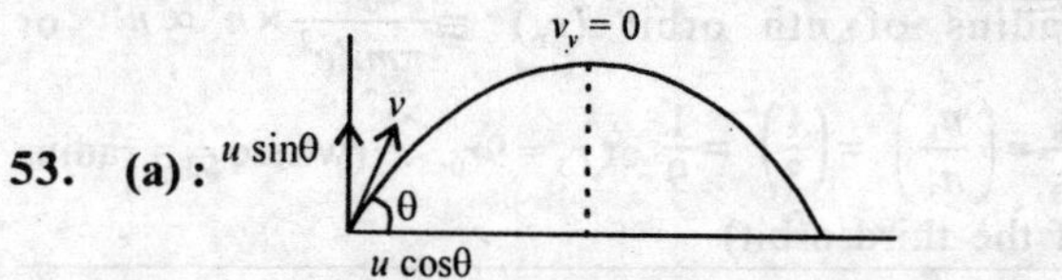

At the topmost point vertical component of velocity = 0

Let time taken to reach the topmost point = T, then

$v_y = 0 = u \sin\theta - gT$

$\Rightarrow T = \frac{u \sin\theta}{g}$

$\therefore$ Total time of flight $= 2T = \frac{2u \sin\theta}{g}$

$\therefore$ Range, $R = u \cos\theta \times \frac{2u \sin\theta}{g} = \frac{u^2 \sin 2\theta}{g}$

$\therefore$ For R to be maximum, $\sin 2\theta = 1$

$\Rightarrow 2\theta = 90° \Rightarrow \theta = 45°$

54. (b) : Sound waves are longitudinal in nature and light waves are transverse in character. Moreover light wave is electromagnetic in nature. That's why light waves do not need a material medium for its propagation.

55. (a)

56. (a) : In both the cases of the cycle and the car, it is the centripetal acceleration towards the centre which provides the necessary frictional force in a turning so that there is no skidding. In the case of the cyclist, as the centre of gravity of the system (cycle + cyclist) goes through the cyclist, the whole, system leans towards the centre of the arc. But in case of the car, the centre of gravity does not pass through a person sitting in the car. That's why due to inertia, that person leans outwards.

57. (c) : As both the electron and the proton enters the electric field with equal energies, the electron will finally traverse a more curved path than the proton as the electron is lighter than the proton, because of which the acceleration of the electron will be much more than that of the proton.

+

$\frac{1}{2}mv^2$ e p

–

58. (d) : If the ice cap of the poles melts, ice will flow towards the equator, and will increase the moment of inertia of the earth thereby decreasing its frequency of rotation. Due to decrease of the frequency of rotation, the day length increases.

59. (a) : The energy gap between the valance and the conduction band is very small, so by raising the temperature we can get more electrons flipping from valance to conduction bond thereby increasing the carriers of electricity in the semiconductors. That's why in semiconductors we have negative temperature coefficient of resistance and so the resistance decreases with temperature.

60. (a) : As the free falling body has an acceleration

equal to 'g', the effective acceleration due to gravity for the pendulum is $g_{eff} = 0$

$\therefore$ Time period $T = 2\pi\sqrt{\frac{l}{g_{eff}}} = \infty$.

CHEMISTRY

61. **(d)** : According to Heisenberg's uncertainity principle,

$\Delta x \times \Delta v = \frac{h}{4\pi}$

Δx = uncertainity in position

Δv = uncertainity in velocity

h = Planck's constant (6.63×10^{-34} Js)

62. **(d)** : $CH_3COOH \xrightarrow{NaOH/CaO} CH_4 + Na_2CO_3$

When sodium salt of carboxylic acids are heated with (NaOH + CaO), alkane is obtained with one less carbon atom than the acid, and the process is called decarboxylation.

63. **(d)** : Magnalium : 95% Al, 5% Mg. It is used in the construction of airships, balance and pistons of motor engine.

Duralumin : 95% Al, 4% Cu, 0.5% Mg, 0.5% Mn. It is used in aeroplanes and automobile parts.

64. **(b)** : If Principle quantum number (n) is 2,

orbitals possible = $2s, 2p_x, 2p_y, 2p_z$

total = 4 (*i.e.* $n^2 = 4$)

If $n = 3$,

Orbitals possible, one s, three p-orbitals and fine d-orbitals total = 9 (*i.e.* $n^2 = 9$)

65. **(d)** : pH = $-\log [H^+]$

$\Rightarrow 2 = -\log [H^+]_1$, and $6 = -\log [H^+]_2$

$\Rightarrow \frac{\log[H^+]_1}{\log[H^+]_2} = \frac{10^{-2}}{10^{-6}} = 10^4 = 10{,}000$

Therefore, acidity is more in pH=2 than pH=6 by an order of 10,000.

66. **(b)** : As, $\frac{P^0 - P}{P^0} = \frac{\frac{w}{m}}{\frac{w}{m} + \frac{W}{M}}$

P^0 = vap. pressure of pure component

P = vap. pressure in solution

w = mass of solute, m = mol. wt. of solute

W = mass of solvent, M = mol. wt. of solvent

$\Rightarrow \frac{121.8 - 120.2}{121.8} = \frac{\frac{15}{m}}{\frac{250}{78}}$

$\Rightarrow m = 356.7$ g

67. **(c)** : Yellow colour is due to the formation of CrO_4^{2-} ion.

$Cr(OH)_3 + NaOH + Na_2O_2 \rightarrow Na_2CrO_4 + 2H_2O$

68. **(a)** : According to Bronsted theory, acid is a substance that can release protons while base are those that accept protons.

69. **(c)** : Lithium aluminium hydride is a strong reducing agent. ($LiAlH_4$)

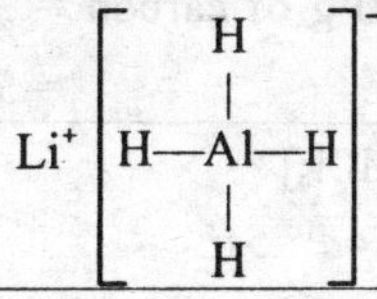

$$Li^+\left[\begin{array}{c} H \\ | \\ H-Al-H \\ | \\ H \end{array}\right]^-$$

70. **(b)** : $C_6H_5COCl \xrightarrow[(H)]{Pd/BaSO_4} C_6H_5CHO$

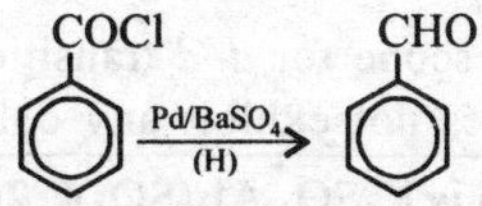

This reaction is called Rosenmund reaction.

71. **(c)** : H_2S is the group reagent for II and IV group of basic radicals (cations). So with $COCl_2$ (no metal here), no metallic sulphide will be produced.

72. **(d)** : As there is no lone pair on boron in BCl_3, therefore no repulsion takes place. But there is a lone pair on nitrogen in NCl_3. Therefore repulsion takes place. Thus BCl_3 is planar molecule but NCl_3 is pyramidal molecule.

73. **(a)** : Conformers are obtained by rotating molecules around σ–bonds between C-atoms.

e.g. $CH_3 - CH_2 - CH_2 - CH_3$

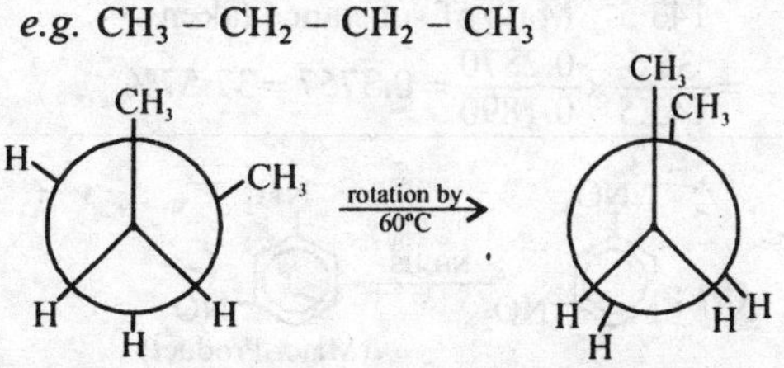

CH₃, H, CH₃, H, H, H — rotation by 60°C → CH₃, CH₃, H, H, H, H

Gauche conformer Eclipsed conformer

74. **(d)** : Nylon–66 is prepared from monomers, adipic acid and hexamethylene diamine by condensation process.

$H_2N - (CH_2)_6 - NH_2 + HOOC - (CH_2)_6 - COOH \rightarrow$

$$\left[NH - (CH_2)_6 - NH - CO - (CH_2)_6 - CO \right]_n$$

Nylon–66

75. **(a)** : $H_2(g) + I_2(g) \rightarrow 2HI(g)$

Δn = no. of product speices – no. of reactant species

$= 2 - (1 + 1) = 0$

As $\Delta H = \Delta E + \Delta n\, RT$

$\Rightarrow \Delta H = \Delta E + 0 \times RT \quad \Rightarrow \Delta H = \Delta E$

76. (a) : 1 carat = 200 mg

0.5 carat = 100 mg

1 mole of C-atoms weight = 12 g

$\Rightarrow$ 12 g of carbon = 6.023×10^{23} C-atoms

$$\Rightarrow \quad 100 \text{ g of carbon} = \frac{6.023\times10^{23}\times100}{12\times1000} = 5.02\times10^{21}$$

77. (b) : $Na_2[CdCl_4]$

Cd : $4d^{10}\,5s^2$

Cd^{2+} : $4d^{10}$

As there is no scope for *d–d* transition in Cd^{2+} ion, therefore, it does not exhibit any colour.

78. (b) : Potash alum is $K_2SO_4.Al_2(SO_4)_3.\ 24H_2O$. It is used for disinfectant purposes.

79. (b) : Aromatic compounds are characterised by their unusual stability, delocalisation of π–electrons in a planar ring. They undergo substitution reactions more favourably than addition reaction these properties are not present in cyclohexane.

80. (c) : Given : Mass of the compound = 0.189 g and mass of AgCl = 0.287 g. Equivalent weight of chlorine is 35.5 and equivalent weight of AgCl is 143.5. Therefore percentage of chlorine

$$= \frac{35.5}{143.5}\times\frac{\text{Mass of AgCl formed}}{\text{Mass of substance taken}}$$

$$= \frac{35.5}{143.5}\times\frac{0.2870}{0.1890} = 0.3757 = 37.57\%.$$

81. (b) : m-dinitrobenzene ($C_6H_4(NO_2)_2$) $\xrightarrow[\Delta]{\overset{\oplus}{N}H_4\overset{\ominus}{HS}}$ m-nitroaniline (NH_2, NO_2)
(Major Product)

82. (c) : $R-CH_2-CH_2OH \xrightarrow{PBr_3} R-CH_2CH_2Br \xrightarrow{KCN}$

$R-CH_2CH_2CN \xrightarrow[H_2O]{H^+} R-CH_2CH_2-COOH$

This is called upgradation reaction.

83. (c) : Glycerine is

1 CH_2OH
|
2 CHOH
|
3 CH_2OH

1 and 3 C-atoms are primary.
2 is secondary C-atom.

84. (a) : $Q = It$

$= 5 \times 200 = 1000$ coulombs

Charge carried by 1 electron $= 1.6\times10^{-19}$C.

$$\Rightarrow \text{No. of electrons for 1000 C} = \frac{1000}{1.6\times10^{-19}} = 6.241\times10^{21}$$

85. (c) : All the alcohols are water soluble due to the formation of extensive Hydrogen bonding between water molecules and alcohol molecules. Lower alcohols are highly soluble in water and their solubility decreases with an increase in the molecular weight.

86. (d) : Steam distillation is employed as there is a large difference between boiling points of ortho and para-nitrophenols. This is due to the presence of intra molecular H-bonding in the case of o-nitrophenol (so low b.p.) and intermolecular H-bonding in p-nitrophenol (so high b.p.)

87. (a) : Radioactive substances usually emit α-rays ($_2^4$He numbers), β-ray (electrons) or γ-rays or sometimes positrons ($_1^0\beta$).

88. (c) : Copper and zinc are the components of brass.

89. (d) : $CaC_2 + 2H_2O \rightarrow Ca(OH)_2 + C_2H_2$

mol. wt. → 64 g

$\Rightarrow$ 64 g $CaC_2 \equiv$ 26 g C_2H_2

$$\Rightarrow \quad 64100 \text{ g } CaC_2 \equiv \frac{26}{64}\times 64100 \text{ g } C_2H_2$$

$\equiv 26040.625$ g C_2H_2

$\equiv 26.04$ Kg C_2H_2

$C_2H_2 + H_2 \longrightarrow C_2H_4$

Mol. wt. 26 g 28 g

$\Rightarrow$ 26 g $C_2H_2 \equiv$ 28 g C_2H_4

$$\Rightarrow \quad 26.04 \text{ Kg } C_2H_2 \equiv \frac{28}{26}\times 26.04 \text{ Kg } C_2H_4$$

$\equiv 28.04$ Kg C_2H_4

$nC_2H_4 \rightarrow (CH_2–CH_2)_n$

Therefore, amount of polythene obtained is 28.04Kg.

90. (a) : According to Charles' and Boyle's Law,

$$\frac{P_1V_1}{T_1} = \frac{P_2V_2}{T_2}$$

$$\Rightarrow \frac{620\times300}{300} = \frac{640\times V_2}{320}$$

$\Rightarrow V_2 = 310$ cc

91. **(b) :** $2Cu^{2+} + 2I^- \rightarrow Cu_2I_2 + I_2 \uparrow$

$2S_2O_3^{2-} + I_2 \rightarrow S_4O_6^{2-} + 2I^-$
(thiosulphate)

Iodometric titration involves the evolution of iodine immediately before adding thiosulphate solution.

92. **(a) :** I^- ion can act as Lewis base *i.e.* it can donate electron pair to some species *e.g.* I_2. The electron donor species are termed as Lewis base.

$I^- + I_2 \rightarrow I_3$

93. **(c) :** Enthalpy change (ΔH) is a state function so it does not depend on the path taken by the reaction, It depend only on the difference of final and initial values of enthalpy change.

94. **(a) :** $NH_3 + 3Cl_2 \rightarrow NCl_3 + 3HCl$.

NCl_3 is an explosive material.

95. **(d) :**

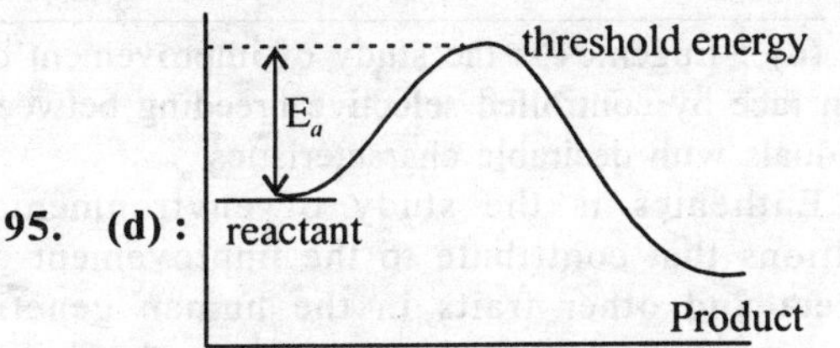

E_a = Activation energy

96. **(b) :** $R - NH_2 + HO - NO \longrightarrow R - OH + N_2 + H_2O$
(HO – NO: Nitrous acid)

97. **(a) :** $BaCl_2\,(0.5M) + H_2SO_4\,(1M) \rightarrow BaSO_4\downarrow + 2HCl$

As Ba^{2+} ion concentration is only 0.5M, therefore only 0.5M of $BaSO_4$ can be precipitated.

98. **(c) :** α, ω-Dihalides when treated with sodium or zinc form cyclo-alkanes. Reaction is called Freund reaction.

$$CH_2\begin{matrix} \diagup CH_2-Br \\ \diagdown CH_2-Br \end{matrix} + Zn \xrightarrow{NaI} CH_2\begin{matrix} \diagup CH_2 \\ \diagdown CH_2 \end{matrix} \text{ or } \triangle$$

Cyclo propane

99. **(d) :** Charge = Current × time

$= 9.95 \times 10 \times 60$

$= 5970\ C$

$\therefore$ 5970 C deposites 3 g of metal

$\Rightarrow$ 96500 C will deposite $= \frac{3}{5970} \times 96500$ g metal

$= 48.49$ g metal

Therefore equivalent weight is 48.49 g

100. **(d) :** Potassium diclromate : $K_2Cr_2O_7$

Let the Oxidation state of Cr be x

$\Rightarrow \quad 2 \times (+1) + 2x + 7 \times (-2) = 0$

$\Rightarrow \quad x = +6.$

101. **(a) :** compressibility factor is defined as :

$$Z = \frac{PV}{(PV)ideal} = \frac{PV}{nRT}$$

for non ideal gases, $Z \neq 1$
for ideal gases, $Z = 1$

102. **(b) :** Molality is not effected by temperature as molality is not involved with volume (volume changes with temperature).

$$\text{Molality} = \frac{\text{moles of solute}}{\text{Weight of solvent (Kg)}}$$

103. **(c) :** $NaNO_3 + AgCl \rightarrow AgNO_3 + NaCl$

$NH_4OH + AgCl \rightarrow Ag(NH_3)_2Cl + 2H_2O$

$Na_2S_2O_3 + AgCl \rightarrow Ag_2S_2O_3 + 2NaCl$

104. **(d) :** Cl, OH and NH_2 groups are all o/p directing while COOH group is a srong *m*-directing agent (due to its electron withdrawing effect).

105. **(a) :** de Broglie proposed the relation :

$\lambda = \frac{h}{mv}$ $\quad \lambda$ = wavelength

mv = momentum of particle.

106. **(d) :** Equilibrium constant

$$\frac{[C_2H_6]}{[C_2H_4][H_2]} = \frac{\text{mole.litre}^{-1}}{(\text{mole.litre}^{-1}).(\text{mole.litre}^{-1})}$$

$$= \frac{1}{\text{mole.litre}^{-1}} = \frac{\text{litre}}{\text{mole}}$$

107. **(d) :** $CH_3 - CH_2 - C \equiv CH \xrightarrow[\text{KMnO}_4]{\text{Cold alkaline}}$

$CH_3 - CH_2 - COOH + HCOOH$

108. **(c) :** Neon : $1s^2, 2s^2, 2p^6$

Excited state of Neon can be represented as :

$1s^2, 2s^2, 2p^5, 3s^1$

109. **(b) :** Visible spectrum ranges from 4000Å to 7000Å.

110. **(d) :** $S + 3/2\ O_2 \longrightarrow SO_3 + 2x$ kcal

$SO_3 \longrightarrow SO_2 + 1/2\ O_2 \longrightarrow SO_3 + y$ kcal

$\therefore$ Heat of formation of SO_2 in equal to $2x - y$ kcal.

111. **(d) :** The bond angle of PBr_3 is lesser than PH_3 but the bond angle of NBr_3 is greater than NH_3.

Size of Br is larger than hydrogen.

112. **(a) :** NaOH is a strong electrolyte and decomposes fully in solution into its ions.

$NaOH \rightarrow Na^+ + OH^-$

Due to high availability of OH^- ions, both strong acids HNO_3 and HCl are neutralised with equal ease. So equal heat of neutralisation for both.

113. **(b) :** Gibbs free energy (ΔG) is given by :

$\Delta G = \Delta H - T\Delta S$

In chemical systems, the reaction moves in a direction in which there is decrease in free energy *i.e.* $\Delta G = -ve$.

Also, decrease in free energy is a measure of the maximum useful work that can be obtained from a reaction. But the reacton can be exotheremic or endothermic *e.g.* water evaporation is endothermic but it is a spontaneous process (*i.e.* $\Delta G = -ve$)

114. **(b) :** Liquid ammonia is used in refrigeration on account of its large heat of evaporation.

115. **(c) :** Tungsten is a transistor element and is very hard due to high metallic bonding.

Tungsten (*W*); Z = 74; $5d^5\ 6s^1$

116. **(a) :** Hydrogen (Z = 1); $1s^1$

This single electron can be expected to go in higher energy levels and when de-excited it gives out different spectral lines *e.g.* Balmer, paschen, etc.

117. **(d) :** Be (Z = 4); $1s^2, 2s^2$

B (Z = 5); $1s^2, 2s^2, 2p^1$

Ionisation potential of Be is greater than that of B as first electron released from Be is from *s*-orbital while it is from *p*-orbital in B.

118. **(a) :** NO_3^- : N → $2s^2$ [⇅] $2p^3$ [↿|↿|↿]   [O ← N (–O)(=O)]

Hybridisation is sp^2 here and therefore planar structure is expected.

$NH_3 : 1s^2, 2s^2, 2p^3$

Hybridisation is sp^3, therefore tetrahedral structure is expected but there is pyramical structure as lone pair of electron occupy one of the corners of tetrahedral.

N (lone pair), H H H

119. **(b) :** Due to the absence of unpaired electron in NO^+ and N_2, both are diamagnetic

$[:N = O]^+$; $:N \equiv N:$

total no. of e^- in NO = 6 + 8 = 14

total no. of e^- in N_2 = 7 + 7 = 14

Therefore, both are isoelectronic.

120. **(a) :** The large sized sulphate anion (SO_4^{2-}) is stabilised better by a large sized cation. So the stability of sulphates down the group, increases. In other words lattice energy is more down the group.

BIOLOGY

121. **(a) :** NO is physiologically ubiquitous as a potent vasodilator. It is produced and rceycled in the respiratory tract to regulate the air way. NO has much higher affinity for haemoglobin than CO_2 and O_2. It has no direct reaction with O_2. Thus it does not impede O_2 transport.

122. **(d) :** Eugenics is the study of improvement of human race by controlled selective breeding between individuals with desirable characteristics.

Euthenics is the study of environmental conditions that contribute to the improvement of intellect and other traits in the human genetic engineering. Obstetrics is the science connected with care of women before, during and after childbirth.

123. **(a) :** As a result of nucleic acid digestion, nitrogenous organic bases-purines (adenine and guanine) and pyrimidines (cytosine, thymine and uracil) are absorbed from intestine into the blood. Most of these are excreted out. In man, purines are changed to uric acid for excretion.

124. **(b) :** Positron Emission Tomographic Scanning (PET) is computerised imaging technique. It gives quantitative information on the metabolic and physiological process of tissue and organs.

125. **(c) :** Phenylketonuria and Alkaptonuria both are inborn errors (congenital) of metabolism. Phenylketonuria is due to accumulation of phenylpyruvic acid and causes mental disorders. Alkaptonuria is the lack of ability to breakdown homogentisic acid into acetoacetic acid. Due to accumulation of homogentisic acid, the urine of patients suffering from this disease turns black as soon as it comes in contact with air.

126. **(d)**

127. **(c)** Growth curve is the graphic representation of the total growth against time. If total growth (of

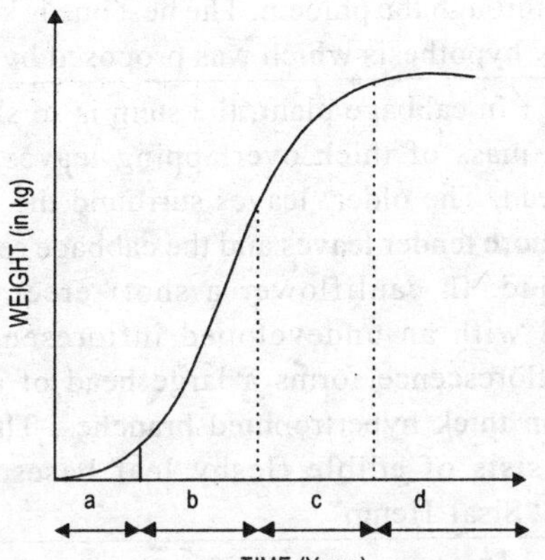

A typical sigmoid growth curve for higher animals including man. (a) Lag phase; (b) log phase; (c) phase of diminishing growth; (d) steady phase.

an organism or population) against time is drawn an S - shaped or sigmoid curve is obtained. It consists of four parts - lag phase, log phase (exponential phase), phase of diminishing growth and stationary phase (steady growth for organs or organisms of indefinite growth). Growth is slow in the lag phase, rapid during log or exponential phase, slow again during the phase of diminishing growth.

128. (d) : Prolactin is a lactogenic hormone produced by the anterior lobe of pituitary gland. It stimulates milk production in cow.

129. (c) Diphtheria is an acute infectious disease caused by *Corynebacterium diphtheriae* and its toxin. If primarily affect the membrane of the nose, throat or larynx and marked by formation of a gray - white pseudomembrane, with fever, pain and in the laryngeal form, aphonia and respiratory obstruction. Tuberculosis is caused by *Mycobacterium tuberculae* and marked by formation of tubercles and causes necrosis in tissue of any organ. Tetanus is an acute, often fatal disease marked by tonic muscular spasm and hyper-reflexia, resulting in lockjaw, generalized muscle spasm, opisthotonus and seizures. It is caused by the neurotoxin. Pertussis is whooping cough.

130. (b) : Ora serrata is a part of third wall of retina of eye. It is composed of neural tissue containing the receptor cells. The posterior part of the retina which ends at the ciliary body along an irregular line is termed as *ora serrata.*

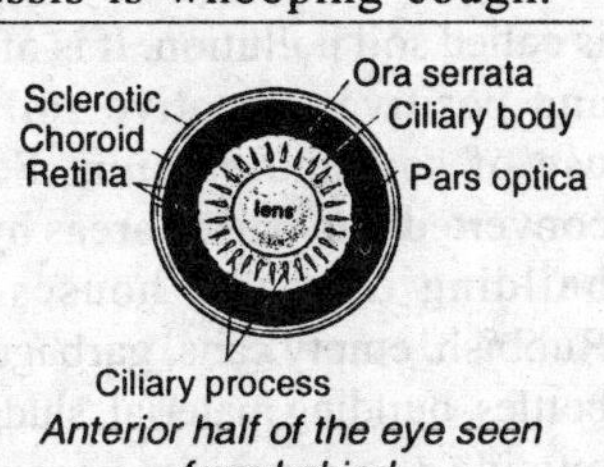

Anterior half of the eye seen from behind.

131. (c) : Colour - blindness is a sex linked disease which is linked to X - chromosome. Cretinism is arrested physical and mental development with dystrophy of bones and soft tissues, due to congenital lack of thyroid secretion. Night - blindness is caused by deficiency of vitamin A. Anaemia is caused due to iron deficiency.

132. (b) : Chloragogen cells (yellow cells) of earthworm are star-shaped, small sized cells storing food. They also help in exertion. Thus it is analogous to liver of higher vertebrates.

133. (c) : Colostrum is maternal milk of mammal formed during the first few days after the birth. It is particularly rich in proteins, including antibodies.

134. (c) Klinefelter's syndrome is characterized by trisomy (XXY). These are male individuals, who are phenotypically fairly normal but have a very low sperm count and, are therefore sterile. As the syndrome has two X chromosomes, one barr body is seen in this case.

135. (d) : The preparation of sperm before penetration of ovum is called capacitation. During this time coating substances of the sperm, especially acrosome is removed and the sperm becomes ready to receive the signal from ovulated egg. After this penetration occurs.

136. (b) : Plasmin is the proteolytic enzyme found in plasma which can digest many proteins through the process of hydrolysis. Plasmin (also known as fibrinolysin) is the active component of fibrinolytic system. This enzyme lyses fibrin and fibrinogen degrading products. Plasmin is formed by its active precursor plasminogen.

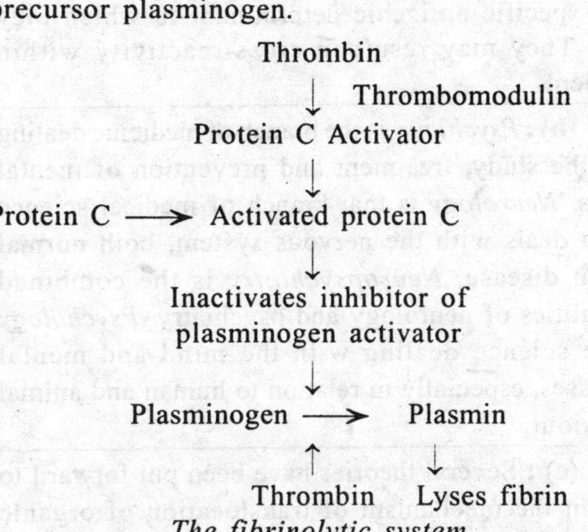

The fibrinolytic system

137. (b)

138. (b) : Juvenile hormone is secreted by corpora allata, a retrocerebral complex present in insect brain. Chemically it is an unsaponifiable, nonsterolic lipid. This hormone regulates morphogenesis and so promotes metamorphosis, *i.e.* development of the larva into adult through pupal stage.

139. (b) : Flight feathers of wings of birds are termed as pinions or remiges of quills wing. They are present at the base of quill or flight feathers.

140. (c) : Metamorphosis in frog is regulated by thyroid activity. During metamorphosis changes occur in heart, lung and intestine, but the nervous system remains the same after metamorphosis. It undergoes least changes however, brain acquires its normal shape and size during metamorphosis.

141. (b) : 1.34 ml of oxygen is present in one gram of haemoglobin *i.e.* each gram of haemoglobin can combine maximally with 1.34 ml of O_2; normally, there are 12–15 gm haemoglobin per dl of blood.

142. (c) : Otoconium are minute particles, composed chiefly of calcium carbonate, found in otolithic membrane on surface of maculae of inner ear.

143. (c) : Any persistent fear of a specific stimulus or object or situation is called phobia. Fear due to pain is called algophobia. Pathophobia is phobia or fear of contracting sexually transmitted disease. Myaphobia is a paradigm created from the misuse of fitness language that translates into a fear of muscle. Haematophobia is fear of blood.

144. (c) : Antiserum contains antibodies. The term antiserum is applied to materials prepared in animals. Antiserum is a serum containing antibodies with affinity for a specific antigenic determinant to which they bind. They may result in cross-reactivity within recipient.

145. (b) : *Psychiatry* is the branch of medicine dealing with the study, treatment and prevention of mental illness. *Neurology* is that branch of medical science which deals with the nervous system, both normal and in disease. *Neuropsychiatry* is the combined specialities of neurology and psychiatry. *Psychology* is the science dealing with the mind and mental processes, especially in relation to human and animal behaviour.

146. (c) : Several theories have been put forward to explain the mechanism of translocation of organic nutrients through the phloem. The best one is known as mass flow hypothesis which was proposed by Munch.

147. (a) : In cabbage plant, the stem is so short that the great mass of thick overlapping leaves tend to form a head. The older leaves surround the younger smaller, more tender leaves and the cabbage resembles a huge bud. In cauliflower a short erect stem is produced with an undeveloped infloresence. The whole inflorescence forms a large head of abortive flowers on thick hypertrophied branches. The onion bulb consists of edible fleshy leaf bases. Agave provides "Sisal Hemp".

148. (a) : It is an example of test cross. Test cross is a cross to know whether an individual is homozygous or heterozygous for the dominant character. When double heterozygote(for eg. TtRr) crossed with double recessive (ttrr), the ratio will be 1:1:1:1.

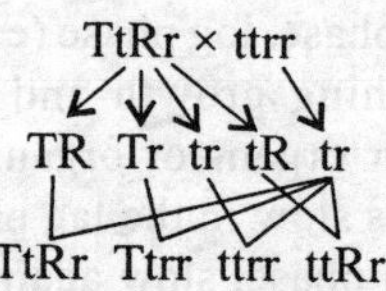

149. (a) : The upper surface of leaf blade or lamina of "Sundew" bears a number (100 - 200) of club - shaped hair or tentacles. Their tips are swollen, glandular and reddish. The glandular heads of the tentacles secrete a thick sticky juice which shines in the sun like dew drops.An insect which happens to touch the head of the tentacle is stuck by its juice. *Aldrovanda* bears whorls of specialised leaves with broad - winged petioles, two lobed winged lamina bearing curved marginal teeth, a number of sensitive trigger hair and colourless digestive glands. The upper surface of each lamina lobe in *Dionaea* contains 3 sensitive spines and a number of red coloured digestive glands.

150 (a) : Unfavourable reiteration of soil by addition or removal of substances and factors which decrease soil productivity, quality of plants and ground water is called soil pollution. It is of two main types : negative and positive. Negative soil pollution includes over use of soil and erosion. Fertile land is also being converted into barren areas by unplanned urbanisation, building of roads, houses or industrial complex. Rubbish, empty cans, garbage, broken furniture, empty bottles, building material, sludge, ash, etc. are all dumped outside the town on vacant lands which not only become barren but also make the nearby lands so.

Positive pollution is a polluction casued by (i) pesticides, herbicides and fumigants (ii) chemical fertilizers and (iii) air pollutants washed down from atmosphere through rain. Excessive use of chemical fertilizers causes soil deterioration through the decrease in natural bacterial population and destruction of crumb structure. The salt content of the soil is also bound to increase with continuous use of fertilizers. Addition of industrial wastes come under positive pollution.

151. (d) : Perisperm is persisting nucellus in the seeds.

152. (b) : Chapparal is a broad - leaved evergreen shrub forest of hard and thick - leaved small trees and shrubs which usually contain resin but are resistant to fires. Both plants and animals are adapted to long droughts. Steppes are grasslands of Eurasia. Temperate deciduous forest has dominant climax vegetation consisting of broad - leaved hardwood trees like Oak, Elm, Maple, Birch, Beech, Hickory, Magnolias, etc. Tropical deciduous forest is dominated by trees, e.g. *Dalbergia, Bombax, Butea, Shorea,* etc.

153. (a) : The primitive atmosphere contained gases like CO_2, CO, N, H_2, etc. Water vapour and metallic carbides reacted to form the first organic compound, methane (CH_4). It is suggested that simple one called organisms somewhat similar to today's cyanobacteria (blue green algae) were present on earth about 3600 million years ago. With the addition of oxygen into the atmosphere, methane and ammonia began to disappear as they got oxidised forming CO_2 and N_2 respectively. The reaction of oxidaton of CH_4 is.

$$CH_4 + 2O_2 \rightarrow CO_2 + 2H_2O$$

154. (d) : The genes involved in quantitative inheritance is called polygenic gene or polygenes. Quantitative inheritance is a type of inheritance controlled by one or more genes in which the dominant allele expressing a part or unit of the trait, the full trait being shown only when all the dominant alleles are present. The gene having a multiple phenotypic effect because of its ability to control expression of a number of characters is called pleiotropic gene.

155. (c) : *Gambusia* feeds on the larva of *Anopheles* mosquitoes. *Anopheles* is the carrier of malarial parasite, *Plasmodium*. Thus, *Gambusia,* is used to control *Anopheles* population and hence, malaria.

156. (b) : Plants that utilize primarily RuBP to fix CO_2, which results in the formation of the three - carbon compound (3 - PGA), are called C_3 plants. Hatch and Slack proposed a new pathway of CO_2 fixation *via* the carboxylation of Phosphoenol Pyruvate (PEP). Because the products are four carbon compounds (oxaloacetic, malic and aspartic acids), plants exhibiting this pathway are referred as C_4 plants. Ribulose diphosphate is the first acceptor of CO_2 in C_3 plants and phosphoenol pyruvate is the first acceptor of CO_2 in C_4 plants. In C_3 plants fixation of one molecule of CO_2 uses 3 ATP and 2 NADPH, whereas in C_4 plants fixation of one molecule of CO_2 uses 5 ATP and 2 NADPH.

157. (c) : In xerophytic plants, stems are flattened (e.g. *Opuntia, Muhlenbeckia*) or cylindrical *(e.g. Euphorbia royleana, E. tirucalli*). Green stems of unlimited growth in such plants have taken over the function of photosynthesis. True leaves are caducous. Formation of phylloclades helps the plant to grow in dry habitats because transpiration is little from the stem.

158. (c) : Biosphere or living mantle is the habitable part of earth and its atmosphere which is composed of both biotic and abiotic components. Biosphere has three subdivisions:-

(i) *Lithosphere* - It is the solid or dry crust of the earth that forms the continents and other land masses.

(ii) *Hydrosphere* - It is the liquid mantle of the earth present in oceans, seas, lakes, ponds, rivers, ground etc.

(iii) *Atmosphere* - It is the gaseous mantle that envelopes the biosphere and overlies both lithosphere as well as hydrosphere.

159. (a), (d) : The red and blue biliproteins, called phycoerythrins and phycocyanins, respectively, are found in algae. They both are called phycobilins. The phycobilins are active in the transfer of light energy to chlorophyll for utilization in the process of photosynthesis. The phycocyanins and phycoerythrins effectively absorb light over range of wavelengths that cannot be absorbed by chlorophyll. Thus, they prevents chlorophyll from long and direct illumination and also from its photo oxidation.

160. (b) : In the sporophyte of *Dryopteris*, the sporangia are usually grouped together in sori. In sporangia each spore mother cell finally undergoes the reduction division (meiosis) to form four haploid spores. Spores under favourable conditions germinate to gametophyte (prothallus). Prothallus is haploid.

161. (b) : When fossil fuels are burnt, S and N are oxidized and there is a build - up in the atmospheric CO_2 and the oxides of S and N, which lead to acid - base interaction. The acidity of the rain water is mainly caused by H_2SO_4 and NHO_3.

162. (b) : Autoradiography is the study of fate of labelled precursors and intermediate metabolites by knowing the movement of radioactivity with the help of photographic films and emulsions at short intervals. Tritiated hydrogen (^3H) and carbon - labelled (^{14}C) compounds of thymidine, uridine and amino acids are used to study synthesis of DNA, RNA and proteins respectively. Cellular fractionation is rupturing cells, separation and suspension of cell constituents. Phase contrast microscope is useful in observing components of living cells and their processes. Tissue culture is a technique of growing cells, tissue and other structures on artificial medium under controlled aseptic conditions inside special containers.

163. (c) : The common wheat is hexaploid with $2n = 42$ and is derived from three diploid species : (i) AA = *Triticum aegilopoides* (2n = 14), (ii) BB = *Aegilops spelloides* ($2n$ = 14), (iii) DD = *Aegilops squarrosa*. The hexaploid wheat therefore, is designated as AABBDD, the tetraploid (2n = 28) as AABB and diploid ($2n$ = 14) as DD.

164. (a) : It is as dihybrid cross.

Ccpp × ccPp

The genotype of colourless flowers will be ccpp.

We know that Ccpp × ccPp

Male gametes are Cpcp

Female gemetes are cPcp

Hence, ratio =

1(colour) : 3 (white)

i.e. 25% coloured flower.

	Cp	cp
cP	CcPp colour	cPcp white
cp	Cpcp white	cpcp white

165. (b)

166. (b) : A species may include sexually as well as apomictically (asexually) reproducing individuals. Fragmentation is vegetative means of reproduction in lower plants. Self - fertilization is the case in which fusion occurs between male and female gametes from same individual.

167. (d) : After M - phase (mitotic phase) a cell may either enter interphase or G_o phase. G_o phase is the stage when cell cycle is arrested. Therefore, further divisions stop.

168. (b) : The gene which inhibits or suppresses the expression of a nonallelic gene is known as epistatic gene. Epistasis reduces the number of phenotypes appearing in the F_2 generation of dihybrid cross. Thus instead of normal 9:3:3:1 dihybrid ratio, epistasis may result in a ratio of 9:3:4 (recessive epistasis), 12:3:1 (dominant epistasis), 13:3 (dominant recessive epistasis) or 9:7 (double recessive epistasis) etc.

169. (d) : All characters of options (a, b and c) are similar to family solanaceae. Gynoecium of Solanaceae is obliquely placed. Ovary becomes 2 - celled or sometimes 4 - celled owing to the development of a false septum. Ovary is superior.

170. (c) : Phytoalexins are non - specific fungitoxic substances, generally phenolic in nature, synthesized *de novo* or in greatly increased concentraton by plants in response to infection by fungi. Phytotron is building in which plants can be grown on a large scale in a range of rigidly controlled conditions of light, temperature of air and soil, humidity and composition of air, water and nutrient content of soil etc. Phytotoxins are toxic substances produced by plants,e.g. Azadirachtin, Rotenones, Aflatoxin, etc. Phytol is a hydrocarbon.

171. (d) : Absorbed alcohol is carried directly to the liver, where it becomes the preferred fuel. Use of moderate amounts of alcohol does not cause liver damage, provided adequate nutrition is maintained.The liver becomes enlarged, yellow, greasy and firm. Hepatocytes are distended by large fat globules which push the hepatocyte nucleus against the cell membrane. Accumulation of fat in the liver of the alcoholic person results from the combination of impaired fatty acid oxidation, increased uptake and esterification of fatty acids to form triglycerides (fats) and diminished lipoprotein biosynthesis and secrection, it means there is increase in the fat synthesis in the liver.

172. (d) : Ovaries secrete steroid hormones or female sex hormones like estrogen and progesterone which are mainly responsible for the controlling of total menstrual cycle. Ovariectomy means total removal of ovary from the body. Thus no hormones would be secreted from ovary and menstrual cycle may be stopped.

173. (b) : Cold blooded animals have no fat layer. The skin of cold-blooded animal is devoid of any fat layer because temperature regulation-the important function of fat layer, is not necessary here. But fat bodies are present in front of each testis. They are reserves of nourishment and cold-blooded animals may use them in hibernation.

174. (b) : In morula stage, the cells divide without any increase in size and becomes a solid mass of cells. Zona pellucida remains undivided till cleavage is complete. After damage it breaks down and morula formation starts.

175. (a) : The ascending limb of Henle's loop is impermeable to water so no water is reabsorbed with solutes (it is known as diluting segment). Due to which nephric filtrate become hypotonic in ascending limb. On the other side, descending limb is not permeable to Na^+ and other solutes. But it is very permeable to water, making more water absorption from the solution, thus, the filtrate becomes hypertonic to plasma.

176. (b) : There are no stomata in the epidermal layer of the leaves of submerged water plant. If at all present, they are nonfunctional. The leaf epidermis either lacks cuticle or it is feebly developed, thus permittng easy absorption of salts dissolved in water and gaseous exchange. Similarly the thin cuticle and epidermis of submerged organs presumbly allow free passage of dissolved organs and CO_2, there is evidence that all epidermal cells are not equally permeable to dissolved salts.

177. (a) : Cutinization involves the transformation of cellulose or pectic substances of the primary or secondary wall into cutin, which forms a continuous layer, called the cuticle. It generally forms the skin or outermost covering of the stem, leaves and some fruits. It is impermeable to water and pathogens.

178. (b) : There are three codons UAA, UAG and UGA which are designated as termination codons. UAA (also known as ochre), UAG (also known as *amber*) and UGA (also known as opal) are three codons whcih whenever present in mRNA, would bring about termination of polypeptide chain which would then be released from ribosome. *m* - RNA has a "termination codon" region which consists of UAA, UAG or UGA.

179. (d) : Plasmids are small, circular, double - stranded, self - replicating additional or extra chromosomal DNA elements which are commonaly found in bacteria (prokaryote).

180. (d) The plants where the usual sexual reproduction has been completely replaced by a type of asexual reproduction are called apomictic,and phenomenon is apomixis. Apomixis offers the possibility of indefinite multipliction of specially favourable biotypes without any variation due to segregation or recombination.

GENERAL KNOWLEDGE

181. (b)

182. (b) : There are seven tombs built by Quatab Shahi near the Golkunda fort, which are situated in Hyderabad.

183. (c)

184. (a) : Hippocrates (460-370 B.C) was a Greek-physician, dedicated to the cause of medical science. He is known as the father of medicine. Rules of conduct for doctors are based on Hippocratic Oath.

185. (a)

186. (d) : Comets are the long tails stars. Halley's comet is the most famous comet which is seen after every 76 years. Last time, it was seen in 1986. Therefore it will be seen next in 2062.

187. (b)

188. (a) : Deep-Blue is a computerized chess system having very high speed and very large memory. Recently this system defeated the world champion of chess.

189. (a)

190. (d) : As Dachigam Sanctuary in Kashmir is popular for hangul or Kashmir stag.

191. (b)

192. (a) : Saeed Anwar, a left handed opening batsman of Pakistan, who scored 194 runs against India in Chennai in May 1997. He has the highest score in a one day cricket match.

193. (c)

194. (d) : Olympic Games were not played in the years 1916, 1940 and 1944 due to world-war.

195. (a)

196. (b) : The first and the ninth Asian Games were held in March 1951 (New Delhi) and in 1982 (New Delhi) respectively.

197. (c)

198. (d) : The Principality of Liechtenstein is situated between Switzerland and Austria.

199. (d)

200. (d) : 'Future Shock' is a science fiction which was written by Alwyn Toffler.

❖ ❖ ❖

SOLVED PAPER
AIIMS - 1998

Time : 3½ Hours Max. Marks : 200

PHYSICS

1. If the equation for the displacement of a particle moving on a circular path is given by $(\theta) = 2t^3 + 0.5$ where θ is in radians and t in seconds, then the angular velocity of the particleat $t = 2$sec, is
(a) 24 rad/sec (b) 12 rad/sec
(c) 8 rad/sec (d) 36 rad/sec

2. A body is projected at such an angle that the horizontal range is three times the greatest height. The angle of projection, is
(a) 42°8′ (b) 33°7′
(c) 25°8′ (d) 53°8′

3. The dimensions of angular velocity, is
(a) $[M^0L^0T^{-1}]$ (b) $M^2L^0T^{-1}]$
(c) $[MLT^{-2}]$ (d) $[ML^2T^{-2}]$

4. If the water falls from a dam into a turbine wheel 19.6 m below then the velocity of water at the turbine, is (Take g = 9.8 m/s²)
(a) 39.2 m/s (b) 19.6 m/s
(c) 9.8 m/s (d) 98.0 m/s

5. A bullet is fired from a rifle. If the rifle recoils freely, then the kinetic energy of the rifle, is
(a) same as that of the bullet
(b) more than that of the bullet
(c) less than that of the bullet
(d) equal or less than that of the bullet

6. In an elliptically polarised light, the amplitude of the vibrations
(a) remains constant
(b) changes in direction only
(c) changes in magnitude only
(d) both (b) and (c)

7. The astronomical telescope consists of objective and eye-piece. The focal length of the objective, is
(a) shorter than that of the eye-piece
(b) greater than that of the eye-piece
(c) equal to that of the eye-piece
(d) five times shorter than that of the eye-piece

8. When hydrogen atom is in its first excited level, its radius, is
(a) twice (b) half
(c) same (d) four times

9. If a simple pendulum oscillates with an amplitude of 50 mm and time period of 2 sec, then its maximum velocity, is
(a) 0.8 m/s (b) 0.15 m/s
(c) 0.10 m/s (d) 0.16 m/s

10. What is the current (I) in the circuit, as shown in figure
(a) 1.2 A
(b) 0.5 A
(c) 1 A
(d) 2 A

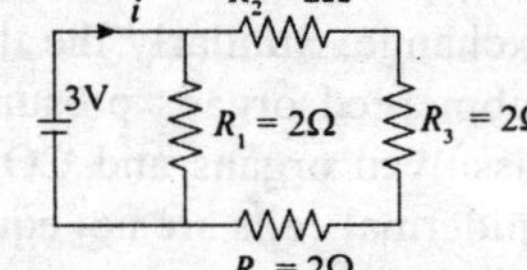

11. Which of the following is not dependent on the intensity of incident radiation in a photo-electric experiment?
(a) stopping potential
(b) amount of photoelectric current
(c) work function of the surface
(d) maximum kinetic energy of photoelectrons

12. What is the area of the plates of a 3 F parallel plate capacitor, if the separation between the plates is 5 mm?
(a) 9.281×10^9 m² (b) 4.529×10^9 m²
(c) 1.694×10^9 m² (d) 12.981×10^9 m²

13. A spring 40 mm long is stretched by the application of a force. If 10 N force required to stretch the spring through 1 mm, then work done in stretching the spring through 40 mm, is
(a) 23 J (b) 68 J
(c) 84 J (d) 8 J

14. The waves in which the particles of the medium vibrate in a direction perpendicular to the direction of wave motion is known as

(a) propagated waves (b) longitudinal waves
(c) transverse wave (d) none of these

15. A sample of gas expands from volume V_1 to V_2. The amount of work done by the gas is greatest, when the expansion, is
(a) adiabatic (b) isobaric
(c) isothermal (d) equal in all cases

16. According to Maxwell's hypothesis, a changing electric field gives rise to
(a) magnetic field (b) electric current
(c) an e.m.f. (d) pressure radiant

17. If the radioactive decay constant of radium is 1.07×10^{-4} per year, then its half-life period is approximately equal to
(a) 6476 years (b) 7000 years
(c) 8900 years (d) 2520 years

18. If the kinetic energy of a body becomes four times of its initial value, then new momentum will
(a) become four times, its initial value
(b) become three times, its initial value
(c) become twice its initial value
(d) ramains constant

19. A quanity of heat required to change the unit mass of a solid substance, from solid state to liquid state, while the temperature remains constant, is known as
(a) hoar frost (b) sublimation
(c) latent heat (d) latent heat of fusion

20. Domain formation is the necessary feature of
(a) ferromagnetism (b) paramagnetism
(c) diamagnetism (d) all of these

21. A body of mass 5 kg is moving in a circle of radius 1 m with an angular velocity of 2 radian/sec. The centripetal force, is
(a) 30 N (b) 20 N
(c) 10 N (d) 40 N

22. The absolute zero is the temperature at which
(a) molecular motion ceases
(b) all substances exist in solid state
(c) water freezes (d) none of these

23. The best material for the core of a transformer, is
(a) hard steel (b) mild steel
(c) stainless steel (d) soft iron

24. Standing waves are produced in 10 m long stretched string. If the string vibrates in 5 segments and wave velocity is 20m/s, its frequency is
(a) 5 Hz (b) 4 Hz
(c) 2 Hz (d) 10 Hz

25. The kinetic energy of an electron, which is accelerated in the potential difference of 100 V, is
(a) 416.6 cal (b) 1.6×10^4 J
(c) 1.6×10^{-17} J (d) 6.636 cal

26. Newton's formula for the velocity of sound in gases, is
(a) $v = \sqrt{\frac{2p}{\rho}}$ (b) $v = \sqrt{\frac{p}{\rho}}$
(c) $v = \sqrt{\frac{\rho}{p}}$ (d) $v = \frac{3}{2}\sqrt{\frac{p}{\rho}}$

27. Light appears to travel in a straight line, because
(a) its wavelength is very small
(b) it is not absorbed by surrounding
(c) its velocity is very large
(d) it is reflected by surrounding

28. Gravitational mass is proportional to gravitational
(a) intensity (b) force
(c) field (d) all of these

29. If the period of oscillation of mass (M) suspended from a spring is 2 sec, then the period of mass 4 M will be
(a) $3T$ (b) $2T$
(c) T (d) $4T$

30. The number of waves, contained in unit length of the medium, is called
(a) wave pulse (b) wave number
(c) elastic wave
(d) electromagnetic wave

31. Longitudinal strain is possible in
(a) gases (b) liquids
(c) solids (d) all of these

32. A Centigrade and a Fahrenheit thermometer are dipped in boiling water. The water temperature is lowered until the Fahrenheit thermometer registers 140°. The fall in temperature as registered by the Centigrade thermometer will be
(a) 60° (b) 40°
(c) 30° (d) 80°

33. Electroplating does not help in
(a) metals to become hard
(b) shining appearance
(c) fine finish to be surface
(d) protect metal againt corrosion

34. What is the relative humidity on a day, when partial pressure of water vapour is 0.012×10^5 Pa and temperature is 12°C? The vapour pressure of water at this temperature is 0.016×10^5Pa
(a) 68% (b) 52%
(c) 25% (d) 75%

35. Heat travels through vaccum by
(a) radiation (b) convection
(c) conduction (d) both (a) and (b)

36. Rocket engines lift a rocket from the earth surface, because hot gases with high velocity
(a) react against the rocket and push it up
(b) push against the air
(c) push against the earth
(d) heat up the air which lifts the rocket

37. A person using a lens as a simple microscope sees an
(a) upright virtual image
(b) inverted real magnified image
(c) inverted virtual image
(d) upright real magnified image

38. 'Mirage' is a phenomenone due to
(a) total internal reflection of light
(b) refraction of light
(c) reflection of light (d) diffraction of light

39. The rate of diffusion, is
(a) equal in solids, liquids and gases
(b) faster in liquids than in solids and gases
(c) faster in solids than in liquids and gasas
(d) faster in gases than liquids and solids

40. A transformer works on the principle of
(a) mutual induction (b) invertor
(c) convertor (d) self-induction

41. If a person with a spring balance and a body hanging from it goes up and up in an aeroplane, then the reading of the weight of the body as indicated by the spring balance, will
(a) first increase and then decrease
(b) go on decreasing
(c) go on increasing
(d) remain the same

42. On a cold morning, a metal surface will feel colder to touch than a wooden surfaces, because
(a) metal has low specific heat
(b) metal has high thermal conductivity
(c) metal has high specific heat
(d) metal has low thermal conductivity

43. Woollen clothes keep the body warm, because wool
(a) decreases the temperature
(b) increases the temperature of body
(c) is a bad conductor
(d) all of these

44. 'Stem corrections' in platinum resistance thermometres are eliminated by the use of
(a) compensating leads
(b) electrodes (c) cells
(d) none of these

45. Lines of force, due to earth's horizontal magnetic field, are
(a) concentric circles (b) curved lines
(c) elliptical (d) parallel & straight

46. If the luminous intensity of a unidirectional bulb is 100 candela, then total luminous flux emitted from the bulb, is
(a) 1256 lumen (b) 986 lumen
(c) 861 lumen (d) 1561 lumen

47. If the metal bob of a simple pendulum is replaced by a wooden bob, then its time period will
(a) remain the same (b) decrease
(c) increase (d) first (b) then (c)

48. The rain drops are spherical in shape due to
(a) thrust on drop (b) surface tension
(c) viscosity (d) residual pressure

49. A body can be negatively charged by
(a) giving some protons to it
(b) removing some electrons from it
(c) giving excess of electrons to it
(d) removing some neutrons from it

50. Electric potential of earth is taken to be zero, because earth is a good
(a) semi-conductor (b) conductor
(c) insulator (d) dielectric

Directions for Q. 51 to 60: *These questions consist of two statements each, printed as Assertion and Reason. While answering these questions you are required to* *choose any one of the following four responses.*

(a) It both Assertion and Reason are true and the Reason is a correct explanation of the Assertion.

(b) If both Assertion and Reason are true but Reason is not a correct explanation of the Assertion.

(c) If Assertion is true but the Reason is false

(d) If both Assertion and Reason are flase.

51. Assertion: A pulsar is a source of radiowaves that vary in intensity at regular intervals.
Reason: A pulsar is a rotating neutron star.

52. *Assertion:* A laser beam of 0.2 W can drill holes through a metal sheet whereas a 1000 W torch-light cannot.
Reason: The frequency of laser light in much higher than that of torch light.

53. *Assertion:* A body can have acceleration even if its velocity is zero at a given instant of time.
Reason: A body is momentarily at rest when it reverses its direction of motion.

54. *Assertion:* Virtual images are always erect.
Reason: Virtual images are formed by diverging lenses only.

55. *Assertion:* The ratio C_p/C_v for a diatomic gas is more than that for a monotomic gas.
Reason: The molecules of a monotomic gas have more degree of freedom than those of a diatomic gas.

56. *Assertion:* In series LCR circuit, the resonance is equal and opposite to the capacitive reactance.
Reason: At resonance the inductive reactance is equal and opposite to the capacitive reactance

57. Assertion: Radio waves can be polarised.
Reason: Sound waves in air are longitudinal in nature.

58. *Assertion:* In series LCR circuit, the resonance occurs at one frequency only.
Reason: At resonance the inductive reactance is equal and opposite to the capacitive reactance.

59. *Assertion:* Newton's rings are formed in the reflected system. When the space between the lens and the glass plate is filled with a liquid of refractive index greater than that of glass, the central spot of the pattern is bright.
Reason: This is because the reflections in these cases will be from a denser to a rarer medium and the two interfering rays are reflected under similar conditions.

60. *Assertion:* Corpuscular theory fails in explaining the velocities of light in air and water.
Reason: According to corpuscular theory, light should travel faster in denser media than in rarer media.

CHEMISTRY

61. Which of the following information can be obtained on the basis of Le Chatelier's principle?
(a) equilibrum constant of a chemical reaction
(b) dissociation constant of a weak acid
(c) entropy change in a reaction
(d) shift in equilibrium position on changing value of a constant

62. Which of the following is the most electropositive element?
(a) phosphorus (b) magnesium
(c) aluminium (d) sulphur

63. Which of the following explains the sequence of filling the electrons in different shells?
(a) Aufbau principle (b) Octate rule
(c) Hund's rule (d) all of these

64. The oxidation numbers of hydrogen in KH, MgH_2 and NaH are respectively
(a) + 2, + 1 and – 2 (b) + 1, + 1 and + 1
(c) – 1, – 1 and – 1 (d) – 2, – 3 and – 1

65. Which of the following does not show hydrogen bondin;
(a) N_2O (b) H_2O
(c) H_2S (d) Fe_3O_4

66. In the gas equation: PV = nRT
(a) V is the volume of one mole of the gas
(b) n no. of moles of the gas have volume V
(c) n is the number of molecules of the gas
(d) P is the pressure of one mole of the gas

67. A first order reaction, which is 30% complete in 30 minutes has a half-life period of
(a) 102.2 min (b) 58.2 min
(c) 24.2 min (d) 120.2 min

68. The physical adsorption of gases on the solid surface is due to
(a) van der Waals forces
(b) covalent bonding
(c) hydrogen bonding

(d) all of these

69. Which of the following salt has the same value of Vant's Hoff factor as that of $K_3[Fe(CN)_6]$?
(a) Na_2SO_4 (b) $Al(NO_3)_3$
(c) $Al_2(SO_4)_3$ (d) Fe_3O_4

70. Which of the following substances is used, in the laboratory, for fast drying of neutral gases?
(a) sodium sulphate
(b) phosphorus pentoxide
(c) sodium phosphate
(d) anhydrous calcium chloride

71. The equivalent weight of an acid is equal to
(a) molecular weight/basicity
(b) melecular weight × basicity
(c) molecular weight × acidity
(d) molecular weight/acidity

72. When the hybridization state of carbon atom changes from sp^3, sp^2 and sp, the angle between the hybridized orbitals
(a) decreases considerably
(b) increase progressively
(c) decreases gradually
(d) all of these

73. The most reactive compound, for the electrophilic nitration, is
(a) benzoic acid (b) nitrobenzene
(c) benzene (d) toluene

74. Hess' law is applicable for the determination of heat of
(a) transition (b) formation
(c) reaction (d) all of these

75. Which of the following has been universally accepted as a reference electrode at all temperatures and has been assigned a value of zero volt?
(a) platinum electrode
(b) copper electrode
(c) graphite electrode
(d) standard hydrogen electrode

76. The purification of alumina is called
(a) Baeyer's process (b) Bosch process
(c) Castuer process (d) Hoop's process

77. The boiling point of water (100°C) becomes 100.52°C, if 3 grams of a non-volatile solute is dissolved in 200 ml of water. The moleular weight of solute is (if K_b for water is = 0.6 K/m)
(a) 17.3 $g.mol^{-1}$ (b) 15.4 $g.mol^{-1}$
(c) 12.2 $g.mol^{-1}$ (d) 20.4 $g.mol^{-1}$

78. The product obtained when acetic acid is treated with phosphorus trichloride, is
(a) $CH_3-\overset{O}{\overset{||}{C}}-Cl$ (b) $CH_3-\overset{O}{\overset{||}{C}}-OCl$
(c) $CH_3-\overset{O}{\overset{||}{C}}-O-PCl_2$
(d) $CH_3-CH_2-\overset{O}{\overset{||}{C}}-OH$.

79. Which of the following is the main cause of late discovery of neutron?
(a) neutron in nucleus moves very fast
(b) neutron is highly unstable particle
(c) neutron is chargeless particle
(d) all of these

80. Which one of the following is used to make 'non-stick' cookware?
(a) poly-ethylene
(b) polytetrafluoroethylene
(c) polystyrene
(d) none of these

81. The reaction: benzene + methyl halide $\xrightarrow{\text{Anhy.AlCl}_3}$ Toluence, is known as
(a) Perkin's reaction (b) Wurtz reaction
(c) Kolbe's reaction (d) Friedel craft reaction

82. Ratio of the energy of a photon wavelengths 3000 Å and 6000 Å is
(a) 1 : 3 (b) 1 : 2
(c) 2 : 1 (d) 1 : 6

83. If a compound, on analysis was found to contain C = 18.5%, H = 1.55%, Cl = 55.04% and O = 24.81%, then its empirical formula is
(a) C_2H_2OCl (b) CH_2ClO
(c) CHClO (d) $ClCH_2O$

84. What is the oxidation number of sulphur in $Na_2S_4O_6$?
(a) $\frac{3}{5}$ (b) $\frac{3}{2}$
(c) $\frac{2}{5}$ (d) $\frac{5}{2}$

85. Nitrosoamines ($R_2N-N=O$) are soluble in water.

On heating them with concentrated H_2SO_4, they give secondary amines. This reaction is called
(a) Sandmeyer's reaction
(b) Fittig's reaction
(c) Perkin reaction
(d) Liebermann nitroso reaction

86. Acetamide is treated separately with the following reagent. Which one of these would give methylamine?
(a) Br_2 + NaOH (b) NaOH + Br_2
(c) KOH + Br_2 (d) none of these

87. The ionic product of water at 25°C is 10^{-14}. Its ionic product at 90°C will be
(a) 1×10^{-14} (b) 1×10^{-12}
(c) 1×10^{-20} (d) 1×10^{-16}

88. Ethanol and dimethyl ether form a pair of functional isomers. The boiling point of ethanol is higher than that of dimethyl ether, due to the presence of
(a) CH_3-group in ethanol
(b) H-bonding in dimethyl ether
(c) H-bonding in ethanol
(d) CH_3-group in dimethyl ether

89. The IUPAC name of the compound

$$CH_3—\underset{\displaystyle OH}{\underset{|}{C}H} = CH—CH_2—COOH$$

(a) 4-hydroxy-4-pentenoic acid
(b) 4-hydroxy-3-pentenoic acid
(c) hydroxy pentenoic acid
(d) 4-hydroxy-4-methyl-3-ene-pentanoic acid

90. Baeyer's reagent is used in the laboratory for
(a) detection of glucose
(b) reduction process
(c) oxidation process
(d) detection of double bond

91. The functional group, which is found in amino acid, is
(a) – CH_3 group (b) – NH_2 group
(c) – COOH group
(d) both (b) and (c)

92. Principal quantum number of an atom is related to the
(a) orbital angular momentum
(b) spin angular momentum
(c) size of the orbital
(d) orientation of the orbital in space

93. A certain current liberated 0.504 g of hydrogen in 2 hours. How many grams of copper can be liberated by the same current flowing for the same time in copper sulphate solution
(a) 31.8 g (b) 16.0 g
(c) 12.7 g (d) 63.5 g

94. The solubility of $BaSO_4$, in water, is 2.33×10^{-3} gram/litre. Its solubility product will be (molecular weight of $BaSO_4$ = 233)
(a) 1×10^{-15} (b) 1×10^{-10}
(c) 1×10^{-5} (d) 1×10^{-20}

95. The reaction of primary amine with chloroform and ethanolic KOH, is called
(a) Reimer-Tiemann reaction
(b) Kolbe's reaction
(c) carbylamine reaction
(d) none of these

96. The rate constant of a reaction is 0.69×10^{-2} min^{-1} and the initial concentration is 0.2 mol L^{-1}. The half-life period is
(a) 800 sec (b) 600 sec
(c) 400 sec (d) 6024 sec

97. One gram mole of a gas at N.T.P. occupies 22.4 litres. This fact was derived from
(a) law of gaseous volumes
(b) Dalton's atomic theory
(c) Avogadro's hypothesis
(d) law of constant proportions

98. An acyl halide is formed when PCl_5 reacts with
(a) amide (b) alcohol
(c) acid (d) ester

99. In the reaction: $4\,Fe + 3\,O_2 \rightleftharpoons 4\,Fe^{3+} + 6\,O_2^{2-}$ which of the following statement is incorrect?
(a) metallic iron is a reducing agent
(b) Fe^{3+} is an oxidising agent
(c) it is a redox reaction
(d) metallic iron is reduced to Fe^{3+}

100. If enthalpies of formation for $C_2H_{4\,(g)}$, $CO_{2\,(g)}$ and $H_2O_{\,(l)}$ at 25°C and 1 atm pressure are 52, – 394 and – 286 kJ/mol respectively, then enthalpy of combustion of $C_2H_{4\,(g)}$ will be
(a) – 141.2 kJ/mol (b) + 14.2 kJ/mol
(c) + 141.2 kJ/mol (d) – 1412 kJ/mol

101. A compound with empirical formula CH_2O has a vapour density of 30. Its molecular formula is
(a) $C_3H_6O_3$ (b) $C_2H_4O_2$

(c) $C_2H_2O_2$ (d) $C_6H_{12}O_6$

102. An equilibrium mixture of the reaction $2H_2S_{(g)} \rightleftharpoons 2H_{2(g)} + S_{2(g)}$, had 0.5 mole H_2S, 0.10 mole H_2 and 0.4 mole S_2 in one litre vessel. The value of equilibrium constant (K) in mole litre^{-1} is

(a) 0.016 (b) 0.008
(c) 0.004 (d) 0.160

103. Which of the following compounds is 2-bromotoluene?

(a) 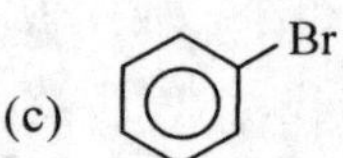 (b) CH_2Br

(c) Br (d) Br, Br

104. At what pressure will a quantity of gas, which occupies 100 ml at a pressure of 720 mm, occupy a volume of 84 ml

(a) 820.20 mm (b) 784.15 mm
(c) 736.18 mm (d) 857.14 mm

105. Which of the following elements are analogous to the lanthanides?

(a) carbides (b) borides
(c) actinides (d) hydrides

106. In an endothermic reaction, the value of change in enthalpy (ΔH) is

(a) zero (b) negative
(c) positive (d) either (b) or (c)

107. Which one of the following shows maximum paramagnetic character?

(a) $[Fe(CN)_6]^{3-}$ (b) $[Fe(CN)_6]^{4-}$
(c) $[Cr(H_2O)_6]^{3+}$ (d) $[Cu(H_2O)_6]^{2+}$

108. The specific conductance of a N/10 KCl at 25°C is 0.0112 ohm^{-1} cm^{-1}. The resistance of cell containing solution at the same temperature was found to be 55 ohms. The cell constant will be

(a) 6.16 cm^{-1} (b) 0.616 cm^{-1}
(c) 0.0616 cm^{-1} (d) 616 cm^{-1}

109. Plank's constant has the same dimension as that of

(a) radiant energy (b) work
(c) power
(d) angular momentum

110. Which of the following is the most stable alkene?

(a) $RCH_2 = CH_2R$ (b) $RCH = CHR$
(c) $R_2C = CR_2$ (d) $CH_2 = CH_2$

Directions for Q. 111 to 120: *These questions consist of two statements each, printed as Assertion and Reason. While answering these questions you are required to choose any one of the following four responses.*

(a) It both Assertion and Reason are true and the Reason is a correct explanation of the Assertion.
(b) If both Assertion and Reason are true but Reason is not a correct explanation of the Assertion.
(c) If Assertion is true but the Reason is false.
(d) If both Assertion and Reason is false.

111. *Assertion:* The energy of an electron is largely determined by its principal quantum number.
Reason: The principal quantum number (n) is a measure of the most probable distance of finding the electrons around the nucleus.

112. *Assertion:* The of a gas does not change, when it undergoes an adiabatic expansion.
Reason: During an adiabatic process, the container should be a perfect conductor.

113. *Assertion:* The 19th electron in potassium atom enters into the 4s-orbital and not into the 3d-orbital.
Reason: (n + 1) rule is followed for determining the orbitals of the lowest energy state

114. *Assertion:* For an ideal gas, at constant temperature, the product of the pressure and volume is a constant.
Reason: The mean square velocity of the molecules is inversely proportional to mass.

115. *Assertion:* Heat energy is completely transformed into work during the isothermal expansion of a gas.
Reason: During an isothermal process, the changes in internal energy of a gas due to decrease in pressure is nullified by the changes due to increase in volume.

116. *Assertion:* Both chlorine and sulphur dioxide act as bleaching agents.
Reason: Chlorine bleaches by vigorous exidation, while sulphur dioxide bleaches by mild reduction.

117. *Assertion:* A solution of sucrose in water is dextro-rotatory. But on hydrolysis in the presence of a little hydrocholoric acid, it becomes laevorotatory.
Reason: Sucrose on hydrolysis gives unequal

amounts of glucose and fructose. As a result of this, change in sign of rotation is observed.

118. *Assertion*: Di-nitrogen in chemically unreactive at ordinary temperature and is very stable.
Reason: The bond dissociation energy is 946 kJ mol^{-1}

119. *Assertion:* Bond order in a molecule, which can assume any value positive or negative, integral or fractional including zero.
Reason: Bond order depends on the number of electrons in the bonding and antibonding orbitals

120. *Assertion:* Alkali metals impart colour to the flame.
Reason: Their ionisation energies are low.

BIOLOGY

121. Photorespiration, usually occurs in
(a) one-cell organelles only
(b) two-cell organelles
(c) three-cell organelles
(d) four-cell organelles.

122. In *Selaginella*, reduction division occurs during the formation of
(a) sperms (b) microspores only
(c) megaspores only (d) both (b) and (c).

123. The term chromatophore was coined by
(a) Schmitz (b) Comparethi
(c) W. Pfeiffer
(d) Singer and Nicholsan

124. The sphere of living matter together with water, air and soil on the surface of earth is called
(a) atmosphere (b) hydrosphere
(c) lithosphere (d) biosphere.

125. Which type of cancer is found in lymph nodes and spleen?
(a) carcinoma (b) sarcoma
(c) leukaemia (d) lymphoma.

126. Which of the following terms is not concerned with genetic recombination in bacteria?
(a) Transformation (b) Transduction
(c) Translation (d) Conjugation.

127. The process of the escape of liquid from the tip of uninjured leaf is called
(a) guttation (b) transpiration
(c) evaporation (d) evapo-transpiration

128. Moderate rainfall during summer produces
(a) desert (b) grasslands
(c) scrub forests (d) deciduous forests.

129. Phenomenon of Industrial melanism demonstrates
(a) natural selection (b) induced mutation
(c) geographical isolation
(d) reproductive isolation.

130. When the gametophyte is not formed by spores but by any other part of sporophyte, it is known as
(a) multispory (b) polyspory
(c) apospory (d) germination.

131. Middle piece of a mammalian sperm contains
(a) nucleus (b) centriole
(c) mitochondria (d) vacuole.

132. The black pigment in the eye, which reduces the internal reflection, is located in
(a) retina (b) iris
(c) sclerotic (d) cornea.

133. The placenta of human beings belong to the category of
(a) haemo-chorialis (b) syndesmo-chorialis
(c) endothelio-chorialis
(d) epithelio-chorialis.

134. Antiserum contain
(a) anitgens (b) leucocytes
(c) antibodies (d) none of these.

135. A mature ligule, having a prominent basal portion, is called
(a) trichocyst (b) heterocyst
(c) rhizophore (d) Glossopodium.

136. Pollination by snail and slug is known as
(a) ornithophilous (b) chiropterophilous
(c) entomophilous (d) malacophilous.

137. Which of the following RNAs picks up specific amino acid from amino acid pool in the cytoplasm to ribosome during protein synthesis?
(a) t-RNA (b) m-RNA
(c) r-RNA (d) all of these.

138. Primitive types of stomata are found in the
(a) apophysis of capsule
(b) leaves of moss plants
(c) axes of the moss plant
(d) all of these.

139. Single filament of Nostoc without mucilage sheath is known as
(a) mycelium (b) colony
(c) trichome (d) hyphae.

140. Secretion of which of the following is under neurosecretory nerve axons?
(a) Pineal (b) Adrenal cortex
(c) Anterior pituitary (d) Posterior pituitary.

141. Sensation of stomach pain is due to
(a) interoceptors (b) exteroceptors
(c) proprioceptors (d) teloreceptors.

142. Addison's disease results from
(a) hyposecretion of adrenal
(b) hypertrophy of gonads
(c) hyperactivity of cells of Leydig
(d) none of these.

143. Galapagos islands are associated with the name of
(a) Wallace (b) Malthus
(c) Darwin (d) Lamarck.

144. Pacinian corpuscles occur in the skin of certain parts of body in mammals. These are
(a) type of glands (b) pain receptors
(c) naked tactile receptors
(d) encapsulated pressure receptors.

145. Which of the following disease is due to an allergic reaction?
(a) Goitre (b) Enteric fever
(c) Skin cancer (d) Hay fever.

146. Sympathetic nerves in mammals arise from
(a) sacral-region (b) cervical region
(c) thoraco-lumbar region
(d) 3rd, 7th, 9th and 10th cranial nerves.

147. In nucleoplasm, a conspicuous body of spherical shape attached to a particular chromosome on a definite position is called
(a) plasmid (b) karyolymph
(c) nucleolus (d) nuclear reticulum.

148. Which of the follwing is dissolved in water for making Bordeaux mixture?
(a) calcium chloride (b) copper sulphate
(c) sodium chloride (d) none of these.

149. A plant cell has potential to develop into full plant. This property of the plant cell is called
(a) tissue culture (b) totipotency
(c) pleuripotency (d) gene cloning.

150. The relationship in an ecosystem can be depicted in
(a) pyramid of energy
(b) pyramid of biomass
(c) pyramid of numbers
(d) all of these.

151. The proper scientific name of cellobiose is
(a) 4-O-β-D-glucopyranosyl-D-α-glucopyranose
(b) 8-O-β-D-glucopyranosyl-D-glucose
(c) $4NH_2SO_4$-β-D-reductase
(d) $6NH_2PO_4$-α-D-reductase.

152. The plant material, which is widely used in the preparation of culture medium, is
(a) *Cycas revoluta* (b) *Cocos nucifera*
(c) *Pinus longifolia* (d) *Borassus flabellifer*.

153. The chief function of pholem is the conduction of
(a) food (b) mineral
(c) water (d) air.

154. Phytotron is a device by which
(a) mutations are produced in plants
(b) plants are grown in controlled environment
(c) protons are liberated
(d) leaf fall occurs on abscission layer.

155. Which of the following is nongenetic, and is utilised for protein synthesis?
(a) *t*-RNA (b) Z-RNA
(c) *m*-RNA (d) none of these.

156. Which of the following is not correctly matched?
(a) Root knot disease–*Meloidogyne javanica*
(b) Smut of bajra–*Tolysporium penicillariae*
(c) Covered smut of barley–*Ustilago nuda*
(d) Late blight of potato–*Phytophthora infestans*.

157. Passive immunity is defined as immunity
(a) inherited from the parents
(b) achieved through vaccination
(c) acquired through first exposure to the disease
(d) achieved through the sera of other animals enriched in anitbodies.

158. The structure, which remains unchanged during metamorphosis of frog's tadpole, is
(a) lung (b) heart
(c) intestine (d) nervous system.

159. Cells of deiter occur in
(a) utriculus (b) retina of eyes
(c) organ of corti (d) sebaceous glands.

160. The cells named podocytes occur in
(a) glomerulus of kidney
(b) wall of capillaries
(c) neck region of nephrons
(d) large intestine.

161. Malathion, parathion and fenitrothion belong to group of
(a) triazines (b) carbamates
(c) pyretheroids (d) organophosphate.

162. Immidiately after ovulation, the mammalian egg is covered by a membrane known as
(a) chorion (b) zona pellucida
(c) corona radiata (d) vitelline membrane.

163. Treatment with 'Alloxan' destroys
(a) STH cells
(b) β-cells of islets of Langerhans
(c) cells of Sertoli (d) cells of Leydig.

164. Distance between two linked genes upon a chromosome is measured in cross over units, is
(a) ratio of crossing over between them
(b) cross-over value
(c) number of other genes between them
(d) none of these.

165. The genes, which are confined to differential region of Y-chromosome only, are called
(a) mutant (b) autosomal
(c) holandric (d) sex-linked.

166. Eggs having yolk in their centre of cytoplasm in peripheral layer, are called
(a) isolecithal (b) microlecithal
(c) centrolecithal (d) telolecithal.

167. Arbor vitae is composed of
(a) grey matter (b) neuroglial cells
(c) white matter (d) both (a) and (c).

168. Termination of gastrulation is marked by
(a) obliteration of archenteron
(b) closure of neural tube
(c) obliteration of blastocoel
(d) closure of blastocoel.

169. Mechanism of uric acid excretion in a nephron, is
(a) osmosis (b) diffusion
(c) secretion (d) ultrafiltration.

170. Most primitive living mammals, which provide an evidence of organic evolution from geographical distribution are found in
(a) China (b) India
(c) Australia (d) Africa.

Directions: *These questions consist of two statements each, printed as Assertion and Reason. While answering these questions you are required to choose any one of the following four responses.*

(a) If both Assertion and Reason are true and the Reason is a correct explanation of the Assertion.
(b) If both Assertion and Reason are true, but Reason is not a correct explanation of the Assertion.
(c) If Assertion is true, but the Reason is false.
(d) If Assertion is false and Reason is true.

171. *Assertion* : Transmission of the nerve impulse across a synapse is accomplished by neurotransmitters.
Reason : Transmission across a synapse usually requires neuro-transmitters because there is small space. i.e., synaptic cleft, that separates one neuron from another.

172. *Assertion* : All terrestrial mammals are air breathers.
Reason : Because of terrestrial habitat, they have well-developed lungs for air breathing.

173. *Assertion* : There is no chance of transmission of malaria to man on the bite of a male *Anopheles* mosquito.
Reason : It carries a non-virulent strain of *Plasmodium*.

174. *Assertion* : Thiamin deficiency results in beri-beri causing paralysis.
Reason : People eating raw fish may also suffer from paralysis due to the dificiency of vitamin B_1. Cooked fish has no such effect.

175. *Assertion* : Minerals are not part of biologically active substances.
Reason : Some individuals suffer anaemia due to the deficiency of iron.

176. *Assertion* : Winged bean is widely cultivated throughout India.
Reason : The protein content in the seeds of winged bean is low.

177. *Assertion* : Meiotic division results in the production of four dissimilar cells.
Reason : Synapses occurs during zygotene of meiosis.

178. *Assertion* : Auxillary buds, in actively growing herbaceous plants generally remain dormant.
Reason : This is due to apical dominance which is under the influence of auxins.

179. *Assertion* : Lysosomes help in the process of photorespiration.
Reason : Lysosomes have acidic enzymes.

180. *Assertion* : Endomycorrhiza of forest trees contribute to the efficient nutrient cycling in tropical forest ecosystems.

Reason : The fungi that form endomycorrhizal associations with plants store nutrient ions and make them available to the host plants.

GENERAL KNOWLEDGE

181. The simon-commission came in which of the following year?
(a) 1939 (b) 1927
(c) 1942 (d) 1932.

182. At present, the total membership of Lok Sabha is
(a) 527 (b) 552
(c) 521 (d) 545.

183. 'JAVA' is a
(a) American intelligence agency
(b) name of tribes, who lives in the interior part of Orissa
(c) computer programming language
(d) none of these.

184. National Housing Bank is a subsidiary of
(a) I.C.I.C.I. (b) S.B.I.
(c) R.B.I. (d) I.D.B.I.

185. 'Frank Worrell' was associated with which of the following sport?
(a) cricket (b) hockey
(c) swimming (d) football.

186. What is Nikkie?
(a) a private firm situated in Japan
(b) currency of Korea
(c) index of share prices in Tokyo stock exchange
(d) rate of interest of fered by Bank of Tokyo.

187. The largest airport in the word in situated in
(a) Saudi Arabia (b) USSR
(c) Denmark (d) USA.

188. Swami Vivekanand was born in which of the following year?
(a) 1897 (b) 1863
(c) 1902 (d) 1892.

189. The Commonwealth games of 1998 were hosted by
(a) England (b) Singapore
(c) Australia (d) Malaysia.

190. Which of the following state, becomes the 22nd state of Indian Union ?
(a) Meghalaya (b) Sikkim
(c) Arunachal Pradesh (d) Tripura.

191. 'Sambalpur' is situated on the bank in which of the following river?
(a) Sarya (b) Jamuna
(c) Mahanadi (d) Saráswati.

192. The dynasty of Bahadur Shah (II) Jafar was in
(a) 1857 to 1862 A.D.
(b) 1837 to 1857 A.D.
(c) 1800 to 1829 A.D.
(d) 1658 to 1707 A.D.

193. Sixth five-year plan to promote significant expansion of employment opportunities was scheduled in the year of
(a) 1974-79 (b) 1961-66
(c) 1980-85 (d) 1969-74.

194. Hindi Day is observed on
(a) 29th August (b) 12 April
(c) 14th September (d) 2 May.

195. 'Lira' is the currency of which of the following country?
(a) Turkey (b) Spain
(c) Philippines (d) Vietnam.

196. Sixty first amendment in the constitution, states about
(a) reducing the voting age from 21 years to 18 years
(b) extended president rule in Punjab
(c) increasing the ceilling of profession tax
(d) reservation of seats for scheduled castes and scheduled tribes in parliament.

197. Which of the following book is written by Sarojini Naidu?
(a) Broken wing (b) Chitra
(c) Great Tragedy (d) Gandevta.

198. India's multi-target surface-to-air missile is known as
(a) Akash (b) Nag
(c) Prithvi (d) Agni.

199. Which of the following is the biggest cave temple in India?
(a) Tuljapur (b) Ajanta
(c) Parli (d) Ellora.

200. Beighton cup in India is associated with
(a) volley ball (b) cricket
(c) basket ball (d) hockey.

❖ ❖ ❖

SOLUTIONS

PHYSICS

1. **(a) :** Angular velocity, $\omega = \frac{d\theta}{dt} = 6t^2$

at $t = 2$ sec

$w = 6 \times 4 = 24$ rad/sec.

2. **(d) :** Let the body be projected at an angle θ with initial speed u.

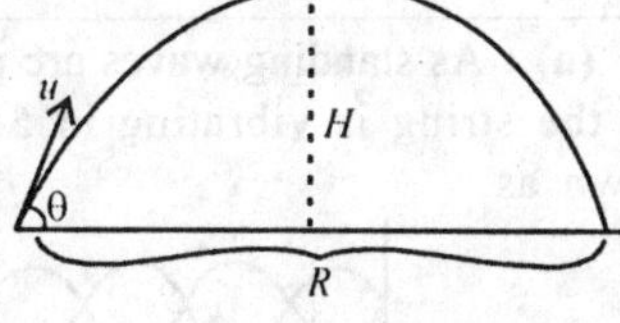

Then the maximum height attained by the body is given by

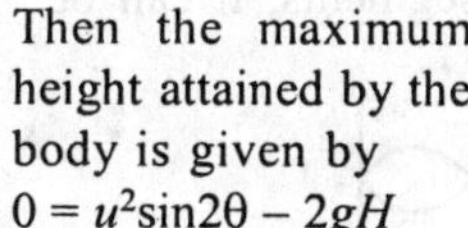

$0 = u^2\sin 2\theta - 2gH$

$\Rightarrow H = \frac{u^2\sin^2\theta}{2g}$

And the range of the projectile

$$R = \frac{u^2\sin 2\theta}{g} = \frac{2u^2\sin\theta\cos\theta}{g}$$

Now given

$$R = 3H \Rightarrow \frac{2u^2\sin\theta\cos\theta}{g} = \frac{3\times u^2\sin^2\theta}{2g}$$

$$\Rightarrow \frac{\sin\theta}{\cos\theta} = \tan\theta = \frac{4}{3}$$

$$\Rightarrow \theta = \tan^{-1}\left(\frac{4}{3}\right) = 53°8'.$$

3. **(a) :** The angular velocity is given by

$$\omega = \frac{2\pi}{T}$$

$\therefore [\omega] = [T^{-1}] = [M^oL^oT^{-1}]$

4. **(b) :** As the water falls freely from a height 19.6 m, so the velocity of water at the turbine is

$$v = \sqrt{2gh} = \sqrt{2\times 9.8\times 19.6} = 19.6 \text{ m/s}$$

5. **(c) :** Let the mass of the bullet be m and that of the rifle be M. Initially both are at rest. Hence the total linear momentum of the system = 0.

Now, after the bullet is fired, let the velocity of the bullet be v and the recoil speed of the rifle be V, then from law of conservation of linear momentum,

$mv - MV = 0$

$$\Rightarrow V = \frac{mv}{M}$$

The KE of the rifle is

$$KE_r = \frac{1}{2}MV^2 = \frac{1}{2}M\frac{m^2v^2}{M^2}$$

$$= \frac{m}{M}\frac{1}{2}mv^2$$

$$= \frac{m}{M}(KE_b)$$

$\because \quad m < M$

$\therefore \quad KE_r < KE_b$

$\therefore$ Kinetic energy of the rifle is less than that of the bullet.

6. **(c)**

7. **(b) :** The focal length of the objective is greater than that of the eye piece so that the image formed by the objective lie in the focal plane of the eye piece. Then the eye piece forms a magnified virtual image of this image.

8. **(d) :** We know that the radii of different orbits of the hydrogen atom are given by

$r_n = n^2a_0$ where a_0=radius of the ground state orbit

$\therefore r_n \propto n^2$

$\therefore$ When the hydrogen atom is in first excited state (*i.e.*, $n = 2$), its radius is 4 times.

9. **(d) :** Given : time period $T = 2$ sec

amplitude of pendulum $A = 50$ mm $= 0.05$ m

We know that the velocity of a simple pendulum undergoing SHM is given by

$$v = \omega\sqrt{A^2 - x^2} = \frac{2\pi}{T}\sqrt{A^2 - x^2}$$

$\therefore \quad v_{max} = \frac{2\pi}{T}\sqrt{A^2 - 0^2}$ ($\because$ maximum velocity occurs at $x = 0$)

$\therefore \quad v_{max} = \frac{2\pi}{T}\times 0.05$

$= 0.16$ m/s

10. **(d) :** As R_2, R_3 and R_4 are in series, their equivalent resistance is $R_2 + R_3 + R_4 = 6\ \Omega$. Now the 6 Ω resistance is in parallel with $R_1 = 2\ \Omega$ whose equivalent risistance will be

$$\frac{2\times 6}{2+6} = \frac{3}{2}\Omega$$

3V ½Ω

$\therefore$ The current through the circuit, $i = \frac{3}{3/2} = 2$ A

11. (a), (c), (d) : The stopping potential, work function of the surface and maximum kinetic energy of photoelectrons do not depend upon the intensity of light used.

12. (c) : Let the area be A

The separation between the plates $d = 5$ mm $= 0.005$ m

We know capacitance $C = \frac{\varepsilon_0 A}{d}$

$$\Rightarrow A = \frac{Cd}{\varepsilon_0}$$
$$= 4\pi \times 3 \times 0.005 \times 9 \times 10^9$$
$$= 1.69 \times 10^9 \text{ m}^2$$

13. (d): Force applied $F = 10$ N

Stretching in the spring $x = 1$ mm $= 0.001$ m

$\therefore$ spring constant $k = \frac{F}{x} = \frac{10}{0.001} = 10^4$

Now the spring is stratched through a distance

$x_1 = 40$ mm
$= 0.04$ m

The force required to stretch it through x_1 is $F_1 = kx_1$

$\therefore$ The work done by this force

$$W = \frac{1}{2}kx_1^2$$
$$= \frac{1}{2} \times 10^4 \times 0.04 \times 0.04$$
$$= \frac{1}{2} \times 16 = 8 \text{ J}$$

14. (c)

15. (c) : We know from first law of thermodynamics that $\Delta Q = \Delta U + \Delta W$ where ΔQ is the heat supplied, ΔU the increas in the internal energy and ΔW is the work done by the gas. Now at constant temperature *i.e.* in isothermal process, $\Delta U = 0$. Hence $\Delta Q = \Delta W$, that maximum work done is possible in isothermal expansion.

16. (a)

17. (a) : Radioactive decay constant $\lambda = 1.07 \times 10^{-4}$/year

$$\therefore \text{ Half life } T_{1/2} = \frac{0.693}{\lambda} = \frac{0.693}{1.07 \times 10^{-4}}$$
$$= 6.476 \times 10^3 \text{ years}$$

18. (c) : The kinetic energy of a body of mass m and velocity v is $E = \frac{1}{2}mv^2 = \frac{p^2}{2m}$ where $p = mv =$ momentum of the body

$$\therefore \frac{p^2}{E} = 2m = \text{constant} \quad \because m = \text{constant}$$
$$\therefore \frac{p_1^2}{E_1} = \frac{p_2^2}{E_2}$$

Now, $E_2 = 4E_1$

$$\therefore \frac{p_1^2}{p_2^2} = \frac{1}{4} \Rightarrow \frac{p_1}{p_2} = \frac{1}{2} \Rightarrow p_2 = 2p_1$$

19. (d) 20. (a)

21. (b): Given, mass of body $m = 5$ kg

radius of circle $r = 1$ m

angular velocity $\omega = 2$ rad/s

$\therefore$ The centripetal force $F_C = mr\omega^2$

$= 5 \times 1 \times 2^2 = 20$ N

22. (a) : At absolute zero of temperature, all translational motion of molecules cease.

23. (d)

24. (a) : As standing waves are produced in the string and the string is vibrating in 5 segments, it can be shown as

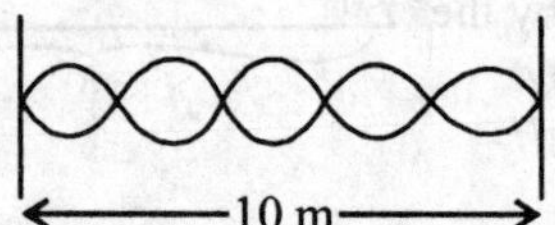

$$\therefore 5\frac{\lambda}{2} = 10$$
$$\Rightarrow \lambda = 4 \text{ m}$$

Given, the velocity of the wave $v = 20$ m/s

$\therefore$ Frequency $\upsilon = \frac{v}{\lambda} = \frac{20}{4} = 5 \text{ s}^{-1} = 5$ Hz

25. (c) : The kinetic energy of the electron, accelerated in the potential of 100 V is

E = 100 eV
$= 100 \times 1.6 \times 10^{-19}$ J $= 1.6 \times 10^{-17}$ J

26. (b) 27. (a) 28. (b)

29. (b) : Considering the mass to be undergoing SHM, the time period of oscillation is given by

$$T = 2\pi\sqrt{\frac{m}{K}}$$

In the first case $m = M$

$$\therefore T = 2\pi\sqrt{\frac{M}{K}}$$

In the second case $m = 4M$

$$\therefore T = 2\pi\sqrt{\frac{4m}{K}} = 2 \times 2\pi\sqrt{\frac{M}{K}} = 2T$$

30. (b) 31. (c)

32. (b) : We have $\frac{C}{100} = \frac{F-32}{180}$ where C = temperature in centigrade scale. F = temperature in °F

Now if $F = 140°$ then

$$C = \frac{100}{180} \times (140 - 32) = 60^\circ$$

The boiling point of water is 100°C

∴ The fall in temperature = 100°C – 60°C = 40°C

33. (a)

34. (d) : Given that standard vapour pressure at 12°C $= 0.016 \times 10^5$ Pa.

The partial pressure of water vapour at 12°C is $= 0.012 \times 10^5$ Pa

$$\therefore \text{R.H.} = \frac{\text{Vapour pressure of air}}{\text{SVP at the same temperature}}$$

$$= \frac{0.012 \times 10^5}{0.016 \times 10^5} = 0.75 = 75\%$$

35. (a) : Heat travels through vacuum by radiation.

36. (a) : Rocket propulsion is based on the principle of Newton's third law, that is every action has equal and opposite reaction.

37. (a) :

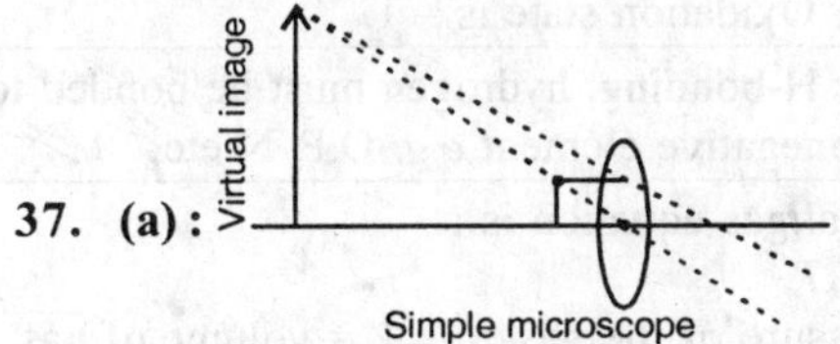

Simple microscope

A simple microscope produces an enlarged and exact but virtual image of the object.

38. (a) : Mirage is a phenomenon observed due to the total internal reflection of light when light travels from a denser medium to a rarer medium. When the angle of incidence of light is more than the critical angle for the two adjacent media, the light gets totally internally reflected.

39. (d) : The rate of diffusion is faster in gases as compared to solids and liquids.

40. (a) : A transformer has got one primary coil, the change of current in which produces an induced emf in the secondary coil. Hence it is based on the principle of mutual induction.

41. (b) : As the person goes up and up above the earth's surface, the acceleration due to gravity decreases. That's why the reading on the spring balance will go on decreasing.

42. (b) : The body temperature during winter is more than the surrounding temperature of our atmosphere. And so the temperature of the wood or the metal surface is at a lower temperature than the body. Now when we touch the wood or the metal surface, because of the temperature difference, heat flow will take palce from our body to wood or metal surface. As the metal surface has got a high thermal condiuctivity than wood, the heat flow from our body to metal surface is faster and so we feel colder to touch the metal surface than a wooden one.

43. (c) : Wool being a bad conductor of heat due to the presence of the air gaps in it and so it does not let our body temperature decrease through conduction. That's why it keeps our body warm.

44. (a) **45. (d)**

46. (a) : We know that the flux is given by

$$\phi = 4\pi I$$
$$= 4\pi \times 100 = 1256 \text{ lumen}$$

47. (a) : We know that the time period of a simple pendulum is given by $T = 2\pi\sqrt{\frac{l}{g}}$, which is independent of the mass of the bob.

Therefore if we replace the metal bob of the simple pendulum with a wooden bob, the time period of the pendulum remains the same.

48. (b) : Because of surface tension, a liquid surface tends to have the minimum area possible. And as for a given volume the surface of a sphere has got the minimum area, the rain drops take a spherical shape.

49. (c) **50. (d)** **51. (b)**

52. (c) : A laser is a highly monochromatic and near-perfect parallel beam of light, due to which the beam can be focussed by a converging lens to a very small spot. As the intensity of the beam is too high, it can drill holes through a metal sheet even if the power is 0.2 W. But even a torch-light of 1000 W power cannot drill holes in such a metal sheet, because the light is less intense and the beam is not parallel.

53. (b) : A body can have acceleration even if its velocity is zero. We can see it as follows –

By definition, acceleration $a = \frac{dv}{dt}$

$$\Rightarrow dv = a\,dt$$
$$\Rightarrow \int dv = \int a\,dt$$
$$\Rightarrow v = at + C$$

where C is a constant

Now we can have a constant C in such a way that

$$at + C = 0$$

or $a = -\frac{C}{t}$

That is, we can have velocity $v = 0$ at an instant when the acceleration is non-zero.

54. (c) : It is not necessory that virtual images are possible only by diverging lenses.

55. (d) : The ratio $\frac{C_P}{C_V}$ is given by,

$\gamma = \frac{C_P}{C_V} = 1 + \frac{2}{n}$ where n is the number of degrees of freedom. Since the number of degrees of freedom for monatomic gas (3) is less than that of diatomic gas (5), $\gamma_{monatomic} > \gamma_{diatomic}$.

56. (d)

57. (b) : As radio waves are electromagnetic waves, they can be polarized.

58. (a) : For resonance to occur, the net reactance of the circuit should be zero. Hence in that condition $X_C - X_L = 0$

$$\therefore \frac{1}{\omega C} - \omega L = 0$$

$$\Rightarrow \omega L = \frac{1}{\omega C} \Rightarrow \omega^2 = \frac{1}{LC}$$

$$\Rightarrow \omega = \frac{1}{\sqrt{LC}}$$

$$\Rightarrow f = \frac{1}{2\pi\sqrt{LC}}$$

Hence resonance occurs at a single frequency and at resonance the inductive reactance is equal and opposite to the capacitive reactance.

59. (c)

60. (a) : According to Newton's corpuscular theory of light, Newton explained refraction as being due to the attraction of the light particles by the particles of the medium making the light ray bend in the boundary. But if this were the case, the velocity of light in a denser medium should have been more than that in a rarer medium. But this is not actually so. The velocity of light in air is more than that in water.

CHEMISTRY

61. (a) : According to Le-Chatelier principal, if a system at equilibrium is subjected to change of concentrations, pressure or temperature, the equilibrium shifts in the direction that tends to undo the effect. So the equilibrium constant of reaction can be calculated.

62. (b) : Sulphur and phosphorus are nonmetals they have very low electropositivity. As aluminium have got one extra-nuclear charge than Mg, it has lesser electropositive character than Mg [due to greater pull exerted by Nucleus on e^-].

63. (a) : According to Aufbau principle, the subshell with minimum energy is filled up first and when this obtains maximum quota of electronss, then the next subshell of higher energy starts filling. So subshell with lowest $(n + l)$ value is filled first. Sequence comes out to be : $1s, 2s, 2p, 3s, 3p, 4s, 3d, 4p, 5s, 4d, 5p, 6s, 4f$ etc.

64. (c) : Hydrogen is present as hydride ion in these molecules *i.e.* Oxidation state is – 1.

65. (c) : For H-bonding, hydrogen must be bonded to highly electronegative element *e.g.* O,F, N etc.

66. (c) : Ideal gas equation is :

$PV = nRT$

P = Pressure of the gas; V = volume of gas

n = no. of moleculas of gas; R = gas constant

T = temperature

67. (b) : For first order reaction

$$t = \frac{1}{K}\log\frac{a}{a-x}$$

$$\frac{t_{30\%}}{t_{50\%}} = \frac{\frac{1}{K}\times 2.303\times\log\frac{100}{100-30}}{\frac{1}{K}\times 2.303\times\log\frac{100}{100-50}}$$

$$\frac{30}{t_{1/2}} = \frac{\log\frac{10}{7}}{\log 2}$$

$$\frac{30}{t_{1/2}} = \frac{0.1549}{0.3010}$$

$$t_{1/2} = \frac{0.3010\times 30}{0.1549} = 58.2 \text{ min}$$

68. (a) : In physical adsorption, gases are held on solid surfaces by weak van der Waal's forces. It is not specific and reversible also.

69. (b) : $K_3[(FeCN)_6]$ on ionisation gives 4 species ($3K^+$ and 1 $[Fe(CN)_6]^{3-}$) and $Al(NO_3)_3$ also gives 4 species ($1Al^{3+}$ and $3NO_3^-$), thus both will have same value of Van't Hoff factor.

70. (a) : Anhydrous sodium sulphate absorbs moisture very efficiently.

71. (a) : Equivalent mass of an acid is defined as the number of parts by mass of it which contains 1.008 parts by mass of replaceable hydrogen or it in the quantity of the acid by mass that supplies one mole of H^+ ions.

$$\text{Eq. mass of acid} = \frac{\text{Molecular mass of the acid}}{\text{Number of replaceable H atoms}}$$

$$= \frac{\text{Molecular mass of the acid}}{\text{Basicity of the acid}}$$

72. (b) : In sp^3 hybridisation, bond angle is – 109ºC
In sp^2 hybridisation, bond angle is – 120ºC
In sp^3 hybridisation, bond angle is – 180ºC

73. (d) : Methyl group is an electron releasing group due to which there is greater electron density in the ring, due to which electrophile attach is favoured.

[Resonance structures of toluene: CH_3 on benzene ↔ ring with $\overset{+}{C}H_3$ and negative charge ↔ ... ↔ ...]

74. (d) : According to this law, the total enthalpy change is independent of intermediate steps involved in the change. It depends only on initial and final values of enthalpy change. So it can be used for the calculation of heat of formation, reaction or transition.

75. (d) : Hydrogen electrode is the primary standard electrode. The hydrogen electrode can act as cathode or anode with respect to other electrode.

$H_2 \rightarrow 2H^+ + 2e^-$ (Anode)

$2H^+ + 2e^- \rightarrow H_2$ (cathode)

76. (a) : Baeyer's process is mainly applied to bauxite ore containing ferric oxide as chief impurity. It can be represented by following reaction sequence.

Bauxite ore $\xrightarrow{\text{Roasting}}$ to convent FeO to Fe_2O_3

$$\text{Roasted ore} + NaOH \xrightarrow[80\text{ atm.}]{150^\circ C} NaAlO_2 \xrightarrow[\text{in } Al(OH)_3]{\text{Hydrolysis}} Al(OH)_3\downarrow + NaOH$$

(NaOH recycled)

77. (a) : As deration in boilding point is given by :

$\Delta T = K_b \times$ molality

Putting the various values, we get :

$$100.52 - 100.00 = 0.6 \times \frac{3/M}{200/1000}$$

$\Rightarrow M = 17.3 \text{ g mol}^{-1}$

78. (a) : Phosphorus trichloride is a chlorinating agent which converts acid to its corresponding acid chloride.

79. (b) : Neutron in free state immediatly decomposes to proton and electron which makes its detection very difficults outside the nucleus.

$${}_0^1n \rightarrow {}_1^1p + {}_{-1}^{0}e$$

80 (b) : Polytetra fluoroethylene is prepared by polymerisation of tetra fluoroethylene.

$$nCF_2{=}CF_2 \xrightarrow{(NH_4)_2S_2O_8} (CF_2 - CF_2)_n$$

This polymer is chemically inert and heat resistant polymer. It is very tough and electrical resistant.

81. (d) : Benzene reacts with methyl iodide in the presence of anhydrous $AlCl_3$ to form toluene. Reaction is called as friedel crafts reaction. It is used for alkylation and acylation of benzene nucleus.

$CH_3I + AlCl_3 \rightarrow CH^+_3\,[AlCl_3I]^-$

$$\overset{+}{CH_3} + C_6H_6 \xrightarrow{(AlCl_3I)^-} C_6H_5CH_3 + HI + AlCl_3$$

Electrophile

82. (b) : Energy of a photon is given by :

$$E = h\nu = \frac{hc}{\lambda}$$

$$\frac{E_1(3000^\circ A)}{E_2(6000^\circ A)} = \frac{hc/3000}{hc/6000} = \frac{2}{1}$$

83. (c) :

Elements	%	At. mass	Relative No. of atom	Simplest ratio of atoms
C	18.5	12	$\frac{18.5}{12}=1.542$	1
H	1.55	1	$\frac{1.55}{1}=1.55$	1
Cl	55.04	35.5	$\frac{55.04}{35.5}=1.55$	1
O	24.81	16	$\frac{24.16}{16}=1.538$	1

Therefore, empirical formula of the compound is CHClO.

84. (d) : Let oxidation state of S be x.

$\therefore \quad 2 \times (+1) + 4x + 6 \times (-2) = 0$

$\Rightarrow \quad 2 + 4x - 12 = 0 \quad \Rightarrow x = \frac{+5}{2}$

85. (d) : Nitrosoamines are prepared from secondary

amines with nitrous acid.

$HO-NO+H^+ \rightleftharpoons H_2O+NO^+$

$R_2NH+NO^+ \rightleftharpoons R_2NH^+NO \rightarrow R_2N-NO+H^+$

Nitrosoamines are readily hydrolysed to the amines by boiling with concentrated H_2SO_4 (or dil.HCl)

$R_2N-NO+H_2O \xrightarrow[\text{or } H_2SO_4]{HCl} R_2NH+HNO_2$

The above reaction is known as Liebermann's nitroso reaction and it is used for detection of secondary amine.

86. (a) : The reaction involved is called as Hoffmann's bromamide reaction.

$R-\overset{O}{\overset{\|}{C}}-NH_2 \xrightarrow{Br_2/KOH} R-NH_2+12\ KBr+K_2CO_3+2H_2O$

Mechanism involved is :

$R-\overset{O}{\overset{\|}{C}}-NH_2 \xrightarrow{Br_2} R-\overset{O}{\overset{\|}{C}}-NH-Br \xrightarrow{KOH}$

$R-\overset{O}{\overset{\|}{C}}-\overset{-}{N}-Br \xrightarrow{-Br^-} (R-\overset{O}{\overset{\|}{C}}-\ddot{N}) \rightarrow R-N=C=O \rightarrow R-NH_2+CO_2$

87. (a) : The product of H^+ and OH^- ions in water at a particular temperature is known as Ionic product of water. It is denoted as K_w.

$K_w=[H^+][OH^-]$

The value of K_w increase with the increase of temperature *i.e.* concentration of H^+ and OH^- ions increase with increase of temperature, but it still exists in the range of 10^{-14}

e.g. 25ºC 1.00×10^{-14}

100ºC 7.50×10^{-14}

88. (c) : Ethanol : Ch_3CH_2OH; Dimethyl ether : MeOMe there is extensive Hydrogen bonding in ethanol due to the presence of –OH groups, while it is not possible in dimethyl ether (no –OH group available) another Hydrogen bonding leads to greater boiling point.

89. (b):

$\overset{5}{CH_3}-\overset{4}{\underset{OH}{\underset{|}{C}}H}=\overset{3}{CH}-\overset{2}{CH_2}-\overset{1}{COOH}$

Therefore, IUPAC name is

4–hydroxy–3–penten–1–oic acid.

90 (d) : Baeyer's reagent is alkaline $KMnO_4$ solution and it is used for oxidation at double bonds *e.g.*

$CH_2=CH_2 \xrightarrow[KMnO_4]{\text{Alkaline}} \begin{array}{l} CH_2-OH \\ | \\ CH_2-OH \end{array}$

This reaction is used as a test for unsaturated compounds.

91. (d) : Amino acids are the building blocks for proteins, chemically they consist of two functional groups *i.e.* $-NH_2$ and –COOH groups. *e.g.*

Glycine : H_2N-CH_2-COOH

92. (c) : Principle Quantum number (n) represent the name, size and energy of the shell to which the electron belongs. Higher the value of 'n' greater is the distance of the shell from the nucleus.

93. (c) : $\dfrac{\text{mass of Hydrogen}}{\text{mass of copper}}$

$=\dfrac{\text{Equivalent mass of Hydrogen}}{\text{Equivalent mass of copper}}$

$\Rightarrow \dfrac{0.504}{\text{mass of copper}}=\dfrac{1}{63.5/2}$

$\Rightarrow$ Mass of copper deposited = 16.0 g

94. (d) : Solubility of $BaSO_4$ in gL^{-1} $=2.33\times10^{-3}$

" " " mol L^{-1} $=\dfrac{2.33}{233}\times10^{-3}$

$=10^{-5}$

Now, $BaSO_4 \rightleftharpoons Ba^{2+}+SO_4^{2-}$

Solubility s s s s

$\therefore$ Solubility Product $=[Ba^{2+}][SO_4^{2-}]$

$=s^2$

$=(10^{-5})^2$

$=10^{-10}$

95. (c) : 1º amines on heating with $CHCl_3$ and alcoholic KOH forms isocyanides (or carbylamine) which posses bad smell. This reaction is known as carbylamine reaction and used for detection of 1º amines.

$C_6H_5NH_2 + CHCl_3 + KOH\ alc. \rightarrow C_6H_5NC$

Isocyanide

96. (d) : Rate constant $=0.69\times10^{-2}\ min^{-1}$

This unit (*i.e.* min^{-1}) is characteristics of first order reaction. For first order reaction, half life time is given as :

$t_{½}=\dfrac{0.693}{k_1}=\dfrac{0.693}{0.69\times10^{-2}}=1.004\times10^2$ min.

$t_{½}=100.4$ min $=6024$

97. (c) : According to ideal gas equation,

$PV=nRT$

Putting the standard conditions, *i.e.* $P=1$ atm,

$n = 1$ mole, $R = 0.0821$ L atm K^{-1}, mol^{-1}, T = 273K

$$V = \frac{nRT}{P} = \frac{1\text{mole} \times 0.0821 \text{ L atm K}^{-1}\text{ mol}^{-1} \times 273K}{1 \text{ atm}}$$

V = 22.4

98. (c) : Acid halides are formed when PCl_5 reacts with carboxylic acids. *e.g.*

$$CH_3COOH + PCl_5 \rightarrow CH_3COCl + POCl_3 + HCl$$

99. (d) : $4Fe + 3O_2 \rightleftharpoons 4Fe^{3+} + 6O_2^{2-}$

In this redox reaction, Iron is acting as a reducing agent (as it is giving out electrons) *i.e.* $Fe \rightarrow Fe^{3+} + 3e^-$

As Fe is readily converted to Fe^{3+} therefore it is oxidised.

100. (d) : $2C(s) + 2H_2 \rightarrow C_2H_4(g)$; $\Delta H_1 = 52$ KJ/mole ..(1)

$C(s) + O_2(g) \rightarrow CO_2(g)$, $\Delta H_2 = -394$ KJ/mole .....(2)

$H_2(g) + \frac{1}{2}O_2(g) \rightarrow H_2O(l)$, $\Delta H_3 = -286$ KJ/mole.....(3)

The combustion of C_2H_4 can be written as :

$C_2H_4(g) \rightarrow 2C(s) + 2H_2$, $\Delta H_1 = -52$ KJ/mole

$2C(s) + 2O_2(g) \rightarrow 2CO_2(g)$, $\Delta H_2 = -2 \times 394$

$2H_2(g) + O_2(g) \rightarrow 2H_2O(l)$, $\Delta H_3 = -2 \times 286$

$\Rightarrow \Delta H = -52 - 2 \times 394 - 2 \times 286 = -1412$ KJ/mole

101. (b) : Molecular mass = 2 × vapour density

= 2 × 30 = 60

Empirical mass = 12 + 2 + 16 = 30

$\Rightarrow n = \frac{60}{30} = 2$

$\Rightarrow$ Molecular formula is $(CH_2O)_2 \equiv C_2H_4O_2$

102. (a) : $2H_2S(g) \rightleftharpoons 2H_2(g) + S_2(g)$

Equilibrium constant is,

$$K = \frac{[H_2]^2[S_2]}{[H_2S]^2} = \frac{[0.1]^2[0.4]}{[0.5]^2}$$

$= 0.016$ mol L^{-1}

103. (a) : Toluene is methyl benzene (benzene ring with CH_3)

$\therefore$ 2–bromo toluene is 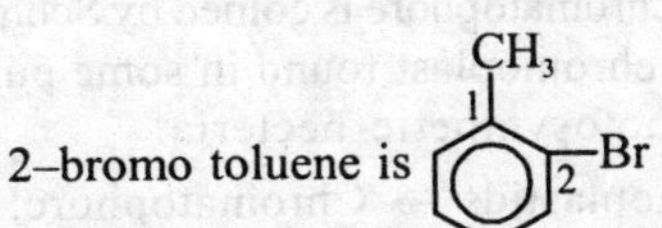

104. (d) : According to Boyle's law,

$$P_1V_1 = P_2V_2$$

Putting values here, we get;

$100 \times 720 = P_2 \times 84$

$\Rightarrow P_2 = 857.14$ mm

105. (c) : Lanthanides and Activides are called as the inner-transition metals lanthanide series consists of 4*f*–metals white actinides series consists of 5*f*–metals.

106. (c) : In an endothermic reaction, enthalpy for the product is higher than that of reactants.

$\therefore \Delta H = \Delta H$ (products) – ΔH(reactant) = +ve

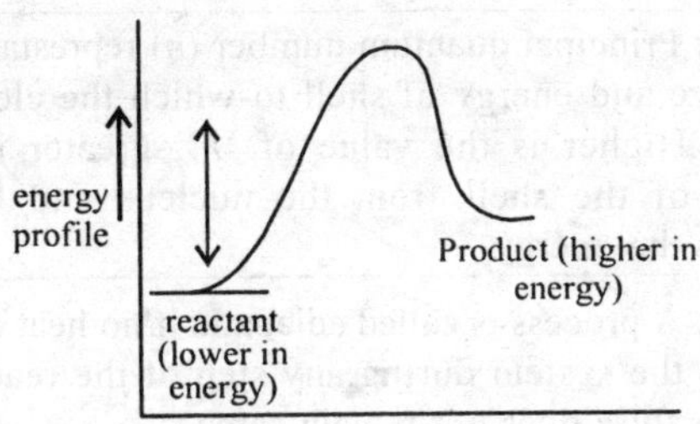

107. (c) : $[Fe(CN)_6]^{3-}$: Fe^{3+}; 3d: [1][1][1][1][1] 4s: [ ]

Due to strong ligand *i.e.* cyanide ion, 3d electrons pair up .

$[Fe(CN)_6]^{3-} \rightarrow$ 3d: [⥮][⥮][1][××][××] 4s: [××] 4p: [××][××][××]

so only one unpaired electron.

$[Fe(CN)_6]^{4-}$; Fe^{2+} : 3d: [⥮][1][1][1][1] 4s: [ ]

Due to strong ligand CN, e^- pair up

$[Fe(CN)6]^{4-} \rightarrow$ [⥮][⥮][⥮][××][××] [××] [××][××][××]

$\therefore$ No unpaired electron

$[Cr(H_2O)_6]^{3+}$ Cr^{3+} : 3d: [1][1][1][ ][ ] 4s: [ ]

As H_2O is weak ligand, no pairity of electron takes place.

$[Cr(H_2O)_6]^{3+} \rightarrow$ 3d: [1][1][1][××][××] 4s: [××] 4p: [××][××][××]

$\therefore$ Three unpaired electrons.

$[Cu(H_2O)_6]^{2+}$ Cu^{2+} : 3d: [⥮][⥮][⥮][⥮][1] 4s: [ ]

only one unpaired electron.

108. (c) : We known that

specific conductance = Cell constant × conductance

$\Rightarrow$ Cell constant = Resitances × sp. conductance

$= 55 \times 0.0112$

$= 0.616\ cm^{-1}$

109. (d) : Planck's constant, $h = 6.63 \times 10^{-34}$ Js

Also, $E = h\nu$

$\Rightarrow h$ = Energy × time

= Force × L × T

$= MLT^{-2} \times L \times T = ML^2T^{-1}$

Angular momentum, $L = mvr$

$= M \times LT^{-1} \times L = ML^2 T^{-1}$

Therefore both has same dimension.

110. (d) : Alkenes are reactive due to the presence of double bond. The π–electrons are loosely held and are therefore, earily polaisable. So more the number of e^{-1} releasing alkyl group on the double bond, lesser is the stability.

111. (a) : Principal quantum number (n) represtant the name, size and energy of shell to which the electron belongs. Higher is the value of 'n', greater is the distance of thc shell from the nucleus and hence greater is the energy.

112. (d) : A process is called adiabatic if no heat enters or leaves the system during any step of the reaction. So temperature does not remain same.

113. (a) : According to Aufbau principle, the unfilled shell with lowest ($n + l$) value will be filled first. Therefore, 4s orbital is filled first then 3d orbital.

for 4s - obital, $(n + l) = 4 + 0 = 4$

for 3d - orbital, $(n + l) = 3 + 2 = 5$

114. (b) : The ideal gas equation is

$PV = nRT$ where; P = pressure

V = volume; T = temperature

R = universal gas constant

n = no. of moles

Now if T = constant, then; PV = constant

115. (a) : In an isothermal expansion, temperature is maintained constant so internal energy change is zero. $(\Delta E = 0)$.

According to first law of thermodynamic,

$\Delta E = q + w;$ q = heat , w = work done

$\Rightarrow$ $q = -w$

This shows that work is done by the system at the expense of heat absorbed.

116. (c) : SO_2 in presence of moisture acts as a bleaching agent. This is due to the reducing nature of SO_2. But bleaching action is only temporary.

$SO_2 + 2H_2O \rightarrow H_2SO_4 + 2[H]$

Similarily, Cl_2 in presence of moisture give out nascent, oxygen and cause bleaching.

$Cl_2 + H_2O \rightarrow 2HCl + [O]$

here bleaching action is permanent.

117. (c) : The hydrolysis of sucrose by boiling with a mineral acid (HCl), produces a mixture of equal molecules of D-glucose and D-fructose. Sucrose solution is dextrorotary, specific rotation = + 66.5°. But on hydrolysis, it becomes laevorotatory. The specific rotation of D – glucose is + 52° and of D – fructose is –92°. Therefore, the net specific rotation of an equimolar mixture of both is :

$\frac{+52^\circ - 92^\circ}{2} = -20^\circ$ $\therefore$ laevorotatory

118. (a) : The N_2 moleculer contains a triple bond N≡N with a short bond length of 1.09Å. This bond is very stable and the dissociation energy is very high (946 KJ mol^{-1}). This N_2 is inert at room temperature.

119. (d) : Bond order is the half of the difference between bonding and anti-bonding electrons. *i.e.*

$$\text{B.O.} = \frac{1}{2}\left[\left(\begin{matrix}\text{Number of } e^- \text{in} \\ \text{bonding M.O.}\end{matrix}\right)\right] - \left[\left(\begin{matrix}\text{Number of } e^- \text{in} \\ \text{antibonding M.O.}\end{matrix}\right)\right]$$

Greater the order, greater is the stability in the molecule.

120. (a) : Alkali metals have very low value of Ionisation energy as compared to other metals. So alkali metals easily get excited and impart to flame.

BIOLOGY

121.(c) : At high light intensity, high O_2 and high temperature, the mesophyll cells in the leaves of all C_3 plants exhibit high rates of photorespiration. C_3 plants, however, exhibit low rates of photorespiration. Phosphoglycolic acid is formed from RuBP in chloroplasts and it is then converted to glycolic acid. Glycolic acid translocates to a peroxisome. Within this cytoplasmic organelle, glycolic acid is oxidized to produce glyoxylic acid and hydrogen peroxide (H_2O_2). The glyoxylic acid is converted to the amino acid glycine with the liberation of O_2. Two glycine molecules react to produce serine and CO_2. In a mitochondrion the serine is metabolized to carbohydrates or incorporated into proteins.

122.(d) : In *Selaginella*, reduction division (meiosis) takes place both in microspore mother cell and megaspore mother cell, which forms haploid microspores and megaspores, respectively.

123.(a) : The term chromatophore is coined by Schmitz. This is one type of chromoplast found in some purple and non-purple photosynthetic becteria.

Plastids → Chromoplastids → Chromatophore.

124.(d) : The sphere of living matter together with water, air and soil on the surface of earth is called biosphere. Atmosphere is the gaseous envelope surrounding a planet. Hydrosphere is the part of the earth composed of water and lithosphere is the crust and mantle (solid portion) of earth.

125.(d) : Carcinoma is a malignant neoplasm of epithelial origin. It is a tumor that arises in the tissues that line the body's organ like nose, colon, breast, prostate, urinary bladder or ureter.

Leukaemias are cancers of the blood or blood forming organs. Sarcoma are tumors that originate in mesodermal tissue like bone, connective tissue, muscle, cartilage or fat. Lymphomas affect the lymphatic system, a network of vessels and nodes that acts as the body's filter.

126.(c) : *Recombination* is the process by which a recombinant chromosome is formed from two different parental cells. Three processes that lead to the formation of recombinant chromosames are known to occur in bacteria. *Transformation* is the transfer of genetic information through the agency of free DNA. *Transduction* is the transfer of a portion of the DNA from one bacterium or makes physical contact with a female or recipient bacterium and transforms genetic elements into it.

Translation is not concerned with the bacterial genetic recombination. It is a step in protein synthesis.

127.(a) : The loss or excretion of water in the form of liquid droplets from the leaves and other parts of an uninjured or intact plant is called guttation. Guttation takes place through special structures called hydathodes.

128.(b) : Moderate rainfall during summer produces grasslands. In desert, the rainfall is less than 10 inches which is very less for any type of vegetation. In tropical as well as temperate regions, the rainfall is suitable for grassland formation. In scrub forest, summer is dry and rainfall occurs in winter. In deciduous forest, leaves are fallen only once yearly.

129.(a) : Industrial melanism is an adaptation where the moths living in the industrial areas developed melanin pigments to match their body with the surroundings. It provides an excellent instance of operation of selection in natural conditions (natural selection). It first occured in Britain.

130.(c) : Apospory is a phenomenon in which a somatic cell in the nucellus directly forms a gametophyte (*i.e.* embryosac) without-meiosis. Such gametophytes are diploid.

131.(c) : Middle piece of a mammalian sperm contains mitochondria. It is well-developed and numerous. Nucleus is present at the sperm head or acrosome. Centriole is present at the neck region.

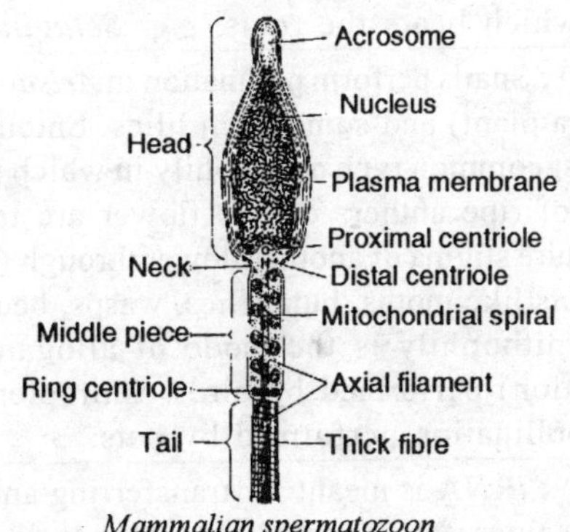

Mammalian spermatozoon

132.(a) : The black pigment in the eye, which reduces the internal reflection is known as retina. It is the innermost coat of the eyeball and it is a thin, light sensitive nervous layer. The external coat of the eyeball is known as sclerotic but in front of the sclerotic, there is a transparent connective tissue called cornea. Iris is the pigmented part present in front of choroid.

133.(a) : The placenta of human beings belongs to the category of *haemo-chorialis*. In this, maternal blood baths foetal chorionic villi directly. In *syndesmo chorialis* placenta, the foetal and maternal components are fused so intimately as to result in a destruction of the uterine epithelium. In *endothelio chorialis* placenta, the uterine mucosa is reduced and the chorionic epithelium comes in contact with the endothelial wall of maternal (uterine) blood vessel. *Epithelio chorialis* type of placenta is of most primitive type.

134.(c) : Antiserum contains antibodies. The term antiserum is applied to materials prepared in animals. Antiserum is a serum containing antibodies with affinity for a specific antigenic determinant. They may result in cross-reactivity with recipient.

135.(d) : Ligule is a membranous, narrow outgrowths from the base of the leaves on the adaxial surface of some Lycophyta *e.g. Selaginella*. Ligule is usually inserted by a comparatively stout foot, the glossopodium in a definite socket, the ligular pit. Trichocysts are found in a member of dinoflagellates. Heterocyst is found in blue green algae, whose function

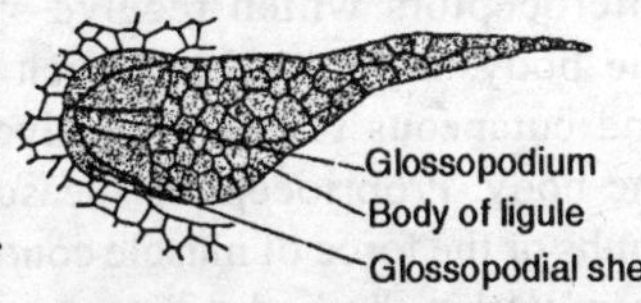

Vertical section of a ligule of *Selaginells kraussiana* passing through the sheath.

is to fix atmospheric nitrogen. Rhizophore is a leafless branch, intermediate in character between root and stem, which bears the roots, *e.g. Selaginella.*

136.(d) : Snails perform pollination in *Arisaema* (snake or cobra plant) and some arum lilies. Entomophily is the most common type of zoophily in which the pollen grains of ripe anthers of one flower are transferred to a mature stigma of another flower through the agency of insects like moths, butterflies, wasps, bees, beetles etc. Ornithophily is the mode of allogamy (cross pollination) performed by birds. Chiropterophily is cross pollination performed by bats.

137.(a) : *t*RNA is meant for transferring amino acids to ribosomes for synthesis of polypeptides. There are different *t*RNAs for different amino acids. Some amino acids can, however, be picked up by 2–6 *t*RNA. *m*RNA brings instructions from the DNA for the formation of a particular type of polypeptide. *r*RNAs help *t*RNA and *m*RNA in the synthesis of proteins over the ribosomes.

138.(a) : The stomata are found in the capsule of mosses. Each stoma leads into an air space below called the substomatal cavity.

139.(c) : In blue green algae (cyanophyta), filament consisting uniseriate or multiseriate chain of cells called as trichomes. Mycelium is a collective term used for mass of hyphae that constitutes vegetative part of a fungus. Hypha is filament of a fungus thallus colonies are formed by aggregation of many individuals.

140.(d) : Secretion of posterior pituitary is under neurosecretory nerve axons. Neurosecretory neurons are glandular, unmyelinated secretory cells with two functions. One of which is to synthesize and release neurohormones either directly into the general circulation (as in the case of neurosecretory neurons of the pars nervosa) or into a portal system.

141.(a) : Sensation of stomach pain is due to interoceptors which receive stimuli from inside of the body. Exteroceptors, such as the eye, ear, taste and cutaneous reaptors, receive stimuli from outside the body. Proprioceptors measure the position of the limbs or the force of muscle contraction, receive stimuli from within the body. Teloreceptor is a sensory nerve terminal which is sensitive to stimuli originating at a distance, such nerve endings exist in the eyes, nerves and nose

142.(a) : Addison's disease results from hyposecretion of adrenal. Addison's disease is a severe or total deficiency of the hormones made in the adrenal cortex, caused by a destruction in the adrenal cortex. Classical Addison's disease results from a loss of both cortisol and aldosterone secretion due to the almost total destrution of both adrenal glands.

143.(c) : Galapagos islands are a chain of 14 islands in the pacific ocean on the west coast of South America Charles Darwin visited these islands during his famous voyage on HMS Beagle (name of his ship) in 1835. The flora and fauna of these islands resemble with those of the South American mainland with which the Galapagos islands were once connected. However birds of Galapagos islands (also called as Darwin's finches) do not resemble the birds of South America.

144.(d) : Pacinian corpuscles occur in the skin of certain parts of the body in mammals. There are encapsulated pressure receptor. Pacinian corpuscles are very rapid adapting pressure receptors in subcutaneous adipose tissue of both hairy and hairless vertebrate skin. They are also found in joint capsules, tendons etc.

145.(d) : Excess of pollen causes allergic reactions in several human beings. The common reactions are also collectively called *hay fever.* The important allergic pollen belong to *Amaranthus spinosus, Chenopodium album, Cynodon, Dactylon, Ricinus communis, Sorghum vulgare, Prosopis chilensis.*

146.(c) : Sympathetic nerves in mammals arise from thoraco-lumber region. Nerves of the sympathetic system originate within the spinal cord of the thoracic and lumbar segments, but beyond the vertebrae each departs from the cord and turns ventrally in a short, white ramus to enter a sympathetic ganglion.

147.(c) : Nucleolus is a naked, round or slightly irregular structure which is attached to the chromatin at a specific region called nucleolar organiser region. Plasmids are additional rings of DNA in bacteria which can replicate independently. Karyolymph or nucleoplasm is a transparent, semifluid and colloidal substance which fills the nucleus.

148.(b) : The first pesticide was discovered by Millardet in 1882. It is known as Bordeaux mixture. In 1878 Millardet of the university of Bordeaux, France, found that downy mildew of grape-vine orchards was absent in areas where the plants were sprayed with copper sulphate alone or mixed with lime to prevent pilferage.

149.(b) : Totipotency or cellular totipotency is the ability of a living somatic nucleated cell to form the complete organism. Theoretically all somatic cells should be totipotent since they carry the full gene complement of the individual. Tissue culture is the technique of maintaining and growing plant cells, tissues or organs aseptically on artificial medium in suitable containers under controlled environmental conditions.

150.(d) : The relationship in an ecosystem can be depicted in pyramid of energy, pyramid of biomass, pyramid of numbers etc. *Pyramid of number* depicts the number of individual organisms at different trophic levels of food chain. The biomass of the members of the food chain present at any one time forms the *pyramid of biomass.* When production is considered in terms of energy, the pyramid indicates the amount of energy flow at each level. This is called *pyramid of energy.*

151.(a) : Cellobiose is the repeating disaccharide unit of cellulose having the glycosidic linkage β $(1\rightarrow4)$; its full name is thus 4–O–β–D–glucopyranosyl D–α– glucopyranose.

152.(b) : Milk of coconut or coconut water (liquid endosperm) may be widely used in culture medium because it contains several plant growth substances. It can be extracted easily.

153.(a) : Phloem is a complex plant tissue which transports organic food inside the body of the plant.

154.(b) : Phytotron is building in which plants can be grown on a large scale in a range of rigidly controlled conditions of light, temperature of air and soil, humidity and composition of air water and nutrient content of soil etc. Individual controlled environment chambers, a common feature of most botanical laboratories, provide more limited, small scale control of environment. Both types of facility can be of immense value in experimental investigations of plant growth.

155.(c) : *m*RNA is messenger RNA which brings coded information from DNA and takes part in its translation by bringing amino acids in a particular sequence during the synthesis of polypeptide. However, the codon of *m*RNA are not recognised by amino acids but by anticodons of their adaptor molecules (*t*RNA→aa–*t*RNAs). Translation occurs over the ribosomes. The same *m*RNA may be used again and again. In the form of polysome, it can help in synthesis of a number of copies simultaneously.

156.(c) : The root knot nematodes, *Meloidogyne sppare* are the most dominant group of plant parasitic nematodes in almost every vegetable field and cause enormous losses every year in the nursery. The common species are *Meloidogyne arenaria, M. incognita* and *M. javanica.* The pathogen responsible for smut of Bajra is *Tolyposporium penicillariae. Ustilago hordei* causes covered smut of barley and *Ustilago nuda* causes loose smut of Barley. The causal organism of late blight of potato is *Phytophthora infestens.*

157.(d) : Passive immunity is defined as immunity achieved through the sera of other animals enriched in antibodies. It is resistance, based on antibodies preformed in another host. Administration of antibody against diphtheria, tetanus, botulism etc. makes large amounts of antitoxin immediately available to neutralize the toxins. The main advantage of this is the prompt availibility of large amount of antibody. *e.g.* Tetanus, rabies, hepatitis etc.

158.(d) : The structure, which remains unchanged during metamorphosis in frog's tadpole, is nervous system. Metamorphosis in frog is a thyroxin mediated process during which changes occur in the structure of lung, heart and intestine, but there is no such a severe change in nervous system. Only, brain acquires its normal shape and size.

159.(c) : Cells of deiter occur in organ of Corti. These are the supporting cells present in three rows in organ of corti. It also appears to contribute lesser amount of collagen to the tectorial membrane. Deiter cells

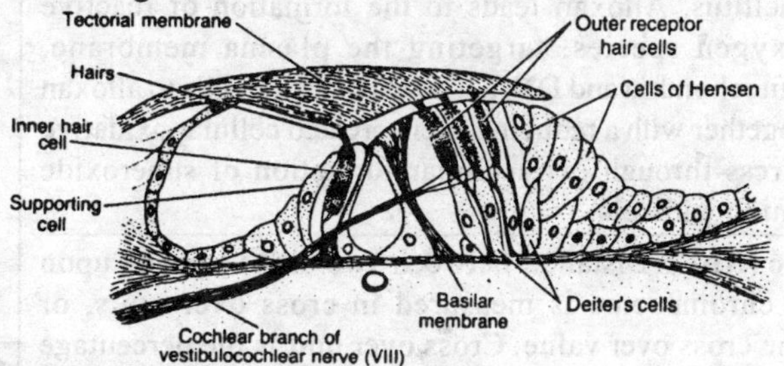

Organ of Corti

present towards the cochlea forms the rods of corti. Its main function is to hold the organ of corti together.

160.(a) : The cells named podocytes occur in glomerulus of kidney. Podocytes play an important role in glomerular differentiation. The podocyte forms the filtration barrier in the glomerulus. In addition podocytes have a role in the characteristic arrangement of cytoskeletal proteins and intermediate filaments in the formation of foot processes.

161.(d) : Organophosphates are organic esters of phosphoric acid and its derivatives. The important organophosphates used as pesticides include malathion, parathion and fenitrothion. Malathion is an ingredient of finit (flit).

162.(c) : Just after ovulation, the layer forms around the ovum is called corona radiata. It is formed by the granulosa cells of cumulus oophorus. It probably increases the likelihood that the ovum will be picked up in the uterine tube.

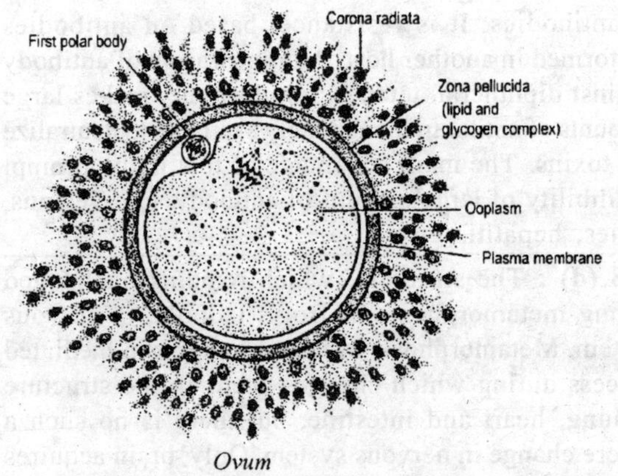

Ovum

163.(b) : Tratment with "Alloxan" destroys β cells of islets of Langerhans.

Alloxan induces damage and death of pancreatic islet cells thus causing insulin dependent diabetes mellitus. Alloxan leads to the formation of reactive oxygen species, targeting the plasma membrane, mitochondria and DNA. The exposure of cells to alloxan together with a reducing agent created cellular oxidative stress through extracellular formation of superoxide anion radicals.

164.(b) : Distance between two linked genes upon a chromosome is measured in cross over units, or the cross over value. Cross over unit is the percentage of meiotic products that are recombinant in an organism heterozygous at each of two linked loci. In diploid organisms, most easily measured method is by crossing the double heterozygote to the double recessive. The percentage can never exceed 50%. This value gives the map distance between the two loci, used in chromosome mapping.

165.(b) : The genes present on the differential region of Y-chromosome are called holandric genes. They are passed directly from male parent to male offspring. Gene which has undergone mutation within the particular stock of organisms is called mutant gene. Chromosome which is not a sex chromosome is called autosomal chromosome. Sex-linked genes are genes having special distribution with reference to sex as a result of being carried on the X–chromosome.

166.(c) : Eggs having yolk in their centre of cytoplasm in peripheral layer, are called *centrolecithal.* It is found in some insect and Hydrozoa. In microlecithal eggs, the amount of yolk is so little that it is found scattered almost uniformaly throughout the egg cytoplasm. Such eggs with evenly distributed yolk in ooplasm is called *isolecithal. Microlecithal* eggs are with very small amount of yolk and *telolecithal* eggs have a polarised distribution of yolk.

167.(d) : Arbor vitae is tree like disposition of the gray and white matter in the cerebellum.

168.(c) : Termination of gastrulation is marked by obliteration of blastocoel. Gastrulation is an embryonic process that ensembles of processes during post-cleavage early development which when completed has brought the cells that will form the various organs to the places where those organs are to be formed. At the termination of gastrulation, archenteron is formed at the place of blastocoel.

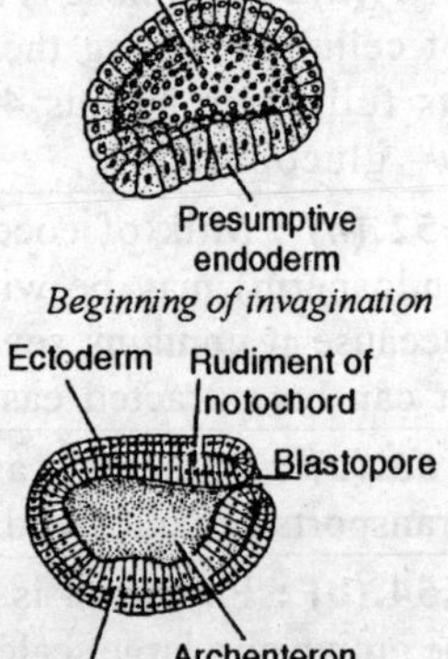

Beginning of invagination

Completed gastrula

169.(c) : Mechanism of uric acid excretion in a nephron is secretion. As blood passes through the kidneys, the nephrons clear the plasma of some substances (*e.g.* urea/uric acid) while simultaneously retaining other, essential substances (water). Substances to be excreted are removed by glomerular filtration and renal tubular secretion and passed into the urine. Secretion refers to the transport of solutes from the peritubular capillaries to the tubular lumens.

170.(a) : Most primitive living mammals, which provide an evidence of organic evolution from geographical distribution are found in China.

171.(a) : Transmission of the nerve impulse across synapse is accomplished by neurotransmitter. Transmission across a synapse usually requires neurotransmmitters because there is small space *i.e.* synaptic cleft separates one neuron from another. Most synaptic transmission is carried by a chemical called neurotransmitter. There are low molecular mass substances released in minute amounts at interneural,

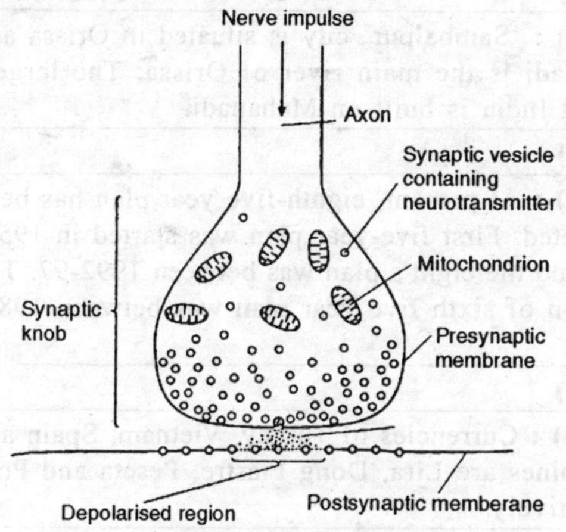

Structure of a synapse

neuromascular and neuroglandular substances. Most wide spread transmitter is acetylcholine.

172. (a) : All terrestrial mammals are air breathers. Because of terrestrial habitat, they have well developed lungs for air breathing. As external respiration takes place in terrestrial animals, three conditions are necessary for this purpose, (i) there should be a large vascular surface with thin blood capillaries, (ii) The membrane of the respiratory surface should be thin and should remain moist (iii) there should be a respiratory pigment and a respiratory medium. All these purposes are successfully served by lungs. Thus well developed lungs make the terrestrial animals air breathers.

173. (c) : There is no chance of transmission of malaria to man on the bite of a male *Anopheles* mosquito. The mouthparts of male mosquito is organised in such a manner that they can't suck the human blood. They feed mainly on the leaf and fruit juices. Thus spreading malaria through male *Anopheles* is next to impossible.

174. (c) : Thiamin deficiency results in beri-beri causing paralysis.

Thiamin or vitamin B_1 is an antineuritic vitamin. Its deficiency causes beri-beri which is characterised by loss of apetite and weight, retarded growth, degeneration of nerves and muscle atrophy, thus in acute cases leads to paralysis.

175. (d) : There are important roles of many minerals as the biologically active substances in the sodium, chlorine, potassium, calcium, phosphorus, iron, iodine, copper, zinc, cobalt etc.

As for example, deficiency of iron in some persons leads to anaemia. Deficiency of iodine leads to goitre and deficiency of fluorine leads to dental caries, thus each of the minerals perform specific role in the body. Their deficiency or excess may evolve several symptoms.

176. (c) : *Psophocarpus tetragonolobus* (winged bean) is a nitrogen fixing herbaceous bean found in tropical Asia. It is also called as Goa bean. All parts of the plant are edible and rich in portein. Ripe seeds are roasted and eaten like peanuts. They contain 34-40% protein and 18% oil. Their nutritive value is similar to that of soyabeans.

177. (b) : Meiosis is a double division which occurs in a diploid cell (or nucleus) and gives rise to four haploid cells (or nuclei), each having half the number of chromosomes as compared to the parent cell. While mitosis give rise to two daughter cells, which are identical to each other as well as to the parent cell. Meiosis gives rise to four daughter cells. These four cells, though resemble each other with respect to chromosome number, they differ, since paternal and maternal chromosomes would reassort during first division and these would give rise to new types due to exchange of chromosome segments. Synapsis occurs during zygotene of meiosis. The two homologous chromosomes get attached to each other, and the process of attachment is known as synapsis. It produces a complex known as synaptinemal complex.

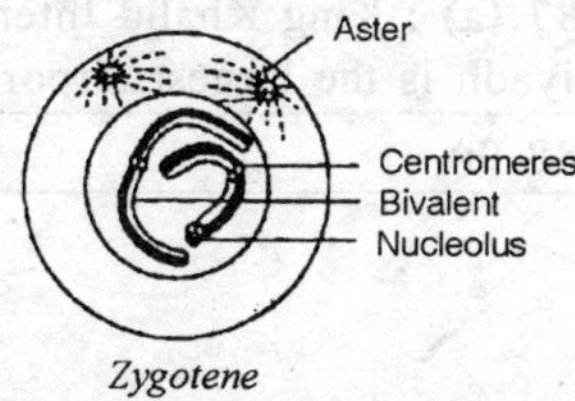

Zygotene

178. (a) : Apical dominance is the phenomenon by which presence of apical bud does not allow the nearby lateral buds (auxillary buds) to grow. When the apical bud is removed, the auxillary buds sprout.

179. (d) : Lysosomes are found in animal cells whereas photorespiration is the process occurs in plant cell. Lysosomes are small vesicles which are bounded by a single membrance and contain hydrolytic enzymes in the form of minute crystalline or semicrystalline granules of 5–8 nm. They are also called acid hydrolases because these digestive enzymes usually function in acidic medium or pH less than 7.

180.(a) : The fungi of endotrophic mycorrhiza invade the cells of the root cortex, with a portion lying externally as a loose mass of hyphae in the soil. These mycorrhizas are found in the families of Ericales, Orchidaceae and Gentiaceae. Mycorrhizas cause considerable stimulation to growth in nutrient deficient soils. The greatest stimulation occurs in the uptake of phosphates. Mycorrhizas can take up phosphate at that low concentrations at which they are unavailable to non-mycorrhizal roots.

GENERAL KNOWLEDGE

181.(b) : In 1927, the British government announced the appointment of a statutory commission. The purpose of which was to probe in functioning of the reforms to be introduced in India by the act of 1899.

182.(d)

183.(c) : 'JAVA' is a computer programming language which is very useful in computer networking.

184.(c)

185.(a) : 'Frank Worrell' was associated with cricket and he was playing from the West Indies side.

186.(c)

187.(a) : King Khalid International Airport outside Riyadh is the largest airport in the World.

188.(b)

189.(d) : Commonwealth games 1998 were hosted at Kualalampur, the capital of Malaysia. The participants are the countries, who are the member of the common wealth, the erstwhile colonies of England.

190.(b)

191.(c) : 'Sambalpur' city is situated in Orissa and Mahanadi is the main river of Orissa. The largest dam of India is built on Mahanadi.

192.(b)

193.(c) : At present, eighth-five year plan has been completed. First five-year plan was started in 1951-1956 and the eight's plan was between 1992-97. The duration of sixth five year plan was between 1980-85.

194.(c)

195.(a) : Currencies of Turkey, Vietnam, Spain and Philippines are Lira, Dong Piastre, Peseta and Peso respectively.

196. (a)

197. (a) : Broken wing, Chitra, Gandevta and Great Tragedy was written by Sarojini Naidu, Rabinder Nath Tagore, Tara Shankar and Z.A. Bhutto respectively.

198. (a)

199. (d) : 'Ellora' is the biggest and one of the oldest evidence of ancient culture and traditions. It is situated near Aurangabad (Maharashtra).

200. (d)

SOLVED PAPER
AIIMS - 1999

Time : 3½ Hours | Max. Marks : 200

PHYSICS

1. The reaction responsible for the production of light energy from the sun is
(a) fission (b) nuclear
(c) fusion (d) none of these.

2. In Young's experiment, the monochromatic light is used to illuminate two slits A and B as shown. Interference fringes are observed on a screen placed in front of the slits. Now if a thin glass plate is placed normally in the path of beam coming from the slit A, then

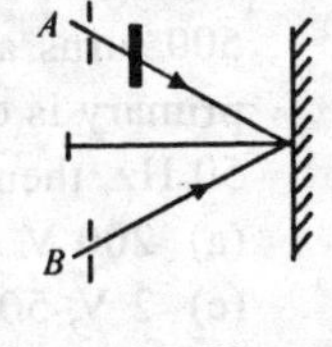

(a) fringe width will decrease
(b) fringes will disappear
(c) fringe width will increase
(d) there will be no change in fringe width.

3. A charged particle enters in a magnetic field H with its initial velocity making an angle of 45° with H. The path of the particle will be
(a) an ellipse (b) a straight line
(c) a circle (d) a helical.

4. Diode is used as a/an
(a) rectifier (b) oscillator
(c) amplifier (d) modulator.

5. In n-type semiconductors, majority charge carriers are
(a) protons (b) holes
(c) neutrons (d) electrons.

6. When n-p-n transistor is used as an amplifier, then
(a) holes move from emitter to base
(b) electrons move from base to collector
(c) holes move from base to emitter
(d) electrons move from collector to base.

7. Two identical galvanometers are converted into an ammeter and a milliammeter. The shunt, which has more resistance due to the current passing through the coil will be
(a) less (b) equal
(c) more (d) zero.

8. Energy is not carried by which of the following wave?
(a) electromagnetic (b) transverse
(c) stationary (d) progressive.

9. A choke coil has
(a) low inductance and high resistance
(b) high inductance and low resistance
(c) low inductance and low resistance
(d) high inductance and high resistance.

10. In the figure, the equivalent resistance between the points A and B is
(a) 8 Ω
(b) 6 Ω
(c) 2 Ω
(d) 4 Ω.

$R_2 = 4\ \Omega$, $R_1 = 2\ \Omega$, $R_4 = 2\ \Omega$, $R_3 = 4\ \Omega$, A, B

11. Boolean algebra is essentially based on
(a) truth (b) numbers
(c) symbol (d) logic.

12. A triode valve has an amplification factor of 20 and its plate is given a potential of 300 V. What should be the grid voltage to reduce the plate-current to zero?
(a) 15 V (b) 8 V
(c) 25 V (d) 12 V.

13. Which of the following is used as a moderator in nuclear reaction?
(a) plutonium (b) cadmium
(c) uranium (d) heavy water.

14. When cathode rays strike a metal target of high melting point with a very high velocity, then which of the following are produced?
(a) α-rays (b) ultrasonic waves
(c) X-rays (d) γ-waves.

15. According to the Bohr theory, relation between main quantum number n and radius of orbit r is

(a) $r \propto n$ (b) $r \propto 1/n$
(c) $r \propto n^2$ (d) $r \propto 1/n^2$.

16. Two identical conductors of copper and aluminium are placed in an identical electric field. The magnitude of induced charge in the aluminium will be
(a) greater than in copper
(b) zero
(c) less than in copper
(d) equal to that in copper.

17. The number of electrons for one coulomb of charge is
(a) 6.25×10^{23} (b) 6.25×10^{21}
(c) 6.25×10^{19} (d) 6.25×10^{18}.

18. Relation between critical angle of water and the glass is
(a) $C_w = C_g = 0$ (b) $C_w = C_g$
(c) $C_w > C_g$ (d) $C_w < C_g$.

19. SONAR emits which of the following waves?
(a) ultrasound (b) radio
(c) light (d) none of these.

20. If a magnetic material, moves from stronger to weaker parts of a magnetic field, then it is known as
(a) paramagnetic (b) ferromagnetic
(c) diamagnetic (d) ani-ferromagnetic.

21. Angle of dip is 90° at
(a) equator (b) poles
(c) both (a) and (b) (d) none of these.

22. If the rotational velocity of a dynamo armature is doubled, then the induced e.m.f. will become
(a) half (b) two times
(c) four times (d) unchanged.

23. Which of the following quantity is increased in a step-down transformer?
(a) voltage (b) current
(c) power (d) frequency.

24. Quantity that remains unchanged in a transformer is
(a) voltage (b) frequency
(c) current (d) none of these.

25. At a common temperature, a block of wood and a block of metal feel equally cool or hot. The temperatures of metal and wood are
(a) less than the temperature of the body
(b) equal to the temperature of the body
(c) greater than the temperature of the body
(d) either (a) or (c).

26. Interference occurs in which of the following waves?
(a) transverse (b) longitudinal
(c) electromagnetic (d) all of these.

27. Sky appears to be blue in clear atmosphere due to light's
(a) scattering (b) diffraction
(c) dispersion (d) all of these.

28. The primary winding of a transformer has 500 turns and its secondary has 5000 turns. If primary is connected to a.c. supply of 20 V and 50 Hz, then secondary will have an output of
(a) 200 V, 50 Hz (b) 2 V, 5 Hz
(c) 2 V, 50 Hz (d) 200 V, 500 Hz.

29. When a magnetic substance is heated, then it
(a) remains the same
(b) loses its magnetism
(c) becomes a strong magnet
(d) either (a) or (c).

30. The north pole of a magnet is brought near a metallic ring. The direction of the induced current in the ring will be
(a) towards south (b) towards north
(c) anti-clockwise (d) clockwise.

31. If vibrations of a string are to be increased by a factor two, then tension in the string must be made
(a) four times (b) half
(c) twice (d) eight times.

32. The average kinetic energy of a gas molecules at 27°C is 6.21×10^{-21} J. Its average kinetic energy at 227°C will be
(a) 10.35×10^{-21} J (b) 52.2×10^{-21} J
(c) 5.22×10^{-21} J (d) 11.35×10^{-21} J.

33. In an adiabatic process, the quantity which remains constant is
(a) pressure
(b) volume
(c) temperature
(d) total heat of the system.

34. If a cyclist moving with a speed of 4.9 m/s on a level road can take a sharp circular turn of radius 4 m, then coefficient of friction between the cycle tyres and road is
(a) 0.51 (b) 0.41
(c) 0.71 (d) 0.61.

35. A particle executes simple harmonic motion with an angular velocity and maximum acceleration of 3.5 rad/sec and 7.5 m/s^2 respectively. Amplitude of the oscillation is
(a) 0.36 (b) 0.28
(c) 0.61 (d) 0.53.

36. A particle of mass m moving with velocity v colloids with a stationary particle of mass $2m$. The speed of the system, after collision, will be
(a) $v/2$ (b) $2v$
(c) $v/3$ (d) $3v$.

37. A stretched rubber has
(a) increased kinetic energy
(b) increased potential energy
(c) decreased kinetic energy
(d) decreased potential energy.

38. Velocity of a body on reaching the point, from which it was projected upwards, is
(a) $v = 2u$ (b) $v = 0$
(c) $v = 0.5u$ (d) $v = u$.

39. If $\vec{P}\cdot\vec{Q} = PQ$, then the angles between $\vec{P}$ and $\vec{Q}$ is
(a) 45° (b) 30°
(c) 60° (d) 0°.

40. How many significant figures are there in 30.00?
(a) 2 (b) 4
(c) 3 (d) 1.

41. Dimensions $[ML^{-1}T^{-1}]$ are related to
(a) torque
(b) work
(c) energy
(d) coefficient of viscosity.

42. The resistance of a galvanometer is 50 Ω and the current required to give full scale deflection is 100 μA. In order to convert into an ammeter for reading upto 10 A, it is necessary to put a resistance of
(a) 5×10^{-5} Ω (b) 5×10^{-3} Ω
(c) 5×10^{-2} Ω (d) 5×10^{-4} Ω.

43. A horizontal platform with an object placed on it is executing SHM in the vertical direction. The amplitude of oscillation is 3.92×10^{-3} m. What must be the least period of these oscillations, so that the object is not detached from the platform?
(a) 0.1556 sec (b) 0.1456 sec
(c) 0.1356 sec (d) 0.1256 sec.

44. Which of the following affects the elasticity of a substance?
(a) impurity of substance
(b) hammering and annaling
(c) change in temperature
(d) all of these.

45. For a particle executing simple harmonic motion, which of the following statements is not correct?
(a) restoring force is maximum at the extreme positions
(b) total energy of the particle always remains the same
(c) restoring force is always directed towards a fixed point
(d) acceleration of the particle is maximum at the equilibrium position.

46. A resonance air column of length 20 cm resonates with a tuning fork of frequency 450 Hz. Ignoring the correction, the velocity of sound in air will be
(a) 920 m/s (b) 720 m/s
(c) 820 m/s (d) 360 m/s.

47. A boy carrying a box on his head is walking on a level road from one place to another on a straight road is doing no work. The statement is
(a) partly correct (b) correct
(c) incorrect (d) insufficient data.

48. When a solid is converted into a gas, directly by heating, then this process is known as
(a) condensation (b) vapourisation
(c) boiling (d) sublimation.

49. The moment of inertia of a regular circular disc of mass 0.4 kg and radius 100 cm about an axis perpendicular to the plane of the disc and passing through its centre is
(a) 0.02 kg-m^2 (b) 0.002 kg-m^2
(c) 0.2 kg-m^2 (d) 2 kg-m^2.

50. Escape velocity of a body when projected from the earth's surface is 11.2 km/s. If it is projected at an angle of 50° from the horizontal, the escape

velocity will be
(a) 11.6 km/s (b) 12.8 km/s
(c) 11.2 km/s (d) 16.2 km/s.

Directions. Q. 51 to 60 : *These questions consist of two statements each, printed as Assertion (A) and Reason (R). While answering these questions you are required to choose any one of the following four responses.*
(a) If both A and R are true, and R is a correct explanation of the A.
(b) If both A and R are true, but R is not a correct explanation of the A.
(c) If A is true, but R is false.
(d) If both A and R are false.

51. *Assertion:* Two adjacent conductors, carrying the same positive charge have a potential difference between them.
Reason: The potential to which a conductor is raised depends upon the charge.

52. *Assertion:* Electrons move away from a region of lower potential to a region of higher potential.
Reason: Since an electron has a negative charge.

53. *Assertion :* The radiation from the sun's surface varies as the fourth power of its absolute temperature.
Reason: The sun is not a black body.

54. *Assertion :* The second postulate of special relativity refers to the velocity of light in vacuum.
Reason: Cerenkov radiation results when particles move through transparent matter at a speed greater than the speed of light in that medium. T is does not violate the second postulate of special relativity.

55. *Assertion :* The kinetic energy of the emitted photo-electrons changes only with a change in the frequency of the incident radiations.
Reason: The kinetic energy of photo-electrons emitted by a photo-sensitive surface depends upon the intensity of the incident radiation.

56. *Assertion:* A hydrogen filled balloon stops rising after it has attained a certain height in the sky.
Reason: The atmospheric pressure decreases with height and becomes zero when maximum height is attained.

57. *Assertion:* Only a change in magnetic flux will maintain an induced current in the coil.
Reason: The presence of large magnetic flux through a coil maintains a current in the coil if the circuit is continuous.

58. *Assertion :* Rydberg's constant varies with the mass number of a given element.
Reason: The reduced mass of the electron is dependent on the mass of the nucleus only.

59. *Assertion:* On a rainy day, it is difficult to drive a car or bus at high speed.
Reason: The value of coefficient of friction is lowered due to wetting of the surface.

60. *Assertion :* Isotopes of an element can be separated by using a mass spectrometer.
Reason: Separation of isotopes is possible because of the difference in electron numbers of isotopes.

CHEMISTRY

61. Atomic orbitals of carbon in carbon dioxide are
(a) sp^2-hybridised (b) sp^3d-hybridised
(c) sp-hybridised (d) sp^3-hybridised.

62. If 300 ml of a gas at 27°C is cooled to 7°C at constant pressure, its final volume will be
(a) 350 ml (b) 540 ml
(c) 135 ml (d) 280 ml.

63. Which of the following will not undergo hydrolysis in water?
(a) ammonium sulphate
(b) sodium sulphate
(c) calcium sulphate
(d) all the salts will hydrolyse.

64. Which of the following statement is true for an electrochemical cell?
(a) H_2 is anode and Cu is cathode
(b) H_2 is cathode and Cu is anode
(c) reduction occurs at H_2 electrode
(d) oxidation occurs at Cu electrode.

65. The radii of F, F^-, O and O^{-2} are in the order of
(a) $O^{2-} > O > F^- > F$ (b) $F^- > O^{2-} > F > O$
(c) $O^{2-} > F^- > F > O$ (d) $O^{2-} > F^- > O > F$.

66. In the reaction:

Phenol $\xrightarrow[CHCl_3]{NaOH}$ A $\xrightarrow{H^+}$ B, B is identified as
(a) benzaldehyde (b) benzene
(c) benzoic acid (d) salicyaldehyde

67. Which of the following has maximum ionisation potential?

(a) Na (b) K
(c) Be (d) Mg.

68. The size of colloidal particle is
(a) 10^{-12} to 10^{-19} m
(b) 10^{-3} to 10^{-9} m
(c) 10^{-9} to 10^{-12} m (d) 10^{-6} to 10^{-9} m.

69. The solubility in water of sulphates down the Be group is Be > Mg > Ca > Sr > Ba. This is due to
(a) higher co-ordination number
(b) high ionisation number
(c) increasing in melting point
(d) all of these.

70. $C_6H_6 \xrightarrow[H_2SO_4]{HNO_3} X \xrightarrow[FeCl_3]{Cl_2} Y$. In the above sequence Y can be
(a) 3-nitrochlorobenzene
(b) 1-nitrochlorobenzene
(c) 4-nitrochlorobenzene
(d) none of these.

71. Which of the following is the best scientific method to test presence of water in a liquid?
(a) use of litmus paper
(b) taste
(c) smell
(d) use of anhydrous copper sulphate.

72. Which of the following are ${}_{16}S^{32}$ and ${}_{15}Pb^{31}$?
(a) isotopes (b) isotones
(c) isobars (d) isomers.

73. Which of the following exhibits the weakest intermolecular forces?
(a) He (b) HCl
(c) NH_3 (d) H_2O.

74. Which of the following does not show electrical conduction?
(a) diamond (b) graphite
(c) sodium (d) potassium.

75. Which of the following transition element shows the highest oxidation state?
(a) Fe (b) Cr
(c) Mn (d) V.

76. The equivalent weight of phosphoric acid (H_3PO_4) in the reaction:
$NaOH + H_3PO_4 \rightarrow NaH_2PO_4 + H_2O$ is
(a) 25 (b) 49
(c) 59 (d) 98.

77. Vinegar is
(a) HCOOH (b) HCHO
(c) CH_3CHO (d) CH_3COOH.

78. Which of the following is a colligative property?
(a) surface tension (b) viscosity
(c) refractive index
(d) osmotic pressure.

79. What is the amount of chlorine evolved, when 2 A of current is passed for 30 minutes in an aqueous solution of NaCl?
(a) 9.81 g (b) 1.32 g
(c) 4.56 g (d) 12.6 g.

80. Pressure in a mixture of 4 g of O_2 and 2 g of H_2 confined in a bulb of 1 litre at 0°C is
(a) 45.215 atm (b) 31.205 atm
(c) 25.215 atm (d) 15.210 atm.

81. The specific conductivity of N/10 KCl solution at 20°C is 0.0212 ohm^{-1} cm^{-1} and the resistance of cell containing this solution at 20° C is 55 ohm. The cell constant is
(a) 2.173 cm^{-1} (b) 1.166 cm^{-1}
(c) 4.616 cm^{-1} (d) 3.324 cm^{-1}.

82. If magnesium atom having atomic number 12 has an isotope with mass number 26, then the number of protons, neutrons and electrons respectively of the atom are
(a) 12, 14, 12 (b) 12, 12, 14
(c) 14, 12, 12 (d) 12, 12, 12.

83. Which of the following compound will not give Cannizzaro's reaction?
(a) $(Me)_3CCHO$ (b) HCHO
(c) CH_3CHO (d) C_6H_5CHO.

84. The rate constant of a first order reaction is 3×10^{-6} per sec. If the initial concentration is 0.10 M, the initial rate of reaction is
(a) 3×10^{-6} Ms^{-1} (b) 3×10^{-5} Ms^{-1}
(c) 3×10^{-8} Ms^{-1} (d) 3×10^{-7} Ms^{-1}.

85. Which oxide of nitrogen is obtained on heating ammonium nitrate at 250°C?
(a) nitrous oxide
(b) nitric oxide
(c) nitrogen dioxide
(d) dinitrogen tetraoxide.

86. Half-life of radium is 1580 years. Its average life will be
(a) 2.275×10^3 years (b) 2.5×10^3 years
(c) 8.825×10^2 years (d) 11.832×10^3 years.

87. The empirical formula of a compound is CH_2O. Its molecular weight is 180. The molecular formula of the compound is
(a) C_4HO_4 (b) $C_5H_{10}O_5$
(c) $C_3H_6O_3$ (d) $C_6H_{12}O_6$.

88. Principal, azimuthal and magnetic quantum numbers are respectively related to
(a) shape, size and orientation
(b) size, shape and orientation
(c) size, orientation and shape
(d) none of these.

89. The common molecular formula for disaccharide is
(a) $C_{12}H_{22}O_{11}$ (b) $C_{10}H_{18}O_8$
(c) $C_{10}H_{20}O_{10}$ (d) $C_{18}H_{22}O_{11}$.

90. Toluene can be oxidised to benzoic acid by
(a) H_2SO_4 (b) $KMnO_4$
(c) $K_2Cr_2O_7$ (d) both (b) and (c).

91. Sodium metal crystallises as a body centred cubic lattice with the cell edge 4.29 Å. What is the radius of sodium atom (in cm)?
(a) 9.312×10^{-7} (b) 1.857×10^{-8}
(c) 2.371×10^{-7} (d) 3.817×10^{-8}.

92. Beilstein test is used for the detection of
(a) Cl (b) Na
(c) N_2 (d) CO_2.

93. Which of the following atoms would be paramagnetic?
(a) Zn (b) Be
(c) Ca (d) N.

94. The weight of a molecule of the compound $C_{60}H_{122}$ is
(a) 5.025×10^{23} g (b) 16.023×10^{23} g
(c) 1.4×10^{-21} g (d) 1.09×10^{-21} g.

95. Which of the following is the correct statement for PH_3?
(a) it is less poisonous than NH_3
(b) it is less basic than NH_3
(c) electronegativity of PH_3 is $>NH_3$
(d) it does not show reducing properties.

96. $CuSO_4$ reacts with KCN solution and forms
(a) $K_3[Cu(CN)_4]$ (b) Cu(CN)
(c) $Cu(CN)_2$ (d) $K_4[Cu(CN)_6]$.

97. Density ratio of O_2 and H_2 is 16 : 1. The ratio of their r.m.s velocities will be
(a) 1 : 4 (b) 1 : 16
(c) 4 : 1 (d) 16 : 1.

98. Which of the following equation does not obey the law of conservation of mass?
(a) $4H + O_2 \rightarrow 2H_2O$ (b) $H_2 + O \rightarrow 2H_2O$
(c) $2H + O_2 \rightarrow H_2O$ (d) both (b) and (c).

99. If benzene reacts with Cl_2 in presence of ultraviolet light then which of the following is formed?
(a) CCl_4 (b) C_6Cl_6
(c) C_6H_5Cl (d) $C_6H_6Cl_6$.

100. Which of the following is the strongest acid?
(a) HClO (b) $HClO_3$
(c) $HClO_2$ (d) $HClO_4$.

101. Benzaldehyde can be prepared by the hydrolysis of
(a) benzyl chloride
(b) benzotrichloride
(c) banzal chloride (d) benzo nitrite.

102. Which of the following metal is present in brass, bronze and german-silver?
(a) Cu (b) Na
(c) Mg (d) Al.

103. The propene reacts with HBr to form
(a) hexane (b) bromopropane
(c) propane (d) ethane.

104. The correct order of the increasing ionic character is
(a) $BeCl_2 < MgCl_2 < BaCl_2 < CaCl_2$
(b) $BeCl_2 < MgCl_2 < CaCl_2 < BaCl_2$
(c) $BeCl_2 < BaCl_2 < MgCl_2 < CaCl_2$
(d) $BaCl_2 < CaCl_2 < MgCl_2 < BeCl_2$.

105. The meta-directing group in the following is
(a) OH (b) NH_2
(c) CH_3 (d) NO_2.

106. Internal energy does not include
(a) rotational energy (b) vibrational energy
(c) nuclear energy
(d) energy gravitational pull.

107. The specific heat of a metal is 0.16. Its approximate atomic weight would be
(a) 40 (b) 16
(c) 32 (d) 64.

108. The vapour pressure of benzene at a certain temperature is 640 mm of Hg. A non-volatile and non-electrolyte solid weighing 2.175 g is added to 39.08 g of benzene. The vapour pressure of the solution is 600 mm of Hg. What is the molecular weight of solid substance?
(a) 69.60 (b) 49.59
(c) 59.60 (d) 108.30.

109. Which among the following has the largest dipole moment?
(a) HI (b) H_2O
(c) NH_3 (d) SO_3.

110. Oxidation state of osmium (Os) in OsO_4 is
(a) +4 (b) +6
(c) +7 (d) +8.

Directions. Q. 111 to 120 : *These questions consist of two statements each, printed as Assertion (A) and Reason (R). While answering these questions you are required to choose any one of the following four responses.*
(a) If both A and R are true, and R is a correct explanation of the A.
(b) If both A and R are true, but R is not a correct explanation of the A.
(c) If A is true, but R is false.
(d) If both A and R are false.

111. *Assertion:* Xenon forms fluorides.
Reason: Because 5d-orbitals are available for valence shell expansion.

112. *Assertion:* Identification of cathode and anode is done by the use of a thermometer.
Reason: Higher is the value of reduction potential, greater would be its reducing power.

113. *Assertion:* Zinc displaces copper from copper sulphate solution.
Reason: The $E°_{298}$ of Zn is -0.76 volts and that of Cu is +0.34 volts.

114. *Assertion:* Reaction of conc. H_2SO_4 on NaBr and NaI does not give HBr and HI.
Reason: HBr and HI are oxidised by conc. H_2SO_4 to Br_2 and I_2.

115. *Assertion:* Taillag of mercury occurs on passing ozone through it.
Reason: Due to oxidation of mercury.

116. *Assertion:* Bond order can assume any value number including zero.
Reason: Higher the bond order, shorter is bond length and greater is bond energy.

117. *Assertion:* The dipole moment helps to predict whether a molecule is polar or nonpolar.
Reason: The dipole moment helps to predict geometry of molecules.

118. *Assertion:* Lower aldehydes and ketones are soluble in water but the solubility decreases as the molecular masses increase.
Reason: Distinction between aldehydes and ketones can be made by Tollen's test.

119. *Assertion:* The term tautomerism was introduced by Maxwell in order to explain the chemical reactivity of a substance according to two possible structures
Reason: Metamers can also be chain isomers or position isomers.

120. *Assertion:* Equivalent conductance of all electrolytes decreases with increasing concentration.
Reason: Lesser number of ions are available per g equivalent at higher concentration.

BIOLOGY

121. Which of the following chambers of the heart has the thickest muscular wall?
(a) left atrium (b) right atrium
(c) right ventricle (d) left ventricle.

122. Which gland plays a key role in metamorphosis of frog's tadpole?
(a) thymus (b) thyroid
(c) pancreas (d) adrenal.

123. Weberian ossicles are found in
(a) fishes (b) frogs
(c) snakes (d) birds.

124. Inflammatory response, in allergy, is caused by the release of
(a) histamines (b) antigen
(c) antibodies (d) prothrombin.

125. XO-chromosomal abnormality in human beings causes
(a) Turner's syndrome
(b) Down's syndrome
(c) Klinefelter's syndrome
(d) none of these.

126. If a person is injured, he should be given blood. Which of the following blood groups should be given without checking the patient's own blood group?
(a) B (b) A
(c) AB (d) O.

127. Which of the following hormones is a derivative of amino acid?
(a) prostaglandin (b) progesterone
(c) epinephrine (d) estrogen.

128. Liver in our body stores
(a) vitamin D (b) vitamin A
(c) vitamin B_{12} (d) all of these.

129. Cumulus covers
(a) ovum (b) ovary
(c) embryo (d) all of these.

130. The function of renin is
(a) stimulation of corpus luteum
(b) vasodilation
(c) to reduce blood pressure
(d) degradation of angiotensinogen.

131. Which of the following is the example of conditioned reflex?
(a) hand withdraws when piered with a needle
(b) eyes closed, when anything enter into it
(c) during digestion food goes forward in alimentary canal
(d) trained dog salivates when you ring a bell.

132. The heartbeat increases at the time of interview due to
(a) secretion of adrenaline
(b) corticotrophic hormone
(c) hyper secretion of renin
(d) autidiuretic hormone secretion.

133. The component of blood which prevents its coagulation in the blood vessels is
(a) haemoglobin (b) plasma
(c) thrombin (d) heparin.

134. Conn's disease is caused by the over-secretion of
(a) aldosterone (b) ADH
(c) ACTH (d) none of these.

135. The extra embryonic membranes of mammalian embryo are derived from
(a) inner cell mass (b) formative cells
(c) trophblast (d) follicle cells.

136. Which one of the following is true during ageing?
(a) increasing in calcium content of arteries and cartilage
(b) decrease in blood urea and GFR
(c) decrease in cholesterol content of cornea and lens
(d) decrease in calcium content of arteries and cartilage.

137. The end-product of ornithine cycle is
(a) carbon dioxide (b) uric acid
(c) urea (d) ammonia.

138. Wings of pigeon, mosquito and bat show
(a) divergent evolution
(b) atavism
(c) convergent evolution
(d) all of these.

139. First step of utilisation of glucose in metabolism is
(a) glycogen (b) ATP
(c) pyruvic acid
(d) glucose-6-phosphate.

140. *Otorhinolaryngology* is the study of
(a) bird's anatomy (b) ENT
(c) brain cells (d) locomotory system.

141. If one strand of DNA has the nitrogenous base sequence ATGCTTGA, the sequence in the complementary strand will be
(a) TAGGTAGT
(b) TACGTACT
(c) TACGAACT (d) TCCGAACT.

142. When a bacteriophage, in its lytic phase, carries some of the bacterium partially digested chromosome with it to another host cell, the process is called
(a) generalised transduction
(b) conjugation
(c) transformation
(d) specialised transduction.

143. Restriction endonucleases are utilised in genetic engineering as
(a) molecular scalpers for cutting DNA at specific sites
(b) molecular builder of nucleotides
(c) molecular degradation to DNA break up
(d) molecular cement for combining DNA bits into long chains.

144. The major component of bacterial cell wall is a polymer called
(a) chitin (b) xylan
(c) cellulose (d) peptidoglycan.

145. Bryophytes are not characterised by
(a) vascular tissues
(b) well-developed root system
(c) alternation of generation
(d) presence of chlorophyll.

146. Hormogonia are the vegetative reproductive structures of
(a) *Oscillatoria*
(b) *Ulothrix*
(c) *Spirogyra*
(d) *Chlamydomonas*.

147. The protein coat of virus is called
(a) capsomeres (b) prions
(c) viriod (d) capsid.

148. The organelle found between cell wall of two cells is called
(a) lomasome (b) lysosome
(c) microsome (d) middle lamella.

149. The *correct* sequence in cell cycle is
(a) $S - M - G_1 - G_2$ (b) $S - G_1 - G_2 - M$
(c) $G_1 - S - G_2 - M$ (d) $M - G_1 - G_2 - S$.

150. Sporogony of malarial parasite occurs in
(a) stomach wall of mosquito
(b) salivary glands of mosquito
(c) RBCs of man
(d) liver of man.

151. In spermatogenesis, the acrosome of sperm is formed by
(a) golgi complex (b) mitochondria
(c) lysosome (d) nucleus.

152. Paired spermathecae occur in *Pheretima* in which of the following segments?
(a) 6, 7, 8, 9 (b) 4, 5, 6, 7
(c) 5, 6, 7, 8 (d) 3, 4, 5, 6.

153. Kidney of adult reptiles are
(a) metanephric (b) mesonephric
(c) protonephric (d) all of these.

154. The familiar disease Amoebiasis is caused by
(a) *Taenia solium*
(b) *Wuchereria bancrofti*
(c) *Entamoeba histolytica*
(d) *Ascaris lumbricoides*.

155. Secondary phloem remains functional generally
(a) less than 1 year
(b) more than 1 year
(c) for 1 year
(d) as long as plant lives.

156. The movement of lamina lobe of Dionaea is
(a) thigmonastic (b) photonastic
(c) seismonastic (d) thermonastic.

157. Casparian strips are the characteristics of
(a) cortex (b) endodermis
(c) pericycle (d) pith.

158. The crystals of calcium carbonate, which appear like a bunch of grapes in epidermal cells of the leaves of some plants, are called
(a) sphaeraphides (b) raphides
(c) otoliths (d) cystoliths.

159. Anemophilous flowers have
(a) small, smooth stigma
(b) coloured flower
(c) sessile stigma
(d) large feathery stigma.

160. The root cell of wheat plant has 42 chromosomes. What would be the number of chromosomes in the synergid cell?
(a) 21 (b) 7
(d) 28 (d) 14.

161. The high energy bonds of ATP are between
(a) C – O (b) O – P
(c) C – N (d) C – C.

162. Which of the following is responsible for the mechanical support, protein synthesis and enzyme transport?
(a) cell membrane
(b) mitochondria
(c) dictyosome
(d) endoplasmic reticulum.

163. The vascular cambium and cork cambium are the examples of
(a) apical meristem
(b) lateral meristem
(c) intercalary meristem
(d) elements of xylem and phloem.

164. Crop rotation is used by farmers to increase
(a) nitrogenous content of soil
(b) organic content of soil
(c) soil fertility
(d) all of these.

165. The food chain, in which micro-organisms break-down the energy rich compounds synthesises by producers is called
(a) ecosystem
(b) detritus food chain
(c) parasitic food chain
(d) predator food chain.

166. Obligate parasites are those organisms which
(a) live only on living host
(b) are essentially parasites but can also become saprophyte
(c) live only on dead and decaying organic matter
(d) are essentially saprophytes but can also becomes parasites.

167. If a homozygous red-flowered plant is crossed with a homozygous white-flowered plant, the offsprings will be
(a) half-white flowered
(b) half red-flowered
(c) all white-flowered
(d) all red-flowered.

168. Nitrous acid causes mutation by
(a) acting as a base analogue
(b) addition of a base pair
(c) hydrolysing base sugar linkage
(d) removing amino group from the bases.

169. Ficus is an example of which kind of inflorescence?
(a) raceme (b) spike
(c) cyathium (d) hypanthodium.

170. Which of the following reduces plant growth and induces dormancy?
(a) cytokinin (b) auxin
(c) xylene (d) abscisic acid.

Directions. Q. 171 to 180 : *These questions consist of two statements each, printed as Assertion (A) and Reason (R). While answering these questions you are required to choose any one of the following four responses.*
(a) If both A and R are true, and R is a correct explanation of the A.
(b) If both A and R are true, but R is not a correct explanation of the A.
(c) If A is true, but R is false.
(d) If both A and R are false.

171. *Assertion:* If you burn a plant, its nitrogen component is given off as ammonia and other gases.
Reason: Hydroponics does not allow plants to grow well if they are supplied with all the mineral nutrients they need.

172. *Assertion:* Co-enzyme is a non-protein group without which certain enzymes are inactive or incomplete.
Reason: Co-enzymes not only provide a point of attachment of the chemical group being transformed but also influence the properties of the group.

173. *Assertion:* Soil particles, particularly clay and organic matter in soil, contain negative charges that attract positively-charged ions such as Ca^{++}, K^{+} and Mg^{++}.
Reason: This attraction keeps these ions at a soil level where they are available to plants.

174. *Assertion:* Wax, resin and suberin coating on the surface of plant parts reduce the rate of transpiration.
Reason: These adaptations are found mostly in xerophytes.

175. *Assertion:* Light is very important external factor of transpiration.
Reason: Light induces stomatal opening and darkness stomatal closure. Thus the rate of transpiration increased in light and decreases in dark.

176. *Assertion:* Rhizobial aggregates have been observed at distinct sites on curled root hairs.
Reason: The infection thread is formed by a process of invagination of the hair cell walls in the region of curling.

177. *Assertion:* It is the brain, not the sense organs, that interprets the stimulus.
Reason: Sense organs are transducers. They transform the energy of a stimulus to the energy of nerve impulses.

178. *Assertion:* Adenine cannot pair with cytosine.
Reason: Because there would be two hydrogen atoms one at the bonding positions and none at the other.

179. *Asserion:* Cartilage (protein matrix) and bone (calcium matrix) are rigid connective tissues.
Reason: Blood is connective tissue in which plasma is the matrix.

180. *Assertion:* Hair cells on the basilar membrane (organ of corti) are responsible for hearing
Reason: Pressure waves, which begin at the oval windows, cause the basilar membrane to vibrate so that the cilia of the hair cells touch the tectorial membrane. This causes the hair cells to initiate nerve impulses, which are carried by the auditory nerve to the brain.

GENERAL KNOWLEDGE

181. Seoul is the capital of
(a) Japan (b) South Korea
(c) Afganisthan (d) Philippines.

182. The Nobel Prize for physiology and Medicine for the year 1998 was given for the discovery of
(a) invading germs (b) prion
(c) viagra (d) streptomycin.

183. AIDS is caused by
(a) helminth (b) streptomycin
(c) virus (d) bacteria.

184. Hirakund dam is constructed on which of the following rivers?
(a) Ganga (b) Kosi
(c) Sutlej (d) Mahanadi.

185. Which of the following is a cave temple in India?
(a) Ellora (b) Mahabalipuram
(c) Perli (d) Tuljapur.

186. The person who served as the President of India twice, was
(a) Dr. Zakir hussain (b) V.V. Giri
(c) S. Radhakrishnan (d) Dr. Rajendra Prasad.

187. How many countries have adopted the Euro currency?
(a) 7 (b) 6
(c) 9 (d) 11.

188. Which of the following is responsible for the disease 'dropsy'?
(a) *Brassica oleracea*
(b) *Argemone maxicana*
(c) *Brassica compestris*
(d) *Oenothera lamarckiana.*

189. Who won the Filmfare Award for Best Feature Film in 1998?
(a) *Satya*
(b) *Zakhmi*
(c) *Ziddi*
(d) *Kuch Kuch Hota Hai.*

190. Hari Prasad Chaurasia is related to which of the following instruments?
(a) Table (b) Santoor
(c) Flute (d) Violin.

191. Fundamental duties were introduced in the Constitution by the
(a) 40th Amendment (b) 42nd Amendment
(c) 48th Amendment (d) 53rd Amendment.

192. In which country did tea originate?
(a) England (b) India
(c) Thailand (d) China.

193. The great anthology of poems Madhushala was composed by

(a) Mahadevi verma
(b) Mulk Raj Anand
(c) Surendra Sharma
(d) Harvansh Rai Bachchan.

194. Ecology is the branch of science, which deals with
(a) soil's surface
(b) human anatomy
(c) cell structure
(d) balance of nature.

195. Which of the following countries is not a member of SAARC?
(a) Nepal (b) Myanmar
(c) Maldives (d) Bangladesh.

196. Which of the following vitamins is required in bone formation?
(a) B (b) A
(c) C (d) D.

197. The dance of India which contains solo performance is
(a) *Dandia* (b) *Disco*
(c) *Bhangra* (d) *Bharatnatyam.*

198. The Fifth Pay Commission was headed by Justice
(a) Anand (b) Pandian
(c) Ahmad (d) Vadhwa.

199. Which of the following pairs is incorrect?
(a) Abdul Fazal - Author
(b) Kapil - Cricket
(c) Feroz Gandhi - Politics
(d) M.F. Hussain - Actor.

200. Which of the following missiles of India has the longest range?
(a) *Akash* (b) *Pinaka*
(c) *Prithvi* (d) both (a) and (b).

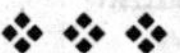

SOLUTIONS

PHYSICS

1. **(c)** : As the interior of the sun is at a very high temperature (of the order of 8000 K), nuclear fusion is the highly possible reaction taking place inside the sun to produce energy.

2. **(d)** : Suppose S_1 and S_2 are the slits at a distance d from each other. Distance of screen be D. Let P be a point where there is a bright fringe. A glass plate is placed in the path of the ray from S_1 to P.
We know that the path difference between the rays in absence of glass plate is $\Delta x = S_2P - S_1P = \frac{dy}{D}$
In presence of the glass plate, the optical path length of the ray from S_1 to P will be different. The total optical path length for this ray is given by

$$S_1P - t + \mu t$$
$$= S_1P + (\mu - 1)t$$

Where μ is the refractive index of the glass plate and t is its thickness.
Hence the new path difference is given by

$$\Delta x' = S_2P - [S_1P + (\mu - 1)t]$$
$$= \Delta x - (\mu - 1)t$$
$$= \frac{dy}{D} - (\mu - 1)t$$

For a bright fringe, $\Delta x' = n\lambda$
and $y = yn$ = distance of the bright fringe from the central fringe

$$\therefore \frac{dy_n}{D} - (\mu - 1)t = n\lambda$$
$$\Rightarrow y_n = \frac{D}{d}[(\mu - 1)t + n\lambda]$$
$$\therefore y_{n+1} - y_n = \omega = \frac{D\lambda}{d}$$

Hence the fringe width remains constant.

3. **(d)** : When a charged particle enters a magnetic field, the particle experiences a Lorentz force given by $\vec{F} = q(\vec{v} \times \vec{B})$, which act in a direction perpendicular to both $\vec{v}$ and $\vec{B}$. Now since the initial velocity of the particle makes an angle 45° with the magnetic field, it will be having a velocity component parallel to $\vec{B}$ and another component perpendicular to $\vec{B}$. The parallel component of velocity is going to experience no force, so it will remain the same but as the perpendicular component will experience a constant force in the normal plane, hence the particle will finally move in a helical path.

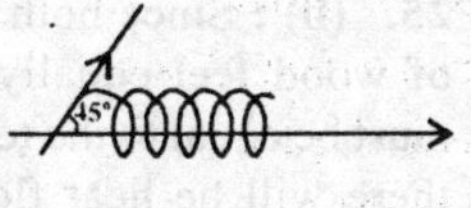

4. **(a)** : Diode is a device which allows to pass a current only when it is forward baised. That's why if we use one alternating voltage source instead of a battery, during the negative cycles the diode will be reverse biased and will not allow the current to flow. Hence it can be used as a rectifier.

(Forward bias of diode)

5. **(d)** : N–type semiconductors are those formed by doping the intrinsic semiconductor with an element which has got more outer most shell electrons than the parent instrinsic semiconductor. When this sort of an element is used for doping, we get more free electrons in the semiconductor and so the majority charge carriers is electrons.

6. **(b)** 7. **(c)**

8. **(c)** : The stationary or standing wave is a superposition of two waves of equal amplitude and frequency moving in opposite direction to each other and so there is no movement of the particles of the medium. That's why there is no transfer of energy in the case of standing waves.

9. **(b)** : A choke will has got high inductance and low resistance. Since an inductor is a non-resistive device, it does not consume any power in the form of heat like a resistance. That's why we use a low resistance and a high inductance in a choke to save power.

10. **(b)** : Since the resistances R_2 and R_3 are in parallel, their equivalent resistance will be $R_{23} = \frac{4 \times 4}{2 \times 4} = 2\ \Omega$
Now the equivalent circuit will be

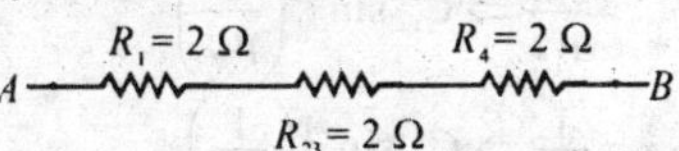

There are three resistances in series. Therefore the equivalent resistance will be $R_{AB} = 2 + 2 + 2 = 6\ \Omega$.

11. (d)

12. (a) : To reduce the plate current to zero V_P should be reduced to zero. Hence for $I_P = 0$.

$\Delta V_P = 0 - 300$
$= -300$ V

We know that amplification factor,

$$\mu = \left(\frac{\Delta V_P}{\Delta V_G}\right)_{\Delta I_P = \text{constant}}$$

$$\therefore \Delta V_G = \frac{\Delta V_P}{\mu}$$

$$= -\frac{300}{20}$$

$$= -15$$

$\therefore$ Required Grid voltage is -15 V.

13. (d)

14. (c) : When fast cathode rays strike a metal surface with high melting point, the cathode rays might transfer its K.E. to an electron in an inner shell, which eventually might come out of the metal surface. Due to the vacancy created in an inner orbit, some outer orbit electron might jump down to fill up the gap thereby emitting some electromagnetic radiation known as x-rays.

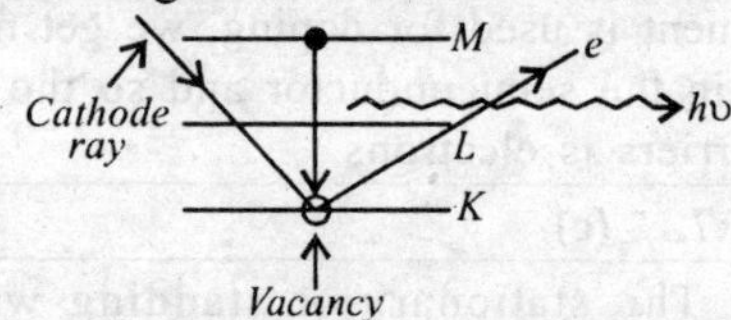

15. (c) : We know that the radius of the nth orbit of a hydrogen like atom/ion is given by

$r_n = n^2 a_0$ where

a_0 = Bohr radius = radius of the ground state of the hydrogen atom

$\therefore r_n \propto n^2$

16. (d)

17. (d) : We know that

$1 \text{ e} = 1.6 \times 10^{-19}$ C

$$\Rightarrow 1\text{C} = \frac{1}{1.6 \times 10^{-19}} = 6.25 \times 10^{18} \text{ electrons}$$

18. (c) : We know that the critical angle for water and glass are given by,

$$\sin C_w = \frac{1}{\mu_w} \Rightarrow C_w \sin^{-1}\left(\frac{1}{\mu_w}\right)$$

$$\sin C_g = \frac{1}{\mu_g} \Rightarrow C_g \sin^{-1}\left(\frac{1}{\mu_g}\right)$$

since $\mu_w < \mu_g$

$$\Rightarrow \frac{1}{\mu_w} > \frac{1}{\mu_g}$$

$$\Rightarrow \sin^{-1}\left(\frac{1}{\mu_w}\right) > \sin^{-1}\left(\frac{1}{\mu_g}\right)$$

$$\therefore C_w > C_g$$

19. (a) 20. (c) 21. (b)

22. (b) : If A is the area of the coil, there are N turns in the coil, ω being the angular velocity of the armature, then the flux through each turn in time t is given by

$$\phi = BA \cos \omega t$$

Using Faraday's Law, the emf induced in each turn of the coil is

$$-\frac{d\phi}{dt} = BA\omega \sin\omega t$$

The total induced emf in the coil

$$\varepsilon = NBA\omega \sin\omega t$$

Now if we double ω, ε will be doubled.

23. (b) : In a step-down transformer, the voltage in the secondary is less than the voltage in the primary circuit. That is $\varepsilon_2 < \varepsilon_1$. Since we know for an ideal transformer

$$\varepsilon_2 i_2 = \varepsilon_1 i_1$$

$$\Rightarrow i_2 = \frac{\varepsilon_1}{\varepsilon_2} i_1$$

$$\Rightarrow i_2 > i_1$$

$\therefore$ The current in the secondary increases.

24. (a) : The idea behind a transformer is to supply the power generated by a power plant to the users without much loss of energy. Since the power plants are normally situated for away from the users, it needs to carry the power for several hundred kilometers through transmission lines. But in so doing, lot of energy is wasted in the form of joule heating i^2Rt. So in this situation we use a transformer to step-up the voltage, so that the current decreases, thereby decreasing the joule heating also. And finally we use a step-down transfomer to reduce the voltage and increase the current, so that the power transferred remains the same.

25. (b) : Since both the block of metal and the block of wood feel equally cold or hot, their temperatures must be equal to the temperature of the body. Otherwise there will be heat flow between the body and either of the blocks. And as the thermal conductivity of the metal is more than that of the wood, it would either feel more hot or more cold than that the block of wood.

26. (d) : Interference is a characteristic of all wave motion, any sort of wave can show interference phenomenon.

27. (a) : On a clear atomsphere, the scattering centres are mainly the air molecules whose dimension is of the order of the wavelenth of light. We know that amount of scattering is proportional to $\frac{1}{\lambda^4}$. Hence red light is the least scattered and more scattering occurs towards the blue end of the spectrum. And on a clear day, as light (blue end) is scattered uniformaly, the sky appears blue.

28. (a) : Given :

Number of turns in the primary $N_1 = 500$

Number of turns in the secondary $N_2 = 5000$

Input voltage $V_1 = 20\text{V}$

Output voltage $V_2 = ?$

We know that

$$|V_2| = \frac{N_2}{N_1} V_1$$

$$= \frac{5000}{500} \times 20 = 200 \text{ V}$$

As in a transfomer the output frequency of the ac supply remains the same as that of the input supply, the frequency of the output current will be 50 Hz.

29. (b)

30. (c) : When the north pole of a magent is brought near a metallic ring, the induced current produced in the ring will be such that it opposes the growth of current in the ring. That's why by Lenz's law, there must be a magnetic north pole created in the ring so that it can repel the approaching north pole.

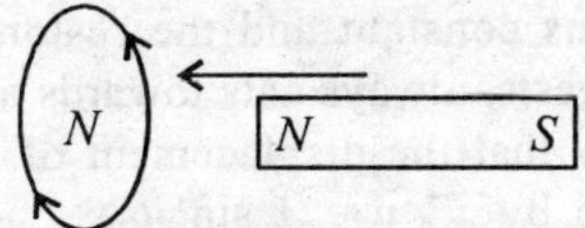

Now the direction of the current will be clockwise if we view it from behind the ring and it wil be anticlockwise if we view it from above.

31. (a) : We know that the frequency of a mechanical wave created in a string is given by

$$\upsilon = \frac{1}{2\pi}\sqrt{\frac{T}{m}}$$

$\therefore$ To double the vibrations, tension T has to be raised by a factor of 4.

32. (a) : We know that the K.E of one mole of a gas molecules at a temperature T is given by $K = \frac{3}{2}KT$

Now, $T_1 = 27°\text{C} = 300\ K$

$K_1 = 6.21 \times 10^{-21}$ J

$T_2 = 227°\text{C} = 500\ K$

$K_2 = ?$

We have, $\frac{K_1}{K_2} = \frac{T_1}{T_2} \Rightarrow K_2 = \frac{T_1}{T_2} \times K_1 = \frac{500}{300} \times 6.21 \times 10^{-21}$

$= 10.35 \times 10^{-21}$ J

33. (d) : Adiabatic processes are those in which there is no transfer of energy between the system and the surrounding. Therefore the total heat of the system remains conserved in an adiabatic process.

34. (d) : We know that while a cyclist moving with a speed v takes a sharp turn on a circular track of radius r, the coefficient of friction is given by

$$\mu = \tan\theta = \frac{v^2}{rg}$$

Here $v = 4.9$ m/s

$r = 4$ m

and $g = 9.8\ \text{m/s}^2$

$$\therefore \mu = \frac{4.9 \times 4.9}{4 \times 9.8} = 0.61$$

35. (c) : The angular velocity $\omega = 3.5$ red/sec

maximum acceleration $a_{max} = 7.5\ \text{m/s}^2$

We know for a SHM, the displacement

$$x = A \sin\omega t$$

$$\therefore \quad v = \frac{dx}{dt} = A\omega \cos\omega t$$

$$\therefore \quad a = \frac{dv}{dt} = -A\omega^2 \sin\omega t$$

$\therefore$ Maximum acceleration

$$|a_{max}| = A\omega^2$$

Now $A\omega^2 = 7.5$

$$\Rightarrow \quad A = \frac{7.5}{\omega^2}$$

$$= \frac{7.5}{(3.5)^2} = 0.6$$

$\therefore$ Amplitude $= 0.6$

36. (c) : $\overset{m}{\text{O}} \xrightarrow{v\rightarrow} \underset{2m}{\overset{v=0}{\text{O}}}$

Here $m_1 = m$

$m_2 = 2m$

$v_1 = v$

$v_2 = 0$

Let the speed of the system after collison $= v$

Using the principle of conservation of linear momentum

$$m_1v_1 + m_2v_2 = (m_1 + m_2)v'$$

$$\Rightarrow v' = \frac{mv + 2m \times 0}{m + 2m} = \frac{mv}{3m} = \frac{v}{3}$$

37. (b)

38. (d) : Let the intial *velocity of* the body = u And final velocity at the intial point be v. Now the potential energy of the body at the point of projection is the same in both the upward and the downward journey. Since the total energy of the system has to be conserved, the kinetic energies at that point must also be the same in both the journeys

$$\therefore \frac{1}{2}mv^2 = \frac{1}{2}mu^2 \Rightarrow v = u$$

39. (d) : $\vec{P}\cdot\vec{Q} = PQ$

$$\Rightarrow PQ\cos\theta = PQ$$

$$\Rightarrow \cos\theta = 1$$

$$\Rightarrow \theta = 0^\circ$$

40. (b)

41. (d) : Torque is defined as

$$\vec{\tau} = \vec{r} \times \vec{F}$$

$\therefore$ Dimensions of torque $[\tau] = [r] \times [F]$

$= [L] \times [MLT^{-2}]$

$= [ML^2T^{-2}]$

Similarly for work and energy the dimensions are same as that of torque *i.e.* $[ML^2T^{-2}]$

Now for viscosity, we know that

$$F = 6\pi\eta r v$$

$$\Rightarrow \eta = \frac{F}{6\pi r v}$$

$$\therefore [\eta] = \frac{F}{[r][v]} = \frac{[MLT^{-2}]}{[L][LT^{-1}]}$$

$$= [ML^{-1}T^{-1}]$$

$\therefore$ The given dimensions are related to the coefficient of viscosity.

42. (d) : The resistance of the galvanometer $G = 50\ \Omega$ The current required for a full scale diflection $I_{FS} = 100\ \mu$ A

$\therefore$ The voltage applied across the galvanometer

$$E = 50 \times 100 \times 10^{-6}$$

$$= 5 \times 10^{-3}\ \text{V} = 5\ \text{mV}$$

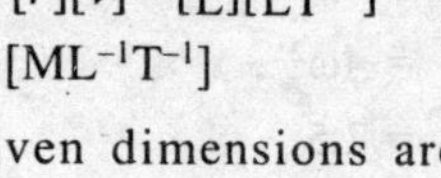

Now to convert this galvanometer into an ammeter we need to put a shunt S in parallel with the galvanometer. The total resistance will be determined by the maximum current read by the ammeter which is 10 A

$$\therefore R = \frac{E}{I} = \frac{5 \times 10^{-3}}{10} = 5 \times 10^{-4}\Omega$$

We can find S from the relation

$$\frac{1}{R} = \frac{1}{S} + \frac{1}{G}$$

$$\Rightarrow \frac{1}{S} = \frac{1}{R} - \frac{1}{G} = \frac{1}{5 \times 10^{-4}} - \frac{1}{50}$$

$$= \frac{10^5}{50} - \frac{1}{50} \cong \frac{10^5}{50}$$

$$\therefore S = \frac{50}{10^5} = 5 \times 10^{-4}\ \Omega$$

43. (d) : As the platform is executing SHM, its time period will be minimum when it has the maximum acceleration. We know that in SHM, the maximum acceleration is given by

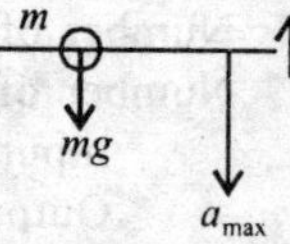

$$a_{max} = \omega^2 A$$

Now if the body is not to be detached from the platform, a_{max} should be less than the acceleration due to gravity. In the limiting case,

$$a_{max} = g$$

$$\Rightarrow \omega^2 A = g$$

$$\frac{4\pi^2 A}{T^2} = g$$

$$\Rightarrow T = 2\pi\sqrt{\frac{A}{g}} = 2\pi \times \sqrt{\frac{3.92 \times 10^{-4}}{9.8}}$$

$$\therefore T_{min} = 0.1256\ \text{sec.}$$

44. (d)

45. (d) : The restoring force in a SHM is given by $F = -Kx \Rightarrow$ if x is maximum F is also maximum. Hence the restoring force is maximum at the extreme positions. In SHM the total energy of the particle always remains constant and the restoring force as the name suggests, always acts towards a fixed point.

We know that the displacement of a particle in SHM is given by $y = A\sin\omega t$

$$\Rightarrow v = \frac{dy}{dt} = A\omega\cos\omega t$$

$$\therefore a = \frac{dy}{dt} = -A\omega^2\sin\omega t$$

$$\therefore \frac{a^2}{A^2\omega^4} + \frac{v^2}{A^2\omega^2} = 1 \Rightarrow a^2 = \omega^2[A^2\omega^2 - v^2]$$

From this expression, it is clear that if v is maximum a is minimum and if v is minimum, a is maximum. As in the equilibrium position, the velocity is maximum, the acceleration is going to be minimum. Hence expression (d) is incorrect.

46. (d) : We know that the minimum length of the air column in a resonance tube corresponds to the fundamental mode of vibrations. Hence by ignoring end correction.

$$l = \frac{\lambda}{4}$$

$$\Rightarrow \lambda = 4l = 4 \times 20 = 80 \text{ cm} = 0.8 \text{ m}$$

Resonant frequency $\upsilon = 450$ Hz

$\therefore$ Speed of sound $\quad v = \nu\lambda$

$$= 450 \times 0.8 = 360 \text{ m/s}$$

47. (b) : We know that the work done is product of the force and the displacement caused by the force on the body along the direction of the force. But here as the weight of the body is not causing any displacement, work done is zero.

48. (d)

49. (c) : The moment of inertia of a disc of radius R about an axis perpendicular to the disc and passing through the centre is given by

$$I = \frac{1}{2}MR^2$$

$$= \frac{1}{2} \times 0.4 \times 1^2 = 0.2 \text{ Kg m}^2$$

50. (c) : The escape velocity of a body projected from the earth's surface is independent of the angle of projection. Hence the escape velocity of the body projected at an angle 50° will also be 11.2 km/s

51. (b) : Let us consider two spherical shells of radii r_1 and r_2 which are possessing the same positive charge Q. Therefore the potential on the surface of each conductor will be

$$V_1 = \frac{KQ}{r_1}$$

$$V_2 = \frac{KQ}{r_2}$$

Since $r_1 \neq r_2$, $V_1 \neq V_2$ and consequently there will be a potential difference between the two conductors.

52. (a) : V_1 (A) —— E ——> V_2 (B), $V_1 > V_2$

Suppose A and B are two regions having potentials V_1 and V_2 such that $V_1 > V_2$. So the electric field will be set up from A to B (*i.e.* from higher potential to lower potential). Now since the electron has got a negative charge, the force experienced by the electron will be in a direction opposite to the direction of the electric field. Hence the electrons move from a region of lower potential to a region of higher potential due to their negative charges.

53. (c) : At as high a temperatrue as 6000 K, the sun acts like a perfect blackbody emitting complete radiation. That's why the radiation coming from the sun's surface follows Stefen's law which states that the energy radiated per unit area per unit time varies as the fourth power of absolute temperature, *i.e.*

$$E = \sigma T^4$$

54. (b) : The second postulate of special theory of relativity states that no material particle can cross the speed of light in vacuum. Cerenkov radiation occurs when some particles move through a transparent medium such as water with a speed more than the speed of light in the medium. So the existence of Cerenkov radiation tells us that the speed of light in a transparent medium can be crossed by a material particle in some circumstances. But this does not violate the second postulate of special theory of relativity as it deals with the speed in vacuum.

55. (c) : Einstein's photoelectric equation states that

$$h\upsilon = h\upsilon_0 + KE_{max}$$

$$\Rightarrow KE_{max} = h\upsilon - h\upsilon_0 = h\upsilon - W$$

Where $W = h\upsilon_0$ = work function of the material

Therefore we see that the maximum kinetic energy of the emitted photoelctrons depends directly on the frequency of the incident radiations. It does not depend upon the intensity of the light used.

56. (b) : The atmospheric pressure is due to the force exerted by the atmosphere on the region below it. But a hydrogen filled balloon rises up in the atmosphere due to density difference only. As the density of hydrogen gas is less than that of air, the hydrogen filled balloon rises up in the air. But as we know that density of air also keeps on decreasing as we move up, so there will be a point up in the atmosphere where the rising balloon will find that its density is same as that of the surrounding atmosphere. As there is no density difference between the balloon and the atomsphere, the balloon will stop rising.

57. (c) : Induced current (emf) in a coil is directly propertional to the rate of change of magnetic flux linked with the coil. If there is no change in the flux, there is no induced current also.

58. (d) : We know that the Rydberg constant is given

by $R = \frac{13.6\text{eV}}{hc}$, which is independent of the mass number of an element.

The electron does not have a reduced mass. It is defined only for a system of masses.

59. (a) : On a rainy day, due to wetness of the surface, the coefficient of friction becomes lowered which might very easily lead to skidding of a bus or car. That's why it is difficult to run a bus or a car with high speed on a rainy day.

60. (c) : Isotopes have same number of electrons and protons but different neutron number. That's why the mass number of isotopes are different and can be separated by using a mass spectrometer.

CHEMISTRY

61. (c) : $C_{\text{excited state}} = 2s^1\,2p_x^{\,1}\,p_y^{\,1}\,p_z^{\,1}$

$O_{\text{ground state}} = 2s^2\,2p_x^{\,2}\,p_y^{\,1}\,p_z^{\,1}$

In the formation of CO_2 molecule, hybridization of orbitals of carbon occurs only to a limited extent involving only one *s* and one *p* orbital and gives rise to *sp* hybridization.

62. (d) : According to Charles' law,

$$\frac{V_1}{T_1} = \frac{V_2}{T_2}$$

$\Rightarrow$ putting the given values :

$$\frac{300\text{ ml}}{300\text{ K}} = \frac{V_2}{280} \Rightarrow V_2 = 280\text{ ml}$$

63. (b) : Ammonium sulphate and sodium sulphate readily hydrolysed in water. Calcium sulphate is sparingly soluble.

64. (a) : As Cu is below hydrogen in the Electrochemical series. Hydrogen is oxidised at anode and comes out as H_2 while Cu is reduced at the cathode.

$2H^+ + 2e^- \rightarrow H_2$, E° = 0.0 volt

$Cu^{2+} + 2e^- \rightarrow Cu$, E° = 0.337 volt

65. (d) : We know that anion is always larger than the corresponding atom therefore $F^- > F$ and $O^{2-} > O$.

Also, in a period, size of the atom decreases from left to right due to greater force of attraction exerted correct order is :

$$O^{2-} > F^- > O > F$$

66. (d) : The given reaction is Riemer-Tiemann reaction.

$$\text{C}_6\text{H}_5\text{OH} \xrightarrow[\text{CHCl}_3]{\text{NaOH}} o\text{-HOC}_6\text{H}_4\text{CHCl}_2 \xrightarrow[\text{H}_2\text{O}]{\text{H}^+} o\text{-HOC}_6\text{H}_4\text{CHO}$$

Salicyldehyde

$$\text{C}_6\text{H}_5\text{OH} \xrightarrow[\text{CHCl}_3]{\text{NaOH}} o\text{-HOC}_6\text{H}_4\text{CCl}_3 \xrightarrow[\text{NaH}_2\text{O}]{\text{H}^+} o\text{-HOC}_6\text{H}_4\text{COOH}$$

Salicylic acid

67. (c) : Alkali metals have lower ionisation potential than alkaline earth metals due to the extra nuclear charge in alkaline earth metals (which pulls e^- inwards). Also, Mg has got lower ionisation potential than Be as electron to be removed from Mg is present in one shell outwards than in Be.

68. (d) : A system is said to be in colloidal state if particles of one or more components have the size range 10^{-6} to 10^{-9}m. In other words, the colloidal solution is a heterogeneous dispersion of solute particles of size ranging between 10^{-6} to 10^{-9} m into a solvent. Particles are visible only with an ultramicroscope.

69. (a) : In the alkaline earth metal group the lower metals have high heat of hydration than the larger ones due to the fact heat of hydration is higher for small sized highly charged cations. So solubility of sulphate of these metals decrease down the group.

70 (a) : $$\text{C}_6\text{H}_6 \xrightarrow[\text{H}_2\text{SO}_4]{\text{HNO}_3} \underset{(x)}{\text{C}_6\text{H}_5\text{NO}_2} \xrightarrow[\text{FeCl}_3]{\text{Cl}_2} \underset{(y)}{m\text{-ClC}_6\text{H}_4\text{NO}_2}$$

$(HNO_3 + H_2SO_4)$ reagent is the agent for nitration in aromatic rings.

$$HNO_3 + 2H_2SO_4 \rightarrow NO_2^+ + HSO_4^- + H_3O^+$$

$$\text{C}_6\text{H}_6 + \overset{\oplus}{\text{NO}_2} \longrightarrow [\text{C}_6\text{H}_6\text{NO}_2]^{\oplus} \xrightarrow{-\text{H}^+} \text{C}_6\text{H}_5\text{NO}_2$$

NO_2 group is a meta directing group so chlorine atom goes to meta position of the ring.

71. (d) :

$$CuSO_4.5H_2O \rightleftharpoons CuSO_4.3H_2O \rightleftharpoons CuSO_4.H_2O \rightleftharpoons CuSO_4$$

Blue　　Pale blue　　Bluish white　White

So interaction of water in a liquid with copper sulphate will produce blue colour so water can be detected.

72. (b) : Isotones are the nucleus that have same number of neutrons in them.

$_{16}S^{32}$: number of neutrons = 32 – 16 = 16

$_{15}P^{31}$: number of neutrons = 31 – 15 = 16

73. (a) : He is a noble gas. Weak van der waal's forces operate between the gaseous molecules of Helium. In NH_3, H_2O and HCl, there is strong Hydrogen bonding between the molecules.

74. (a) : Potassium and Sodium are metals so have mobile electrons. In graphite, each of the C-atom is covalently bonded to three other C-atoms so one valence electron is available for electrical and thermal conduction there is no mobile electron present in diamond as each C-atom is bonded to four other C-atoms by covalent bond.

75. (c) : Mn shows highest oxidation state of +7. *i.e.* $KMnO_4$

Mn (Z = 25) : 4s [⇅] 3d[5] [1|1|1|1|1] (ground state)

Mn (excited) : [1] [1|1|1|1|1] [1]

76. (d) : The given reaction is :

$NaOH + H_3PO_4 \rightarrow NaH_2PO_4 + H_2O$

Molecular mass of H_3PO_4 is 98. As there is only one electron change involved therefore, equivalent weight of H_3PO_4 in this reaction is, $\frac{98}{1} = 98$

77. (d) : Vinegar is 6–10% aqueous solution of acetic acid. It is obtained by fermentation of liquors containing ethyl alcohol.

78. (d) : Colligative properties are those properties that depend only on the number of particles (ions, atoms, molecules) present in the solution e.g. elevation in boiling point, depression in freezing point, osmotic pressure etc.

79. (b) : As $Q = It$

$\Rightarrow$ Total charge carried $= 2 \times 30 \times 60 = 3600$ C

Now,

96500 C of charge deposites 35.5 g chlorine

$\Rightarrow$ 3600 C of charge will deposite

$$= \frac{35.5}{96500} \times 3600 = 1.32 \text{ g}$$

80. (c) : Moles of oxygen, $n_{O_2} = \frac{4}{32} = 0.125$ mol

Moes of Hydrogen, $n_{H_2} = \frac{2}{2} = 1.00$ mol

Temperature = 273 K, volume = 1 Litre

$$\Rightarrow \text{Total pressure} = \frac{(n_{O_2} + n_{H_2}) \times RT}{V}$$

$$= \frac{1.125 \times 0.0821 \times 273}{1} = 25.215 \text{ atm.}$$

81. (b) : We know that

specific conductance = cell constant × conductance

$\Rightarrow$ Cell constant = Resistance × specific conductance

$= 0.0212 \times 55$

$= 1.166 \text{ cm}^{-1}$

82. (a) : Isotopes are nuclei that have same atomic number but different atomic mass.

$\therefore$ Atomic number of the isotope = 12

$\Rightarrow$ Number of electrons and protons = 12

Number of neutrons = At. mass – Atomic no. = 26 – 12 = 14

83. (c) : Cannizaro reaction is given by those aldehydes and ketones which do not contain any α–hydrogens

$Me-C(Me)_2-CHO$ (Me—C(Me)(Me)—CHO), $CH_2 = O$, $C_6H_5 - CHO$

No α–hydrogen atom is present.

84. (d) : For first order reaction,

rate = rate constant × concentration of reactant

$\therefore$ Initial rate = rate constant × Initial concentration

$= 3 \times 10^{-6} \times 0.10 = 3 \times 10^{-7}$ M s^{-1}

85. (a) : On heating Ammonium nitrate,

$NH_4NO_3 \rightarrow N_2O + 2H_2O$

Nitrous oxide is evolved.

86. (a) : Average life = half life × 1.44

$= 1580 \times 1.44$

$= 2275.2$

$= 2.275 \times 10^3$ years.

87. (d) : Empirical formula of compound is CH_2O

Empirical mass = 12 + 2 + 16 = 30

Molecular weight of compound = 180

As, $n = \frac{\text{molecular mass}}{\text{empirical mass}} = \frac{180}{30} = 6$

Therefore, Molecular formula of compound is $(CH_2O)_6 = C_6H_{12}O_6$

88. (b) : Principle quantum number (n) represents the name, size and energy of the shell of the electron. $n = 1, 2, 3, 4$ ......

Azimuthal quantum number (l) describes the spatial distribution of electron cloud and angular momentum.

Magnetic quantum number (m) describes the possible orientations of orbitals.

89. (a) : Molecular formula for monosaccaride (*e.g.* glucose, fructose) is given by : $C_6H_{12}O_6$. Therefore, molecular formula for the disacchorides is $C_{12}H_{22}O_{11}$.
As $2C_6H_{12}O_6 \rightarrow C_{12}H_{22}O_{11} + H_2O$

90. (d) : $C_6H_5CH_3 \xrightarrow[\text{or } K_2Cr_2O_7]{KMnO_4} C_6H_5COOH$

Both $KMnO_4$ and $K_2Cr_2O_7$ are strong oxidising agents therefore can oxidise any alkyl benzene to benzoic acid.

91. (b) : In body centred cubic crystals,

$$\text{radius} = \frac{\sqrt{3}}{4} \times \text{edge length}$$
$$= \frac{\sqrt{3}}{4} \times 4.29 \times 10^{-8} \text{ cm}$$
$$= 1.8576 \times 10^{-8} \text{ cm}$$

92. (a) : Beilstein's test : A small quantity of organic compound is taken on the flattened end of Cu wire and introduced in the flame. A green or blue colour indicates halogens.

93. (d) : N (Z = 7) : $1s^2$ [↑↓] $2s^2$ [↑↓] $2p^3$ [↑][↑][↑]

Due to the presence of three unpaired electrons, N atom will be paramagnetic in nature.

94. (c) : Molecular weight of $C_{60}H_{122} = 60\times12+1\times122 = 842$

$\therefore$ Weight of 1 mole of $C_{60}H_{122}$ molecules = 842 g
or Weight of 6.023×10^{23} molecules = 842 g

$\Rightarrow$ Weight of 1 molecule of $C_{60}H_{122} = \frac{842}{6.023\times10^{23}}$ g $= 1.4 \times 10^{-21}$ g

95. (b) : Nitrogen is more electronegative than the phosphorus atom. In NH_3, nitrogen attracts the bonded pair of elctron between N and H atoms towards it, and this effect is more in NH_3 than in PH_3. Due to this effect, the lone pair of electrons in NH_3 can participate more than that of PH_3.

96. (a) : $CuSO_4 + 2KCN \rightarrow Cu(CN)_2 + K_2SO_4$
$2Cu(CN)_2 \rightarrow Cu_2(CN)_2 + (CN)_2$
$Cu_2(CN)_2 + 6KCN \rightarrow 2K_3Cu\,(CN)_4$
$2CuSO_4 + 10KCN \rightarrow 2K_3Cu(CN)_4 + 2K_2SO_4 + (CN)_2$

97. (a) : The root mean square velocity is defined as the square of different velocities possessed by molecules of a gas at a given temperature.

$$V_{rms} = \sqrt{\frac{3kT}{m}} \Rightarrow V_{rms} \propto \frac{1}{\sqrt{m}}$$

m = mass of gas molecules

$$\text{density} = \frac{\text{mass}}{\text{volume}}$$

$$\Rightarrow V_{rms} \propto \frac{1}{\sqrt{\text{density}}}$$

$$\Rightarrow \frac{V_{rms}(O_2)}{V_{rms}(H_2)} = \sqrt{\frac{\text{density of } H_2}{\text{density of } O_2}} = \sqrt{\frac{1}{16}} = \frac{1}{4}$$

98. (d) : According to law of conservation of mass in all chemical changes the total mass of the system remains constant or in a chemical reaction, mass is neither created nor destroyed. This law was proposed by Lavoisier and tested by Landolt.

But in (b) and (c), mass of reactants is not equal to the mass of products.

99. (d) : Benzene $+ Cl_2 \xrightarrow{UV}$ Gammexane ($C_6H_6Cl_6$)

100.(d) : More the number of oxygen atoms attached to the central atom, more is the electron withdrawal effect towards oxygen atom, which in turn makes central atom electron deficient so the hydrogen attached becomes more and more acidic with increasing number of oxygen atoms.

101.(c) : $C_6H_5CHCl_2$ (Benzal chloride) $\xrightarrow[H^+]{H_2O}$ $C_6H_5CH{=}O$ (Benzaldehyde) $+ 2HCl$

102.(a) : Brass is an alloy of Cu and Zn. Bronze is an alloy of Cu and Sn. German-silver is an alloy of Cu, Zn and Ni.

103.(b) : HBr adds on the double bond of propene according to Markownikoff's rule.

$CH_3CH{=}CH_2 + HBr \rightarrow CH_3{-}CH(Br){-}CH_2(H) \equiv CH_3\,CH(Br).CH_3$

Propene → 2–Bromopropane

104.(b) : In the alkaline earth metal group, down the group as the size increases the ability to lose electrons *i.e.* ionic character increases. The smaller metal require more ionisation potential for cation formation.

105. (d) : NO_2 group is the electron withdrawing group due to which electron density in the ring decreases. Therefore meta positions are preferred over orto / para positions.

106. (d) : Every substance is associated with a definite amount of energy which depends upon its chemical nature as well as on its temperature, pressure and volume. This energy is called as internal energy and it includes translational, rotational and vibrational energy of the molecule.

107. (a) : According to Dulong Petit's law :

Atomic weight × specific heat = 6.4

$$\text{Atomic weight} = \frac{6.4}{0.16} = 40$$

108. (a) : Relative lowering of vapour pressure is given by :

$$\frac{P^0 - P_s}{P^0} = X_A \,;\; X_A = \text{mole fraction of solute}$$

P^0 = vapour pressure of pure solvent

P_s = vapour pressure of solution

$$\Rightarrow \frac{39.08/78}{39.08/78 + 2.175/M_A} \Rightarrow M_A = 69.60$$

109. (b) : Dipole moment in the molecule depends upon the charge and the distance between the charges.

As oxygen is more electronegative than nitrogen, iodine or sulphur, it will have greater dipole moment.

110. (d) : OsO_4, Let oxidation state of Os be x.

$$x + 4 \times (-2) = 0 \Rightarrow x = +8$$

111. (b) : Xenon belongs to noble gases which are considered to be very unreactive. In xenon atom, the ionisation potential of Xe to lose one electron was found to be nearly equivalent that of $O_2 \rightarrow O_2^+ + e^-$. Also, due to the presence of empty 5*d*–orbitals, electrons can be excited and higher valency of xenon can be produced. *e.g.* XeF_2, XeF_4, XeF_6 etc.

112. (d) : Identification of cathode and anode is done by using ammeter. The liberated electrons at the anode after oxidation flow to the cathode side of cell. So the 'positive electricity' flow from cathode to the anode.

113. (a) : $Zn + Cu^{2+}_{(aq)} \rightarrow Zn^{2+}_{(aq)} + Cu$

$$E^\circ_{Cu^{2+}/Cu} = 0.34v, \quad E^\circ_{Zn^{2+}/Zn} = -0.76v$$

The above values show that zinc will release electrons and copper will like to get reduced.

114. (a) : H_2SO_4 when react with NaBr and NaI, give out Br_2 and I_2 as concentrated H_2SO_4 is a strong oxidising agent.

115. (a) : When mercury is exposed to ozone it get superficially oxidised and loses its meniscus and stitches to the glass.

116. (b) : Bond order

$$= \frac{1}{2}\left[\begin{matrix}\text{No. of bonding} \\ \text{orbital electrons}\end{matrix} - \begin{matrix}\text{No. of antibonding} \\ \text{orbital elctrons}\end{matrix}\right].$$ The bond order zero indicates that the bond does not exist.

117. (a) : The linear triatomic molecules of the type B–A–B *e.g.* CO_2 have no dipole moment, not because the individual C=O bonds are non-polar but because the two bond moments (polarity) cancel each other. Therefore, geometry of molecules can be predicted by the value of dipole moment.

118. (b) : Lower aldehydes and ketones are soluble in water due to polar effect of >C = O which makes hydrogen bonds with water molecules. As the size of the aldehydes and ketones increases the hydrophobic part i.e., alkyl chain increases which weakens the H-bond formations with H_2O molecules and decreases the solubility.

119. (c) : Metamers differ in nature of alkyl groups attached to the same functional group.

e.g. $CH_3—O—C_3H_7$ (Methyl propyl ether) $C_2H_5—O—C_2H_5$ (Diethyl ether)

120. (a) : Equivalent conductance is defined as the conducting power of all the ions produced by one equivalent in a given solution. Therefore, at higher concentrations, degree of dissociation of electrolyte is less. Degree of dissociation can be increased by dilution.

BIOLOGY

121. (d) : In vertebrate heart, the walls of ventricle are thicker than the walls of auricle. Wall of left ventricle ia three times thicker than that of right ventricle. This is so because it receive a large amount of oxygenated blood from lungs and pumps that with great force to all visceral organs and parts of body through aorta.

122. (b) : Thyroid glands play a key role in metamorphosis of frog's tadpole. Metamorphosis is profound changes of form during development from larva to adult animal. The process of metamorphosis is essentially under hormonal control. Hormones from the hypothalamus (*e.g.* TSH or thyroid stimulating hormone) and the thyroid gland regulate the process of metamorphosis. Thyroxine hormone affects the tissues directly, causing the degeneration and necrosis of some cells and stimulating the growth and differentiation of others.

123. (a) : Weberian ossicles are found in fishes. The chewing construction with the rotating skull renders a single Weberian ossicle counecting the sound receiving swimming bladder and internal ear. This is a series of four or five modified vertebrae connecting thc swimbladder and the inner ear.

124. (a) : Inflammatory response, in allergy is caused by histamines. The presence of foreign body such as bacteria within the body provokes a protective in flammatory response. Histamine increases the capillary permeability.

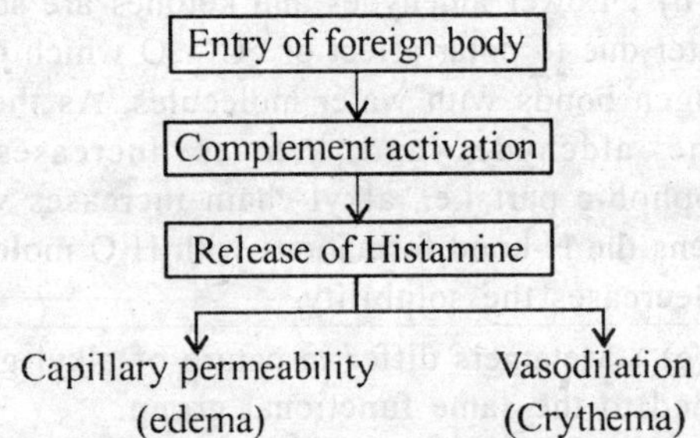

125. (a) : Turner's syndrome is characterised by the monosomy of XO type. These are immature sterile females with webbed neck. Klinefelter's syndrome is characterised by trisomy (XXY). These are male individuals, who are phenotypically fairly normal but have a fairly low sperm count and therefore sterile. Down's syndrome is caused due to the presence of extra chromosome 21 (in trisomy 21) i.e. The patients suffering from Down's syndrome is called mongolian idiot.

126. (d) : It a person is injured, he should be given blood. The blood group O should be given without checking the patients own blood group. Blood group O has anti A and anti B antibodies in serum but no antigens. Due to the absence of antigens, O blood group can be recognised as the universal donor.

127. (c) : Epinephrine is the derivative of amino acid. Epinephrine is formed by the hydroxylation and decarboxylation of the amino acids phenylalanine and tyrosine.

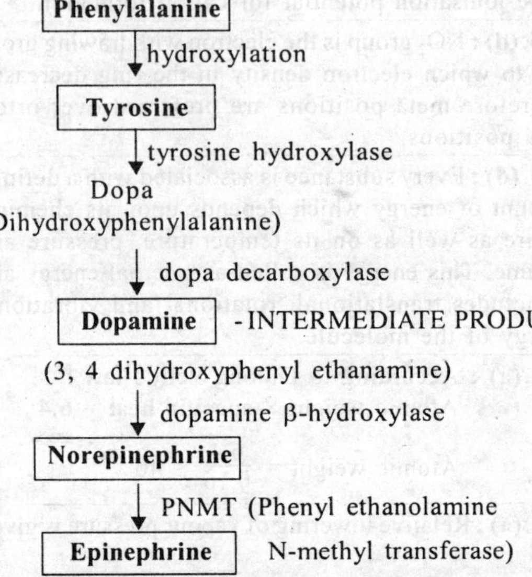

Biosynthetic pathway of Epinephrine

Progesterone, estrogen and prostaglandin can be derived from cholesterol and fatty acid respectively.

128. (b) : Liver in our body stores vitamin A. The fat soluble vitamin A may be stored in large amounts and this gives them the potential to cause toxicity if consumed in high amounts. Retinol or vitamin A is synthesized by the liver and thus it is stored by the liver.

129. (a) : Cumulus covers ovum. Within the mature follicle, the ovum is surrounded by a group of granulosa cells known as cumulus (cumuloophorus). The follicular epithelial cells are known as granulosa cells.

130. (d) : The function of renin is degradation of angiotensinogen. When the blood pressure falls the hormone renin secreted by juxtaglomerular cells of kidney plays an important role in reabsorption of sodium. Renin on reaching the blood, changes angiotensinogen (inactive compound released from liver) of plasma into angiotensin II via angiotensin I

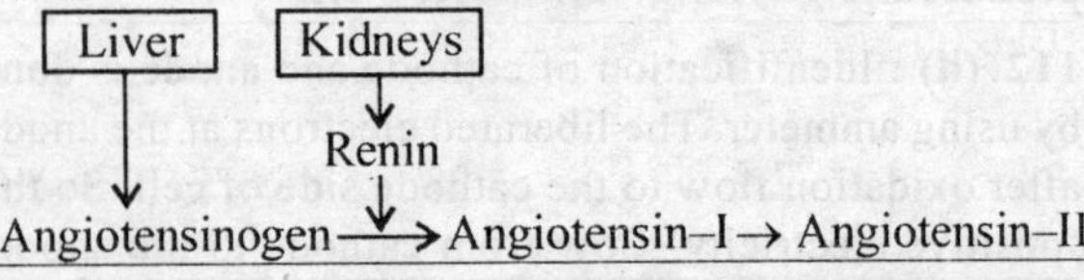

131. (d) : Trained dog salivates when you ring a bell is the example of conditioned reflex. It is also called acquired reflexes. It is not inborn, but acquired and dependent on past experience, training and learning *i.e.* adopted during the course of lifetime.

132. (a) : The heartbeat increases at the time of interview due to secretion of adrenaline. Adrenaline is a stress hormone. At the time of interview, the candidate suffers from anxiety or tension, this leads to the extra production and secretion of adrenaline.

133. (d) : Heparin prevents blood coagulation in the blood vessels. It is a product of most cells. It is an anticoagulant, blocking conversion of prothrombin to thrombin. Haemoglobin is the blood pigment necessary for oxygen transport. Plasma is the component of blood. Thrombin is the product of blood clotting.

134. (a) : Conn's disease is caused by the over secretion of aldosterone.

It is a disease of the adrenal glands involving excess production of a hormone, aldosterone. It is a cause of high blood pressure. Other symptoms may occur because high aldosterone levels in the blood act on the kidney.

135. (c) : The extra embryonic membranes of mammalian embryo are derived from trophoblast. After the cleavage of the zygote, blastocyst is formed. Then, trophoblast, the epithelial layer surrounding the blastocyst is formed. This trophoblast cells are destined to form most of the extra embryonic membrane in mammals.

136. (a) : Ageing is associated both with calcium deficiency, due to low dietary intake and decreased intestinal absorption, and with vitamin D deficiency, secondary to depletion of body stores resulting from inadequate exposure to sunlight.

The consequences of calcium deficiency might thus include not only osteoporosis, but also arteriosclerosis and hypertension due to the increase of calcium in the vascular wall, amyotrophic lateral sclerosis and senile dementia due to calcium deposition in the central nervous system, and a decrease in cellular function, because of blunting of the difference in extracellular-intracellular calcium, leading to diabetes mellitus, immune deficiency and other disorders.

137. (c) : The end-product of ornithine cycle is urea.

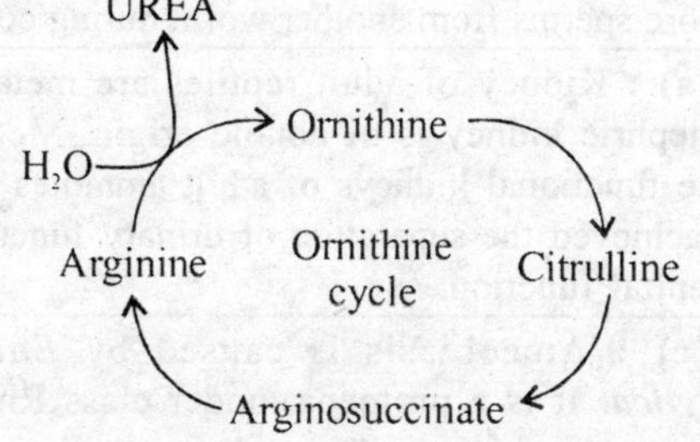

Most of the NH_4^+ formed by deamination of amino acids in the liver is converted to urea, and the urea is excreted in the urine. The synthesis of urea via ornithine cycle involves conversion of the amino acid ornithine to citrulline and then to arginine, following which urea is split off and ornithine is regenerated.

138. (a) : Wings of pigeon, mosquito and bat show divergent evolution. It is the evolutionary process resulting in dissimilarity in structural features of organisms that occupy similar habitat.

Atavism is the regaining of same structures after a certain gap of few generations.

139. (d) : First step of utiliZation of glucose in metabolism is glucose - 6 - phosphate. It is the first step of glycolysis. According to the Embden Meyerhof -Parnas scheme, the conversation would be like.

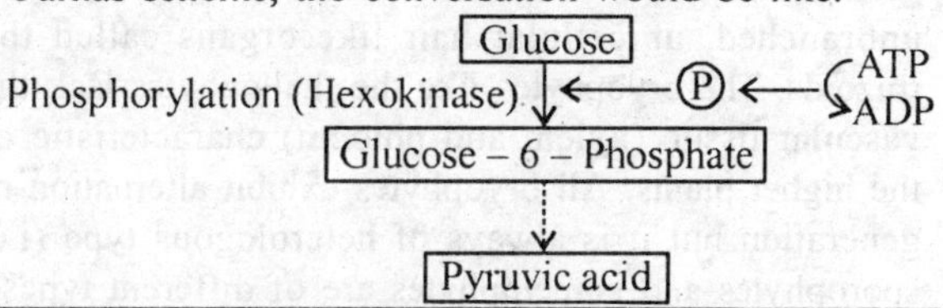

140. (b) : Otorhinolaryngology is the study of ENT that means ear, nose and throat.

141. (c) : If one strand of DNA has the nitrogenous base sequence ATGCTTGA, the sequence in the complementary strand will be

```
A T G C T T G A
| | | | | | | |
T A C G A A C T
```

As A binds, with T and G binds with C we get the result TACGAACT.

142. (a) : When certain proviruses turn into virulent viruses thereby causing lysis of host cell, they may carry with them segments of host's DNA. It such virus particles carrying a segment of DNA from one host infects another host which is different than the first one, the latter may inherit some of the properties of the properties of the former host due to transfer of DNA segment through infecting phase. This phenomenon of transfer of genetic material from one bacterial strain to another through the agency of virus is called transduction. In conjugation, genetic material is transferred through a conjugation tube, when two strains come in contact. In transformation, genetic material is released from one strain and a part may be acquired from another strain, which thus gets transformed without coming in contact with the other strain.

143. (a) : Endonucleases are very specific and cut DNA at very specific nucleotide sequences. They are popularly called restriction enzymes, because their action is restricted to only very specific sequences which exhibit a two-fold symmetry as follows :

AAG CTT
TTC GAA

144. (d) : Bacterial cell wall is the outer rigid covering of the cell which provides shape and protection to the protoplasm. Bacterial wall contains peptidoglycan and diominopimelic acid. Peptidoglycan consists of two linked molecules, acetyl glucosamine an acetyl muramic acid.

145. (a) & (b) : The plant body of bryophytes lacks the true roots, stem or leaves. It grows prostrate on the ground and is attached to the substratum by delicate, unbranched, unicellular hair like organs called the rhizoids. The bryophytes like the thallophytes lack the vascular tissue (xylem and phloem) characteristic of the higher plants. All bryophytes exhibit alternation of generation but it is always of heterologous type (i.e. sporophytes and gametophytes are of different types). Gametophytes of bryophyte are green, leafy individual and due to presence of chlorophyll they are autotrophic in nature. The sporophyte is dependent for its nutrient wholly or partially on the gametophyte plant to which it is attached organically throughout its life.

146. (a)

147. (d) : The mature virus particle (Singular unit virion) consists of an outer, inert, non-genetic protein coat or shell which surrounds and protects the genetic material or nucleic acid forming the core. The protein coat is called capsid. the capsid is made up of numerous small subunits called the capsomeres.

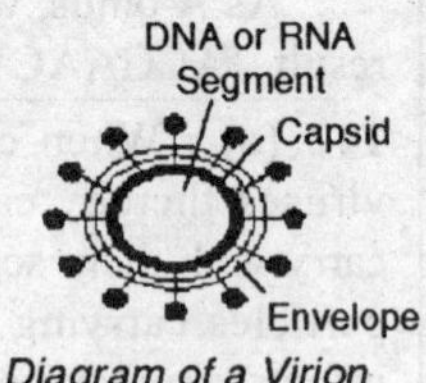

Diagram of a Virion

148. (d) : Middle lamella is a thin, amorphous and cementing layer between two adjacent cells Lomasomes are plasmalemma foldings found in fungal cells below the wall. Lysosomes are small vesicles which are bounded by a single membrane and contain hydrolytic enzymes. Microsomes are particals isolated from cytoplasm for biochemical study by mechanically centrifuging the result.

149. (c) : Cell cycle consists of two states, a long non-dividing growing I-phase and a short dividing M-phase. I-phase (interphase) is divisible into three stages, G_1, S and G_2. Therefore, there are following stages in cell cycle

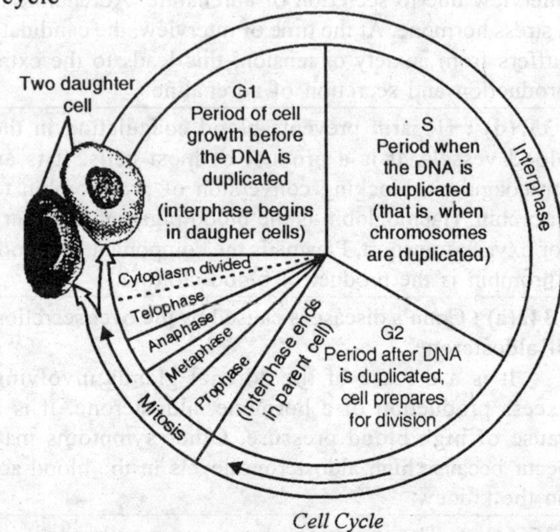

Cell Cycle

(i) G_1 – phase – first growth phase or post mitotic gap phase.
(ii) S – phase – synthetic phase
(iii) G_2 – phase – second growth phase or pre-mitotic gap phase
(iv) M– phase (mitotic phase)

150. (a) : Sporogony of malarial parasites occur in stomach wall of mosquito. It is an asexual multiplication phase. The nucleus of the oocyst divides and followed by cytoplasmic division, several sporozoites are formed. This is the infective stage, when a mosquito bites a man, thousands of sporozoites enter into the blood of the man.

151. (a) : In spermatogenesis, the acrosome of sperm is formed by golgi complex. Acrosome is a part of sperm head. This acrosome is formed by a special granule secreted by golgi body. The acrosome contains all the enzymes present in golgi complex.

152. (a) : Paired spermathecae occur in 6, 7, 8, 9 segments of *Pheretima.* These are four pairs of small flask shaped structures. Their function is to receive and store sperms from another worm during copulation.

153. (a) : Kidney of adult reptiles are metanephric. Metanephric kidney is of double origin. Metanephric are the functional kidneys of adult amniotes and they have achieved the separation of urinary function from the genital function.

154. (c) : Ameobiasis is caused by *Entamoeba histolytica.* It is a protozoa, under class Rhizopoda, order Amoebida. *Taenia solium* causes Cestodiasis, Cysticercosis. *Wuchereria bancrofti* causes Filariasis, *Ascaris lumbricoides* causes Ascariasis.

155. (c) : Secondary phloem is made up of the same type of cells as are found in the primary phloem (metaphloem) - sieve tubes, companion cells tubes become non functional by development of a pad of wall material over the seive phloem fibres and phloem parenchyma. The sieve plates. It generally happens at the end of a growing season. Such a nonfunctional phloem may get crushed during the next growing season due to the expanding cylinder of newly formed secondary xylem and phloem.

156. (a) : *Dionaea* is an American herb that possesses a rosette of long-petioled leaves. The upper surface of each lamina lobe contains 3 sensitive spines and a number of red-coloured digestive glands. If an insect happens to touch a senstitive spine twice in quick succession, the two lobes of the lamina fold rapidly. Bending of sensitive spines after coming in contact with an insect is thigmonastic. Opening and closing of flowers in response to light and darkness is alled photonasty. Seismonasty is shown by *Mimosa.* A response to temperature changes is termed as thermonasty

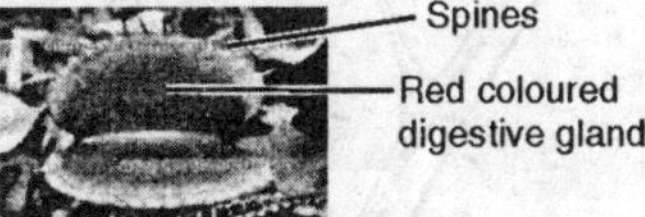

Dionaea showing two lobes of lamina

157. (b) : Endodermis is a single layer of compactly arranged cells which are generally parenchymatous, but have distinct wall characteristics. Caspary (1865–66) recognised a band of the wall material in the radial and transverse walls of endodermis. This particular wall material is chemically different from the rest of the wall. It is known as *casparian strip or band.* It is believed to be made of suberin.

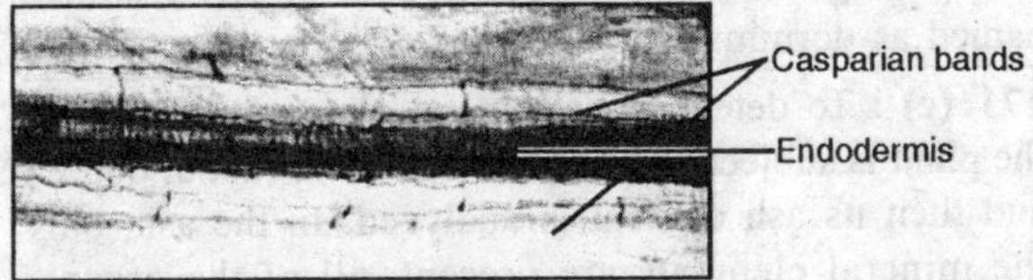

158. (d) : Calcium carbonate crystals have been reported from within the cells of Banyan leaf (*Ficus benghalensis*) and some members of the families *Acanthaceae, cucurbitacae, Urticaceae,* etc. In the leaf of Banyan they have been seen to occur in grape-like clusters hanging from a stalk that is attached to the cell wall. The name cystolith is given to such a cluster. Some cells contain star-shaped aggregation of crystals of calcium oxalate, which are known as *sphaeraphides*. Raphide is needle-shaped crystals of calcium oxalate occurring in bundles in certain plant cells. Otolith is gronule of calcium carbonate in vertebrate inner ear.

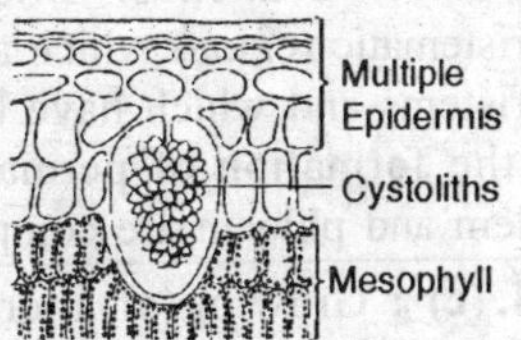

Epidermis in Ficus showing cystoliths

159. (d) : In anemophilous flowers, stigma is hairy, feathery or branched to catch the wind-borne pollen grains.

160. (a) : The female gametophyte, also called embryo sac, is mostly a 7-celled and eight nucleated structure. The micropylar end of the central cell is occupied by the egg apparatus, comprising an egg cell and two synergids, and at its chalazal end three antipodal cells are present. Cells of the egg apparatus and the antipodal cells are uninucleate and haploid whereas the central cell is binucleate or diploid.

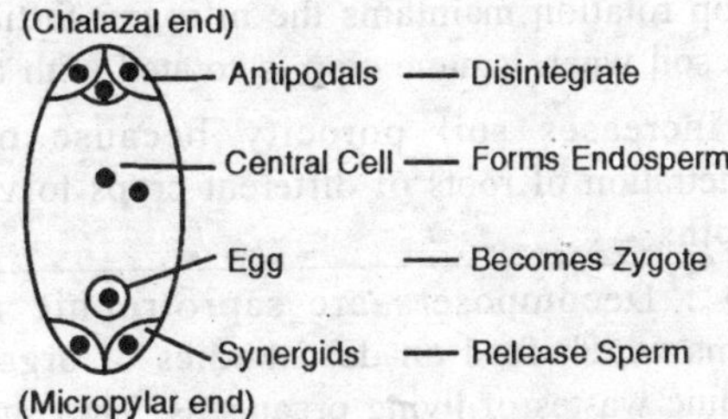

Angiospermic Embryo sac

161. (b) : High-energy phosphate bonds are universally symbolized by the symbol~ and high energy phosphate groups as ~ P. ATP can be designated as A–R~P~P~P. ADP as A–R–P~P. In other words, the ADP–ATP system is carrier of phosphoryl ($-PO_2^{2-}$) groups from high energy phosphate compounds.

162. (d) : Endoplasmic reticulum functions as cytoskeleton or intracellular and ultrastuctural skeletal framework by providing mechanical support to colloidal cytoplasmic matrix. Proteins and enzymes synthesised by ribosomes enter the channels of rough endoplasmic reticulum both for intracellular use as well as extracellular transport.

163. (b) : The secondary meristems are usually lateral. They give rise to secondary tissues that constitute secondary growth. The common examples are vascular cambium of the root (derived from conjunctive parenchyma), interfascicular vascular cambium, cork cambium, wound cambium and accessory cambia. The apical meristems are present at the tips of stem, root and their branches. Intercalary meristems are meristematic regions which are derived from the apical meristems and which have been separated from them by the formation of permanent tissues in between. Xylem and phloem are complex permanent tissues.

164. (c) : Growing of alternate crops in the similar seasons on the same piece of land is called crop rotation. Crop rotation is helpful in improvement of soil fertility because of the following reasons.

(i) It decreases the chances of soil borne diseases because the pathogens are unable to find the same host next year.

(ii) It avoids deficiency of minerals from one level because the roots of different crops penetrate to different depths in the soil.

(iii) Crop rotation maintains the nitrogen fertility of the soil when legume crop is rotated with others.

(iv) It increases soil porocity because of the penetration of roots of different crops to various depths.

165. (b) : Decomposers are saprotrophic micro organisms which feed on dead bodies of organisms and organic wastes of living organisms. They are also called detrivores. They brings mineralisation (the digested form of organic matter is partly absorbed by micro organisms for their own assimilation. The remaining adds raw materials and minerals back into the substratum. The phenomenon is called mineralisation).

166. (a) : Obligate parasites can grow only upon suitable living host tissues. The best examples of obligate parasites are the downy and powdery mildews.

167. (d) : The red colour of flower dominates upon white colour of flower. In the present varieties both parents are of pure variety, therefore, the offsprings will be all red flowered as shown below :

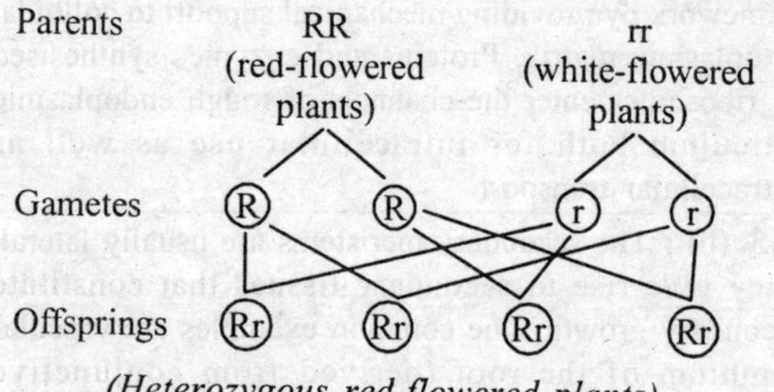

(Heterozygous red-flowered plants)

168. (d) : Nitrous acid deaminates with decreasing frequency, the bases G, C and A in DNA and with equal frequencies in RNA. HNO_2 deaminates adenine (A) to hypoxanthine (H) : Cytosine (C) to uracil (U) and guanine (G) to xanthine (X). It pairs with C; U pairs with A and X pairs with C.

169. (d) : When the fleshy receptacle forms a hollow cavity with an apical opening guarded by scales, and the flowers are borne on the inner wall of the cavity,

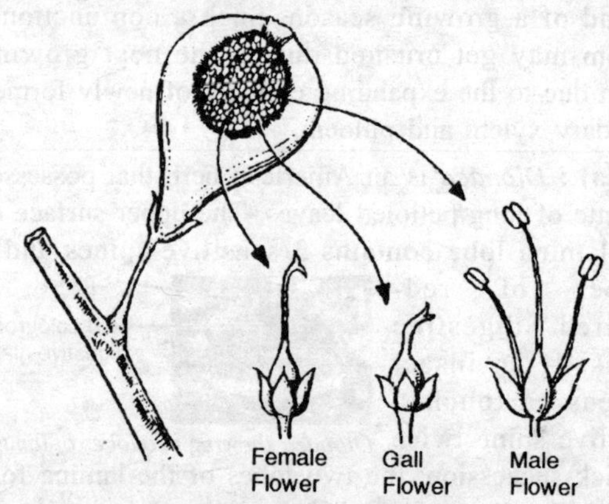

Hypanthodium inflorescence (Ficus)

the inflorescence is a hypanthodium, as in *Ficus* (*e.g.* banyan, fig. peepul, etc.). Here the female flowers develop at the base of the cavity and the male flowers higher up towards the apical pore.

170. (d) : Abscisic acid induces dormancy of buds towards the approach of winter. Seed dormancy is mainly caused by abscisic acid. Because of its action in inducing dormancy, abscisic acid or ABA is also named as dormin.

171. (c) : To detect some mineral elements of a plant, the plant is subjected to high temperature (about 600ºC) and then its ash content is analyzed. In the ash, only the mineral elements are present, all of the organic compounds have been decomposed and passed off in the form of gases. The primary elements (carbon, hydrogen and oxygen) are therefore given off as CO_2, water vapour and oxygen. We cannot accurately detect the element nitrogen with this method since some of it is given off in the form of ammonium or nitrogen gas. The method of growing plants in aqueous nutrient solutions as employed by Sacks and Knob is used experimentally and commercially today and is known as hydroponic culture.

172. (a) : Some enzymes depend for activity only on their structure as proteins, while others require in addition nonprotein structures, or cofactor for activity. The cofactor may be either a metal ion or a complex organic molecule called a coenzyme usually function as intermediary carriers of electrons or of specific atoms or functional groups that are transferred in the overall enzymatic reaction.

173. (b) : Mineral matter occurs in the form of particles in soil. The particles are irregular in outline and enclose spaces for circulation of air and water. Depending upon their size, mineral particles of the soil are called sand, slit and clay. Clay particles are chemically active. Water and chemical nutrients are abundant. Soil is the source of a number of essential elements to the plants. They are called plant nutrients or essential mineral elements.

174. (b) : Wax is often secreted in the form of grains, plates or rods on the surface of cuticle. It forms characteristic *glaucous*, "bloom" on the surface of leaves and fruits. Oil and resins are often abundantly developed *e.g. Pinus* suberin prevents evaporation of water from inner tissues of plants.

175. (a) : In the majority of plants stomata open in the presence of light and close in darkness. A strong light further increases transpiration probably due to its heating effect. Because most of the transpiration occurs through stomata, the rate of transpiration falls down appreciably in the darkness.

176. (a) : The symbiotic relationship between legumes and *Rhizobium* seems to be species–specific. The accumulation of soil bacteria in the vicinity of plant roots occur especially roots of legume plants. This accumulation probably occurs because plant roots excrete certain growth factors into the soil. Then the bacteria either penetrate the relatively soft root hair tip or invade damaged or broken root hairs and progress in an infection thread through the cortex tissue to the immediate area of the endodermis and pericycle. Cell divisions commence in the endolermis and pericycle area and the nodule grows rapidly and pushes its way to the surface of the root.

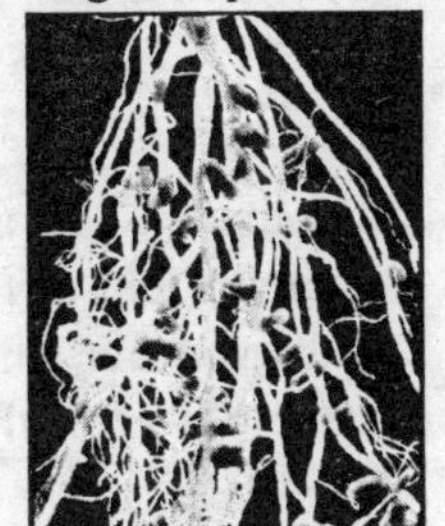

Root nodules showing association of Rhizobium with root of leguminous plant

177. (a) : It is the co-ordinated process by which stimulus passes to the brain via sense organs or sensory receptors. These receptors are transducers that convert various form of energy in the environment into action potentials in neurons. The form of energy converted by the receptors include, mechanical, thermal, electromagnetic and chemical energy. Information about the internal and external environment reaches to the sensory receptors which in turn after getting adequate stimulus, transfer it to the brain through nerve impluses. Then the brain gives response for the stimulus.

178. (c) : The purine and pyrimidine bases pair only in certain combinations. Adenine pairs with thymine (A:T) and guanine with cytosine (G:C). Adenine and thymine are joined by two hydrogen bonds through atoms attached to positions 6' and 1'. Cytosine and guanine are joined by three hydrogen bonds through positions 6', 1' and 2'.

179. (b) : Cartilage and bone are rigid connective tissues because in cartilage, protein is the matrix and in bone calcium is the matrix both of which are solid structures. On the other hand blood is the connective tissue. Where plasma is the matrix which is mainly the liquid component having some blood cells in it.

180. (a) : Hair cells on the basilar membrane is responsible for hearing. In the cochlear duct of the internal ear, the basilar papilla forms a basilar membrane with hair cells constituting an organ of corti, the fibres are embeded in a tectorial membrane lying above the organ of Corti which is sensitive to vibrations of high frequency. The mechanism is as follow

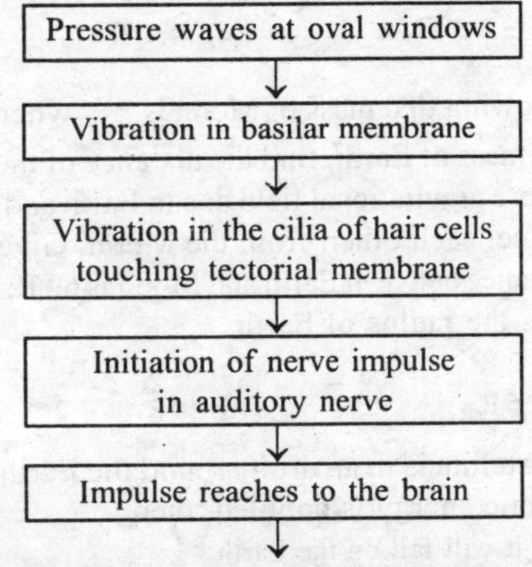

GENERAL KNOWLEDGE

181. (b)	**182. (c)**	**183. (c)**	**184. (d)**	**185. (a)**
186. (d)	**187. (d)**	**188. (b)**	**189. (d)**	**190. (a)**
191. (b)	**192. (d)**	**193. (d)**	**194. (d)**	**195. (b)**
196. (d)	**197. (d)**	**198. (b)**	**199. (d)**	**200. (c)**

❖ ❖ ❖

SOLVED PAPER
AIIMS - 2000

Time : 3½ Hours

Max. Marks : 200

PHYSICS

1. A body is allowed to slide down a frictionless track freely under gravity. The track ends in a semicircular shaped part of diameter D. What should be the height (minimum) from which the body must fall so that it completes the circle.
(a) $\frac{4}{5}D$ (b) $\frac{5}{4}D$
(c) D (d) 2D.

2. What is the dimensional formula of gravitational constant G?
(a) $M^{-1}L^3T^{-2}$ (b) $M^{-2}L^3T^{-2}$
(c) $M^{-1}L^2T^{-2}$ (d) $M^{-1}L^3T^{-1}$.

3. A body of mass 5 kg has momentum of 10 kg m/s. When a force of 0.2 N is applied on it for 10 seconds, what is the change in its kinetic energy?
(a) 1.1 J (b) 2.2 J
(c) 3.3 J (d) 4.4 J.

4. Knowing that mass of Moon is $\frac{M}{81}$ where M is the mass of Earth, find the distance of the point where gravitational field due to Earth and Moon cancel each other, from the Moon. Given that distance between Earth and Moon is 60 R, where R is the radius of Earth.
(a) 2 R (b) 4 R
(c) 6 R (d) 8 R.

5. A satellite is in an orbit around the Earth; if its kinetic energy is doubled, then
(a) it will fall on the Earth
(b) it will rotate with a greater speed
(c) it will maintain its path
(d) it will escape out of Earth's gravitational field.

6. For an electron in the second orbit of hydrogen, what is the moment of momentum as per the Bohr's model?
(a) $2\pi h$ (b) πh
(c) $\frac{h}{\pi}$ (d) $\frac{2h}{\pi}$

7. Half life of a substance is 20 minutes. What is the time between 33% decay and 67% decay?
(a) 40 minutes (b) 20 minutes
(c) 30 minutes (d) 25 minutes.

8. When a ray of light enters a glass slab, then
(a) its frequency and velocity changes
(b) only frequency changes
(c) its frequency and wavelength changes
(d) its frequency does not change.

9. Match the elements of table I and table II.

Table I	Table II
1. Myopia	(i) Bifocal lens
2. Hypermetropia	(ii) Cylindrical lens
3. Presbyopia	(iii) Concave lens
4. Astigmatism	(iv) Convex lens

(a) 1 - iii, 2 - iv, 3 - i, 4 - ii
(b) 1 - iv, 2 - iii, 3 - i, 4 - ii
(c) 1 - i, 2 - ii, 3 - iii, 4 - iv
(d) 1 - ii, 2 - iv, 3 - i, 4 - iii.

10. A doctor advices a patient to use spectacles with a convex lens of focal length 40 cms in contact with a concave lens of focal length 25 cms. What is the power of the resultant combination?
(a) 1.5 D (b) –1.5 D
(c) 6.5 D (d) –6.5 D.

11. Turn ratio in a step-up transformer is 1 : 2. If a Lechlanche cell of 1.5 V is connected across the input, what is the voltage across the output?
(a) 1.5 V (b) 0.0 V
(c) 3 V (d) 0.75 V.

12. The Sun emits a light with maximum wavelength 510 nm while another star x emits a light with

maximum wavelength of 350 nm. What is the ratio of surface temperature of the Sun and the star x?

(a) 1.45 (b) 0.68
(c) 0.46 (d) 2.1.

13. Surface temperature of star A and B are 727°C and 327°C respectively. What is the ratio $H_A : H_B$ for the heat radiated per second by the two stars?

(a) 5 : 3 (b) 25 : 9
(c) 625 : 81 (d) 125 : 27.

14. Ratio of intensities of two waves is 9 : 1. If these two are superimposed, what is the ratio of maximum and minimum intensities?

(a) 9 : 1 (b) 3 : 1
(c) 4 : 1 (d) 5 : 3.

15. Which of the following is true?

(a) Momentum is conserved in all collisions but kinetic energy is conserved only in inelastic collisions.
(b) Neither momentum nor kinetic energy is conserved in inelastic collisions.
(c) Momentum is conserved in all collisions but not kinetic energy.
(d) Both momentum and kinetic energy are conserved in all collisions.

16. Two resistance filaments of same length are connected first in series and then in parallel. Find the ratio of power dissipated in both cases assuming that equal current flows in the main circuit.

(a) 1 : 4 (b) 4 : 1
(c) 1 : 2 (d) 2 : 1.

17. Given a number of capacitors labelled as 8 μF, 250 V. Find the minimum number of capacitors needed to get an arrangement equivalent to 16 μF, 1000 V.

(a) 4 (b) 16
(c) 32 (d) 64.

18. A rod of length 1.4 m and negligible mass has two masses of 0.3 kg and 0.7 kg tied to its two ends. Find the location of the point on this rod where the rotational energy is minimum when the rod is rotated about that point.

(a) 0.98 m from 0.3 kg (b) 0.98 m from 0.7 kg
(c) 0.7 m from 0.3 kg (d) 0.7 m from 0.7 kg.

19. What accounts for the flow of charge carriers in forward and reverse biasing of silicon p - n diode?

(a) drift in forward bias and diffusion in reverse bias
(b) drift in reverse bias and diffusion in forward bias
(c) drift in both reverse and forward bias
(d) diffusion in both forward and reverse bias.

20. A 60 W incandescent lamp operates at 120 V. The number of electrons passing through the filament per second will be

(a) 1.61×10^{12} (b) 3.12×10^{18}
(c) 7.21×10^{12} (d) 12.40×10^{13}.

21. Given a current carrying wire of non uniform cross section. Which of the following is constant throughout the length of the wire?

(a) current, electric field and drift speed
(b) drift speed only
(c) current and drift speed
(d) current only.

22. An insulated charged sphere of radius 5 cms has a potential of 10 V at the surface. What is the potential at centre?

(a) 10 V (b) zero
(c) same as that at 5 cms from the surface
(d) same as that at 25 cms from the surface.

23. A body is projected from the ground with some angle to the horizontal. What happens to the angular momentum about the initial position in this motion?

(a) decreases (b) increases
(c) remains same
(d) first increases and then decreases.

24. What should be the amount of current through the ring of radius 5 cms so that field in the centre is with earth's magnetic field of 7×10^{-9} Wb/m² is

(a) 0.5 A (b) 0.28 A
(c) 2.8 A (d) none.

25. Which of the following statements is not correct about the magnetic field?

(a) magnetic lines of force don't cut each other
(b) inside the magnet the lines go from north to

south pole of the magnet
(c) the magnetic lines form a closed loop
(d) tangents to the magnetic lines give the direction of the magnetic field.

26. Let E_a be the electric field due to a dipole in its axial plane distant l and let E_q be the field in the equitorial plane distant l′. The relation between E_a and E_q is
(a) $E_a = E_q$ (b) $E_a = 2\ E_q$
(c) $E_q = 2\ E_a$ (d) $E_a = 3E_q$.

27. Particle nature and wave nature of electromagnetic waves and electrons can be shown by
(a) electron has small mass, deflected by the metal sheet
(b) X-ray is diffracted, reflected by thick metal sheet
(c) light is refracted and diffracted
(d) light is polarised and refracted.

28. A light of intensity I_0 passes through a material of thickness d. The resultant intensity is
(a) $I = I_0\ e^{-d\lambda}$ (b) $I = I_0\ (1 - e^{-d\lambda})$
(c) $I = I_0\ e^{-d/\lambda}$ (d) $I = I_0\ (1 - e^{-d/\lambda})$.
(λ being the wavelength of light)

29. A light wave moves from air to glass with frequency υ and wavelength λ. Then
(a) υ changes
(b) υ does not change, λ change.
(c) λ does not change
(d) υ and λ changes.

30. A man waves his arms while walking. This is
(a) to keep constant velocity
(b) to ease the tension
(c) to increase the velocity
(d) to balance the effect of earth's gravity.

31. A transverse stationary wave passes through a string with the equation $y = 10 \sin\pi(0.02x - 2.00t)$ where x is in meters and t in seconds. The maximum velocity of the particles in wave motion is
(a) 63 (b) 78
(c) 100 (d) 121.

32. Seven capacitors each of capacitance 2 mF are to be connected to obtain a capacitance of 10/11 mF. Which of the following combination is possible?
(a) 5 in parallel, 2 in series
(b) 4 in parallel, 3 in series
(c) 3 in parallel, 4 in series
(d) 2 in parallel, 5 in series.

33. In a series *LCR* circuit the voltage across resistance, capacitance and inductance is 10 V each. If the capacitance is short circuited, the voltage across the inductance will be
(a) $\frac{10}{\sqrt{2}}$ V (b) 10 V
(c) $10\sqrt{2}$ V (d) 20 V.

34. Eddy currents are produced when
(a) a metal is kept in varying magnetic field
(b) a metal is kept in the steady magnetic field
(c) a circular coil is placed in a magnetic field
(d) through a circular coil current is passed.

35. A moving coil galvanometer has a resistance of 900 Ω. In order to send only 10% of the main current through this galvanometer, the resistance of the required shunt is
(a) 0.9 Ω (b) 100 Ω
(c) 405 Ω (d) 90 Ω.

36. Force between two identical bar magnets whose centres are *r* metre apart is 4.8 N when their axes are in the same line. If separation is increased to 2*r*, the force between them is reduced to
(a) 2.4 N (b) 0.6 N
(c) 1.2 N (d) 0.3 N.

37. Which of the following statements is true?
(a) The presence of a large magnetic flux through a coil maintains a current in the coil if the circuit is continuous.
(b) A coil of a metal wire kept stationary in a non-uniform magnetic field has an emf induced in it.
(c) A charged particle enters a region of uniform magnetic field at an angle of 85° to the magnetic lines of force; the path of the particle is a circle.
(d) There is no change in the energy of a charged particle moving in a magnetic field although a magnetic force is acting on it.

38. The resistance between the terminal points A and B of the given infinitely long circuit will be

(a) $\sqrt{3}-1$

(b) $1-\sqrt{3}$

(c) $1+\sqrt{3}$

(d) $2+\sqrt{3}$.

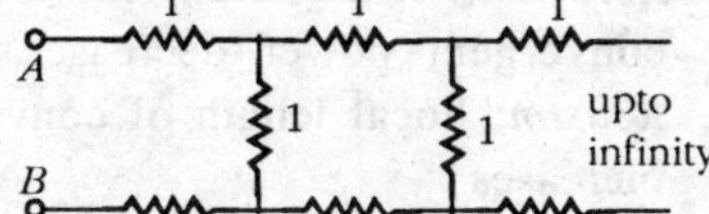

39. Potential energy of equal +ve charge 1 μC held 1 m apart in air is

(a) 1 J (b) 9×10^{-3} eV

(c) zero (d) 9×10^{-3} J.

40. In a Neon discharge tube 2.9×10^{18} Ne^+ ions move to the right each second, while 1.2×10^{18} electrons move to the left per second, electron charge is 1.6×10^{-19} C. The current in the discharge tube is

(a) 1 A towards right

(b) 0.66 A towards right

(c) 0.66 A towards left

(d) zero.

41. The earth's magnetic induction at a certain point is 7×10^{-5} Wb/m². This is to be annulled by the magnetic induction at the centre of a circular conducting loop of radius 5 cm. The required current in the loop is

(a) 0.56 A (b) 5.6 A

(c) 0.28 A (d) 2.8 A.

42. The self-induced e.m.f. in closing a d.c. current circuit is e_c, in breaking it is e_b and the e.m.f. of the source is e_0, then

(a) $e_c > e_0 > e_b$ (b) $e_c < e_0 < e_b$

(c) $e_c < e_b < e_0$ (d) $e_c = e_b < e_0$.

43. Electric potential V at any point x, y, z in space is given by $V = 6z^2$. The value of the electric field at the point (2, –1, 3) is

(a) 24 (b) –12

(c) –36 (d) 12.

44. The increase in internal energy of a system is equal to the work done on the system. Which process does the system undergo?

(a) isochoric (b) adiabatic

(c) isobaric (d) isothermal.

45. A flask containing air at 27°C is corked up at atmospheric pressure. The cork can be forced out by a pressure of 2.5 atmosphere. To what temperature the flask should be heated to do that?

(a) 150 K (b) 300 K

(c) 600 K (d) 750 K.

46. A body of mass 20.00 g has volume 5.0 cm³. The maximum possible error in the measurement of mass and volume respectively are 0.01 and 0.1 cm³. The percentage error in the density will be nearest to

(a) 1% (b) 2%

(c) 11% (d) 25%.

47. A good photographic print is obtained by an exposure of 2 seconds at a distance of 1 m from the lamp. How much time will be required to get equally good result at a distance 2 m from the same lamp?

(a) 1 second (b) 2 second

(c) 4 second (d) 8 second.

48. Two spheres of equal mass collide with the collision being absolutely elastic but not central. Then the angle between the velocities (θ) must be

(a) $\theta = 180°$ (b) $\theta \leq 180°$

(c) $90° \leq \theta \leq 180°$ (d) $\theta = 90°$.

49. A column of mercury of length h = 10 cm is contained in the middle of a narrow horizontal tube of length 1 m closed at ends. The air in both halves of the tube is under a pressure of P_0 = 76 cm of mercury. The tube is now slowly made vertical. The distance moved by mercury will be

(a) 4.5 cm (b) 3.0 cm

(c) 2.5 cm (d) 1.2 cm.

50. A simple pendulum has a bob suspended by an inextensible thread of length 1 metre from a point A of suspension. At the extreme position of oscil!ation, the thread is suddenly caught by a peg at a point B distant (1/4) m from A and the bob begins to oscillate in the new condition. The change in frequency of oscillation of the pendulum is approximately given by (g = 10 m/s²).

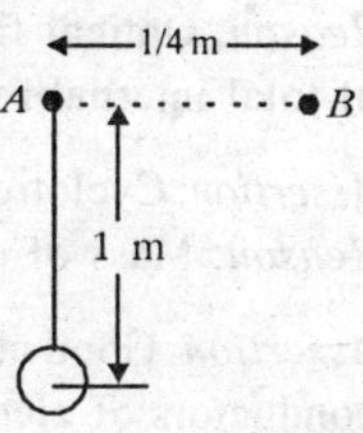

(a) $\frac{\sqrt{10}}{2}$ hertz (b) $\frac{1}{4\sqrt{10}}$ hertz

(c) $\frac{\sqrt{10}}{3}$ hertz (d) $\frac{1}{\sqrt{10}}$ hertz.

Directions :*The following questions consists of two statements, one labelled as Assertion (A) and the other labelled as Reason (R). You are to examine these two statements carefully and decide if the Assertion A and the Reason R are individually true and if so, whether the Reason is a correct explanation of the Assertion. Select your answers to these items using the codes given below:*

(a) Both A and R are true and R is the correct explanation of A.

(b) Both A and R are true but R is not the correct explanation of A.

(c) A is true but R is false.

(d) A is false but R is true.

51. *Assertion*: Density of all the nuclei is same.
Reason: Radius of nucleus is directely proportional to the cube root of mass number.

52. *Assertion*: Danger signals are made of red colour.
Reason: Velocity of red light is maximum and thus more visibility in dark.

53. *Assertion*: Current and time both have direction as well as magnitude but still are not considered vector.
Reason: They do not follow laws of vector addition.

54. *Assertion*: If polar ice melts, days will be longer.
Reason: Moment of inertia increases and thus angular velocity decreases.

55. *Assertion*: Endoscopy involves use of optical fibres to study internal organs
Reason: Optical fibres are based on phenomena of total internal reflection.

56. *Assertion*: Cyclotron does not accelerate electrons.
Reason: Mass of electrons is very small.

57. *Assertion*: Good conductors of heat are also good conductors of electricity and vice versa.
Reason: Mainly electrons are responsible for these conductions.

58. *Assertion*: Air at some distance above the fire is hotter than the same distance below it.
Reason: Air surrounding the fire carries heat upwards.

59. *Assertion*: If a convex lens is kept in water its convergent power decreases.
Reason: Focal length of convex lens in water increases.

60. *Assertion:* If current is flowing through a machine of iron eddy currents are produced.
Reason: Change in magnetic flux through an area causes eddy currents.

CHEMISTRY

61. Oxidation state of sulphur in S_8, H_2S and S_2F_2 is

(a) 0, −2, −1 (b) 0, +2, −1

(c) 1, −2, +1 (d) 0, −2, +1.

62. Which of the following is paramagnetic?

(a) NO_2 (b) N_2O

(c) N_2O_3 (d) N_2O_5.

63. $CuSO_4$ dissolves in NH_3 due to the formation of

(a) $Cu(OH)_2$ (b) $Cu[(NH_3)_4]SO_4$

(c) $Cu[(NH_3)_4(OH)_2]$ (d) CuO.

64. 12 g of an alkaline earth metal gives 14.8 gm of its nitride. Atomic weight of the metal is

(a) 12 (b) 20

(c) 40 (d) 14.8.

65. Which of the following has a tendency for covalent compound formation?

(a) Na (b) Mg

(c) Ca (d) Ba.

66. A gas z is bubbled through a solution containing x^- and y^-. If the reduction potential are in the order x > y > z, then

(a) y will oxidise z and not x

(b) y will oxidise x and not z

(c) y will oxidise both x and z

(d) y will reduce both x and z.

67. A molecule contains atoms x and y so that x occurs at the corners of the cube while y at the face centre. The formula of the molecule can be

(a) xy_3 (b) x_3y

(c) xy_2 (d) x_2y.

68. Which of the following is true about ClO_2?

(a) it is paramagnetic
(b) it dimerises in liquid phase
(c) it is an linear molecule
(d) it is very reactive.

69. The formula of microcosmic salt and the product obtained by heating it is
(a) $Na(NH_4)PO_4$; $NaPO_3$
(b) $Na(NH_4)_2HPO_4$; $NaPO_3$
(c) $Na(NH_4)HPO_4$; $NaPO_4$
(d) $Na(NH_4)HPO_4$; $NaPO_3$.

70. CO_2 is liberated on adding sodium carbonate to a carboxylic acid. The carbon of CO_2 comes from
(a) carboxylic group (b) carbonate
(c) alkyl group (d) methyl.

71. Which is not hydrolysed:
(a) PCl_3 (b) NCl_3
(c) $AsCl_3$ (d) $SnCl_3$.

72. In dichromate dimer
(a) 4 Cr – O bonds are equal
(b) 6 Cr – O bonds are equal
(c) all Cr – O bonds are equal
(d) all Cr – O bonds are unequal.

73. Which of the following don't act as Lewis acid?
(a) BF_3 (b) $SnCl_4$
(c) CCl_4 (d) SF_3.

74. The percentage of CH_4 in coal gas is
(a) 10-15% (b) 25-35%
(c) 2-5% (d) 35-50%.

75. The enthalpy change for the following reaction $NaOH_{(aq)} + HCl_{(aq)} \rightarrow NaCl_{(aq)} + H_2O_{(l)}$ is –57 kJ. Predict the value of the enthalpy change in the following reaction.
$Ba(OH)_2 + H_2SO_{4(aq)} \rightarrow BaSO_{4(s)} + 2H_2O_{(l)}$
(a) –57 kJ (b) –76 kJ
(c) –114 kJ (d) –228 kJ.

76. Which of the following 0.1 M solution will show maximum boiling point?
(a) sodium chloride (b) copper chloride
(c) magnesium sulphate
(d) chromium sulphate.

77. In the formation of $[Ni(CN)_4]^{2-}$, the type of hybridisation involved is
(a) sp^2 (b) sp^3d
(c) dsp^2 (d) sp^3d.

78. The unit in which the solubility product of barium phosphate is expressed as
(a) $mol^2\ dm^{-6}$ (b) $mol^3\ dm^{-9}$
(c) $mol^4\ dm^{-12}$ (d) $mol^5\ dm^{-15}$.

79. Helium atom is two times heavier than a hydrogen molecule. At 298 K, the average kinetic energy of the helium atom is
(a) two times that of a hydrogen molecule
(b) same as that of a hydrogen molecule
(c) four times that of a hydrogen molecule
(d) half that of a hydrogen molecule.

80. The boiling point of CCl_4 is higher than that of $CHCl_3$ because
(a) $CHCl_3$ forms hydrogen bonds
(b) CCl_4 is highly soluble in water
(c) CCl_4 has strong van der Waal's forces of attraction than $CHCl_3$
(d) CCl_4 is more ionic than $CHCl_3$.

81. Salicylic acid is prepared from phenol by
(a) Reimer - Tiemann reaction
(b) Kolbe's synthesis
(c) Gattermann's reaction
(d) None of the above.

82. The salient feature of the theory of absolute reaction rates is the
(a) formation of activated complex
(b) collision of the reactant molecules
(c) matching potential energy of the reactant molecules
(d) decrease of entropy of the reactant molecules.

83. Portland cement contains the following amount of CaO
(a) 5-15% (b) 20-35%
(c) 50-60% (d) 70-80%.

84. In dichromate dimer
(a) 4 Cr – O bonds are equal
(b) 6 Cr – O bonds are equal
(c) all Cr – O bonds are equal
(d) all Cr – O bonds are unequal.

85. Acetamide and ethylamine can be distinguished by reacting with

(a) dilute HCl and heat
(b) NaOH solution and heat
(c) acidified $KMnO_4$ (d) Br_2 water.

86. A vessel of one litre capacity containing 1 mole of SO_3 is heated till a state of equilibrium is attained.

$$2SO_{3\,(g)} \rightleftharpoons 2SO_{2\,(g)} + O_{2\,(g)}.$$

At equilibrium, 0.6 moles of SO_2 had formed. The value of equilibrium constant is
(a) 0.18 (b) 0.36
(c) 0.45 (d) 0.68.

87. Gasoline is a mixture of hydrocarbons containing
(a) C_3 to C_5 carbon atoms
(b) C_7 to C_9 carbon atoms
(c) C_{12} to C_{16} carbon atoms
(d) C_{14} to C_{18} carbon atoms.

88. Identify the product in the reaction.

$$C_6H_6 \xrightarrow[\text{Reflux}]{HNO_3/H_2SO_4} \text{intermediate compound} \xrightarrow{Sn/HCl} \text{product.}$$

(a) $C_2H_5NO_2$ (b) $C_6H_4(NO_2)_2$

(c) 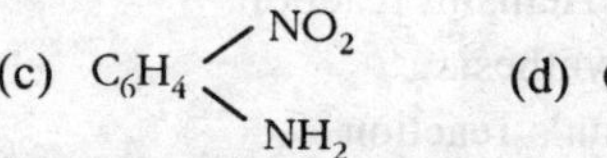

(d) $C_6H_4(NH_2)_2$

89. *Tempering* steel is a process of heating
(a) steel in contact with carbon and quenching it
(b) steel in the presence of ammonia and quenching it
(c) the hardened steel to a temperature below redness and cooling it slowly
(d) steel to bright redness and quenching it.

90. Which of the following ions in aqueous solution is the best conductor of electricity?
(a) Li^+ (b) Na^+
(c) Mg^{2+} (d) Cs^+.

91. If the r.m.s. speed of a gas molecule at 27°C is $100\sqrt{2}$ ms^{-1} the r.m.s. speed at 327°C would be
(a) 100 ms^{-1} (b) 200 ms^{-1}
(c) 300 ms^{-1} (d) 400 ms^{-1}.

92. Sodium thiosulphate is used in photography to
(a) reduce AgBr grains to metallic Ag
(b) dissolve out Ag produced by reduction
(c) remove unaffected AgBr in the photographic film or plate
(d) none of these.

93. Nitrogen and oxygen exist as diatomic but their cogeners are P_4 and S_8 respectively. This is due to
(a) phosphorus and sulphur are solids
(b) phosphorus and sulphur polymerise as soon as they are formed
(c) phosphorus and sulphur catenate due to the existence of *d*-orbitals and form strainless structures
(d) none of these.

94. The IUPAC name of $CH \equiv C - CH = CH{\cdot}CH_3$ is
(a) pent-1-yn-3ene (b) pent-3, ene-1, yne
(c) pent-2-ene-4 yne (d) 3-ene-pent-1 yne.

95. The AsF_5 molecule is trigonal pyramidal. The hybrid orbitals used by the As atoms for bonding are
(a) $d_{x^2-y^2}, d_{z^2}, s, px, py$
(b) d_{xy}, s, p_x, p_y, p_z
(c) $s, p_x, p_y, p_z, d_{z^2}$
(d) $d_{x^2-y^2}, s, p_x, p_y, p_z$.

96. Which one of the following is the correct order of the size of iodine species?
(a) $I > I^- > I^+$ (b) $I > I^+ > I^-$
(c) $I^+ > I^- > I$ (d) $I^- > I > I^+$.

97. Philosopher's wool when heated with BaO at 1100°C gives a compound. Identify the compound.
(a) $BaZnO_2$ (b) $Ba + ZnO_2$
(c) $BaCdO_2$ (d) $BaO_2 + Zn$.

98. The pH value of 0.1 M NaOH solution is (when there is a given reaction $[H^+][OH^-] = 10^{-14}$)
(a) 13 (b) 12
(c) 11 (d) 2.

99. Which of the following have nonlinear structure?
(a) $Ag(NH_3)_2^+$ (b) $HgCl_2$
(c) $SnCl_2$ (d) $BeCl_2$.

100. Identify the transition element:
(a) $1s^2, 2s^22p^6, 3s^23p^6, 4s^2$
(b) $1s^2, 2s^22p^6, 3s^23p^63d^{10}, 4s^24p^1$
(c) $1s^2, 2s^22p^6, 3s^23p^63d^{10}, 4s^24p^6$
(d) $1s^2, 2s^22p^6, 3s^23p^63d^2, 4s^2$.

101. The edge length of face centred unit cube cell is 508 pm. If the radius of the cation is 110 pm, the radius of the anion is
(a) 288 pm (b) 398 pm
(c) 144 pm (d) 618 pm.

102. A certain aqueous solution of $FeCl_3$ [formula mass = 162] has a density of 1.1 g/mL and contains 20.0% $FeCl_3$. Molar concentration of this solution is

(a) 0.028 (b) 0.163
(c) 1.357 (d) 1.47.

103. The combustion enthalpies of carbon, hydrogen and methane are –395.5 kJ mol^{-1}, –284.8 kJ mol^{1} and –890.4 kJ mol^{-1} respectively at 25°C. The value of standard formation enthalpies of methane at that temperature is

(a) 890.4 kJ mol^{-1} (b) –298.8 kJ mol^{-1}
(c) –74.7 kJ mol^{-1} (d) –107.7 kJ mol^{-1}.

104. The following nuclear transmition

$^{23}_{11}Na + ^{1}_{1}H \rightarrow ^{32}_{12}Mg + ^{1}_{0}n$

belongs to

(a) (n, L) type (b) (p, n) type
(c) (L, n) type (d) (d, p) type.

105. Baking soda or baking powder is

(a) washing soda (b) caustic soda
(c) soda ash
(d) sodium bicarbonate.

106. NaOH is prepared by the electrolysis of

(a) aqueous solution of sodium chloride with platinum electrode
(b) sodium chloride solution with graphite anode and iron cathode
(c) sodium carbonate with platinum electrodes
(d) sodium carbonate with nickel electrodes.

107. The process associated with sodium carbonate manufacture is known as .... process.

(a) Chamber (b) Haber
(c) Le-Blanc (d) Castner.

108. Identify the correct statement:

(a) Elemental sodium can be prepared and isolated by electrolysing an aqueous solution of sodium chloride.
(b) Elemental sodium is a strong oxidising agent.
(c) Elemental sodium is insoluble in ammonia.
(d) Elemental sodium is easily oxidised.

109. An ore of potassium is

(a) carnallite (b) cryolite
(c) bauxite (d) dolomite.

110. Which has lowest thermal stability?

(a) Li_2CO_3 (b) Na_2CO_3
(c) K_2CO_3 (d) Rb_2CO_3.

Directions : *The following questions consists of two statements, one labelled as Assertion (A) and the other labelled as Reason (R). You are to examine these two statements carefully and decide if the Aseertion A and the Reason R are individually true and if so, whether the Reason is a correct explanation of the Assertion. Select your answers to these items using the codes given below:*

(a) Both A and R are true and R is the correct explanation of A.
(b) Both A and R are true but R is not the correct explanation of A.
(c) A is true but R is false.
(d) A is false but R is true.

111. *Assertion:* Formic acid reduces mercuric chloride to mercurous chloride on heating, while acetic acid does not.
Reason: Formic acid is stronger than acetic acid.

112. *Assertion:* Bond order can have positive, negative or fractional value.
Reason: Bond order depends upon the bonding and antibonding orbital electrons.

113. *Assertion:* H_3PO_3 is dibasic acid.
Reason: Two hydrogen atoms are directly attached to the P.

114. *Assertion:* Heat of neutralization for both HNO_3 and HCl with NaOH is 53.7 KJ/mole.
Reason: NaOH is a strong electrolyte/base.

115. *Assertion:* Pb^{4+} can be reduced easily to Pb^{2+}.
Reason: Pb^{2+} is paramagnetic.

116. *Assertion:* Maleic acid shows geometrical isomerism.
Reason: It has –C = C– bond.

117. *Assertion:* 0.1 M solution of glucose has same increment in the freezing point than 0.1 M solution of urea.
Reason: K_f for both has same value.

118. *Assertion:* When an atom in group 1A of the periodic table undergoes radioactive decay by emitting a positron, the resulting element belongs to zero group.

Reason: When an atom emits a positron, its atomic number increases by one unit.

119. *Assertion:* Alkenes and cycloalkanes series of hydrocarbons have same general formula.
Reason: Either insertion of a double bond or formation of a ring reduce the number of hydrogen atoms of corresponding alkane by 2.

120. *Assertion:* The carbon atoms of the benzene ring may be numbered for identification of substituent groups, just as a continuous chains of carbon atoms are numbered.
Reason: Smallest set of numbers designating the substituents is the preferred set.

BIOLOGY

121. Which of the following organism is found in lymph nodes?
(a) *Plasmodium* (b) *Wuchereria*
(c) *Taenia* (d) *Diplococcus*.

122. "Gametes are never hybrid". This is a statement of
(a) law of dominance
(b) law of independent assortment
(c) law of segregation
(d) law of random fertilisation.

123. Mendel was not able to say anything about recombination and crossing over because
(a) he did not have a large and strong microscope
(b) he chose only pure type
(c) traits he chose, were not linked and present on different chromosomes or were far apart
(d) traits he chose had no genes.

124. Sprain is due to excessive pulling of
(a) tendon (b) muscle
(c) ligament (d) neurons.

125. A man suddenly sees a tiger. His heart beat goes up, blood pressure increases, etc. Which hormone is released at this time in his body.
(a) parathormone (b) corticoid
(c) adrenaline (d) thyroxine.

126. A scientist wants to study the viral effects on plants. Which of the following part of the plant should he exclude?
(a) phloem (b) pith
(c) cortex (d) shoot apex.

127. A man has enlarged breasts, sparse hair on body and sex compliment as XXY. He then suffers from
(a) Down's syndrome (b) Klinefelters syndrome
(c) Edward's syndrome (d) Turner's syndrome.

128. "They have raised cheek bones, oblique eyes and yellowish skin colours". Here they refers to
(a) Adrenoids (b) Negroids
(c) Mongoloids (d) Africans.

129. Urea is transported by
(a) plasma (b) RBC
(c) blood plasma (d) WBC.

130. In fast swimming fishes, propulsion is due to
(a) pelvic fin (b) pectoral fin
(c) dorsal fin (d) caudal fin.

131. While dissecting a rat, when you are pinning the rat in the dissecting tray, which side should face you?
(a) dorsal (b) ventral
(c) anterior (d) lateral.

132. The molecule which mainly absorb light energy and convert it to chemical energy in photosynthesis are
(a) chlorophyll (b) chlorophyll *a*
(c) chlorophyll *b* (d) xanthophyll.

133. Apical dominance can be overcome by application of
(a) auxin (b) cytokinin
(c) florigen (d) gibberellin.

134. Thickening of arteries due to cholesterol deposition is
(a) arteriosclerosis (b) rheumatic heart
(c) blood pressure (d) cardiac arrest.

135. Blood vessels in *Pheretima*, which have valves are
(a) dorsal (b) ventral
(c) integumentary (d) lateral.

136. Rate of transpiration can be measured by
(a) Ganong's potometer (b) porometer
(c) auxanometer (d) respirometer.

137. If we take food rich in lime juice, then
(a) action of ptyalin on starch is enhanced
(b) action of ptyalin on starch is reduced
(c) action of ptyalin on starch is unaffected
(d) action of ptyalin on starch stops.

138. Why do we move our hands while walking?

(a) to relieve our tension
(b) to walk faster
(c) to maintain equilibrium against force of gravity
(d) to increase blood circulation.

139. Transverse section of a plant is stained with safranin and fast green. What is the colour of the phloem?
(a) red (b) green
(c) pink (d) orange.

140. Gene which suppresses other gene's activity but does not lie on the same locus is called as
(a) epistatic (b) supplementary
(c) hypostatic (d) codominant.

141. Resolving limit of our eye is
(a) 1′ (b) 1″
(c) 1/60′ (d) 1/60″.

142. Root cap is formed by
(a) dermatogen (b) calyptrogen
(c) vascular cambium (d) wound cambium.

143. Amniocentesis is
(a) digestion of amino acid
(b) conversion of glucose to amino acids
(c) taking out of cells near the foetus
(d) killing of child before birth.

144. Malignant tertian malaria is caused by
(a) *Plasmodium vivax* (b) *P. ovale*
(c) *P. falciparum* (d) *P. malariae*.

145. A bacterial cell divides once every minute and it takes 1 hour to fill a cup. How much time will it take to fill half the cup?
(a) 30 minutes (b) 60 minutes
(c) 29 minutes (d) 59 minutes.

146. In 1929, a scientist discovered an antibiotic which was found very effective. The name of the scientist and the antibiotic, respectively are
(a) Alexander Fleming, Penicillin
(b) Alexander Fleming, Streptomycin
(c) Alexander, Penicillin
(d) None of the above.

147. Albinism and phenylketonuria are disorders due to
(a) recessive autosomal genes
(b) dominant autosomal genes
(c) recessive sex genes
(d) dominant sex genes.

148. A man has a wound. Normally a bleeding wound develops a clot and flow of blood stops. If this does not happen to the man, then he probably suffers from
(a) AIDS (b) tetanus
(c) haemophilia (d) malaria.

149. Which of the following is the best way to determine paternity?
(a) protein analysis
(b) chromosome counting
(c) DNA finger printing
(d) gene counting.

150. Coiling of a tendril around a support is an example of
(a) photonasty (b) thigmonasty
(c) nyctinasty (d) hydronasty.

151. You met a person who has bulging/protruding eyes, tachycardia and higher body temperature. He suffered from
(a) hyperthyroidism (b) acromegaly
(c) diabetes (d) cretinism.

152. One of the possible early sources of energy were/was
(a) CO_2 (b) chlorophyll
(c) green plants
(d) UV rays and lightening.

153. The limiting factor in nitrification of soil is
(a) soil nature (pH) (b) light
(c) temperature (d) air.

154. Colchicine inhibits
(a) prophase (b) anaphase
(c) interphase (d) spindle formation.

155. Blood pressure is measured by
(a) sphymogmanometer (b) stethoscope
(c) electrocardiogram (d) phonocardiogram.

156. The most important source of energy on earth is
(a) ATP molecules (b) chlorophyll
(c) xanthophyll (d) carotenoids.

157. Sexual reproduction in which DNA of bacteria is transferred to another by the help of bacteriophage is
(a) transformation (b) transduction
(c) transcription (d) conjugation.

158. A person is suffering from impaired nervous

system and madness after prolonged consumption of polluted water. Which metal is responsible?
(a) Hg (b) Ca
(c) Mn (d) Pb.

159. Body temperature of cold blooded animals
(a) is constant
(b) fluctuates with surrounding temperature
(c) becomes very low at times
(d) is very cold.

160. Plants can be cultivated in soil less medium where all required nutrients are supplied from the outside in water solution, this method comes under
(a) water culture (b) hydroponics
(c) hybrid culture (d) critical culture media.

161. A part of brain of frog is removed which helps it to respire and locomote. The removed part of brain is
(a) medulla oblongata (b) diencephalon
(c) cerebellum (d) cerebral hemisphere.

162. Which enzyme digests peptides releasing amino acid one by one?
(a) pepsin (b) trypsin
(c) peptidases (d) aminopeptidase.

163. Cyanobacteria helps farmers by
(a) reducing the alkanity of the soil
(b) reducing the acidity of the soil
(c) neutralising the alkanity of the soil
(d) water logging.

164. A person having parkinson's disease shows defective action of which neutrotransmitter in brain
(a) dopamine (b) seratonin
(c) noradrenaline (d) eukalphia.

165. Most of the plants cultivated in agriculture are actually belonging to the succession level
(a) early 1° succession (b) late 1° succession
(c) early 2° succession (d) late 2° succession.

166. A plant has a butterfly shaped flower with one standard two wing like and two keel petals. The plant belongs to the family
(a) papilionaceae (b) compositae
(c) malvaceae (d) rubiaceae.

167. The part of cauliflower that we eat is
(a) stem (b) leaf
(c) flower (d) inflorescence.

168. The vacuoles are surrounded by a thin membrane called
(a) plasmodesmata (b) hydathodes
(c) tonoplast (d) both (b) and (c).

169. Pneumolaxis and inhibitory centres are associated with
(a) breathing (b) respiration
(c) digestion (d) sleeping.

170. The conidiophores of *Pencillium* are
(a) uninucleate and colourless
(b) uninucleate and pigmented
(c) binuclcate and pigmented
(d) binucleate and pigmented.

Directions : *The following questions consists of two statements, one labelled as Assertion (A) and the other labelled as Reason (R). You are to examine these two statements carefully and decide if the Assertion A and the Reason R are individually true and if so, whether the Reason is a correct explanation of the Assertion. Select your answers to these items using the codes given below:*
(a) Both A and R are true and R is the correct explanation of A.
(b) Both A and R are true but R is not the correct explanation of A.
(c) A is true but R is false.
(d) A is false and R is true.

171. *Assertion:* Hearing aids help the hearing impaired to hear.
Reason: They make sound travel through skull bones.

172. *Assertion:* Cyanobacteria are photosynthetic, blue green algae with all the prokaryotic structures.
Reason: They are green due to presence of chloroplasts.

173. *Assertion:* Plants also have hormones called as phytohormones.
Reason: They increase the rate of reactions and thus always accelerate growth and other related changes.

174. *Assertion:* Leguminous plants are best preferred for rotation of crops.
Reason: They have root nodules which have nitrogen fixing bacterium *Clostridium*.

175. *Assertion:* Cancer is contagious and cells can spread from one person to other.
Reason: Cancerous cells are highly dedifferentiated cells.

176. *Assertion:* Fruit juices taste bitter on being kept for some time.
Reason: Microorganisms of the air spoil it quickly.

177. *Assertion:* Amphibians have evolved from fishes.
Reason: Take the example of the fossil *Archaeopteryx*.

178. *Assertion:* Vascular cambium is considered as lateral meristem.
Reason: It gives rise to lateral shoots.

179. *Assertion:* Person with blood group AB can take blood from any other person.
Reason: Blood group incompatibility is due to antigen -antibody reaction. Blood group AB has no antibody and thus the antigen of the other group is not affected.

180. *Assertion:* Snakes exposed to gamma rays become non poisonous.
Reason: Poisonous snakes have poison glands and a pair of poison fangs. They are affected by gamma rays.

GENERAL KNOWLEDGE

181. India's one billionth baby was born on 12, May 2000 in
(a) Safdurjung Hospital, New Delhi
(b) Maternity Hospital, Bombay
(c) Christian Medical College, Vellore
(d) City Hospital, Chennai.

182. *Abhigyan Shakuntalam* has been written by
(a) Tulsidas (b) Kalidasa
(c) Valmiki (d) Kabir.

183. Who is the chairman of Censor Board of India?
(a) Shatrughan Sinha
(b) Mala Sinha
(c) Asha Parekh
(d) Rajesh Khanna.

184. In India, whose sign is found on currency note?
(a) President of India
(b) Finance Minister
(c) Prime Minister
(d) Governer, Reserve Bank.

185. Who won the wimbeldon women's singles 99?
(a) Stephy Graph
(b) Lindsy Devenporti
(c) Martina Hingris
(d) Martina Navratilova.

186. Gyanpeeth award' 98 was honoured to
(a) Gireesh Karnad (b) Arundhathi Roy
(c) Asha Sharan Devi (d) A.B. Vajpayee.

187. Full form of "SAARC"
(a) South Asian Association for Regional Coordination
(b) South Asian Association for Regional Cooperation
(c) South African Agriculture Research Council
(d) South Asia And Rest Countries.

188. Suez canal joints
(a) Red sea and Dead sea
(b) Red sea and Mediteranian sea
(c) Dead sea and Mediteranian sea
(d) Pacific and Atlantic sea.

189. Full form of "http"
(a) hyper text transfer programme
(b) hyper text transfer protocol
(c) hyper text transfer protocol
(d) high tech. testing protocol.

190. First surface to surface missile test fired in India
(a) Prithvi (b) Agni
(c) Rohini (d) Naga.

191. What are bulls in stock market?
(a) stock brokers (b) steady games
(c) big losses (d) big gains.

192. What is fiscal deficit?
(a) same as budget deficit
(b) difference between expenditure and revenue earned
(c) annual debt
(d) repayed debts and their interests.

193. What is the full form of DOT?
(a) Direct Observation Treatment
(b) Distant Observation Treatment

(c) Domestic Oral Treatment
(d) Duel Oriented Treatment.

194. Which Indian city is known as 'Space City"?
(a) Hyderabad
(b) Ahmedabad
(c) Bangalore
(d) Thiruvananthapuram

195. Dronacharya Award is given to
(a) Teachers
(b) Sports coaches
(c) Retired sports persons
(d) National Champion in Archery

196. Who wrote 'Sare Jahan Se Achchha Hindostan Hamara'?
(a) Ram Prasad Bismil
(b) Iqbal
(c) Rabindra Nath Tagore
(d) Bankim Chandra Chatterjee.

197. Which is the highest gallantry award ?
(a) Ashoka Chakra
(b) Param Vir Chakra
(c) Mahavir Chakra
(d) None of these.

198. At what temperature do both the Centigrade and Fahrenheit thermometers show the same reading?
(a) -20^0 (b) -40^0
(c) 42^0 (d) O^o

199. Dr. C.V. Raman was awarded Nobel Prize in
(a) Physics (b) Medicine
(c) Chemistry (d) Literature.

200. Greenhouse effect means
(a) trapping of solar energy due to atmospheric carbon dioxide
(b) pollution in the tropical region
(c) trapping of solar energy due to Nitrogen in atmosphere
(d) planting of green trees.

❖ ❖ ❖

SOLUTIONS

PHYSICS

1. **(b)** : For the body to complete the vertical circle, the speed at the bottom of the circular track must equal $\sqrt{5gR}$, where R is the radius of the circle. If the body falls through a height h until it reaches the bottom of the track,

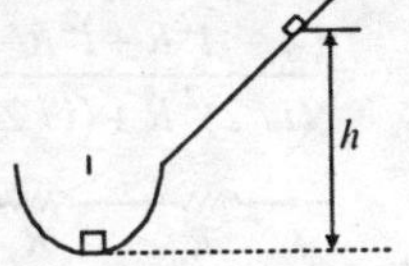

$$\sqrt{5g\frac{D}{2}} = \sqrt{2gh} \text{ (From energy conservation)}$$

or, $h = \frac{5D}{4}$.

2. **(a)** : Gravitational constant comes in the formula

$$F = \frac{Gm_1m_2}{r^2} \text{ or } G = \frac{Fr^2}{m_1m_2} = \frac{\text{kg}\frac{\text{meter}}{\text{sec}^2}(\text{meter})^2}{\text{kg}^2}$$

$\equiv \text{kg}^{-1} (\text{meter})^3(\text{sec})^{-2} \equiv M^{-1}L^3T^{-2}$.

3. **(d)** : $u = \frac{p}{m} = \frac{10}{5} = 2$ m/s, $a = \frac{0.2}{5}$ m/s^2

$v = u + at = 2 + \frac{0.2}{5} \times 10 = 2.4$ m/s.

$\Delta K = \frac{1}{2} mv^2 - \frac{1}{2} mu^2 = \frac{1}{2} \times 5 \times (2.4)^2 - \frac{1}{2} \times 5 \times 2^2$

$= 4.4$ J.

4. **(c)** : Let C be the point where the gravitational field due to earth and the moon be equal. C is at a distance x from the moon and $(60R - x)$ from the earth. We know that the gravitational field at a distance r from mass M is given by

$E = G\frac{M}{r^2}$

60R
C
(60R–x) x
Earth Moon

In our case
$E_1 = E_2$

$\Rightarrow G\frac{M}{(60R-x)^2} = G\frac{\frac{M}{81}}{x^2}$

$\Rightarrow 81x^2 = (60R - x)^2$

$\Rightarrow (9x)^2 = (60R - x)^2$

$\therefore 9x = \pm (60R - x)$

$\therefore 9x = 60R - x$ or $9x = x - 60R$

$\Rightarrow 10x = 60R$ or $8x = -60R$

$\Rightarrow x = 6R$ or $x = -\frac{60}{8}R$

which is not possible as distance cannot be negative.

5. **(d)** : On doubling the kinetic energy, the velocity becomes $\sqrt{2}$ times the initial velocity. As the escape velocity is $\sqrt{2}$ times that of the orbital velocity, the satellite will escape out of the earth's gravitational field.

The orbital velocity is given by

$v_o = \sqrt{\frac{GM}{R}}$

K.E. $K = \frac{1}{2} mv_o^2 \Rightarrow v_o = \sqrt{\frac{2K}{m}}$

if *K.E.* is doubled, then

$v'_o = \sqrt{\frac{2\times 2K}{m}} = \sqrt{2}\sqrt{\frac{2K}{m}} = \sqrt{2}\, v_o$

Since escape velocity $v_e = \sqrt{\frac{2GM}{R}} = \sqrt{2}\, v_o$.

6. **(c)** : As per Bohr's model of hydrogen atom, the angular momentum of the electron in allowed orbits is given by $L = \frac{nh}{2\pi}$, $n = 1, 2, 3,.....$

For the second orbit $n = 2$, $L = 2\frac{h}{2\pi} = \frac{h}{\pi}$.

7. **(b)** : Let N_0 be the number of nuclei at the beginning. Number of undecayed nuclei after 33% decay = 0.67 N_0

Number of undecayed nuclei after 67% decay = 0.33 N_0

Also $0.33 N_0 \approx \frac{0.67N_0}{2}$. And in one half life the number of undecayed nuclei becomes half.

Exact calculation :

Let number of nucler at the beginning = N_0

Let the time required for 33% decay = t_1

Then $0.67\, N_0 = N_0\, e^{-\lambda t_1}$

$\Rightarrow e^{-\lambda t_1} = 0.67$ ....(1)

Time required for 67% decay = t_2

$\therefore e^{-\lambda t_2} = 0.33$ ....(2)

[Since after 33% decay, 67% will remain and after 67% decay, 33% will remain].

$\therefore \quad (2) \div (1) \Rightarrow e^{-\lambda(t_2 - t_1)} = \frac{0.33}{0.67} = \frac{1}{2}$

$\therefore \quad -\lambda\,(t_2 - t_1) - ln\left(\frac{1}{2}\right)$

$\therefore \quad t_2 - t_1 = -\frac{ln\left(\frac{1}{2}\right)}{\lambda} = -\frac{ln\left(\frac{1}{2}\right) \times T_{½}}{0.693}$

$= -\frac{ln\left(\frac{1}{2}\right) \times 20}{-ln\left(\frac{1}{2}\right)}$ = 20 minutes

8. (d) : When a ray of light enters a glass-slab its frequency does not change. This is because frequency is the property of the source emitting the radiation. And once the light is emitted, its frequency remains same in all the media it propagates through.

9. (b) : For myopia (shortsightedness) a convex lens is used. For hypermetropia, we need concave or diverging lens for the ray of light to be focused on the retina. For presbyopia bifocal lens is used and astigmatism is cleared with cylindrical lenses. Therefore the correct alternative is (b)

10. (b) : Power of the resultant combination is given by

$$P = P_1 + P_2$$

First lens is a convex lens with power

$$P_1 = +\frac{1}{0.40} = +\,2.5 \text{ D}$$

The second lens is a concave lens with power

$$P_2 = -\frac{1}{0.25} = -\,4 \text{ D}$$

$\therefore$ The total power of the combination

$$P = P_1 + P_2 = 2.5 - 4 = -\,1.5 \text{ D}$$

11. (b) : Transformers are used for stepping-up or stepping down an A.C current (A.C voltage source).

Leclanche cell gives a D.C. voltage. As the input from a Leclanche cell does not change with time, the magnetic flux linked with the secondary also does not change and hence the induced *emf* is zero. Hence the output will be zero.

12. (b) : From Wien displacement Law,

$\lambda_m T \cong$ constant

$\therefore 510 \times T_{sun} = 350 \times T_{star}$ or $\frac{T_{sun}}{T_{star}} = \frac{350}{510} = 0.68$.

13. (c) : $\frac{H_A}{H_B} = \left(\frac{T_A}{T_B}\right)^4 = \left(\frac{727+273}{327+273}\right)^4 = \frac{625}{81}$.

14. (c) : Ratio of the intensities = 9 : 1

$\therefore$ Ratio of the amplitudes = 3 : 1

On superposition,

$$\frac{\text{Maximum Intensity}}{\text{Minimum Intensity}} = \frac{(3+1)^2}{(3-1)^2} = 4:1.$$

15. (c) : As there is no external force acting on the system, the momentum of the system remains conserved in a collision but the kinetic energy is conserved only in elastic collisions.

16. (b) : Required ratio

$$= \frac{i^2R + i^2R}{(i/2)^2R + (i/2)^2R} = 4:1.$$

Series Combination

Parallel Combination

17. (c) : Let *m* capacitors are joined in series and *n* such groups are joined in parallel.

So, $C = 8/m$ and $C_{equi.} = n \times \frac{8}{m} = 16$

or, $n = 2m$.

Potential of arrangement, $mV = 1000$

or, $m = \frac{1000}{250} = 4. \quad \therefore \quad n = 2 \times 4 = 8.$

So, total number of capacitors required

$= nm = 8 \times 4 = 32.$

18. (a) : For the rotational energy to be minimum the moment of inertia of the system about the axis through the point must be minimum. If this point in at a distance of x from 0.3 kg mass, $I = 0.3x^2 + 0.7(1.4 - x)^2$

$\frac{dI}{dx} = 0$ gives $x = 0.98$ m.

19. (b)

20. (b) : The power of the incandescent lamp $P = 60$ W

Operating voltage V = 120 V

$\therefore$ Current through the filament $I = \frac{P}{V} = \frac{60}{120} = \frac{1}{2}$ A

Now $Q = I \times t$

For $t = 1$ sec, $Q = I = \frac{1}{2}$ C

$\Rightarrow \quad ne = \frac{1}{2}$

where e = electronic charge, and n = number of electrons.

$\therefore n = \frac{1}{2e} = \frac{1}{2 \times 1.6 \times 10^{-19}} = 3.12 \times 10^{18}$

21. (d) : In steady state condition the current at each cross-section will be the same. Drift velocity and electric field depend on the current density, $\bar{M}$ which varies from one cross-section to another.

22. (a) : Each point of the sphere must be at the same

potential and at any point interior to the sphere, the potential is same as that at the surface.

23. (b) : About point O, the angular momentum of the projectile is in clockwise sense. The torque on the projectile about point O (moment of mg) is also in clockwise sense. Hence the angular momentum increases.

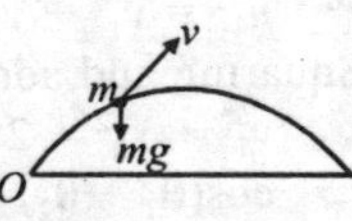

24. (d) : Given that the field at the centre of the ring $B = 7 \times 10^{-9}$ Wb/m²

We know that $B = \dfrac{\mu_0 I}{2r}$

$$\Rightarrow I = \frac{2Br}{\mu_0}$$

$$= \frac{2\times 7\times 10^{-9}\times 0.05}{4\pi\times 10^{-7}}$$

$$= 5.57 \times 10^{-4} \text{ A}$$

25. (b) : Inside the magnet the lines go from south pole to the north pole.

26. (b) : $E_{\text{axial}} = \dfrac{1}{4\pi\varepsilon_0}\dfrac{2p}{r^3}$; $E_{\text{equatorial}} = \dfrac{1}{4\pi\varepsilon_0}\dfrac{p}{r^3}$.

$\therefore E_a = 2E_{\text{eq}}$.

27. (d)

28. (c) : Alternatives (a) and (b) are dimensionally incorrect. When $d \to 0, I \to I_0$. Alternative (c) meets this requirement.

29. (b) : υ does not change, λ changes. The frequency υ is a property of the source of radiation but λ is a function of the refractive index of the medium.

30. (d) : Due to waving of the arms, the centre of gravity remains at a comfortable position, so it helps to walk comfortably.

31. (a) : $y = 10 \sin\pi(0.02x - 2.00t)$

$$\frac{\partial y}{\partial t} = -20\pi \cos \pi(0.02x - 2.00t)$$

$$\left(\frac{\partial y}{\partial t}\right)_{\max} = 20\pi = 63 \text{ units.}$$

32. (a) : 5 capacitors in parallel gives 5×2 mF = 10 mF.

The 2 capacitors in series give 1 mF.

When they are connected in series, total capacitance will be $\dfrac{10\times 1}{10+1} = \dfrac{10}{11}$ mF.

33. (a) : Since voltage across L, C and R is same, equal to 10 V, therefore $R = X_L = X_C$.

Also total voltage in the circuit is

$$I\,[R^2 + (X_L - X_C)^2]^{1/2} = I\,R = 10 \text{ V}.$$

When capacitor is short circuited current in the circuit

$$I = \frac{10}{(R^2 + X_L{}^2)^{1/2}} = \frac{10}{\sqrt{2}\,R}.$$

Potential drop across inductance

$$= IX_L = IR = 10/\sqrt{2} \text{ V}.$$

34. (a) : Suppose a metal plate is kept in a magnetic field. On the surface of the metal plate, we can imagine a loop, which will be associated with a magnetic flux due to the magnetic field. As the magnetic field is changing, there is change of magnetic flux through this loop and so an electric current is going to be induced in the loop, which is known as the eddy current.

35. (b) :

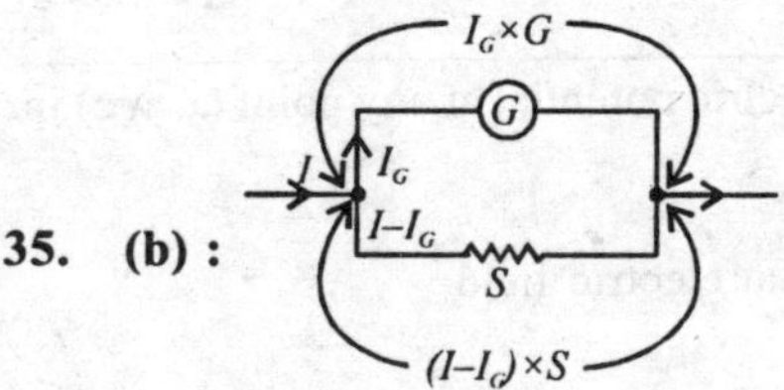

Here $I_g = I/10$. Now $I_g G = (I - I_g)\,S$.

$$\therefore \quad S = \frac{I_g G}{I - I_g}.$$

In this case $G = 900\ \Omega$. Hence $S = 100\ \Omega$.

36. (d) : In magnetic dipole, Force $\propto 1/r^4$

$$\therefore \quad \text{New force} = \frac{4.8}{2^4} = \frac{4.8}{16} = 0.3 \text{ N}.$$

37. (b) : Non-uniform magnetic field causes change in flux.

38. (c) : The equivalent circuit may be shown as :

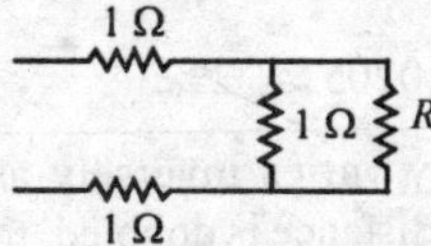

where R may be treated as the total resistance.

Hence $1 + \dfrac{1\times R}{1+R} + 1 = R$.

This gives $R = 1 \pm \sqrt{3}$.

Since $1 - \sqrt{3}$ gives –ve value,

therefore $R = 1 + \sqrt{3}$.

39. (d) : The potential energy is given by

$$U_P = \frac{1}{4\pi\varepsilon_0}\times\frac{q_1 q_2}{r}$$

$$= 9 \times 10^9 \times \frac{1\times 10^{-6}\times 1\times 10^{-6}}{1}$$

$$= 9 \times 10^{-3} \text{ J}$$

40. (b) : Charge on ions = $2.9 \times 10^{18} \times 1.6 \times 10^{-19}$ C
Charge on electrons = $1.2 \times 10^{18} \times 1.6 \times 10^{-19}$ C
Total charge = $4.1 \times 1.6 \times 10^{-1}$ C
$= 6.56 \times 10^{-1}$ C = 0.66 C.

$$\text{Current} = \frac{\text{Charge}}{\text{Time}} = \frac{0.66\,(\text{C})}{1\,(\text{s})} = 0.66 \text{ A}.$$

The direction of current in a circuit is, by convention, taken along the direction in which positive charges flow. Hence the current in the discharge tube flows towards right.

41. (b) : $H = 7 \times 10^{-5} = \frac{\mu_0}{4\pi}\frac{2\pi I}{R}$

Here R = 5 cm = 0.05 m and $\frac{\mu_0}{4\pi} = 10^{-7}$.
Hence I = 5.6 A.

42. (c)

43. (c) : The electric potential at any point (x, y, z) in space is given as

$V = 6Z^2$

We know that electric field

$\vec{E} = -\vec{\Delta}V$

$$\Rightarrow \quad \vec{E} = -\left[\frac{\partial V}{\partial x}\hat{i} + \frac{\partial V}{\partial y}\hat{j} + \frac{\partial V}{\partial z}\hat{k}\right] = -12Z\,\hat{k}$$

$\therefore E(2, -1, 3) = -12 \times 3 = -36$

44. (b) : First law of thermodynamics gives
$\Delta Q = \Delta U + \Delta W$. Here $\Delta U = -\Delta W$.
Hence $\Delta Q = 0$. Therefore the process is adiabatic.

45. (d) : $\frac{P_1}{T_1} = \frac{P_2}{T_2}$. Here $P_1 = 1, P_2 = 2.5, T_1 = 300$ K.
This gives T_2 = 750 K.

46. (b) : $\rho = M/V$. Hence $\frac{\Delta\rho}{\rho} = \frac{\Delta M}{M} + \frac{\Delta V}{V}$

$$= \frac{0.01}{20.00} + \frac{0.1}{5.0} = 0.0205 \cong 2\%.$$

47. (d) : Intensity varies inversely as the square of the distance. When distance is doubled, the time required for good print will be 4 times.

48. (d) : Since the given collision is elastic, so we can use both. The principles of conservation of linear momentum and conservation of kinetic energy. And as the mass of the two bodies are equal and considering one body to be initially at rest, we have

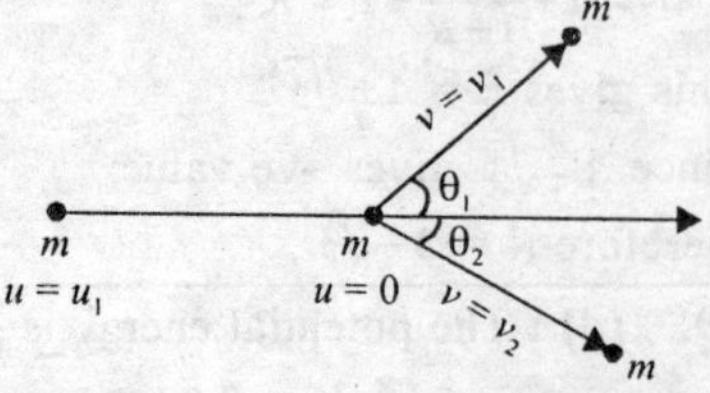

$u_1 = v_1\cos\theta_1 + v_2\cos\theta_2$ ... (i)

$v_1\sin\theta_1 = v_2\sin\theta_2$

$\Rightarrow v_1\sin\theta_1 - v_2\sin\theta_2 = 0$ ... (ii)

$u_1^2 = v_1^2 + v_2^2$ ... (iii)

Squaring and adding (i) and (ii), we have

$v_1^2 + v_2^2 + 2v_1v_2(\cos\theta_1\cos\theta_2 - \sin\theta_1\sin\theta_2) = u_1^2$

$\Rightarrow \cos(\theta_1 + \theta_2) = 0$ using (iii)

$\Rightarrow \cos\theta = 0$ where $\theta = \theta_1 + \theta_2$

$\Rightarrow \theta = 90°$.

49. (b) :

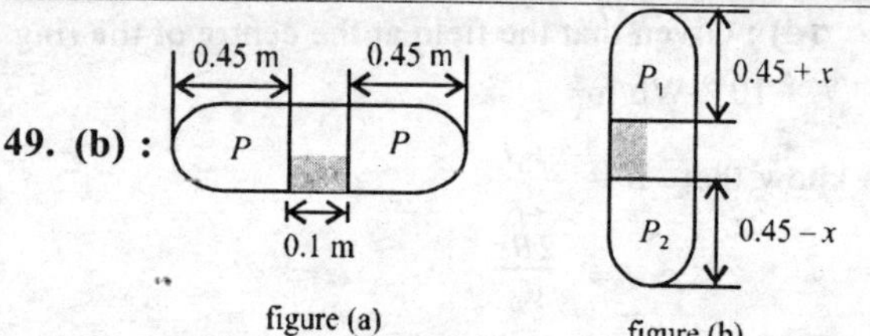

Figure (a) shows the horizontal position and figure (b) shows the vertical position of the tube.
When the tube is horizontal, the volume of air at the two sides of mercury column = $0.45 \times \alpha$, where α is the area of cross-section of the tube.
The pressure of air at each side = 76 cm of Hg
= 0.76 m of Hg
Now, for the vertical position of the tube, let the mercury be displaced by x metre.
Then, the volume of the air at the upper part
$= (0.45 + x)\alpha$
If the new pressure of air at the upper part be p_1, then from Boyle's law, we get

$0.76 \times 0.45 \times \alpha = p_1 \times (0.45 + x) \times \alpha$

or, $P_1 = \frac{0.76 \times 0.45}{0.45 + x}$ ... (i)

Volume of air at the lower part of the tube = $(0.45 - x)\alpha$
If the new pressure of air at this part be p_2, then applying Boyle's law, we get

$0.76 \times 0.45 \times \alpha = p_2 \times (0.45 - x) \times \alpha$

or, $P_2 = \frac{0.76 \times 0.45}{0.45 - x}$ ... (ii)

Now, obviously, $p_2 > p_1$ and the difference in pressure between the lower and upper parts of the tube, *i.e.* $(p_2 - p_1)$ will be due to the mercury column of 0.1 m in its vertical position.

$\therefore p_2 - p_1 = 0.1$ ... (iii)

From (i) and (ii), we get

$$p_2 - p_1 = \frac{0.76 \times 0.45}{0.45 - x} - \frac{0.76 \times 0.45}{0.45 + x}$$

$$= \frac{(0.76 \times 0.45)(0.45 + x) - (0.76 \times 0.45)(0.45 - x)}{(0.45)^2 - x^2}$$

$$= \frac{0.76 \times 0.45 \times 2x}{(0.45)^2 - x^2} \quad \text{... (iv)}$$

Now, from (iii) and (iv), we get

$$\frac{0.76\times 0.45\times 2x}{(0.45)^2 - x^2} = 0.1$$

or, $x^2 + 6.84x - 0.2025 = 0$

or, $x = \frac{-6.84 \pm \sqrt{(6.84)^2 - 4\times 1\times(0-0.2025)}}{2\times 1}$

or, $x = 0.029, -6.87$.

Negative value of x is discarded as it is absurd.

$\therefore \quad x = 0.029 = 2.9$ cm.

So, mercury will be displaced by 2.9 cm (nearly).

50. (b) : Length of the pendulum is $l = 1$ m.

$\therefore$ Time period $T = 2\pi\sqrt{\frac{l}{g}} = 2\pi\sqrt{\frac{1}{10}}$

$\therefore$ Frequency $f = \frac{1}{T} = \frac{1}{2\pi}\sqrt{10} = 0.5032$ Hz.

Now since the pendulum thread is caught by a thread 1/4 m from the original point of suspension, so the new length of the pendulum is

$$l' = 1 - \frac{1}{4} = \frac{3}{4} \text{ m}$$

$\therefore$ Time period, $T' = 2\pi\sqrt{\frac{3/4}{10}}$

$\therefore$ Frequency $f' = \frac{1}{2\pi}\sqrt{\frac{10}{3/4}} = \frac{2}{\sqrt{3}}\frac{1}{2\pi}\sqrt{10} = 0.5811$ Hz.

$\therefore$ Change in frequency, $\Delta f = 0.5811 - 0.5032$
$= 0.0779$ Hz.

51. (a) : Experimentally, it is found that the average radius of a nuleus is given by

$R = R_0 A^{1/3}$ where

$R_0 = 1.1 \times 10^{-15}$ m $= 1.1$ fm

and A = mass number

The volume of a nucleus is

$$V = \frac{4}{3}\pi R^3 = \frac{4}{3}\pi R_0^3 A.$$

Now as the masses of a proton and a neutron are roughly equal, say m, the mass of a nucleus is also roughly proportional to the mass number A, $M=mA$

Hence density within a nucleus $\rho = M/V = \frac{mA}{\frac{4}{3}\pi R_0^3 A}$

$= \frac{m}{\frac{4}{3}\pi R_0^3}$ is independent of the mass number A.

52. (c) : Red colour is always used for danger signals, because as red colour is having the longest wavelength, it is the least scattered. So, this signal can be seen from a very long distance.

53. (a) : A physical quantity to be treated as a vector, it is necessary for it to have both magnitude and direction. But this is not a sufficient condition for the physical quantity to be treated as a vector. A vector quantity has to follow the laws of vector addition. That's why, even though current and time have both magnitude and direction, they are not considered as vectors.

54. (a) : As the polar ice melts, it will flow towards the equator thereby increasing the moment of inertia of earth. Hence the angular velocity decreases. So, the day length will become longer.

55. (a)

56. (d) : Any charged particle can be accelerated with the help of a cyclotron but in the case of an electron, being very light, the process of accelerating the electron with a cyclotron is relativistically unfavourable. Very easily it will attain a velocity at which it will show relativistic effects.

57. (a) : Metals are good conductors of electricity. It is because of the presence of a large number of free electrons in metals. And for metals electrons are the main cause for thermal conduction. That's why all good conductors of heat are also good conductors of electricity.

58. (a) : The air surrounding the fire becomes hot and its density decreases. That's why this less dense air rises up and the cold air comes down. So below the fire, only cold air can be present.

59. (a) : The focal length of a lens in a medium of refractive index μ_m is given by

$$\frac{1}{f_m} = \left(\frac{\mu - \mu_m}{\mu_m}\right)\left(\frac{1}{R_1} - \frac{1}{R_2}\right)$$ where μ is the refractive index of glass.

In air

$$\frac{1}{f_a} = (\mu - 1)\left(\frac{1}{R_1} - \frac{1}{R_2}\right)$$

From these two expressions it is clear that

$$f_m > f_a$$

That is the focal length of the convex lens in water increases thereby reducing its convergent power.

60. (d) : Eddy currents are produced when a metal sheet is placed in a changing magnetic field. In the metal sheet, we can consider closed loops as shown in the figure, through which an induced current flows due to a change of magnetic flux. This current is called eddy current and it gives rise to loss of thermal energy.

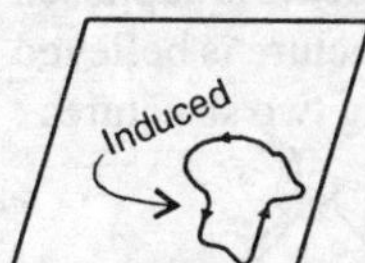

CHEMISTRY

61. (d) : Oxidation state of S in $S_8 = 0$

Oxidation state of S in $H_2S \Rightarrow +2 + x = 0$

$\Rightarrow x = -2$

Oxidation state of S in $S_2F_2 \Rightarrow 2x + 2(-1) = 0$

$\Rightarrow x = +1$

62. (a) : NO_2 is paramagnetic due to the presence of unpaired electron on the nitrogen atom.

63. (c) : $NH_3 + H_2O \rightarrow NH_4OH$

$CuSO_4 + NH_4OH \rightarrow Cu(OH)_2 + (NH_4)_2SO_4$

$Cu(OH)_2 + 2NH_4OH + (NH_4)_2SO_4 \rightarrow [Cu(NH_2)_4]\ SO_4 + 4H_2O$

Tetrammine cupric sulphate

The complex is called as Schotzer's reagent which is used for dissolving cellulose in the manufacture of artificial silk.

64. (c) Let the alkaline earth metal be A

$\therefore \quad 3A + N_2 \rightarrow A_3N_2$

$$\Rightarrow \frac{\text{Molecular mass of compd.}}{\text{Atomic mass of metal}} = \frac{\text{Wt. of compd.}}{\text{Wt. of metal}}$$

Let Atomic mass of metal be x

$\Rightarrow$ Molecular mass of compound $= 3x + 28$

$$\Rightarrow \frac{3x+28}{3x} = \frac{14.8}{12} \Rightarrow x = 40$$

65. (b) : Mg has a greater covalent compound forming tendency than Na, Ca and Ba.

This is due to the small size and strong positive nuclear charge attraction due to which ion formation involve higher energies.

66. (a) : More is the value of reduction potential, more is the tendency to get reduced. So as z gas has lowest reduction potential, therefore, z will be oxidised easily.

67. (a) . x atoms are at the corners of the cube, therefore,

number of x-atoms per unit cell $= \frac{1}{8} \times 8 = 1$

y-atoms are at the face centre of cube

$\therefore$ Number of y-atoms per unit cell $= \frac{1}{2} \times 6 = 3$

$\Rightarrow$ The formula of the molecule is xy_3

68. (a) : ClO_2 molecule has an angular structure with O–Cl–O bond angle of 117.6°. The molecule is supposed to contain a three electron bond. Its structure is believed to be a resonance hybrid of the following two structures :

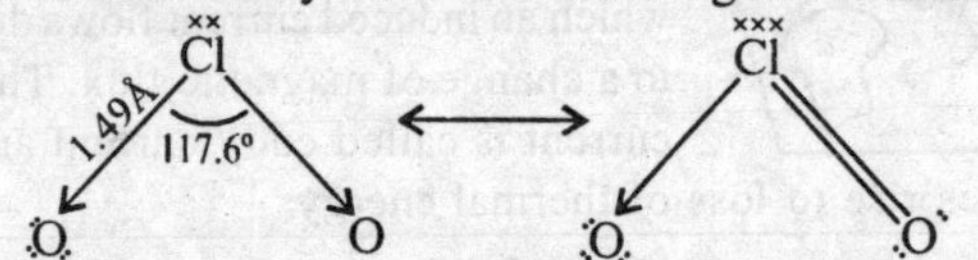

The structure arises from sp^3d hybridisation of Cl–atom. The molecule is paramagnetic due to the presence of three electron bond.

69. (d) : Microcosmic salt is $Na(NH_4)HPO_4$.

$Na(NH_4)HPO_4 \xrightarrow{\Delta} NaPO_3 + H_2O + NH_3$

It is prepared by :

$NH_4Cl + Na_2HPO_4 + 4H_2O \rightarrow Na(NH_4)HPO_4.4H_2O + NaCl$

70. (b) : Carboxylic acids react with carbonates forming corresponding salts thus evolutation of CO_2 must be from carbonates.

$2RCOOH + Na_2CO_3 \rightarrow 2RCOONa + H_2O + CO_2 \uparrow$

71. (b) : NCl_3 cannot be hydrolysed as there is no vacant d-orbitals available. All other group V elements can expand their coordination sphere due to the availability of vacant orbital.

72. (c) : Dichromate has the following structure,

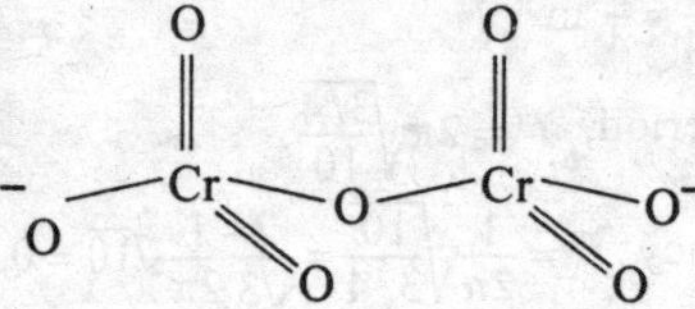

Therefore, all the Cr – O bond lengths are found to be equal.

73. (c) : Lewis acids are those molecules which can accept electron pair and those who can donate electron pairs are called Lewis base.

CCl_4 molecule does not have any vacant orbital where it can accept pair of electrons so CCl_4 cannot act as Lewis acid.

74. (b) : Methane is also called as Marsh gas as it is found in marshy areas. In coal gas methane composition ranges from 25 to 35%.

75. (c) : $Ba(OH)_2 + H_2SO_{4(aq)} \rightarrow BaSO_{4(s)} + 2H_2O_{(l)}$

In this reaction, neutralisation of dibasic acid by $Ba(OH)_2$ base is happening. So neutralisation reactions involving two protons should be about double as that of neutralisation reactions involving one proton.

76. (d) : Sodium chloride ; NaCl

Copper chloride ; Cu_2Cl_2

Magnesium sulphate ; $MgSO_4$

Chromium sulphate ; $Cr_2(SO_4)_3$

As maximum number of particles (*i.e.* ions) will be obtained when $Cr_2(SO_4)_3$ is dissolved in water.

Therefore, maximum boiling point will be observed in this case as elevation in boiling point is a colligative property and depends on the number of particles.

77. (c) : Ni : [⥮|⥮|⥮|1|1] $3d^8$ [⥮] $4s^2$

Ni^{2+} : [⥮|⥮|⥮|1|1] $3d^8$ [ ] $4s^0$

$[Ni(CN)_4^{2-}]$: [⥮|⥮|⥮|⥮|xx] $3d$ [xx] $4s$ [xx|xx|] $4p$

⇒ Hybridisation is dsp^2.

78. (d) : Barium phosphate when dissolved in water:

$Ba_3(PO_4)_2 \rightarrow 3Ba^{2+} + 2PO_4^{3-}$

Let the solubility of $Ba_3(PO_4)_2$ be s mol dm^{-3}

⇒ Solubility product = $(Ba^{2+})^3 (PO_4^{3-})^2$

$= s^5$ mol^5 dm^{-15}

79. (b) : Average kinetic energy per mole does not depend on the nature of the gas, it depends only on temperatrue.

Average kinetic energy per molecule = $\frac{3}{2}kT$

k = Boltzman constant, T = temperature.

80. (c) : CCl_4 and $CHCl_3$ (structures)

There is a stronger van der Waal's forces of attraction between the moleculer in CCl_4 compound than in $CHCl_3$.

81. (a) : Phenol $\xrightarrow[NaOH]{CCl_4}$ Salicylic Acid

Reaction is called as Riemer-Tiemann reaction. It involves the attack of dichloro carbene on benzene ring.

82. (a) : According to Absolute reaction rate theory, the bimolecular reaction between the two molecules A_2 and B_2 passes through the formation of the so called activated complex, which then decomposes to yield product AB.

$$A_2 + B_2 \rightleftharpoons (A_2B_2)^{\#} \rightarrow 2AB$$

83. (c) : Composition of portland cement is as follows:

Calcium oxide	CaO	61.5%
Silica	SiO_2	22.5%
Alumina	Al_2O_3	7.5%
Magnesium oxide	MgO	2.5%
Ferric oxide	Fe_2O_3	2.0%
Potassium oxide	K_2O	1.5%
Sulphur trioxide	SO_3	1.0%
Sodium oxide	NaO_2	1.5%

84. (c) : $^{-}O-Cr(=O)_2-O-Cr(=O)_2-O^{-}$ (Dichromate ion $Cr_2O_7^{2-}$)

85. (b) : Acetamide in the presence of NaOH and heat changes to acetic acid while ethylamine does not undergo any reaction.

$CH_3CONH_2 \rightarrow CH_3COOH + NH_3 \uparrow$
acetamide

86. (d) : $2SO_3(g) \rightleftharpoons 2SO_2(g) + O_2(g)$

Inital conc. → 1.0 mole 0.0 mole 0.0 mole

Equilibrium → 0.4 mole 0.6 mole 0.3 mole

⇒ Equilibrium constant is given by :

$$K = \frac{[SO_2]^2[O_2]}{[SO_3]^2} = \frac{(0.6)^2(0.3)}{(0.4)^2} = 0.75$$

87. (b)

88. (d) : Benzene $\xrightarrow[reflux]{HNO_3/H_2SO_4}$ m-dinitro benzene $\xrightarrow{Sn/HCl}$ 3-amino aniline

89. (c) : Tempering of steel is a process of heating the steel to a temperature below redness and then cooling it slowly. A thin film of the oxide is formed on the surface of steel.

90. (d) : As small compact cations are solvated more in the solution which cause their ionic mobility to slow down. Li^+, Mg^{2+} and Na^+ are heavily solvated, so lesser ionic mobility.

91. (b) : Root mean square velocity is given by :

$$V_{rms} = \sqrt{\frac{3kT}{m}} \Rightarrow V_{rms} \propto \sqrt{T}$$

$$\Rightarrow \frac{V_{rms}\text{ (at 27° C)}}{V_{rms}\text{ (at 327° C)}} = \sqrt{\frac{(27+273)K}{(327+273)K}} = \sqrt{\frac{300}{600}} = \frac{1}{\sqrt{2}}$$

$\therefore$ V_{rms} (at 327°C) = $100\sqrt{2} \times \sqrt{2} = 200$ ms^{-1}

92. (c) : In photography, AgBr is mainly used as the light sensitive material. The unchanged AgBr after devoloping the film is treated with $Na_2S_2O_3$ to solution. Solution of sodium thiosulphate is used as fixer and forms a soluble complex with silver halide.

$$AgBr + 2Na_2S_2O_3 \rightarrow Na_3[Ag(S_2O_3)_2] + NaBr$$

93. (c) : As nitrogen and oxygen atoms are small and highly electronegative with no vacant *d*-orbitals available for bonding multiple bonds are formed between oxygen-oxygen and nitrogen-nitrogen atoms.

$N \equiv N \quad O = O$

As the size of P and S atoms is large so multiple bonds are not strong enough, also catenation is possible due to vacant *d*-orbitals.

94. (b) :

$$\overset{1}{C}H \equiv \overset{2}{C} - \overset{3}{C}H = \overset{4}{C}H - \overset{5}{C}H_3$$

IUPAC name : Pent–3–ene–1–yne.

95. (c) : As : [⥮] [1|1|1] [1| | | |]

Hybridisation involved is sp^3d involving *s*, p_x, p_y, p_z and d_{z^2}.

96. (d) : Anions are always larger as compared to the corresponding parent atom as the effective nuclear force of attraction decreases per electron while on losing an electron (cation formation) size shrinking as effective nuclear charge increases per electron.

97. (a) : When Philosopher's wool (*i.e.* ZnO) is heated with BaO at 1100°C, It gives BaO + ZnO $\rightarrow$ $BaZnO_2$.

98. (a) : $[H^+][OH^-] = 10^{-14}$

Concentration of OH^- *i.e.* $[OH^-]$ in 0.1 M NaOH solution, $[OH^-] = 10^{-1}$ M

$\Rightarrow [H^+] = \dfrac{10^{-14}}{10^{-1}} = 10^{-13}$

$\Rightarrow pH = -\log[H^+] = 13$

99. (c) : $SnCl_2$ is non linear due to the presence of lone pair of electrons on the ccentral tin atom.

Cl–Sn(:)–Cl (bent structure with lone pair on Sn)

100. (d) : Transition elements are those elements which posses partly filled *d*-subshells in their elementary form or their commonly occurring ions *i.e.* $(n-1)d^{1-10}\,ns^{1-2}$.

101. (c) : In face centred unit cubic cell, the edge length can be written as :

$a = 2(r_+ + r_-)$

a = edge length, r_+ = radius of cation

r_- = radius of anion

$\Rightarrow 508 = 2(110 + r_-) \Rightarrow r_- = 144$ pm

102. (c) : 20% $FeCl_3$ solution means 100 g of solution contains 20 g $FeCl_3$.

$\Rightarrow$ Volume of 100 g solution $= \dfrac{100\text{ g}}{1.1\text{ g/mL}} = 90.91$ mL

moles of 20 g $FeCl_3 = \dfrac{20}{162} = 0.1234$ mole

$\Rightarrow$ Molar concentration of solution

$= \dfrac{0.1234}{90.91} \times 1000$

$= 1.357$ M

103. (c) : Combustion of carbon;

$C(s) + O_2(s) \rightarrow CO_2(g);\ \Delta H_1 = -395.5$ kJ/mol

Combustion of Hydrogen;

$H_2(g) + \frac{1}{2}O_2(s) \rightarrow H_2O(g);\ \Delta H_2 = -284.8$ kJ/mol

Combustion of Methane;

$CH_4(g) + 2O_2(g) \rightarrow CO_2 + 2H_2O;\ \Delta H_3 = -890.4$

Formation of Methane;

$C(s) + 2H_2(g) \rightarrow CH_4(g);\ \Delta H = ?$

From the above equations,

$\Delta H = \Delta H_1 + 2\Delta H_2 - \Delta H_3$

$= -395.5 - 2 \times 284.8 + 890.4$

$= -74.7$ kJ/mole

104. (b) : ${}^{23}_{11}Na + {}^{1}_{1}H \rightarrow {}^{32}_{12}Mg + {}^{1}_{0}n$

${}^{1}_{1}H$ represents proton (or *p*)

${}^{1}_{0}n$ represents neutron (or *n*)

The reaction is of (*p*, *n*) type.

105. (d) : Baking soda is sodium bicarbonate ($NaHCO_3$). It is obtained as the intermediate product in the solvay ammonia soda process. Normal carbonate can be changed bicarbonate by passing CO_2 through its saturated solution.

$$Na_2CO_3 + H_2O + CO_2 \rightarrow 2NaHCO_3.$$

106. (b) : A sodium chloride solution contains Na^+, Cl^-, H^+ and OH^- ions. On passing electricity, Na^+ and H^+ move toward cathode and Cl^- and OH^- ions towards anode. The discharge potintial of H^+ is less than Na^+, therefore hydrogen ions get discharged easily similarly at anode, Cl^- ions easily discharged as Cl_2. Solution becomes rise in Na^+ and OH^- ions.

107. (c) : Le-Blanc process : It involves the following steps :

$NaCl + H_2SO_4 \rightarrow NaHSO_4 + HCl$

$NaHSO_4 + NaCl \rightarrow Na_2SO_4 + HCl$

$Na_2SO_4 + CaCO_3 + 4C \rightarrow Na_2CO_3 + CaS + 4CO$

(coke) Black

Na_2CO_3 is separated from CaS by dissolving it in water.

108. (d) : Elemental sodium can lose electrons very easily so it acts as strong reducing agent.

$Na_{(s)} \rightarrow Na^+ + e^-$

It dissolves in liquid ammonia giving out a conducting and reducing solution. It cannot be prepared by electrolysing sodium chloride solution in water as sodium reacts violently with water.

109. (a) : Carnallite ore is $KCl.MgCl_2.6H_2O$.

110. (a) : Since the alkali metals are highly electropositive, their carbonates are highly stable towards heat. As the electropositivety increases down the group, the stability is in order of :

$Cs_2CO_3 > Rb_2CO_3 > K_2CO_3 > Na_2CO_3 > Li_2CO_3$

Lithium carbonate decomposes on heating.

111. (b) : Formic acid behaves as reducing agent as it is oxidised to an unstable acid. Carbonic acid, which decomposes into CO_2 and H_2O.

$HCOOH + 2HgCl_2 \rightarrow Hg_2Cl_2 + CO_2 + 2HCl$

$HCOOH + Hg_2Cl_2 \rightarrow CO_2 + 2HCl + 2Hg$

(Black)

Acetic acid remains unaffected by mercuric chloride, as it does not show reducing properties.

112. (a) : Bond order is the half of the difference between bonding and anti-bonding electrons. Bond order =

$$\frac{1}{2}\left[\left(\begin{array}{c}\text{no. of } e^- \text{ in}\\ \text{bonding M.O.}\end{array}\right) - \left(\begin{array}{c}\text{no. of } e^- \text{ in}\\ \text{antibonding M.O.}\end{array}\right)\right]$$

Higher the value of bond order, stronger is the bond.

113. (c) : Structure of H_3PO_3 is :

$$\begin{array}{c} O \\ \| \\ H - P - OH \\ | \\ OH \end{array}$$

Due to the presence of two hydroxyl protons, H_3PO_3 is dibasic acid.

114. (a) : NaOH is strong electrolyte and dissociates fully in solution into its ions.

115. (b) : When ns^2 electrons of outermost shell do not participate in bonding, it is called inert pair effect. Since the inert pair effect increases down the group, therefore pb^{2+} compounds are more stable than pb^{4+} compounds. Pb^{4+} compounds thus, act as oxidizing agent.

116. (a) : Geometrical isomerism is possible when different groups are attached to the double bonded carbon atoms. *e.g.* Maleic acid and Fumaric acid are geometrical isomers.

$$\begin{array}{c} H - C - COOH \\ \| \\ H - C - COOH \end{array} \qquad \begin{array}{c} HOOC - C - H \\ \| \\ H - C - COOH \end{array}$$

(Cis–form) (Maleic acid) (trans–form) (Fumaric acid)

117. (a) : Depression in freezing point is a colligative property, depends on the number of particles present in the solution. As both 0.1 M solution of Glucose and 0.1 M solution of urea contain same number of moles (number of particles) therefore, both have same K_f.

118. (c) : Positron emission :

$${}^b_aX \rightarrow {}^b_{a-1}X + {}^0_1\beta$$

positron

Therefore, after positron emission, atomic number of the atom decreases by one and mass number remains uneffected.

119. (a) : Alkenes have general formula as C_nH_{2n} same as that of cycloalkanes.

e.f. $CH_3CH = CHCH_3 \Rightarrow C_4H_8 \ (\equiv C_nH_{2n})$

2–butene

$$\begin{array}{c} CH_2 - CH_2 \\ | \quad\quad | \\ CH_2 - CH_2 \end{array} \Rightarrow C_4H_8 \ (= C_nH_{2n})$$

Cyclobutane

120. (b) : Nomenclature in benzene ring :

(Benzene ring numbered 1–6)

For only one substituent, no numbering is required.

For two substituents on the ring, numbering is done to sure that the smallest total of the positions is there.

(Ring with CH_3 at 1 and CH_3 at 3; alternate numbering 1′–6′)

1, 3–dimethyl benzene is prefered as it corresponds to smallest total of number of positions.

BIOLOGY

121. (b) : *Wuchereria,* the causative agent of filariasis is found in lymph nodes. The embryos or micro-filariae passing through the lymph nodes, find their way into the main lymphatic duct and go to circulatory system. But the adult worms harbour the lymphatic system, they settle down at some spot–inguinal, scrotal and abdominal lymphatics. *Plasmodium,* causative agent of malaria can be found in human R.B.C., liver etc. *Taenia* causing cysticercosis found in small intestine (mainly) in man. *Diplococcus,* producing pneumonia, in man is found in lung, blood etc.

122. (c) : "Gametes are never hybrid". This is a statement of law of segregation.

Mendel's principle of segregation is inherent in the results of Mendel. Though in F_1, the dominant phenotype appears, the recessive phenotype is not lost but reappears in F_2. This suggested that there is no blending of Mendelian factors in F_1, but that they stay together and only one is expressed. At the time of the formation of gametes, these two factors obviously separate or regregate, otherwise recessive type will not appear in F_1. The gametes which are formed are always pure for a particular character. A gamete may carry either the dominant or the recessive factor but not both. This is why it is called either as "principle of segregation" or as "law of purity of gametes."

123. (c) : Mendel was not able to say anything about recombination and crossing over because traits he chose, were not linked and present on different chromosomes or were far apart.

(i) In each of the seven pairs of character, studied by Mendel, there are only 2 alternative forms for each character–one dominant over the other. The independent assortment of characters is based on independent assortment of non-homologous chromosome. But for recombination and crossing over to occur the linked genes should be present in homologous chromosome. Thus crossing over and recombination are the deviation of Mendel's law.

124. (c) : Sprain is due to excessive pulling of ligament. A sprain is a stretch or tear in the ligament resulting from a sudden movement that causes the neck to extend to an extreme position.

125. (c) : A man suddenly sees a tiger. His heart beat goes up, blood pressure increases, etc. Adrenaline is released at this time in his body. Increased adrenal medullary secretion in the part of the diffused sympathetic discharge provoked in emergency situations. Thus a man, after being excited starts to secrete adrenaline in large amount. It increases blood sugar, and blood lactic acid levels, along with these it increases heat production, metabolic rate and body temperature. Its coordinated actions help the body reactions in stress. This is why adrenal medulla is sometimes called the gland for 'fight, fright and flight'.

126. (d) : Apical meristems or shoot tip meristems are always free of viral infections, therefore, for virus-free cultures shoot tips are preferred in tissue culture.

127. (b) : A man has enlarged breasts, sparse hair on body and sex compliment as XXY. He then suffers from Klinefelters syndnome. It is a disease due to chromosomal aberration. Klinefelters syndrome is characterised by trisomic (XXY) male. These are male individulas which are phenotypically fairly normal but have a very low sperm count and are therefore sterile. Chromosome constituents of Klinefelters syndrome are following :

Sex chromosome	*Sex*	*Phenotype*
XXY (trisomic)	male	Klinefelter's syndrome
XXYY (tetrasomic)	male	Klinefelter's syndrome
XXXY (tetrasomic)	male	Extreme Klinefelter's syndrome
XXXXY (pentasomic)	male	Extreme Klinefelter's syndrome

128. (c) : "They have raised cheek bones, oblique eyes and yellowish skin colours". Here they refer to mongoloids. This syndrome was described by Langdon-Down in 1866 and was popularly called mongolian idiots or Down's syndrome. Trisomy 21 is responsible for it. Phenotypic abnormalities associated with this syndrome resembles mongoloids-thus called mongolian idiots. The features are slant of eyes, thick tongue, sagging mouth, unusual palm and feet, obesity and slow mental growth. The life expectancy of these idiots is about 8 to 12 years.

129. (c) : Urea is transported by blood plasma. Urea present in the urine is the ultimate product of excretion. Excretion or renal clearance is done through the blood plasma. Not only urea, but creatine, insulin all are transported by the blood plasma.

130. (d) : In fast swimming fishes, propulsion is due to caudal fin. Caudal fin has an important role in fish movement. As they pass backward, a progressively greater transverse amplitude of the waves propel them forward. One wave created due to caudal fin is followed by the another and so an. This transmits a backward momentum to push the water backwards. Thus the whole body operates as a single self propelling system, and the fish is thrust forward.

131. (b) : While dissecting a rat, at the time of pinning in the dissecting tray, ventral side of the rat should face the person dissecting it. As rat is a chordate (vertebrate), it has its nerve cord at dorsal position. To keep the nerve cord intact (because, if dissection affects the nervous system, whole body system would be disturbed) dissection is not done dorsally, but it is done ventrally.

132. (b) : The transfer of light energy may be from one chlorophyll *a* molecule to another, from chlorophyll *b* to chlorophyll *a*, from carotenoids to chlorophyll *a* or from phycobilins to chlorophyll *a*. Chlorophyll *a* shows the two photo systems PS I and PS II. Chlorophyll *a* exists in two forms, one form with an absorption maximum at 673 nm (chl. *a* 673) and the other with an absorption maximum at 683 nm (chl *a* 683).

133. (b) : Presence of cytokinin in an area causes preferential movement of nutrients towards it when applied to lateral buds, they help in their growth despite the presence of apical bud. They thus act antagonistically to auxin which promotes apical dominance.

134. (a) : Thickening of arteries due to cholesterol deposition is arteriosclerosis. This extremely widespread disease predisposes to myocardial infarction, cerebral thrombosis, and other serious illness. It is characterized by infiltration of cholesterol and appearance of foam cells in certain lesions of the arterial wall, distorting the vessels and making them rigid.

135. (a) : Blood vessels of *Pheretima,* which have valves are dorsal. Dorsal blood vessel in *Pheretima* is situated mid dorsally. It has a thick, mascular wall. Blood passes from backward to forward direction. To prevent the backward flow of the blood, valves are present infront of each septum.

136. (a) : *Ganong's potometer* is an apparatus for measuring the rate of transpiration. *Porometer* is an apparatus for knowing the relative sizes of stomata. *Auxanometer* is used to measure plant growth. *Respirometer* is used to measure the rate of respiration.

137. (b) : If we take food rich in lime juice, then action of ptyalin on starch is reduced. Starch is attacked by ptyalin, the α –amylase in saliva. However, the optimal pH for this enzyme is 6.7 and its action is inhibited by the additon of lime juice. Because, lime juice makes the medium more acidic which is not suitable for ptyalin action.

138. (c) : We move our hands while walking. We do so to maintain equilibrium against force of gravity. Body has to maintain a balance at the time of walking, otherwise there would be a chance to fall down. Gravitational force always acts on our body and attracts the body towards it. Thus there is a downward force acting on the body. To reduce the force and to maintain a balance while walking, movement of hands is necessary.

139. (c) : Pink is the colour of safranin. Plant cell walls are stained with safranin.

140. (a) : The phenomenon by which a gene suppresses the phenotypic expression of a nonallelic gene is called epistasis. The alleles which do not show dominant recessive relationship and are able to express themselves independently when present together are called codominant alleles. Supplementary genes are a pair of nonallelic genes, one of which produces its effect independently in the dominant state while the dominant allele of the second gene is without any independent effect but is able to modify the effect of the former to produce a new trait.

141. (a) : Resolving power is the ability to distinguish two close points as distinct points. Human eye has a resolving power of 1 minute (1′).

142. (b) : The root cap if it is independent in origin arises from a special layer called the calyptrogen. In case it is not independent in origin, it arises from the dermatogen.

143. (c) : Aminocentesis is taking out of cells near the foetus. It is a technique of drawing amniotic fluid and testing it to find out the sex and disorders of the foetus. The amniotic fluid is usually taken in the 14th or 15th week after conception. It prevents accidental damage of the foetus and placenta. Nowadays, this technique has been banned because of its misuse by some persons.

144. (c) : Malignant tertian malaria is caused by *P. falciparum.* It is also known as pernicious malaria. The fever cycle is 48 hours. The fever is often fatal to the patient as it affects the brain. Its incidence follows that of *P. vivax.*

145. (d) : Bacteria becomes double in every minute. Therefore, in 59th minute, they must be present in half cup and in next minute by their doubling the cup become full of them.

146. (a) : The role of fungi in producing antibiotic substances was first established by Sir Alexander Fleming in 1929. He extracted the great antibiotic drug penicillin from *Penicillium notatum*.

147. (a) : Genes control various traits in an organism through a control exercise on the developmental process. If genes are recessive, they fail to perform the function. Phenylketonuria and albinism is caused due to presence of recessive autosomal genes. *Phenylketonuria* is due to accumulation of phenylpyruvic acid and causes mental disorders. *Albinism* is due to absence of melanin pigment and individuals suffering with this disease are incapable of converting dihydroxyphenylalanine into melanin.

148. (c)

149. (c) : DNA finger printing is the best way to determine paternity. Polymorphism at the DNA level is a genetic variation that is being used to advantage. DNA fingerprinting tooks directly at persons genetic make up. The test is done by extracting DNA from the nuclei of white blood cells, spermatozoa or hair follicle cells. Every individuals has unique band pattern. Paternity is determined by comparing the accused man's DNA fingerprint with that of the child.

150. (b) : Bending of tendrils after coming in contact of support is called *thigmonasty.* Opening and closing of flowers in response to light and darkness is called *photonasty,* e.g. *Calendula.* Greater growth on one side causes the organ to bend to the opposite side, *e.g.* circinate coiling and opening of fern leaf are called nyctinasty. Hydronasty is the nastic movement in which the stimulus is water.

151. (a) : A person suffering from hyperthyroidism has bulging/protruding eyes, tachycardia and higher body temperature. It is also known as thyrotoxicosis. Besides the mentioned symptoms, hyperthyroidism has a considerable load on cardiovascular system. Graves' disease and Hashimoto thyroiditis are also due to hyperthyroidism.

152. (d) : In primitive atmosphere, the external sources of energy were – (i) solar radiations such as ultra-violet light, X-rays, etc., (ii) energy from electrical discharges like lightening, (iii) high energy radiations are other sources of energies.

153. (a) : Molecular hydrogen acts as a specific inhibitor of nitrogen fixation.

154. (d) : Colchicine inhibits metaphase. Colchicine inhibits the formation of mitotic spindles and are used to increase the percentage of metaphase cells for chromosome analysis. Metaphase arresting solution is effective with bone marrows, difficult tumor samples and problematic tissues.

155. (a) : Blood pressure is measured by sphygmomano meter. Two curved metal tubes are opened by a rubber pressure pad. The device has a registering manometer. *Stethoscope* is used to measure pulse rate. *Electrocardiogram* is an electrical recording of heart and is used to investigate heart disease. *Phonocardiogram* is a recording of heart sounds, which leaves a permanent record in the form of a tracing recorded on paper.

156. (a) : The ATP-ADP system functions as a carrier of chemical energy because ADP is able to accept a phosphate group during coupled energy-yielding reaction of catabolism and the ATP so formed is able to donate its terminal phosphate group in coupled energy-requiring reactions.

157. (b) : In *transduction,* a virus (bacteriophage) when released from a host bacterial strain may carry with it a part of genetic material of the host strain and may transfer it to another strain, which in turn is infected by this virus. In *transformation,* genetic material is released from one strain and a part may be acquired from another strain, which thus gets transformed without coming in contact with the other strain. In *conjugation* genetic material is transferred through a conjugation tube, when two strains come in contact. In *transcription* *m*RNAs are formed from DNA.

158. (d) : A person is suffering from impaired nervous system and madness after prolonged consumption of polluted water. Studies on the effects of lead in human especially in children have demonstrated a relationship between exposure to lead and a variety of adverse health effects. These effects include impaired mental and physical development, decreased heme biosynthesis, elevated hearing threshold and decreased serum levels of Vit D. The neurotoxicity of lead is of particular concern.

159. (b) : Body temperature of cold blooded animals fluctuates with surrounding temperature. Cold blooded animals do not have any temperature regulating mechanism or homeostasis. Thus their body temperature fluctuate with the environmental temperature. It is seen mostly in lower group of vertebrates. They make their own physiological mechanism (like hibernation/diapause) to get rid of the extremity of temperature.

160. (b) : The method of growing plants in aqueous

nutrient solutions as employed by Sacks and Knop is used experimentally and commercially today and is known as hydroponic culture.

161. (a) : A part of brain of frog which helps to respire and locomote is called medulla oblongata. It is a part of hind brain. Diencephalon helps in metabolism of carbohydrate, fat and proteins. The temperature and reproductive activity of the body are also controlled by it. Cerebellum helps in maintaining equilibrium. Cerebral hemispheres help in controlling intelligence, memory, thought etc.

162. (c) : Peptidase digests the peptide bond. Endopeptidase can split certain peptide linkages at any point in a peptide chain, in contrast to the exopeptidases, which can split only terminal peptide bonds.

163. (b) : Cyanobacteria fix atmospheric nitrogen to nitrogen oxides (nitrate and nitrites). These oxides reduce the acidity of soil.

164. (a) : Parkinson's disease is a progressive neuro-degenerative disorder which affects movement or control of movements. The causes of Parkinson's is not completely understood but a known cause is the degeneration of a group of nerves in the centre of the brain. These nerves produce a chemical messenger called dopamine. When 80% of dopamine is lost, the symptoms of the disease is produced.

165. (d) : Succession starting on a site previously occupied by a community forest clearcut or abundoned crop field, for example is known as secondary succession.

166. (a) : Corolla is papilionaceous, petals 5, the posterior odd petal (outer most) is called standard, two lateral ones the wings and the two anterior ones fused to form a keel or carina (a boat-shaped structure).

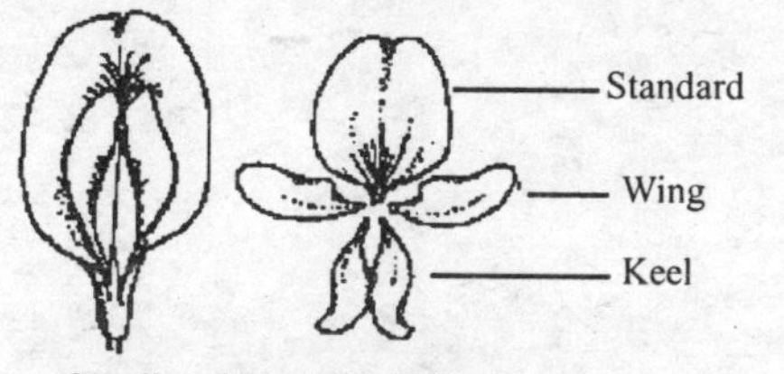

Corolla of family Palpilonaceae

167. (d) : Cauliflower is an example of inflorescenc with condensed shoot. All florets are edible.

168. (c) : Tonoplast is inner plasma-memberane enclosing vacuole. Plasmodesmata is extremely fine cytoplasmic threads one to few tenths of a micrometer wide passing through walls of living plant cells and connecting cytoplasm of adjacent cells. Hydathode is water-excreting gland occurring on the edges or tips of leaves of many plants. These perform guttation.

169. (a) : Pneumolaxis and inhibitory centres are associated with breathing. Pneumolaxis centre is pons. Stimulation inhibits inspiratory centre activity thereby control rate and depth of ventilation. This area is important for regulating the amount of air one takes in with each breath.

170. (b)

171. (c) : Hearing aids help the hearing impaired to hear. Hearing impairment means deafness. It can be classified as conductive loss of hearing which occurs when bones of the middle ear do not function properly and sensorineural deafness which results from long exposure to excessive noise levels. The function of hearing aid is to remove these difficulty by acting on those specific areas.

172. (c) : Cyanobacteria are autotrophic in nature. Photosynthetic pigments include chlorophyll *a* carotenoids and phycobilins. Photosynthetic thylakoids occur freely in the outer part of protoplast called chromoplasm. Cyanobacteria are prokaryotic due to lack of membrane bound cell organelles and distinct nucleus.

173. (c) : Growth regulators are organic subst
other than nutrients, which in low concentrat
growth, differentiation and developm
or inhibiting the same. Plant grow
called phytohormones. Technic
a chemical substance produ
translocated to another regi
physiological reactions w

174. (c) : Usually
rice, millets etc. a
Gram, Pea, Pul
etc. Legumi
nodules c
Rhizobi
salts
as

o
a c
repro

and programmed manner, the cell continues to divide and multiple abnormally, until a detectable lump of tumor develops.

176. (c) : Spoilage of fruit juice occurs due to fermentation. Fermentation is the major energy yielding process of several different microorganisms. They are capable of existing and breaking down organic compounds in the absence of oxygen.

177. (c) : Amphibians have evolved from fishes but *Archaeopteryx* can not give any proof in favour of this. *Archaeopteryx* is the connecting link between birds and reptiles. The class Amphibia includes all those animals which live partly in fresh water as well as partly on land. They are the lowest and earliest tetrapods which first of all successfully descended on land from some fish like ancestors possibly in Devonian time. They are characterised by their outstanding features and thus stand in between the fishes and reptiles.

178. (d) : Secondary vascular tissues are formed by vascular combium. Vascular combium is produced by two types of meristems, fascicular or intrafascicular and interfascicular cambium. Only one type of primary lateral meristem is found in plants. It is interfascicular cambium.

179. (a) : Person with blood group AB can take blood from any other person. Blood group incompatibility is due to antigen antibody reaction. Blood group AB has no anitibody and thus the antigen of the other group is not affected. On the other hand group AB blood, with both A and B antigens can be given safely only to group AB people.

180. (b)

GENERAL KNOWLEDGE

181. (a)	**182. (b)**	**183. (c)**	**184. (d)**
185. (b)	**186. (a)**	**187. (b)**	**188. (b)**
189. (c)	**190. (a)**	**191. (b)**	**192. (b)**
193. (a)	**194. (c)**	**195. (b)**	**196. (b)**
197. (b)	**198. (b)**	**199. (a)**	**200. (a)**

SOLVED PAPER
AIIMS - 2001

Time : 3½ Hours Max. Marks : 200

PHYSICS

1. Two coherent monochromatic light beams of amplitude 3 and 5 units are superposed. The maximum and minimum possible intensities in the resulting beams are in the ratio
(a) 4 : 2 (b) 16 : 1
(c) 8 : 2 (d) 4 : 2.

2. Two masses are attached to a rod end to end. If torque is applied they rotate with angular acceleration α. If their distances are doubled and same torque is applied, then they move with angular acceleration
(a) 4α (b) α
(c) 3α (d) α/4.

3. A particle is revolving in a circle of radius R. If the force acting on it is inversely proportional to R, then the time period is proportional to
(a) R (b) R^2
(c) $1/R$ (d) $1/R^2$.

4. At a place earth's magnetic field, 5×10^5 Wb/m^2 is acting perpendicular to a coil of radius R = 5 cm. If $\mu_0/4\pi = 10^{-7}$, then how much current is induced in circular loop?
(a) 0.2 A (b) 0 A
(c) 4 A (d) 40 A.

5. An engine is working. It takes 100 calories of heat from source and leaves 80 calories of heat to sink. If the temperature of source is 127°C, then temperature of sink is
(a) 147°C (b) 47°C
(c) 100°C (d) 47 K.

6. Speed in kilometer per hour in S.I. unit is represented as
(a) KMPH (b) Kmhr^{-1}
(c) Kmh^{-1} (d) kilometer/hour.

7. Colour of a star depends upon
(a) luminosity (b) temperature
(c) brightness (d) all of these.

8. Dimension of resistivity is
(a) $ML^2T^{-2}I^{-1}$ (b) $ML^3T^{-3}I^{-2}$
(c) $ML^3T^{-2}I^{-1}$ (d) $ML^2T^{-2}I^{-2}$.

9. If mass of an atom is M moving with speed v, what will be its speed after the emission of an α-particle if speed of α-particle is zero ?
(a) $\frac{Mv}{M+2}$ (b) $\frac{Mv}{M-4}$
(c) $\frac{Mv}{M+4}$ (d) $\frac{M-4}{Mv}$

10. If electron is moving from A to B in wire AB, then current induced in the coil is

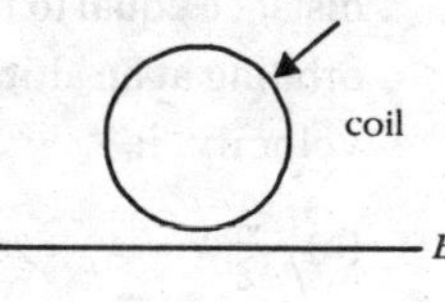

(a) anticlockwise (b) clockwise
(c) arbitrary direction
(d) no current will be induced.

11. A wire of length l carries a steady current. It is bent first to form a circular plane loop of one turn. The magnetic field at the centre of the loop is B. The same length is now bent more sharply to give a double loop of smaller radius. The magnetic field at the centre caused by the same is
(a) B (b) $B/4$
(c) $4B$ (d) $B/2$.

12. A metal rod consumes power P on passing current. If it is cut into two half and joined in parallel, it will consume power
(a) P (b) $2P$
(c) $4P$ (d) $P/4$.

13. A body of mass M moving with velocity V

explodes into two equal parts. If one comes to rest and the other body moves with velocity v, what would be the value of v ?

(a) V (b) $V/\sqrt{2}$
(c) $4V$ (d) $2V$.

14. Which of the following physical quantities do not have same dimensions?

(a) pressure and stress
(b) tension and surface tension
(c) strain and angle (d) energy and work.

15. A solid sphere and a hollow sphere are heated the same temperature. Point out the true statement.

(a) hollow sphere cools more quickly.
(b) both hollow and solid sphere cools equally.
(c) solid sphere cools more quickly.
(d) none of the statement is true.

16. The orbital velocity of an artificial satellite in a circular orbit above the earth's surface at a distance equal to radius of earth is v. For a satellite orbiting at an altitude half of earth's radius, orbital velocity is

(a) $\frac{3}{2}v$ (b) $\sqrt{3/2}\ v$
(c) $2/\sqrt{3}\ v$ (d) $\frac{2}{3}v$.

17. The time period of a simple pendulum is T remaining at rest inside a lift. Find the time period of pendulum when lift starts to move up with an acceleration of $g/4$.

(a) T (b) $T/2$
(c) $2T/5$ (d) $2T/\sqrt{5}$.

18. 1 Kcal of heat flowing through a rod of iron. When the rod is cut down to 4 pieces then what will be the heat flowing through each piece having same differential temperature?

(a) 1/2 Kcal (b) 1/4 Kcal
(c) 1 Kcal (d) 1/15 Kcal.

19. From the given figure find the frequency of oscillation of the mass m.

(a) $n = \frac{1}{2\pi}\sqrt{\frac{K}{m}}$ (b) $n = \frac{1}{2\pi}\sqrt{\frac{K^2}{2m}}$
(c) $n = 2\pi\sqrt{\frac{m}{2K}}$ (d) $n = \frac{1}{2\pi}\sqrt{\frac{K}{2m}}$.

20. From the figure find the capacitance of the capacitor?

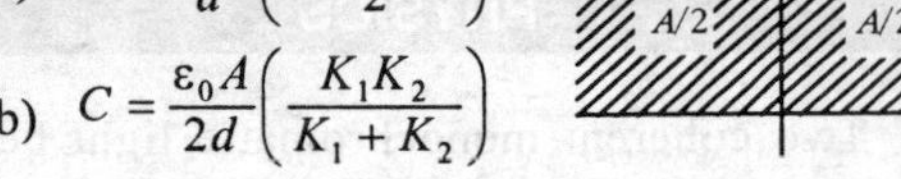

(a) $C = \frac{\varepsilon_0 A}{d}\left(\frac{K_1+K_2}{2}\right)$
(b) $C = \frac{\varepsilon_0 A}{2d}\left(\frac{K_1K_2}{K_1+K_2}\right)$
(c) $C = \frac{\varepsilon_0 A}{d}\left(\frac{K_1}{K_2}\right)$
(d) $C = \frac{\varepsilon_0 A}{d}\left(\frac{2K_1K_2}{K_1+K_2}\right)$.

21. S.I. unit of velocity is

(a) m/s (b) m sec^{-1}
(c) m hr^{-1} (d) m/hr.

22. Mass of the proton is 1840 times that of electron. It is accelerated through a potential difference of 1 V. Find its kinetic energy.

(a) 6 eV (b) 2 eV
(c) 10 eV (d) 1 eV.

23. Two spheres of same metal have radii a and b. They have been connected to a conducting wire. Find the ratio of the electric field intensity upon them.

(a) a/b (b) b/a
(c) b^2/a (d) b^2/a^2.

24. The work function of a metal is 3.4 eV. If the frequency of incident radiation is increased to twice, then the work function of the metal becomes

(a) 3.4 eV (b) 7.2 eV
(c) 6.8 eV (d) 1.7 eV.

25. If red light is replaced by white light then width of diffraction pattern will

(a) increases (b) decreases
(c) a central white band is obtained
(d) no effect.

26. Maximum energy transfer for an elastic collision will occur if one body is at rest when

(a) $m_1 = m_2$ (b) $m_2 = \frac{1}{2} m_1$
(c) $m_1 >> m_2$ (d) $m_2 >> m_1$.

27. Which of the following is path dependent?
(a) U (b) PdV
(c) P (d) V.

28. If fundamental frequency is 50 and next successive frequencies are 150 and 250 then it is
(a) a pipe closed at both end
(b) a pipe closed at one end
(c) an open pipe (d) a stretched pipe.

29. If in a circuit current lags behind EMF by $\pi/2$. Then it is a/an
(a) resistor circuit (b) capacitor
(c) inductor circuit (d) CR circuit.

30. In Planck's oscillator energy is given as

$$E = \frac{hv}{\exp\left(\frac{h\upsilon}{Kt} - 1\right)}$$

If $K = 0$, then energy would be
(a) $h\upsilon$ (b) 0
(c) Kt (d) ∞.

31. Temperature of the star is determined by
(a) distance (b) colour
(c) size (d) none of these.

32. If hot water is mixed with cold water
(a) temperature first increases then become constant
(b) temperature first decreases then become constant
(c) increases continuously
(d) first it is uncertain then become constant.

33. For liquid to rise in a capillary tube, the angle of contact should be
(a) acute (b) obtuse
(c) right (d) none of these.

34. Escape velocity of a rocket is 11.2 km/sec. It is released at an angle of 45°. Its escape velocity is
(a) 11.2 m/sec (b) $11.2\sqrt{2}$ km/sec
(c) 11.2 km/sec (d) 22.3 km/sec.

35. X-ray beams are affected by
(a) electric field (b) magnetic field
(c) both (a) and (b) (d) none of these.

36. The heat produced in a long wire is characterised by resistance, current and time through which the current passes. If the errors in measuring these quantities are respectively 1%, 2% and 1%, then total error in calculating the energy produced is
(a) 4% (b) 6%
(c) 4/3% (d) 8%.

37. If a unit positive charge is taken from one point to another over an equipotential surface, then
(a) work is done on the charge
(b) work is done by the charge
(c) work done is constant
(d) no work is done.

38. Figure shows the electric lines of forces emerging from a charged body. If the electric field at A and B are E_A and E_B respectively and if the displacement between A and B is r, then
(a) $E_A > E_B$ (b) $E_A < E_B$
(c) $E_A = E_B / r$ (d) $E_A = E_B / r^2$.

39. A charge is placed at the centre of cube of side a then flux linked with one of its given faces will be
(a) $\frac{Q}{\varepsilon_0}$ (b) $\frac{Q}{6\varepsilon_0}$
(c) $\frac{Q}{\varepsilon_0 a^2}$ (d) $\frac{Q}{4\pi\varepsilon_0 a^2}$.

40. A small piece of metal wire is dragged across the gap between the pole pieces of a magnet in 0.4 sec. If magnetic flux between the pole pieces is known to be 8×10^{-4} Wb, then induced emf in the wire, is
(a) 4×10^{-3} V (b) 8×10^{-3} V
(c) 2×10^{-3} V (d) 6×10^{-3} V.

41. If the earth is treated as a sphere of radius R and mass M, its angular momentum about the axis of its rotation with period T, is
(a) $\frac{MR^2T}{2\pi}$ (b) $\frac{4\pi MR^2}{5T}$
(c) $\frac{\pi MR^3}{T}$ (d) $\frac{2\pi MR^2}{T}$

42. Antimony and Bismuth are usually used in thermocouple, because
(a) a constant thermo e.m.f. is produced
(b) higher thermo e.m.f. is produced
(c) a negative thermo e.m.f. is produced
(d) lower thermo e.m.f. is produced.

43. A constant pressure air thermometer gave a reading of 47.5 units of volume when immersed in ice-cold water, and 67 units in a boiling liquid. The boiling point of the liquid, is
(a) 125°C (b) 100°C
(c) 135°C (d) 112°C.

44. Two particles are seen to collide and move jointly together after the collision. During such a collision, for the total system,
(a) both the mechanical energy and the linear momentum are conserved
(b) linear momentum is conserved but not the mechanical energy
(c) neither the mechanical energy nor the linear momentum is conserved
(d) mechanical energy is conserved but not the linear momentum.

45. A body weighed 250 N on the surface assuming the earth to be a sphere of uniform mass density, how much would it weigh half way down to the centre of the earth?
(a) 195 N (b) 240 N
(c) 125 N (d) 210 N.

46. For an enclosure maintained at 1000 K, the maximum radiation occurs at wavelength λ_m. If the temperature is raised to 2000 K, the peak will shift to
(a) $\frac{5}{2}\lambda_m$ (b) $\frac{1}{2}\lambda_m$
(c) $\frac{7}{2}\lambda_m$ (d) $\frac{3}{2}\lambda_m$.

47. A certain radioactive element has a half-life of 20 years. If we have a block with 10 g of the element in it, after how many years will there be just 2.5 g of the element in the block?
(a) 80 years (b) 40 years
(c) 100 years (d) 60 years.

48. What is the dimensional formula for the gravitational constant ?
(a) $[M^{-1}L^3T^{-2}]$ (b) $[M^{-1}L^3T^{-1}]$
(c) $[M^{-2}L^3T^{-2}]$ (d) $[M^{-2}L^{-1}T^3]$.

49. The equivalent resistance between A and C of the given circuit, is 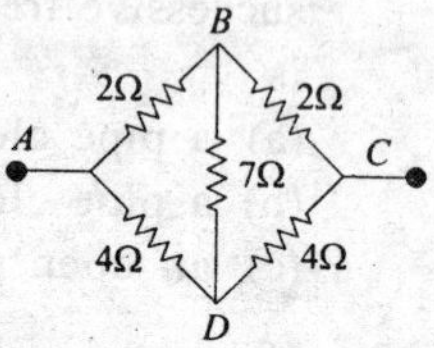
(a) 8 Ω
(b) $\frac{32}{12}\Omega$
(c) $\frac{4}{3}\Omega$ (d) $\frac{8}{3}\Omega$.

50. A source of frequency 240 Hz is moving towards an observer with a velocity of 20 m/s. The observer is now moving towards the source with a velocity of 20 m/s. Apparent frequency heard by observer, if velocity of sound is 340 m/s, is
(a) 268 Hz (b) 270 Hz
(c) 360 Hz (d) 240 Hz.

Directions for Questions 51-60 : In each of the following questions, a statement of Assertion (A) is given and a corresponding statement of Reason (R) is given just below it. Of the statements, mark the correct answer as -
(a) If both A and and R are true and R is the correct explanation of A.
(b) If both A and R are true but R is not the correct explanation of A.
(c) If A is true but R is false.
(d) If A is false but R is true.

51. *Assertion* (A) : Centripetal force does no work.
Reason (R) : Force and displacement are perpendicular to each other.

52. *Assertion* (A) : Skiers uses air glasses.
Reason (R) : Light reflected by snow is partially polarised.

53. *Assertion* (A) : LASER is used to measure distant object as moon.
Reason (R) : They are highly coherent source of light.

54. *Assertion* (A) : Work done in uniform circular motion is zero.
Reason (R) : Force is always directed along displacement.

55. *Assertion* (A) : At pole value of acceleration due to gravity (g) is greater than that of equator.
Reason (R) : Earth rotates on its axis in addition to revolving round the sun.

56. *Assertion* (A) : During reverse biasing a diode doesn't conduct current.
Reason (R) : It narrows the depletion layer.

57. *Assertion* (A) : On increasing the frequency of light larger number of photoelectrons are emitted.
Reason (R) : The number of electrons emitted depends on the intensity of incident light.

58. *Assertion* (A) : Soldiers are asked to break steps while crossing the bridge.
Reason (R) : The frequency of thick marching may be equal to the natural frequency of bridge and may lead to resonance which can break the bridge.

59. *Assertion* (A) : The time period of revolution of a satellite around a planet is directly proportional to the radius of the orbit of the satellite.
Reason (R) : Artificial satellite do not follow Kepler's laws of planatary motion.

60. *Assertion*: Electric appliances with metallic body *e.g.*, heaters, presses etc., have three pin connections, whereas an electric bulb has a two pin connection.
Reason: Three pin connections reduce heating of connecting cables.

CHEMISTRY

61. Which of the following is aromatic?

(a) 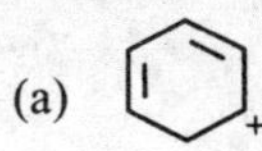 (b) 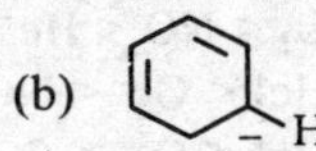

(c) 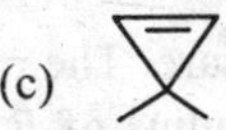 (d) 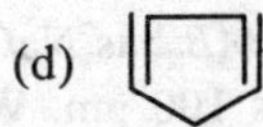

62. Which of the following is most stable carbocation?
(a) CH_3^+ (b) $CH_3CH_2\overset{+}{C}H_2$
(c) $CH_3\overset{+}{C}H_2CH_3$ (d) $CH_3-\overset{+}{C}H(CH_3)-CH_3$

63. Hybridisation in CH_3, $\overset{+}{C}H_3$ and $\overset{-}{C}H_3$ are respectively
(a) sp^2, sp^2, sp^3 (b) sp^2, sp^3, sp^3
(c) sp^3, sp^3, sp^2 (d) sp^3, sp^2, sp^2.

64. In the following reaction order, B is
$$CH_3CH_2-COOH \xrightarrow{P/Br_2} A \xrightarrow[H^+]{\text{alc. KOH}} B$$
(a) $CH_2=CH-COOH$
(b) $CH_2-CH(Br)-COOH$ (c) CH_3CH_2COBr
(d) CH_3CH_2OH.

65. Which of the following arrangement is possible?

	n	l	m	s
(a)	5	2	2	$+\frac{1}{2}$
(b)	2	2	0	$-\frac{1}{2}$
(c)	3	-2	1	$+\frac{1}{2}$
(d)	0	0	1	$+\frac{1}{2}$.

66. Strongest acid among the following is
(a) acetic acid (b) FCH_2COOH
(c) $F_2CHCOOH$ (d) F_3CCOOH.

67. Which of the following is strongest Bronsted base?
(a) ClO^- (b) ClO_2^-
(c) ClO_3^- (d) ClO_4^-.

68. Which of the following has highest hydration energy?
(a) $MgCl_2$ (b) $CaCl_2$
(c) $BaCl_2$ (d) $SrCl_2$.

69. In which of the following $p\pi$ - $d\pi$ bonding is possible?
(a) CO_3^{2-} (b) PO_4^{3-}
(c) NO_3^- (d) NO_2^-.

70. Which of the following is always feasible?
(a) $\Delta H = T\Delta S$
(b) ΔH (+ve), $T\Delta S$ (−ve) and $\Delta H > T\Delta S$
(c) ΔH (−ve), $T\Delta S$ (+ve) and $\Delta H < T\Delta S$
(d) ΔH (−ve), $T\Delta S$ (−ve) and $\Delta H > T\Delta S$.

71. Given that $C + O_2 \rightarrow CO_2$; $\Delta H° = -a$ kJ.
$2CO + O_2 \rightarrow 2CO_2$; $\Delta H° = -b$ kJ
The heat of formation of CO is
(a) $b - 2a$ (b) $\frac{2a-b}{2}$
(c) $\frac{b-2a}{2}$ (d) $2a - b$.

72. Which of the following hydrogen halide is most

basic?
(a) HF (b) HCl
(c) HBr (d) HI.

73. Which of the following is soluble in water?
(a) Be (b) Sr
(c) Mg (d) Ba.

74. When the temperature of reactions will increase then the effect on pH value will
(a) increase (b) decrease
(c) first increases then decreases
(d) remains same.

75. Hardest compound of boron is
(a) magnesium boride
(b) aluminium boride
(c) boron nitride (d) boron carbide.

76. Which of the following has highest second ionization energy?
(a) Ni (b) V
(c) Cr (d) Mn.

77. Smallest intermolecular distance is found in
(a) O_2 (b) O_2^{+2}
(c) O_2^- (d) O_2^{-2}.

78. The pH of aqueous solution of ammonium formate is
(pK_a of HCOOH = 3.8 and pK_b of NH_3 = 4.8)
(a) 7 (b) 6.0
(c) 6.5 (d) 8.9.

79. Which azide is explosive?
(a) $Ba(N_3)_2$ (b) NaN_3
(c) KN_3 (d) Mg_3N_2.

80. dsp^2 hybridisation is found in
(a) $[NiCl_4]^{2-}$ (b) $[COCl_4]^{2-}$
(c) $[CuCl_4]^{3-}$ (d) $[CuCl_4]^{2-}$.

81. Which of the following order of basic strength is correct?
(a) $NH_3 < NH_2OH < HN_3 < NH_2–NH_2$
(b) $NH_2OH < HN_3 < NH_2–NH_2 < NH_3$
(c) $HN_3 < NH_3 < NH_2OH < NH_2–NH_2$
(d) $HN_3 < NH_2OH < NH_2–NH_2 < NH_3$.

82. A packet of colloidal system is taken in which colloidal particles are still. Two electrodes are taken in system and voltage is applied so that liquid medium moves under the influence of electric field. This phenomenon is called
(a) dorn effect (b) electroosmosis
(c) electrophoresis (d) electrodialysis.

83. Which one forms KHX_2 type compound?
(a) HF (b) HCl
(c) HI (d) HBr.

84. Rate determining step in nitration of benzene is
(a) formation of NO_2^+
(b) formation of carbocation
(c) replacement of H atom
(d) none of these.

85. Which of the following is stable (inert) to fire?
(a) CCl_4 (b) C_2H_5OH
(c) CH_4 (d) C_4H_{10}.

86. The pH value of decinormal solution of NH_4OH which is 20% ionised is
(a) 12.95 (b) 12.30
(c) 14.70 (d) 13.30.

87. The composition of carnalite is
(a) $KCl{\cdot}MgCl_2{\cdot}6H_2O$ (b) $Na_2Al_2O_3$
(c) Fe_3O_4 (d) Na_3AlF_6.

88. A spoon to be electroplated with gold should be
(a) cathode (b) anode
(c) electrolyte (d) none of these.

89. Which of the following option w.r.t. increasing bond order is correct ?
(a) $NO < C_2 < O_2^- < He^+$
(b) $C_2 < NO < He^+ < O_2^-$
(c) $He^+ < O_2^- < NO < C_2$
(d) $He^+ < O_2^- < C_2 < NO$.

90. A solid AB has NaCl type structure. The radius of A^+ is 100 pm. What is the radius of B^-?
(a) 190.47 (b) 540.13
(c) 525 (d) 78.12.

91. Correct equation of Freundrich isotherm is
(a) $\log\left(\frac{x}{m}\right) = \log K + \frac{1}{n}\log C$
(b) $\log\left(\frac{m}{x}\right) = \log K + \frac{1}{n}\log C$

(c) $\log\left(\frac{x}{m}\right) = \log C + \frac{1}{K}\log C$

(d) $\log\left(\frac{x}{m}\right) = \log C + \frac{1}{n}\log K$.

92. Crystalline solids have
(a) short range order (b) long range order
(c) anisotropic distribution
(d) no order.

93. How many electrons are delivered at the cathode during electrolysis by a current of 1 A in 60 seconds
(a) 3.74×10^{20} (b) 6.0×10^{23}
(c) 7.48×10^{21} (d) 6.0×10^{20}.

94. In which of the following reaction $K_p > K_c$?
(a) $PCl_3 + Cl_2 \rightarrow PCl_5$ (b) $H_2 + I_2 \rightarrow 2HI$
(c) $2SO_3 \rightarrow O_2 + 2\ SO_2$
(d) $N_2 + 3H_2 \rightarrow 2NH_3$.

95. The IUPAC name of the compound having the formula CCl_3CH_2CHO is
(a) 2, 2, 2-trichloropropanal
(b) 1, 1, 1-trichloropropanal
(c) 3, 3, 3-trichloropropanal
(d) 1, 2, 1-dichloromethanal.

96. Which of the following molecule or ions is a bidentate ligand ?
(a) $C_2O_4^{2-}$ (b) Br_2^+
(c) CH_3NH_2 (d) $CH_3\text{-}C \equiv N$.

97. The number of electrons required to deposit 1 gm equivalent aluminium (atomic wt. = 27) from a solution of aluminium chloride will be
(a) 3 (b) 1
(c) 4 (d) 2.

98. Which of the following is a characteristic of a reversible reaction ?
(a) it never proceeds to completion
(b) it can be influenced by a catalyst
(c) it proceeds only in forward direction
(d) number of moles of reactants and products are equal.

99. How many litres of ammonia gas at S.T.P. would be needed to prepare 100 ml of 2.5 M ammonium hydroxide solution ?
(a) 5.6 lit (b) 0.056 lit
(c) 11.2 lit (d) 0.56 lit.

100. The equilibrium constant of a reaction is 300. If the volume of a reaction flask is trippled, the equilibrium constant will be
(a) 300 (b) 100
(c) 600 (d) 150.

101. Which of the following is the correct sequence of atomic weights of the given elements ?
(a) Ni > Co > Fe (b) Fe > Co > Ni
(c) Co > Fe > Ni (d) Co > Ni > Fe.

102. The aqueous solution of which of the following salt will have the lowest pH ?
(a) $NaClO_3$ (b) $NaClO$
(c) $NaClO_4$ (d) $NaClO_2$.

103. Which of the following alkanes is optically active?
(a) 3-methyl hexane (b) propane
(c) 2, 3, 4-trimethyl pentane
(d) 2-methyl butane.

104. A solution with pH = 2 is more acidic than one with a pH = 6, by a factor
(a) 4000 (b) 5000
(c) 8000 (d) 10 000

105. Vapour pressure of benzene at 30°C is 121.8 mm. When 15 g of a non-volatile solute is dissolved in 250 g of benzene, its vapour pressure is decreased to 120.2 mm. The molecular weight of the solute is
(a) 35.67 g (b) 356.7 g
(c) 432.8 g (d) 502.7 g

106. The BCl_3 is a planar molecule where as NCl_3 is pyramidal, because
(a) B–Cl bond is more polar than N–Cl bond
(b) N–Cl bond is more covalent than B–Cl bond
(c) nitrogen atom is smaller than boron atoms
(d) BCl_3 has no lone pair but NCl_3 has a lone pair of electrons

107. Which of the following compound is not coloured?
(a) $Na_2[CuCl_4]$ (b) $Na_2[CdCl_4]$
(c) $K_4[Fe(CN)_6]$ (d) $K_3[Fe(CN)_6]$

108. If 0.189 g of a chlorine containing organic compound gave 0.287 g of silver chloride, then the percentage of chlorine in the organic compound is

(a) 35.47 (b) 35.57
(c) 37.57 (d) 45.37

109. Which of the following statements is not true about alcohols?
(a) lower alochols have fiery taste and strong smell
(b) as molecular mass increases the boiling point increases
(c) lower alcohols are water insoluble and their solubility increases with molecular weight
(d) lower alcohols are water soluble and their solubility decreases with molecular weight

110. The electronic configuration $1s^2 2s^2 2p^5 3s^1$ shows
(a) ground state of fluorine atom
(b) excited state of fluorine atom
(c) excited state of neon atom
(d) excited state of ion O_2^-

Directions for Questions 111-120 : In each of the following questions, a statement of *Assertion (A)* is given and a corresponding statement of *Reason (R)* is given just below it. Of the statements, mark the correct answer as -
(a) If both A and and R are true and R is the correct explanation of A.
(b) If both A and R are true but R is not the correct explanation of A.
(c) If A is true but R is false.
(d) If A is false but R is true.

111. *Assertion (A)* : Relative strength of acids can be known by knowing the value of dissociation constant.
Reason (R) : It gives the value of H^+ dissolved in solution.

112. *Assertion (A) : o*-nitrophenol is more volatile than *p*-nitrophenol.
Reason (R) : Intramolecular hydrogen bonding is present in *o*-nitrophenol while intermolecular H - bonding is in *p*-nitrophenol.

113. *Assertion (A) :* CH_3OCH_3 and C_2H_5OH has comparable molecular weight but boiling point of C_2H_5OH is more than dimethyl ether.
Reason (R) : C_2H_5OH forms intermolecular H-bonding while CH_3OCH_3 forms intramolecular H-bonding.

114. *Assertion (A) :* $CHCl_3$ and CH_3OH are miscible.
Reason (R) : One of them is polar.

115. *Assertion (A) :* In some cases oxygen shows positive oxidation number though it is an electronegative element.
Reason (R) : Fluorine is more electronegative than oxygen.

116. *Assertion (A) :* B_2H_6, Si_2H_6 are said to have similar structure.
Reason (R) : They have same number of σ and π bonds.

117. *Assertion (A) :* Hydrogen nuclei combines to form helium nuclei then energy is released
Reason (R) : Binding energy/nucleon of He is greater than hydrogen.

118. *Assertion (A) :* Water is used as a moderator in nuclear reactor.
Reason (R) : Moderator is a light substance that absorb neutrons.

119. *Assertion*: Ionisation potential of B (atomic no.4) is less than Be (atomic no. 5).
Reason: The first electron released from Be is of *p*-orbital but that from B is of *s*-orbital.

120. *Assertion*: Na_2SO_4 is soluble in water while $BaSO_4$ is not.
Reason: Lattice energy of $BaSO_4$ exceeds its hydration energy.

BIOLOGY

121. If a stimulus, several times greater than the threshold stimulus is provided to a muscle fibre, it will:-
(a) contract with a larger force
(b) contract wih a smaller force
(c) contract with the same force
(d) undergo tetany.

122. During the cell cycle, 2 molecules of DNA are present in a chromosome in the:-
(a) G_1 phase
(b) beginning of S phase
(c) G_2 phase (d) end of M phase.

123. Barr Body is found in the cytoplasm during:-
(a) interphase in cell of female mammal
(b) interphase in cell of male mammal

(c) prophase in cell of female mammal
(d) prophase in cell of male mammal.

124. The respiratory centre in the brain is stimulated by:-
(a) CO_2 concentration in venous blood
(b) O_2 concentration in artery blood
(c) CO_2 concentration in artery blood
(d) O_2 concentration in venous blood.

125. Cocaine is a stimulant, which may cause addiction. It is an alkaloid obtained from:-
(a) *Eucalyptus* (b) *Erythroxylon*
(c) *Rauwolfia* (d) *Papaver*.

126. Some students, during a study, caught, marked and released 80 fishes in a pond. Later 100 fishes were caught at random. Among these 40 were found to be marked. What is the approximate number of fishes in the pond?
(a) 50 (b) 100
(c) 200 (d) 4000.

127. Which of these are considered most essential in the origin of life?
(a) enzymes (b) nucleic acids
(c) carbohydrates (d) proteins.

128. Wooden doors swell up and get stuck during the rainy season. This is due to the phenomenon of:-
(a) imbibition (b) endosmosis
(c) capillarity (d) deplasmolysis.

129. Which of these are most widely used in Genetic Engineering?
(a) plastid (b) plasmid
(c) mitochondria (d) ribosome.

130. Which floral family has (9) + 1 arrangement of anthers in the androecium
(a) malvaceae (b) rutaceae
(c) fabaceae (d) caesalpinaceae.

131. The ratio in a dihybrid test cross between two individuals is given by:-
(a) 2:1 (b) 1:2:1
(c) 3:1 (d) 1:1:1:1.

132. Porous wood contains:-
(a) vessels (b) fibres only
(c) tracheids (d) sieve tubes.

133. A human RBC is placed in 1.5% salt solution. It will:-
(a) swell up (b) shrink
(c) remain unaffected (d) burst.

134. A frog has its brain crushed. But when pinched on the leg, The leg draws away. It is an example of:-
(a) neurotransmitter induced response.
(b) simple reflex (c) conditioned reflex
(d) automated motor response.

135. Which of the following is an egg laying mammal:-
(a) kangaroo (b) *Platypus*
(c) penguin (d) whale.

136. In RNA thiamine is replaced by:-
(a) uracil (b) adenine
(c) thiamine (d) guanine.

137. All veins carries deoxygenated blood except:-
(a) pulmonary veins (b) hepatic vein
(c) hepatic portal vein (d) renal artery.

138. Genetic drift operates only in:-
(a) island population (b) smaller population
(c) larger population
(d) Mendelian population.

139. Which of the following pesticides is an acetylcholinesterase inhibitor?
(a) aldrin (b) BHC
(c) endosulfan (d) malathion.

140. The sphere of living matter together with water, air and soil on the surface of earth is called-
(a) atomosphere (b) hydrosphere
(c) lithosphere (d) biosphere.

141. Photorespiration, usually occurs in-
(a) one-cell organelles
(b) two cell organelles
(c) three cell organelles
(d) four cell organelles.

142. Clove is a part of
(a) flower
(b) thalamus of a flower
(c) auxillary bud (d) seed.

143. Velamen is a specialized tissue found in
(a) aerial roots of *Orchids*
(b) succulent leaves
(c) pneumatophores (d) stilt roots.

144. Hydroponics is
(a) cultivation of plants in water
(b) growth of plants towards water

(c) growth of plants away from water
(d) soil-less cultivation of plants.

145. Coconut's Husk fibre coir of commerce is extracted from
(a) epicarp (b) mesocarp
(c) endocarp (d) seed coat.

146. Induction of flowering by low temperature in plants is
(a) cryobiology (b) vernalization
(c) phototropism (d) pruning.

147. Viral diseases have no cure because
(a) viruses have no cell wall
(b) viruses can multiply repeatedly within the host cell
(c) presence of capsid
(d) virus possesses no cytoplasm.

148. Tadpoles can be made to grow in size by:-
(a) injecting thyroxine hormone
(b) feeding the eggs of other frogs
(c) injecting gonadotrophic hormones
(d) providing them with suitable climatic conditions.

149. Sella Turcica is found:-
(a) in bones (b) in joints.
(c) nearby pituitary (d) nearby thyroid.

150. Class Crustacea have following features
(a) cephalothorax, book lungs, chitinous exoskeleton
(b) head and thorax, biramous appendages, book lungs
(c) head and thorax, book lungs, chitinous exoskeleton
(d) cephalothorax, biramous appendages, gills.

151. Chloromycetin is obtained from
(a) *Streptomycetin venezualae*
(b) *Streptomycetin remosus*
(c) *Bacillus subtilis*
(d) *Clostridium botulimin.*

152. Mutualism is found in
(a) hermit crab and sea anemone
(b) butterfly and flower
(c) zoochlorellae and Hydra
(c) *E.coli* and man.

153. In respiration from 180g of glucose which of the following is formed
(a) 264gm CO_2 + 190gm H_2O + 391 Kcal
(b) 264gm CO_2 + 108gm H_2O + 686 Kcal
(c) 390gm CO_2 + 108gm H_2O + 686 Kcal
(d) 390gm CO_2 + 264gm H_2O + 391 Kcal.

154. Extranuclear genes occurs in
(a) plastids - and not inherited
(b) plasmid - and not inherited
(c) mitochondria - and inherited by female
(d) mitochondria - and inherited by male.

155. In plants, water moves from
(a) less negative to more negative gradient
(b) more negative to less negative gradient
(c) same gradients
(d) none of the above.

156. Stomata opens
(a) in day time - for gaseous exchange
(b) in day time - no gaseous exchange
(c) in night time only - for gaseous exchange
(d) in night time only - no gaseous exchange.

157. Identify the correct statement
(a) in amniotes last nerve is spinal accessory
(b) in non-amniotes last nerve is vagus
(c) optic is shortest nerve
(d) olfactory nerves has mixed fibres.

158. Which of the following is wrongly matched?
(a) haemoglobin in mammals - RBC
(b) haemozoin - *Plasmodium* cytoplasm
(c) haemocyanin - prawn
(d) haemoglobin dissolved in blood - *Pheretima*

159. Which of the following is non- pathogenic bacteria of colon?
(a) *Escherichia coli* (b) *Balantidium coli*
(c) *Entamoeba coli*
(d) *Enterobius vermicularis.*

160. During which of the following formation free nuclear division occurs?
(a) flower (b) endosperm
(c) gametes (d) fruit.

161. Some Gram -ve bacteria have peptidoglycan and an extra layer of
(a) lipo-polysaccharide
(b) lipo-protein
(c) protein (d) both (a) and (c).

162. Which of the following is correct about nematocyst?

(a) it can be re-used
(b) its ejection is conditioned reflex
(c) it is ejected on contact and pierce the prey
(d) due to which other *Hydra* doesn't come in contact with it.

163. Which of the following statements about phytochrome is true?
(a) P_r absorbs yellow light and becomes P_{fr}
(b) P_r absorbs red light and becomes P_{fr}
(c) P_{fr} absorbs red light and becomes P_r
(d) P_{fr} absorbs yellow light and becomes P_r.

164. Blackmann's law is related to
(a) respiration (b) transpiration
(c) root pressure (d) photosynthesis.

165. An oocyte is released from the ovary under the influence of LH
(a) after completing meiosis and before polar bodies are released
(b) after completing meiosis I and before release of polar bodies
(c) after completing meiosis
(d) after completing meiosis I and after release of polar bodies.

166. Classical experiment to prove essentiality of CO_2 for photosynthesis was given by
(a) Arnon (b) Von Moll
(c) Calvin *et al* (d) Hill

167. Which of the following statements are correct regarding short day plants (SDPs)?
(a) they are apt to flower in the fall
(b) they are the same as long as long day plants
(c) they do not have a critical photoperiod
(d) all of the above are correct

168. In prokaryotes, genetic recombination can occur during
(a) transduction (b) transformation
(c) conjugation (d) all of these

169. Photosynthetic bacteria do not contain
(a) quantasome (b) PS-I and PS-II
(c) PS-II (d) PS-I

170. Which is Indian dwarf wheat
(a) *T. dicoccum* (b) *T. sphaerococcum*
(c) *T. twigidum* (d) *T. aestivum*

Directions to Q. 171 to Q. 180 : *The following questions consists of an Assertion (A) and reason (R). Select the correct answer from the following.*
(a) if both A and R are true and R is the Correct explantion of A
(b) if both A and R are true and R is not the correct explanation of A
(c) if A is true but R false
(d) A is false but R is true.

171. *Assertion* : Stomata remain open during day.
Reason : Stomata help in exchange of gases.

172. *Assertion* : Among the land animals, the Cheetah can run fastest over the ground.
Reason : The Cheetah uses its powerful forelimbs to push itself forward during running.

173. *Assertion* : Wounds heal slowly due to vitamin C deficiency.
Reason : Vitamin C is essential for collagen formation

174. *Assertion* : A plant girdled upto bast will die.
Reason : Water transportation will cease.

175. *Assertion* : Phenylketonuria is a disease in which excretion of phenylalanine occurs in urine.
Reason : It is due to dietary imbalance.

176. *Assertion* : Salamander, *Sphenodon* are classified as amphibian.
Reason : Their skin is naked, moist and glandular

177. *Assertion* : *Watson* and *Crick* provided experimental proof of semiconservative nature of DNA relication.
Reason : DNA polymerase binds nucleotides in replication.

178. *Assertion* : DNA code does not copied in the synthesis of transfer RNA.
Reason : Transfer RNA move out of the nucleus and after attaching on the ribosomes, form the template.

179. *Assertion* : Monocot stem bear collateral open vascular bundles.
Reason : If cambium is absent such vascular bundles are called closed type.

180. *Assertion* : Plasma membrane is exceedingly thin and not visible as a separate layer.
Reason : It appears merely as a surface layer of cytoplasm.

GENERAL KNOWLEDGE

181. Recent earthquake in Bhuj was measured by which of the following instrument?
(a) sonometer (b) chromatograph
(c) protarograph (d) seismograph.

182. Alzeimer's day is celebrated in which month?
(a) August (b) September
(c) 5th June (d) December.

183. Which of the following enquired 'Tehelka'.com defence dealing case?
(a) retired supreme court judge
(b) high court judge
(c) combined parliament committee
(d) supreme court judge.

184. Who is the chairman of Rajya Sabha of India?
(a) Speaker (b) President
(c) Vice President (d) Governor.

185. Which of the following cricketer batted in matches as - from opener to 9th down?
(a) Sanjay Manjarekar (b) Lala Amarnath
(c) Sunil Gavaskar (d) Vinu Mankad.

186. Next olympic will be held in
(a) Sydney - 2004 (b) London - 2004
(c) New York - 2004 (d) Athens - 2004.

187. Which of the following language is not followed in UN?
(a) Spain (b) Arabic
(c) French (d) German.

188. When was song 'Jana gana mana' adopted as the National Anthem of India?
(a) 14th August 1947 (b) 24th January 1950
(c) 15th August 1947 (d) 26th January 1950

189. Miss Universe recently was held in
(a) Paris (b) New York
(c) London (d) Peurto rico.

190. Highest peak in India is
(a) K_2 (b) Everest
(c) Nanda Devi (d) Kanchanchanga.

191. Which religion is followed by maximum people in the world?
(a) Christianity (b) Buddhism
(c) Islam (d) Hindustani.

192. Leiberhan commision is set out for
(a) Tehelka dispute (b) Jharkhand dispute
(c) Bharatpur arms export
(d) Ayodhya disputes.

193. Head of Army, Air Force and Navy are respectively
(a) General, Air Chief Marshall, Admiral
(b) General, Admiral, Air Chief Marshall
(c) Admiral, Air Chief Marshall, General
(d) Major General, Admiral, Air Chief Marshall.

194. Which of the following is wrong about PIN code?
(a) it consists of six digits.
(b) first digit represent any of six zones.
(c) second and third digit represent sub zones.
(d) last three digits shows specific region.

195. Which of the following is not a function of Reserve Bank of India?
(a) to catch fake currency note
(b) to maintain the value of rupee
(c) to regulate the flow of credit
(d) it has supervisory power over other banks.

196. Present President of USA is
(a) George Bush (b) Bill Clinton
(c) Al gore (d) Tony Blair.

197. Which of the following is not matched?
(a) Badminton - Santosh Trophy
(b) Cricket - Durand Cup
(c) Hockey - Agha Khan Cup
(c) Tennis - Hens Irish Cup.

198. Which of the following official document is related with India?
(a) green paper
(b) white paper (c) yellow book
(d) blue book.

199. 'Adi Granth' was written by
(a) Guru Gobind Singh
(b) Guru Arjun Dev
(c) Guru Teg Bahadur
(d) Guru Nanak Dev.

200. The capital of Lakshadweep, is
(a) Kavaratti (b) Port Blair
(c) Kohima (d) Silvasa.

❖❖❖

SOLUTIONS

PHYSICS

1. **(b)** : It is given that the amplitudes A_1 and A_2 are in the ratio $\frac{A_1}{A_2}=\frac{3}{5}$

∴ After superposition the maximum and minimum intensities will be in the ratio

$$\frac{I_{max}}{I_{min}}=\frac{(A_1+A_2)^2}{(A_1-A_2)^2}=\frac{(3+5)^2}{(3-5)^2}=\frac{8^2}{(-2)^2}=\frac{64}{4}=\frac{16}{1}$$

2. **(d)** : m_1 ← R → C_1 ← R → m_2 (axis of rotation)

Suppose the masses m_1 and m_2 are attached to the ends of a massless rod. C_1 is the axis of rotation which is at a distance R from each of the masses.

∴ the moment of inertia of the system,

$$I = m_1R^2 + m_2R^2 = (m_1 + m_2)R^2$$

Now if the distance between the masses is doubled, then the moment of inertia

$$I' = m_1(2R)^2 + m_2(2R)^2 = (m_1 + m_2)4R^2$$

Since the same torque is applied in both the cases,

$$\tau = I\alpha = I'\alpha'$$

$$\Rightarrow \alpha'=\frac{I\alpha}{I'}=\frac{(m_1+m_2)R^2\alpha}{(m_1+m_2)4R^2}=\frac{\alpha}{4}$$

3. **(a)** : Given that the force is inversely proportional to R

i.e. $F \propto \frac{1}{R}$

or $F=\frac{k}{R}$ ... (i)

or $mRw^2=\frac{k}{R}$

or $w^2=\frac{k}{mR^2}$

∴ $w^2 \propto \frac{1}{R^2}$

⇒ $w \propto \frac{1}{R}$

⇒ $\frac{2\pi}{T} \propto \frac{1}{R}$

⇒ $T \propto R$

4. **(b)** : As the earth's magnetic field is acting perpendicular to the coil and as here is no charge of magnetic flux through the coil, the current induced in the coil is zero.

5. **(b)** : Heat taken from source Q_1 = 100 cal

Heat left to sink Q_2 = 80 cal

∴ efficiency of the engine $\eta=1-\frac{Q_2}{Q_1}=1-\frac{80}{100}$ = 20%

Temperature of the source T_1 = 127ºC = 400 K

Temperature of the sink T_2 = ?

We know that

$$\eta = 1-\frac{T_2}{T_1}$$

$$\Rightarrow 0.2 = 1-\frac{T_2}{400}$$

$$\Rightarrow \frac{T_2}{400} = 1-0.2 = 0.8$$

$$\Rightarrow T_2 = 320\ K = 47^\circ C$$

6. **(b)** 7. **(b)**

8. **(c)** : By definition

$$R = \rho\frac{l}{A}$$

$$\Rightarrow \rho = \frac{RA}{l}=\frac{\frac{V}{I}A}{l}=\frac{VA}{Il}$$

$$\therefore [\rho] = \frac{[V][A]}{[I][l]}$$

$$= \frac{ML^2T^{-2}L^2}{IL}=[ML^3T^{-2}I^{-1}]$$

9. **(b)** : M ($v \rightarrow$) ——→ O (α, $v = 0$) ——→ $M-4$

Applying the principle of momentum conservation,

$Mv = (M - 4)v'$ [$\because$ the speed of the α-particle is zero]

$\Rightarrow \quad v' = \dfrac{Mv}{M-4}$

10. (d) : Due to the current flowing in the wire, there is no change of magnetic flux linked with the wire and so there is no induced current.

11. (c) : The wire of length l is bent to from a circular loop, so $2\pi r = l$

$$\Rightarrow r = \frac{l}{2\pi}$$

The magnetic field at the centre of the loop is

$$B = \frac{\mu_0 I}{2r} = \frac{\mu_0 I \times 2\pi}{2l}$$

Now the same length of the wire is bent to from a double loop

$\therefore 2 \times 2\pi r' = l$

$$\Rightarrow r' = \frac{l}{4\pi}$$

And the magnetic field at the centre

$$B' = \frac{\mu_0 I \times 2}{2 \times r'} = \frac{2\mu_0 I}{2 \times \frac{l}{4\pi}} = \frac{2 \times 4\pi\mu I}{2l}$$

$$\therefore \frac{B'}{B} = 4 \Rightarrow B' = 4B$$

12. (c) : Let the resistance of the rod be R. If the rod is divided into two equal parts, then each part of the rod will have a resistance of $R/2$. Now these two parts of the rod are connected in parallel and a voltage V is applied across them. Hence the total power consumed is

$$P' = \frac{V^2}{R/2} + \frac{V^2}{R/2} = 4\frac{V^2}{R} = 4P \text{ where}$$

$P = \dfrac{V^2}{R}$ is the power consumed by the original rod when voltage V is applied across it.

13. (d) : [diagram: mass M moving with velocity V; after explosion two masses $M/2$ with $v = 0$ and $v = v$]

Before explosion, the total momentum of the system $= MV$

After explosion, the total momentum of the system

$$= \frac{M}{2} \times 0 + \frac{M}{2} \times v = \frac{Mv}{2}$$

From the principal of momentum conservation,

$$MV = \frac{Mv}{2}$$

$\Rightarrow \quad v = 2V$

14. (b) : Pressure and stress both have the dimensions of Force/area. Strain and angle are both dimensionsless. Energy and work have the same dimensions force × distance.

Tension and surface tension refer to two different physical quantities and their dimensions are different. Tension is a force and surface tension is force per unit length.

15. (c) : The solid sphere cools more quickly because the thermal conductivity of the solid sphere is more than that of the hollow sphere.

16. (c) : The satellite is moving at an attitude above the surface equal to the radius of the earth R.

$$\therefore \quad \frac{mv_0^2}{2R} = G\frac{Mm}{4R^2}$$

$$\Rightarrow v_0 = \sqrt{\frac{GM}{2R}}$$

Now if the satellite moves at an attitude equal to $R/2$ then,

$$\frac{mv_0'^2}{3R/2} = G\frac{Mm}{9 \times (R/2)^2}$$

$$\Rightarrow \quad v_0'^2 = \frac{2}{3}\cdot\frac{GM}{R}$$

$$\Rightarrow \quad v'_0 = \frac{\sqrt{2}}{\sqrt{3}}\sqrt{\frac{GM}{R}} = \frac{\sqrt{2}}{\sqrt{3}}v_0\sqrt{2}$$

$$= \frac{\sqrt{4}}{\sqrt{3}}v_0 = \frac{2}{\sqrt{3}}v_0$$

17. (d) : When the lift is at rest, the time period of the simple pendulum is $T = 2\pi\sqrt{\dfrac{l}{g}}$

Now, if the lift is moving up with an acceleration $\dfrac{g}{4}$ then the effective acceleration due to gravity

$$g' = g + \frac{g}{4} = \frac{5g}{4}$$

$$\therefore \text{ Time period } T' = 2\pi\sqrt{\frac{l}{g'}}$$

$$= 2\pi\sqrt{\frac{l}{5g/4}}$$

$$= \frac{2}{\sqrt{5}} \times 2\pi\sqrt{\frac{l}{g}} = \frac{2}{\sqrt{5}}T$$

18. (c) : We know that the heat flowing through a conductor is given by

$$\frac{Q}{t} = -KA\left(\frac{d\theta}{dx}\right)$$

$$\Rightarrow Q = -KA\left(\frac{d\theta}{dx}\right)t$$

Where K = thermal conductivity of the material

A = area of cross-section

$\frac{d\theta}{dx}$ = temperature gradient

t = time

Now if we cut the rod into 4 pieces, A remains same K remains same, $\frac{d\theta}{dx}$ is said to be same, so for same time t, Q is going to be same as earlier.

19. (a) :

If we pull the mass m towards right by a distance x then the restoring force it experiences is

$$F = -kx$$

$$\Rightarrow \quad m\frac{d^2x}{dt^2} = -kx$$

$$\Rightarrow \frac{d^2x}{dt^2} + \frac{k}{m}x = 0 \Rightarrow \frac{d^2x}{dt^2} + \omega^2 x = 0$$

Where $\omega = \sqrt{\frac{x}{m}}$

$$\Rightarrow \quad \frac{2\pi}{T} = \sqrt{\frac{x}{m}}$$

$$\Rightarrow \quad n = \frac{1}{2\pi}\sqrt{\frac{x}{m}}$$

20. (b) : The given capacitor can be viewed as a series combination of two capacitors C_1 and C_2 where

$$C_1 = \frac{\varepsilon_0 K_1 A/2}{d}; \qquad C_2 = \frac{\varepsilon_0 K_2 A/2}{d}$$

where d is the separation between the plates,

$\therefore$ The effective capacitance

$$C = \frac{C_1 C_2}{C_1 + C_2}$$

$$= \frac{\frac{\varepsilon_0 K_1 A/2}{d} \times \frac{\varepsilon_0 K_2 A/2}{d}}{\frac{\varepsilon_0 K_1 A/2}{d} + \frac{\varepsilon_0 K_2 A/2}{d}} = \frac{\left(\frac{\varepsilon_0 A}{2d}\right)^2 K_1 K_2}{\left(\frac{\varepsilon_0 A}{2d}\right)(K_1 + K_2)}$$

$$= \frac{\varepsilon_0 A}{2d}\left(\frac{K_1 K_2}{K_1 + K_2}\right)$$

21. (b)

22. (d) : The charge on a proton = e. Hence when the proton is accelerated through a potential difference of 1V, its K.E. = 1eV.

23. (d) : Since both the metal spheres are connected to the same conducting wire, both of them will be having same charge on them. Let the charge on each of them be q.

Then, the electric field intensities are given by,

$$E_a = \frac{kq}{a^2}, \quad E_b = \frac{kq}{b^2}$$

$$\therefore \quad \frac{E_a}{E_b} = \frac{b^2}{a^2}$$

24. (a) : The work fuction of a metal is an inherent property of the metal itself and it does not change with the frequency of the incident light.

25. (c) : Since white light is not monochromatic, so we obtain a central white bond instead of getting fringes or a diffraction pattern.

26. (a) : During elastic collision between two equal masses, the velocity of the two bodies get interchanged. So if one body is at rest, energy transfer will be maximum for $m_1 = m_2$.

27. (b)

28. (b) : For a pipe closed at one end, the frequencies are odd multiples of the fundamental frequencies.

29. (c) :

Figure shows a purely inductive circuit, in which a sinusoidal emf is applied. The induced emf across the inductor is $-L\frac{di}{dt}$ so that from Kirchhoffi's law,

$$\varepsilon_0 \sin\omega t - L\frac{di}{dt} = 0$$

$$\Rightarrow \frac{di}{dt} = \frac{\varepsilon_0}{L}\sin\omega t$$

$$\text{or } i = -\frac{\varepsilon_0}{\omega L}\cos\omega t + C$$

The constant C can be shown to be zero from the fact that, the emf being sinusoidal, the current should also be so, and the average current over one time period has to be zero.

$$\therefore i = -\frac{\varepsilon_0}{\omega L}\cos\omega t \quad \text{or} \quad i = \frac{\varepsilon_0}{\omega L}\sin(\omega t - \pi/2)$$

which shows that the current lags behind the emf by a phase of $\pi/2$.

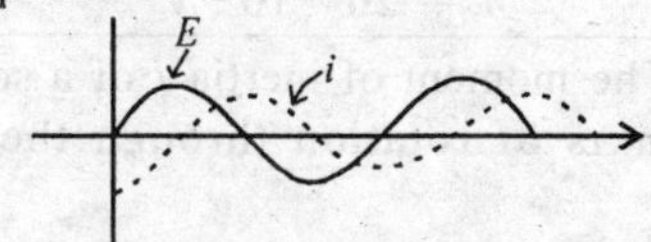

30. (b)

31. (b) : We know from Wien's displacement law that

$\lambda_m T = b$, where

λ_m = wavelength of light emitted with maximum intensity.

T = Temperature of the star

$\therefore$ From the colour (wavelength) of the emitted light, we can determine the temperature of the star.

32. (b) 33. (a)

34. (c) : The escape velocity is independent of the angle of projection. So, the escape velocity of the rocket remains same.

35. (d)

36. (b) : The heat produced in a wire due to current flow is given by

$$H = I^2Rt$$

$$\therefore \quad \frac{\Delta H}{H} = \frac{2\Delta I}{I} + \frac{\Delta R}{R} + \frac{\Delta t}{t}$$

$$= 2 \times 0.02 + 0.01 + 0.01 = 0.06 = 6\%$$

37. (d) : Since the potential at each point of an equipotential surface is the same, the potential does not change while we move a unit positive charge from one point to another. Therefore work done in the process is zero.

38. (a) : Since the density of the electric lines of force at A is more than that at B, the electric field at A, $E_A > E_B$ (elecric field at B).

39. (b) : Gauss's law tells that the total flux through an area enclosing a charge Q is $\frac{Q}{\varepsilon_0}$. Now as the cube is having six faces and as we can assume a symmetrical distribution of fluxes among its faces, the flux associated with one of its faces is $\frac{Q}{6\varepsilon_0}$.

40. (c) : The charge of flux through the metal wire

$\Delta\phi = 8 \times 10^{-4}$ Wb

Time taken $\Delta t = 0.4$ sec

$$\therefore \text{ Induced emf. } \quad e = \frac{\Delta\phi}{\Delta t}$$

$$= \frac{8 \times 10^{-4}}{0.4}$$

$$= 20 \times 10^{-3} \text{ V}$$

41. (b) : The moment of inertia I of a solid sphere about the axis of rotation through the centre is

$$I = \frac{2}{5} MR^2$$

$$\therefore \text{ Angular momentum } L = I\omega = \frac{2}{5} MR^2 \times \frac{2\pi}{T}$$

$= \frac{4\pi MR^2}{5T}$ where T = time period of rotation.

42. (b)

43. (d) : A constant pressure air-thermometer is based on the law

$$\frac{V_1}{T_1} = \frac{V_2}{T_2} \quad \Rightarrow \frac{T_2}{V_1} = \frac{V_2}{V_1}$$

Here it is given that $V_1 = 47.5$

$V_2 = 67$

$T_1 = 0°\text{C} = 273$ K

$$\therefore \quad T_2 = 273 \times \frac{67}{47.5} = 385.07 \text{ K}$$

$$= 112°\text{C}$$

44. (b) : This is a case of a totally inelastic collision, in which linear momentum is conserved but the total mechanical energy is not conserved.

45. (c) :

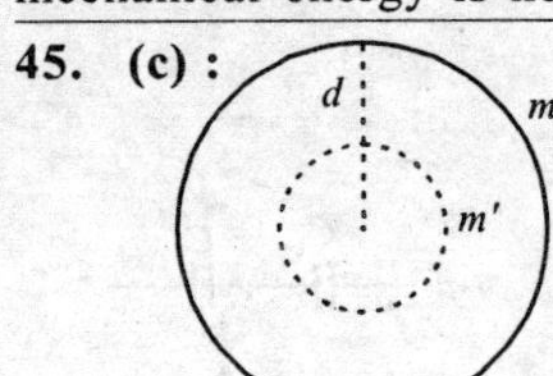

At a depth d below the surface of the earth,

$$mg' = G\frac{M'm}{(R-d)^2}$$

$$M' = \frac{4}{3}\pi (R-d)^3\rho$$

$$\Rightarrow g' = \frac{GM'}{(R-d)^2}$$

$$= \frac{4}{3} G\pi (R-d)\rho$$

If $d = \frac{R}{2}$ then

$$g' = \frac{4}{3} G\pi \rho = \frac{2\pi GR\rho}{3}$$

On the surface of the earth

$$g = \frac{Gm}{RV} = \frac{4}{3}\pi GR\rho$$

$$\therefore \quad g' = \frac{g}{2}$$

$\therefore$ The body weighed 250 N on the surface of the earth would weigh $\frac{1}{2} \times 250 = 125$ N, half way down towards the centre of the earth.

46. (b) : We know from Wien's displacement law,

$$\lambda_m T = \text{constant}$$

$$\therefore \quad \lambda_m T_1 = \lambda'_m T_2$$

$$\Rightarrow \quad \lambda'_m = \frac{\lambda_m T_1}{T_2} = \frac{\lambda_m \times 1000}{2000} = \frac{\lambda_m}{2}$$

47. (b) : $T_{½} = 20$ years

$N_0 = 10$ g

$N = 2.5$ g

$$N = N_0 e^{-\lambda t} \qquad \lambda = \frac{0.693}{T_{½}}$$

$$\Rightarrow \quad e^{-\lambda t} = \ln\left(\frac{N}{N_0}\right)$$

$$\Rightarrow \quad t = \frac{1}{\lambda}\ \ln\left(\frac{N_0}{N}\right) = \frac{T_{½}}{0.693} \times \ln\left(\frac{N_0}{N}\right)$$

$$= \frac{20}{0.693} \times \ln\left(\frac{10}{2.5}\right) = 40 \text{ years}$$

48. (a)

49. (b), (d) : The given circuit is a balanced Wheatstone bridge circuit. So, the resistance 7 Ω may be regulated. Therefore, we have the equivalent circuit as,

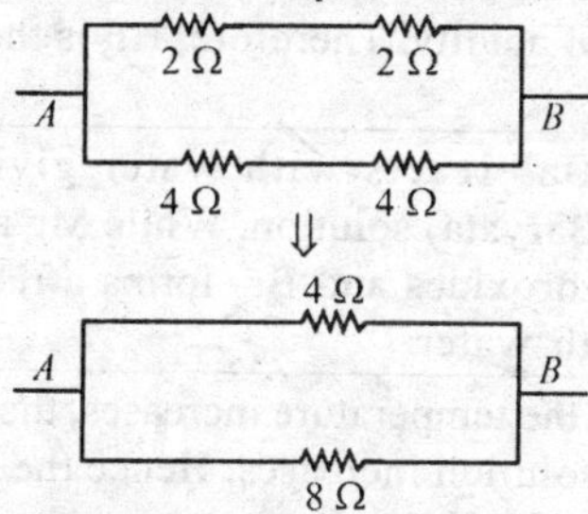

∴ The quivalent resistance between A and B is

$$R = \frac{4 \times 8}{4+8} = \frac{32}{12} = \frac{8}{3}\ \Omega$$

50. (b) : Frequency of source $n = 240$ Hz

Velocity of source $v_s = 20$ m/s

Velocity of observer $v_0 = 20$ m/s

Velocity of sound $v = 340$ m/s

Given both the source and the observer are moving towards each other. Hence the apparent frequency of the source is,

$$n' = n\left[\frac{v + v_0}{v - v_s}\right]$$

$$= 240 \times \left[\frac{340+20}{340-20}\right]$$

$$= 240 \times \frac{360}{320} = 270 \text{ Hz}$$

51. (a) : Since centripetal force is perpendicular to the displacement of the body, ,work done is zero as

$$W = \vec{F}.\vec{d} = Fd\cos\theta$$

52. (a)

53. (a) : As LASER is highly monochromatic and highly coherent, we can send a LASER beam to the moon, from where it comes back reflected without much loss of intensity. That's why the large distances can be measured accurately with the help of LASER.

54. (c) : In uniform circular motion, the force is always directed perpendicular to the displacement.

55. (a) : Because of the rotation of the earth, the value of acceleration due to gravity changes. Due to this rotation, the value of 'g' becomes minimum at the equator and maximum at the poles.

56. (c) : During reverse biasing, the depletion layer widens, and so there is more resistance for an electron or a hole to cross that layer to conduct current.

57. (d) 58. (a)

59. (c) : Kepler's laws are the general rules for all planetary motions. Hence artificial satellites showed also follow the same laws.

60. (c) : The third pin is used for grounding purposes so that it leaves the user safe while handling the appliance by making the extra charge on it get discharged.

CHEMISTRY

61. (b) : Aromaticity can be predicted by the use of Huckle's rule which says that $(4n + 2)$ π–electrons are required in delocalisation system to give it aromaticity.

$(4n + 2)$ π electrons means 2, 6, 10 .....π electrons.

Here total number of electrons available for delocalisation = 6

∴ It is expected to be aromatic.

62. (d) : Carbocation is more stable if it is bonded to electron relasing group which somewhat stabilise the carbocation. So more the number of electron releasing groups, more is the stability.

$\overset{+}{C}H_3$ $\quad CH_3 \rightarrow \overset{+}{C}H_2 \quad CH_3 \rightarrow \overset{+}{C}H \leftarrow CH_3 \quad CH_3 \rightarrow \overset{+}{C} \leftarrow CH_3$ (with CH_3 below, arrow pointing up to C)

(least stable) (most stable)

63. (a) : CH_3 (methyl free radical) has planar structure with sp^2 hybridisation of 'C' atom. The odd electron is present in unhybridised $2p_z$ orbital.

$\overset{\oplus}{C}H_3$ (methyl carbonium ion) has also trigonal planar structure (sp^2).

$\overset{\ominus}{C}H_3$ (methyl carbanion ion) has tetrahedral structure (sp^3) and one of the hybrid orbital contains the lone pair of electrons.

64. (a) :

$$CH_3-CH_2-COOH \xrightarrow{P/Br_2} CH_3-\underset{Br}{CH}-COOH \xrightarrow[H^+]{alc.\ KOH}$$

$$CH_2 = CH - COOH + HBr$$

$P + Br_2$ is brominating agent that brominates the α–position. The product then undergo dehydrohalogenation in the pressure of alcoholic potassium hydroxides.

65. (a) : When $n = 5$, then $l = 0, 1, 2, 3, 4$.
Again when $l = 2$, then $m = -2, -1, 0, +1, +2$.
The 's' value can be $\pm 1/2$
Hence the arrangement, $n = 5, l = 2, m = 2, s = +1/2$ is possible for an electron.

66. (d) : Fluorine is a highly electronegative element, it withdraws electron from the neighbouring atoms. Therefore, more is the number of fluorine atoms attached, greater will be the acidity of the molecules. *e.g.* FCH_2COOH is more acidic than CH_3COOH. Therefore, correct order of acidity is :

$$CF_3COOH > CF_2HCOOH > FCH_2COOH > CH_3COOH$$

67. (a) : $HClO_4$ is the strongest acid among $HClO$, $HClO_2$, $HClO_3$ and $HClO_4$ as more the number of oxygen atoms attached, more is the acidity of the molecule order of acidity is :

$$HClO < HClO_2 < HClO_3 < HClO_4$$

So the conjugate base order will be just the reverse:

$$ClO^- > ClO_2^- > ClO_3^- > ClO_4^-$$

68. (a) : Smaller sized and highly charged metal atoms have higher hydration energy. In the alkaline earth metal, the hydration energy for the compact and charged ions is greater than the large sized charged ions. Therefore, order of hydration energy in this group is $Be^{2+} > Mg^{2+} > Ca^{2+} > Sr^{2+} > Ba^{2+}$

69. (b) : Carbon, oxygen and nitrogen atoms do not have any d-orbital available. Therefore, in CO_2^{2-}, NO_2^- and NO_3^-, there is no possibility of p_π–d_π type of bonding.

In PO_4^{3-} phosphorus atom have vacant d-orbital available which is used to form p_π–d_π type of bonding with p-orbital of oxygen atom.

70. (c) : Feasibility of reaction is determined by free energy change value (ΔG). ΔG is given by gibbs – Helmhots equation :

$$\Delta G = \Delta H - T\Delta S$$

Reaction is feasible if ΔG value is negative. Therefore, if ΔH is negative and $T\Delta S$ is positive then the ΔG will always be feasible.

71. (c) : $C + O_2 \rightarrow CO_2$; $\Delta H° = -a$ kJ
$2CO + O_2 \rightarrow 2CO_2$; $\Delta H° = -b$ kJ

Formation of CO can be written as :

$$C + \frac{1}{2}O_2 \rightarrow CO\ ;\ \Delta H° = ?$$

Adding equation : $C + O_2 \rightarrow CO_2$; $\Delta H° = -a$ kJ

$$CO_2 \rightarrow CO + \frac{1}{2}O_2\ ;\ \Delta H° = \frac{b}{2}\text{ kJ}$$

We get $\Delta H°_f(CO) = \frac{b}{2} - a = \frac{b-2a}{2}$

72. (a) : The bond strength H-X decreases from HF to HI. Thus HF is the most stable and hence weakest acid while is least stable and most acidic. In aqueous solutions, HF is only slightly ionised but HCl, HBr and HI are almost completely ionised. As basicity is the reverse of acidity. Therefore, HF is the most basic of all H-X.

73. (d) : 'Ba' reacts with water giving soluble hydroxide (Baryata) solution. While Mg and Sr forms insoluble hydroxides and Br_2 forms a reddish brown solution with water.

74. (d) : As the temperature increases, the dissociation of water in solution increases. Hence the H^+ ion conc. increases and pH of the solution decreases with increase in temperature.

75. (d) : Boron carbide is written as B_4C. It is produced by reducing B_2O_3 with C at 1600° C. Fibres of B_3C have an enormous tensile strength and are used to make bullet-proof clothing.

76. (c) : Electronic configuration for chromium is :
${}_{24}Cr \rightarrow 1s^2\,2s^2\,2p^6\,3s^2\,3p^6\,3d^5\,4s^1$

After ionisation of $4s$ electron the next electron which will be ionised is from $3d$ orbital. As $3d^5$ electronic configuration, therefore is stable. Hence, the second ionisation of Cr will require much greater ionisation energy than the expected one.

77. (b) : In O_2, the bond order = 2
In O_2^{+2}, the bond order = 2.5
In O_2^-, the bond order = 1.5
In O_2^{-2}, the bond order = 1
As the bond order in O_2^{+2} is highest, so its internuclear distance is smallest.

78. (c) : For a salt of weak acid and weak base, its

$$pH = 7 + \frac{1}{2}pK_a - \frac{1}{2}pK_b$$

$= 7 + \frac{1}{2} \times 3.8 - \frac{1}{2} \times 4.8 = 6.5$

79. (a) : Ionic azides are usually much more stable e.g. KN_3, NaN_3 and Mg_3N_2 than the covalent azides. Covalent azides are used as detonators and explosives *e.g.* $Ba(N_3)_2$.

80. (b) : Electronic configuration of Co :

Co (Z = 27) : $4s^2\ 3d^7$

Co^{2+} : $3d^7$

$[CoCl_4]$: ⇅ ⇅ ⇅ 1 xx | xx | xx xx (3d, 4s, 4p)

Therefore, hybridisation is dsp^2 and structure is square planar.

81. (b) : Basicity in nitrogen compounds is attributed to the availability of lone pair of electrons. The order of availability of e^- pair on N-atom is :

$NH_3 > NH_2\ NH_2 > HN_3 > NH_2OH$.

Therefore, same is the order of basicity of these compounds.

82. (b) : Electron osmosis – when electro phoresis of dispersed particles in a colloidal system is presented by some smitable means, it is observed that the dispersion medium it self begins to move in an electric field. This phenomenon is called as electro-osmosis.

83. (a) : Hydrogen fluoride is an associated molecule and can be represented by H_2F_2. This is due to the fact that strong Hydrogen bonding exist between the molecules. (as F is highly electronegative element)

$H_2F_2 + KF \rightarrow KHF_2 + HF$

84. (b) : The nitration of benzene takes places in three steps, *i.e.*

(i) Generation of electrophile (NO_2^+)

(ii) Attack of an electrophile to benzene ring forming the carbocation

(iii) Loss of proton from carbocation giving nitrobenzene.

The attack of electrophile to benzene ring giving a carbocation is the slowest and rate determining step.

85. (a) : CCl_4 is non-inflammable due to strong C—Cl bonds in it. Therefore it is inert to fire and used as a fire-extinguisher under the name of pyrene.

86. (b) : Concentration of NH_4OH solution = 0.1 N

Concentration of OH^- ions in solution,

$[OH^-] = 20\%$ of 0.1 N $= \frac{20}{100} \times 0.1$

$= 0.02$ N

$\Rightarrow$ pOH $= -\log[OH^-] = -\log(0.02)$

$= 2 - 0.301$

$\Rightarrow$ pH $= 14 -$ pOH $= 12.30$

87. (a) : carnallite is ore of potassium and its formula is $KCl.\ MgCl_2.6H_2O$.

88. (a) : Standard Electrode potential for Gold is

$Au^{3+} + 3e^- \rightleftharpoons Au,$

is 1.50 volt. therefore, gold get easily reduced. So to electroplate gold on the spoon, spoon should be made cathode as reduction takes place on cathode.

89. (d) : Bond order of the molecules :

$O_2 : KK(\sigma 2s)^2 (\sigma^* 2s)^2 (\sigma 2p_x)^2 (\pi 2p_y)^2 (\pi 2p_z)^2 (\pi^* 2p_y)^2 (\pi 2p_z)^1$

Bond order of $O_2^- = \frac{1}{2}(8-5) = 1.5$

$He_2^+ : (\sigma\ 1s)^2 (\sigma^*\ 1s)^1$

Bond order of $He_2^+ = \frac{1}{2}(2-1) = 0.5$

$C_2 : Kk(\sigma\ 2s)^2 (\sigma^*\ 2s)^2 (\sigma 2p_x)^2 (\pi 2p_y)^1 (\pi 2p_z)^1$

Bond order $= \frac{1}{2}(6-2) = 2.0$

$NO : Kk\ (\sigma 2s)^2 (\sigma^*\ 2s)^2 (\sigma 2p_x)^2 (\pi^2 p_y)^2 (\pi^2 p_z)^2 (\sigma^* 2p_x)^1$

Bond order $= \frac{1}{2}(8-3) = 2.5$

90. (a) : NaCl type structure is also called face centred cubic lattice. Here the radius ratio (r_c/r_a) ranges from 0.414 to 0.732.

radius ratio $= \frac{r_c}{r_a} = \frac{\text{radius of cation}}{\text{radius of anion}}$

$\Rightarrow$ radius of anion $(B^-) = \frac{\text{radius of } A^+}{\text{radius ratio}}$

$= \frac{100}{0.414}$ to $\frac{100}{0.732}$

$= 241.5$ to 136.6.

91. (a) : Freundlich gave an empirical relationship between the quantity of gas adsorbed by unit mass of solid adsorbent and concentration at a particular temperature.

$\log x/m = \log K + \frac{1}{n} \log C$

x = mass of gas adsorbed, m = mass of adsorbent

C = concentration, k, n = constants.

92. (c) : Crystalline solids are anisotropic therefore their physical properties *e.g.* electrical conductivity, thermal conductivity, refractive index are the different in different directions. But amorphous solids, liquids and gases are isotropic (*i.e.* same physical properties in all directions).

93. (a) : Charge = current × time

Charge, Q = 1A × 60 sec

= 60 coulumb

Now,

96500 C charge is carried by 6.023×10^{23} electron

$\Rightarrow$ 60 C charge $= \frac{6.023\times10^{23}}{96500} \times 60$ electrons

$= 3.74 \times 10^{20}$ electrons

94. (c) : $K_p = K_c\,(RT)^{\Delta n}$

Δn = change in number of moles

If Δn = positive then K_p will be greater than K_c.

$PCl_3 + Cl_2 \rightarrow PCl_5$, $\Delta n = 1-2 = -1$; $K_p < K_c$

$H_2 + I_2 \rightarrow 2HI$, $\Delta n = 0$; $K_p = K_c$

$2SO_3 \rightarrow O_2 + 2SO_2$, $\Delta n = 1$; $K_p > K_c$

$N_2 + 3H_2 \rightarrow 2NH_3$; $\Delta n = -2$; $K_p < K_c$

95. (c) : $Cl-\overset{3}{C}(Cl)_2-\overset{2}{CH_2}-\overset{1}{CHO}$

Therefore IUPAC name is 3,3,3 – trichloropropanal.

96. (a) : Bidentate ligands are those ligand which can coordinate to metal atom by two donor atoms. *e.g.*

CH_2-NH_2 / CH_2-NH_2 (ethylenediamine) and oxalate: $O=C-O^-$ / $O=C-O^-$

97. (a) : $Al^{3+} + 3e^- \rightarrow Al$

Therefore, number of electrons required to deposite 1 gm equivelent of aluminium is three mole.

98. (b) : Reversible reactions are those reaction in which there is equilibrium established at every infinitesimal step. But the rate of forward and rate of backward reaction can be influenced (or speed up) by the use of catalyst.

99. (a) : Molecular weight of NH_4OH = 35

Now,

35 g of NH_4OH is needed to prepare 1 M solution in 1 litre

$\Rightarrow$ 35 g NH_4OH is 1 L solution ≡ 1 molar solution

$\Rightarrow$ 2.5×35 g NH_4OH is 1 L solution ≡ 2.5 molar solution

$\Rightarrow \frac{2.5\times35}{10}$ g NH_4OH is 100 L solution ≡ 2.5 molar solution

$\Rightarrow$ 8.75 g NH_4OH was dissolved.

$NH_3 + H_2O \rightarrow NH_4OH$

For 35 g NH_4OH, NH_3 needed = 22.4 L at S.T.P

$\Rightarrow$ for 8.75 g NH_4OH, NH_3 needed $= \frac{22.4}{35} \times 8.75$ L

= 5.6 L

100. (a) : The equilibrium constant is not affected by changing the volume of the whole reaction flask.

101. (d) : Fe (Z = 26) ; Atomic weight = 55.85

Co (Z = 27) ; Atomic weight = 58.93

Ni (Z = 28) ; Atomic weight = 58.69

The correct order of Atomic weights is

CO > Ni > Fe

102. (c) : $NaClO_4 \rightarrow Na^+ + ClO_4^-$

$NaClO_3 \rightarrow Na^+ + ClO_3^-$

$NaClO_2 \rightarrow Na^+ + ClO_2^-$

$NaClO \rightarrow Na^+ + ClO^-$

In aqueous solution, these compounds decompose into ions. ClO_4^- will most easily abstract proton from water molecules. So it will be most acidic.

103. (a) : 3–methylhexane is

$CH_3-CH_2-CH_2-\overset{*}{C}H(CH_3)-CH_2-CH_3$

C* = chiral carbon atom (due to which the compound is optically active).

104. (d) : pH = – log[H⁺]

$\Rightarrow$ pH = 2 $\Rightarrow$ $[H^+]$ for pH = 2 = 10^{-2}

pH = 6 $\Rightarrow$ $[H^+]$ for pH = 6 = 10^{-6}

$\Rightarrow \frac{10^{-2}}{10^{-6}} = 10^4 = 10{,}000$

105. (b) : Relative lowering of vapour pressure is given by :

$$\frac{P^0 - P}{P^0} = \frac{w/m}{w/m + W/M}$$

Where, P^0 = Vapour pressure of pure solvent

P = Vapour pressure of solution

w = mass of slute

m = molecular mass of solute

W = mass of solvent

M = molecular mass of solvent.

For dilute solution

$$\Rightarrow \frac{121.8-120.2}{121.8} = \frac{15/m}{250/78} \Rightarrow m = 356.265$$

106. (d) : BCl_3 : [1×] [1×|1×|] (Central Borm atom)
2s 2p

No lone pair of electron is available in BCl_3.

NCl_3 : [1↓] [1×|1×|1×] (Central N-atom)
2s 2p

One lone pair of electron is available on N-atoms, it occupies a corner in the tetrahedral arrangement. Therefore, NCl_3 appears pyramidal in shape.

107. (a) : $Na_2[CuCl_4]$
Oxidation state of copper = + 2
Electronic configuration of $Cu^{2+} \Rightarrow 3d^9$
As there is no *d–d* transition possible, the molecule is not coloured.

108. (c) : Organic compound → Comp. + AgCl
0.189 g 0.287 g

$$\text{Percentage of chlorine in AgCl} = \frac{35.5}{143.35} \times 100 = 24.76\%$$

$$\text{Weight of chlorine in 0.287 g AgCl} = \frac{24.76}{100} \times 0.287 = .07106 \text{ g}$$

$$\text{Percentage of chlorine in 0.189 g} = \frac{.07106}{0.189} \times 100 = 37.598\%$$

109. (c) : All the alcohols are water soluble as alcohol molecules forms extensive hydrogen bonding with the water molecules.

110. (c) : The ground state electronic configuration of neon atom (Z = 10) is :
$1s^2, 2s^2, 2p^6$
Therefore first excited state of Neon will be :
$1s^2, 2s^2, 2p^5, 3s^1$

111. (a) : Dissociation consant for :

$$HA \rightleftharpoons H^+ + A^-$$

Can be given as :

$$K_s = \frac{[H^+][A^-]}{[HA]}$$

Therefore, we can say that dissociation constant is a measure of its ability to furnish protons in the solution.

112. (a) : *p*-nitrophenol has higher boiling point than *o*-nitrophenol, because intermolecular hydrogen bonding present in *p*-nitrophenol is responsible for it. But intramolecular hydrogen bonding in *o*-nitrophenol does not effect boiling point.

113. (c) : Due to the presence of hydroxyl group (–OH), there is extensive hydrogen bonding between the ethanol molecales (C_2H_5OH). But there is no such Hydrogen bonding in Dimethyl ether (due to absence of –OH group). So boiling point of Dimethyl ether is much lower than ethanol.

114. (a) : $CHCl_3$ and CH_3—OH are miscible due to intermolecular van der Waal's force of attraction. However CH_3OH is polar and $CHCl_3$ is non-polar.

115. (a) : Oxygen is the most electronegative element after fluorine. Therefore, in the componds between oxygen and fluorine, oxygen is found to show positive oxidation state.
e.g. OF_2 : Oxygen difluoride.
Oxidation state of oxygen here is +2.

116. (d) : B_2H_6 is an electron deficient compound. B_2H_6 contain some unusual bonds which are called as 2-electron, 3-centre bonds.

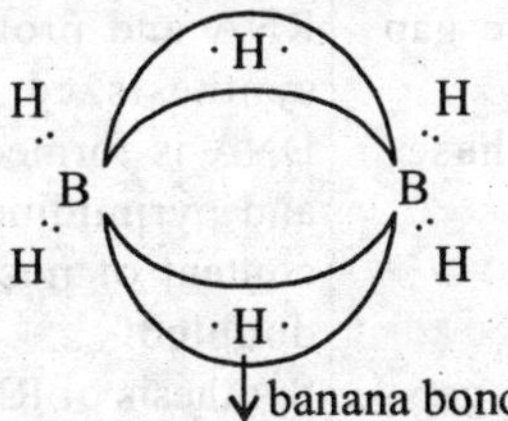

Si_2H_6 is called disilane.

$$\begin{array}{c} H \quad H \\ | \quad\; | \\ H-Si-Si-H \\ | \quad\; | \\ H \quad H \end{array}$$

117. (a) : A nuclear reaction in which two lighter nuclei are fused together to form a heavier nuclei is called nuclear fusion. In such a process, more stable nuclei come into existence binding energy per nucleon increases. Fusion reactions are highly exothermic because of loss of mass during fusion. *e.g.*

$${}_1^2H + {}_1^2H \rightarrow {}_2^4He + 24.9 \text{ MeV}$$

118. (a) : Heavy water is used as a moderator in nuclear reactors to absorb high speed neutrons. So that they slow down the rate of nuclear reaction.

119. (d) : Electronic configuration of Berylium and Boron is given as :
Be (Z = 4) : $1s^2, 2s^2$
Be (Z = 5) : $1s^2, 2s^2, 2p^1$

Ionisatin potential of Be is greater than that of Boron as first electron released from Be is from *s*-orbital while it is from *p*-orbital in Boron.

120. (a) : The large sized sulphate anion (SO_4^{2-}) is stabilised better by a large sized cation. So the stability of sulphates down the group increases so the lattice energy is more in $BaSO_4$ than in Na_2SO_4.

BIOLOGY

121. (c) : A muscle fibre would contract only when it receives stimulation of certain intensity called threshold stimulus. Response of a muscle fibre to a stimulus is not proportionate to its intensity. It is absent when the intensity is subliminal. Muscle fibre contracts to the maximum whether the stimulus has threshold value or supra–liminal value.

122. (b) : Cell cycle is a series of cyclic changes through which a cell passes during its growth and divisions. In the cell cycle, the resting stage or interphase can be divided into three periods.

Periods of Interphase	*Function*
G_1/post-mitotic gap phase	RNA and proteins synthesiszed
S/Synthetic phase	DNA is formed from purines and pyrimidines. The DNA content of nucleus would be doubled.
G_2/Pre mitotic gap phase	Synthesis of RNA and protein continues, but DNA synthesis stops

123. (a) : Barrbody is also known as sex chromatin, X chromatin. Barr body is partially inactivated and development of this facultative heterochromatin occurs in one of the two X chromosomes in interphase nuclei. Any of the two X–chromosomes can become heterochromatic.

124. (b) : Respiratory centre controls the rate of respiration. Respiratory centre is located in medulla oblongata and pons. It has the following components (i) inspiratory area – connected to inspiratory muscles, (ii) Pneumotaxic area, (iii) Expiratory area, (iv) chemosensitive area. Chemoreceptors located on carotid and aortic bodies are sensitive to oxygen deficiency in arterial blood. They send information to respiratory centre.

125. (b) : Cocaine is a natural alkaloid obtained from leaves of *Erthyroxylon coca*. Its chemical formula is $C_{17}H_{21}NO_4$. It is a powerful CNS stimulant. It causes lack of sleep and loss of appetite.

126. (c) : According to Petersons Mark and Recapture Method, the population (P) is given by

$$P = m(r + u)/r$$

where m = number of marked fishes

r = number of marked fishes recaptured

u = number of unmarked fishes captured.

$P = m(r + u)/r$ $\quad m = 80$

$= \frac{80(40+60)}{40}$ $\quad r = 40$

$= 200$ $\quad u = (100 - 40) = 60$

127. (c) : In the primordial hot soup, simple organic molecules reacted amongst themselves to form heavier and larger molecules. When temperature of the earth cooled down to 1000°C or even lower a variety of simple hydrocarbons are formed. First, small chain compounds of C, H and O were formed from hydroxy derivatives. Some of the nucleotides came to have more phosphates and functioned as energy suppliers. Nucleotides underwent polymerization to form nucleic acids, DNA and RNA. Later enzymes and coenzymes came into existence.

128. (a) : Jamming of wooden frames during rains is caused by swelling of wood due to imbibition. (The absorption of water by the solid particles of a substance without forming a solution is called imbibition).

129. (b) : Plastids are semiautonomous cell organelles. They take part in storage and synthesis of organic compounds. Mitochondria are called the power houses of the cell as they are the centres of Krebs cycle or respiration liberating the maximum amount of energy. Ribosomes are submicroscopic polypeptide manufacturing naked granular nucleoprotein cell organelles.

Plasmids are defined as autonomous elements, whose genomes exist in the cell as the extrachromosomal unit. These are the chromosomal element found in bacteria. Plasmids are used as cloning vectors, due to their increased yield potential.

130. (c) : In Fabaceae stamens have diadelphous arrangement i.e. (9) + 1. In total these are 10 in number.

131. (d) : Test cross is a cross to know the genotype of the individual. The individual is crossed with recessive parent. The dihybrid test cross ratio is 1:1:1:1.

The characters under consideration is tall white and dwarf black.

Gametes of TtWw = TW, Tw, tW, tw

Gametes of ttww = tw

♂/♀	tw	tw	tw	tw
TW	TtWw	TtWw	TtWw	TtWw
Tw	Ttww	Ttww	Ttww	Ttww
tW	ttWw	ttWw	ttWw	ttWw
tw	ttww	ttww	ttww	ttww

Thus the ratio of TtWw : Ttww : ttWw : ttww : is 1 : 1 : 1 : 1

132. **(a) :** Porous wood possesses abundant vessels. Due to the presence of vessels, the hardwoods are also called porous wood.

133. **(b) :** For human RBC, 0.9% salt solution is isotonic. Hence a medium of 1.5 % salt solution would be hypertonic i.e. more concentrated. Hence the RBC will shrink due to exosmosis.

134. **(b) :** A simple reflex action is a nerve mediated spontaneous automatic and involuntary response to a stimulus acting on a specific receptor without consulting the will of the animal. Conditioned reflexes are those reflex actions that are not present at birth but develop later in life through learning, habit, experience or regular association of an indifferent stimulus with unconditioned stimulus.

135. **(b) :** Duck billed platypus is an egg laying mammal. It is a monotreme.

136. **(a) :** In RNA, thymine is replaced by uracil.

137. **(a) :** Pulmonary veins carry oxygenated blood from the lungs to the left atrium of the heart. Hepatic portal vein forms the hepatic portal system. It enters liver and breaks into capillaries. The renal artery branches out from the dorsal aorta and supplies blood to the kidney.

138. **(b) :** Some evolution occurs by random fluctuations in gene frequency called genetic drift. Such fluctuations are more likely to occur in a small population. Given frequency in small population changes by chance.

139. **(d) :** Organophosphates (Malathion) kills insects by inhibiting enzyme cholinesterase. It is carbamates. They are the organic esters of the carbonic acid. In their structure, they are quite similar to acetylcholine and, therefore have strong affinity for the enzyme *acetylcholinesterase*, and inhibits its activity.

140. **(d) :** Biosphere is the living mantle or biologically inhabited part of earth along with its abiotic or physiochemical component. Biosphere consists of three interacting subdivisions – atmosphere, lithosphere and hydrosphere. Atmosphere is the transparent gaseous mantle surrounding the earth. Lithosphere is the outer solid crust of earth. Hydrosphere is liquid mantle of earth.

141. **(c) :** In photorespiration uptake of oxygen and evolution of carbondioxide are light dependent. RuBP carboxylase act as RuBP oxygenase. It occurs in chloroplast and require the help of peroxisomes and mitochondria.

142. **(a) :** Cloves are unopened floral buds of *Syzygium aromaticum*.

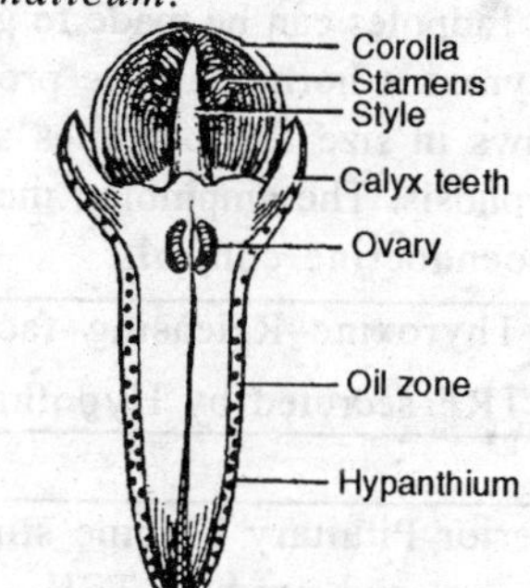

Diagrammatic longitudinal section through a clove flower bud

143. **(a) :** Velamen is a dead spongy tissue present in epiphytic roots (hygroscopic roots). With the help of velamen, these roots are able to absorb water from moist atmosphere, dew and rain.

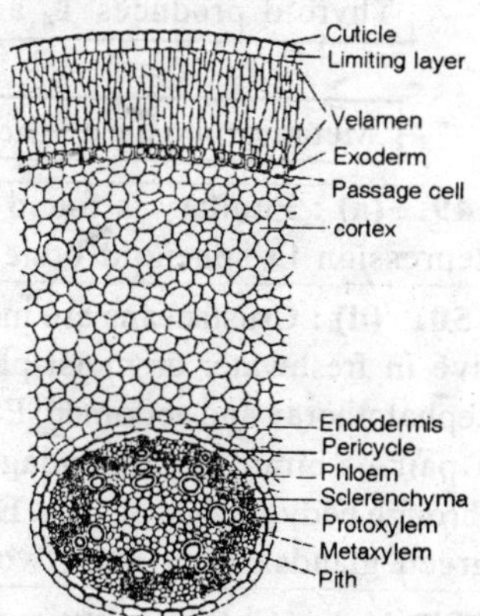

Detailed structure of a portion of T.S. of orchid root

144. **(d) :** Hydroponics is soilless cultivation of plants by placing the roots in the nutrient solution. Goerick (1940) used the term hydroponics to refer the growth of plants in water and sand culture.

145. **(b) :** Commercial coir is obtained from the fibrous husk (mesocarp) of fruits of coconut palm. The fibre is valued for its lightness, elasticity, exceedingly high resistance to mechanical wear and dampness.

146. **(b) :** Vernalization is a process of shortening of the juvenile or vegetative phase and hastening flowering by a previous cold treatment. The term vernalization was coined by Lysenko (1928).

147. (b) : Viruses have the strong reproductive capacity within the host body, thus when viral disease occurs, several copies of that virus are produced in the body and cure by taking medicines is almost impossible. Only, body's own immunity can destroy them. Viruses cause a number of infectious human diseases like common cold, yellow fever, rabies, cancer, AIDS etc.

148. (a) : Tadpoles can be made to grow in size by injecting thyroxine hormone. The process by which tadpole grows in size and becomes adult is known as metamorphosis. The amphibian metamorphosis is under neuroendocrine control.

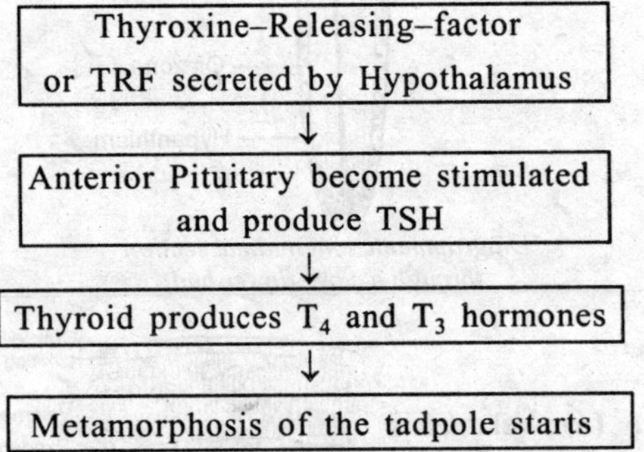

149. (a) : Pituitary is found in sella turcica. It is a depression in sphenoid bone of cranial cavity.

150. (d) : Crustaceans are mostly marine but a few live in freshwater or moist places. Body consists of cephalothorax and abdomen. Each body segment bears a pair of biramous appendages. Respiration occurs through body surface or gills. Excretion occurs through green glands. They bear two pairs of antennae.

151. (a) : Chloromycetin or chloramphenicol is obtained from *Streptomyces venezuelae* and *S. lavendulae*.

Maximum number of antibiotics are produced by mycelial bacteria known as actinomycetes.

152. (c) : Mutualism is an obligatory positive interspecific interaction strongly beneficial to both species. The unicellular photosynthetic plants, called *Zoochlorellae* live symbiotically in the outer tissues of coelenterates. Algae are photosynthetic and produce oxygen and nitrogenous compounds beneficial to hosts and in exchange they obtain materials like carbon dioxide and nitrogenous wastes released by metabolism of host animals. The relationship between hermit crab and sea anemone is an example of commensalism.

153. (b) : In respiration, from 180 gm of glucose 264 gm CO_2 + 108 gm H_2O + 686 Kcal energy is formed.

$C_6H_{12}O_6 + 6O_2 \rightarrow 6CO_2 + 6H_2O + 686$ Kcal

Atomic weight of C = 12, H = 1, O = 16

$C_6H_{12}O_6 = (12 \times 6 + 12 \times 1 + 16 \times 6)$
$= 180$ gm

$6CO_2 = 6\,(12 + 16 \times 2)$
$= 264$ gm

$6H_2O = 6\,(2 \times 1 + 16)$
$= 108$ gm

$\therefore$ From 1 molecule or 180 gm of glucose, through respiration, 264 gm CO_2, 108 gm H_2O and 686 Kcal energy are formed.

154. (c) : Cytoplasmic inheritance or non chromosomal (extranuclear) inheritance is the passage of traits from parents to offspring through structures present inside cytoplasm of contributing gametes. The genes controlling cytoplasmic inheritance are called plasma genes or extra nuclear genes. These occur in plastids, mitochondria, plasmids. Cytoplasmic inheritance is usually uniparental. It is also called maternal inheritance as zygote receives its cytoplasm from ovum.

155. (a) : Water always moves from the area of high water potential to the area of low water potential i.e., from less negative potential to more negative potential.

156. (a) : Stomata are meant for gaseous exchange but are also the main source of transpiration. In majority of plants stomata open in the presence of light and close in darkness.

157. (b) : 10 pairs of cranial nerves are present in anamniotes (fishes and amphibians) and 12 pairs occur in amniotes (reptiles, birds and mammals). In anamniotes the cranial nerves are – Olfactory, Optic, Occulomotor, Trochlear, Trigeminal, Abducens, Facial, Auditory, Glossopharyngeal and Vagus. In amniotes two more cranial nerves, Spinal accessory and Hypoglossal nerves are present in addition to the above ten.

158. (c) : In arthropods like prawn, the blood is colourless and contains WBCs only. The blue respiratory pigment, haemocyanin is present in the blood of molluscs. The RBCs of mammals contain the red pigment haemoglobin which carries oxygen.

159. (a) : *Escherichia coli* is the non-pathogenic bacteria of colon. It is the motile or non-motile organism which lives in the intestine of humans as the part of normal flora. One of the characterisitcs of *Escherichia coli* is the production of bacteriocins (colieins), a specific type of metabolite which is not only lethal to the organism of the same species but also to related organisms.

Balantidium coli results in inflammation of alimentary tract. *Entamoeba coli* causes amoebic dysentery. *Enterobius vermicularis* infection is known as oxyuriasis or enterobiosis.

160. (b) : In Nuclear endosperm the primary endosperm nucleus divides repeatedly without wall formation produce a large number of free nuclei. It is most common type of endosperm. It is named so because it contains free nuclei in the beginning.

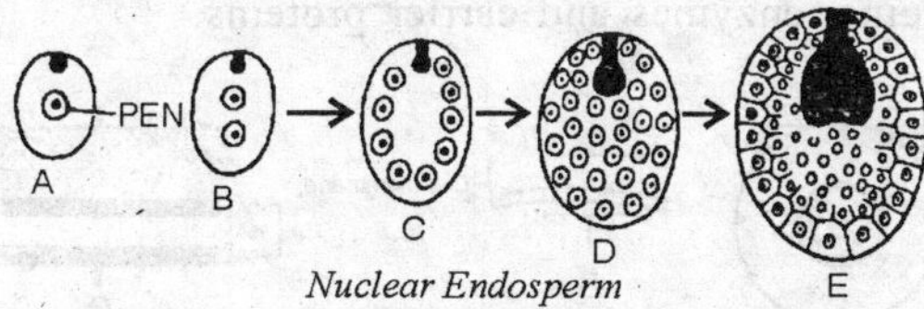

Nuclear Endosperm

161. (c) : Cell wall is two layered and wavy in Gram (-) bacteria. The wall contains peptidoglycan in the inner layer. The outer layer has lipopolysaccharides, proteins and phospholipids.

162. (c) : Nematocysts are the stinging cells and are the organs of offence and defence of coelenterates, Nematocyst contains a poisonous proteinaceous fluid hypnotoxin along tube which injects the fluid into the victim. Nematocysts are activated in response to chemicals secreted by prey. They explode after coming in contact with the prey.

163. (b) : Phytochrome is an amorphous photoreceptor chromoprotein. It exists in two interconvertible forms i.e., P_r and P_{fr}.

$$P_r \text{ (inactive)} \underset{\substack{\text{far red} \\ \textbf{(in dark)}}}{\overset{\text{Red light}}{\rightleftharpoons}} P_{fr} \text{ (active)}$$

164. (d) : Blackmann formulated the principle of limiting factors. He studied the effect of CO_2 concentration, light intensity and temperature on the rate of photosynthesis.

165. (b) : Graafian follicle develops under influence of FSH of anterior pituitary. Its follicular cells secrete estrogen. Rising level of estrogen decreases production of FSH, and stimulates secretion of LH. The two cause mature graafian follicle to release the ovum.

166. (c) : *Calvin et al* while working on *Chlorella* found that carbon dioxide fixes during dark phase of photosynthesis. 6 molecules of CO_2 combines with 6 RuBP and after a chain of reaction form one molecule of glucose (six calvin cycle are required for the production of one glucose molecule).

167. (a)

168 (b) : In prokaryotes meiosis is absent due to absence of gamete formation. But there occurs genetic recombination through following three processes :

Transduction, Tranformation and conjugation (for more details please refer solution no. 157 of AIIMS 2000).

170. (a)

171. (b) : The opening and closing of stomata is a function of turgor changes in guard cells. In light malic acid produce in guard cells, which dissociates into hydrogen and malate ions, resulting in intake of K^+ ions through H^+–K^+ ion exchange. There is increase in concentration of K^+ and malate ions in guard cells, endosmosis of water into guard cells resulting in increased turgor pressure which results in stomatal opening.

Stomata are chiefly concerned with gaseous exchange during photosynthesis and respiration and water loss through transpiration.

172. (a) : Cheetah is the most successful among quadrapedal animals. Because of its specially developed forelimbs and bodyshape, it acquires the power of fastest running over the ground. During running, it uses its powerful forelimbs to push itself forward.

173. (a) : Wounds heal slowly due to vitamin deficiency. The best characterized function of vitamin C is the synthesis of collagen connective tissue protein at the level of hydroxylation of prolyl and lysyl residues of procollagen. Thus vitamin C is important for tissue healing. Patients with peptic ulcers will heal faster on vitamin C than those with extra vitamin C.

174 (c) : A plant girdled upto bast will show the sign of degradation because of the non transportation of the solute which occurs through phloem (bast). Water transportation will case if the xylem portion is girdled.

Girdled bast
↓ stop
Solute translocation
↓ results
death of root
↓ hence
death of plant

175 (c) : Phenylketonuria is the inborn error in metabolism. This disease is associated with metabolic breakdown of phenylalanine. The disease occurs due to accumulation of phenylpyruvic acid and causes mental disorders.

176. (d) : Salamander is a semiterrestrial lizard like tailed carnivorous and nocturnal amphibian. Sphenodon is a burrowing, carnivorous and nocturnal reptile. It is regarded as a living fossil.

177. (d) : Watson and Crick suggested that replication of DNA is semiconservative. Semiconservative nature of DNA replication was proved by Messelson and Stahl by using heavy isotope of nitrogen (15N).

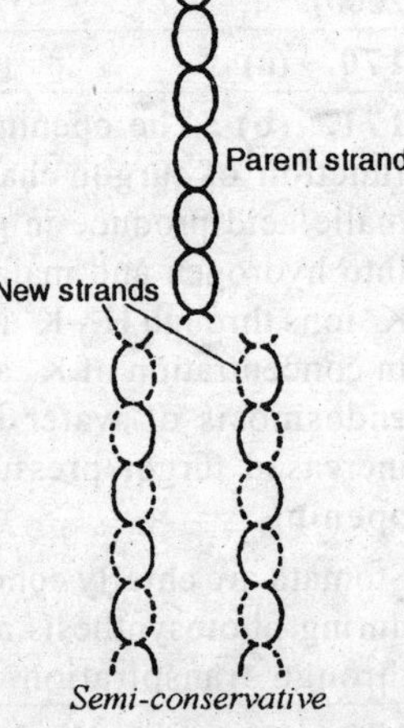

Semi-conservative

DNA polymerase III establishes phosphodiester linkages between the adjacent deoxyribonucleoside phosphate in presence of ATP/GTP, TPP and Mg^{2+}. It produces a new strand of DNA. DNA polymerase binds nucleotides in 5'–3' direction.

178. (c) : *t*RNA is synthesized in the nucleus as a DNA template. Only 0.025% of DNA codes for *t*RNA. *t*RNA is an exception to other cellular RNAs in that a part of its ribonucleotide sequence (–CCA) is added after it comes off the DNA template *t*RNA is formed from only a small part of DNA molecule. Therefore, it does not show any obvious base relationship to DNA.

179 (d) : Monocot stem bear collateral closed vascular bundle. In monocot stem cambium is absent and such vasular bundle is called closed type.

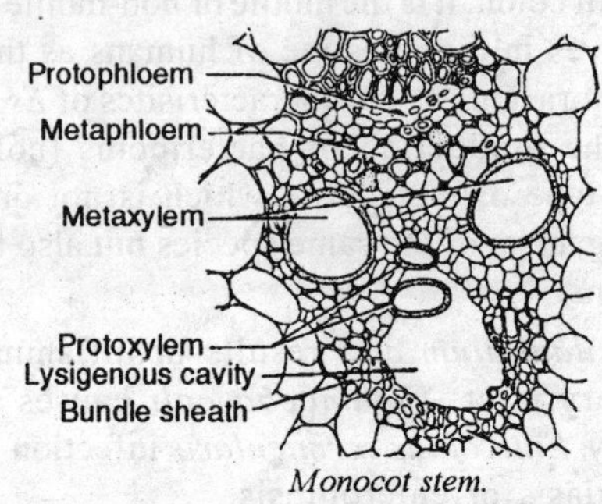

Monocot stem.

180. (a) : All cells are bounded by a thin membrane called the plasmalemma. This membrane is not seen under light microscope as separate layer. It has no cell cement and thus it is very thin. It has structural proteins, enzymes and carrier proteins.

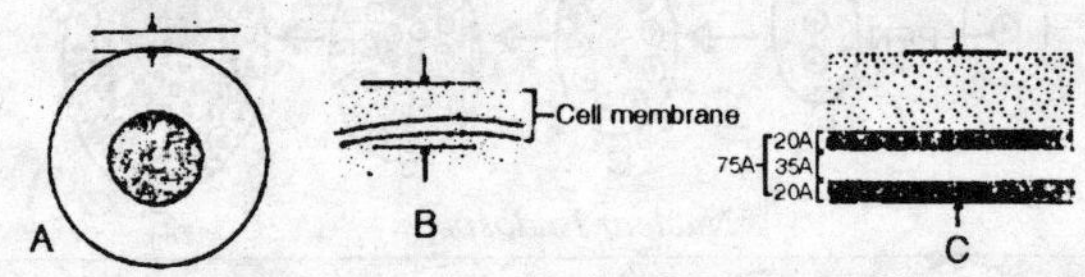

The cell membrane : (A) Light microscope view. (B) and (C) Electron microscope views.

GENERAL KNOWLEDGE

181.	(d)	**182.**	(b)
183.	(a)	**184.**	(c)
185.	(d)	**186.**	(d)
187.	(d)	**188.**	(b)
189.	(d)	**190.**	(a)
191.	(a)	**192.**	(d)
193.	(a)	**194.**	(b)
195.	(a)	**196.**	(b)
197.	(b)	**198.**	(b)
199.	(b)	**200.**	(a)

❖ ❖ ❖

SOLVED PAPER
AIIMS - 2002

Time : 3½ Hours Max. Marks : 200

PHYSICS

1. Length cannot be measure by
(a) fermi (b) micron
(c) debye (d) light year.

2. The dimension of torque is
(a) $[MT^{-2}]$ (b) $[ML^{-1}T^{-1}]$
(c) $[ML^2T^{-2}]$ (d) $[ML^3T^{-3}]$.

3. If vectors $\vec{P} = a\hat{i} + a\hat{j} + 3\hat{k}$ and $Q = a\hat{i} - 2\hat{j} - \hat{k}$ are perpendicular to each other, then the positive value of a is
(a) 3 (b) 1
(c) 2 (d) 0.

4. Three different objects m_1, m_2 and m_3 are allowed to fall from rest and from the same point O along three different frictionless paths. The speeds of the three objects, on reaching the ground, will be in the ratio of
(a) $m_1 : m_2 : m_3$ (b) 1 : 1 : 1
(c) $m_1 : 2m_2 : 3m_3$ (d) $\frac{1}{m_1} : \frac{1}{m_2} : \frac{1}{m_3}$.

5. A particle starts from rest and has an acceleration of 2 m/s² for 10 sec. After that, it travels for 30 sec with constant speed and then undergoes a retardation of 4 m/s² and comes back to rest. The total distance covered by the particle is
(a) 650 m (b) 750 m
(c) 700 m (d) 800 m.

6. Hubble's law is related with
(a) comet (b) speed of galaxy
(c) black hole (d) planetary motion.

7. At 0 K temperature, a p-type semiconductor
(a) does not have any charge carriers
(b) has few holes but no free electrons
(c) has few holes and few free electrons
(d) has equal number of holes and free electrons.

8. The potential barrier, in the depletion layer, is due to
(a) ions (b) electrons
(c) holes (d) forbidden band.

9. The speed of an electron having a wavelength of 10^{-10} m is
(a) 7.25×10^6 m/s (b) 5.25×10^6 m/s
(c) 6.26×10^6 m/s (d) 4.24×10^6 m/s.

10. An electron having charge e and mass m is moving in a uniform electric field E. Its acceleration will be
(a) $\frac{e^2}{m}$ (b) $\frac{eE}{m}$
(c) $\frac{eE^2}{m}$ (d) $\frac{mE}{e}$.

11. In the given figure, the capacitance C_1, C_3, C_4, C_5 have a capacitance 4 μF each. If the capacitor C_2 has a capacitance 10 μF, then effective capacitance between A and B will be

(a) 2 μF (b) 6 μF
(c) 4 μF (d) 8 μF.

12. An electric bulb marked 40 W and 200 V, is used in a circuit of supply voltage 100 V. Now its power is
(a) 100 W (b) 20 W
(c) 40 W (d) 10 W.

13. The magnetic needle of a tangent galvanometer is deflected at an angle 30° due to a magnet. The horizontal component of earth's magnetic field 0.34 × 10^{-4} T is along the plane of the coil. The magnetic intensity is
(a) 1.96×10^{-4} T (b) 1.96×10^4 T
(c) 1.96×10^{-5} T (d) 1.96×10^5 T.

14. The coefficient of mutual inductance, when magnetic flux changes by 2×10^{-2} Wb and current changes by 0.01 A is
(a) 2 H (b) 4 H
(c) 3 H (d) 8 H.

15. Light propagates rectilinearly because of its
(a) frequency (b) velocity
(c) wavelength (d) wave nature.

16. Brilliance of diamond is due to
(a) shape (b) reflection
(c) cutting
(d) total internal reflection.

17. Velocity of light is equal to
(a) $\sqrt{\varepsilon_0\mu_0}$ (b) $\sqrt{\varepsilon_0/\mu_0}$
(c) ε_0/μ_0 (d) $\sqrt{\frac{1}{\varepsilon_0\mu_0}}$.

18. The Cauchy's dispersion formula is
(a) $n = A + B\lambda^{-2} + C\lambda^{-4}$
(b) $n = A + B\lambda^{-2} + C\lambda^{4}$
(c) $n = A + B\lambda^{2} + C\lambda^{-4}$
(d) $n = A + B\lambda^{2} + C\lambda^{4}$.

19. Golden view of sea shell is due to
(a) diffraction (b) polarisation
(c) dispersion (d) reflection.

20. At the uppermost point of a projectile, its velocity and acceleration are at an angle of
(a) 0° (b) 90°
(c) 45° (d) 180°.

21. The kinetic energy of a body becomes four times its initial value. The new linear momentum will be
(a) same as the initial value
(b) four times of the initial value
(c) twice of the initial value
(d) eight times of the initial value.

22. The angular momentum of a moving body remains constant if
(a) net external force is applied
(b) net external torque is applied
(c) net pressure is applied
(d) net external torque is not applied.

23. The force of gravitation is
(a) repulsive
(b) conservative
(c) electrostatic
(d) non-conservative.

24. Kepler's second law is based on
(a) Newton's first law
(b) special theory of relativity
(c) Newton's second law
(d) conservation of angular momentum.

25. A conducting sphere of radius 10 cm is charged with 10 μC. Another uncharged sphere of radius 20 cm is allowed to touch it for some time. After that if the spheres are separated, then surface density of charges on the spheres will be in the ratio of
(a) 1 : 4 (b) 1 : 2
(c) 1 : 3 (d) 1 : 1.

26. What is the path difference for destructive interference?
(a) $n\lambda$ (b) $\frac{(n+1)\lambda}{2}$
(c) $n(\lambda + 1)$ (d) $\frac{(2n+1)\lambda}{2}$.

27. A siren emitting sound of frequency 800 Hz is going away from a static listener with a speed of 30 m/s. Frequency of the sound to be heard by the listener is (Take velocity of sound as 300 m/s)
(a) 733.3 Hz (b) 481.2 Hz
(c) 644.8 Hz (d) 286.5 Hz.

28. A string in a musical instrument is 50 cm long and its fundamental frequency is 800 Hz. If a frequency of 1000 Hz is to be produced, then required length of string is
(a) 62.5 cm (b) 40 cm
(c) 50 cm (d) 37.5 cm.

29. If equation of sound wave is
$y = 0.0015\sin(62.4x + 316t)$,
then its wavelength will be
(a) 0.2 unit (b) 0.3 unit
(c) 0.1 unit (d) 2 unit.

30. The graph between wave number ($\bar{\nu}$) and angular frequency (ω) is

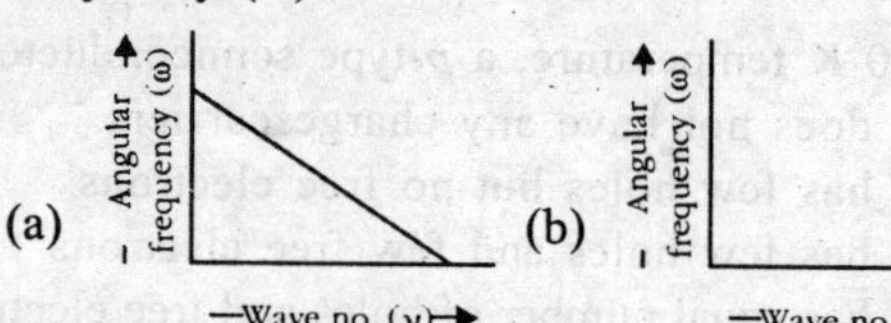

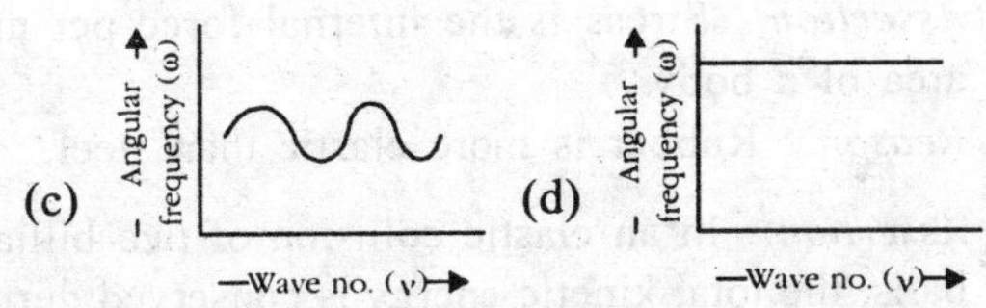

31. If v_0 be the orbital velocity of a satellite in a circular orbit close to the earth's surface and v_e is the escape velocity from the earth, then relation between the two is

(a) $v_o = v_e$ (b) $v_e = \sqrt{3}v_o$

(c) $v_e = \sqrt{2}v_o$ (d) $v_e = 2v_o$.

32. The breaking stress of a wire depends upon

(a) length of the wire

(b) material of the wire

(c) radius of the wire

(d) shape of the cross-section.

33. The density of a substance at 0°C is 10 g/cc and at 100°C, its density is 9.7 g/cc. The coefficient of linear expansion of the substance is

(a) 10^{-4} (b) 10^{-2}

(c) 10^{-3} (d) 10^{2}.

34. Scent sprayer is based on

(a) Charle's law (b) Archimedes principle

(c) Boyle's law (d) Bernoulli's theorem.

35. According to Wein's displacement law

(a) λT = constant (b) λ/T = constant

(c) $\lambda \propto (1/T)$ (d) both (b) and (c).

36. A black body is at a temperature 300 K. It emits energy at a rate, which is proportional to

(a) 300 (b) $(300)^3$

(c) $(300)^2$ (d) $(300)^4$.

37. The latent heat of vapourisation of water is 2240 J. If the work done in the process of vapourisation of 1 g is 168 J, then increase in internal energy is

(a) 2408 J (b) 2072 J

(c) 2240 J (d) 1904 J.

38. The velocities of sound at the same temperature in two monoatomic gases of densities ρ_1 and ρ_2 are v_1 and v_2 respectively. If $\rho_1/\rho_2 = 4$, then the value of v_1/v_2 is

(a) 1/4 (b) 2

(c) 1/2 (d) 4.

39. The property utilized in the manufacture of lead shots is

(a) specific weight of liquid lead

(b) compressibility of liquid lead

(c) specific gravity of liquid lead

(d) surface tension of liquid lead.

40. When a wire is stretched and its radius becomes $r/2$, then its resistance will be

(a) $16R$ (b) $2R$

(c) $4R$ (d) 0.

Directions for Q. 41 to 60 : *These questions consist of two statements each, printed as Assertion and Reason. While answering these questions you are required to choose any one of the following four responses.*

(a) *If both the assertion and reason are true and reason is a correct explanation of the assertion.*

(b) *If both assertion and reason are true but assertion is not a correct explanation of the assertion.*

(c) *If the assertion is true but the reason is false.*

(d) *If both assertion and reason are false.*

41. *Assertion :* Planet is a heavenly body revolving round the sun.

Reason : Star is luminous body made of gaseous material.

42. *Assertion :* Coloured spectrum is seen when we look through a muslin cloth.

Reason : It is due to the diffraction of white light on passing through fine slits.

43. *Assertion :* When tiny circular obstacle is placed in the path of light from some distance, a bright spot is seen at the centre of the shadow of the obstacle.

Reason : Destructive interference occurs at the centre of the shadow.

44. *Assertion :* The quantity L/R possesses dimension of time.

Reason : To reduce the rate of increase of current through a solenoid, we should increase the time constant (L/R).

45. *Assertion :* In a simple battery circuit, the point of the lowest potential is positive terminal of the battery.

Reason : The current flows towards the point of the higher potential, as it does in such a circuit from the negative to the positive terminal.

46. *Assertion :* We use a thick wire in the secondary of a step down transformer to reduce the production heat.
Reason : When the plane of the armature is parallel to the line of force of magnetic field, the magnitude of induced e.m.f. is maximum.

47. *Assertion :* We cannot think of a magnetic field configuration with three poles.
Reason : A bar magnet does exert a torque on itself due to its own field.

48. *Assertion :* Thin films such a soap bubble or a thin layer of oil on water show beautiful colours when illuminated by white light.
Reason : It happens due to the interference of light reflected from the upper surface of the thin film.

49. *Assertion :* Quasar emits radiowaves more than radio galaxy.
Reason : Quasar has very small size.

50. *Assertion :* S.I. units are logical and coherent.
Reason : S.I. system of units is a rationalised system.

51. *Assertion :* It is difficult to move a cycle along the road with its brakes on.
Reason : Sliding friction is greater than rolling friction.

52. *Assertion :* Faraday's laws are consequences of conservation of energy.
Reason : In a purely resistive A.C. circuit, the current lags behind the e.m.f. in phase.

53. *Assertion :* The flash of lightening is seen before the sound of thunder is heard.
Reason : Speed of sound is greater than speed of light.

54. *Assertion :* Blue star is at high temperature than red star.
Reason : Wein's displacement law states that $T \propto (1/\lambda_m)$.

55. *Assertion :* The time-period of pendulum, on a satellite orbiting the earth is infinity.
Reason : Time-period of a pendulum is inversely proportional to $\sqrt{g}$.

56. *Assertion :* Stress is the internal force per unit area of a body.
Reason : Rubber is more elastic than steel.

57. *Assertion :* In an elastic collision of two billiard balls, the total kinetic energy is conserved during the short time of oscillation of the balls (i.e. when they are in contact).
Reason : Energy spent against friction does not follow the law of conservation of energy.

58. *Assertion :* The earth without its atmosphere would be inhospitably cold.
Reason : All heat would escape in the absence of atmosphere.

59. *Assertion :* In simple harmonic motion, the motion is to and fro and periodic.
Reason : Velocity of the particle $(v) = \omega\sqrt{k^2 - x^2}$ (where x is the displacement).

60. *Assertion :* Woolen clothes keep the body warm in winter.
Reason : Air is a bad conductor of heat.

CHEMISTRY

61. Methyl orange is the example of which type of dye?
(a) acid dye (b) mordant dye
(c) azo dye (d) both (a) and (c).

62. Enzymes with two sites are called
(a) apoenzyme (b) allosteric enzyme
(c) holoenzyme (d) conjugate enzyme.

63. Teflon is a polymer of
(a) tetrafluoroethylene
(b) tetrabromoethylene
(c) tetraiodoethylene
(d) tetrachloroethylene.

64. Lucas test is used for the determination of
(a) alcohols (b) alkyl halides
(c) phenols (d) aldehydes.

65. Which of the following is involved in Sandmayer's reaction?
(a) ferrous salt (b) diazonium salt
(c) ammonium salt (d) cupromonium salt.

66. The weight of one molecule of a compound $C_{60}H_{122}$ is

(a) 1.2×10^{-20} g (b) 5.025×10^{23} g
(c) 1.4×10^{-21} g (d) 6.023×10^{23} g.

67. Which of the following is not an ore of iron?
(a) limonite (b) caniterite
(c) magnetite (d) none of these.

68. If P is pressure and ρ is density of a gas, then P and ρ are related as
(a) $P \propto \rho$ (b) $P \propto (1/\rho)$
(c) $P \propto \rho^2$ (d) $P \propto (1/\rho^2)$.

69. Quantum numbers of an atom can be defined on the basis of
(a) Hund's rule
(b) Pauli's exclusion principle
(c) Aufbau's principle
(d) Heisenberg's uncertainty principle.

70. Which of the following has maximum energy?

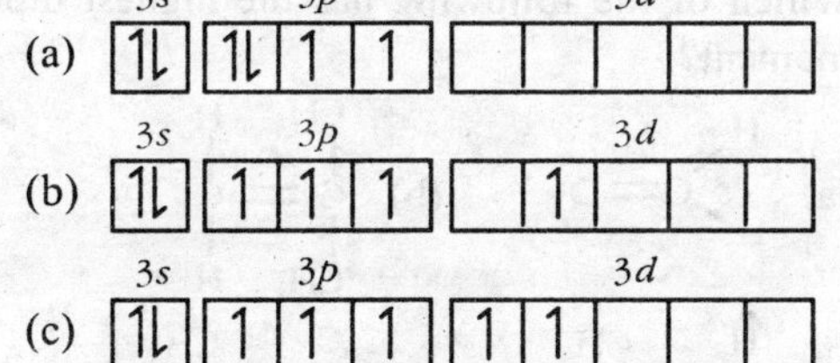

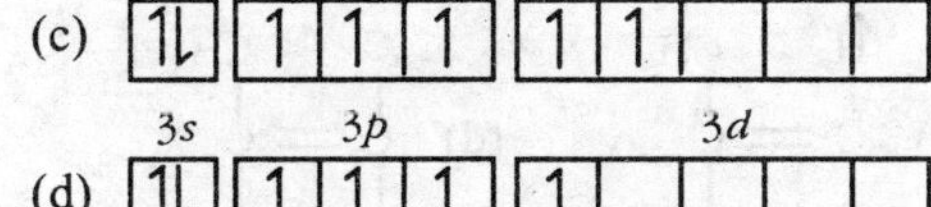

71. The intermediate formed in aldol condensation is
(a) aldol (b) carbanion
(c) alcohol (d) α-hydrogen ester.

72. The compound most suitable for the preparation of cyanohydrin is
(a) C_2H_5COOH (b) $C_6H_5NH_2$
(c) $C_2H_5COC_2H_5$ (d) $C_2H_5 - C_2H_5$.

73. In the reaction :
$C_6H_5CHO + C_6H_5NH_2 \rightarrow C_6H_5N = HCC_6H_5 + H_2O$,
the compound $C_6H_5N = HCC_6H_5$ is known as
(a) aldol (b) Schiff's base
(c) Schiff's reagent (d) Benedict's reagent.

74. Action of acetylene on dilute H_2SO_4 gives
(a) acetic acid
(b) acetaldehyde
(c) acetone
(d) acetoacetic ester.

75. CH_3COCH_3 can be converted to $CH_3CH_2CH_3$ by the action of
(a) HIO_3 (b) HNO_3
(c) HI (d) H_3PO_3.

76. At 80°C, distilled water has concentration equal to 1×10^{-6} mole/litre. The value of K_w at this temperature will be
(a) 1×10^{-6} (b) 1×10^{-12}
(c) 1×10^{-9} (d) 1×10^{-15}.

77. The pH of solution containing 0.10 M sodium acetate and 0.03 M acetic acid is
(pK_a for $CH_3COOH = 4.57$)
(a) 4.09 (b) 6.09
(c) 5.09 (d) 7.09.

78. Oxidation state of Fe in Fe_3O_4 is
(a) 3/2 (b) 5/4
(c) 4/5 (d) 8/3.

79. For the reaction :

$$H_2 + Cl_2 \xrightarrow{\text{sunlight}} 2HCl$$

the order of reaction is
(a) 0 (b) 2
(c) 1 (d) 3.

80. The correct order of solubility in water for He, Ne, Ar, Kr, Xe is
(a) He > Ne > Ar > Kr > Xe
(b) Xe > Kr > Ar > Ne > He
(c) Ne > Ar > Kr > He > Xe
(d) Ar > Ne > He > Kr > Xe.

81. Spectrum of Li^{2+} is similar to that of
(a) H (b) Be
(c) He (d) Ne.

82. IUPAC name of $CH_3 - \underset{(CH_2CH_3)}{\underset{|}{CH}} - CH_2 - \underset{CN}{\underset{|}{CH}} - CH_3$ is
(a) 2-cyano, 3-methylhexane
(b) 2-dimethyl, 4-cyanopentane
(c) 3-methyl, 5-cyanohexane
(d) 2-cyano, 3-methylhexane.

83. Which of the following molecule has highest bond energy?
(a) F – F (b) N – N
(c) C – C (d) O – O.

84. The heat of neutralization of a strong base and a strong acid is 57 kJ. The heat released when 0.5 mole of HNO_3 solution is added to 0.20 moles of NaOH solution, is
(a) 11.4 kJ (b) 34.7 kJ
(c) 23.5 kJ (d) 58.8 kJ.

85. The solubility of CuBr is 2×10^{-4} mol/L at 25°C. The K_{sp} value for CuBr is
(a) 4×10^{-8} mol^2 L^{-2} (b) 4×10^{-4} mol^2 L^{-2}
(c) 4×10^{-11} mol^2 L^{-2} (d) 4×10^{-15} mol^2 L^{-2}.

86. Schottky defect defines imperfection in the lattice structure of a
(a) solid (b) gas
(c) liquid (d) plasma.

87. An AB_2 type structure is found in
(a) NaCl (b) CaF_2
(C) Al_2O_3 (d) N_2O.

88. Azimuthal quantum number defines
(a) *e*/*m* ratio of electron
(b) angular momentum of electron
(c) spin of electron
(d) magnetic momentum of electron.

89. Which of the following does not have valence electron in 3d-subshell?
(a) Fe (III) (b) Cr (I)
(c) Mn (II) (d) P (0).

90. The reaction:

$$C_2H_5OH + SOCl_2 \xrightarrow{\text{Pyridine}} C_2H_5Cl + SO_2 + HCl$$

is known as
(a) Kharasch effect
(b) Williamson's synthesis
(c) Darzen's procedure
(d) Hunsdiecker reaction.

91. Which of the following compound is a tribasic acid?
(a) H_3PO_2 (b) H_3PO_4
(c) H_3PO_3 (d) $H_4P_2O_7$.

92. Thermite is a mixture of iron oxide and
(a) zinc powder
(b) potassium metal
(c) sodium shavings
(d) aluminium powder.

93. Which of the following reaction produces hydrogen?
(a) $Mg + H_2O$ (b) $H_2S_4O_8 + H_2O$
(c) $BaO_2 + HCl$ (d) $Na_2O_2 + 2HCl$.

94. An element (atomic mass 100 g/mol) having BCC structure has unit cell edge 400 pm. The density of element is (No. of atom in BCC (Z) = 2).
(a) 2.144 g/cm³ (b) 7.289 g/cm³
(c) 5.188 g/cm³ (d) 10.376 g/cm³.

95. The size of colloidal particle is
(a) 10^{-3} to 10^{-9} m (b) 10^{-9} to 10^{-12} m
(c) 10^{-6} to 10^{-9} m (d) 10^{-12} to 10^{-19} m.

96. Which of the following is a chiral compound?
(a) hexane (b) *n*-butane
(c) methane
(d) 2,3,4-trimethyl hexane.

97. Which of the following has the highest dipole moment?

(a) $H_2C=O$ (b) $(CH_3)_2C=CH_2$

(c) 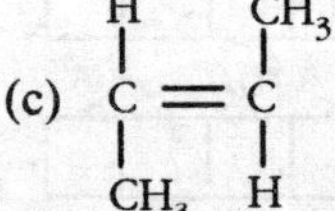 (d) 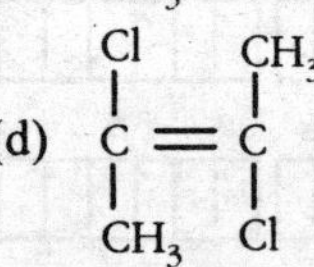

98. The length of C – C bond in benzene is
(a) 1.22 Å (b) 1.54 Å
(c) 1.39 Å (d) 1.56 Å.

99. The number of σ- and π-bonds present in pent-4-ene, 1-yne is
(a) 10, 3 (b) 4, 9
(c) 3, 10 (d) 9, 4.

100. Which of the following is most stable?
(a) 1-butene (b) 1-pentene
(c) 2-butene (d) 2-pentene.

Direction for Q. 101 to 120 : *These questions consist of two statements each, printed as Assertion and Reason. While answering these questions you are required to choose any one of the following four responses.*
(a) *If both assertion and reason are true and reason is a correct explanation of the assertion.*

(b) *If both the assertion and reason are true but the reason is not a correct explanation of the assertion.*
(c) *If the assertion is true but the reason is false.*
(d) *If both the assertion and reason are false.*

101. *Assertion* : During an adiabatic process, heat energy is not exchanged between system and its surroundings.
Reason : The temperature of a gas increases when it undergoes an adiabatic expansion.

102. *Assertion* : Potassium and caesium are used in photo-electric cells.
Reason : Potassium and caesium emit electrons on exposure to light.

103. *Assertion* : Physical absorption of molecules takes place on surface only.
Reason : In this process, the bonds of the absorbed molecules are broken.

104. *Assertion* : Boiling and melting points of amides are higher than corresponding acids.
Reason : It is due to strong intermolecular hydrogen bonding in their molecules.

105. *Assertion* : Stannous chloride gives grey precipitate with mercuric chloride, but stannic chloride does not do so.
Reason : Stannous chloride is a powerful oxidising agent which oxidises mercuric chloride to metallic mercury.

106. *Assertion* : DNA molecules and RNA molecules are found in the nucleus of a cell.
Reason : On heating, the enzymes do not lose their specific activity.

107. *Assertion* : All halogens are coloured.
Reason : The halogens absorb visible light.

108. *Assertion* : F – F bond has low bond dissociation energy.
Reason : The fluorine has lower reactivity.

109. *Assertion* : Phenol is a weak acid than ethanol.
Reason : Groups with +M effect and –I effect decrease acidity at *m*-position.

110. *Assertion* : Ethers behave as bases in the presence of mineral acids.
Reason : It is due to the presence of lone pair of electrons on the oxygen.

111. *Assertion* : For Balmer series of hydrogen spectrum, the value $n_1 = 2$ and $n_2 = 3, 4, 5$.
Reason : The value of *n* for a line in Balmer series of hydrogen spectrum having the highest wave length is 4 and 6.

112. *Assertion* : An increase in surface area increases the rate of evaporation.
Reason : Stronger the inter-molecular attractive forces, fast is the rate of evaporation at a given temperature.

113. *Assertion* : Diamond is a bad conductor.
Reason : Graphite is a good conductor.

114. *Assertion* : Atoms can neither be created nor destroyed.
Reason : Under similar condition of temperature and pressure, equal volume of gases does not contain equal number of atoms.

115. *Assertion* : Mass and volume are extensive properties.
Reason : Mass/volume is also an extensive parameter.

116. *Assertion* : Absolute values of internal energy of substances can not be determined.
Reason : It is impossible to determine exact values of constituent energies of the substances.

117. *Assertion* : Cuprous ion (Cu^+) is colourless whereas cupric ion (Cu^{++}) is blue in the aqueous solution.
Reason : Cuprous ion (Cu^+) has unpaired electrons while cupric ion (Cu^{++}) does not.

118. *Assertion* : Dinegative anion of oxygen (O^{2-}) is quite common but dinegative anion of sulphur (S^{2-}) is less common.
Reason : Covalency of oxygen is two.

119. *Assertion* : Sigma (σ) is a strong bond, while pi (π) is a weak bond.
Reason : Atoms rotate freely about pi (π) bond.

120. *Assertion* : Absorption spectrum consists of some bright lines separated by dark spaces.
Reason : Emission spectrum consists of dark lines.

BIOLOGY

121. Which of the following displays immune tolerance?
(a) B-cells (b) α-cells
(c) T-cells (d) both (a) and (c).

122. Cyclosporine is used as
(a) allergic eczema
(b) immunodepressant
(c) prophylactic for viruses
(d) prophyacetic for marasmus.

123. The cranial capacity was largest among the
(a) Peking man (b) Java ape man
(c) African man (d) Neanderthal man.

124. A point mutation comprising the substitution of a purine by pyrimidine is called
(a) transition (b) translocation
(c) deletion (d) transversion.

125. Which of the following teeth are lophodont?
(a) incisor and canine
(b) canine and premolar
(c) premolar and molar
(d) premolar and incisor.

126. The photorespiratory carbon-oxidation cycle involves the interaction of
(a) chloroplast (b) mitochondria
(c) peroxisomes (d) all of these.

127. Which of the following is related to glycosylation of protein?
(a) lysosome (b) mitochondria
(c) peroxisome
(d) rough endoplasmic reticulum.

128. Frameshift mutation occurs when
(a) base is deleted
(b) base is deleted or added
(c) base is added
(d) anticodons are not present.

129. A chromosome carrying the centromere at one of the ends is called
(a) acentric (b) apocentric
(c) telocentric (d) metacentric.

130. Glycolysis is found in cytoplasm of virtually all types of aerobic/anaerobic cells. In this process, glucose is converted into a compound which is
(a) PEP (b) acetyl CoA
(c) pyruvic acid (d) citric acid.

131. Excretion in cockroach takes place by
(a) nephridium (b) parotid gland
(c) coxal glands (d) malpighian tubules.

132. Ambulacral grooves are absent in the living forms of the class
(a) crinoidea (b) asteroidea
(c) ophiuroidea (d) echinodermata.

133. The ganglia of sympathetic and the central nervous system in frog develops from the
(a) neural cell
(b) neural plate cells
(c) notochordal cells
(d) neural crest cells.

134. Lysis of foreign cell is mediated through
(a) IgM only (b) IgM and IgG
(c) IgA only (d) IgD and IgE.

135. Which of the following digestive juices have the minimum pH?
(a) bile (b) gastric juice
(c) saliva (d) pancreatic juice.

136. Introduction of foreign genes for improving genotype is
(a) biotechnology (b) vernalization
(c) tissue culture
(d) genetic engineering.

137. Pure line breed refers to
(a) heterozygosity only
(b) heterozygosity and linkage
(c) homozygosity only
(d) homozygosity and self assortment.

138. If a homozygous red flowered plant is crossed with a homozygous white flowered plant, the off-spring would be
(a) half red-flowered
(b) all red flowered
(c) half white-flowered
(d) half pink-flowered.

139. Bud dormancy is induced by
(a) ABA (b) ethylene
(c) IAA (d) gibberellic acid.

140. Xenia and metaxenia terms are related with
(a) pollen culture (b) xylem and phloem
(c) only endosperm
(d) pollen and endosperm.

141. Algae are useful because they
(a) are large in number
(b) are used in alcoholic fermentation
(c) purify the atmosphere
(d) are used in study of photosynthesis.

142. The plant body of moss (*Funaria*) is
(a) completely sporophyte
(b) predominantly sporophyte with gametophyte
(c) completely gametophyte
(d) predominantly gametophyte with sporophyte.

143. Elater mechanism for seed dispersal is exhibited by
(a) *Riccia* (b) *Dryopteris*
(c) *Funaria* (d) *Marchantia*.

144. Megasporophyll of *Cycas* has the same nature as
(a) stamen (b) petal
(c) sepal (d) carpel.

145. When the filament runs along the back of anther, it is called
(a) adnate (b) longitudinal
(c) versatile (d) syngenecious.

146. If turgor pressure becomes equal to the wall pressure, then
(a) water leaves the cell
(b) water enters the cell
(c) no exchange of water takes place
(d) solute goes from the cell into water.

147. Passage cells are found in
(a) dicot stem (b) monocot root
(c) ariel root (d) monocot stem.

148. Green mufler is used against which type of pollution ?
(a) air (b) soil
(c) water (d) noise.

149. The abundance of a species population within its habitat is called
(a) niche density (b) relative density
(c) regional density (d) absolute density.

150. Which of the following structure helps in the respiration of lichens?
(a) soredia (b) isidia
(c) cyphella (d) cephalodia.

151. In *Entamoeba histolytica*, the presence of chromatid bodies is characteristic of
(a) precystic stage
(b) mature quadrinucleate stage
(c) trophozoite stages
(d) mature binucleate stage.

152. What is left, when bath-sponges dries up?
(a) spicules (b) tentacles
(c) holdfast (d) spongin fibres.

153. *Hydra* receives impulses and stimuli through
(a) nerve net (b) nematocytes
(c) sensory cells (d) neuron cells.

154. Adults of *Wuchereria bancrofti* attacks
(a) excretory system
(b) nervous system
(c) blood circulation
(d) lymph vessels.

155. The sites of the first, second and third moulting of the *Ascaris* larva are
(a) soil, lung and intestine
(b) liver, stomach and intestine
(c) soil, alveoli and lung
(d) soil, intestine and lungs.

156. Wobble hypothesis was given by
(a) R.W. Holley (b) M. Nirenberg
(c) H.G. Khorana (d) F.H.C. Crick.

157. Which of the following are uricotelic animals?
(a) rohu and frog (b) camel and frog
(c) lizard and crow
(d) earthworm and eagle.

158. Curdling of milk in small intestine occurs due to the action of
(a) rennin (b) erypsine
(c) trypsin (d) chymotrypsin.

159. The vitamin nicotinamide can be synthesized in our body from
(a) tyrosine (b) tryptophan
(c) valine (d) phenyl alanine.

160. Which of the following would not give Fehling's test ?

(a) glucose (b) sucrose
(c) fructose (d) lactose.

Directions for Q. 161 to 180 : *These questions consists of two statements each, printed as assertion and reason. While answering these questions you are required to choose any one of the following four responses.*

(a) *If both the assertion and reason are true and reason is a correct explanation of the assertion.*
(b) *If both the assertion and reason are true but reason is not a correct explanation of the assertion.*
(c) *If the assertion is true but reason is false.*
(d) *If both the assertion and reason are false.*

161. *Assertion :* Study of biology requires basic knowledge of chemistry and physics.
Reason : Living organisms are made up of atoms and molecules which follow chemical and physical laws.

162. *Assertion :* Living organisms are regarded as closed systems.
Reason : Energy of living organisms cannot be lost or gained from the environment.

163. *Assertion :* Death is regarded as the most important regulatory process on earth.
Reason : It avoids over-crowding, caused by continuous reproduction.

164. *Assertion :* WBCs accumulate at the site of wounds by diapedesis.
Reason : It is the squeezing of leucocytes from the endothelium.

165. *Assertion :* Specilization of cells is advantageous for the organism.
Reason : It increases the operational efficiency of an organism.

166. *Assertion :* The imbalance in the concentration of Na^+, K^+ and proteins generates the resting potential.
Reason : To maintain the unequal distribution of Na^+ and K^+, the neurons use electrical energy.

167. *Assertion :* The regulation of RBC production is accompanied by the kidneys.
Reason : Erythropoietin hormone circulates to the red bone marrow, where it increases stem cell mitosis and speeds up the development of RBCs.

168. *Assertion :* Lateral line system is found in fishes and aquatic larval amphibians.
Reason : Lateral line system has receptors which are the clusters of sensory cells derived from ectoderm.

169. *Assertion :* Histamine is involved in allergic and inflammatory reactions.
Reason : Histamine is a vasodilator.

170. *Assertion :* The number of cells in a multicellular organism is inversely proportional to the size of body.
Reason : All the cells in the biological world are of same size.

171. *Assertion :* Systematics is the branch of biology that deals with classification of living organism.
Reason : The aim of classification is to group the organisms in an orderly manner.

172. *Assertion :* The megaspore mother cell undergoes mitosis to produce four megaspores.
Reason : Megaspore mother cells and the megaspores are both haploid.

173. *Assertion :* In bacteria, photosynthesis occurs by utilizing wavelengths longer than 700 nm.
Reason : Here the reaction centre is B-890.

174. *Assertion :* The two cotyledons in the seed are the embryonic leaves.
Reason : The embryo contains radicle and plumule.

175. *Assertion :* The collenchyma is thick walled living tissue.
Reason : The collenchyma is thickened due to the deposition of pectin.

176. *Assertion :* Clones are a group of organism of identical genotype, produced by same kind of sexual reproduction and same sexual processes.
Reason : These are prepared by a group of cells descended from many cells or by inbreeding of a completely heterozygous line.

177. *Assertion :* It is important that the organisms should have cell.
Reason : A cell keeps its chemical composition steady within its boundary.

178. *Assertion :* Plasmids are single stranded extra-chromosomal DNA.

Reason : Plasmids are possessed by eukaryotic cells.

179. *Assertion :* The *m*RNA attaches itself to the ribosome via its 3′ end.

Reason : The *m*RNA has F-capsular nucleotide and bases of lagging sequence.

180. *Assertion :* When six molecules of carbon dioxide participate in photosynthesis, 12 molecules of NADPH + H^+ and 18 ATP are used up, forming one hexose molecule.

Reason : The photosynthetic light reaction results in the formation of ATP and $NADPH_2$.

GENERAL KNOWLEDGE

181. Highest city of the world is in
(a) Tibet (b) China
(c) Japan (d) Mexico

182. Which of the following mountain is found in Tibet ?
(a) Mt. Kailas (b) Mt. Everest
(c) Dholagiri (d) Mt. Abu

183. 1st successful Indian expedition to Annapurna-I was undertaken in which year ?
(a) 1998 (b) 2001
(c) 1999 (d) 2002

184. Copper T is an IUCD used in
(a) preventing fertilization by blocking the sperms from getting to the fallopian tube
(b) prevents ovulation
(c) preventing fertilized eggs from implanting in the endometrium lining
(d) none of the above

185. Who was first to take 350 wickets in test matches ?
(a) Dennis Lillee (b) Courtney Walsh
(c) Kapil Dev (d) Richard Hadley

186. Which of these lines is the closest border lines ?
(a) Durand line & Mc Mohan line
(b) Radcliff line & Mc Mohan line
(c) Durand line & Radcliff line
(d) none of the above

187. M.M.Joshi is .... speaker of Loksabha
(a) 9th (b) 10th
(c) 11th (d) 12th

188. 1st artificial satellite to go round the earth ?
(a) Sputnik – I (b) Apollo – II
(c) Aryabhatta (d) Rohini

189. "Shades of sword" is written by
(a) M.J.Akbar (b) Sanjay Khan
(c) Khushwant Singh (d) Tariq

190. Only bengali film to be produced by Raj Kapoor
(a) Nala Damayanti (b) Jamai Sasthi
(c) Ramrajya (d) Indrasabha

191. ISO mark related to health services
(a) 9001 (b) 9003
(c) 9002 (d) 9004

192. 'Day for the care of aged'
(a) 1st October (b) 5th October
(c) 16th October (d) 24th October

193. 'Dirty snowballs" refers to
(a) meteorites (b) asteroid
(c) comets (d) old space craft

194. Surrogate motherhood refers to
(a) one who donates ovum
(b) bearing child of some one else after the ovum is fertilized by artificial insemination
(c) step mother (d) none of these

195. "Ad hoc" means
(a) for the time being
(b) for a fixed period of time
(c) for specific purpose
(d) none of these

196. Shakespeare's sonnet has .... lines
(a) 9 (b) 14
(c) 24 (d) 12

197. Bill for right to pets to be introduced first in
(a) Britain (b) US
(c) Canada (d) India

198. Mount Kamet found in which country
(a) Tibet (b) India
(c) China (d) Mexico

199. Number of females/males in India
(a) 933 (b) 930
(c) 927 (d) 940

200. When was the golden jubilee of Indian Parliament celebrated?
(a) 1st Jan. 1997 (b) 15th Aug. 1997
(c) 26th Jan. 2002 (d) 13th May 2002.

❖❖❖

SOLUTIONS

PHYSICS

1. **(c) :** Debye is the unit of electric dipole moment. Therefore length cannot be measured by debye.

2. **(c) :** Torque, τ = force × distance.
Therefore dimension of torque = dimensions of force × dimensions of distance = $[MLT^{-2}]$ $[L]$ = $[ML^2T^{-2}]$.

3. **(a) :** Vector $\vec{P} = a\hat{i} + a\hat{j} + 3k$
and vector $\vec{Q} = a\hat{i} - 2\hat{j} - \hat{k}$.
If two vectors are perpendicular to each other, then

$$\vec{P} \cdot \vec{Q} = 0 \text{ or } (a\hat{i} + a\hat{j} + 3\hat{k}) \cdot (a\hat{i} - 2\hat{j} - \hat{k}) = 0$$

or $a^2 - 2a - 3 = 0$.
Solving this quadratic equation, we get a = 3 or −1. Therefore positive value of a is 3.

4. **(b) :** As the speed of an object, falling freely under gravity, depends only upon its height from which it is allowed to fall and not upon its mass. Since the paths are frictionless and all the objects are falling through the same vertical height, therefore their speeds on reaching the ground must be same. Or ratio of their speeds = 1 : 1 : 1.

5. **(b) :** Initial velocity (u) = 0,
Acceleration (a_1) = 2 m/s² and time during acceleration (t_1) = 10 sec.
Time during constant velocity (t_2) = 30 sec and retardation (a_2) = −4 m/s² (−ve sign due to retardation).
Distance covered by the particle during acceleration,

$$s_1 = ut_1 + \frac{1}{2}a_1t_1^2 = (0 \times 10) + \frac{1}{2} \times 2 \times (10)^2$$
$$= 100 \text{ m} \quad \text{... (i)}$$

And velocity of the particle at the end of acceleration,

$$v = u + a_1t_1 = 0 + (2 \times 10) = 20 \text{ m/s.}$$

Therefore distance covered by the particle during constant velocity (s_2) = $v \times t_2$

$$= 20 \times 30 = 600 \text{ m} \quad \text{... (ii)}$$

Relation for the distance covered by the particle during retardation (s_3) is $v^2 = u^2 + 2a_2s_3$
or, $(0)^2 = (20)^2 + 2 \times (-4) \times s_3 = 400 - 8s_3$
or, $s_3 = 400/8 = 50$ m ... (iii)
Therefore total distance covered by the particle

$$s = s_1 + s_2 + s_3 = 100 + 600 + 50 = 750 \text{ m.}$$

6. **(b) :** From Hubble law, speed of a galaxy (v) = Hr (where H = Hubble constant and r is its distance from earth). Thus Hubble's law is related with the speed of the galaxy.

7. **(b) :** At 0 K temperature, a pure semiconductor behaves as an insulator, because it has a few holes in its valence band. But there is no free electron in this state.

8. **(a) :** The depletion layer is the region at the junction of a diode which is devoid of ions. Therefore the potential barrier in the depletion layer is due to ions.

9. **(a) :** Wavelength (λ) = 10^{-10} m.
Velocity of the electron, $v = h/m\lambda$

$$= \frac{6.6 \times 10^{-34}}{(9.1 \times 10^{-31})(10^{-10})} = 7.25 \times 10^6 \text{ m/s.}$$

where m = mass of electron equal to 9.1×10^{-31} kg and h is Planck constant equal to 6.6×10^{-34} J-s.

10. **(b) :** Charge on electron = e
Mass of electron = m and intensity of uniform electric field = E.
Acceleration of the electron,

$$a = \frac{\text{Force on the electron}}{\text{Mass of electron}}$$
$$= \frac{\text{Electric charge} \times \text{electric field}}{\text{Mass of electron}} = \frac{eE}{m}.$$

11. **(c) :** Capacitance of capacitors C_1, C_3, C_4, C_5 = 4 μF each and capacitance of capacitor C_2 = 10 μF. If a battery is applied across A and B, the points b and c will be at the same potential (since $C_1 = C_4 = C_3 = C_5$ = 4 μF). Therefore no charge flows through C_2. We have the capacitors C_1 and C_5 in series. Therefore their equivalent capacitance,

$$C' = \frac{C_1 \times C_5}{C_1 + C_5} = \frac{4 \times 4}{4 + 4} = 2\,\mu\text{F}.$$

Similarly, C_4 and C_3 are in series. Therefore their equivalent capacitance,

$$C'' = \frac{C_3 \times C_4}{C_3 + C_4} = \frac{4 \times 4}{4 + 4} = 2\,\mu\text{F}.$$

Now C' and C'' are in parallel. Therefore effective capacitance between A and B

$= C' + C'' = 2 + 2 = 4$ μF.

12. (d) : Actual power of bulb (P_1) = 40 W
Actual voltage of bulb (V_1) = 200 V and supply voltage (V_2) = 100 V.

Power (P) = $\frac{V^2}{R} \propto V^2$. Therefore $\frac{P_1}{P_2} = \frac{V_1^2}{V_2^2}$

or, $\frac{40}{P_2} = \frac{(200)^2}{(100)^2} = 4$ or $P_2 = \frac{40}{4} = 10$ W

(where P_2 = power when voltage is 100 V).

13. (c) : Angle through which magnet is deflected (θ) = 30° and horizontal magnetic field (B_H)=0.34×10^{-4} T.
Magnetic intensity = $B_H \tan\theta = 0.34 \times 10^{-4} \times \tan 30°$
$= (0.34 \times 10^{-4}) \times 0.577 = 1.96 \times 10^{-5}$ T.

14. (a) : Change in magnetic flux (ϕ) = 2×10^{-2} Wb and change in current (I) = 0.01 A.
Change in magnetic flux, $\phi = 2 \times 10^{-2} = MI$

$= M \times 0.01$ or $M = \frac{2\times10^{-2}}{0.01} = 2$ H

(where M = coefficient of mutual inductance).

15. (d) : Light propagates rectilinearly. But it can take a slight turn at obstacles. This property of light is due to its wave nature.

16. (d) : Total internal reflection can occur only when a ray is incident on the surface of a medium whose refractive index is smaller than that of the medium in which the ray is travelling. Since the refractive index of air is 1.00029 and that of diamond is 2.42, therefore brilliance of diamond is due to total internal reflection.

17. (d) : Relation for velocity of light (c) = $\sqrt{\frac{1}{\varepsilon_0\mu_0}}$
(where ε_0 = permittivity constant equal to 8.85×10^{-12} F/m and μ_0 = permeability constant equal to 1.26×10^{-6} H/m.

Numerically velocity of light (c) = $\sqrt{\frac{1}{\varepsilon_0\mu_0}}$

$= \sqrt{\frac{1}{(8.85\times10^{-12})\times(1.26\times10^{-6})}} \approx 3\times10^8$ m/s.

18. (a) : The Cauchy's dispersion formula represents the dispersion of most of the substances with considerable accuracy. Also from the Cauchy's dispersion formula if n is refractive index and A, B and C are constants, then $n = A + B\lambda^{-2} + C\lambda^{-4}$.

19. (b) : When a ray of light falls on sea shell, then its small amount first gets refracted (slightly polarised) and then almost gets reflected back (fully polarised). That is why, view of sea shell is golden due to polarisation.

20. (b) : At the uppermost point of a projectile, the vertical component of the velocity of projection becomes zero, while the horizontal component remains constant. And the acceleration (due to gravity) is always vertically downwards. Therefore at the uppermost point of a projectile, its velocity and acceleration are at an angle of 90°.

21. (c) : Initial kinetic energy (E_1) = E and final kinetic energy (E_2) = $4E$.

Kinetic energy of a body is $\frac{1}{2}mv^2$

Since the value of m remains constant, therefore for the kinetic energy to be 4 times, the new value of velocity (v) should be 2 times the initial value.
Initial linear momentum (p_1) = mv.
Therefore new linear momentum (p_2) = $m \times 2v$
$= 2\,mv = 2p_1$.

22. (d) : When the net external torque acting on a system is zero, the total angular momentum of the system remains constant. Therefore the angular momentum of a moving body remains constant if net external torque is not applied.

23. (b) : Earth behaves as a huge magnet and has a tendency to attract all the objects due to gravitational force. Therefore gravitational force is a conservative force.

24. (d) : Kepler's second law states that the line between a planet and the sun sweeps out equal areas in equal times. Kepler's second law is based on law of conservation of angular momentum.

25. (b) : Radius of conducting sphere (R_1) = 10 cm charge on the conducting sphere = 10 μC and radius of uncharged sphere (R_2) = 20 cm
For a spherical conductor, the density of charge is proportional to its radius. Therefore ratio of density of charges of the spheres will be 1 : 2.

26. (d) : If the waves interfere destructively, then path difference is given by $\frac{\lambda}{2}, \frac{3\lambda}{2}, \frac{5\lambda}{2}$ etc.
Therefore path difference of a destructive interference

is $\frac{(2n+1)\lambda}{2}$ (where n = 1, 2, 3, ...) etc.

27. (a) : Frequency of siren (υ) = 800 Hz
Speed of siren (v_s) = $v - v_o$ = 30 m/s
Velocity of listener (v_o) = 0 and velocity of sound (v) = 330 m/s.
From the Doppler's law, frequency heard from siren when it is going away from a listener is

$$= \left(\frac{v - v_0}{v + v_s}\right) \times \upsilon = \left(\frac{330 - 0}{330 + 30}\right) \times 800 = 733.3 \text{ Hz}.$$

28. (b) : Initial length of string (l_1) = 50 cm = 0.5 m
Initial fundamental frequency (n_1) = 800 Hz and final frequency (n_2) = 1000 Hz.

Frequency of vibration of the string, $n = \frac{1}{2l}\sqrt{\frac{T}{m}} \propto \frac{1}{l}$

$$\therefore \frac{n_1}{n_2} = \frac{l_2}{l_1} \text{ or } l_2 = \frac{n_1 \times l_1}{n_2} = \frac{800 \times 50}{1000} = 40 \text{ cm}.$$

(where l_2 = final length of the string).

29. (c) : Equation of sound wave is

$$y = 0.0015 \sin(62.4x + 316t).$$

Standard equation of a sound wave is

$$y = A \sin 2\pi\left[\frac{x}{\lambda} + \frac{t}{T}\right].$$

Comparing the given equation with the standard equation, we get

$$2\pi/\lambda = 62.4 \text{ or, } \lambda = \frac{2\pi}{62.4} = 0.1 \text{ unit.}$$

(where λ = wavelength of the wave)

30. (a) : Wave number, $\bar{v} = \frac{1}{\text{Angular frequency } (\omega)}$
The graph between wave number ($\bar{v}$) and angular frequency (ω) is a straight line which always satisfies the equation $y = mx + c$, where m is slope of the line but not equal to zero. Therefore graph is a straight line as shown in option (a).

31. (c) : Orbital velocity of satellite = v_o and escape velocity from the earth = v_e.
We have orbital velocity (v_o) = $\sqrt{gR}$
and escape velocity (v_e) = $\sqrt{2gR}$
Therefore ratio of orbital velocity to escape velocity

$$\frac{v_o}{v_e} = \sqrt{\frac{gR}{2gR}} = \frac{1}{\sqrt{2}} \text{ or } v_e = \sqrt{2}v_o.$$

32. (b) : The stress at which rupture occurs in a material is called its breaking stress. It depends on the material of the wire.

33. (a) : Initial temperature (T_1) = 0°C
Initial density (ρ_1) = 10 g/cc
Final temperature (T_2) = 100°C and
Final density (ρ_2) = 9.7 g/cc.

Coefficient of volumetric expansion (α_v) = $\frac{\Delta\rho}{\rho_1 \times \Delta T}$

$$= \frac{\rho_1 - \rho_2}{\rho_1(T_2 - T_1)} = \frac{10 - 9.7}{10(100 - 0)} = \frac{0.3}{1000} = 3 \times 10^{-4}.$$

Therefore coefficient of linear expansion,

$$\alpha_1 = \frac{\alpha_v}{3} = \frac{3 \times 10^{-4}}{3} = 10^{-4}.$$

34. (d) : A scent sprayer is an example of fall in pressure due to increase in velocity. Also as per Bernoulli's theorem that datum head, pressure head and velocity head of a flowing liquid is constant. Therefore scent sprayer is based on Bernoulli's theorem.

35. (a, c) : Wien's displacement law states that the absolute temperature of a black body and the peak wavelength of its radiations are inversely proportional. *i.e.* $\lambda \propto 1/T$ or λT = constant.

36. (d) : Temperature of a black body (T) = 300 K. Stefan's law of radiation states that energy emitted by the black body (E) $\propto T^4 \propto (300)^4$.

37. (b) : Latent heat of vapourisation of water (L) = 2240 J, mass of the water (m) = 1 g and work done (dW) = 168 J.
From first law of thermodynamics, heat supplied in vapourisation (dQ) = $mL = dU + dW$
or $1 \times 2240 = dU + 168$
or $dU = 2240 - 168 = 2072$ J
(where dU = increase in internal energy).

38. (c) : Velocity of sound in the gas of density ρ_1 is v_1 and velocity of sound in the gas of density ρ_2 is v_2.
Velocity of sound in gas, $v = \sqrt{\frac{\gamma P}{\rho}} \propto \sqrt{\frac{1}{\rho}}$.

Therefore $\frac{v_1}{v_2} = \sqrt{\frac{\rho_2}{\rho_1}} = \sqrt{\frac{1}{4}} = \frac{1}{2}$.

39. (d) : The property utilized in the manufacture of lead shots is surface tension of liquid lead. In this process, molten lead is made to pass through a sieve from a high tower and allowed to fall in water. The molten lead particles, while descending, assume a spherical shape and solidify in this form, before falling into water.

40. (a) : Initial radius of wire, $r_1 = r$ and final radius of wire, $r_2 = r/2 = 0.5r$.

Since volume of the wire after stretch remains constant, therefore $l_1A_1 = l_2A_2$

or $\frac{l_1}{l_2} = \frac{A_2}{A_1} = \frac{r_2^2}{r_1^2} = \left(\frac{0.5r}{r}\right)^2 = \frac{1}{4}$.

The resistance $(R) = \rho\frac{l}{A} \propto \frac{l}{A}$.

Therefore $\frac{R_1}{R_2} = \frac{l_1}{l_2} \times \frac{A_2}{A_1} = \frac{1}{4} \times \frac{1}{4} = \frac{1}{16}$

or $R_2 = 16R_1 = 16R$.

41. (b) : A heavenly body revolving round the sun is called a planet and there are nine planets in our solar system. A heavenly body, made of gaseous material and luminous due to its own energy, is called a star. The sun is also a star and is nearest to earth.

42. (a) : The coloured spectrum is due to diffraction of white light on passing through fine slits made by fine threads in the muslin cloth.

43. (c) : The waves diffracted from the edges of circular obstacle, placed in the path of light, interfere constructively at the centre of the shadow resulting in the formation of a bright spot.

44. (c) : Induced e.m.f. $(\varepsilon) = \frac{Ldi}{dt}$

and current $(i) = \frac{\varepsilon}{R} = \frac{1}{R} \times \frac{Ldi}{dt}$

or, $\frac{L}{R} = \frac{idt}{di} = \frac{\text{current} \times \text{time}}{\text{current}} = \text{time}$.

In order to increase the rate of increase of current through a solenoid, we increase the time constant (L/R). Since L of the given solenoid is constant, therefore we use a high resistance in series with it.

45. (d) : In a battery circuit, the point of lowest potential is the negative terminal of the battery. And the current flows from higher potential to lower potential.

46. (b) : A step-down transformer converts electrical energy from a high voltage to one at a low voltage. Accordingly the current in the secondary will be larger than that in the primary. In order to produce less heat in the secondary, we use a wire of lesser resistance i.e. thick wire. We also know that when the plane of the armature is parallel to the lines of force of magnetic field, the rate of change of magnetic flux linked with it is maximum. Therefore the e.m.f. induced in the armature in this orientation is maximum.

47. (d) : Magnetic poles always exist in pairs. However, one can imagine magnetic field configuration with three poles. When north poles of two magnets or south poles of two magnets are glued together, they provide a three pole field configuration. Also a bar magnet does not exert a torque on itself due to its own field.

48. (c) : The beautiful colours are seen on account of interference of light reflected from the upper and the lower surfaces of the thin film. As conditions for constructive and destructive interference depend upon the wavelength of light, therefore coloured interference fringes are observed.

49. (b) : A quasar is a very big source of radio waves and its size is very small as compared to the size of a galaxy. A radio galaxy emits radio waves which lie in the range 10^{30} to 10^{38} watt. A quasar emits radio waves which lie in the range of 10^{37} to 10^{38} watt.

50. (b) : A coherent system means a system based on a certain set of basic units from which all derived units are obtained by multiplication or division without introducing numerical factors. In S.I. system of units, heat energy, electric energy and mechanical energy are measured in joule (J). But in C.G.S. system, they have different units.

51. (a) : When brakes are on, there is no rolling of the wheels and the wheels slide. The sliding friction is greater than the rolling friction. Thus it is difficult to move a cycle along the road with its breaks on.

52. (c) : Faraday's laws involve conservation of mechanical energy into electrical energy. This is in accordance with the law of conservation of energy. We also know that in pure resistance, the e.m.f. is in phase with the current.

53. (c) : The speed of sound is 340 m/s and speed of light is 3×10^8 m/s in air. Thus flash of lightening is seen before the sound of thunder is heard.

54. (a) : From Wien's displacement law, temperature $(T) \propto 1/\lambda_m$ (where λ_m is the maximum wavelength). Thus temperature of a body is inversely proportional to the wavelength. Since blue star has smaller wavelength and red star has maximum wavelength, therefore blue star is at higher temperature then red star.

55. (a) : Time-period of simple pendulum, $T = 2\pi\sqrt{\frac{l}{g}}$

Thus time-period is inversely proportional to $\sqrt{g}$ (where g is acceleration due to gravity). And as the value of g on a satellite is zero, therefore time-period of pendulum is infinity.

56. (b) : Stress is the internal force per unit area of a body. If the same force is applied to the rubber and steel, then strain in rubber is more. It means the rubber is more elastic than steel.

57. (d) : The billiard balls in an elastic collision are in a deformed state. And their total energy is in the form of P.E. and K.E. Thus K.E. is less than the total energy. The energy spent against friction is dissipated in the form of heat which is not available for doing work.

58. (a) : Heat radiated out by earth is reflected back by the atmosphere. In the absence of atmosphere, all the heat will escape from earth's surface which will make the earth inhospitably cold. The atmosphere helps in maintaining the temperature through convection of heat.

59. (b) : A particle is said to execute simple harmonic motion, if it moves to and fro about a fixed point under the action of a restoring force which is directly proportional to its displacement from the fixed point and is always directed towards the fixed point. Also the velocity of the particle when its displacement is x, $v = \omega\sqrt{k^2 - x^2}$.

60. (a) : Woolen fibres enclose a large amount of air in them. Both wool and air are the bad conductors of heat and their coefficient of thermal conductivity is small. Thus they prevent any loss of heat from our body.

CHEMISTRY

61. (d) : Methyl orange belongs to the group of azo dyes. It is also acidic in nature due to presence of sulphonic group.

$$HO_3S-C_6H_4-N{=}N-C_6H_4-N(CH_3)_2$$

Methyl orange

62. (b) : Enzymes with two active sites are called allosteric enzymes. One of these sites is the catalytic site for the concerned reaction. Other site may be the site for inhibition of catalysis by enzyme or to activate the enzyme further.

63. (a) : Teflon is polytetrafluoro ethylene and it is prepared from tatrafluoro ethylene by heating under pressure in the presence of ammonium peroxydisulphate.

$$nCF_2 = CF_2 \xrightarrow[\text{high pressure}]{(NH_4)_2S_2O_8} (CF_2 - CF_2)_n$$

It is chemically inert and heat resistant polymer.

64. (a) : Lucas test – Alcohol reacts with concentrated hydrochloric acid in presence of anhydrous $ZnCl_2$ to form alkyl halides. The three type of alcohols undergo this reaction at different rates. Order of rate of reaction is : tertiary > secondary > primary.

$$R-OH + HCl \xrightarrow{ZnCl_2} \underset{\text{Alkyl chloride}}{R-Cl} + H_2O$$

65. (b) : Aryl halides can be prepared by the decomposition of aryl diazonium salts in presence of copper halides solution dissolved in the corresponding halogen acid, the diazo group is replaced by a halogen atom. This reaction is known as Sandmeyer reaction.

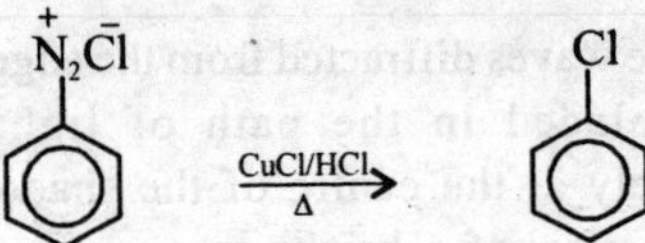

Diazonium salts Chloro benzene

66. (c) : Molecular weight of $C_{60}H_{122} = 60\times12+1\times122 = 842$

$\therefore$ Weight of 1 mole of $C_{60}H_{122}$ molecules = 842 g

$\Rightarrow$ Weight of 6.023×10^{23} molecules = 842 g

$\Rightarrow$ Weight of 1 molecule $= \dfrac{842}{6.023\times10^{23}} = 1.4 \times 10^{-21}$ g

67. (b) : Magnetite – Fe_2O_3
Limonite – $FeO(OH)$
Caniterite is not an iron ore.

68. (a) : Ideal gas equation is given as :
$PV = nRT$
P = Pressure of gas, V = volume of gas
n = moles of gas, R = gas constant
T = temperature

$\Rightarrow PV = \dfrac{w}{M}RT$ w = mass of gags
M = Molecular mass of gas

$$P = \left(\frac{w}{V}\right)\frac{RT}{M} \Rightarrow P = \rho\frac{RT}{M}$$

$$\left(\text{As } \rho = \frac{w}{V}\right)$$

$\Rightarrow P \propto \rho$

69. **(b) :** Each electron in an atom is designated by a set of four quantum numbers. According to Pauli's exclusion principle, no two electron in an atom have same values of all the four quantum numbers. Therefore consequently, an orbital accommodates two electrons with opposite spins, there two electron have the same value of quantum number '*n*', '*l*' and '*m*' but value of '*s*' will be different.

70. **(c) :** The order of increasing energy of the subatomic orbitals is $s < p < d < f$. The energy in excited state is more than that in the ground state. Since option (c) is in an excited state, therefore it has maximum energy.

71. **(b) :** Aldol condensation : when a carbonyl compound containing α-hydrogen is treated with a base, first of all carbanion is formed.

e.g. $CH_3CHO \xrightarrow[NaOH]{OH^-} \overset{\ominus}{C}H_2-CHO$

$$\overset{\ominus}{C}H_2CHO + CH_3-CH{=}O \longrightarrow CH_3-\underset{\underset{O^-}{|}}{CH}-CH_2-CHO \xrightarrow{H^+}$$

$$CH_3-\underset{\underset{OH}{|}}{CH}-CH_2-CHO \quad \text{(Aldol)}$$

72. **(c) :** Cyanohydrin can be prepared easily by the reaction of HCN with carbonyl compounds (*i.e.* Ketones)

$$\underset{\text{Ketone}}{(C_2H_5)_2C=O} \xrightarrow{HCN} \underset{\text{Cyanohydrin}}{(C_2H_5)_2C(OH)CN}$$

73. **(b) :** In the given reaction aldehyde (C_6H_5CHO) reacts with aniline ($C_6H_5NH_2$), they form amine ($C_6H_5-N=CHC_6H_5$) which is known as Schiff's base.

74. **(b) :** Acetylene is converted to acetaldehyde when acetylene is treated with dil. H_2SO_4 and small amount of $HgSO_4$.

$$\underset{\text{Acetylene}}{CH\equiv CH} + H_2O \xrightarrow[Hg^{2+}]{\text{Dil. } H_2SO_4} \underset{\text{acetaldehyde}}{CH_3-CHO}$$

75. **(c) :** CH_3COCH_3 can be converted to $CH_3CH_2CH_3$ by reduction process in which the ketone is heated with hydroiodic acid and red phosphorus.

$$CH_3COCH_3 + HI \xrightarrow{P} CH_3CH_2CH_3$$

76. **(b) :** $[H_3O^+] = 1\times10^{-6}$ mol L^{-1}

or $[H^+] = 1\times10^{-6}$ mol L^{-1}

As for distilled water $[H^+] = [OH^-]$

$[H^+] = [OH^-] = 1\times10^{-6}$ mol L^{-1}

$K_w = [H^+][OH^-]$

$= 10^{-12}$ mol^2 L^{-2}

77. **(c) :** According to Henderson's equation,

$$pH = pk_a + \log\frac{[\text{salt}]}{[\text{acid}]}$$

$$CH_3COOH + NaOH \rightarrow CH_3COONa + H_2O$$

Putting the values, we get :

$$pH = 4.57 + \log\frac{0.10}{0.03}$$

$\Rightarrow \quad pH = 5.09$

78. **(d) :** Let the oxidation state of Fe be x

$\Rightarrow \quad 3x + 4(-2) = 0$

$\Rightarrow \quad x = +\frac{8}{3}$

79. **(a) :** Photochemical reaction between H_2 and Cl_2 is zero order reaction, the concentration of gases per unit volume in the gaseous phase will not change with time, although the quantities will change.

80. **(b) :** As the size of the noble gas atoms increases down the group, the polarisation of the electron cloud becomes easier. So heavier noble gas atoms are easily polarised in polar water.

81. **(a) :** Number of electrons in Li^{2+} is one similar to the hydrogen atom. One electron system shows similar kind of spectra. Many electron system spectra is complex due to inter-electronic repulsions.

82. **(c) :** $CH_3-\overset{3}{\underset{\underset{2\,CH_2CH_3^{\,1}}{|}}{CH}}-\overset{4}{CH_2}-\overset{5}{\underset{\underset{CN}{|}}{CH}}-\overset{6}{CH_3}$

Therefore, IUPAC name is 3-methyl - 5-cyano hexane.

83. **(c) :** The bond energies of F – F, C – C, N – N and O – O bonds are 33, 80, 39 and 34.2 kJ/mole respectively. Therefore molecule of C – C has the highest bond energy.

84. **(a) :** Heat of neutralization (ΔH) = 57 kJ, volume of HNO_3 = 0.5 mole and volume of NaOH = 0.2 mole. When HNO_3 solution is added to NaOH solution, then 0.2 mole of HNO_3 solution will combine with 0.2 mole of OH^- ions of NaOH solution.

∴ Heat released = ΔH × 0.2 = 57 × 0.2 = 11.4 kJ.

85. **(a) :** $CuBr \rightarrow Cu^+ + Br^-$

Solubility of CuBr is 2×10^{-4} mol L^{-1}

Therefore, solubility of $Cu^+ = 2\times10^{-4}$ mol L^{-1}

$\Rightarrow$ Solubility product $= 2\times10^{-4}\times2\times10^{-4}$

$= 4\times10^{-8}$ mol$^2L^{-2}$

86. **(a) :** Schottky defect – If some of the lattice points are unoccupied, called vacancies or holes, the lattice becomes defective. Equal number of cations and anions usually absent so that the crystal remains neutral.

87. **(b) :** For an AB_2 type structure, the equivalent equation at equilibrium is

$$AB_2 \rightleftharpoons A^{2+} + 2B^-.$$

For CaF_2, the equivalent equation at equilibrium is

$$CaF_2 \rightleftharpoons Ca^{2+} + 2F^-.$$

Therefore CaF_2 has an AB_2 type structure.

88. **(b) :** Azimuthal quantum number defines the spatial distribution of electron cloud and angular mementum.

e.g. $l = 0$, s – subsehll
$l = 1$, p – subshell
$l = 2$, d – subshell

Orbital angular momentum of an electron is calculated using the expression.

$$= \sqrt{l(l+1)}\frac{h}{2\pi}$$

89. **(d) :** Phosphorus (P) has electronic configuration $1s^2, 2s^2, 2p^6, 3s^2, 3p^3$

Therefore, no valence electron is present in the $3d$-subshell.

Fe (III) has electronic configuration : $3d^5 4s^0$

Cr(I) : $3d^5\ 4s^0$

Mn (II) : $3d^5\ 4s^0$

90. **(c) :** Derzen's method : Alkyl halides are prepared when thionyl chloride and alcohols are refulxed in presence of pyridine.

$$R-OH + SOCl_2 \xrightarrow[\text{reflux}]{\text{Py}} R-Cl + SO_2 + HCl.$$

Byproducts of this reaction are gases (SO_2, HCl) so can be easily removed from the reaction mixture.

91. **(b) :** H_3PO_4 is a tetrahedral structure molecule. It contains three –OH group so that three protons can be released. So it acts as a tribasic acid.

(H_3PO_4) (tribasic acid) — $P(=O)(OH)_3$

(H_3PO_3) (dibasic acid) — $HP(=O)(OH)_2$

(H_3PO_2) (monobasic acid) — $H_2P(=O)(OH)$

$(HO)_2P(=O)-O-P(=O)(OH)_2$ $H_4P_2O_7$ (tetra basic acid)

92. **(d) :** Thermite process involved the reduction metal oxides by the use of aluminium powder.

$$Fe_2O_3 + 2Al \rightarrow Al_2O_3 + 2Fe$$

93. **(a) :** Alkali and alkaline earth metals react with water to produce hydrogen gas and metal hydroxide. This is due to their high electropositive character.

$$2Na + 2H_2O \rightarrow 2NaOH + H_2$$
$$Mg + 2H_2O \rightarrow Mg(OH)_2 + H_2$$

94. **(c) :** Atomic mass of element = 100 g/mol

Cell edge = 400 pm = $400 \times 10^{-12} = 4 \times 10^{-10}$

and number of atoms in BCC (Z) = 2.

As the atomic mass of the metal is 100 gm/mol, therefore

$$\text{mass of each atom } (m) = \frac{100}{6.023 \times 10^{23}} = 16.6 \times 10^{-23} \text{ g.}$$

The volume of unit cell = $(4 \times 10^{-8})^3 = 64 \times 10^{-24}$ cm^3.

And mass of unit cell = $Z \times m$

$= 2 \times (16.6 \times 10^{-23}) = 33.2 \times 10^{-23}$ g.

$$\text{Therefore density of element} = \frac{\text{Mass of unit cell}}{\text{Volume of unit cell}}$$

$$= \frac{33.2 \times 10^{-23}}{64 \times 10^{-24}} \approx 5.188 \text{ g/cm}^3.$$

95. **(c) :** A system is said to be in colloidal state if particles of one or more components have the same size range 10^{-6} m to 10^{-9} m. In other words, the colloidal solution is a heterogenous dispersion of solute particles size ranging from 10^{-6} m into the solvent. Particles are visible only with an ultra microscope.

96. **(d) :** Chiral compound contains one or more 'Chiral' carbon atoms. Chiral carbon atoms usually are bonded to four different atoms or group of atoms.

$CH_3-CH_2-CH_2-CH_2-CH_2-CH_3$ (hexane)
(Achiral)

CH_4 (Methane)
(Achiral)

$CH_3-CH_2-CH_2-CH_3$ (n-butane)
(Achiral)

$CH_3-CH(CH_3)-CH(CH_3)-CH(CH_3)-CH_2-CH_3$
(Chiral)
2, 3, 4-trimethyl hexane

97. **(a) :** $H_2C \overset{\rightarrow}{=} O$

The electronegative oxygen atom is a strong electron withdrawing group. So there is polarity in the carbonyl compounds. This polarity is even greater than in the asymmetric alkene.

$CH_3 \searrow C=C \nearrow H$, $CH_3 \nearrow$ $\searrow H$ $\quad$ $CH_3 \searrow C=C \nearrow H$, $H \nearrow$ $\searrow CH_3$ $\quad$ $Cl \searrow C=C \nearrow CH_3$, $CH_3 \nearrow$ $\searrow Cl$

(some polarity) (Polarity is compensated) (Polarity cancels out)

98. **(c)** : The bond length C – C (single bond as in ethane) is 1.54 Å and C = C (double bond as in ethene is 1.33 Å. The carbonte carbon bond length in benzene has been found to be 1.39Å which lies between single and double bond length value.

99. **(a)** : Pent - 4 - en - 1 - yne

$$\overset{1}{CH} \equiv \overset{2}{C} - \overset{3}{CH_2} - \overset{4}{CH} = \overset{5}{CH_2}$$

No. of (σ) bonds – 4 (C–C) + 6(C–H) = 10
No. of π- bonds – 1 (C=C) + 2(C≡C) = 3

100. **(d)** :

$CH_3–CH=CH–CH_3$ (2-butene) $\quad$ $CH_3–CH_2–CH=CH_2$ (1-butene)

$CH_3–CH_2–CH_2–CH=CH_2$ (1-pentene) $\quad$ $CH_3–CH_2–CH=CH–CH_3$ (2-pentene)

Acording to Saytzeff rule, stability of alkenes depends upon the substitution on C=C bond. More of substitution by alkyl group, the more stable is the alkene.

101. **(c)** : In adiabatic process, no heat enters or leaves the system. The system is completely insulated from its surroundings. From first law of thermodynamics, change in internal energy,

$$\Delta E = q - W = 0 - W = -W.$$

Since the work is done at the expense of internal energy, therefore internal energy of the system decreases and hence temperature of the gas falls.

102. **(a)** : The valence shell electron in the alkali metals is so loosely held that even the low energy photons (light) can eject this electron from the metal surface. This phenomenon is called as photoelectric effect. K and Cs are used in photoelectric cells which are sensitive to blue light.

103. **(c)** : In physical absorption, the substance absorbed is retained not only on the surface but also more or less uniformly distributed throughout the entire body. And absorbed molecules are not broken under ordinary conditions.

104. **(a)** : Amides are $R - CONH_2$

Acids are $R - COOH$

Due to the presence of $-NH_2$ group in amides there is stronger hydrogen bonding between the amide molecules than between the acid molecules. Some acids are rather present in dimers form due to the presence of intra molecular hydrogen bonding.

$$R-C\begin{matrix} \nearrow O\cdots H-O \searrow \\ \searrow O-H\cdots O \nearrow \end{matrix}C-R$$

105. **(c)** : $SnCl_2$ (stannous chloride) on reaction with mercuric chloride ($HgCl_2$), oxidises to $SnCl_4$ (stannic chloride)

$$SnCl_2 + 2HgCl_2 \rightarrow SnCl_4 + \underset{\text{(Greyish)}}{Hg_2Cl_2}$$

So in this reaction, stannous chloride is acting as reducing agent that reduces Hg(II) to Hg(I) and then to Hg(0)

$$SnCl_2 + Hg_2Cl_2 \rightarrow 2Hg + SnCl_4.$$

106. **(d)** : In the cell, DNA molecules (*i.e.* Deoxyribose Nucleic acid) are present predominatly in the nucleus, some DNA is also present in the mitochondria in Eukaryotes.

RNA molecules (*i.e.* Ribose nucleic acid) are present in cytoplasm of the eukaryotes and in nucleus in some prokaryotes and virus.

107. **(a)** : All the halogens are coloured. The colour deepens with the rise of atomic number from fluorine to iodine.

The colour is due to the absorption of energy from visible light by their molecules or excitation of outer electrons to higher energy levels.

F	Cl	Br	I
Light yellow	Yellow green	Reddish brown	Deep violet.

108. **(c)** : Lower velue of bond dissociation energy of fluorine is due to the high inter electronic repulsions between non-bonding electrons of the 2*p*-orbital of small sized fluorine. As a result F–F bond is weaker as comparison to Cl–Cl and Br–Br bonds.

Bond dissociation energy

F–F	38 K cal/mole
Cl–Cl	57 K cal/mole
Br–Br	45.5 K cal/mole
I–I	35.6 K cal/mole

109. **(d)** : Phenol is a stronger acid than the ethanol. This is due to the resonance stabilisaton of the phenolate ion which is produced after deprotonation.

OH (phenol) $\underset{}{\overset{-H^+}{\rightleftharpoons}}$ O⊖ ⟷ O ⟷ O ⟷ O

But there is no such stabilisation in the case of ethanol

$$C_2H_5OH \rightleftharpoons C_2H_5O^- + H^+$$

The groups with +M and –I effect decrease the acidity at p-position, but at m-position the acidity is increased due to –I-effect.

110. **(a) :** Due to the presence of lone pair of electrons on oxygen atom, ethers behave as base and form stable oxonium salts with mineral acids.

$$C_2H_5-\ddot{O}-C_2H_5 + HCl \rightarrow C_2H_5-\overset{\oplus}{\underset{H}{O}}-C_2H_5\ \overset{\ominus}{Cl}$$

Diethyl oxonium Chloride

111. **(c) :** The wavelength of the line can be calculated by the Ritz formula :

$$\frac{1}{\lambda} = R\left(\frac{1}{n_1^2} - \frac{1}{n_2^2}\right), \quad \text{R = Rydberg constant}$$

Therefore, for calculating highest wavelength in Balmer series ($n_1 = 2$), n_2 should be 3,4,5.

112. **(c) :** More is the surface area, fast is the rate of evaporation at a given temperature this is due to the fact that more surface area means more number of molecules at the surface which can then be evaporated easily. Strong inter-molecular forces of attraction slows down the rate of evaporation.

113. **(b) :** In diamond, each carbon atom is in sp^3 hybridised state and linked to four other carbon atoms tetraherally by covalent bonds. Since there is no mobile electron present, diamond is bad conductor of heat and electricity.

In graphite each carbon atom is in sp^2 hybridised state and is linked to three other carbon atoms in a hexagonal planar structure. The π–electrons are free to move throughout the entire layers, therefore graphite is good conductor of heat and electricity.

114. **(c) :** Atoms can neither be created nor destroyed. This is the statement of law of conservation of mass.

Under similar conditions of temperature and pressure, equal volume of gases contain equal number of atoms.

As, $PV = nRT$ (Ideal gas equation)

If, for Ist case, $P_1V_1 = n_1RT_1$

for IInd case, $P_2V_2 = n_2RT_2$

$$\Rightarrow \frac{P_1V_1}{P_2V_2} = \frac{n_1RT_1}{n_2RT_2} \Rightarrow n_1 = n_2$$

115. **(c) :** Extensive properties are dependent upon the amount of the substance. *.e.g.* mass, volume etc.

Intensive properties are independent of the amount of the substance. *e.g.* temperature, density.

116. **(a) :** Internal energy is given by :

$$E = E_{translational} + E_{rotaional} + E_{vibrational} + E_{bonding} + E_{electronic}$$

Accurate measurement of some forms of energy which contribute to the absolute value of internal energy for a given substance in a given state is impossible. So difference of the initial state and final state is calculated and is denoted by

$$\Delta E = E_f - E_i$$

117. **(c) :** Cuprous ions (Cu^+) is colourless because it has no unpaired electrons in the 3*d* sub-shell as it has $3d^{10}$ configuration. The cupric ion (Cu^{++}) has one unpaired electron as it has configuration $3d^9$. By absorbing the visible light, the unpaired electron can migrate from one set of *d*-orbitals to another under the applied field of water molecules. Hence cupric ion (Cu^{++}) in aqueous solution shows blue colour.

118. **(b) :** Oxygen is second most electronegative element after fluorine. So it can easily gain electrons to form dinegative anion (O^{2-}) while sulphur is not so electronegative element as oxygen.

119. **(c) :** Sigma bonding involves end to end overlapping of the two atomic orbitals *e.g.* between *s* and *s*, *s* and *p* and *p* and *p* orbitals.

Pi bonding (π) involves sidewise overlapping of the two atomic orbitals *e.g.* between *p* and *p* orbitals.

Overlapping of orbitals is more effective in σ bonding than in π–bonding. Due to the geometry of overlapping or orbitals, rotation of one atom is not possible around π–bonds.

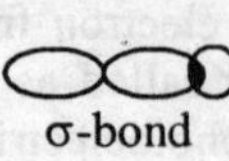
σ-bond

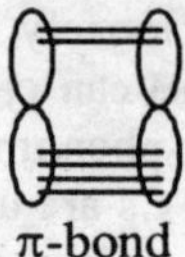
π-bond

120. **(d) :** Absorption spectrum is produced when white light is passed through a substance and transmitted light is analysed by a spectrograph. The dark spaces corresponds to the light radiation absorbed by the substance. And emission spectrum is produced by analysing the radiant energy emitted by an excited substance by a spectrograph. Thus discontinuous spectra consisting of a series of sharp lines and separated by dark bands are obtained.

BIOLOGY

121. **(d) :** Immune tolerance is acquired as an inability to react to particular self or non-self antigens. Both B-cells and T-cells display tolerance, generally to their specific antigen classes. Basically B-cells form a part of the humoral immune system and T-cells form a part of the cell-mediated immune system.

122. **(b) :** Cyclosporine is used as immunodepressant. This drug is derived from a fungus and is used to prevent rejection of kidney, heart and liver transplants. Cyclosporine inhibits the activity of helper T-cells.

123. **(d) :** *Neanderthal* man was the first human fossils discovered in 1856 having a cranial capacity of 1400 cc. African man (*Australopithecus*) was discovered in 1924 having a cranial capacity of 300-500 cc. Java ape man (*Pithecanthropus erectus*) discovered in 1920 and its cranial capacity was 900 cc whereas Peking man (*Sinanthropus pekinensis*) was discovered in 1924 and its cranial capacity was 1075 cc. These show that *Neanderthal* man has the largest cranial capacity.

124. **(d) :** Transversion are those base replacement where a purine is replaced by a pyrimidine and *vice versa*. It means that CG can be replaced by GC and *vice versa*. Similarly AT can be replaced by TA and *vice versa*.

125. **(c) :** The premolars and molars are called cheek teeth. These are also called lophodont teeth. Their free ends are flattened and bear transverse ridges to crush and grind the food.

126. **(d) :** The substrate for photorespiration is glycollate formed in chloroplasts. It changes enzymatically into glyoxylate inside peroxisomes where it is further converted into glycine. The glycine changes to serine inside the mitochondria.

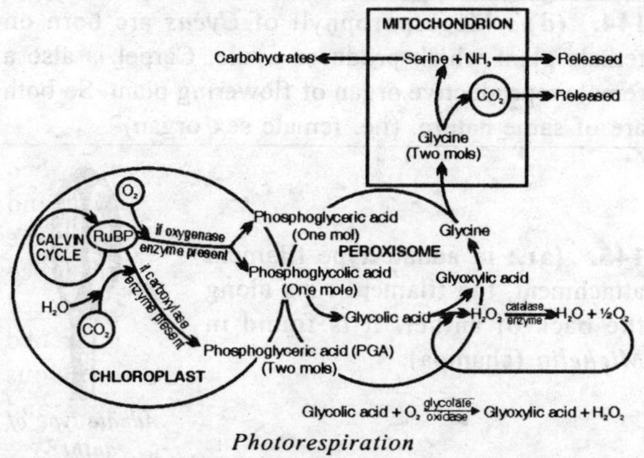

Photorespiration

127. **(d) :** Glycosylation is bonding of sugar residue to another organic compound. Glycoprotein are formed in the lumen of rough endoplasmic reticulum, but may subsequently be modified in the lumen of the golgi aparatus, where other amino acids of the protein may become glycosylated.

128. **(b) :** Frameshift mutation occurs when one or more nucleotides are either added or deleted from DNA. The result of such mutation is nonfunctioning of protein because the the sequence of codons is altered. Example of frameshift mutation due to deletion.

Original (wild type) message or reading frame

CAT GAT CAT GAT CAT GAT CAT

Deletion

CAT GAT ATG ATC ATG ATC AT

Message out of frame

129. **(c) :** If centromere is truly terminal, i.e. situated at the tip of chromosome, the chromosome is said to be telocentric. Telocentric chromosome are very rare.

Telocentric chromosome

130. **(c) :** In glycolysis one molecule of hexose sugar (glucose/fructose), a 6C-compound is splitted to form two molecules of a 3C-compound, pyruvic acid ($CH_3COCOOH$).

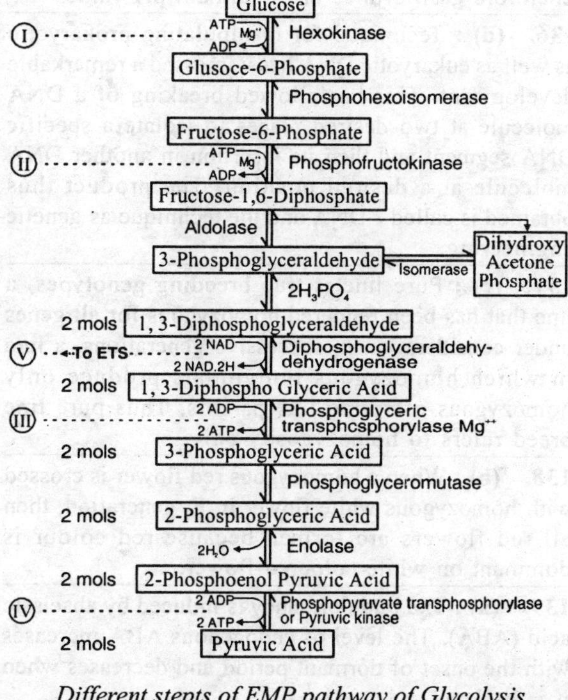

Different stepts of EMP pathway of Glycolysis

131. (d) : In cockroach, excretion is mainly performed by one or two pairs of malpighian tubules. One of this pair opens into the middle region of intestine and other pair of coxal glands are located in prosoma and opens at bases of fifth walking legs.

132. (c) : Ambulacral grooves are found in the arms of an echinoderms lined by tube feet. Ambulacral grooves are absent in ophiuroidea which are covered by ossicles.

133. (d) : In frog, all nerve cells connecting to central nervous system (brain and spinal cord) with receptor and effectors constitute the peripheral nervous system. Some small masses of nerve cell bodies are called ganglia. They develop neural crest cells in frog.

134. (b) : Lysis is the death and subsequent breakdown of a cell. Under normal conditions such cells are engulfed by phagocytes and degraded by their lysosome. Lysis of foreign cell is mediated through IgM and IgG. These are called immunoglobulins.

135. (b) : Bile is alkaline viscous fluid, yellow to green in colour and having a pH of 7.8-8.6. Saliva is secreted by salivary gland and its pH is about 6.8. Gastric juice is secreted by the gastric gland in stomach and its pH value is 1-2.5 and pancreatic juice is colourless watery fluid and slightly alkaline. Its pH is 7.5-8.0. Therefore gastric juice has minimum pH value.

136. (d) : Technique for manipulating prokaryotic as well as eukaryotic DNA has witnessed a remarkable development. This has allowed breaking of a DNA molecule at two desired places to isolate a specific DNA segment and then its insertion in another DNA molecule at a desired position. The product thus obtained is called *r* DNA and the technique as genetic engineering.

137. (c) : Pure line is true breeding genotypes, a line that has been rendered homozygous for all genes under consideration in successive generations, a line in which homozygous individuals produce only homozygous offspring like parents. Thus pure line breed refers to homozygosity only.

138. (b) : When a homozygous red flower is crossed with homozygous white flower in F_1 generation, then all red flowers are formed because red colour is dominant on white coloured flower.

139. (a) : The bud dormancy is induced by abscissic acid (ABA). The level of endogenous ABA increases with the onset of dormant period and decreases when it is broken.

140. (d) : The effect of pollen on endosperm is called xenia whereas pollen of stomatic cell lying outside the endosperm is known as metaxenia.

141. (c) : Maximum solar energy is trapped by algae and hence they evolve maximum amount of oxygen by the process of photosynthesis. Therefore algae are useful because they purify the atmosphere by releasing oxygen.

142. (d) : The gametophytic generation represents the dominant phase in the life cycle of bryophytes. The sporophyte phase is dependent on the gametophyte. That is why, the plant body of *Funaria* is predominantly gametophytic generation with sporophyte.

143. (d) : *Marchantia* is a liverwort. Its sporophyte contains elongated cells with spiral thickenings on its wall called elaters. These elaters are hygroscopic in nature. The resulting twisting movement helps in dispersal of spores.

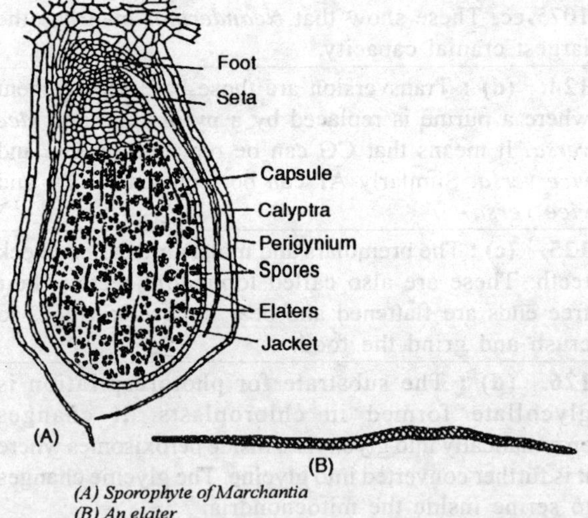

(A) Sporophyte of Marchantia
(B) An elater

144. (d) : Megasporophyll of *Cycas* are born on female plant which produces ovule. Carpel is also a female reproductive organ of flowering plant. So both are of same nature. (i.e. female sex organ).

145. (a) : In adnate type filament attachment, the filament runs along the back of anther. It is found in *Michelia* (champa).

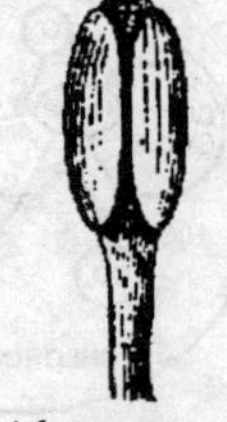

Adnate type of anther

146. (c) : The pressure that develops in a cell from time to time due to osmotic diffusion of water molecules into a cell that causes stretching of the cell wall is

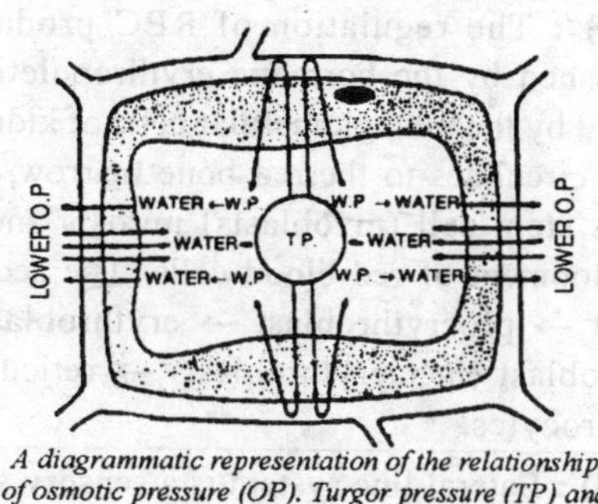

A diagrammatic representation of the relationship of osmotic pressure (OP). Turgor pressure (TP) and wall pressure (WP) the state of final equilibrium.

called turgor pressure. Due to turgor pressure, rigid cell wall offers resistance. This resistance works in a direction opposite to turgor pressure. But it is equal to turgor pressure and is called wall pressure. In this condition, no exchange of water takes place.

147. (b) : Passage cells are found in monocot root.

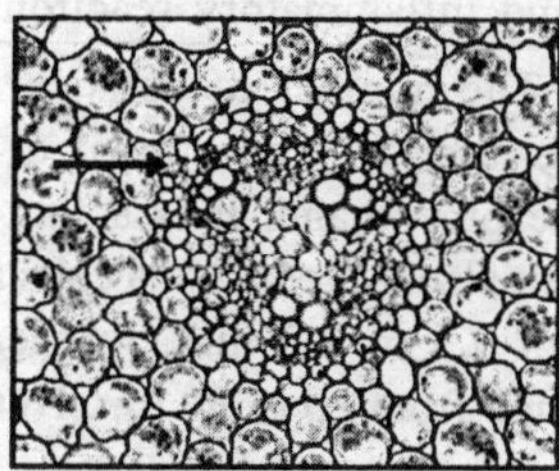
The arrow indicates a non lignified "passage cell" in the endodermis

It is an unthickened cell in the endodermis of a root, found opposite to the protoxylem element through which solutions can diffuse in the transverse direction.

148. (d) : Green plants are being planted around the road side to check the noise pollution. This is known as green muffler. Noise pollution is measured in decibels.

149. (a) : The functional role of a species in the community including activities and relationship is called niche. Niche is the social position held by an organism with respect to its associates. The abundance of a species population within its habitat is called niche density.

150. (c) : Cyphella are small depressions or cavity like opening into the medulla on the ventral surface

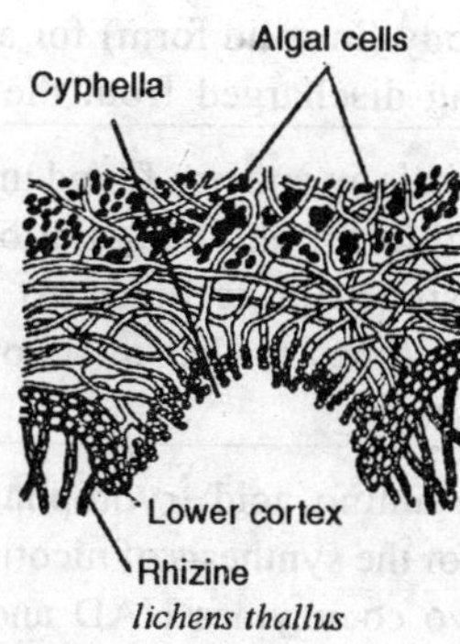

lichens thallus

of the thallus of certain lichens. They perform respiratory functions.

151. (a) : In *Entamoeba histolytica*, the precystic or minute forms encyst only in the lumen of the intestine. In precystic stage, the chromatid bodies are found which disappear as the cysts mature.

152. (d) : *Euspongia* or *Spongia* is also called bath sponges. When it dries up, only its skeleton is left which is made up of spongin fibre.

153. (c) : In *Hydra* sensory cells are found in the gastrodermis. They are supposed to be stimulated by the entry of the prey into the gastrovascular cavity.

154. (d) : *Wuchereria bancrofti* is a dreaded human parasite. It is digenetic parasite completing its life cycle in two hosts, the final host is man harbouring the adult worm. The adult worms live coiled up in the gland and lymph vessels of man.

155. (c) : The development of *Ascaris* larva takes place outside the body of host in soil and their cleavage starts in shelled eggs. First moulting takes place in soil in shelled egg whereas second and third moulting takes place in alveoli and lung respectively. The final moulting takes place in intestine.

156. (d) : The triplet code is a degenerate one with many codons than the number of amino acid types coded. An explanation for this degeneracy is provided by the Wobble hypothesis proposed by F.H.C. Crick in 1966.

157. (c) : Uricotelic animals (living in dry conditions) are those animals which excrete uric acid as their excretory product *e.g.* lizard and crow. These animals conserve water in their bodies and synthesize crystals of uric acids from ammonia. These crystals can be retained in the body (in solid form) for a considerable time before being discharged from the body.

158. (a) : Rennin is an enzyme found in gastric juices and are responsible for the coagulation of milk. It acts by hydrolysing peptide links. At 37°C, rennin can coagulate 10^7 times to that of its own weight of milk in ten minutes.

159. (b) : The amino acid tryptophan serves as a source material for the synthesis of nicotinamide which in turn forms two coenzymes NAD and NADP with metabolic roles.

160. (b) : Fehling's test is given only by reducing sugars. When Fehling's solution is added to any reducing sugar then a red precipitate is formed which shows that reduction has taken place. Sucrose does not give this test.

161. (a) : The advancement in the field of biology has reached to such an extent that it requires the basic knowledge of chemistry, physics and other basic sciences. It is a fact that living organisms are made up of atoms and molecules which follow chemical and physical laws. Therefore knowledge of chemistry and physics is essential.

162. (d) : Living organisms are regarded as open system as they can loose or gain the mass or energy from the surrounding environment. All living organisms restore their lost energy either from the sunlight or indirectly from the food material.

163. (a) : Death is regarded as the most important regulatory process on earth. It reduces the number of individuals in a population and avoids over-crowding caused by continuous reproduction. Over-crowding due to reproduction is countered by death as the ultimate termination of functional life.

164. (b) : During a wound, germs are removed by the process of phagocytosis by WBC. WBCs accumulate at the site of wound by diapedesis. Diapedesis is the squeezing of leucocytes out from the endothelium of capillaries to fight against foreign agent.

165. (a) : Specialization of cells into tissue, organ and organ systems is advantageous for the organism. It increases the operational efficiency through division of labour which avoids duplication of work.

166. (c) : To maintain the unequal distribution of Na^+ and K^+ ion, the neuron uses chemical energy in the form of ATP to actively transport Na^+ ion out of the cell and move K^+ inside the cell.

167. (a) : The regulation of RBC production is accomplished by the hormone erythropoietin which is secreted by the juxtaglomerular cells of kidney. This hormone circulates to the red bone marrow, where it increases stem cell (myoblasts) mitosis and speeds the development of red blood cells. The sequence is myoblast → proerythroblast → erythroblast → normoblast (metaerythroblast) → reticulocyte → erythrocytes.

168. (b) : Lateral line system is a sensory system of fishes and aquatic and larval amphibians whose receptors are clusters of sensory cells derived from ectoderm. These clusters of sensory cells are called neuromast organs.

169. (a) : Histamine is s derivative of the aminoacid histidine produced by damaged cells of vertebrates. When released, it has the effect of dilating capillaries and lowering blood pressure. Histamine is involved in allergic and inflammatory reactions.

170. (d) : The number of cells in a multicellular organism are directly proportional to the size of the body. On the other hand, it is a fact that cells vary greatly in their size. Mycoplasma cells are the smallest, ranging from 0.1 to 0.3 mm, whereas human cells generally range from 20 to 30 μm. Nerve cells are the longest.

171. (b) : Taxonomy or systematics is the branch of biology for the classification of biological world of living organisms. The classification is the grouping of the organisms in an orderly manner. This grouping is based upon similarities and dissimilarities.

172. (d) : The diploid megaspore mother cell has a large nucleus and dense cytoplasm. This cell undergoes mitosis (reduction division) to produce a group of four haploid cells called megaspore.

173. (b) : In bacteria, the reaction centre is B-890 and photosynthesis occurs by utilizing wavelengths longer than 700 nm. The reductant is NADH + H^+. In bacteria, the donor may be hydrogen sulphide or malate or succinate but not water.

174. (b) : In the typical angiospermic plant, cotyledons in the seed are the embryonic leaves. The radicle of the embryo upon the seed germination produces the root system and the plumule produces the shoot system. The radicle and plumule are contained in the embryo.

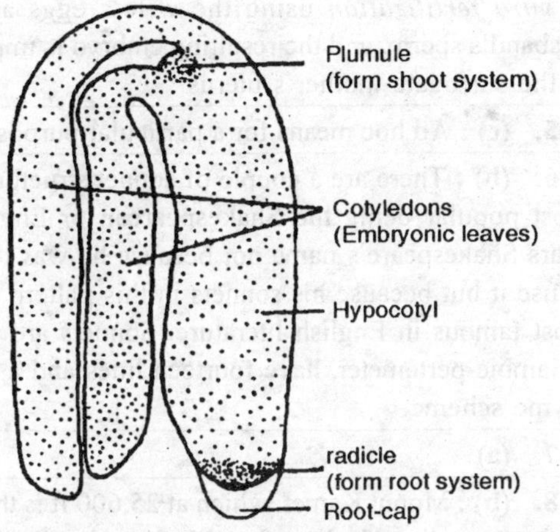

Mature dicotyledonous embryo

175. (a) : Collenchyma is a specialized type of parenchyma which functions as supporting tissue. The cell walls are irregularly thickened due to the deposition of cellulose and pectin. They are living tissue and possess the ability to divide.

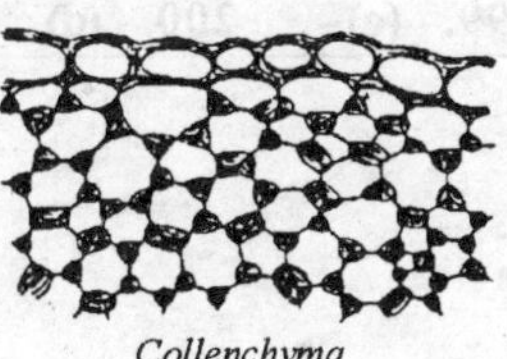
Collenchyma

176. (c) : Clone is a group of cells descended from the same single parent cell. In most of the cases, nucleic acid sequences are said to be cloned when they are inserted into vectors such as plasmids and copied within host cells during gene manipulation.

177. (a) : The metabolic reactions of a living organisms can occur only in a delicately balanced environment in the non-living organisms. The cells are the life supporting chambers which have such a special environment. A living cell keeps its chemical composition steady within its boundary.

178. (c) : Plasmids are found mostly in prokaryotic cells and yeasts. They do not form a part of the normal chromosomal DNA of a cell and capable of replicating independently. It constitutes a form of extra-chromosomal DNA.

179. (d) : The *m*RNA attaches itself to the small subunit (30s) of the ribosome via its 5′ end. This attachment is assisted by the G-cap nucleotide and bases of sequence present on the messenger RNA systems where G-cap is present as in eukaryotes.

180. (b) : When six molecules of carbon dioxide enter calvin cycle, one hexose molecule is formed, whereas 18 ATP and 12 NADPH + H^+ molecules are used up. The light reaction of photosynthesis results in the formation of ATP and $NADPH_2$.

GENERAL KNOWLEDGE

181. (a) : According to The Guinness Book of World Records, the highest town in the world is Wenzhuan, which was founded in 1955 on the Qinghai-Tibet road north of the *Tangla mountain range*. It is 16,730 feet above sea level.

182. (a) : A great mass of black rock soaring to over 22,000 feet, Mt. Kailash has the unique distinction of being the world's most venerated holy place at the same time that it is the least visited. The supremely sacred site of four religions and billions of people, Kailash is seen by no more than a few thousand pilgrims each year. This curious fact is explained by the mountain's remote location in far western Tibet. Dhaulagiri Mountain is in Nepal. Everest was formed about 60 million years ago. It's summit ridge seperates Nepal and Tibet. Mt Abu is in Rajasthan, India.

183. (d) : The Indian Army (Adventure Wing) successfully scaled technically one of the most difficult peaks in the World, the ANNAPURNA-I located at a height of 8091 metre over Central Nepal on May 6, 2002. This was the first ever expedition to this peak by an Indian Team.

184. (a), (c) : *Copper T* is a small device which is placed into the uterine cavity. The vertical and horizontal arms of the IUD contain some copper. The IUD slowly releases copper into the uterine cavity. Copper stops sperm from making their way up through the uterus into the tubes, thus preventing fertilization. If fertilization were to occur, the IUD would prevent the fertilized egg from successfully implanting in the lining of the uterus.

185. (c) **186. (a)**

187. (c) : After the death of GMC Balayogi in helicopter crash, M.M. Joshi was elected as 11th speaker of Loksabha.

188. (a) **189. (a)** **190. (a)**

191. (c)

192. (a) : The Welfare Portfolio Committee in collaboration with the SA Council for the Aged will host a special session in Parliament on 1 October 1996 to celebrate the International Day for the Aged.

The theme of the session, "Connecting the Generations in Praise of Age", aims to strengthen interaction and unity between older persons from various cultural groups, enhance their role in building the new democracy, and sharing between young and old.

193. (c) : Comets described as "big dirty snowballs." The "dirty" part refers to little bits of stone, not unlike sand, embedded in the comet's icy nucleus.

194. (b) : A surrogate mother is a woman who agrees, usually by contract and for a fee, to bear a child for a couple who are childless because the wife is infertile or physically incapable of carrying a developing fetus. Often the surrogate mother is the biological mother of the child, conceiving it by means of *artificial insemination* with sperm from the husband. In gestational surrogacy, the wife is fertile but incapable of carrying a growing fetus; the child is conceived by *in vitro fertilization* using the wife's eggs and her husband's sperm, and the resulting embryo is implanted in the surrogate mother's uterus.

195. (c) : Ad hoc means for a particular purpose only.

196. (b) : There are a couple of sonnet structures, the most popular being the Shakespearean or English. It bears Shakespeare's name not because he was the first to use it but because his sonnets in this pattern are the most famous in English literature. Sonnets are written in iambic pertameter, have fourteen lines and a certain rhyme scheme.

197. (a)

198. (b) : Mount Kamet, which at 25,600 ft is the third highest peak in India after Mt Kanchanjunga and Mt Nanda Devi.

199. (c) **200. (d)**

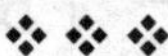

SOLVED PAPER
AIIMS - 2003

Time : 3½ Hours Max. Marks : 200

PHYSICS

1. The velocity with which a projectile must be fired so that it escapes earth's gravitation does not depend on
   (a) mass of the earth
   (b) mass of the projectile
   (c) radius of the projectile's orbit
   (d) gravitational constant.

2. Bernoulli's equation is a consequence of conservation of
   (a) energy (b) linear momentum
   (c) angular momentum (d) mass.

3. A laser beam is used for carrying out surgery because it
   (a) is highly monochromatic
   (b) is highly coherent
   (c) is highly directional
   (d) can be sharply focussed.

4. A wire of length L is drawn such that its diameter is reduced to half of its original diameter. If the initial resistance of the wire were 10 Ω, its new resistance would be
   (a) 40 Ω (b) 80 Ω
   (c) 120 Ω (d) 160 Ω.

5. A proton is about 1840 times heavier than an electron. When it is accelerated by a potential difference of 1 kV, its kinetic energy will be
   (a) 1840 keV (b) 1/1840 keV
   (c) 1 keV (d) 920 keV.

6. An electric dipole placed in a non-uniform electric field experiences
   (a) both a torque and a net force
   (b) only a force but no torque
   (c) only a torque but no net force
   (d) no torque and no net force.

7. In an ideal parallel LC circuit, the capacitor is charged by connecting it to a d.c. source which is then disconnected. The current in the circuit
   (a) becomes zero instantaneously
   (b) grows monotonically
   (c) decays monotonically
   (d) oscillates instantaneously.

8. To a germanium sample, traces of gallium are added as an impurity. The resultant sample would behave like
   (a) a conductor
   (b) a p-type semiconductor
   (c) an n-type semiconductor
   (d) an insulator.

9. A radioactive substance decays to $1/16^{th}$ of its initial activity in 40 days. The half-life of the radioactive substance expressed in days is
   (a) 2.5 (b) 5
   (c) 10 (d) 20.

10. A neutron makes a head-on elastic collision with a stationary deuteron. The fractional energy loss of the neutron in the collision is
   (a) 16/81 (b) 8/9
   (c) 8/27 (d) 2/3.

11. The motion of planets in the solar system is an example of the conservation of
   (a) mass (b) linear momentum
   (c) angular momentum (d) energy.

12. Two small drops of mercury, each of radius R, coalesce to form a single large drop. The ratio of the total surface energies before and after the change is
   (a) $1 : 2^{1/3}$ (b) $2^{1/3} : 1$
   (c) 2 : 1 (d) 1 : 2.

13. A black body, at a temperature of 227°C, radiates heat at a rate of 20 cal m^{-2} s^{-1}. When its temperature is raised to 727°C, the heat radiated by it in cal m^{-2} s^{-1} will be closest to

(a) 40 (b) 160
(c) 320 (d) 640.

14. Two springs of force constants k and $2k$ are connected to a mass as shown in figure. The frequency of oscillation of the mass is

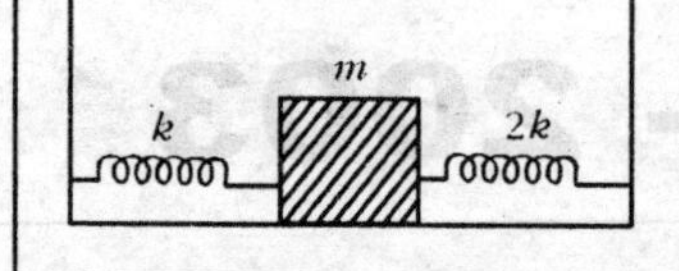

(a) $\frac{1}{2\pi}\sqrt{\frac{k}{m}}$ (b) $\frac{1}{2\pi}\sqrt{\frac{2k}{m}}$
(c) $\frac{1}{2\pi}\sqrt{\frac{3k}{m}}$ (d) $\frac{1}{2\pi}\sqrt{\frac{m}{k}}$

15. When a beam of light is used to determine the position of an object, the maximum accuracy is achieved if the light is
(a) polarised (b) of longer wavelength
(c) of shorter wavelength
(d) of high intensity.

16. A double slit experiment is performed with light of wavelength 500 nm. A thin film of thickness 2 μm and refractive index 1.5 is introduced in the path of the upper beam. The location of the central maximum will
(a) remain unshifted
(b) shift downward by nearly two fringes
(c) shift upward by nearly two fringes
(d) shift downward by 10 fringes.

17. If an electron and a photon propagate in the form of waves having the same wavelength, it implies that they have the same
(a) energy (b) momentum
(c) velocity (d) angular momentum.

18. Characteristic X-rays are produced due to
(a) transfer of momentum in collision of electrons with target atoms
(b) transition of electron from higher to lower electrons orbits in an atom
(c) heating of the target
(d) transfer of energy in collision of electrons with atoms in the target.

19. Three charges are placed at the vertices of an equilateral triangle of side a as shown in the given figure. The force experienced by the charge placed at the vertex A in a direction normal to BC is

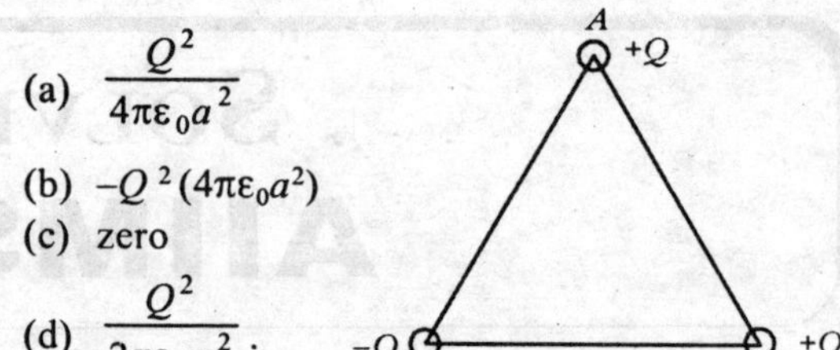

(a) $\frac{Q^2}{4\pi\varepsilon_0 a^2}$
(b) $-Q^2(4\pi\varepsilon_0 a^2)$
(c) zero
(d) $\frac{Q^2}{2\pi\varepsilon_0 a^2}$.

20. A capacitor of capacitance 2 μF is connected in the tank circuit of an oscillator oscillating with a frequency of 1 kHz. If the current flowing in the circuit is 2 mA, the voltage across the capacitor will be
(a) 0.16 V (b) 0.32 V
(c) 79.5 V (d) 159 V.

21. The earth's magnetic field at a given point is 0.5 × 10^{-5} Wb/m^2. This field is to be annulled by magnetic induction at the center of a circular conducting loop of radius 5.0 cm. The current required to be flown in the loop is nearly
(a) 0.2 A (b) 0.4 A
(c) 4 A (d) 40 A.

22. A frog can be levitated in a magnetic field produced by a current in a vertical solenoid placed below the frog. This is possible because the body of the frog behaves as
(a) paramagnetic (b) diamagnetic
(c) ferromagnetic (d) antiferromagnetic.

23. Shown below are the black body radiation curves at temperatures T_1 and T_2 ($T_2 > T_1$). Which of the following plots is correct?

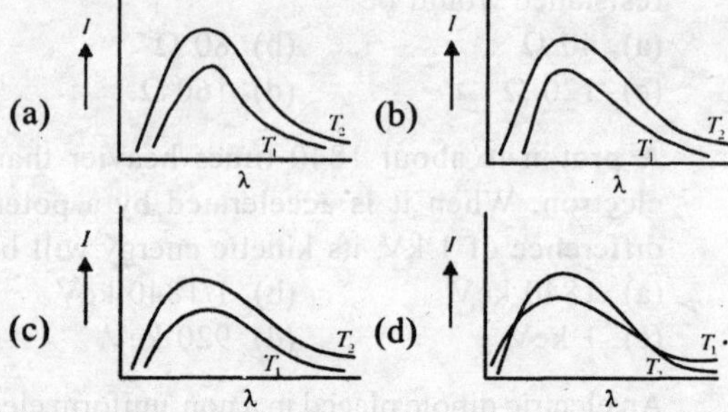

24. Figure shown is a distribution of charges. The flux of electric field due to these charges through the surface S is

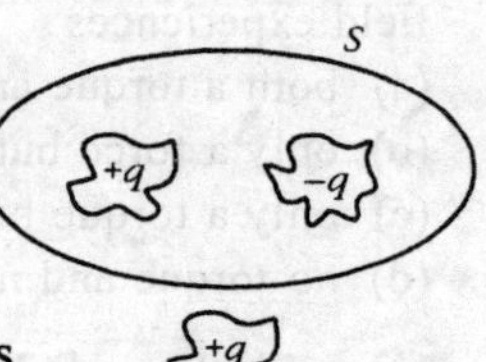

(a) $3q/\varepsilon_0$ (b) $2q/\varepsilon_0$
(c) q/ε_0 (d) zero.

25. In an experiment to find the focal length of a concave mirror a graph is drawn between the magnitudes of u and v. The graph looks like

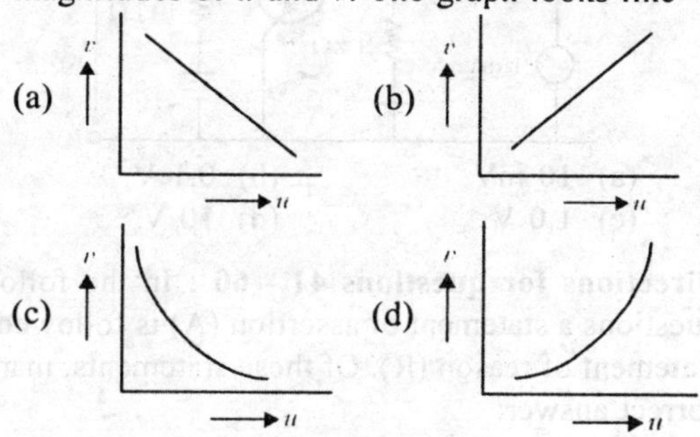

26. Nuclear fusion is possible
(a) only between light nuclei
(b) only between heavy nuclei
(c) between both light and heavy nuclei
(d) only between nuclei which are stable against β-decay.

27. An electron is travelling along the x-direction. It encounters a magnetic field in the y-direction. Its subsequent motion will be
(a) straight line along the x-direction
(b) a circle in the xz plane
(c) a circle in the yz plane
(d) a circle in the xy plane.

28. The difference in lengths of a mean solar day and a sidereal day is about
(a) 1 min (b) 4 min
(c) 15 min (d) 56 min.

29. A body starting from rest moves along a straight line with a constant acceleration. The variation of speed (v) with distance (s) is represented by the graph

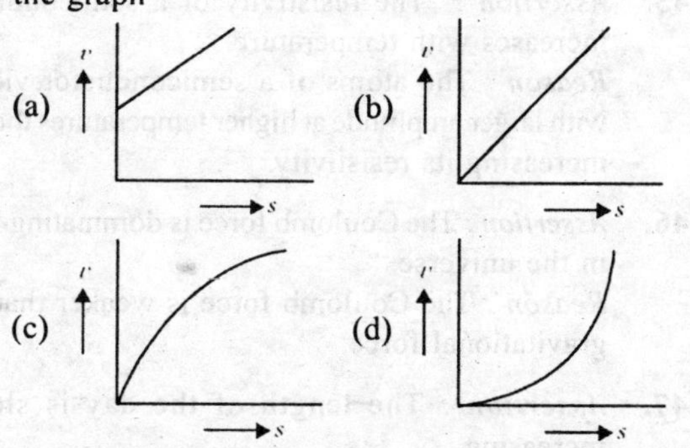

30. A rectangular loop carrying a current i_1, is situated near a long straight wire carrying a steady current i_2. The wire is parallel to one of the sides of the loop and is in the plane of the loop as shown in the figure. Then the current loop will
(a) move away from the wire
(b) move towards the wire
(c) remain stationary
(d) rotate about an axis parallel to the wire.

31. A ball is thrown vertically upwards. Which of the following plots represents the speed-time graph of the ball during its flight if the air resistance is not ignored?

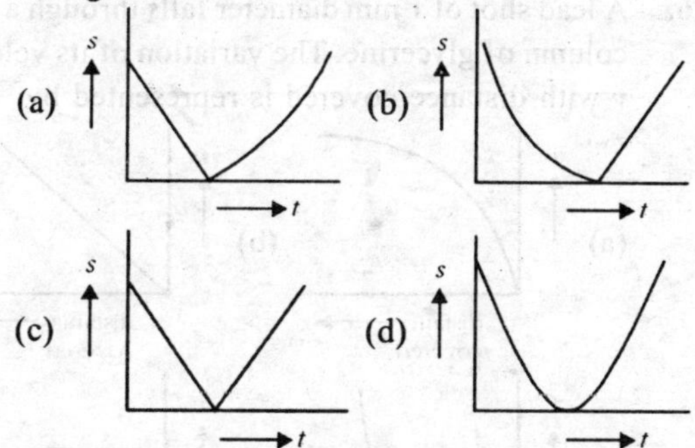

32. Radioactive nuclei that are injected into a patient collect at certain sites within its body, undergoing radioactive decay and emitting electromagnetic radiation. These radiations can then be recorded by a detector. This procedure provides an important diagnostic tool called
(a) gamma camera (b) CAT scan
(c) radiotracer technique
(d) gamma ray spectroscopy.

33. In a material medium, when a positron meets an electron both the particles annihilate leading to the emission of two gamma ray photons. This process forms the basis of an important diagnostic procedure called
(a) MRI (b) PET
(c) CAT (d) SPECT.

34. An astronaut is looking down on earth's surface from a space shuttle at an altitude of 400 km. Assuming that the astronaut's pupil diameter is

5 mm and the wavelength of visible light is 500 nm, the astronaut will be able to resolve linear objects of the size about

(a) 0.5 m (b) 5 m
(c) 50 m (d) 500 m.

35. An earthquake generates both transverse (S) and longitudinal (P) sound waves in the earth. The speed of S waves is about 4.5 km/s and that of P waves is about 8.0 km/s. A seismograph records P and S waves from an earthquake. The first P wave arrives 4.0 min before the first S wave. The epicentre of the earthquake is located at a distance about

(a) 25 km (b) 250 km
(c) 2500 km (d) 5000 km.

36. A lead shot of 1 mm diameter falls through a long column of glycerine. The variation of its velocity v with distance covered is represented by

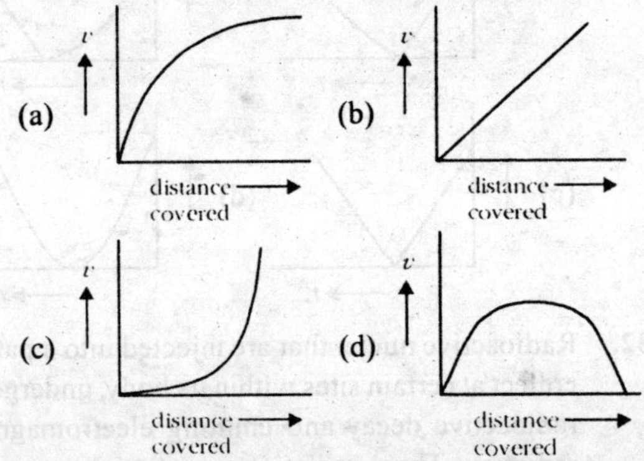

37. The maximum distance upto which TV transmission from a TV tower of height h can be received is proportional to

(a) $h^{1/2}$ (b) h
(c) h (d) h^2.

38. In short wave communication, waves of which of the following frequencies will be reflected back by the ionospheric layer having electron density 10^{11} per m^3?

(a) 2 MHz (b) 10 MHz
(c) 12 MHz (d) 18 MHz.

39. Using mass (M), length (L), time (T) and current (A) as fundamental quantities, the dimension of permeability is

(a) $M^{-1}LT^{-2}A$ (b) $ML^2T^{-2}A^{-1}$
(c) $MLT^{-2}A^{-2}$ (d) $MLT^{-1}A^{-1}$.

40. In the following common emitter configuration an *npn* transistor with current gain $\beta = 100$ is used. The output voltage of the amplifier will be

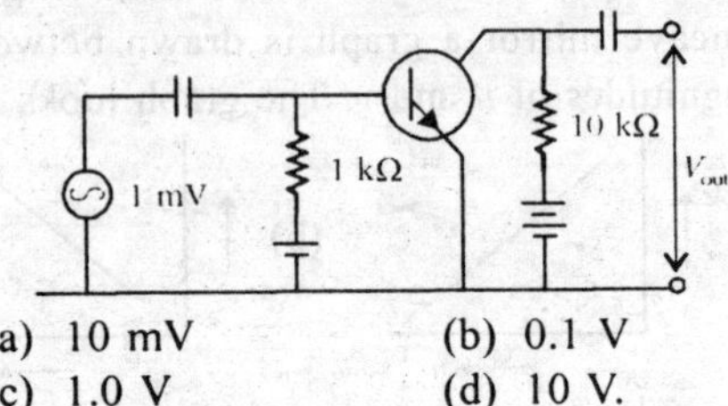

(a) 10 mV (b) 0.1 V
(c) 1.0 V (d) 10 V.

Directions for questions 41 - 60 : In the following questions a statement of assertion (A) is followed by a statement of reason (R). Of these statements, mark the correct answer:

(a) if both assertion and reason are true and the reason is the correct explanation of the assertion
(b) if both assertion and reason are true and the reason is not the correct explanation of the assertion
(c) if assertion is true but reason is false
(d) if both assertion and reason are false statements.

41. *Assertion :* Temperatures near the sea coast are moderate.
Reason : Water has a high thermal conductivity.

42. *Assertion :* The earth is slowing down and as a result the moon is coming nearer to it.
Reason : The angular momentum of the earth moon system is not conserved.

43. *Assertion :* A tube light emits white light.
Reason : Emission of light in a tube takes place at a very high temperature.

44. *Assertion :* Radioactive nuclei emit β^- particles.
Reason : Electrons exist inside the nucleus.

45. *Assertion :* The resistivity of a semiconductor increases with temperature.
Reason : The atoms of a semiconductor vibrate with larger amplitude at higher temperatures thereby increasing its resistivity.

46. *Assertion :* The Coulomb force is dominating force in the universe.
Reason : The Coulomb force is weaker than the gravitational force.

47. *Assertion :* The length of the day is slowly increasing.

Reason : The dominant effect causing a slowdown in the rotation of the earth is the gravitational pull of other planets in the solar system.

48. *Assertion :* Bohr had to postulate that the electrons in stationary orbits around the nucleus do not radiate.
Reason : According to classical physics all moving electrons radiate.

49. *Assertion :* The possibility of an electric bulb fusing is higher at the time of switching on and off.
Reason : Inductive effects produce a surge at the time of switch-off and switch-on.

50. *Assertion :* The stars twinkle while the planets do not.
Reason : The stars are much bigger in size than the planets.

51. *Assertion :* A beam of charged particles is employed in the treatment of cancer.
Reason : Charged particles on passing through a material medium lose their energy by causing ionization of the atoms along their path.

52. *Assertion :* When a beetle moves along the sand within a few tens of centimeters of a sand scorpion, the scorpion immediately turns towards the beetle and dashes towards it.
Reason : When a beetle disturbs the sand, it sends pulses along the sand's surface. One set of pulses is longitudinal while the other set is transverse.

53. *Assertion :* When a bottle of cold carbonated drink is opened, a slight fog forms around the opening.
Reason : Adiabatic expansion of the gas causes lowering of temperature and condensation of water vapours.

54. *Assertion :* The size of a hydrogen balloon increases as it rises in air.
Reason : The material of the balloon can be easily stretched.

55. *Assertion :* Owls can move freely during night.
Reason : They have large number of rods on their retina.

56. *Assertion :* It is hotter over the top of a fire than at the same distance on the sides.
Reason : Air surrounding the fire conducts more heat upwards.

57. *Assertion :* The amplitude of an oscillating pendulum decreases gradually with time.
Reason : The frequency of the pendulum decreases with time.

58. *Assertion :* Microwave communication is preferred over optical communication.
Reason : Microwaves provide large number of channels and bandwidth compared to optical signals.

59. *Assertion :* Neutrons penetrate matter more readily as compared to protons.
Reason : Neutrons are slightly more massive than protons.

60. *Assertion :* In high latitudes one sees colourful curtains of light hanging down from high altitudes.
Reason : The high energy charged particles from the sun are deflected to polar regions by the magnetic field of the earth.

CHEMISTRY

61. The paramagnetic species is
(a) KO_2 (b) SiO_2
(c) TiO_2 (d) BaO_2.

62. The reagent commonly used to determine hardness of water titrimetrically is
(a) oxalic acid
(b) disodium salt of EDTA
(c) sodium citrate (d) sodium thiosulphate.

63. The true statement for the acids of phosphorus, H_3PO_2, H_3PO_3 and H_3PO_4 is
(a) the order of their acidity is $H_3PO_4 > H_3PO_3 > H_3PO_2$
(b) all of them are reducing in nature
(c) all of them are tribasic acids
(d) the geometry of phosphorus is tetrahedral in all the three.

64. The ion which is not tetrahedral in shape is
(a) BF_4^- (b) NH_4^+
(c) $Cu(NH_3)_4^{2+}$ (d) $NiCl_4^{2-}$.

65. The complex used as an anti-cancer agent is
(a) *mer*-$[Co(NH_3)_3Cl_3]$ (b) *cis*-$[PtCl_2(NH_3)_2]$
(c) *cis*-$K_2[PtCl_2Br_2]$ (d) $Na_2[CoCl_4]$.

66. The colourless species is
(a) VCl_3 (b) $VOSO_4$

(c) Na_3VO_4
(d) $[V(H_2O)_6]SO_4 \cdot H_2O$.

67. MnO_4^{2-} (1 mole) in neutral aqueous medium is disproportionated to
(a) 2/3 mole of MnO_4^- and 1/3 mole of MnO_2
(b) 1/3 mole of MnO_4^- and 2/3 mole of MnO_2
(c) 1/3 mole of Mn_2O_7 and 1/3 mole of MnO_2
(d) 2/3 mole of Mn_2O_7 and 1/3 mole of MnO_2.

68. Lanthanide for which +II and +III oxidation states are common is
(a) La (b) Nd
(c) Ce (d) Eu.

69. The mixture of concentrated HCl and HNO_3 made in 3 : 1 ratio contains
(a) ClO_2 (b) NOCl
(c) NCl_3 (d) N_2O_4.

70. On dissolving moderate amount of sodium metal in liquid NH_3 at low temperature, which one of the following does not occur?
(a) blue coloured solution is obtained
(b) Na^+ ions are formed in the solution
(c) liquid NH_3 becomes good conductor of electricity
(d) liquid ammonia remains diamagnetic.

71. The ligand called π acid is
(a) CO (b) NH_3
(c) $C_2O_4^{2-}$ (d) ethylene diamine.

72. The compound used for gravimetric estimation of copper(II) is
(a) $Cu_2(SCN)_2$ (b) Cu_2O
(c) Cu_2I_2 (d) Cu_2CO_3.

73. In the extraction of copper from sulphide ore the metal is formed by reduction of Cu_2O with
(a) FeS (b) CO
(c) Cu_2S (d) SO_2.

74. Among the following the strongest acid is
(a) CH_3COOH (b) C_6H_5COOH
(c) *m*-$CH_3OC_6H_4COOH$
(d) *p*-$CH_3OC_6H_4COOH$.

75. Among the following the weakest base is
(a) $C_6H_5CH_2NH_2$ (b) $C_6H_5CH_2NHCH_3$
(c) $O_2NCH_2NH_2$ (d) CH_3NHCHO.

76. IUPAC name of [cyclohexene ring with CH_3] is
(a) 3-methyl cyclohexene
(b) 1-methyl cyclohex-2-ene
(c) 6-methyl cyclohexene
(d) 1-methyl cyclohex-5-ene.

77. Intermolecular hydrogen bonding is strongest in
(a) methylamine (b) phenol
(c) formaldehyde (d) methanol.

78. The *ortho/para* directing group among the following is
(a) COOH (b) CN
(c) $COCH_3$ (d) $NHCOCH_3$.

79. The treatment of benzene with isobutene in the presence of sulphuric acid gives
(a) *iso*-butyl benzene (b) *tert*-butyl benzene
(c) *n*-butyl benzene (d) no reaction.

80. The most reactive nucleophile among the following is
(a) CH_3O^- (b) $C_6H_5O^-$
(c) $(CH_3)_2CHO^-$ (d) $(CH_3)_3CO^-$.

81. The absolute configuration of the following compound is

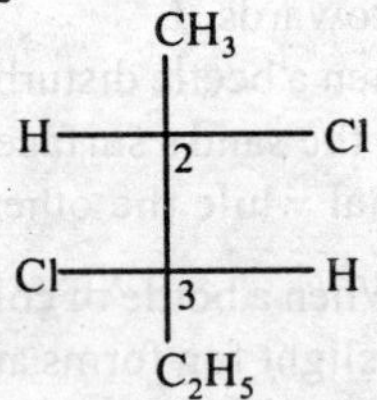

(a) 2 S, 3 R (b) 2 S, 3 S
(c) 2 R, 3 S (d) 2 R, 3 R.

82. Subunits present in haemoglobin are
(a) 2 (b) 3
(c) 4 (d) 5.

83. At higher temperature, iodoform reaction is given by
(a) $CH_3CO_2CH_3$ (b) $CH_3CO_2C_2H_5$
(c) $C_6H_5CO_2CH_3$ (d) $CH_3CO_2C_6H_5$.

84. Among the following, the achiral amino acid is
(a) 2-ethylalanine (b) 2-methylglycine
(c) 2-hydroxymethyl serine
(d) tryptophan.

85. Nitrobenzene gives N-phenylhydroxylamine by
(a) Sn/HCl (b) H_2/Pd-C
(c) Zn/NaOH (d) Zn/NH_4Cl.

86. Propan-1-ol can be prepared from propene by
(a) H_2O/H_2SO_4
(b) $Hg(OAc)_2/H_2O$ followed by $NaBH_4$
(c) B_2H_6 followed by H_2O_2
(d) CH_3CO_2H/H_2SO_4.

87. Which of the following are arranged in the decreasing order of dipole moment?
(a) CH_3Cl, CH_3Br, CH_3F
(b) CH_3Cl, CH_3F, CH_3Br
(c) CH_3Br, CH_3Cl, CH_3F
(d) CH_3Br, CH_3F, CH_3Cl.

88. What is the co-ordination number of sodium in Na_2O?
(a) 6 (b) 4
(c) 8 (d) 2.

89. Which of the following compounds possesses the C – H bond with the lowest bond dissociation energy?
(a) toluene (b) benzene
(c) *n*-pentane
(d) 2,2-dimethylpropane.

90. One gram sample of NH_4NO_3 is decomposed in a bomb calorimeter. The temperature of the calorimeter increases by 6.12 K. The heat capacity of the system is 1.23 kJ/g/deg. What is the molar heat of decomposition for NH_4NO_3?
(a) – 7.53 kJ/mol (b) – 398.1 kJ/mol
(c) – 16.1 kJ/mol (d) – 602 kJ/mol.

91. Which one of the statements given below concerning properties of solutions, describes a colligative effect?
(a) Boiling point of pure water decreases by the addition of ethanol.
(b) Vapour pressure of pure water decreases by the addition of nitric acid.
(c) Vapour pressure of pure benzene decreases by the addition of naphthalene.
(d) Boiling point of pure benzene increases by the addition of toluene.

92. Which of the following reactions is used to make a fuel cell?
(a) $Cd_{(s)} + 2Ni(OH)_{3\,(s)} \rightarrow CdO_{(s)} + 2Ni(OH)_{2\,(s)} + H_2O_{(l)}$
(b) $Pb_{(s)} + PbO_{2\,(s)} + 2H_2SO_{4\,(aq)} \rightarrow 2PbSO_{4\,(s)} + 2H_2O_{(l)}$
(c) $2H_{2\,(g)} + O_{2\,(g)} \rightarrow 2H_2O_{(l)}$
(d) $2Fe_{(s)} + O_{2\,(g)} + 4H^+_{(aq)} \rightarrow 2Fe^{2+}_{(aq)} + 2H_2O_{(l)}$.

93. Which one of the following is not a buffer solution?
(a) 0.8M H_2S + 0.8M KHS
(b) 2M $C_6H_5NH_2$ + 2M $C_6H_5NH_3^+Br^-$
(c) 3M H_2CO_3 + 3M $KHCO_3$
(d) 0.05M $KClO_4$ + 0.05M $HClO_4$.

94. Which one of the following has $\Delta S°$ greater than zero?
(a) $CaO_{(s)} + CO_{2\,(g)} \rightleftharpoons CaCO_{3\,(s)}$
(b) $NaCl_{(aq)} \rightleftharpoons NaCl_{(s)}$
(c) $NaNO_{3\,(s)} \rightleftharpoons Na^+_{(aq)} + NO_3^-{}_{(aq)}$
(d) $N_{2\,(g)} + 3H_{2\,(g)} \rightleftharpoons 2NH_{3\,(g)}$.

95. The quantum number *m* of a free gaseous atom is associated with
(a) the effective volume of the orbital
(b) the shape of the orbital
(c) the spatial orientation of the orbital
(d) the energy of the orbital in the absence of a magnetic field.

96. Which one of the following is not a surfactant?
(a) $CH_3-(CH_2)_{15}-\overset{\overset{\large CH_3}{|}}{\underset{\underset{\large CH_3}{|}}{N^+}}-CH_3Br^-$
(b) $CH_3-(CH_2)_{14}-CH_2-NH_2$
(c) $CH_3-(CH_2)_{16}-CH_2OSO_2^-Na^+$
(d) $OHC-(CH_2)_{14}-CH_2-COO^-Na^+$.

97. Time required to deposit one millimole of aluminium metal by the passage of 9.65 amperes through aqueous solution of aluminium ion is
(a) 30 s (b) 10 s
(c) 30,000 s (d) 10,000 s.

98. In which of the following acid-base titration, pH is greater than 8 at equivalence point?
(a) acetic acid versus ammonia
(b) acetic acid versus sodium hydroxide
(c) hydrochloric acid versus ammonia
(d) hydrochloric acid versus sodium hydroxide.

99. Which of the following is not a green house gas?
(a) carbon dioxide (b) water vapour
(c) methane (d) oxygen.

100. The potential energy diagram for a reaction $R \rightarrow P$ is given in the figure. $\Delta H°$ of the reaction corresponds to the energy

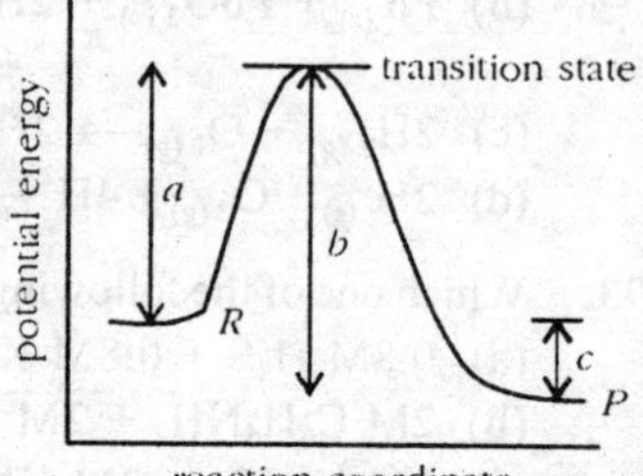

(a) a
(b) b
(c) c
(d) $a + b$.

Directions for questions 101 - 120 : In the following questions a statement of assertion (A) is followed by a statement of reason (R). Of these statements, mark the correct choice:

(a) if both assertion and reason are true and the reason is the correct explanation of the assertion
(b) if both assertion and reason are true and the reason is not the correct explanation of the assertion
(c) if assertion is true but reason is false
(d) if both assertion and reason are false.

101. *Assertion :* Solution of Na_2CrO_4 in water is intensely coloured.
Reason : Oxidation state of Cr in Na_2CrO_4 is +VI.

102. *Assertion :* NF_3 is a weaker ligand than $N(CH_3)_3$.
Reason : NF_3 ionizes to give F^- ions in aqueous solution.

103. *Assertion :* PbI_4 is a stable compound.
Reason : Iodide stabilizes higher oxidation state.

104. *Assertion :* $^{22}_{11}Na$ emits a positron giving $^{22}_{12}Mg$.
Reason : In β^+ emission neutron is transformed into proton.

105. *Assertion :* Barium is not required for normal biological function in human.
Reason : Barium does not show variable oxidation state.

106. *Assertion :* Haemoglobin is an oxygen carrier.
Reason : Oxygen binds as O_2^- to Fe of haemoglobin.

107. *Assertion :* Glycosides are hydrolysed in acidic conditions.
Reason : Glycosides are acetals.

108. *Assertion :* Benzyl bromide when kept in acetone water it produces benzyl alcohol.
Reason : The reaction follows S_N2 mechanism.

109. *Assertion :* Activity of an enzyme is pH dependent.
Reason : Change in pH affects the solubility of the enzyme in water.

110. *Assertion :* Alkyl benzene is not prepared by Friedel-Crafts alkylation of benzene.
Reason : Alkyl halides are less reactive than acyl halides.

111. *Assertion :* Hydroxyketones are not directly used in Grignard reaction.
Reason : Grignard reagents react with hydroxyl group.

112. *Assertion :* *Trans*-2-butene on reaction with Br_2 gives *meso*-2,3-dibromobutane.
Reason : The reaction involves *syn* -addition of bromine.

113. *Assertion :* *Cis*-1,3-dihydroxycyclohexane exists in boat conformation.
Reason : In the chair form, there will not be hydrogen bonding between the two hydroxyl groups.

114. *Assertion :* The increase in internal energy (ΔE) for the vapourization of one mole of water at 1 atm and 373 K is zero.
Reason : For all isothermal processes, $\Delta E = 0$.

115. *Assertion :* $BaCO_3$ is more soluble in HNO_3 than in plain water.
Reason : Carbonate is a weak base and reacts with the H^+ from the strong acid, causing the barium salt to dissociate.

116. *Assertion :* ΔH and ΔE are almost the same for the reaction, $N_{2(g)} + O_{2(g)} \rightleftharpoons 2NO_{(g)}$.
Reason : All reactants and products are gases.

117. *Assertion :* Photochemical smog is produced by nitrogen oxides.
Reason : Vehicular pollution is a major source of nitrogen oxides.

118. *Assertion :* Increasing pressure on pure water decreases its freezing point.
Reason : Density of water is minimum at 273 K.

119. *Assertion :* The micelle formed by sodium stearate in water has $-COO^-$ groups at the surface.

Reason : Surface tension of water is reduced by the addition of stearate.

120. *Assertion* : The O – O bond length in H_2O_2 is shorter than that of O_2F_2.
Reason : H_2O_2 is an ionic compound.

BIOLOGY

121. The crystal of lead zirconate is a key component of :
(a) electroencephalography
(b) electrocardiography
(c) magnetoencephalography
(d) sonography.

122. Which one of the following is a matching pair of a certain body feature and its value/count in a normal human adult?
(a) urea - 5-10 mg/100 ml of blood
(b) blood sugar (fasting) - 80-100 mg/100 ml
(c) total blood volume - 3 - 4 litres
(d) ESR in Wintrobe method - 9-15 mm in males and 20-34 mm in females.

123. Which one of the following pairs of terms / names mean one and the same thing?
(a) gene pool - genome
(b) codon - gene (c) cistron - triplet
(d) DNA fingerprinting - DNA profiling.

124. Which one of the following is a matching pair?
(a) Lubb - sharp closure of AV valves at the beginning of ventricular systole
(b) Dup - sudden opening of semilunar valves at the beginning of ventricular diastole
(c) Pulsation of the radial artery - valves in the blood vessels
(d) Initiation of the heart beat - Purkinje fibres.

125. Mr. X is eating curd/yoghurt. For this food intake in a food chain he should be considered as occupying:
(a) first trophic level (b) second trophic level
(c) third trophic level (d) fourth trophic level.

126. July 11 is observed as:
(a) World population day
(b) No tobacco day
(c) World environment day
(d) World health day.

127. Biological Oxygen Demand (BOD) is a measure of:
(a) industrial wastes poured into water bodies
(b) extent to which water is polluted with organic compounds
(c) amount of carbon monoxide inseparably combined with haemoglobin
(d) amount of oxygen needed by green plants during night.

128. Which one of the following is a sesamoid bone?
(a) pelvis (b) patella
(c) pterygoid (d) pectoral girdle.

129. Both corpus luteum and macula lutea are:
(a) found in human ovaries
(b) a source of hormones
(c) characterized by a yellow colour
(d) contributory in maintaining pregnancy.

130. Photorespiration in C_3 plants starts from:
(a) phosphoglycerate (b) phosphoglycolate
(c) glycerate (d) glycine.

131. Just as *Xenopsylla* is to *Yersenia pestis*, so is:
(a) *Glossina palpalis* to *Wuchereria bancrofti*
(b) *Culex* to *Plasmodium falciparum*
(c) *Homo sapiens* to *Taenia solium*
(d) *Phlebotomus* to *Leishmania donovani*.

132. Continued consumption of a diet rich in butter, red meat and eggs for a long period may lead to:
(a) vitamin toxicity (b) kidney stones
(c) hypercholesterolemia
(d) urine laden with ketone bodies.

133. Drinking of mineral water with very low level of pesticides (about 0.02 ppm) for long periods may:
(a) produce immunity against mosquito
(b) cause leukemia (blood cancer) in most people
(c) cause cancer of the intestine
(d) lead to accumulation of pesticide residues in body fat.

134. A person passes much urine and drinks much water but his blood glucose level is normal. This condition may be the result of :
(a) a reduction in insulin secretion from pancreas
(b) a reduction in vasopressin secretion from posterior pituitary
(c) a fall in the glucose concentration in urine
(d) an increase in secretion of glucagon.

135. What is true about *t*RNA?
(a) it binds with an amino acid at it 3′ end

(b) it has five double stranded regions
(c) it has a codon at one end which recognizes the anticodon on messenger RNA .
(d) it looks like clover leaf in the three dimensional structure.

136. An example of competitive inhibition of an enzyme is the inhibition of:
(a) succinic dehydrogenase by malonic acid
(b) cytochrome oxidase by cyanide
(c) hexokinase by glucose-6-phosphate
(d) carbonic anhydrase by carbon dioxide.

137. Which one of the following is a matching pair of certain organism(s) and the kind of association?
(a) shark and sucker fish - commensalism
(b) algae and fungi in lichens - mutualism
(c) orchids growing on trees - parasitism
(d) cuscuta (dodder) growing in other flowering plants - epiphytism.

138. Photochemical smog formed in congested metropolitan cities mainly consists of :
(a) ozone, peroxyacetyl nitrate and NO_x
(b) smoke, peroxyacetyl nitrate and SO_2
(c) hydrocarbons, SO_2 and CO_2
(d) hydrocarbons, ozone and SO_x.

139. In almost all Indian metropolitan cities like Delhi, the major atmospheric pollutant(s) is/are:
(a) suspended particulate matter (SPM)
(b) oxides of sulphur
(c) carbon dioxide and carbon monoxide
(d) oxides of nitrogen.

140. Excessive stimulation of vagus nerve in humans may lead to:
(a) hoarse voice (b) peptic ulcers
(c) efficient digestion of proteins
(d) irregular contractions of diaphragm.

141. Restriction enzymes:
(a) are endonucleases which cleave DNA at specific sites
(b) make DNA complementary to an existing DNA or RNA
(c) cut or join DNA fragments
(d) are required in vectorless direct gene transfer.

142. The map given below indicates the former and the present distribution of an animal:
Which animal could it be:
(a) Wild ass
(b) Nilgai
(c) Black buck
(d) Lion.

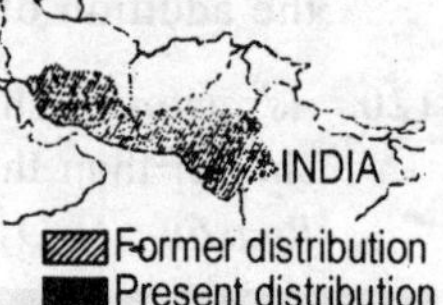

143. Which one of the following correctly represents the manner of replication of DNA?

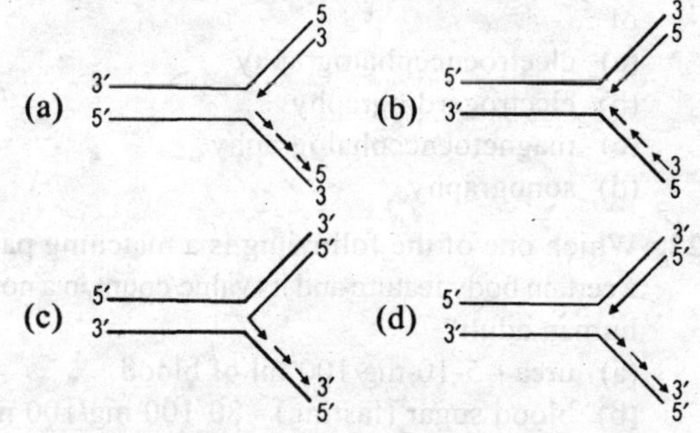

144. Which one of the following codons codes for the same information as UGC?
(a) UGU (b) UGA
(c) UAG (d) UGG.

145. A person is wearing spectacles with concave lenses for correcting vision. While not using the glasses, the image of a distant object in his case will be formed:
(a) on the blind spot (b) behind the retina
(c) in front of the retina (d) on the yellow spot.

146. The early stage human embryo distinctly possesses :
(a) gills (b) gill slits
(c) external ear (pinna) (d) eye brows.

147. The phase of menstrual cycle in humans that last for 7-8 days, is:
(a) follicular phase (b) ovulatory phase
(c) luteal phase (d) menstruation.

148. The source of somatostatin is same as that of:
(a) thyroxine and calcitonin
(b) insulin and glucagon
(c) somatotropin and prolactin
(d) vasopresin and oxytocin.

149. People recovering from long illness are often advised to include the alga *Spirulina* in their diet because it:
(a) makes the food easy to digest

(b) is rich in proteins
(c) has antibiotic properties
(d) restores the intestinal microflora.

150. Viroids have:
(a) single stranded RNA not enclosed by protein coat
(b) single stranded DNA not enclosed by protein coat
(c) double stranded DNA enclosed by protein coat
(d) double stranded RNA enclosed by protein coat.

151. In a dicotyledonous stem, the sequence of tissues from the outside to the inside is:
(a) phellem - pericycle - endodermis - phloem
(b) phellem - phloem - endodermis - pericycle
(c) phellem - endodermis - pericycle - phloem
(d) pericycle - phellem - endodermis - phloem.

152. Hill reaction occurs in:
(a) high altitude plants (b) total darkness
(c) absence of water
(d) presence of ferricyanide.

153. Which one of the following pairs is correctly matched:
(a) *Rhizobium* - Parasite in the roots of leguminous plants
(b) Mycorrhizae - Mineral uptake from soil
(c) Yeast - Production of biogas
(d) Myxomycetes - The disease ring worm.

154. Pollen grains are able to withstand extremes of temperature and dessication because their exine is composed of:
(a) cutin (b) suberin
(c) sporopollenin (d) callose.

155. One of the genes present exclusively on the X-chromosome in humans is concerned with
(a) baldness
(b) red-green colour blindness
(c) facial hair/moustaches in males
(d) night blindness.

156. Which one of the following statements with regard to embryonic development in humans is correct?
(a) cleavage divisions bring about considerable increase in the mass of protoplasm
(b) in the second cleavage division, one of the two blastomeres usually divides a little sooner than the second
(c) with more cleavage divisions, the resultant blastomeres become larger and larger
(d) cleavage division results in a hollow ball of cells called morula.

157. Plasmodesmata connections help in:
(a) cytoplasmic streaming
(b) synchronous mitotic divisions
(c) locomotion of unicellular organism
(d) movement of substances between cells.

158. The quiescent centre in root meristem serves as a
(a) site for storage of food which is utilized during maturation
(b) reservoir of growth hormones
(c) reserve for replenishment of damaged cells of the meristem
(d) region for absorption of water.

159. *Azolla* is used as a biofertilizer because it
(a) multiplies very fast to produce massive biomass
(b) has association of nitrogen - fixing *Rhizobium*
(c) has association of nitrogen - fixing cyanobacteria
(d) has association of mycorrhiza.

160. The plant part which consists of two generations, one within the other, is:
(a) germinated pollen grain (b) embryo
(c) unfertilized ovule (d) seed.

Directions for questions 161 - 180 : In the following questions, a statement of assertion (A) is followed by a statement of reason (R).
(a) *If both Assertion and Reason are true and the reason is the correct explanation of the assertion, then mark (a)*
(b) *If both Assertion and Reason are true but the reason is not the correct explanation of the assertion, then mark (b)*
(c) *If Assertion is true statement but Reason is false, then mark (c)*
(d) *if both Assertion and Reason are false statements, then mark (d).*

161. *Assertion* : Mast cells in the human body release excessive amounts of inflammatory chemicals which cause allergic reactions.
Reason : Allergens in the environment on reaching human body stimulate mast cells in certain individuals.

162. *Assertion* : Use of fertilizers greatly enhances crop productivity.
Reason : Irrigation is very important in increasing crop productivity.

163. *Assertion* : Smaller the organism higher is the rate

of metabolism per gram weight.
Reason : The heart rate of a six month old baby is much higher than that of an old person.

164. *Assertion* : Bats and whales are classified as mammals.
Reason : Bats and whales have four-chambered heart.

165. *Assertion* : Severe Acute Respiratory Syndrome (SARS) originated in China.
Reason : China is the most populated country of the world.

166. *Assertion* : Organochlorine pesticides are organic compounds that have been chlorinated.
Reason : Fenitrothion is one of the organochlorine pesticides.

167. *Assertion* : Holoblastic cleavage with almost equal-sized blastomeres is a characteristic of placental animals.
Reason : Eggs of most mammals, including humans, are of centrolecithal type.

168. *Assertion* : Inhabitants close to very busy airports are likely to experience health hazards.
Reason : Sound level of jet aeroplanes usually exceeds 160 dB.

169. *Assertion* : All birds, except the ones like koel (cuckoo) build nests for retiring and taking rest during night time (day time for nocutrnal)
Reason : Koel lays its eggs in the nests of tailor bird.

170. *Assertion* : Old age is not an illness. It is a continuation of life with decreasing capacity for adaptation.
Reason : Cessation of mitosis is a normal genetically programmed event.

171. *Assertion* : A cell membrane shows fluid behaviour.
Reason : A membrane is a mosaic or composite of diverse lipids and proteins.

172. *Assertion* : In plant tissue culture, somatic embryos can be induced from any plant cell.
Reason : Any viable plant cell can differentiate into somatic embryos.

173. *Assertion* : *Rhoeo* leaves contain anthocyanin pigments in epidermal cells.
Reason : Anthocyanins are accessory photosynthetic pigments.

174. *Assertion* : Water and mineral uptake by root hairs from the soil occurs through apoplast until it reaches endodermis.
Reason : Casparian strips in endodermis are suberized.

175. *Assertion* : Long distance flow of photoassimilates in plants occurs through sieve tubes.
Reason : Mature sieve tubes have parietal cytoplasm and perforated sieve plates.

176. *Assertion* : Many visitors to the hills suffer from skin and respiratory allergy problem.
Reason : Conifer trees produce a large quantity of wind-borne pollen grains.

177. *Assertion* : Yeasts such as *Saccharomyces cerevisiae* are used in baking industry.
Reason : Carbon dioxide produced during fermentation causes bread dough to rise by thermal expansion.

178. *Assertion* : In a food chain members of successive higher levels are fewer in number.
Reason : Number of organisms at any trophic level depends upon the availability of organisms which serve as food at the lower level.

179. *Assertion* : Tropical rain forests are disappearing fastly from developing countries such as India.
Reason : No value is attached to these forests because these are poor in biodiversity.

180. *Assertion* : Leaf butterfly and stick insect show mimicry to dodge their enemies.
Reason : Mimicry is a method to acquire body colour blending with the surroundings.

GENERAL KNOWLEDGE

181. Euthanasia (mercy killing) was first legalized in :
(a) Switzerland
(b) Netherland (Holland)
(c) France (d) Italy.

182. Positron emission tomography (PET) is one of the best methods for functional imaging because :
(a) isotopes of basic body elements are used for imaging
(b) isotopes with long half-lives are used
(c) isotopes with short half-lives are used
(d) positrons are directly involved used in imaging.

183. Magnetic resonance (MR) images are derived from the proton-bearing species present principally from water and :

(a) long alkane chain protons of the fatty acid moieties
(b) short alkane chain protons of the fatty acid moieties
(c) long alkene chain protons of the fatty acid moieties
(d) short alkene chain protons of the fatty acid moieties.

184. The following separation technique depends on the molecular size of the protein:
(a) chromatography on a carboxymethyl (CM) cellulose column
(b) iso-electric focusing
(c) gel filtration chromatography
(d) chromatography on a diethylaminoethyl (DEAE) cellulose column.

185. The approximate number of genes contained in the genome of Kalpana Chawla was:
(a) 40,000 (b) 30,000
(c) 80,000 (d) 1,00,000.

186. In internet what does 'http' mean?
(a) High Transfer Text Protocol
(b) Highest Transfer Text Protocol
(c) Hyper Text Transfer Protocol
(d) Hyper Transfer Text Protocol.

187. The Indian-born US physicist who was awarded the Nobel Prize in Physics for his work on astrophysics is:
(a) H.G. Khorana
(b) Subramanyam Chandrasekhar
(c) Sivaramakrishna Chandrasekhar
(d) C.V. Raman.

188. Which German physicist invented the electron microscope which won him the 1986 Nobel Prize in Physics ?
(a) Ernst Ruska (b) Van't Hoff
(c) J.H.D. Jensen (d) Eugene P. Wigner.

189. Who was the first Indian to be awarded the World Food Prize in 1987?
(a) M.S. Swaminathan (b) Sunderlal Bahuguna
(c) Anna Hazare (d) B.R. Barwale.

190. Thantology is the science that deals with:
(a) death in all its aspects
(b) solving paternity of child
(c) identification of living
(d) detection of lie.

191. What is the disease, Tetanus also known as?
(a) Gangrene (b) Shingles
(c) Lockjaw (d) Whooping cough.

192. When seen from earth, which of the following planet eclipsed (crossed a cross) of the sun on May 7, 2003?
(a) Mercury (b) Uranus
(c) Saturn (d) Jupiter.

193. Israel's Prime Minister Yitshak Rabin won the Nobel Prize for:
(a) peace (b) literature
(c) chemistry (d) economics.

194. Who was the world's first space tourist?
(a) Desmond Rickett (b) Dennis Tito
(c) Igor Kajelinkov (d) Li Wang.

195. Which city was gifted to Charles II by the Portuguese when he married the sister of the King of Portugal in 1662?
(a) Mumbai (b) Paris
(c) Lisbon (d) Castille.

196. How many "World Cultural Heritage Sites" are there in India?
(a) 10 (b) 17
(c) 14 (d) 15.

197. Who is the mother of Bharat in the epic Ramayana?
(a) Kaushalya (b) Sumitra
(c) Urmila (d) Kaikayee.

198. Which is the 'Nawab of Bengal' is supposed to be responsible for 'Black Hole' of Calcutta (Kolkatta)?
(a) Mir Jafer (b) Sirajuddaula
(c) Alivardi Khan (d) Sarfaraj Khan.

199. In which country the 'Dogs' were once worshipped as 'Gods'?
(a) Egypt (b) Greece
(c) Italy (d) Mangolia.

200. From which of the following places the international dateline crosses:
(a) Atlantic ocean (b) Pacific ocean
(c) Greenwich (d) Cape of Good Hope.

❖❖❖

SOLUTIONS

PHYSICS

1. **(b) :** For a projectile to leave the gravitational field of the earth, its kinetic energy would be at least equal to its potential energy. That is

$$\frac{1}{2}mv_e^2 = G\frac{Mm}{R} \Rightarrow v_e = \sqrt{\frac{2GM}{R}}$$

where G is the universal gravitational constant, M is the mass of the earth and R is the radius of the earth. Hence the escape velocity of a projectile is independent of its own mass.

2. **(a)**

3. **(d) :** As the laser beam is highly monochromatic, directional and coherent, it can be sharply focused and that is why it is used for carrying out surgery.

4. **(d) :** Let the original diameter of the wire be D. Therefore the new diameter is $D/2$.

Original area of cross-section is $\frac{\pi D^2}{4}$

and the final area of cross-section is $\frac{\pi D^2}{16}$

The new length of the wire is given by

$$L \times \frac{\pi D^2}{4} = L' \times \frac{\pi D^2}{16} \Rightarrow L' = \frac{16}{4}L = 4L$$

Now, we know that the resistance is given by $R = \rho\frac{L}{A}$.

$$\therefore \quad R' = \rho\frac{L'}{A'} = \rho\frac{4L}{A/4} = 16R.$$

$$\left[\because A' = \frac{\pi D^2}{16} = \frac{A}{4}\right]$$

$$\therefore \quad R' = 16 \times 10 = 160\ \Omega.$$

5. **(c) :** The charge on a proton is equal to e, the electronic charge. The potential difference is $V = 1$ kV. Hence the kinetic energy of the proton is $E = 1$ keV.

6. **(a) :** If an electric dipole is placed in a non-uniform electric field, then the positive and the negative charges of the dipole will experience a net force. And as one end of the dipole is experiencing a force in one direction and the other end in the opposite direction, so the dipole will have a net torque also.

7. **(d) :** When the capacitor is connected to a d.c. source and then disconnected, it gets charged and then it starts discharging through the inductor. An induced emf is produced in the circuit which opposes the growth of current in L. When the capacitor is fully discharged, the electric energy stored in the capacitor (*i.e.* $1/2\, q^2/C$) gets converted fully into magnetic field energy ($1/2\, LI^2$). As soon as the discharge of the capacitor is complete, current stops and the magnetic flux linked with L starts collapsing. Therefore, an induced emf is again developed which starts recharging the capacitor in the opposite direction. When the recharging is completed, all magnetic energy stored in L appears as the electric energy between the plates of the capacitor. The entire process keeps on repeating and the energy taken from the cell keeps on oscillating between C and L. Hence the current in the circuit starts oscillating as soon as the d.c. source charging the capacitor is disconnected.

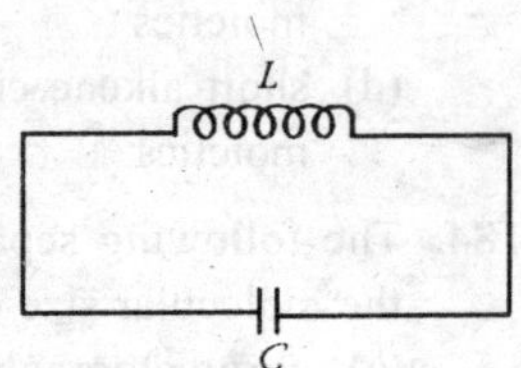

8. **(b) :** An intrinsic germanium have four outer electrons which they use to form bonds with four neighbouring Ge atoms. Gallium, being from group III is having three outer electrons. So when we add gallium atoms into germanium, some gallium atoms have a chance to replace some of the germanium atoms. But with gallium, only three neighbouring Ge atoms can make bonds with Ga. The bond with the fourth neighbouring Ge atom is broken as Ga is having a shortage of one outer electron. The broken bond can be filled up by an electron when the electron gets enough energy to jump from the valence bond creating a hole out there. So, we get a p-type semiconductor.

```
        Ge                    Ge       hole
        |                     |       o
Ge — Ge — Ge           Ge — Ga .  . Ge
        |                     |
        Ge                    Ge
```

9. **(c) :** We know that the activity of radioactive substance, $A = A_0 e^{-\lambda t}$

$\Rightarrow \frac{A}{A_0} = e^{-\lambda t} = e^{-\frac{0.693}{T^{1/2}}t} \quad \left[\because T_{1/2} = \frac{0.693}{\lambda}\right]$

$\Rightarrow \frac{1}{16} = e^{-\frac{0.693\times 40}{T^{1/2}}} \Rightarrow \frac{0.693\times 40}{T_{1/2}} = \ln 16$

$\Rightarrow T_{1/2} = \frac{0.693\times 40}{\ln 16} = 9.997 \approx 10$ days.

10. (b) : (n) ⟶ (D)

One deuteron consists of one proton and one neutron. As the mass of a proton and a neutron is approximately same ($\approx 1.67 \times 10^{-27}$ kg), we assume that the mass of the neutron be m and the mass of the deuteron be $2m$ as the electron mass is negligibly small compared to that of proton and neutron.

Let the initial velocity of the neutron be u. As the deuteron is initially at rest, the final velocity of the neutron is

$$v_1 = \left(\frac{m-2m}{m+2m}\right)u = -\frac{mu}{3m} = -\frac{u}{3}.$$

and the velocity of the deuteron is

$$v_2 = \frac{2m}{m+2m}u = \frac{2}{3}u.$$

Total energy before collision is $E_1 = \frac{1}{2}mu^2$

After collision, the energy gained by the deuteron is

$$E_d = \frac{1}{2}\times(2m)v_2^2 = m\times\left(\frac{2}{3}u\right)^2 = \frac{4}{9}mu^2.$$

E_d is the amount of energy lost by the neutron. Therefore the fractional loss of energy of the neutron is

$$\frac{E_d}{E_1} = \frac{(4/9)mu^2}{(1/2)mu^2} = \frac{8}{9}.$$

11. (c)

12. (b) : Radius of one drop of mercury is R.

$\therefore$ The volume of one drop $= \frac{4}{3}\pi R^3$

$\therefore$ Total volume of the two drops,

$$V = 2\times\frac{4}{3}\pi R^3 = \frac{8}{3}\pi R^3$$

Let the radius of the large drop formed be R'.

The volume of the large drop is also V.

$$\therefore \quad \frac{4}{3}\pi R'^3 = \frac{8}{3}\pi R^3 \Rightarrow R'^3 = 2R^3 \Rightarrow R' = 2^{1/3}R.$$

Now the surface area of the two drops is

$$S_1 = 2\times 4\pi R^2 = 8\pi R^2$$

and the surface area of the resultant drop is

$$S_2 = 4\pi R'^2 = 4\pi 2^{2/3}R^2$$

Let T be the surface tension of mercury. Therefore the surface energy of the two drops before coalescing is

$$U_1 = S_1 T = 8\pi R^2 T$$

and the surface energy after coalescing,

$$U_2 = S_2 T = 2^{2/3}\times 4\pi R^2 T$$

$$\therefore \quad \frac{U_1}{U_2} = \frac{8\pi R^2 T}{2^{2/3}\times 4\pi R^2 T} = \frac{2}{2^{2/3}} = 2^{1/3}$$

13. (c) : The temperature of the black body is

$T_1 = 227°C = 500$ K.

$\therefore$ Using Stefan's law, the rate of heat radiation per unit area per unit time is

$$E_1 = \sigma T^4 \Rightarrow 20 = \sigma(500)^4 \Rightarrow \sigma = \frac{20}{(500)^4}.$$

Now the temperature of the blackbody is raised to

$T_2 = 727°C = 1000$ K

$\therefore$ Rate of heat radiation per unit area

$$E_2 = \sigma T_2^4 = \frac{20}{(500)^4}\times(1000)^4$$

$$= 20\times 2^4 = 320 \text{ cal m}^{-2}\text{ s}^{-1}.$$

14. (c) : Let the mass m be displaced towards right by a distance x. Then the spring 1 will be extended and the spring 2 will be compressed by an amount of x each. The restoring force on mass m due to spring 1 is

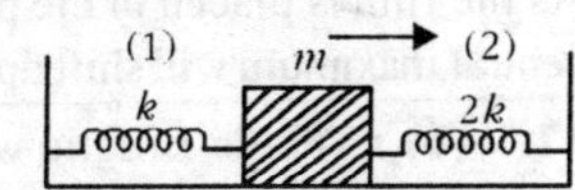

$F_1 = -kx$

And the restoring force due to spring 2 is

$F_2 = -(2k)x$

$\therefore$ Total force on the mass m is

$F = F_1 + F_2 = -kx - 2kx = -3kx$

$$\Rightarrow \quad m\frac{d^2x}{dt^2} = -3kx \Rightarrow \frac{d^2x}{dt^2} + \frac{3k}{m}x = 0$$

$$\Rightarrow \quad \frac{d^2x}{dt^2} + \omega^2 x = 0 \text{ where } \omega^2 = \frac{3k}{m} \Rightarrow \omega = \sqrt{\frac{3k}{m}}$$

$$\Rightarrow \quad f = \frac{\omega}{2\pi} = \frac{1}{2\pi}\sqrt{\frac{3k}{m}}.$$

15. (c) : For maximum accuracy in finding the position of an object using a light beam is achieved, when the light beam used is of shorter wavelength, because if the wavelength is longer, the spread in the wave will be more.

16. (c) : Wavelength $\lambda = 500$ nm $= 500 \times 10^{-9}$ m

Thickness of the film, $t = 2$ μm $= 2 \times 10^{-6}$ m

Refractive index $\mu = 1.5$

When there is no thin film placed in the path of any one of the two beams, the path difference between them is given by dy/D (considering the two beams meetings at a point P). In case we put a thin film in the path of one of the beams, then the optical path of that beam gets longer.

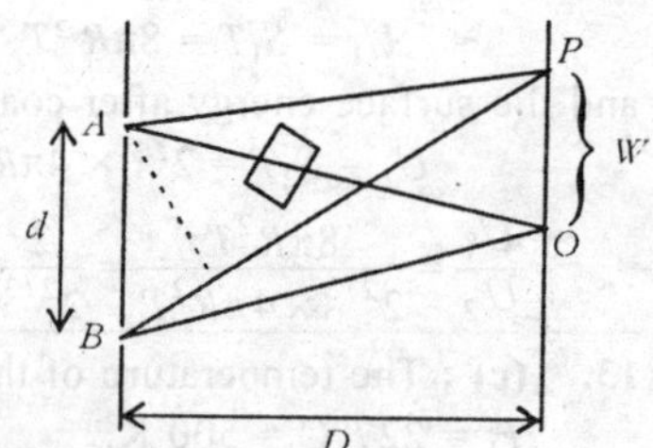

Now for the central maximum, path difference in absence of the film is $\Delta x = 0$. But when we put the film, the path difference becomes

$$\Delta x = \mu t - t = (\mu - 1)t$$
$$= (1.5 - 1) \times 2 \times 10^{-6} = 10^{-6} \text{ m} = 1 \text{ mm}.$$

Now, $\Delta x = \frac{dy}{D} \Rightarrow y = \frac{D}{d}\Delta x = \frac{D}{d} \times 1\,\mu\text{m}$

And the fringe width is given by

$$W = \frac{D\lambda}{d} = \frac{D}{d} \times 500 \times 10^{-9} \text{ m} = \frac{D}{d} \times 0.5 \times 1\,\mu\text{m}$$

$$\therefore \quad y = \frac{D}{d} \times 1\,\mu\text{m} = 2 \times \frac{D}{d} \times \frac{1}{2} \times 1\,\mu\text{m} = 2W.$$

As the film is placed in the path of the upper beam, the central maximum will shift upward by nearly two fringes.

17. (b) : The de-Broglie wavelength of a particle or a photon is given by $\lambda = h/p$ where h is the Planck's constant and p is the momentum. As the electron and the photon are having the same wavelength λ, the momentum of both of them will be the same.

18. (b) : When the high energy electron hits the target and takes out an electron from the inner orbit, there is a possibility of an outer electron to fall down to fill up that vacancy. And when such a transition of electron takes place from a higher energy level to a lower energy level, the difference of energy between the two levels is given off in the form of radiation known as characteristic X-rays.

19. (c) : The force experienced by A due to B is

$$F_1 = \frac{1}{4\pi\varepsilon_0}\frac{QQ}{a^2} \text{ along } \overline{AB} \text{ (attractive)}$$

The force experienced by A due to C is

$$F_2 = \frac{1}{4\pi\varepsilon_0}\frac{Q^2}{a^2} \text{ along}$$

$\overline{CA}$ produced (repulsive)

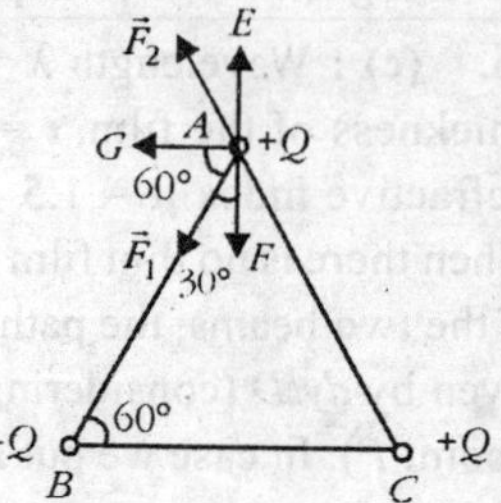

Now the force $\vec{F}_1$ is having a component $F_1 \cos 30°$ along and the force $\vec{F}_2$ is having a component $F_2 \cos 30°$ along $\overline{AE}$. $\overline{AE}$ and $\overline{AF}$ are both normal to $\overline{BC}$ but they are mutually opposite to each other. And as $|\vec{F}_1| = |\vec{F}_2|$, so the forces along $\overline{AE}$ and $\overline{AF}$ will both cancel each other. And so the force experienced by the charge at A in the direction normal to $\overline{BC}$ is zero.

20. (c) : $X_C = \frac{1}{\omega C} = \frac{1}{2\pi f C}$

$$= \frac{1}{2 \times 3.14 \times 1 \times 10^3 \times 2 \times 10^{-6}} = \frac{10^3}{4 \times 3.14}$$

Voltage, $V = i \times X_C = 2 \times 10^{-3} \times \frac{10^{-3}}{4 \times 3.14} = 0.16$ V.

21. (b) : The magnetic field at the centre of a circular loop carrying current I is given by $B = \frac{m_0 I}{2r}$ where r is the radius of the circular loop.

Given that $r = 5.0$ cm $= 0.05$ m.

Now, $B = \frac{\mu_0 I}{2r} = 0.5 \times 10^{-5}$

$$\Rightarrow \quad I = \frac{0.5 \times 10^{-5} \times 2 \times 0.05}{\mu_0} = \frac{0.5 \times 10^{-5} \times 0.1}{4\pi \times 10^{-7}}$$

$= 0.3978 \approx 0.4$ Å.

22. (a) : In the presence of an external magnetic field, the atomic dipoles of paramagnetic substances are aligned along the field. The material gets magnetised and it produces an extra magnetic field in the material in the direction of the field. So for paramagnetic materials, the resultant field is greater than the applied field. As the body of a frog behaves like a paramagnetic substance, the smallest magnetic field on the body of the frog will be strong enough to lift it up.

23. (c) : From Wien's displacement law, we know that, $\lambda_m T =$ constant

which means that as temperature increases then the wavelength having the maximum intensity shifts towards left. Here, $T_2 > T_1$.

$$\therefore \quad \lambda_{m_{T_2}} < \lambda_{m_{T_1}}$$

But in plot (a) $\lambda_{m_{T_2}} = \lambda_{m_{T_1}}$, in plot (b) $\lambda_{m_{T_2}} > \lambda_{m_{T_1}}$ and in plot (d) $\lambda_{m_{T_2}} > \lambda_{m_{T_1}}$. Therefore the correct plot is (c) where $\lambda_{m_{T_2}} < \lambda_{m_{T_1}}$.

24. (d) : According to Gauss's law, the total electric flux through a closed surface is given by

$$\phi = \oint_s \vec{E}\cdot d\vec{s} = \frac{Q}{\varepsilon_0}$$

where Q is the total charge enclosed by the surface. The total charge enclosed by the given surface is $Q = +q - q = 0$. $\therefore$ The total flux $\phi = 0$.

25. **(c)**

26. **(a) :** Nuclear fusion is possible only between light nuclei. The nuclear process of two light nuclei getting close enough to produce a larger nucleus is energetically favourable reaction.

27. **(b) :** We know that the force on a charged particle e due to a magnetic field is given by

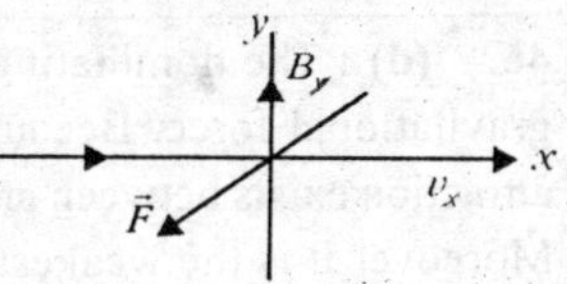

$\vec{F} = e(\vec{v}\times\vec{B})$

Here $\vec{v} = v_x = \hat{i}$ and $\vec{B} = B_y\hat{j}$

$\therefore \quad \vec{F} = ev_x B_y(\hat{i}\times\hat{j}) = ev_x B_y\hat{k}$

Therefore the subsequent motion of the charged particle will be a circle in the xz plane.

28. **(b) :** The sidereal day is about 4 min shorter than our normal solar 24-hour day, to be precise, the difference is 3 min 56 seconds.

29. **(b) :** For a body moving with constant acceleration a, $v = u + at$

Since the body starts from rest, $u = 0$

$\therefore \quad v = at$

which is a straight line passing through the origin. Hence the correct graph is (b).

30. **(b) :** As two like currents attract and unlike currents repel each other, the wire will attract the side A of the loop near the wire and parallel to it and the far side of the loop again parallel to the wire will be repelled. But the force of attraction will be more as that side of the loop is closer to the wire and so effectively the current loop will more towards the wire.

31. **(d) :** During the upward motion the speed of body decreases and will be zero at the highest point (since gravitational force acting downward), afterward the body start downward motion and its speed increases.

32. **(c)** **33.** **(d)**

34. **(c) :** The resolving power of the eye is given by

$R = 1.22\frac{\lambda}{b}\times D$

where λ is the wavelength of light, b is the diameter of the eye lens and D is the distance from the lens at which light is focused.

$D = 400$ km $= 400000$ m, $d = 5$ mm $= 5\times10^{-3}$ m

$\lambda = 500$ nm $= 500\times10^{-9}$ m

$$\therefore \quad R = 1.22\times\frac{500\times10^{-9}\times4\times10^{5}}{5\times10^{-3}} = 48.8 \approx 50 \text{ m.}$$

35. **(c) :** Velocity of the S waves is $v_1 = 4.5$ km/s. The velocity of the P waves is $v_2 = 8.0$ km/s.

Let the time taken by the S and P waves to reach the seismograph be t_1 and t_2. It is given that

$t_1 - t_2 = 4$ min $= 4\times60 = 240$ sec ... (i)

Let the distance of the epicentre (km) be S. Then

$S = v_1t_1 = v_2t_2$

$\Rightarrow \quad 4.5\times t_1 - 8t_2 = 0 \Rightarrow t_2 = \frac{4.5}{8}t_1$ ... (ii)

Using (i) and (ii)

$t_1 - t_2 = 240 \Rightarrow t_1\left(1-\frac{4.5}{8}\right) = 240$

$\Rightarrow \quad t_1 = \frac{240\times8}{3.5} = 548.5$ s.

$\therefore \quad S = v_1t_1 = 4.5\times548.5 = 2468.6 \approx 2500$ km.

36. **(a) :** Initially due to the action of gravity, the lead shot will move with increasing velocity for some time. Then due to the viscosity of the glycerine column, the lead shot will attain a constant terminal velocity. As initially, there is some upthrust on the shot due to glycerine the increase of velocity will not be fully linear. So the variation is shown by plot (a).

37. **(a) :** If the height of the antenna is h, then the maximum distance upto which the TV transmission for a TV tower can be received is proportional to $h^{1/2}$.

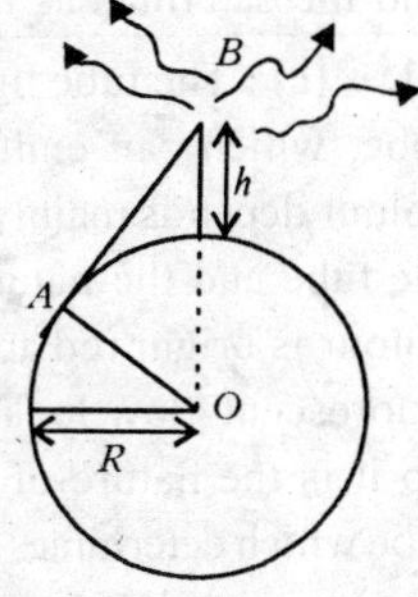

Suppose that the height of the TV antena be h and the radius of the earth be R and $R >> h$. Let A be a receiving station. In the limit $h << R$, we can assume that BA is a tangent to the surface of the earth. Then $\angle BAO = 90°$ and so

$BO^2 = AB^2 + AO^2 \Rightarrow (R+h)^2 = AB^2 + R^2$

$\Rightarrow \quad AB^2 = R^2 + h^2 + 2Rh - R^2 = 2Rh + h^2$

as $h << R$ we neglect h^2 and so

$AB^2 = 2Rh \Rightarrow AB = \sqrt{2Rh}$

$\therefore \quad AB \propto h^{1/2}$.

38. **(a) :** We know that the artificial frequency of a sky wave for reflection from an ionospheric layer of the atmosphere is given by, $\upsilon_c = 9n^{1/2}$
where n is the number density of electrons/m^3.
It is given that $n = 10^{11}/\text{m}^3$

$\therefore \quad \upsilon_c = 9 \times (10^{11})^{1/2} = 2.8 \times 10^6 \text{ Hz} = 2.8 \text{ MHz}.$

Hence the wave of frequency 2 MHz will be reflected back.

39. **(c) :** We know that the force per unit length of a wire carrying current due to another parallel wire carrying current is given by

$$\frac{dF}{dl} = \frac{\mu_0 i_1 i_2}{2\pi d} \Rightarrow \mu_0 = \frac{2\pi d}{i_1 i_2}\frac{dF}{dl}$$

$$\therefore \quad [\mu_0] = \frac{[\text{L}]}{[\text{A}^2]} \cdot \frac{[\text{MLT}^{-2}]}{[\text{L}]}$$

or $[\mu_0] = [\text{MLT}^{-2}]\,[\text{A}^{-2}] = [\text{MLT}^{-2}\text{A}^{-2}]$.

40. **(c) :** We know that the output voltage is given by,

$$v_0 = v_i \times \beta \times \frac{R_L}{R_{BE}}$$

Here, $v_i = 1$ mV, $\beta = 100$

$R_L = 10\ \text{k}\Omega$, $R_{BE} = 1\ \text{k}\Omega$

$$\therefore \quad v_0 = 1 \times 10^{-3} \times 100 \times \frac{10}{1} = 1.0 \text{ V}.$$

41. **(b)**

42. **(d) :** One of the basic requirement of the existence of all planetary motions is the conservation of angular momentum. If this law is violated, then no gravitational law will be able to explain the behaviour of the planets and the satellites as they do.

43. **(c) :** The tube light is nothing but a gas discharge tube, which can emit light of different colours. This colour depends mainly upon the nature of the gas inside the tube and the nature of the glass. For neon gas the colour is bright red and for CO_2 it is bluish. Again the fluorescent glow looks yellowish green for soda glass. So it is the nature of the glass and the gas inside the tube which determines the colour of the fluorescent glow. As argon is filled inside a tube light, the colour of the light is white.

44. **(c) :** Nuclear stability depends upon the ratio of neutron to proton. If the n/p ratio is more than the critical value, then a neutron gets converted into a proton forming a β^- particle in the process.

$$n \rightarrow p + e^-$$

The β^- particle (e^-) is emitted from the nucleus in some radioactive transformation. So electrons do not exist in the nucleus but they result in some nuclear transformation.

45. **(d) :** With the increase of temperature, the average energy exchanged in a collision increases and so more valence electrons can cross the energy gap, thereby increasing the electron-hole pairs. As in a semiconductor, conduction occurs mainly through electron-hole pairs, so conductivity increases with increase of temperature. Which in turn implies that the resistivity of a semiconductor decreases with rise in temperature.

46. **(d) :** The dominating force in the universe is the gravitational force. Because the gravitational force of attraction exists between any two bodies in the universe. Moreover it is the weakest of all the four fundamental forces in nature.

47. **(d) :** Because of the gravitational pull of other planets in the solar system, the earth cannot get slowed down in rotation. Because, if it happens so, it will affect the conservation of angular momentum which is not possible.

48. **(b) :** According to classical physics, all moving charged particle radiate electromagnetic radiation. So moving electrons will also radiate energy. If we see the atomic structure we find that electrons revolve around the nucleus in some particular orbits. Bohr termed these orbits as the stationary orbits as the electrons do not radiate energy as long as they are moving in these orbits. This is one of Bohr's postulates. This postulate is based on the fact that if the moving electrons radiate thereby losing energy, they have got a chance to finally fall back onto the nucleus and the atom will be collapsed.

49. **(a)**

50. **(b) :** This is true that the stars are much bigger in size than the planets. But this is not the reason why the stars twinkle but the planets do not. Actually the planets do not have their own light to twinkle. As the stars have their own light, and as they are very much for away from us, the light coming from the stars has to travel a very long distance and for a very long time to arrive us. And so the light coming from the stars is found to change their intensities continuously and hence the stars are seen to be twinkling.

51. **(b) :** A radiation consists of a beam of charged

particles. Normally the radiation that is used for cancer treatment is a light energy radiation which when imposed upon the cancerous tissues, destroys the cancer cells.

52. (a) : A beetle's motion sends fast longitudinal and slower transverse waves along the sand's surface. The sand scorpion intercepts the longitudinal waves first and learns the direction of the beetle by noting which one of the eight legs of the scorpion is disturbed first by the pulses. Then the scorpion dashes towards the beetle to catch it.

53. (c) **54. (b)**

55. (c) : There are two types of receptors in the eyes. One is called rods and other is cons. The rods are sensitive for dark light. As the owl has large number of cones in its retina and so the owl can move freely in the dark.

56. (c) : When we put a fire in a place, the air above the fire gets heated up. Hot air being light moves up. To fill up the gap cold air from the side of the fire rushes in. As the top of a fire is covered by hot air, it feels hotter over the top of the fire than at the same distance on the sides.

57. (c) : The amplitude of an oscillating pendulum decreases with time because of friction due to air. Frequency of simple pendulum is given by

$$f = \frac{1}{2\pi}\sqrt{\frac{g}{l}}$$

which is independent of amplitude and so even though the frequency remains the same, the amplitude keeps on decreasing till it becomes zero.

58. (d) : The quality of a communication system is determined by its information carrying capacity. The information carrying capacity is directly proportional to its bandwidth. The wider the bandwidth, the greater its information carrying capacity.

As the light frequencies used in optical fibre systems is much larger than the highest frequency microwave transmissions, so the bandwidth in case of optical communication systems is much larger than that in microwave communications. The bandwidth of the optical fibre systems is quite suitable for the present day communication needs and also for the future. That's why optical communication is preferred over microwave communication.

59. (b)

60. (a)

CHEMISTRY

61. (a) : KO_2 is a superoxide of potassium containing superoxide ion, O^{2-} which has a three electron bond. Thus this ion can be represented as $\left[:\ddot{O} \overset{\cdot\cdot\cdot}{—} \ddot{O}:\right]$.

The presence of one unpaired electron in three electron bond makes this ion paramagnetic.

62. (b) : Disodium salt of ethylene diamine tetracetic acid has been used for the estimation of M^{2+} metal ions like Mg^{2+}, Ca^{2+} etc. by complexometric titrations.

In this titration, indicator ions (D^{3-} ions) form red-metal indicator complex, $[MD^-]$ with M^{2+} ions.

(i) $\underset{\text{metal ion (}Mg^{2+}\text{ or }Ca^{2+}\text{)}}{M^{2+}} + \underset{\text{indicator ion (blue)}}{D^{3-}} \xrightleftharpoons{pH\ =\ 10} \underset{\text{Metal indicator complex (red)}}{[M^{2+}D]^-}$

(ii) $\underset{\text{(red)}}{[M^{2+}D]^-} + \underset{\text{EDTA ion}}{EDTA^{4-}} \rightleftharpoons \underset{\text{metal-EDTA complex}}{[M^{2+}(EDTA)]^{2-}} + \underset{\text{(blue)}}{D^{3-}}$

The release of the free indicator ion is marked by a change from red (colour of $[M^{2+}D]^-$ complex) to blue (colour of D^{3-} ion) colour.

63. (d) : H_3PO_2, H_3PO_3 and H_3PO_4 contain one, two and three ionisable hydrogen atoms respectively.

$H_3PO_2 \rightleftharpoons H^+ + H_2PO_2^-$

$H_3PO_3 \rightleftharpoons H^+ + H_2PO_3^- \rightleftharpoons 2H^+ + HPO_3^{2-}$

$H_3PO_4 \rightleftharpoons H^+ + H_2PO_4^- \rightleftharpoons 2H^+ + HPO_4^{2-}$

$\rightleftharpoons 3H^+ + PO_4^{3-}$

But there is very little difference in acidity.

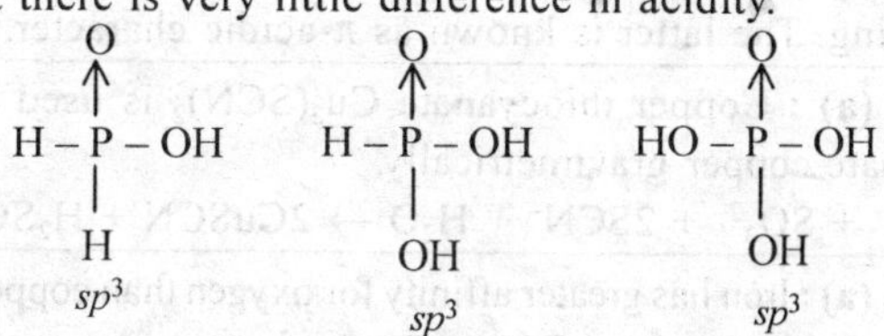

As sp^3 hybridised, therefore all are tetrahedral.

64. (c) : $[Cu(NH_3)_4]^{2+}$

$Cu^{2+} \rightarrow 3d^9\ 4s^0$

	3d					4s	4p		
Cu^{2+}	1l	1l	1l	1l	1				
$[Cu(NH_3)_4]^{2+}$ →	1l	1l	1l	1l	××	××	××	××	1

dsp^2 square planar

One electron is shifted from $3d$ to $4p$ orbital.

65. (b) : *Cis*-$[PtCl_2(NH_3)_2]$ is used as an anti-cancer agent, called as cisplatin and is highly toxic. On injecting, the more reactive Cl groups are lost so the Pt atom bonds to a N atom in guanosine (part of the DNA molecule). Those cells which are undergoing cell division are attacked by cisplatin.

66. (c) : Na_3VO_4 contains colourless ortho-vanadate (VO_4^{3-}) ion.

67. (a) : $3MnO_4^{2-} + 2H_2O \rightarrow MnO_{2\,(s)} + 2MnO_4^- + 4OH^-$

for one mole

$$MnO_4^{2-} + \frac{2}{3}H_2O \rightarrow \frac{1}{3}MnO_{2\,(s)} + \frac{2}{3}MnO_4^- + \frac{4}{3}OH^-$$

68. (d) :

La	– +3
Nd	– +2, +3, +4
Ce	– +3, +4
Eu	– +2, +3

69. (b) : $\underbrace{3HCl + HNO_3}_{\text{aqua regia}} \longrightarrow \underset{\text{nitrosyl chloride}}{NOCl} + 2H_2O + 2Cl$

70. (d) : The alkali metals dissolve in liquid ammonia without evolution of hydrogen. The colour of the dilute solution is blue and are paramagnetic in nature.

$M \rightarrow M^+$ (in liquid ammonia) + e^- (ammoniated)

$M + (x + y)NH_3 \rightarrow [M(NH_3)_x]^+ + e^-(NH_3)_y$

solvated electron

71. (a) : Carbon monoxide is π -acid ligand as it characterises both metal to carbon and carbon to metal bonding. The latter is known as π-acidic character.

72. (a) : Copper thiocyanate $Cu_2(SCN)_2$ is used to estimate copper gravimetrically.

$2Cu^{2+} + SO_3^{2-} + 2SCN^- + H_2O \rightarrow 2CuSCN + H_2SO_4$

73. (a) : Iron has greater affinity for oxygen than copper.

$Cu_2O + FeS \rightarrow FeO + Cu_2S$

$FeO + SiO_2 \rightarrow \underset{\text{(slag)}}{FeSiO_3}$

$2Cu_2S + 3O_2 \rightarrow 2Cu_2O + 2SO_2$

$2Cu_2O + Cu_2S \xrightarrow[\text{reduction}]{\text{auto}} 6Cu + SO_2.$

74. (c) : Benzoic acid (COOH on benzene), p-methoxybenzoic acid (COOH, para-OCH_3), m-methoxybenzoic acid (COOH, meta-OCH_3), CH_3COOH

$K_a : 6.3 \times 10^{-5}$ 3.3×10^{-5} 8.2×10^{-5} 1.75×10^{-5}

– OCH_3 group displays electron withdrawing acid strengthening inductive effect at the *meta* position but at the *para* position, an electron releasing acid weakening resonance effect operates (which at this position outweighs the inductive effect).

75. (c) : – NO_2 group exerts a strong electron withdrawal effect due to which basicity at – N atom decreases.

76. (a) : (cyclohexene ring with CH_3 at position 3; positions 1, 2, 3 marked)

Therefore, IUPAC name is 3-methylcyclohex-1-ene or simply, 3-methylcyclohexene.

77. (d) : Methanol has – OH group due to which there will be more intermolecular hydrogen bonding among the given molecules.

$$\text{- - - H—}\underset{}{\overset{CH_3}{O}}\text{- - - H—}\overset{CH_3}{O}\text{- - - H—}\overset{CH_3}{O}$$

We know that with the increase of electronegativity and decrease in size of the atom to which hydrogen is covalently linked, the strength of the hydrogen bond increases.

78. (d) : For *o*/*p* directing group, there should be partial –ve charge at the *o* and *p* positions.

(Resonance structures of acetanilide: $NHCOCH_3$ on benzene ↔ $\overset{\oplus}{N}HCOCH_3$ with negative charge at ortho ↔ negative charge at para ↔ negative charge at other ortho ↔ etc.)

79. (b) :

$$CH_3-\overset{CH_3}{\overset{|}{C}}=CH_2 + H_2SO_4 \longrightarrow CH_3-\overset{CH_3}{\overset{|}{\underset{\oplus}{C}}}-CH_3$$

isobutene   [3° carbocation]

$$C_6H_6 + CH_3-\overset{CH_3}{\overset{|}{\underset{\oplus}{C}}}-CH_3 \longrightarrow \text{(arenium ion with } H \text{ and } C(CH_3)_3\text{)} \xrightarrow{-H^+} C_6H_5-\overset{CH_3}{\overset{|}{\underset{CH_3}{\underset{|}{C}}}}-CH_3$$

t-butyl benzene

80. **(d) :** More the number of attached methyl groups better is the nucleophilicity due to +I-effect.

81. **(b) :**

$$\begin{array}{c} {}^{1}CH_3 \\ H - \overset{2}{C} - Cl \\ Cl - \overset{3}{C} - H \\ C_2H_5 \end{array}$$

Nomenclature is according to Cahn - Ingold-Prelog method *i.e.*, priority rule.

82. **(c) :** One molecule of haemoglobin has 4 haeme groups, and each of them is capable of taking up one molecule of O_2; therefore, oxyhemoglobin may be depicted as $Hb(O_2)_4$.

83. **(b) :** Only $CH_3COOC_2H_5$ will give ethanol, C_2H_5OH after hydrolysis (which can give positive iodoform test).

$CH_3COOCH_3 \rightarrow CH_3COOH + CH_3OH$

$CH_3COOC_2H_5 \rightarrow CH_3COOH + CH_3CH_2OH$

$C_6H_5COOCH_3 \rightarrow C_6H_5COOH + CH_3OH$

$CH_3COOC_6H_5 \rightarrow CH_3COOH + C_6H_5OH$

84. **(c) :** 2-ethylalanine ; $H_5C_2 - \underset{CH_3}{\overset{NH_2}{C}} - COOH$ (Chiral)

2-methylglycine ; $CH_3 - \underset{H}{\overset{NH_2}{C}} - COOH$ (Chiral)

2-hydroxymethylserine ; $HOCH_2 - \underset{CH_2OH}{\overset{NH_2}{C}} - COOH$ (Achiral)

tryptophan ; (indol-3-yl)$-CH_2 - \underset{H}{\overset{NH_2}{C}} - COOH$ (Chiral)

85. **(d) :** $C_6H_5NO_2 \xrightarrow{Zn/NH_4Cl} C_6H_5NHOH$

86. **(c) :** Hydroboration yields 1° alcohol from alkenes.

$$3CH_3CH{=}CH_2 \xrightarrow[THF]{BH_3\ in} (CH_3CH_2CH_2)_3B$$

$$\xrightarrow{3H_2O_2} \underset{\text{1-propanol}}{3CH_3CH_2CH_2OH} + H_3BO_3$$

87. **(b) :** The values of dipole moments of methyl halides:

CH_3F - 1.51 D ; CH_3Cl - 1.56 D;

CH_3Br - 1.4 D ; CH_3I - 1.29 D

$\therefore$ $CH_3Cl > CH_3F > CH_3Br > CH_3I$.

88. **(b) :** Na_2O has antifluorite structure. O^{2-} ions constitute a ccp lattice and Na^+ ions occupy the tetrahedral voids, each O^{2-} ion is in contact with 8 Na^+ ions and each Na^+ ion is in contact with 4 O^{2-} ions. Thus C.N. of sodium in Na_2O = 4.

89. **(a) :** Bond dissociation energy for C – H are given below in the given molecules.

$C_6H_5CH_3$	- 85 Kcal/mol
C_6H_6	- 110 Kcal/mol
$CH_3CH_2CH_2CH_2CH_3$	- 98 Kcal/mol
$H_3C - \underset{CH_3}{\overset{CH_3}{C}} - CH_3$	- 92 Kcal/mol

90. **(d) :** Heat of decomposition, $\Delta E = m \cdot s \cdot \Delta T$

$= 1 \times 1.23 \times 6.12 = 7.5276$ kJ.

Molar heat of decomposition for NH_4NO_3

$= 7.5276 \times 80 = 602.2$ kJ.

91. **(d) :** Boiling point of a pure solvent increases by increase in number of soluble particles present in it. So by addition of toluene, boiling point of pure benzene increases.

92. **(c) :** Fuel cells are galvanic cells in which chemical energy of fuels is directly converted into electrical energy. e.g., Hydrogen - oxygen fuel cell.

93. **(d) :** Buffer solutions can be obtained by mixing a weak acid with its salt formed with a strong base or by mixing a weak base with its salt formed with a strong acid.

As $HClO_4$ is a strong acid, therefore equimolar mixture of $HClO_4$ and its salt $KClO_4$ is not a buffer solution.

94. **(c) :** Here, the number of product species is greater than the number of reactant species. So it leads to positive value of entropy.

95. **(c) :** This quantum number describes the orientation or distribution of electron cloud.

96. **(b) :** To act as surfactant, there should be both polar and non-polar ends in the molecules.

97. **(b) :** $Al^{3+} + 3e^- \rightarrow Al$

For deposition of 1g equivalent ≡ 96500 C

For deposition of 1 millimole ≡ 96.500 C

As $Q = It \Rightarrow t = \frac{Q}{I} = \frac{96.5}{9.65} = 10$ s.

98. (b) : Acetic acid is a weak acid while sodium hydroxide is a strong base. Therefore at the equivalent point, there will be enough hydroxide ions left.

99. (d) : Carbon dioxide, water vapours and methane are all green house gases.

100. (c) : ΔH = activation energy of forward reaction – activation energy of backward reaction

$\therefore \quad \Delta H = b - a = c.$

101. (a) : Na_2CrO_4 solution in water is yellow in colour, when acidified changes to orange colour (due to the formation of $Cr_2O_7^{2-}$ ions).

$Na_2CrO_4 + H_2SO_4 \rightarrow Na_2Cr_2O_7 + Na_2SO_4 + H_2O$

Oxidation state : Na_2CrO_4

Let oxidation state of Cr be x.

$\Rightarrow \quad 2(+1) + x + 4(-2) = 0 \Rightarrow x = +6.$

102. (c) : Due to high electronegativity of F-atoms, the lone pair of N-atom in NF_3 molecule cannot be ligated easily.

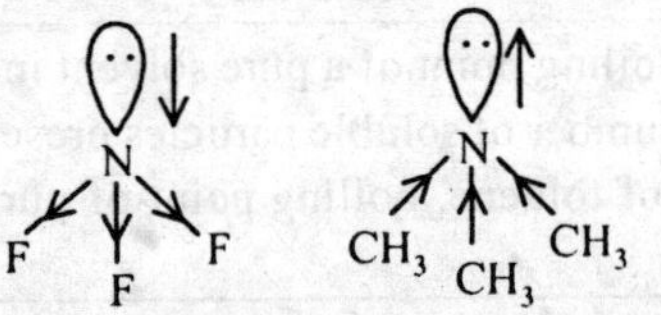

Except, nitrogen fluoride, all other halides hydrolyse in water.

$NCl_3 + 3H_2O \rightarrow NH_3 + 3HClO.$

103. (d) : Due to screening effect, down the group, lower oxidation states become more stable. e.g., Pb(II) is more stable than Pb(IV). But small, highly electronegative elements like F-atoms can somewhat stabilise its higher oxidation state.

104. (d) : ${}_{11}Na^{22} \rightarrow {}_{12}Mg^{22} + {}_{-1}\beta^0$

It involves β-particle emission.

While positron emission is due to the conversion of proton into neutron.

$${}^1_1p \rightarrow {}^1_0n + {}^0_1\beta$$

105. (a) : Ba - (Xe) $6s^2$

It shows oxidation state of +II only.

106. (c) : Haemoglobin is the oxygen carrier in the human blood. It consists of four subunits and one molecule of haemoglobin can carry 4 molecules of O_2. O_2 binds to Fe of heme part.

107. (d) : Glycosides are formed by treating glucose with CH_3OH in the presence of dry HCl gas and can be hydrolysed by strong reagents like HCN, NH_2OH and $C_6H_5NHNH_2$. Also, glycosides are known as hemi-acetals.

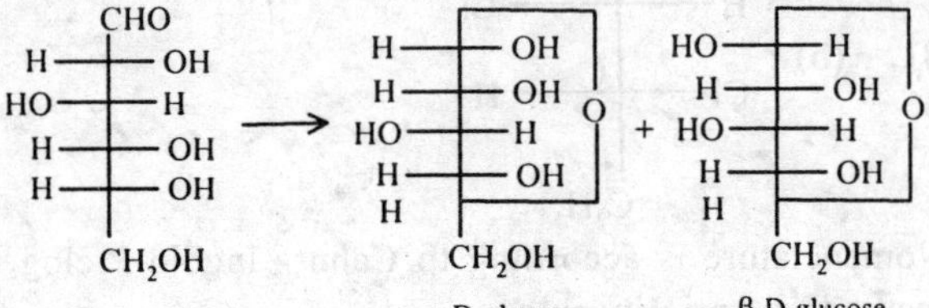

α-D-glucose β-D-glucose (hemi-acetal)

108. (a) : $HO^- + C_6H_5CH_2-Br \xrightarrow{S_N2} [HO^{\delta-}\cdots CH_2(C_6H_5)\cdots Br^{\delta-}] \rightarrow C_6H_5CH_2-OH + Br^-$

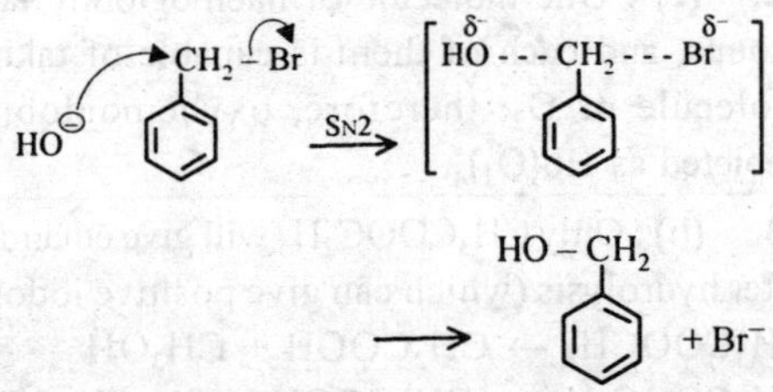

109. (b) : Enzymes are proteins which act as catalyst for bio-chemical reactions. pH affect their activity as protonation-deprotonation may cause denaturation of the protein structure. Solubility is also affected.

110. (b) : The monoalkyl derivative first formed readily undergoes further alkylation at a still greater speed to produce polysubstituted products, and alkyl halide employed may also undergo an isomeric change. Due to these difficulties alkyl benzene is not generally prepared by Friedel-Craft's alkylation of benzene.

111. (a) : Grignard reagents are very reactive. Hence the Grignard reagents will react with hydroxyl group.

112. (c) : With *trans*-2-butene, the product of Br_2 addition is optically inactive due to the formation of symmetric *meso* compounds.

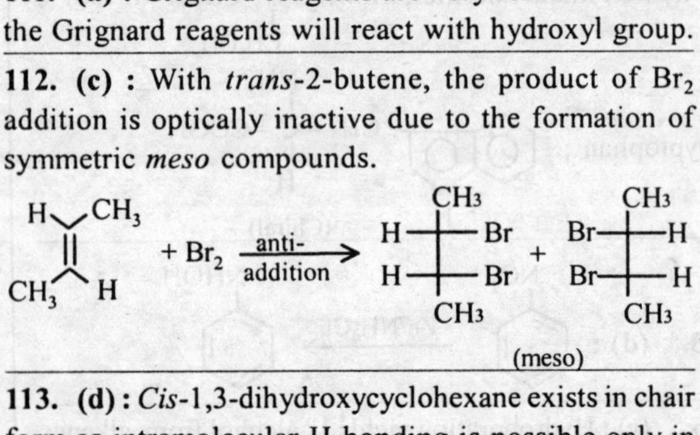

$trans\text{-}CH_3CH{=}CHCH_3 + Br_2 \xrightarrow[\text{addition}]{\text{anti-}}$ (meso)

113. (d) : *Cis*-1,3-dihydroxycyclohexane exists in chair form as intramolecular H-bonding is possible only in chair form.

114. (a) : At 373 K or 100°C, the water starts boiling and at this temperature the vaporization of water is an isothermal process.

The internal energy change (ΔE), depend only on

temperature, it follows that at constant temperature, the internal energy of the gas remains constant, *i.e.* ΔE is zero.

115. (a) : $BaCO_3 + 2HNO_3 \rightarrow Ba(NO_3)_2 + H_2O + CO_2$.

116. (b) : $\Delta H = \Delta E + \Delta nRT$

Δn = change in number of moles of products and reactant species.

$$N_{2\,(g)} + O_{2\,(g)} \rightleftharpoons 2NO_{\,(g)}$$

$\Delta n = 2 - 2 = 0$

$\Delta H = \Delta E + 0 \times RT$ or, $\Delta H = \Delta E$.

117. (b) : NO_2 + U.V. light $\rightarrow$ NO + O

Atomic oxygen produced as above reacts with hydrocarbons to give a variety of free hydrocarbon radicals aldehyde, ketones, O_3, peroxyacetyl nitrate (PAN) etc. PAN mixes with the fog and gets condensed on smoke or dust particles in the air to for a smog which is called photochemical smog.

118. (b) : According to Clapeyron-Clausius equation,

$$\frac{dT}{dP} = \frac{T(V_l - V_s)}{\Delta H_f}$$

Since density of ice is less than that of water, V_s is greater than V_l. In other words, the expression on the right hand side of the above equation is negative. This means that the increase of pressure must lower and decrease of pressure must raise the freezing point.

119. (b) : Micelle is formed if molecules with polar and non-polar ends assemble in bulk to give non-polar interior and polar exterior.

120. (d) : O_2F_2 has the similar structure as that of H_2O_2 but the O – O bond length is shorter in O_2F_2 than in H_2O_2. This is due to the high electronegativity of attached F-atoms.

BIOLOGY

121. (b) : The crystal of lead zirconate is a key component of electrocardiography. It is a piezoelectric material (the material which has a net dipole moment and which can produce electricity when subjected to pressure or stress), crystal or ceramic in nature. The thickness of this material is the critical factor in allowing proper vibrational frequency, most common material used is lead zirconate titanate. Electrocardiography is a commonly used, non-invasive procedure for recording electrical changes in the heart.

122. (b) : Normal blood sugar level in adult human varies from 80-100 mg/100 ml (fasting) to 100-120 mg/100 ml (after meal).

Normal blood urea is 20-40 mg/dl

Total blood volume is 4-5 litres

ESR in wintrobe method is 0-9 mm in male and 0 - 20 mm in female.

123. (d) : Gene pool is the total gene present in a population. Genome is the total genetic constitution of an organism. Codon is the basic unit of genetic code, a sequence of three adjacent nucleotide in DNA or *m*RNA that code for an amino acid. Gene is the basic unit of heredity; a sequence of DNA nucleotide that encodes a protein.

Cistron is a segment of DNA nucleotides that codes for a polypeptide chain. Triplet is a three nucleotides sequence coding for an amino acid.

Therefore, codon ≈ triplet

cistron ≈ gene

DNA fingerprinting is technically called DNA profiling or DNA typing.

124. (a) : The gradually increasing contraction of ventricular muscles during systole first causes the closure of bicuspid and tricuspid valves (AV valves), producing a low-pitched "lubb" sound. Later, it causes the opening of the semilunar valves of systemic and pulmonary aorta. At the end of ventricular systole, semilunar valves shut, producing the second, louder heart sound, the "dup". Thus each heart beat is accompanied by a "lubb-dup" sound.

125. (c) : Mr. X eating curd / yoghurt should be considered as occupying third trophic level. Producers or greeen plants (first trophic level) are consumed by herbivore (second trophic level). And from them curd, yoghurt (made from dairy breed) is consumed by third trophic level like man.

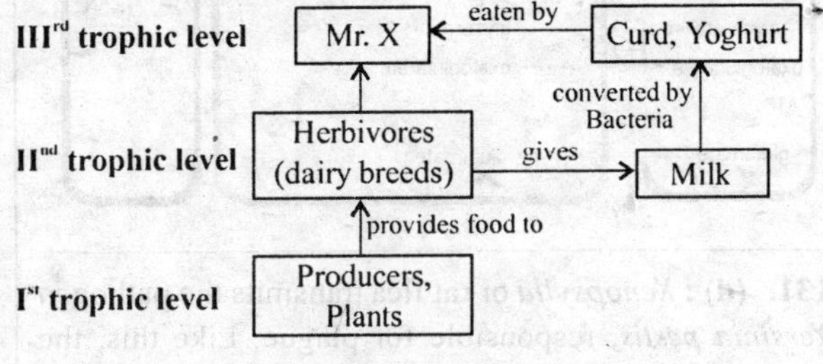

126. (a) : World population day - 11th July

No tobacco day - 31st May

World environment day - 5th June

World health day - 7th April.

127. (b) : To measure water pollution, Biological Oxygen Demand or BOD test is made. In this test, amount of oxygen sufficient to degrade waste organic matter by bacteria in a sample is measured. The more oxygen used up by the bacteria to degrade the organic matter in the sample, the greater the BOD would be.

128. (b) : Patella is a sesamoid bone. Sesamoid bones are formed by ossification of a tendon where the tendon moves over a bony surface.

129. (c) : Both corpus luteum and macula lutea are characterised by a yellow colour. After an egg is released from the ovary, the cells that line the ovarian follicle change shape and colour to become a corpus luteum (yellow body). Macula lutea is the yellowish spot present at the posterior pole of eye. Lutein, zeaxanthin, α-carotene and β-cryptoxanthin are responsible for its yellow colouration.

130. (b) : In the process of photorespiration oxygen combines with RUBP (Ribulose-biphosphate) in chloroplast as following

$$O_2 + RUBP \xrightarrow{\text{Rubisco}} \text{3-Phosphoglycerate} +$$

$$\text{2-Phosphoglycolate} \longrightarrow CO_2$$

Phosphoglycolate enters in peroxisomes and is finally converted to CO_2.

Overview of photorespiration

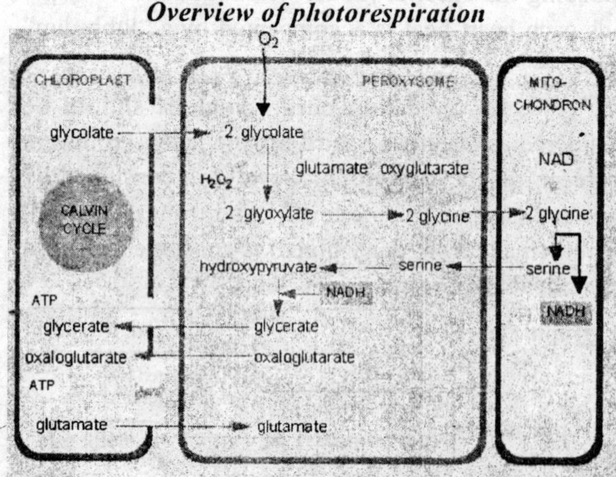

131. (d) : *Xenopsylla* or rat flea transmits the pathogen *Yersinia pestis*, responsible for plague. Like this, the sand fly *Phlebotomus* transmits the protozoa *Leishmania donovani* which is the causative agent of *Kala azar*, oriental sore etc.

132. (c) : Cholesterol is a soft waxy substance that is a natural component of the fats in the blood-stream and in all the cells of the body. In our body 8% to 10% of the saturated fatty acids are coming from animal product, such as butter, egg, red meat. Continued consumption of this type of diet leads to hypercholesterolemia due to the presence of excess amount of saturated fatty acid.

133. (d)

134. (b) : Vasopressin or ADH secreted from posterior pituitary stimulates reabsorption of water by the distal convoluted tubule and the collecting renal tubules and thus regulates urine volume. It has no such important effect on glucose metabolism. Therefore, a person whose blood glucose level is normal, but passes much urine and drinks much water has a reduction in vasopressin secretion which ultimately leads to diabetes insipidus.

135. (a) : *t*RNA has four recognition sites among these one is the amino acid attachment site. It has the amino acid attachment site with the 3′ terminal - CCA sequence.

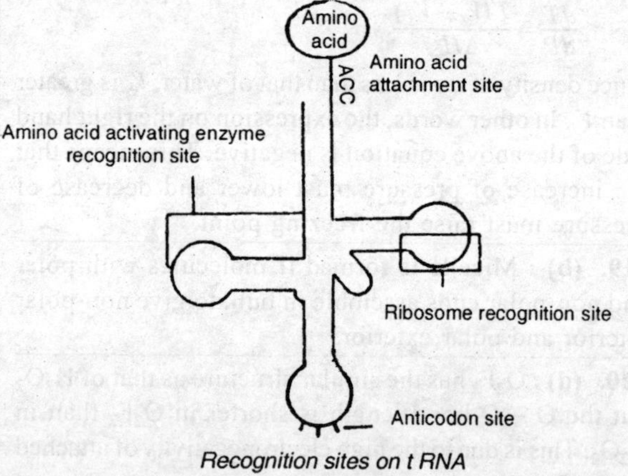

Recognition sites on t RNA

136. (a) : An example of competitive inhibition of an enzyme is the inhibition of succinic dehydrogenase by malonic acid. It is the simple type of competitive inhibition. A competitive inhibitor resembles the substrate and binds to the active site of the enzyme. The substrate is then prevented from binding to the same active site.

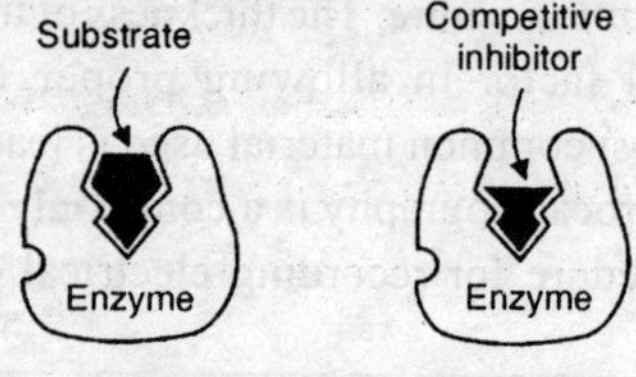

Competitive inhibitor

137. (b) : The association between fungi and algae in lichen is regarded as the true mutual relationship, in which both the partners are benefitted. In lichen, fungus lives on the algae which manufactures food by virtue of the chlorophyll present in its cells, while the algae enjoys the protection afforded by the fungal envelope, to live in very dry conditions.

138. (a) : Photochemical smog mainly consists of ozone, peroxyacetyl nitrate and different oxide of nitrogen and hydrocarbons released from different engines. Nitric oxide (NO) is formed by reaction between oxygen and nitrogen. This reacts with air forming nitrogen dioxide (NO_2). This gas absorbs light due to which nitric oxide (NO) and a molecule of nascent oxygen [O] are formed.

$$NO_2 \longrightarrow NO + [O]$$

This atomic oxygen reacts with unburnt hydrocarbons to give rise to peroxy radicals which after reaction with oxygen form ozone or reacting with NO_2 give rise to peroxyacetyl nitrate (PAN).

139. (a) : In almost all Indian metropolitan cities like Delhi, the major atmospheric pollutants are SO_2, NO_2 and particulate matter in which the SPM (Suspended Particulate Matter) in Delhi's air exceeds the permitted levels by over 100%.

140. (b) : Excessive stimulation of vagus nerve in humans may lead to peptic ulcer. Vagal stimulation increases peristalsis which in excess, secretes more HCl and pepsin from stomach. These causes erosion through protective barrier of mucus and muscularis mucosa into the submucosa which leads to peptic ulcer.

141. (a) : Restriction enzymes are endonucleases which cleave DNA at specific sites. They are originally extracted from the bacterium *E.coli*. Type I restriction enzymes bind to a recognition site of a duplex DNA and cleave one strand only. Type II restriction enzymes are more valuable in gene manipulation and cleave the duplex at specific target sites at or near the binding site.

142. (a) : The wild ass, once widely distributed in north-western arid zone; now confined to Runn of Kutchchh and Pakistan.

143. (d) : Replication takes place discontinuously and short pieces called okazaki fragments are synthesized. One strand may synthesize a continuous strand and the other okazaki fragments, or both strands may synthesize okazaki fragments. Both new strands are synthesized in 5′-3′ direction. Thus one strand is synthesized forwards and the other backwards.

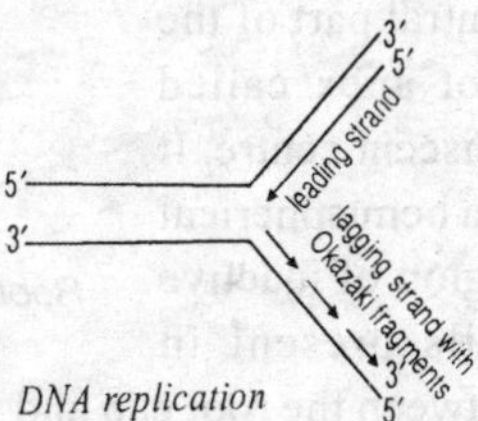

DNA replication

144. (a) : UGU codes for the same information as UGC as both codes for cystine. UGA and UAG are non-sense codons and UGG codes for tryptophan.

145. (c) : As the person uses spectacles having concave lens, he must be suffering from myopia or short-sightedness. Here the eyeballs become elongated, so that parallel rays are focussed in front of retina.

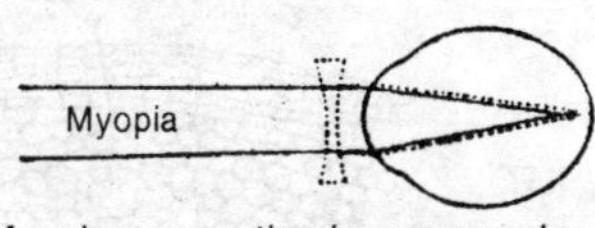

Myopia - correction by concave lens
(Wintom & Bayliss)

146. (b)

147. (b) : The phase of menstrual cycle in humans that last for 7-8 days is ovulatory phase. During this phase production of FSH decreases while that of LH increases which leads to ovulation on about the 14th day. But it may range from 9th to 16th day (approximately).

148. (d) : The source of somatostatin is same that of vasopressin and oxytocin. Somatostatin is produced from hypothalamus (somatostatin neuron) and oxytocin and vasopressin are also produced in the nuclei of hypothalamus, though later they are stored and released from posterior pituitary.

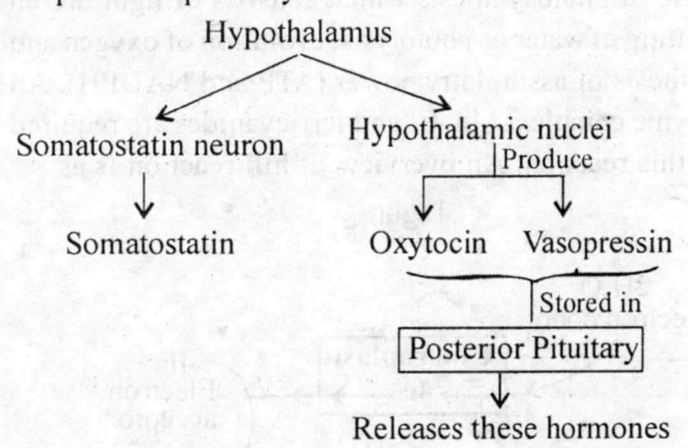

149. (b) : *Spirulina* is a blue-green algae. *Spirulina platensis* is one of the richest source of protein, containing 40-50 percent crude protein on dry weight basis which under favourable condition may reach upto 70 percent. Its protein has balanced composition containing all essential amino-acids and lysine and tryptophan being present in sufficient quantities. *Spirulina* is also rich in vitamins, particularly Vit. B_{12}, which is not common in plant products and contains considerable amounts of fats, carbohydrates and minerals. It's lipids are made up of unsaturated fatty acids that do not form cholesterol.

150. (a) : Viroids are a group of pathogens of some higher plants that are smaller or simpler than any of the known virus. They consist of single stranded linear or circular RNA molecules without a protein coat.

151. (c) :

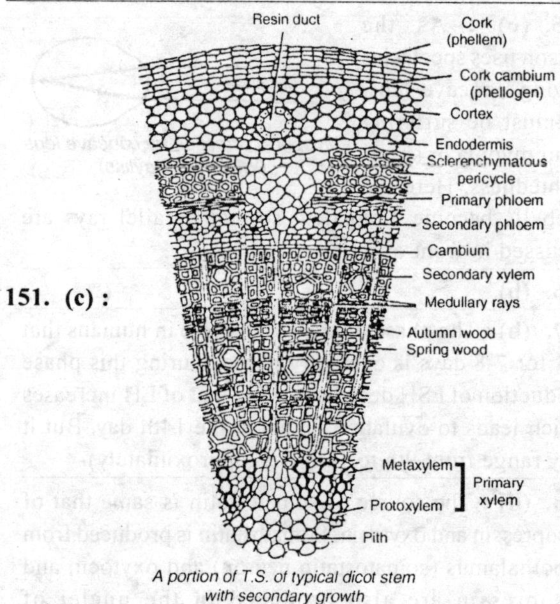

A portion of T.S. of typical dicot stem with secondary growth

152. (d) : Hill reaction is the light phase or photochemical phase of photosynthesis which consists of light driven splitting of water or photolysis, evolution of oxygen and synthesis of assimilatory power (ATP and NADPH). An enzyme complex, Mn, Cl and ferricyanides are required for this reaction. An overview of hill reaction is as

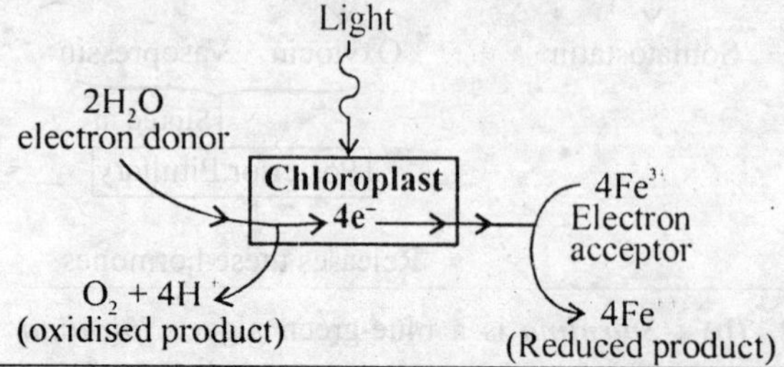

153. (b) : Mycorrhiza is an example of mutualism. It is an association between a fungus and the root of a higher plant. eg., Pine, Birch. The fungus obtains shelter and food from root and helps the root in absorption of water, dissolution and absorption of inorganic nutrients locked in organic matter (especially nitrogen and phosphorus) and protection from other fungi.

154. (c) : Exine is outer layer of pollen grain which is acetolysis resistant layer. It is also resistant to physical and biological degradation. Because of this property of exine, pollen grains are found well preserved for long periods in fossil deposits.

155. (b) : The most common form of red-green colour blindness is an 'X chromosome linked recessive' disorder. The 'red' and 'green' genes are known to reside at the tip of the long arm of the X chromosome. Women have two copies of the X-chromosome, and so they may have normal colour vision, even if they carry one copy of the defective gene. Men have only one X-chromosome, and so will be colour blind.

156. (d) : During the embryonic development in humans, cleavage division results in a hollow ball of cells called morula. Solid mass of 32 cells formed from zygote after successive mitotic division (after 3rd division of cleavage) is called morula.

157. (d) : A characteristic of most plant cells is the presence of cytoplasmic material that establish continuity between adjacent cells. These bridges are called plasmodesmata. These permit the free circulation of fluid, which is essential to the maintenance of plant cell toxicity.

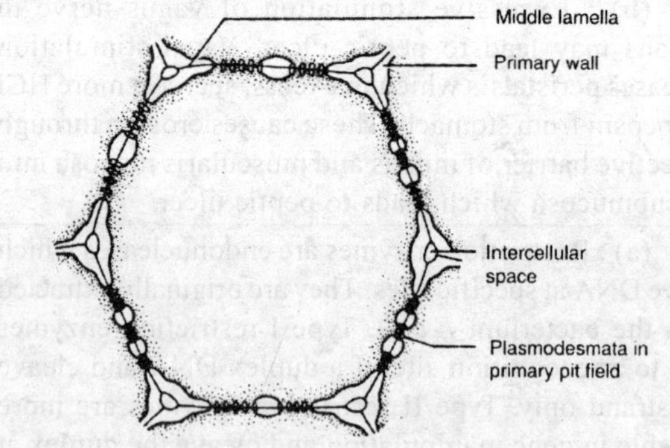

Parenchyma cell with pit fields and plasmodesmata

158. (c) : A zone of inactive cells is present in the central part of the root apex called quiscent centre. It is a hemispherical region of inactive cells present in between the root cap and the active meristematic region of root apex. This zone contains several hundred cells

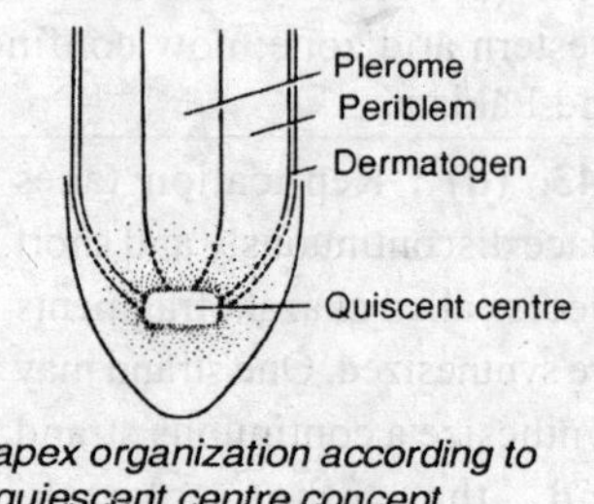

Root apex organization according to quiescent centre concept

which are characterized by having lower concentration of DNA, RNA and protein. The quiescent centre acts as reservoir of cells and becomes active whenever the previously active initials get damaged or during the establishment of the secondary roots.

159. (c) : *Azolla* is a pteridophyte and used as a biofertilizer because it has association with nitrogen-fixing cyanobacteria *Anabaena azollae*.

160. (d)

161. (a) : Mast cells act on body's defense mechanism. When some allergens like different pollutants, smog, smoke, pollen grains etc. come in contact with mast cell, they stimulate the mast cells. The allergic reaction is triggered by cross linking of IgE molecules on the surface of mast cells by allergen. And ultimately mast cells release excessive amounts of inflammatory chemicals which cause allergic reactions.

162. (b) : The direct application of fertilizers to crop or soils is a simple route to increase crop yield.
Average yield per hectare has increased from 1.1 tons in 1950 to 2.3 tons in 1986 by the use of inorganic fertilizers.
Irrigation is very important in increasing crop productivity as water is an essential component of vital activities of a plant.

163. (c) : The basal metabolic rate is defined as the energy requirement of the human body at rest and reflects the caloric needs of the body. BMR can be determined by total body weight and the amount of muscle mass. BMR is inversely related with the weight or volume of an organism, i.e. smaller the organism, higher is the basal metabolic rate and vice versa.
Heart rate of six month old baby is 110-112 beats/min. Though it is higher than normal adult person, but it is lower than the old person. At the age of 60, a man may have maximum heart rate of 160 beats/min (avg 120 beats/min.)

164. (b) : Bats and whales are classified as mammal because they possess the essential mammalian characteristics like presence of milk gland or mammae, presence of pinnae, viviparous nature, hairs on body, presence of diaphragm etc. Though bats and whales have four chambered heart, it cannot be considered as the main characteristic of being mammals because it is also present in some reptiles (e.g. crocodile) and all birds.

165. (b) : SARS, a severe acute type of 'Atypically atypical pneumonia' caused by metapneumo virus (a type of corona virus) was first reported (WHO) in China (Beijing, Guangdong, HongKong, Taiwan etc.) Though China is the most populated country of the world, it is not directly responsible for the origin of SARS. The killer pneumonia virus is responsible for SARS origin.

166. (c) : Organochlorine pesticides are organic compounds or hydrocarbons to which are added several atoms of chlorine through the process called chlorination. Rate of degradation of organochlorines is very low. eg.; DDT, BHC.
Fenitrothion is organophosphate pesticide which is the organic ester of phosphoric acid and its derivatives. These pesticides are very toxic but are not persistant.

167. (c) : In holoblastic cleavage, the cleavage furrows bisect the entire egg, or in other words, entire egg divides by each cleavage furrow. In placental mammals having isolecithal or microlecithal egg, the holoblastic cleavage produces blastomeres of equal or approximately equal size.
Centrolecithal eggs are found in insects and in some hydrozoa. Here, yolk is concentrated at the centre of egg and the cytoplasm is present surrounding it. Meroblastic cleavage occurs in them.

168. (b) : Inhabitants close to very busy airports are likely to experience health hazards. Because maximum acceptable range of sound is 80-90 dB. But in the places like airports this level is always exceeds thus it creates sound pollution and related health hazards like auditory fatigue, deafness etc.
Jet planes generally produce sound above 160 dB which is much more than normal level, thus they also produce sound pollution. But as jet aeroplanes are used for some special purposes, they normally do not land in common (very busy) airports (without emergency). Thus it has no direct relation in causing sound pollution and related hazards in areas nearby very busy airports.

169. (c) : Koel and cuckoo need not build nests because they transfer their responsibilities to build nests, incubate eggs and nurture hatchlings to other birds specially crows. Thus they are called as "brood parasites". Being the brood parasite of the crow, the koel's breeding cycle synchronizes with that of crow. Both the koel's and crow's eggs are grey-green with rusty brown markings. Tailor bird is a garden bird which makes its nest by sewing, it has no direct relation with koel and cuckoo.

170. (c) : Old age is the result of ageing or senescence which may be defined as the progressive deterioration in structure and function of the body cells, tissues, organs and organ systems of the organism with their advancing age. Here, the body's immune system loses its ability to effectively deal with the antigens. This reduces the resistance as well as adaptation of the body. Cessation of mitosis is not as such a genetically programmed event. During ageing, there is a decrease in multiplication of cells, though it differs in various tissues.

171. (a) : The structure of cell membrane can be described by the fluid-mosaic model. The essential feature of fluid-mosaic model (by Singer and Nicolson, 1972) is that cell membranes are considered to be quasifluid structures in which the lipids and proteins are in mosaic manner. The Singer-Nicolson model considered the lipid-protein association (mosaic) to be hydrophobic. The fluidity of the membrane is the result of this hydrophobic interaction, thus a cell membrane shows fluid behaviour.

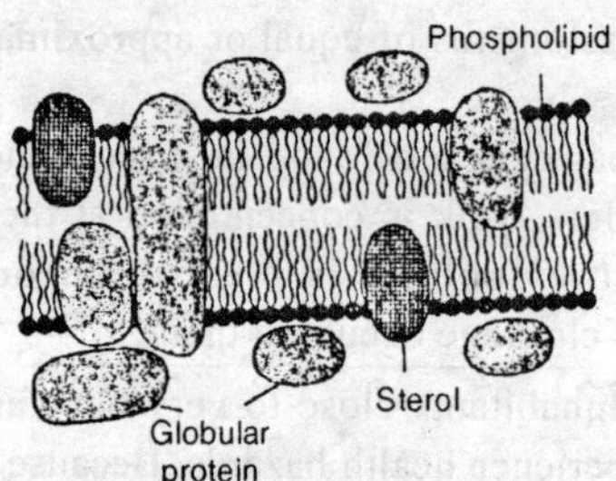

Schematic representation of a section through a eukaryote fluid mosaic membrane

172. (a) : Any viable somatic cell of a plant has the ability to form full fledged plants. This ability of plant cell is known as cellular totipotency.

173. (c) : Anthocyanin is a colouring pigment of certain higher plants that imparts a bluish or reddish colour. Rhoeo leaves contain anthocyanin pigments in epdiermal cells.

174. (b) : The apoplast is the system of adjacent cell walls which is continuous through the plant. As water evaporates from the mesophyll cell walls into the intercellular air spaces, tension develops in the continuous stream of water in the apoplast, and water is drawn through the walls in a mass flow by the cohesion of water molecules. When water moving through spaces in the cell wall reaches the endodermis, it's progress is stopped by a waterproof substance called suberin which is deposited in cell walls in the form of bands called casparian strips. Therefore water and solutes must pass through the cell surface membrane and into the cytoplasm of the cells of the endodermis.

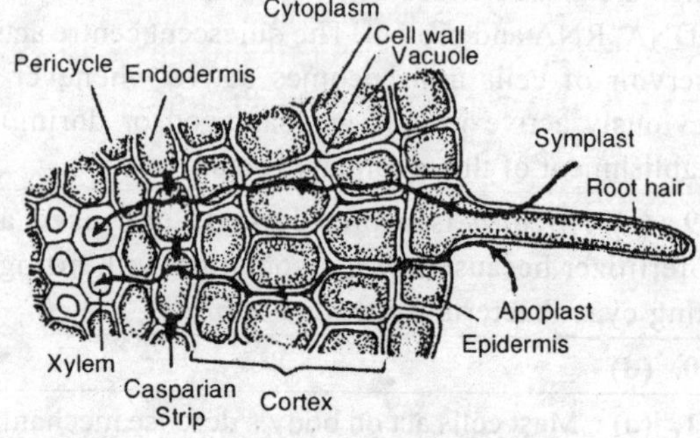

Diagram showing symplast and apoplast pathwaty of water moment in root.

175. (a) : The main function of sieve tube is the transport of food products from green and storage organs of the plant to other organs of the plant. The sieve elements are sieve tubes arranged one above the other and have sieve plates (obligue or transverse perforated septa) on their end walls. The cytoplasm occur in the form of a thin living layer along the inner side of cellulose wall. The nucleus disappears in mature sieve elements.

176. (b) : Some trees of hill like oak, ash, elm, hickory, pecan and mountain cedar produce allergic pollen grains which cause allergy to people. The signs and symptoms of pollen allergy are

- sneezing
- itching eyes, nose and throat
- dark circles under the eyes caused by restricted blood flow near the sinuses
- watering eyes
- conjunctivities

Conifer trees produce a large quantity of wind borne pollen grains because many pollen grains are destroyed in the process of pollination done by wind.

177. (c) : Yeast such as *Saccharomyces cerevisiae* is used in baking industry. The yeast ferments glucose to yield ethyl alcohol and carbon dioxide. This carbon dioxide is used in baking industry for raising dough. Kneading, stretching and folding of the dough develops the protein structure to improve its elastic properties and its ability to hold gas. This improved gluten properties enable better retention of the gases within the dough as the structure expands and the cell walls become thinner.

178. (a) : In a food chain the number of animals and biomass at the lower trophic level is abundant. Successive links of carnivores decrease rapidly in number until there are very few carnivores at the top.

179. (c) : Tropical rain are disappearing fast from developing countries such as India. Forest lands are converting into agricultural and industrial lands to fulfil the requirements of increasing population. Tropical rain forests are rich in biodiversity.

180. (a) :

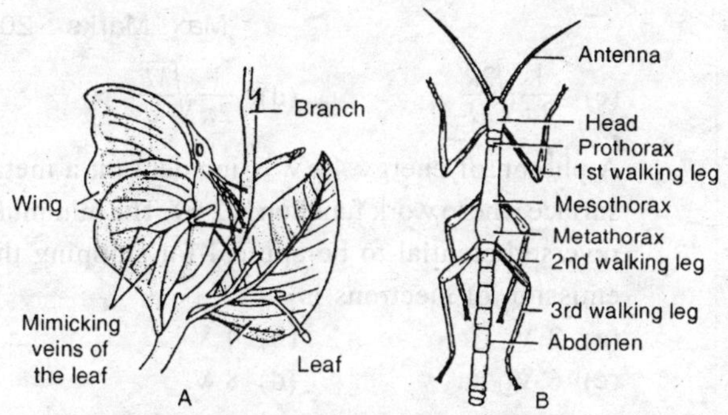

(A) Walking leaf insect (*phyllium*) showing resemblance with a green leaf (an example of concealing mimicry). **(B)** Caterpillar of geometrid moth showing resemblance to a twig.

Mimicry is a process by which two or more organisms independently derive protection from predation. This may be done by acquiring body colour blending with the surrounding or sometimes they bring resemblance to a distasteful, poisonous or harmful organisms. Leaf butterfly and stick insect show the colour of leaf, stem etc. by which they can dodge their enemies and predator.

GENERAL KNOWLEDGE

181. (b)	**182.** (a)
183. (a)	**184.** (c)
185. (b)	**186.** (c)
187. (b)	**188.** (a)
189. (a)	**190.** (a)
191. (c)	**192.** (a)
193. (a)	**194.** (b)
195. (a)	**196.** (b)
197. (d)	**198.** (b)
199. (a)	**200.** (b)

SOLVED PAPER AIIMS - 2004

Time : 3½ Hours Max. Marks : 200

PHYSICS

1. The waves produced by a motorboat sailing in water are
   (a) transverse (b) longitudinal
   (c) longitudinal and transverse
   (d) stationary.

2. In an orbital motion, the angular momentum vector is
   (a) along the radius vector
   (b) parallel to the linear momentum
   (c) in the orbital plane
   (d) perpendicular to the orbital plane.

3. A nucleus of mass number A, originally at rest, emits an α-particle with speed v. The daughter nucleus recoils with a speed
   (a) $\frac{2v}{A+4}$ (b) $\frac{4v}{A+4}$
   (c) $\frac{4v}{A-4}$ (d) $\frac{2v}{A-4}$

4. When an electron-positron pair annihilates, the energy released is about
   (a) 0.8×10^{-13} J (b) 1.6×10^{-13} J
   (c) 3.2×10^{-13} J (d) 4.8×10^{-13} J.

5. A sphere of mass M and radius R is falling in a viscous fluid. The terminal velocity attained by the falling object will be proportional to
   (a) R^2 (b) R
   (c) $1/R$ (d) $1/R^2$.

6. Two springs are connected to a block of mass M placed on a frictionless surface as shown below. If both the springs have a spring constant k, the frequency of oscillation of the block is

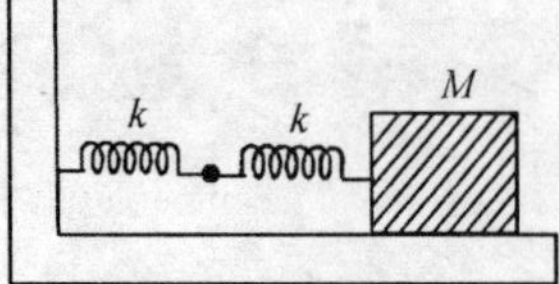

   (a) $\frac{1}{2\pi}\sqrt{\frac{k}{M}}$ (b) $\frac{1}{2\pi}\sqrt{\frac{k}{2M}}$
   (c) $\frac{1}{2\pi}\sqrt{\frac{2k}{M}}$ (d) $\frac{1}{2\pi}\sqrt{\frac{M}{k}}$.

7. A photon of energy 4 eV is incident on a metal surface whose work function is 2 eV. The minimum reverse potential to be applied for stopping the emission of electrons is
   (a) 2 V (b) 4 V
   (c) 6 V (d) 8 V.

8. A proton and an α-particle, moving with the same velocity, enter into a uniform magnetic field, acting normal to the plane of their motion. The ratio of the radii of the circular paths described by the proton and α-particle is
   (a) 1 : 2 (b) 1 : 4
   (c) 1 : 16 (d) 4 : 1.

9. Two parallel beams of positrons moving in the same direction will
   (a) repel each other
   (b) will not interact with each other
   (c) attract each other
   (d) be deflected normal to the plane containing the two beams

10. The electric field due to a uniformly charged sphere of radius R as a function of the distance from its centre is represented graphically by

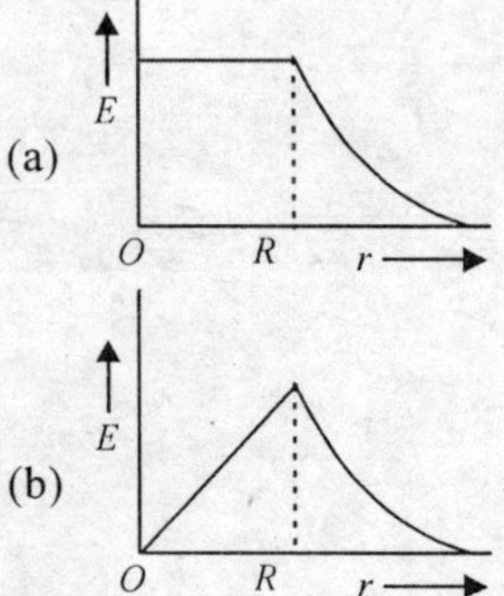

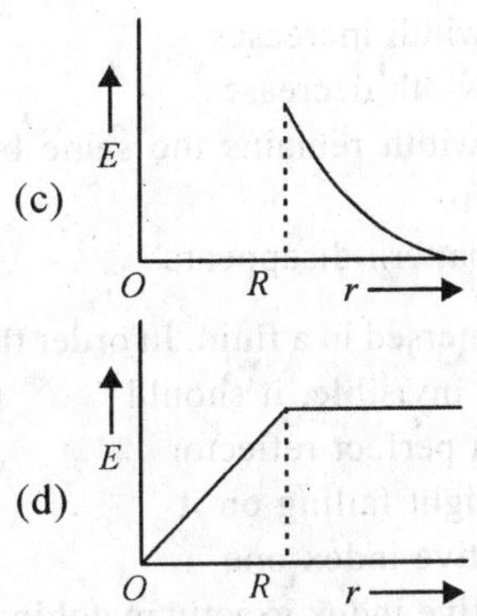

11. Equipotential surfaces associated with an electric field which is increasing in magnitude along the x-direction are
(a) planes parallel to yz-plane
(b) planes parallel to xy-plane
(c) planes parallel to xz-plane
(d) coaxial cylinders of increasing radii around the x-axis.

12. Suppose the sun expands so that its radius becomes 100 times its present radius and its surface temperature becomes half of its present value. The total energy emitted by it then will increase by a factor of
(a) 10^4 (b) 625
(c) 256 (d) 16.

13. The temperature (T) dependence of resistivity (ρ) of a semiconductor is represented by

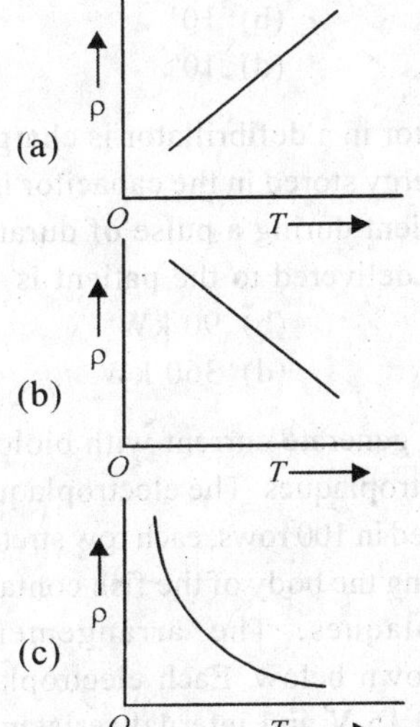

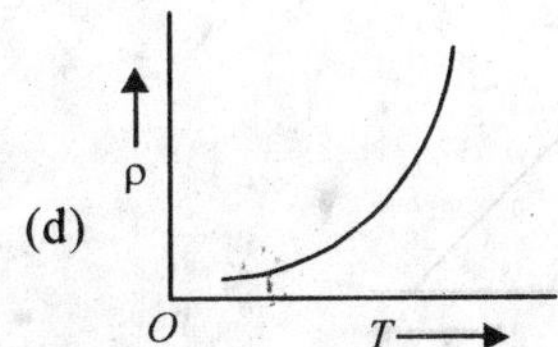

14. In old age arteries carrying blood in the human body become narrow resulting in an increase in the blood pressure. This follows from
(a) Pascal's law (b) Stoke's law
(c) Bernoulli's principle
(d) Archimedes principle.

15. The direction of the angular velocity vector is along
(a) the tangent to the circular path
(b) the inward radius (c) the outward radius
(d) the axis of rotation.

16. A circular coil of radius R carries an electric current. The magnetic field due to the coil at a point on the axis of the coil located at a distance r from the center of the coil, such that $r >> R$, varies as
(a) $1/r$ (b) $1/r^{3/2}$
(c) $1/r^2$ (d) $1/r^3$.

17. Sodium lamps are used in foggy conditions because
(a) yellow light is scattered less by the fog particles
(b) yellow light is scattered more by the fog particles
(c) yellow light is unaffected during its passage through the fog
(d) wavelength of yellow light is the mean of the visible part of the spectrum.

18. The magnetic field due to a straight conductor of uniform cross-section of radius a and carrying a steady current is represented by

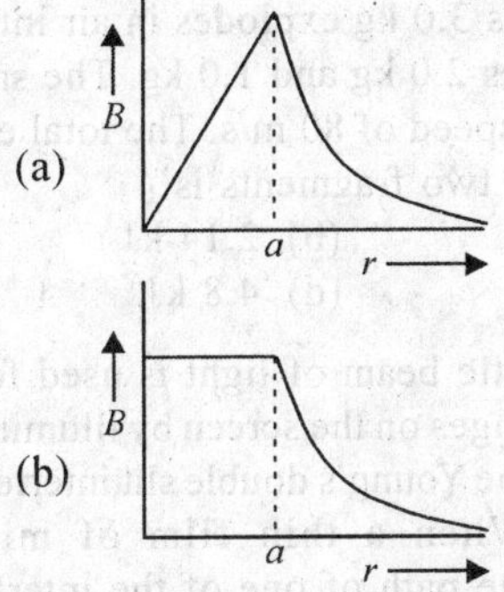

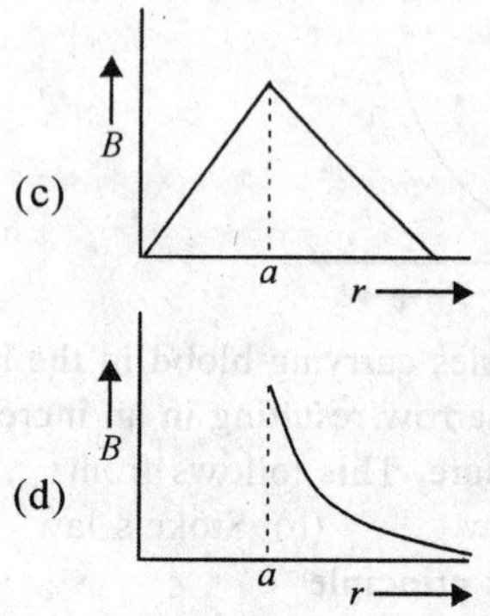

19. Which of the following velocity-time graphs shows a realistic situation for a body in motion?

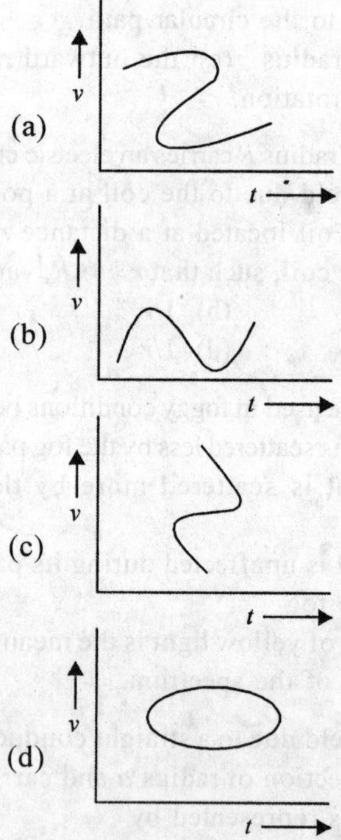

20. A bomb of mass 3.0 kg explodes in air into two pieces of masses 2.0 kg and 1.0 kg. The smaller mass goes at a speed of 80 m/s. The total energy imparted to the two fragments is

(a) 1.07 kJ (b) 2.14 kJ
(c) 2.4 kJ (d) 4.8 kJ.

21. A monochromatic beam of light is used for the formation of fringes on the screen by illuminating the two slits in the Young's double slit interference experiment. When a thin film of mica is interposed in the path of one of the interfering beams then

(a) the fringe width increases
(b) the fringe width decreases
(c) the fringe width remains the same but the pattern shifts
(d) the fringe pattern disappears.

22. An object is immersed in a fluid. In order that the object becomes invisible, it should

(a) behave as a perfect reflector
(b) absorb all light falling on it
(c) have refractive index one
(d) have refractive index exactly matching with that of the surrounding fluid.

23. An organ pipe closed at one end has fundamental frequency of 1500 Hz. The maximum number of overtones generated by this pipe which a normal person can hear is

(a) 14 (b) 13
(c) 6 (d) 9.

24. The Magnetic Resonance Imaging (MRI) is based on the phenomenon of

(a) nuclear magnetic resonance
(b) electron spin resonance
(c) electron paramagnetic resonance
(d) diamagnetism of human tissues.

25. Carbon dating is best suited for determining the age of fossils if their age in years is of the order of

(a) 10^3 (b) 10^4
(c) 10^5 (d) 10^6.

26. A 40 μF capacitor in a defibrillator is charged to 3000 V. The energy stored in the capacitor is sent through the patient during a pulse of duration 2 ms. The power delivered to the patient is

(a) 45 kW (b) 90 kW
(c) 180 kW (d) 360 kW.

27. Eels are able to generate current with biological cells called electroplaques. The electroplaques in an eel are arranged in 100 rows, each row stretching horizontally along the body of the fish containing 5000 electroplaques. The arrangement is suggestively shown below. Each electroplaques has an emf of 0.15 V and internal resistance of 0.25 Ω.

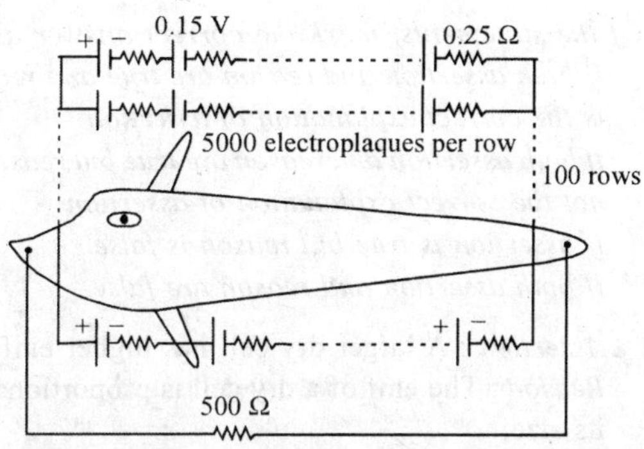

The water surrounding the eel completes a circuit between the head and its tail. If the water surrounding it has a resistance of 500 Ω, the current an eel can produce in water is about

(a) 1.5 A (b) 3.0 A
(c) 15 A (d) 30 A.

28. N moles of a monoatomic gas is carried round the reversible rectangular cycle $ABCDA$ as shown in the diagram. The temperature at A is T_0. The thermodynamic efficiency of the cycle is

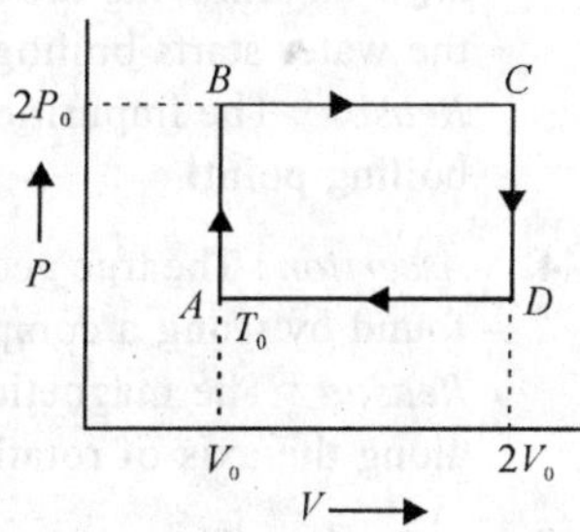

(a) 15% (b) 50%
(c) 20% (d) 25%.

29. Liquid oxygen remains suspended between two pole faces of a magnet because it is

(a) diamagnetic (b) paramagnetic
(c) ferromagnetic (d) antiferromagnetic.

30. An endoscope is employed by a physician to view the internal parts of a body organ. It is based on the principle of

(a) refraction
(b) reflection
(c) total internal reflection
(d) dispersion.

31. We wish to see inside an atom. Assuming the atom to have a diameter of 100 pm, this means that one must be able to resolve a width of say 10 pm. If an electron microscope is used, the minimum electron energy required is about

(a) 1.5 keV (b) 15 keV
(c) 150 keV (d) 1.5 MeV.

32. When a compact disc is illuminated by a source of white light, coloured lines are observed. This is due to

(a) dispersion (b) diffraction
(c) interference (d) refraction.

33. In the basic CsCl crystal structure, Cs^+ and Cl^- ions are arranged in a bcc configuration as shown in the figure. The net electrostatic force exerted by the eight Cs^+ ions on the Cl^- ions is

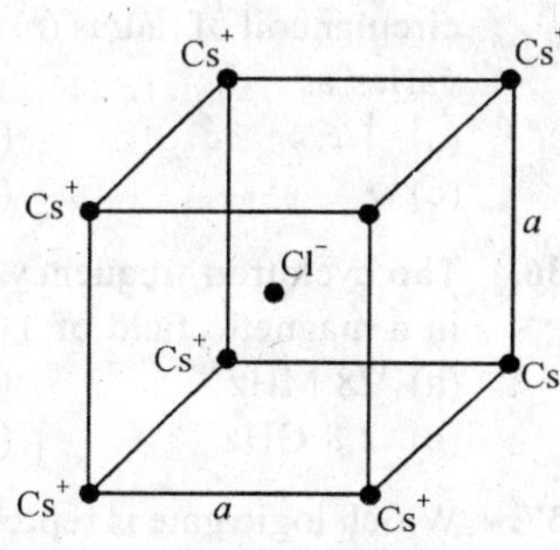

(a) $\frac{1}{4\pi\varepsilon_0}\frac{4e^2}{3a^2}$ (b) $\frac{1}{4\pi\varepsilon_0}\frac{16e^2}{3a^2}$

(c) $\frac{1}{4\pi\varepsilon_0}\frac{32e^2}{3a^2}$ (d) zero.

34. The dependence of binding energy per nucleon, B_N, on the mass number A, is represented by

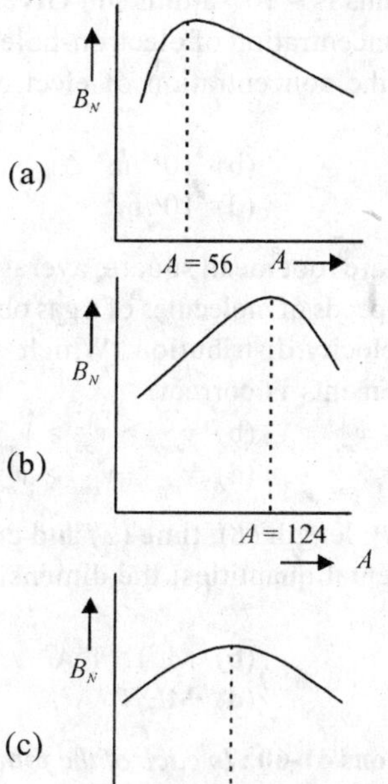

(d) 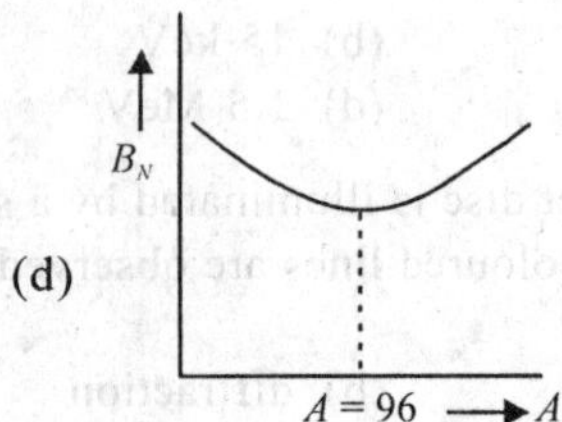

35. The magnetic moment of a current (I) carrying circular coil of radius (r) and number of turns (n) varies as
(a) $1/r^2$ (b) $1/r$
(c) r (d) r^2.

36. The cyclotron frequency of an electron gyrating in a magnetic field of 1 T is approximately
(a) 28 MHz (b) 280 MHz
(c) 2.8 GHz (d) 28 GHz.

37. Which logic gate is represented by the following combination of logic gates?

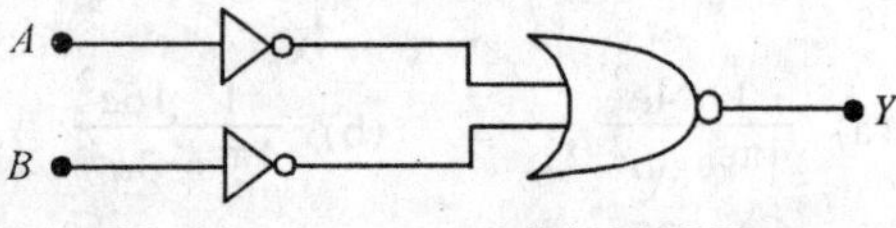

(a) OR (b) NAND
(c) AND (d) NOR.

38. A Ge specimen is doped with Al. The concentration of acceptor atoms is ~ 10^{21} atoms/m^3. Given that the intrinsic concentration of electron-hole pairs is ~ 10^{19}/m^3, the concentration of electrons in the specimen is
(a) 10^{17}/m^3 (b) 10^{15}/m^3
(c) 10^4/m^3 (d) 10^2/m^3.

39. v_{rms}, v_{av} and v_{mp} are root mean square, average and most probable speeds of molecules of a gas obeying Maxwellian velocity distribution. Which of the following statements is correct?
(a) $v_{rms} < v_{av} < v_{mp}$ (b) $v_{rms} > v_{av} > v_{mp}$
(c) $v_{mp} < v_{rms} < v_{av}$ (d) $v_{mp} > v_{rms} > v_{av}$.

40. Using mass (M), length (L), time (T) and current (A) as fundamental quantities, the dimension of permittivity is
(a) $ML^{-2}T^2A$ (b) $M^{-1}L^{-3}T^4A^2$
(c) $MLT^{-2}A$ (d) $ML^2T^{-1}A^2$.

Directions for questions 41-60 : *In each of the following questions, a statement of Assertion (A) is given followed by a corresponding statement of Reason (R) just below it. Of the statements, mark the correct answer as*
(a) If both assertion and reason are true and reason is the correct explanation of assertion
(b) If both assertion and reason are true but reason is not the correct explanation of assertion
(c) If assertion is true but reason is false
(d) If both assertion and reason are false.

41. *Assertion* : A larger dry cell has higher emf.
Reason : The emf of a dry cell is proportional to its size.

42. *Assertion* : A red object appears dark in the yellow light.
Reason : The red colour is scattered less.

43. *Assertion* : In a pressure cooker the water is brought to boil. The cooker is then removed from the stove. Now on removing the lid of the pressure cooker, the water starts boiling again.
Reason : The impurities in water bring down its boiling point.

44. *Assertion* : The true geographic north direction is found by using a compass needle.
Reason : The magnetic meridian of the earth is along the axis of rotation of the earth.

45. *Assertion* : There are very small sporadic changes in the period of rotation of the earth.
Reason : Shifting of large air masses in the earth's atmosphere produce a change in the moment of inertia of the earth causing its period of rotation to change.

46. *Assertion* : In a transistor the base is made thin.
Reason : A thin base makes the transistor stable.

47. *Assertion* : ^{90}Sr from the radioactive fall out from a nuclear bomb ends up in the bones of human beings through the milk consumed by them. It causes impairment of the production of red blood cells.
Reason : The energetics β-particles emitted in the decay of ^{90}Sr damage the bone marrow.

48. *Assertion* : At the first glance, the top surface of the Morpho butterfly's wing appears a beautiful blue-green. If the wing moves the colour changes.
Reason : Different pigments in the wing reflect light at different angles.

49. *Assertion* : A famous painting was painted by not using brush strokes in the usual manner, but rather a myriad of small colour dots. In this painting the colour you see at any given place on the painting changes as you move away.
Reason : The angular separation of adjacent dots changes with the distance from the painting.

50. *Assertion* : A disc-shaped magnet is leviated above a superconducting material that has been cooled by liquid nitrogen.
Reason : Superconductors repel a magnet.

51. *Assertion* : Energy is released in nuclear fission.
Reason : Total binding energy of the fission fragments is larger than the total binding energy of the parent nucleus.

52. *Assertion* : Smaller drops of liquid resist deforming forces better than the larger drops.
Reason : Excess pressure inside a drop is directly proportional to its surface area.

53. *Assertion* : The melting point of ice decreases with increase of pressure.
Reason : Ice contracts on melting.

54. *Assertion* : Heavy water preferred over ordinary water as a moderator in reactors.
Reason : Heavy water, used for slowing down the neutrons, has lesser absorption probability of neutrons than ordinary water.

55. *Assertion* : The driver in a vehicle moving with a constant speed on a straight road is in a non-inertial frame of reference.
Reason : A reference frame in which Newton's laws of motion are applicable is non-inertial.

56. *Assertion* : In He-Ne laser, population inversion takes place between energy levels of neon atoms.
Reason : Helium atoms have a meta-stable energy level.

57. *Assertion* : A transistor amplifier in common emitter configuration has a low input impedence.
Reason : The base to emitter region is forward biased.

58. *Assertion* : Thermodynamic process in nature are irreversible.
Reason : Dissipative effects cannot be eliminated.

59. *Assertion* : Crystalline solids can cause X-rays to diffract.
Reason : Interatomic distance in crystalline solids is of the order of 0.1 nm.

60. *Assertion* : Photoelectric effect demonstrates the wave nature of light.
Reason : The number of photoelectrons is proportional to the frequency of light.

CHEMISTRY

61. Which of the following is only acidic in nature?
(a) $Be(OH)_2$ (b) $Mg(OH)_2$
(c) $B(OH)_3$ (d) $Al(OH)_3$.

62. Which one of the following forms with an excess of CN^- (cyanide) a complex having coordination number two?
(a) Cu^+ (b) Ag^+
(c) Ni^{2+} (d) Fe^{2+}.

63. Which of the following is not considered as an organometallic compound?
(a) *cis*-platin (b) ferrocene
(c) Zeise's salt (d) Grignard reagent.

64. Dimethyl glyoxime gives a red precipitate with Ni^{2+}, which is used for its detection. To get this precipitate readily the best pH range is
(a) < 1 (b) 2 - 3
(c) 3 - 4 (d) 9 - 11.

65. The element which forms oxides in all oxidation states +I to +V is
(a) N (b) P
(c) As (d) Sb.

66. For decolourization of 1 mole of $KMnO_4$, the moles of H_2O_2 required is
(a) 1/2 (b) 3/2
(c) 5/2 (d) 7/2.

67. The statement true for N_3^- is
(a) it has a non-linear structure
(b) it is called pseudohalogen
(c) the formal oxidation state of nitrogen in this anion is –1
(d) it is isoelectronic with NO_2.

68. Which of the following does not have optical isomer?
(a) $[Co(NH_3)_3Cl_3]$ (b) $[Co(en)_3]Cl_3$
(c) $[Co(en)_2Cl_2]Cl$
(d) $[Co(en)(NH_3)_2Cl_2]Cl$.

69. For electron affinity of halogens which of the following is correct?
(a) Br > F (b) F > Cl
(c) Br > Cl (d) F > I.

70. Shape of O_2F_2 is similar to that of
(a) C_2F_2 (b) H_2O_2
(c) H_2F_2 (d) C_2H_2.

71. The liquefied metal expanding on solidification is
(a) Ga (b) Al
(c) Zn (d) Cu.

72. The compound insoluble in water is
(a) mercurous nitrate (b) mercuric nitrate
(c) mercurous chloride
(d) mercurous perchlorate.

73. Which of the following imparts green colour to the burner flame?
(a) $B(OMe)_3$ (b) $Na(OMe)$
(c) $Al(OPr)_3$ (d) $Sn(OH)_2$.

74. The ONO angle is maximum in
(a) NO_3^- (b) NO_2^-
(c) NO_2 (d) NO_2^+.

75. Among the following the dissociation constant is highest for
(a) C_6H_5OH (b) $C_6H_5CH_2OH$
(c) $CH_3C \equiv CH$ (d) $CH_3NH_3^+Cl^-$.

76. The strongest base among the following is
(a) 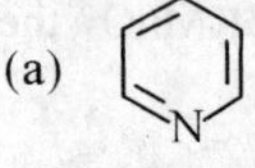

(b) 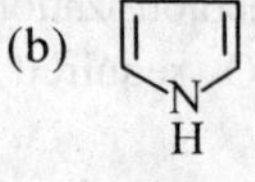

(c) 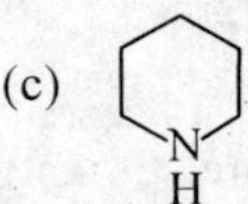

(d) NH_2

77. The compound having only primary hydrogen atoms is
(a) isobutene (b) 2,3-dimethylbutene
(c) cyclohexane (d) propyne.

78. Among the following the aromatic compound is
(a) + (b) +
(c) (d)

79. The dipole moment is the highest for
(a) *trans*-2-butene (b) 1,3-dimethylbenzene
(c) acetophenone (d) ethanol.

80. The geometrical isomerism is shown by
(a) 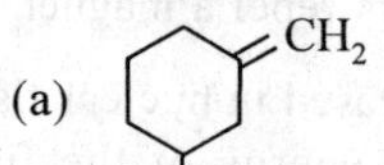

(b) 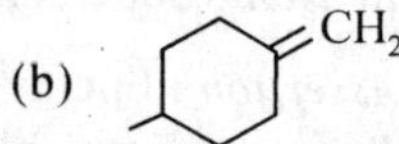

(c) 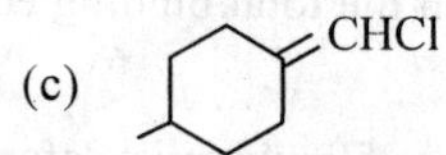

(d) 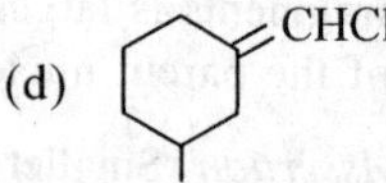

81. The reagent used for the separation of acetaldehyde from acetophenone is
(a) $NaHSO_3$ (b) $C_6H_5NHNH_2$
(c) NH_2OH (d) $NaOH - I_2$.

82. Among the following the most reactive towards alcoholic KOH is
(a) $CH_2 = CHBr$ (b) $CH_3COCH_2CH_2Br$
(c) CH_3CH_2Br (d) $CH_3CH_2CH_2Br$.

83. Among the following, the one which reacts most readily with ethanol is
(a) *p*-nitrobenzyl bromide
(b) *p*-chlorobenzyl bromide
(c) *p*-methoxybenzyl bromide
(d) *p*-methylbenzyl bromide.

84. The nucleic acid base having two possible binding sites is
(a) thymine (b) cytosine
(c) guanine (d) adenine.

85. *o*-Toluic acid on reaction with Br_2 + Fe gives
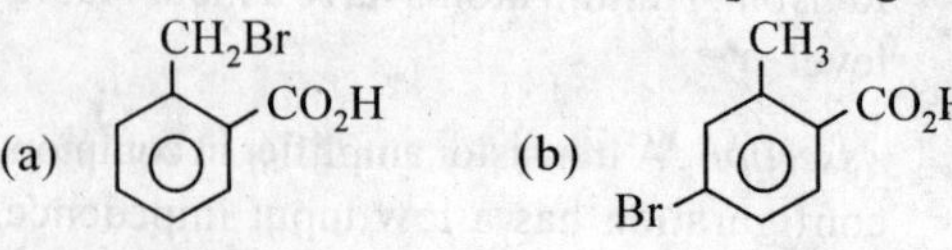

(c) 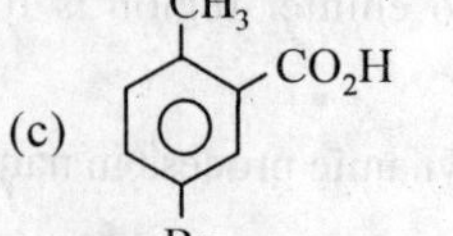

(d) 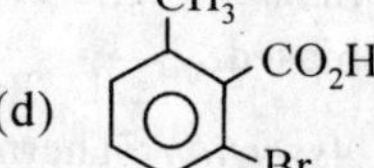

86. Aromatic nitriles (ArCN) are not prepared by reaction:
(a) Ar X + KCN (b) ArN_2^+ + CuCN
(c) $ArCONH_2 + P_2O_5$ (d) $ArCONH_2 + SOCl_2$.

87. Melting points are normally the highest for
(a) tertiary amides (b) secondary amides
(c) primary amides (d) amines.

88. The most suitable reagent for the conversion of $RCH_2OH \rightarrow RCHO$ is
(a) $KMnO_4$ (b) $K_2Cr_2O_7$
(c) CrO_3
(d) PCC (pyridine chloro chromate).

89. Which of the following is arranged in the increasing order of enthalpy of vaporization?
(a) NH_3, PH_3, AsH_3 (b) AsH_3, PH_3, NH_3
(c) NH_3, AsH_3, PH_3 (d) PH_3, AsH_3, NH_3.

90. For principle quantum number $n = 4$, the total number of orbitals having $l = 3$ is
(a) 3 (b) 7
(c) 5 (d) 9.

91. The average osmotic pressure of human blood is 7.8 bar at 37°C. What is the concentration of an aqueous NaCl solution that could be used in the blood stream?
(a) 0.16 mol/L (b) 0.32 mol/L
(c) 0.60 mol/L (d) 0.45 mol/L.

92. How much energy is released when 6 moles of octane is burnt in air? Given ΔH_f° for $CO_{2\,(g)}$, $H_2O_{(g)}$ and $C_8H_{18\,(l)}$ respectively are – 490, –240 and +160 kJ/mol.
(a) – 6.2 kJ (b) – 37.4 kJ
(c) – 35.5 kJ (d) – 20.0 kJ.

93. For the equilibrium $H_2O_{(l)} \rightleftharpoons H_2O_{(g)}$ at 1 atm and 298 K,
(a) standard free energy change is equal to zero ($\Delta G^\circ = 0$)
(b) free energy change is less than zero ($\Delta G < 0$)
(c) standard free energy change is less than zero ($\Delta G^\circ < 0$)
(d) standard free energy change is greater than zero ($\Delta G^\circ > 0$).

94. The crystal system of a compound with unit cell dimensions $a = 0.387$, $b = 0.387$ and $c = 0.504$ nm and $\alpha = \beta = 90°$ and $\gamma = 120°$ is
(a) cubic (b) hexagonal
(c) orthorhombic (d) rhombohedral.

95. What is the pH of 0.01 M glycine solution? For glycine, $Ka_1 = 4.5 \times 10^{-3}$ and $Ka_2 = 1.7 \times 10^{-10}$ at 298 K?
(a) 3.0 (b) 10.0
(c) 6.1 (d) 7.2

96. Of the following which change will shift the reaction towards the product?
$I_{2\,(g)} \rightleftharpoons 2I_{(g)}$, ΔH_r° (298 K) = +150 kJ
(a) increase in concentration of I
(b) decrease in concentration of I_2
(c) increase in temperature
(d) increase in total pressure.

97. Which of the following statements is true for the electrochemical Daniel cell?
(a) Electrons flow from copper electrode to zinc electrode.
(b) Current flows from zinc electrode to copper electrode.
(c) Cations move toward copper electrode.
(d) Cations move toward zinc electrode.

98. Which of the following is a biodegradable polymer?
(a) cellulose (b) polythene
(c) polyvinyl chloride (d) nylon-6.

99. The rate constant k, for the reaction
$$N_2O_{5\,(g)} \rightarrow 2NO_{2\,(g)} + 1/2\, O_{2\,(g)}$$
is $2.3 \times 10^{-2}\ s^{-1}$. Which equation given below describes the change of $[N_2O_5]$ with time? $[N_2O_5]_0$ and $[N_2O_5]_t$ correspond to concentration of N_2O_5 initially and at time t.
(a) $[N_2O_5]_t = [N_2O_5]_0 + kt$
(b) $[N_2O_5]_0 = [N_2O_5]_t\, e^{kt}$
(c) $\log[N_2O_5]_t = \log[N_2O_5]_0 + kt$
(d) $\ln\dfrac{[N_2O_5]_0}{[N_2O_5]_t} = kt$.

100. Ozone in stratosphere is depleted by
(a) CF_2Cl_2 (b) C_7F_{16}
(c) $C_6H_6Cl_6$ (d) C_6F_6.

Directions for Q. 101 to Q. 120 : *In each of the following questions, a statement of Assertion (A) is given followed by a corresponding statement of Reason (R) just below* *it. Of the statements, mark the correct answer as*

(a) *If both assertion and reason are true and reason is the correct explanation of assertion*

(b) *If both assertion and reason are true but reason is not the correct explanation of assertion*

(c) *If assertion is true but reason is false*

(d) *If both assertion and reason are false.*

101. *Assertion* : $HClO_4$ is a stronger acid than $HClO_3$.
Reason : Oxidation state of Cl in $HClO_4$ is +8 and in $HClO_3$ +5.

102. *Assertion* : The free gaseous Cr atom has six unpaired electrons.
Reason : Half-filled *s* orbital has greater stability.

103. *Assertion* : The $[Ni(en)_3]Cl_2$ (en = ethylene diamine) has lower stability than $[Ni(NH_3)_6]Cl_2$.
Reason : In $[Ni(en)_3]Cl_2$ the geometry of Ni is trigonal bipyramidal.

104. *Assertion* : Sb (III) is not precipitated as sulphide when in its alkaline solution H_2S is passed.
Reason : The concentration of S^{2-} ion in alkaline medium is inadequate for precipitation.

105. *Assertion* : Nuclear binding energy per nucleon is in the order - ${}^{9}_{4}Be > {}^{7}_{3}Li > {}^{4}_{2}He$.
Reason : Binding energy per nucleon increases linearly with difference in number of neutrons and protons.

106. *Assertion* : Mg is not present in enamel of human teeth.
Reason : Mg is an essential element for biological functions of human.

107. *Assertion* : Carboxypeptidase is an exopeptidase.
Reason : It cleaves the N-terminal bond.

108. *Assertion* : Sucrose is a non-reducing sugar.
Reason : It has glycosidic linkage.

109. *Assertion* : Isobutanal does not give iodoform test.
Reason : It does not have α-hydrogen.

110. *Assertion* : Styrene on reaction with HBr gives 2-bromo-2-phenylethane.
Reason : Benzyl radical is more stable than alkyl radical.

111. *Assertion* : The pK_a of acetic acid is lower than that of phenol.
Reason : Phenoxide ion is more resonance stabilised.

112. *Assertion* : 2-bromobutane on reaction with sodium ethoxide in ethanol gives 1-butene as a major product.
Reason : 1-butene is more stable than 2-butene.

113. *Assertion* : The major products formed by heating $C_6H_5CH_2OCH_3$ with HI are $C_6H_5CH_2I$ and CH_3OH.
Reason : Benzyl cation is more stable than methyl cation.

114. *Assertion* : Molar entropy of vaporisation of water is different from ethanol.
Reason : Water is more polar than ethanol.

115. *Assertion* : Aqueous gold colloidal solution is red in colour.
Reason : The colour arises due to scattering of light by colloidal gold particles.

116. *Assertion* : Copper metal gets readily corroded is an acidic aqueous solution.
Reason : Free energy change for this process is positive.

117. *Assertion* : Addition of silver ions to a mixture of aqueous sodium chloride and sodium bromide solution will first precipitate AgBr rather than AgCl.
Reason : K_{sp} of AgCl < K_{sp} of AgBr

118. *Assertion* : Alcohols are dehydrated to hydrocarbons in the presence of acidic zeolites.
Reason : Zeolites are porous catalysts.

119. *Assertion* : All F – S – F angle in SF_4 is greater than 90° but less than 180°.
Reason : The lone pair-bond pair repulsion is weaker than bond pair-bond pair repulsion.

120. *Assertion* : Effusion rate of oxygen is smaller than nitrogen.
Reason : Molecular size of nitrogen is smaller than oxygen.

BIOLOGY

121. Cultivation of Bt cotton has been much in the news. The prefix Bt means
(a) "Barium-treated" cotton seeds

(b) "Bigger thread" variety of cotton with better tensile strength
(c) produced by "biotechnology" using restriction enzymes and ligases
(d) carrying an endotoxin gene from *Bacillus thuringienesis*.

122. Which one feature is common to leech, cockroach and scorpion?
(a) nephridia (b) ventral nerve cord
(c) cephalization (d) antennae.

123. Unidirectional transmission of a nerve impulse through nerve fibre is due to the fact that
(a) nerve fibre is insulated by a medullary sheath
(b) sodium pump starts operating only at the cyton and then continues into the nerve fibre
(c) neurotransmitters are released by dendrites and not by axon endings
(d) neurotransmitters are released by the axon endings and not by dendrites.

124. The total number of nitrogenous bases in human genome is estimated to be about
(a) 3.5 million (b) 35 thousand
(c) 35 million (d) 3.1 billion.

125. The Great Barrier Reef along the east coast of Australia can be categorised as
(a) population (b) community
(c) ecosystem (d) biome.

126. Which one of the following is a pair of endangered species?
(a) Garden lizard and Mexican poppy
(b) Rhesus monkey and Sal tree
(c) Indian peacock and carrot grass
(d) Hornbill and Indian aconite.

127. Which one of the following is a matching pair of a drug and its category?
(a) amphetamines - stimulant
(b) lysergic acid dimethyl amide - narcotic
(c) heroin - psychotropic
(d) benzodiazepam - pain killer.

128. In which one of the following pairs the two items mean one and the same thing?
(a) malleus - anvil
(b) SA node - pacemaker
(c) leucocytes - lymphocytes
(d) haemophilia - blood cancer.

129. Which one of the following categories of organisms do not evolve oxygen during photosynthesis?
(a) red algae
(b) photosynthetic bacteria
(c) C_4 plants with Kranz anatomy
(d) blue green algae.

130. A baby has been born with a small tail. It is a case exhibiting
(a) retrogressive evolution
(b) mutation (c) atavism
(d) metamorphosis.

131. Which one of the following is correctly matched regarding an Institute and its location?
(a) National Institute of Virology - Pune
(b) National Institute of Communicable Diseases - Lucknow
(c) Central Drug Research Institute - Kasauli
(d) National Institute of Nutrition - Mumbai.

132. Electron beam therapy is a kind of radiation therapy to treat
(a) enlarged prostrate gland
(b) gall bladder stones by breaking them
(c) certain types of cancer
(d) kidney stones.

133. Severe Acute Respiratory Syndrome (SARS)
(a) is caused by a variant of *Pneumococcus pneumoniae*
(b) is caused by a variant of the common cold virus (corona virus)
(c) is an acute form of asthma
(d) affects non-vegetarians much faster than the vegetarians.

134. Cattle fed with spoilt hay of sweet clover which contains dicumarol
(a) are healthier due to a good diet
(b) catch infections easily
(c) may suffer vitamin K deficiency and prolonged bleeding
(d) may suffer from beri beri due to deficiency of B vitamins.

135. If the Bengal Tiger becomes extinct
(a) hyenas and wolves will become scars
(b) the wild areas will be safe for man and domestic

animals
(c) its gene pool will be lost for ever
(d) the populations of beautiful animals like deers will get stabilized.

136. Nitrogen oxides produced from the emission of automobiles and power plants, are the source of fine air borne particles which lead to
(a) photochemical smog
(b) dry acid deposition
(c) industrial smog
(d) wet acid deposition.

137. A lake with an inflow of domestic sewage rich in organic waste may result in
(a) drying of the lake very soon due to algal bloom
(b) an increased production of fish due to lot of nutrients
(c) death of fish due to lack of oxygen
(d) increased population of aquatic food web organisms.

138. Minamata disease was caused due to the consumption of
(a) sea food containing lot of cadmium
(b) fish contaminated with mercury
(c) oysters with lot of pesticide
(d) sea food contaminated with selenium.

139. An artificial pacemaker is implanted subcutaneously and connected to the heart in patients
(a) having 90% blockage of the three main coronary arteries
(b) having a very high blood pressure
(c) with irregularity in the heart rhythm
(d) suffering from arteriosclerosis.

140. An example of gene therapy is
(a) production of injectable hepatitis B vaccine
(b) production of vaccines in food crops like potatoes which can be eaten
(c) introduction of gene for adenosine deaminase in persons suffering from Severe Combined Immuno-deficiency (SCID)
(d) production of test tube babies by artificial insemination and implantation of fertilized eggs.

141. The pollen tube usually enters the embryo sac
(a) through one of the synergids
(b) by directly penetrating the egg
(c) between one synergid and central cell
(d) by knocking off the antipodal cells.

142. What is the first step in the Southern Blot technique?
(a) denaturation of DNA on the gel for hybridization with specific probe
(b) production of a group of genetically identical cells
(c) digestion of DNA by restriction enzyme
(d) isolation of DNA from a nucleated cell such as the one from the scene of crime.

143. Women who consumed the drug thalidomide for relief from vomiting during early months of pregnancy gave birth to children with
(a) no spleen (b) hare-lip
(c) extra fingers and toes
(d) underdeveloped limbs.

144. Given below is a pedigree chart of a family with five children. It shows the inheritance of attached ear-lobes as opposed to the free ones. The squares represent the male individuals and circles the female individuals.
Which one of the following conclusions drawn is correct?
(a) the parents are homozygous recessive
(b) the trait is Y-linked
(c) the parents are homozygous dominant
(d) the parents are heterozygous.

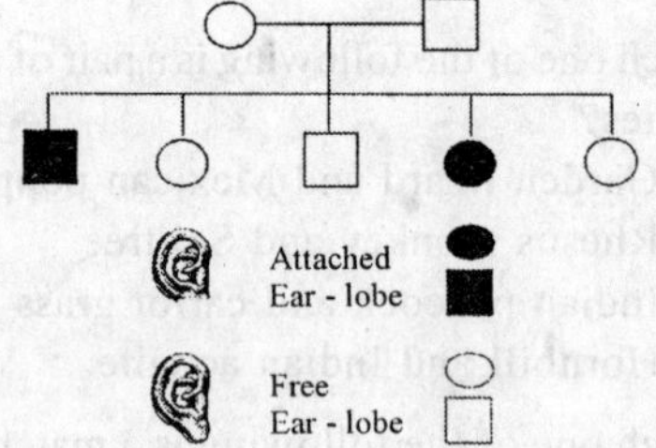

145. Given below is a representation of a kind of chromosomal mutation. What is the kind of mutation represented?

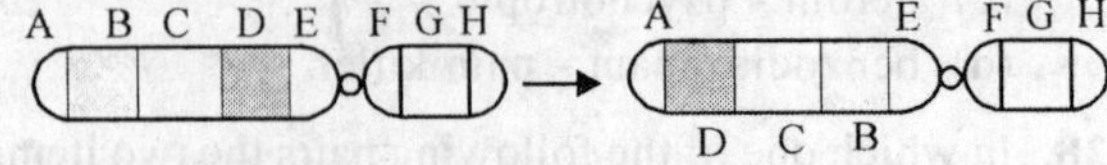

(a) deletion
(b) duplication
(c) inversion
(d) reciprocal translocation.

146. Which one of the following pairs is correctly matched with regard to the codon and the amino acid coded by it?
(a) UUA - valine (b) AAA - lysine
(c) AUG - cysteine (d) CCC - alanine.

147. The treatment of snake-bite by antivenine is an example of
(a) artificially acquired active immunity
(b) artificially acquired passive immunity
(c) naturally acquired passive immunity
(d) specific natural immunity.

148. The bacteria *Pseudomonas* is useful because of its ability to
(a) transfer genes from one plant to another
(b) decompose a variety of organic compounds
(c) fix atmospheric nitrogen in the soil
(d) produce a wide variety of antibiotics.

149. DNA is present in
(a) chromosomes and dictyosomes
(b) chloroplasts and lysosomes
(c) mitochondria and chloroplasts
(d) mitochondria and endoplasmic reticulum.

150. Pruning of plants promotes branching because the axillary buds get sensitized to
(a) ethylene (b) gibberellin
(c) cytokinin (d) indole acetic acid.

151. The sugarcane plant has
(a) dumb-bell shaped guard cells
(b) pentamerous flowers
(c) reticulate venation (d) capsular fruits.

152. Potato and sweet potato
(a) have edible parts which are homologous organs
(b) have edible parts which are analogous organs
(c) have been introduced in India from the same place
(d) are two species of the same genus.

153. In *Ulothrix* meiosis takes place in
(a) cells of the filament
(b) holdfast (c) zygote
(d) zoospores.

154. In a plant organ which is covered by periderm and in which the stomata are absent, some gaseous exchange still takes place through
(a) aerenchyma (b) trichomes
(c) pneumatophores (d) lenticels.

155. Somaclonal variation can be obtained by
(a) application of colchicine
(b) irradiation with gamma rays
(c) tissue culture (d) hybridisation.

156. If the high altitude birds become rare or extinct, the plants which may disappear along with them are
(a) pine (b) oak
(c) orchids (d) rhododendrons.

157. Companion cells in plants are associated with
(a) vessels (b) sperms
(c) sieve elements (d) guard cells.

158. Mossess and ferns are found in moist and shady places because both
(a) require presence of water for fertilization
(b) do not need sunlight for photosynthesis
(c) depend for their nutrition on microorganisms which can survive only at low temperature
(d) cannot compete with sun-loving plants.

159. Cork cambium results in the formation of cork which becomes impermeable to water due to the accumulation of
(a) resins (b) suberin
(c) lignins (d) tannins.

160. How many differcnt types of gametes can be formed by F_1 progeny, resulting from the following cross:

AA BB CC × aa bb cc

(a) 3 (b) 8
(c) 27 (d) 64.

Directions for Q. 161 to Q. 180 : *In each of the following questions, a statement of Assertion (A) is given followed by a corresponding statement of Reason (R) just below it. Of the statements, mark the correct answer as*
(a) *If both Assertion and Reason are true and Reason is the correct explanation of Assertion*
(b) *If both Assertion and Reason are true but Reason is not the correct explanation of Assertion*
(c) *If Assertion is true but Reason is false*
(d) *If both Assertion and Reason are false.*

161. *Assertion* : Agricultural output increased several times after introduction of DDT.
Reason : DDT was the first insecticide used on a wide scale.

162. *Assertion* : Diabetes insipidus is marked by excessive urination and too much thirst of water.

Reason : Anti-diuretic hormone (ADH) is secreted by the posterior lobe of pituitary gland.

163. *Assertion* : Coacervates are believed to be the precursors of life.
Reason : Coacervates were self-duplicating aggregates of proteins surrounded by lipid molecules.

164. *Assertion* : Tapeworm, roundworm and pinworm are endoparasites of human intestine.
Reason : Improperly cooked food is the source of all intestinal infections.

165. *Assertion* : Fish meal is a rich source of protein for cattle and poultry.
Reason : Fish meal is produced from non-edible parts of fishes like fins, tail etc.

166. *Assertion* : Animals adopt different strategies to survive in hostile environment.
Reason : Praying mantis is green in colour which merges with plant foliage.

167. *Assertion* : Among the primates, chimpanzee is the closest relative of the present day humans.
Reason : The banding pattern in the autosome numbers 3 and 6 of man and chimpanzee is remarkably similar.

168. *Assertion* : Dope test is used to estimate the level of blood alcohol by analysing the breath of persons drinking alcohol.
Reason : A drunken person usually feels tense and less talkative.

169. *Assertion* : The honey bee queen copulates only once in her life time.
Reason : The honey bee queen can lay fertilized as well as unfertilized eggs.

170. *Assertion* : From evolutionary point of view, human gestation period is believed to be shortening.
Reason : One major evolutionary trend in humans has been the larger head undergoing relatively faster growth rate in the foetal stage.

171. *Assertion* : Natural selection is the outcome of differences in survival and reproduction among individuals that show variation in one or more traits.
Reason : Adaptive forms of a given trait tend to become more common; less adaptive ones become less common or disappear.

172. *Assertion* : Ginger has a prostrate-growing rhizome.
Reason : Shoot growth is not effected by gravity.

173. *Assertion* : Photomodulation of flowering is a phytochrome - regulated process.
Reason : Active form of phytochrome (Pfr) directly induces floral induction in shoot buds.

174. *Assertion* : Cyclic pathway of photosynthesis first appeared in some eubacterial species.
Reason : Oxygen started accumulating in the atmosphere after the non-cyclic pathway of photosynthesis evolved.

175. *Assertion* : Nitrogen-fixing bacteria in legume root nodules survive in oxygen-depleted cells of nodules.
Reason : Legheamoglobin completely removes oxygen from the nodule cells.

176. *Assertion* : Red algae contribute in producing coral reefs.
Reason : Some red algae secrete and deposit calcium carbonate over their walls.

177. *Assertion* : Insects visit flowers to gather honey.
Reason : Attraction of flowers prevents the insects from damaging other parts of the plant.

178. *Assertion* : Coconut tree is distributed in coastal areas over a large part of the world.
Reason : Coconut fruit can float and get dispersed over thousands of kilometers before losing viability.

179. *Assertion* : Deficiency of sulphur causes chlorosis in plants.
Reason : Sulphur is a constituent of chlorophyll, proteins and nucleic acids.

180. *Assertion* : Cattle breeds can be improved by superovulation and embryo transplantation.
Reason : Superovulation in high milk-yielding cows is induced by hormonal injection.

GENERAL KNOWLEDGE

181. Birbal Sahni was a
(a) zoologist
(b) founder of Central Drug Research Institute
(c) ornithologist (d) paleobotanist.

182. In the year (2003) the chemistry Nobel Prize was awarded to the following work.
(a) aquaporins (b) Na^{++} channels
(c) Ca^{++} channels (d) methyl chavicol.

183. It lives underwater for up to three years as nymph before emerging as a flying insect. Fossils of this

insect dating back about 300 million years have been found.
(a) scorpion fly (b) stone fly
(c) caddis fly (d) may fly.

184. A man-made tunnel in India transfers water from which one river to another?
(a) Narmada to Tapti (b) Betwa to Sone
(c) Beas to Sutlej
(d) Godawari to Krishna.

185. The great Fisher Bank is situated off
(a) the coast of New Foundland
(b) the Chilean coast (c) the Spanish coast
(d) the coast of Great Britain.

186. Which one of the following organisation's iron and steel plant was built to use charcoal as a source of power, to start with, but later switched over to hydroelectricity?
(a) the Tata Iron Steel Company
(b) the Indian Iron and Steel Company
(c) Mysore Iron and Steel Company
(d) Hindustan Steel Limited.

187. Rishikesh is famous for the production of
(a) antibiotics (b) heavy electricals
(c) fertilizers (d) transistorized radios.

188. Rayon fibre is manufactured from
(a) petroleum (b) wood and pulp
(c) chemicals (d) naphtha.

189. Nepanagar is famous for
(a) paper board industries
(b) craft paper industries
(c) carbon paper industries
(d) newsprint paper industries.

190. Since the Britishers wanted India to produce and supply raw materials to feed English factories, they pushed a policy that encouraged cultivation of
(a) jute (b) indigo
(c) cotton (d) commercial crops.

191. Primary sector refers to
(a) industry (b) agriculture
(c) trade (d) banks.

192. Recently there was a report on adverse effect of wearing neck tie. Tight neck tie may cause
(a) glaucoma (b) hypertension
(c) hoarseness of voice(d) hyperthyroidism.

193. The noise produced in office is normally at the level of
(a) 20 db (b) 30 db
(c) 40 db (d) 60 db.

194. In the year 2003 in an eco-marathon contest in Hiroshima the 'Fancy Carol' recorded the mileage of distance per litre of petrol as
(a) 396 km/litre (b) 936 km/litre
(c) 1962 km/litre (d) 3962 km/litre.

195. Dravida Munnetra Kazhakam (DMK) was founded by
(a) M.G. Ramachandran
(b) C.N. Annadurai
(c) Kumar Swami Kamraj
(d) Lalithambika Antharjanam.

196. All of the following won the title of 'Miss World' except
(a) Lara Dutta (b) Aishwarya Rai
(c) Yukta Mukhi (d) Priyanka Chopra.

197. Where is 'Indira Gandhi Rashtriya Uran Akadimi' situated?
(a) Dehradun (b) Raebareli
(c) Allahabad (d) Mussorrie.

198. All of the following are correct about 'Media Lab' except
(a) the third media lab is situated in India
(b) it is supported by government funding
(c) it is interdisciplinary *i.e.* involves sociologists, economists, computer sciences etc.
(d) it plans to produce wearable computer.

199. In the year 2003 which of the following Indian American was honoured by President Bush for his research in automotive technology?
(a) Hiren Gandhi (b) Sabeer Bhatia
(c) Guraj Deshpande (d) Vinod Khosla.

200. Who of the following was a medical doctor?
(a) Samuel Taylor Coleridge
(b) John Webster (c) Somerset Maugham
(d) Thomas Gray.

☺☺☺

SOLUTIONS

PHYSICS

1. **(c) :** The motion of the water boat disturbs the surface of water. Bow waves are generated on the surface. These are transverse waves at the surface. Inside the water, the vibrations of the rudder produces longitudinal waves.

2. **(d) :** In orbital motion, the angular momentum vector is perpendicular to the plane in which the rotational motion take place and its sense is given by the right hand fist rule. When the fingers of right hand fist point in the direction of motion, the thumb is in the direction of $\vec{L}$ (angular momentum).

3. **(c) :** $\underset{\text{(parent nucleus)}}{{}^{A}X} \rightarrow \underset{\text{(daughter nucleus)}}{{}^{A-4}Y} + \alpha^4$

As the parent nucleus is at rest, then according to conservation of momentum.

$\Rightarrow \quad 0 = m_Y v_Y + m_\alpha v_\alpha$

$\Rightarrow \quad 0 = (A-4)v_Y + 4v$

$\Rightarrow \quad v_Y = \frac{4v}{A-4}$, the recoil speed of daughter nucleus.

4. **(b) :** Antiparticles of stable particles (such as the position and the antiproton) are themselves stable. However, when a particle and its antiparticle meet, the annihilation reaction can occur, the particle and antiparticle both vanish and instead two or more photons can be produced. Conservation of energy and momentum require that, neglecting the kinetic energies of the particles, when two photons are emitted each must have an energy equal to the rest mass energy of the particles.
Thus when electron-positron pair annihilate each other, the energy released is equal to rest mass of electron and positron.

$$e^- + e^+ \rightarrow \gamma_1 + \gamma_2$$

$[E_{\gamma_1} = E_{\gamma_2} = 0.511 \text{ MeV} = 0.8 \times 10^{-13} \text{ J}]$

The total energy released $= 1.6 \times 10^{-13}$ J.

5. **(a) :** Stoke's law : $6\pi r\eta v = \frac{4}{3}\pi r^3(\rho - \sigma)g$

$\therefore \quad v \propto r^2$.

As M is given, $\rho = \frac{M}{\frac{4}{3}\pi r^3}$

But as r^3 increases, M also increases and ρ is a constant. σ also is a constant.

$\therefore \quad v$, the terminal velocity $\propto r^2$.

6. **(b) :** The spring constant of spring connected in series is equal to

$$k = \frac{k_1 k_2}{k_1 + k_2} = \frac{k}{2}$$

Thus frequency of oscillation of given system is

$$f = \frac{1}{2\pi}\sqrt{\frac{k}{2m}}.$$

7. **(a) :** When stopping potential is applied no electron will reach the cathode and the current will becomes zero.

$\therefore \quad eV_0 = \frac{1}{2}mv_{max}^2$

Also, $\frac{1}{2}mv_{max}^2 = h\upsilon -$ work function

$= 4 \text{ eV} - 2\text{eV} = 2 \text{ eV}.$

$\Rightarrow \quad eV_0 = 2 \text{ eV} \Rightarrow$ stopping potential $= 2$ V.

8. **(a) :** While describing circular path, the centripetal and centrifugal forces are balancing each other.

$\Rightarrow \quad \frac{mv^2}{r} = qvB$

(as the uniform magnetic field is acting normal to the plane)

$\Rightarrow \quad r = \frac{mv}{qB} \Rightarrow \frac{r_p}{r_\alpha} = \frac{m_p v}{eB} \times \frac{2eB}{m_\alpha v} = \frac{2m_p}{4m_p}$ [as $m_\alpha = 4m_p$]

$\therefore \quad r_p : r_\alpha = 1 : 2.$

9. **(c) :** Two parallel beams of positrons travelling in the same direction is the same as two parallel currents travelling in the same direction. They attract each other.

10. **(b) :** The magnitude of the electric field at a point exterior to the sphere is $\frac{1}{4\pi\varepsilon_0}\frac{Q}{r^2}$.
The magnitude of electric field inside the sphere is given by $\frac{1}{4\pi\varepsilon_0}\frac{Qr}{a^3}$.

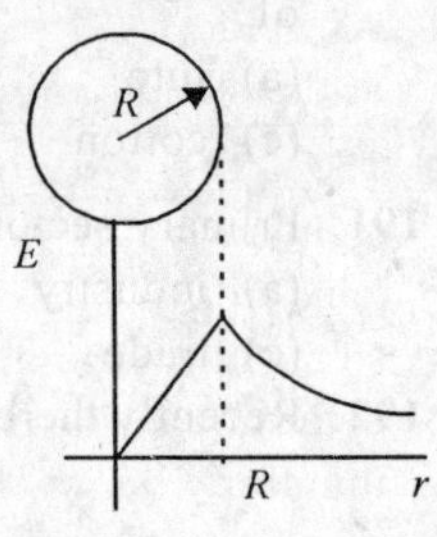

The field is directly proportional to r.

11. **(a) :** Any surface which has same electrostatic potential at every point is called an equipotential surface. Electric field is always perpendicular to an equipotential surface. Therefore x-direction is perpendicular only to yz plane.

12. **(b) :** According to Stefan's law, the radiation energy emitted per second per unit area of a black body $= \sigma T^4$, where σ is called Stefan's constant.

Energy emitted $\propto AT^4 \Rightarrow E \propto 4\pi r^2 T^4$

where A = area of the body, T = temperature in Kelvin. When sun expands such that its radius becomes 100 times its present radius and its surface temperature becomes half. Then energy emitted by it is

$$E \propto 4\pi(100)^2 r^2 \left(\frac{T}{2}\right)^4$$

$$\propto \left(\frac{100}{4}\right)^2 E$$

Total energy emitted will be increased by

$$\frac{E'}{E} = \frac{(100/4)^2 E}{E} = 625.$$

13. **(b) :** The variation of specific resistance with temperature is given by

$$\rho = \rho_0 [1 + \alpha(T - T_0)]$$

where α = temperature coefficient of resistance which is negative for semiconductor.

$$\rho = \rho_0 + \rho_0\alpha(T - T_0)$$

Comaring with straight line equation, $y = mx + c$

$\Rightarrow$ m, slope is negative.

14. **(c) :** According to continuity theorem as

$$av = \text{constant}$$

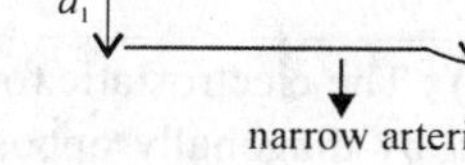

as area increases velocity decreases. So when blood flows from narrow arteries to wider one, velocity decreases. According to Bernoulli's principle,

$$P + \frac{1}{2}\rho v^2 = \text{constant}$$

As velocity decreases, pressure increases. Thus when arteries become narrow, blood pressure increases.

15. **(d) :** According to the right hand rule wrap the right hand around the axis of rotation so that the fingers are pointing in the direction of rotation. The thumb points in the direction of angular velocity.

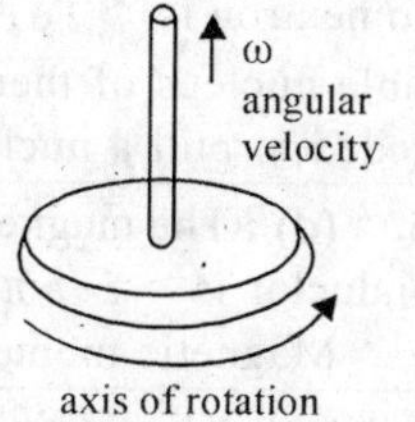

16. **(d) :** Magnetic field at a point on the axis of a loop is given by

$$B = \frac{\mu_0}{4\pi} \frac{2\pi I R^2}{(R^2 + r^2)^{3/2}}$$

When $r >> R$,

$$B = \frac{\mu_0}{4\pi} \frac{2\pi R^2 I}{r^3} = \frac{\mu_0}{2\pi} \frac{AI}{r^3}. \quad \text{Thus, } B \propto (1/r^3).$$

17. **(a) :** Sodium lamp light emits monochromatic light i.e. it is comprised of only one wavelength (deep yellow). This colour is scattered less in the foggy condition while other light sources produce light at many different discrete wavelengths and all provide some degree of colour rendering. Also sodium lamps emit light very near to the peak sensitivity of the human eye under normal viewing conditions.

18. **(a) :** Magnetic field at a point outside the straight conductor is

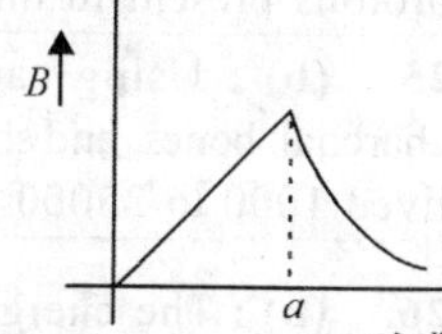

$$B = \frac{\mu_0 I}{2\pi r}$$

i.e. $B \propto (1/r) \quad (r > a)$.

Magnetic field at a point lying inside the conductor is

$$B \propto r \quad (r < a).$$

19. **(b) :** In the other graphs, at a particular time more than one velocity is shown which is not possible in realistic situation.

20. **(d) :** Velocity of second piece can be find out using conservation of momentum.

$$0 = m_1v_1 + m_2v_2 = 2 \times v_1 + 1 \times 80$$

$\Rightarrow \quad v_1 = -40$ m/s.

Negative sign showing that particle is moving in opposite direction of other particle direction.

Energy imparted to the fragments are converted into their kinetic energy.

$$\therefore \quad \text{Total energy} = \frac{1}{2}m_1v_1^2 + \frac{1}{2}m_2v_2^2$$

$$= \frac{1}{2} \times 2 \times 1600 + \frac{1}{2} \times 1 \times 6400$$

$$= 4800 \text{ J} = 4.8 \text{ kJ}.$$

21. **(c) :** The presence of thin mica in the path of one of the interfering beams changes only the path difference between the beams due to which the pattern shifts upwards. But the fringe width remains the same. As mochromatic light is used, one cannot make out which is the central shift as all the fringes are having the same colour and intensity.

22. (d) : If the refractive index of two media are same, the surface of separation does not produce refraction or reflection which helps in visibility.

23. (c) : Human ear can hear frequencies upto 20,000 Hz. So for closed pipe,

overtone, $\upsilon = \frac{nv}{4L} = n \times$ fundamental frequency

$\therefore \quad 20{,}000 = n \times 1500 \quad \Rightarrow \quad n \approx 13.$

Maximum possible harmonics obtained

$= 1, 3, 5, 7, 9, 11, 13 \ldots\ldots\ldots$

Therefore one can hear maximum upto 13th harmonics.

Overtone = 7 – 1 = 6.

24. (a) : MRI is extension of NMR or nuclear magnetic resonance imagning. Magnetic resonance imaging is a noninvasive technique which uses strong magnetic field for generating resonance at low radio frequency in the protons present in the body.

25. (b) : Using carbon dating, samples of wood, charcoal, bones, and shells have been identified as having lived 1000 to 25000 years ago.

26. (b) : The energy stored in capacitor = $\frac{1}{2}CV^2$

$= \frac{1}{2} \times 40 \times 10^{-6} \times (3000)^2$

$= 20 \times 9 \times 10^6 \times 10^{-6} = 180$ J.

The power delivered in 2 ms is

$= \frac{180}{2 \times 10^{-3}} = 90 \times 10^3 \text{ W} = 90 \text{ kW}.$

27. (a) : In each row all the 5000 electroplaques are connected in series.

Therefore, equivalent emf = 0.15 × 5000 = 750 V.

Equivalent resistance = 0.25 × 5000 = 1250 Ω.

All 100 rows are connected in parallel.

Therefore voltage = 750 V.

Equivalent resistance = $\frac{1250}{100} = 12.50\ \Omega$.

Thus resultant circuit of eel becomes

750 V 12.50 Ω

500 Ω

Current across 500 Ω = $\frac{V}{R} = \frac{750}{500 + 12.50} = 1.46$ A

$I \approx 1.5$ A.

28. (b) : At A, temperature = T_0, volume = V_0, pressure - P_0 for n moles of monoatomic gas.

At A, $P_0V_0 = nRT_0$ (cold)

At B, $2P_0V_0 = nRT'_{high} \Rightarrow T' = 2T_0$

Maximum thermal efficiency of the reversible engine of this Carnot's cycle

$= \eta = 1 - \frac{T_C}{T_h} = 1 - \frac{T_0}{2T_0} = \frac{1}{2} = 50\%.$

29. (b) : Molecular bonding of O_2 based on orbitals show that O_2 is paramagnetic, which is true experimentally.

30. (c) : This is made of optical fibres whose interior is coated with a refractive index greater than that of the outer cover, glass.

31. (b) : In electron microscope, electrons are used as the 'light source'. The resolving power of a microscope is approximately equal to that of wavelength of the light used. The de Broglie wavelength λ of a particle is related to its momentum p by

$$\lambda = \frac{h}{p} = \frac{h}{mv}$$

The speed of required electron is

$$v = \frac{h}{m\lambda} = \frac{6.63 \times 10^{-34} \text{ Js}}{9.11 \times 10^{-31} \text{ kg} \cdot 10^{-11} \text{ m}} = 7.28 \times 10^7 \text{ m/s}$$

This corresponds to kinetic energy of $E = \frac{1}{2}mv^2$

$= \frac{1}{2} \times 9.11 \times 10^{-31} \times (7.28 \times 10^7)^2 \times \frac{1 \text{ eV}}{1.6 \times 10^{-19} \text{ J}}$

= 15.1 keV.

32. (b) : In compact disc colour results due to phenomenon of diffraction, in which small ripples on the surface of it break up white light into the colour of rainbow.

33. (d) : The electrostatic force due to one Cs^+ ion is balanced by diagonally opposite other Cs^+. Thus the net electrostatic force on Cl^- ion due to eight Cs^+ ions is zero.

34. (a) : The graph showing that greater the binding energy per nucleon, the more stable the nucleus is. The graph has its maximum of 8.8 MeV/nucleon when the number of nucleons is 56. The nucleus that has 56 protons and neutron is $^{56}_{26}$Fe, an iron isotope. This is the most stable nucleus of them all, since maximum energy is needed to pull a nucleon away from it.

35. (d) : The magnetic moment of a current carrying conductor is $i \cdot n \pi r^2 = niA$.

i.e. Magnetic moment ∝ r^2.

36. (d) : Cyclotron frequency

$$\upsilon = \frac{qB}{2\pi m} = \frac{1.6\times10^{-19}\times1}{2\times3.14\times9.1\times10^{-31}}$$
$$= 28 \times 10^{9}\ \text{Hz} = 28\ \text{GHz}.$$

37. (c) : Truth table

A	B	A'	B'	Y
0	0	1	1	0
0	1	1	0	0
1	0	0	1	0
1	1	0	0	1

Output of this is same as that of AND gate.

38. (a) : When Ge specimen is doped with Al, then concentration of acceptor atoms is also called concentration of holes.

Using formula, $n_i^2 = n_0 p_0$, where

n_i = concentration of electron-hole pair = $10^{19}/\text{m}^3$

n_0 = concentration of electron

p_0 = concentration of holes = 10^{21} atom/m^3

$\Rightarrow \quad (10^{19})^2 = 10^{21} \times n_0 \;\Rightarrow\; n_0 = 10^{17}/\text{m}^3.$

39. (b) : $v_{rms} = \sqrt{\frac{3K_BT}{m}} = 1.73\sqrt{\frac{K_BT}{m}}$

$$v_{av} = \sqrt{\frac{8K_BT}{\pi m}} = 1.60\sqrt{\frac{K_BT}{m}}$$

$$v_{mp} = \sqrt{\frac{2K_BT}{m}} = 1.41\sqrt{\frac{K_BT}{m}}$$

From these equations, $v_{rms} > v_{av} > v_{mp}$.

40. (b) : Force of attraction between two charges is given by

$$F = \frac{1}{4\pi\varepsilon_0}\frac{q_1q_2}{r^2}$$

$$\Rightarrow \quad \varepsilon_0 = \frac{1}{4\pi}\frac{1}{F}\frac{q_1q_2}{r^2} = \frac{\text{A}^2\text{T}^2}{\text{MLT}^{-2}\text{L}^2}$$

(where 4π is dimensionless)

$= \text{M}^{-1}\text{L}^{-3}\text{T}^4\text{A}^2.$

41. (d) : The electrical force of a cell or battery called electromotive force (emf). This force, which makes electrons flow around a circuit. Each kind of cell has a particular emf. The size of a cell has no effect on its emf. The chemicals in the cell determines its emf, but large cells last longer than small cells of same basic type. This means that from a large cell, we get a particular emf for more time as compared to small cell.

42. (b) : A red object reflects red colour from a light falling on it. Thus when this object is viewed in yellow light then it absorbs all yellow light falling on it and appears dark. From Rayleigh's scattering is inversely proportional to λ^4. Red colour has largest wavelength; therefore this colour is scattered least as compared to other colours.

43. (c) : The pressure cooker works on the principle that boiling point of a liquid increases with increase of vapour pressure above the liquid. Water, along with food to be cooked are heated in a closed vessel, so that the confined water vapour raises the superincumbent pressure. As a result, water boils at a temperature higher than 100°C. When the cooker is removed from the stove and the lid is removed, pressure again decreases due to which its boiling point decreases and water starts boiling again.

44. (d) : From the compass we are able to know the direction of the magnetic poles. The north of compass points towards the magnetic south pole. If we know the magnetic declination at that particular place (which is angle between geographic meridian and magnetic meridian) we can easily find out the true geographic north-south direction.

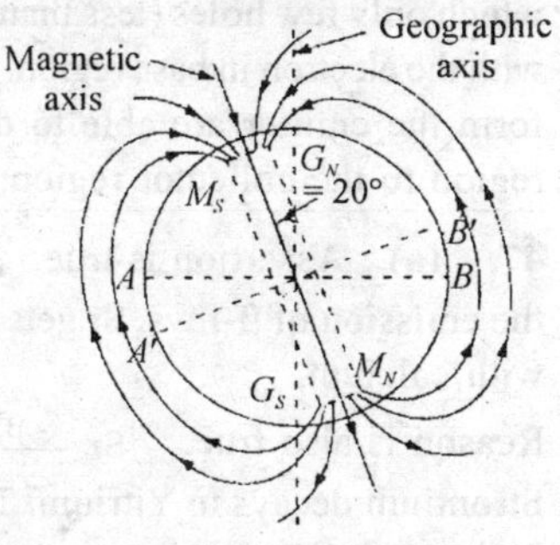

Imaginary lines drawn along the earth's surface in the direction of the horizontal component of the magnetic field of the earth at all points passing through the north and south magnetic poles. This is similar to the longitudes of the earth, which pass through the geographic north and south poles.

45. (a) : Normally when a body is moving in a straight line, whatever be the internal changes, the centre of mass continuous in its trajectory with the same velocity and a system that is rotating continues to rotate with the same angular velocity and changes occur in such a way that the angular momentum is conserved. Classical physics, taking the whole of the earth as a system does not allow sporadic changes in the speed of the earth. However, according to the information on the earth's rotation by U.S. Naval observatory sporadic changes of the speed of rotation of the earth have been observed and this is attributed to the influence of the moon on the tides. This makes it necessary to take the earth and the moon (at least) as one system.

In the reason given, though normally when taking the

earth as a single system, internal changes do not affect the motion, now that one has to take the earth-moon system, the reason that the earth's angular velocity can also change due to the events on earth alone cannot be ruled out. Then the total angular momentum of the earth-moon system will be conserved. The reason is also right, though according to the rules of the game for the 12th class examinations, one can take only the earth as a whole as a system. In that case, both the assertion and reason are wrong.

46. **(c) :** The base is lightly doped and very thin, this constructional feature is key of transistor action due to which only few holes (less than 5%) are able to combine with the electron in base region. Most of the holes coming form the emitter are able to diffuse through the base region to the collector region.

47. **(a) :** Assertion is true. ${}^{90}_{38}\text{Sr}$ decays to ${}^{90}_{39}\text{Y}$ by the emission of β-rays. Sr gets absorbed in bones along with calcium.

Reason is also true. ${}^{90}\text{Sr} \xrightarrow{\beta} {}^{90}\text{Y}$

Strontium decays to Yitrium. This emits β-rays of very high energy. Sr does not emit γ-rays. The damage is by the β-rays only.

48. **(c) :** Many Morpho butterflies are coloured in metallic, shimmering shades of blue and green. These colours are not due to pigmentation but due to iridescence: the extremely fine lamellated scales covering the Morpho's wings reflect incident light repeatedly at successive layers leading to interference effect that depends on both the wavelengths and angle of incidence. Thus the colours produced vary with viewing angle. However they are actually surprisingly uniform, perhaps due to the tetrahedral (diamond-like) structural arrangement of scales or diffraction from overlying cell layers. This structure may be called photonic crystal.

49. **(a) :** For the human eye, the resolving power or angular separation of objects changes as distance from the object changes. Thus when we are close to the painting our eyes can pick out the separate colours of dots. But when we move away from the painting, our eyes blend the dots and we see different colours.

50. **(a) :** Since superconductors exist only below a certain critical temperature and above that temperature they behave like normal materials. When magnet is placed above superconductor and cooled using liquid nitrogen. The induced magnetic field inside the superconductor is exactly equal and opposite in direction to the applied magnetic field, so that they cancel within the super conductor. These poles will repel each other and the force of repulsion is enough to float the magnet.

51. **(a) :** When a heavy nucleus splits into two medium-sized ones, each of the new nuclei will have more binding energy per nucleon than the original nucleus. The extra energy will be given off. *e.g.* if the uranium nucleus ${}^{235}_{92}\text{U}$ is broken into two small nuclei, the binding energy difference per nucleon is about 0.8 MeV. The total energy given off is therefore

$$\frac{0.8\text{ MeV}}{\text{nucleon}} \times 235 \text{ nucleon} = 188 \text{ MeV}$$

52. **(c) :** The excess pressure inside the small drop is large as compared to the large drop because of which smaller drop of liquid resists deforming force better than the large drop.

Excess pressure $= \dfrac{2T}{r}$

where T = surface tension

r = radius of liquid drop.

Therefore excess pressure is inversely proportional to its radius and hence the surface area.

53. **(b) :**

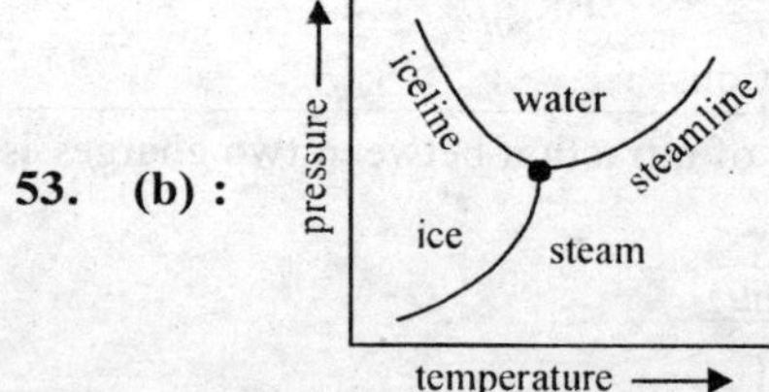

It can be easily seen from the graph that as pressure increases the melting point of ice decreases.

54. **(a) :** A bombarding particle gives up most energy when it makes an elastic collision with a particle of similar mass. For neutrons, hydrogen atoms would be most effective but unfortunately absorption occurs. However, deuterium (heavy water) and carbon (as graphite) are both suitable in which less absorption occurs. Therefore they are used as moderators.

55. **(c) :** If one takes two frames with origin O_1 and O_2 and if a body P is at rest, both according to O_1 as well as O_2. The body is at rest. If the frame is moving with a constant velocity, the same observation will not be made. Therefore a frame moving with a constant velocity cannot be taken as an inertial frame. Assertion

is right.
But the reason given is wrong because the frame on which Newton's laws of motion are applicable is an inertial frame.

56. **(b) :** Helium-neon laser uses a gaseous mixture of helium and neon. An electric discharge in the gas pumps the helium atoms to higher energy level, (which is meta stable energy level).

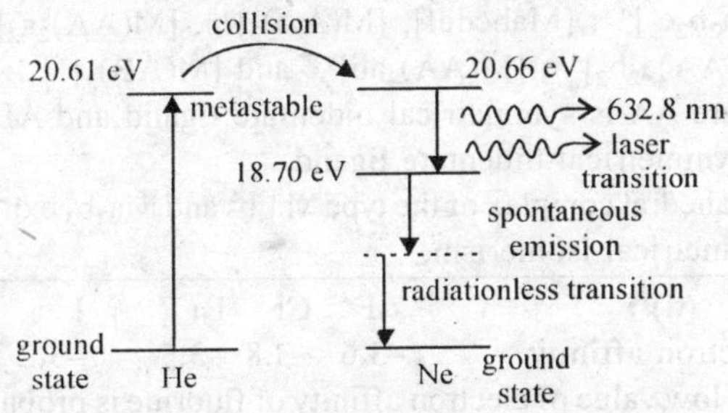

Sequence of transitions in He-Ne laser.

Then these helium atom excite the neon atoms to higher level by collision and produce an inverted population of neon atom which emit radiation when they are stimulated to fall to lower level.

57. **(b) :** Input impedance of common emitter configuration $= \left.\frac{\Delta V_{BE}}{\Delta i_B}\right|_{V_{CE} = \text{constant}}$

where ΔV_{BE} = voltage across base and emitter, Δi_B = base current which is order of few microampere.

Thus input impedance of common emitter is low.

58. **(a) :** In an irreversible process, there always occurs some loss of energy. This is because energy spent in working against the dissipative force is not recovered back. Some irreversible processes occur in nature such as friction where extra work is needed to cancel the effect of friction. Salt dissolves in water but a salt does not separate by itself into pure salt and pure water.

59. **(c) :** For diffraction, the slit width should be of the order of the incident wavelength. The regular spacing of the atoms in crystal is of the order of wavelength of X-rays (0.1 nm) because of which X-rays are diffracted from the crystals.

60. **(d) :** Photoelectric effect can be explained on the basis of quantum theory or particle nature of light where wave nature of light fails to explain the photoelectric effect. The number of photoelectrons is proportional to the intensity of incident light.

$I = nh\upsilon$ where n is the number of photons emitted/absorbed per unit area per second. n and $h\upsilon$ are independent factors.

CHEMISTRY

61. **(c) :** $B(OH)_3$ in aqueous medium coordinates a molecule of water to form the hydrated species $H_2O \rightarrow B(OH)_3$. In this species, B^{3+} ion, because of its small size, exercises a high polarizing power thereby pulling the sigma electron charge of the coordinated O atom towards itself. The coordinated oxygen, in turn, pulls the sigma electron charge of the OH bond of the attached H_2O molecule towards itself. This facilitates the removal of H^+ ion from the O – H bond, as shown below.

$$H_2O \rightarrow B(OH)_3 \rightleftharpoons [B(OH)_4]^- + H^+$$

Thus the solution of $B(OH)_3$ in water acts as a weak acid. That is why it reacts with NaOH solution to produce the sodium salt.

$$B(OH)_3 + NaOH \rightleftharpoons Na^+[B(OH)_4]^-$$
$$\rightleftharpoons \underset{\text{sodium metaborate}}{Na^+ BO_2^-} + 2H_2O$$

62. **(b) :** The total number of points of attachment to the central element is termed the coordination number and this can vary from 2 to as many as 16, but is usually 6. There is no way to predict the coordination number. The arrangement of coordination number 2 is not very common for first row transition metal ion complexes. Some of the best known examples for silver (I). For instance, a method often employed for the detection of chloride ions involves the formation of the linear diamminesilver(I) complex.

The first step is :

$$Ag^+ + Cl^- \rightarrow AgCl \text{ (white ppt.)}$$

and to ensure that the precipitate is really the chloride salt, two further tests must be done:

$$AgCl + 2NH_3 \rightarrow [Ag(NH_3)_2]^+$$

and $[Ag(NH_3)_2]^+ + HNO_3 \rightarrow AgCl$ (ppts.)

The reaction of a bidentate ligand such as

1,2-diaminoethane with Ag^+ does not lead to chelated ring systems, but instead to linear two coordinate complexes. One reason for this is that bidentate ligands can not exist in trans arrangements that is they cannot span 180 degrees.

63. (a) : $\begin{matrix} H_3N & & Cl \\ & Pt & \\ H_3N & & Cl \end{matrix}$ is not an organometallic compound as it does not contain carbon-metal bond. Cisplatin is an inorganic compound, used as anticancer drug and falls into class of DNA damaging agents.

64. (d) : Nickel(II) forms a precipitate with the organic compound dimethylglyoxime, $C_4H_6(NOH)_2$. The formation of the red chelate occurs quantitatively in a solution in which the pH is buffered in the range of 5 to 9. The chelation reaction that occurs is illustrated below.

$$2\,\underset{\text{dimethylglyoxime (DMG)}}{(H_3C)(CH_3)C_2(=N-OH)_2} + Ni^{2+} \xrightarrow{NH_3} \underset{Ni(DMG)_2}{Ni(DMG)_2} + 2H^+$$

Although the loss of one proton occurs from one oxime group (NOH) on each of the two molecules of dimethylglyoxime, the chelation reaction occurs due to donation of the electron pairs on the four nitrogen atoms, not by electrons on the oxygen atoms. The reaction is performed in a solution buffered by either an ammonia or citrate buffer to prevent the pH of the solution from falling below 5. If the pH does become too low the equilibrium of the above reaction favors the formation of nickel(II) ion, causing the dissolution of $Ni(DMG)_2$ back into the mother liquor.

65. (a) : Stability of oxides of higher oxidation states decreases with increasing atomic number.
Nitrogen exhibits a large number of oxidation states such as +1, +2, +3, +4, +5 in N_2O, NO, N_2O_3, N_2O_4 and N_2O_5.

66. (c) : Acidified $KMnO_4$ is decolourised by H_2O_2 in following way.

$$2KMnO_4 + 3H_2SO_4 \rightarrow K_2SO_4 + 2MnSO_4 + 3H_2O + 5O$$
$$5H_2O_2 + 5O \rightarrow 5H_2O + 5O_2$$
$$2KMnO_4 + 3H_2SO_4 + 5H_2O_2 \rightarrow K_2SO_4 + 2MnSO_4 + 8H_2O + 5O_2$$

Thus, for 2 moles of $KMnO_4$ required H_2O_2 = 5
For 1 mole of $KMnO_4$ required H_2O_2 = 5/2 mole.

67. (c) : Azide ion is a linear molecule, it is a pseudo halide and formal oxidation state of N in azide ion is –1.

$$N_3^-;\ :\overset{2-}{N}-\overset{+}{N}\equiv N: \longleftrightarrow :N\equiv\overset{+}{N}-\overset{2-}{N}: \longleftrightarrow \underset{\text{major}}{:N=\overset{+}{N}=N:}$$

68. (a) : Optical isomerism is very common in octahedral complexes of general formulae, $[Ma_2b_2c_2]^{n\pm}$, [Mabcdef], $[M(AA)_3]^{n\pm}$, $[M(AA)_2a_2]^{n\pm}$, $[M(AA)a_2b_2]^{n\pm}$, $[M(AA)_2ab]^{n\pm}$ and $[M(AB)_3]^{n\pm}$, where AA is symmetrical bidentate ligand and AB is unsymmetrical bidentate ligand.
Octahedral complex of the type Ma_4b_2 and Ma_3b_3 exhibit geometrical isomerism.

69. (d) :

	F	Cl	Br	I
Electron affinity	–3.6	–3.8	–3.5	–3.2

The low value of electron affinity of fluorine is probably due to small size of fluorine atom, i.e. electron density is high which hinders the addition of an extra electron.

70. (b) : O_2F_2 and H_2O_2, both have open book type structure.

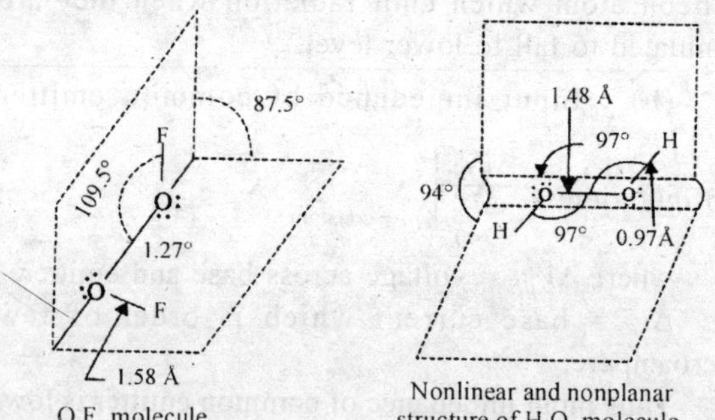

O_2F_2 molecule
Nonlinear and nonplanar structure of H_2O_2 molecule.

In O_2F_2, one O – O bond and two O – F bonds are lying in different planes, *i.e.* this molecule like H_2O_2 has non-linear and non-planar structure.

71. (a) : Gallium is a chemical element in the periodic table that has the symbol Ga and atomic number 31. A rare, soft silvery metallic poor metal, gallium is brittle at low temperature but is liquid above room temperature and can indeed melt in the hand.
Gallium metal expands by 3.1 percent when it solidifies, and therefore should not be stored in either glass or metal containers. Gallium also corrodes most other metals by diffusing into their metal lattice.

72. (c) : According to "solubility rule" following compounds are soluble in water:

(i) All common group IA and NH_4^+ compounds.
(ii) All common NO_3^- (nitrate), CH_3COO^- (acetate), ClO_4^- (perchlorate) compounds
(iii) All common Cl^-, Br^-, I^- compounds, except those of Ag^+, Pb^{2+}, Cu^+ and Hg_2^{2+} (mercurous)
(iv) All common SO_4^{2-} (sulphate) compounds, except those of Ca^{2+}, Sr^{2+}, Ba^{2+} and Pb^{2+}.

73. (a) : The vapours of trialkyl borates $B(OR)_3$ or R_3BO_3 burn with green edged flame. This is the qualitative test of borates.

$$2BO_3^{---} + 3H_2SO_4 \rightarrow 3SO_4^{2-} + \underset{\text{boric acid}}{2H_3BO_3}$$

$$H_3BO_3 + 3ROH \rightarrow R_3BO_3 + 3H_2O$$

74. (d) : The nitrate ion has three resonance structure, with the double bond on a different oxygen for each. In all resonance structures the nitrogen has three bonds, therefore, its hybridisation is sp^2. Each of the oxygen atoms also has sp^2 hybridisation, since the hybridisation is determined by the resonance structure with the double bond, where the oxygen has a double bond and two lone pairs.

The actual geometry of the polyatomic ion is trigonal planar with bond angles of 120°.

120°

NO_2^- : 18 electrons; ideal geometry trigonal planar, sp^2 with bond angle of 116°.

NO_2 : 17 electrons, ideal geometry trigonal planar; sp^2 with bond angle of 134°.

NO_2^+ : 16 electrons; ideal geometry linear ; sp with bond angle of 180°.

$$\ddot{O}=\overset{\oplus}{N}=\ddot{O}$$

75. (d) : $CH_3\overset{+}{N}H_3\overset{-}{Cl}$ is a salt which can be completely ionized in aqueous solution.

76. (c) : The basicity is a measure of a compound's ability to accept a proton (H^+). (b) and (d) are weaker bases as the lone pair are involved in resonance. In (a) carbon adjacent to N is sp^2 hybridised hence is more electronegative therefore, pulls the electron density from nitrogen.

77. (a, d) : A 1° hydrogen atom is one that is bonded to a 1° carbon atom; a 2° hydrogen atom is one that is connected to a 2° carbon atom; etc.

$(H_3C)_2C=CH_2$ (only 1° hydrogen atoms)

$H_3C-HC(CH_3)-C(CH_3)=CH_2$ (vinylic carbon) (1° and 3° H-atoms)

cyclohexane (2° hydrogen atoms)

acetylinic carbon

$CH_3C \equiv CH$ (only 1° hydrogen atoms)

78. (a) : (a) ; $4n + 2 = 2$, $n = 0$ (integer)

(b) ; $4n + 2 = 4$, $n = 0.5$

(c) ; $4n + 2 = 4$, $n = 0.5$

(d) ; $4n + 2 = 4$, $n = 0.5$

Only (a) obeys Huckel's rule.

79. (c) : The value of dipole moment of acetophenone is 3 debye, which is maximum among the given compounds.

80. (d) : In all other compounds the groups present on doubly bonded carbons are identical.

81. (a) : Acetophenone does not give addition reaction with $NaHSO_3$.

82. (d) : In alkyl halides, polarity of C – Br bond increases with increase in chain length.

83. (c) **84. (c)**

85. (c) : $-CH_3$ group is *o*- and *p*- directing group, however $-COOH$ group is meta directing, thus the new entering electrophile occupies the position which should be *m*- with respect to $-COOH$ group and *p*- with respect to $-CH_3$ group.

86. (a)

87. (c) : Melting points are normally higher for primary amides due to presence of hydrogen bonding.

88. (d) : Pyridine chloro chromate (PCC) $[C_5H_5NH^+ClCrO_3^-]$ selectively oxidizes primary alcohols to aldehydes. Secondary alcohols can be oxidized to ketones with PCC.

89. (d)

90. (b) : $n = 4$

$1s^2\, 2s^2\, 2p^6\, 3s^2\, 3p^6\, 3d^{10}\, 4s^2\, 4p^6\, 4d^{10}\, 4f^{14}$

$l = 3$ only for f orbital.

Thus the total number of orbitals for $l = 3$ is equal to 7 (because f contains seven orbitals).

91. (b) : $\pi = CRT$

$$C = \frac{\pi}{RT} = \frac{7.8}{0.082 \times 310} = 0.31 \text{ mol/L}.$$

92. (b) : $C + O_2 \rightarrow CO_2$; $\Delta H_f^\circ = -490$ kJ/mol $\times$ 8

$H_2 + \frac{1}{2}O_2 \rightarrow H_2O$; $\Delta H_f^\circ = -240$ kJ/mol $\times$ 9

$8C + 18H \rightarrow C_8H_{18}$; $\Delta H_f^\circ = +160$ kJ/mol

$$8C + 8O_2 + 9H_2 + \frac{9}{2}O_2 - 8C - 18H \rightarrow 8CO_2 + 9H_2O - C_8H_{18}$$

$$\Delta H_f^\circ = -3920 - 2160 - 160$$

$C_8H_{18} + \frac{25}{2}O_2 \rightarrow 8CO_2 + 9H_2O$; $\Delta H^\circ = 6240$ kJ/mol

ΔH° for 6 moles of octane = 6240 × 6 = 37440 kJ/mol.

93. (b) : $H_2O_{(l)} \rightleftharpoons H_2O_{(g)}$

This is a spontaneous process at standard conditions thus, the standard free energy change must be less then zero, *i.e.* $\Delta G^\circ < 0$.

94. (b) : When $a = b \neq c$, $\alpha = \beta = 90^\circ$, $\gamma = 120^\circ$. The given condition is characteristic of hexagonal system.

95. (c) : $K = Ka_1 \times Ka_2 = 4.5 \times 10^{-3} \times 1.7 \times 10^{-10} = 7.65 \times 10^{-13}$

$$[H^+] = \sqrt{KC} = \sqrt{7.65 \times 10^{-13} \times 0.01} = \sqrt{7.65 \times 10^{-15}} = 0.87 \times 10^{-7}$$

pH = – log 0.87 × 10^{-7} = 7 – 0.93 = 6.07.

96. (c) : The given reaction is endothermic, so on increasing the temperature, it will shift in forward direction.

97. (c) : In Daniel cell, during the passage of electric current through external circuit, electrons flow from the zinc electrode to the copper electrode. At the zinc electrode, the zinc metal is oxidised to Zn^{++} which go into the solution. The electrons released at the electrode travel through the external circuit to the copper electrode where they are used in the reduction of Cu^{2+} ions to metallic copper which is deposited on the electrode.

98. (a) : The substance which is susceptible of degradation by biological processes, as by bacterial or other enzymatic action is known as biodegradable substance.

99. (d) : $k = \frac{1}{t} \ln \frac{a \text{ (initial)}}{a - x \text{ (after time } t)}$

$$k_t = \ln \frac{[N_2O_5]_0}{[N_2O_5]_t}$$

100. (a) : Ozone depletion is caused by a number of pollutants like chlorofluorocarbons (14% of total depletion), nitrogen oxides, sulphur oxides, CCl_4, Cl_2 etc. Maximum ozone depleting potential or OPD is of chlorofluorocarbons (CF_2Cl_2) due to release of chlorine by it. A single chlorine atom converts 1 lakh molecules of ozone to oxygen.

101. (b) : Greater the number of negative atoms present in the oxy-acid make the acid stronger.

In general, the strengths of acids that have general formula, $(HO)_mZO_n$ can be related to the value of n. As the value of n increases, acidic character also increases. The negative atoms draw electrons away from the Z-atom and make it more positive. The Z-atom, therefore, becomes more effective in withdrawing electron density away from the oxygen atom that bonded to hydrogen. In turn, the electrons of H – O bond are drawn more strongly away from the H-atom. The net effect makes it easier from the proton release and increases the acid strength.

102. (c) : $_{24}Cr \rightarrow [Ar]\, 3d^4\, 4s^2$

$Cr \rightarrow [Ar]\, 3d^5\, 4s^1$

Full-filled s-orbital has greater stability.

103. (d) : $[Ni(en)_3]Cl_2$ is a chelating compound and chelated complexes are more stable than similar complexes with unidentate ligands as dissociation of the complex involves breaking of two bonds rather than one.

In $[Ni(en)_3]Cl_2$, Ni with d^8 configuration shows octahedral geometry. Six electrons will occupy the t_{2g} orbitals and two electrons will occupy the e_g orbitals.

104. (c) : Sb(III) is a basic radical of IIB group for which group reagent is H_2S in presence of dilute HCl. It is necessary to maintain the proper hydrogen ion concentration for the precipitation of IInd group cations and to check the precipitation of IV group cations.

105. (d) : Binding energy per nucleon of ${}_3Li^7$ (5.38 MeV) is lesser than ${}_2He^4$ (7.08 MeV) as helium is found to be more stable than Li. As the atomic mass number increases, the binding energy per nucleon decreases. As the atomic number and the atomic mass number increase, the repulsive electrostatic forces within the nucleus increase due to the greater number of protons in the heavy elements. To overcome this increased repulsion, the proportion of neutrons in the nucleus must increase to maintain stability. This increase in the neutron-to-proton ratio only partially compensates for the growing proton-proton repulsive force in the heavier, naturally occurring elements. Because the repulsive forces are increasing, less energy must be supplied, on the average, to remove a nucleon from the nucleus. The BE/A has decreased. The BE/A of a nucleus is an indication of its degree of stability. Generally, the more stable nuclides have higher BE/A than the less stable ones. The increase in BE/A as the atomic mass number decreases from 260 to 60 is the primary reason for the energy liberation in the fission process. The increase in the BE/A as the atomic mass number increases from 1 to 60 is the reason for the energy liberation in the fusion process, which is the opposite reaction of fission.

106. (b) : Enamel, the hardest substance of the body is composed of fluorine not magnesium. Magnesium is an essential element as it acts as a factor of many enzymes of glycolysis and a number of other metaboilic reactions dependent upon ATP.

107. (c) : Carboxypeptidase is an exopeptidase because it breaks the peptide chain at terminal ends. Carboxypeptidase cleaves carboxy-terminal amino acids that have aromatic or branched aliphatic side chains.

108. (a) : Sucrose is a non-reducing sugar as it does not reduce Tollen's or Fehling's reagent, due to absence of free aldehyde or ketone group. It contains stable acetal or ketal structure which cannot be opened into a free carboxyl group.

Sugar is composed of α-D-glucopyranose unit and β-D-fructofuranose unit. These units are joined by α–β-glycosidic linkage between C-1 of the glucose unit and C-2 of the fructose unit.

109. (c) : $(CH_3)_2CH-CHO$

Isobutanal has α-hydrogen atom.

Acetaldehyde, acetone and methyl ketones having CH_3CO group undergo haloform reaction. The hydrogen atoms of the methyl group are first replaced by halogen atoms. This reaction is used as a test of CH_3CO – group. Due to absence of CH_3CO – group isobutanal does not give iodoform test.

110. HBr adds to the double bond of the styrene forming 1-bromo-1-phenylethane.

styrene $\xrightarrow{HBr}$ 1-bromo-1-phenylethane (Br)

This is an example of elimination-addition reaction.

Note : Here given assertion is wrong.

111. (c) : Lower the value of pK_a, more acidic will be the compound. Acetic acid is more acidic than phenol. This indicates that carboxylate ion should be more stable than the phenoxide ion and it is clear that carboxylate ion has more equivalent resonating structures than the phenoxide ion.

112. (d) : 2-bromobutane on reaction with sodium ethoxide in ethanol gives 2-butene as a major product.

$$EtO^- + H-\underset{\displaystyle CH_3}{\underset{|}{CH}}-CH(CH_3)-Br \longrightarrow EtOH + \underset{\displaystyle CH_3}{\underset{|}{CH}}=\overset{\displaystyle CH_3}{\overset{|}{CH}} + Br^-$$

This is according to Saytzeff's rule i.e. the predominant product is the most substituted alkene, i.e. are carrying the largest number of alkyl substituents of hydrogen is eliminated preferentially from the carbon atom joined to the least number of hydrogen atoms.

2-butene is more stable than 1-butene due to presence of large number of hyperconjugating structures in 2-butene.

113. (a) : $C_6H_5CH_2OCH_3 \xrightarrow{H^+} C_6H_5\overset{+}{C}H_2 + CH_3OH$

$$\downarrow I^-$$

$$C_6H_7CH_2I$$

This can be explained on the basis of S_N1 mechanism, the carbonium ion produced being benzylium ion, since this type is more stable than alkylium ion.

114. (b) : Molar entropy of vaporization of water is more than ethanol, as water has greater forces of attraction than ethanol.

115. (a) : The colour of colloidal solution depends on the wavelength of light scattered by the dispersed particles. The wavelength of light further depends on the size and nature of the particles. The colour of colloidal solution also changes with the way the observer receives the light. Finest gold sol is red in colour. As size of the particles increases, it becomes purple, then blue and finally golden yellow.

116. (d) : Copper corrods at negligible rates in unpolluted air, water and deaerated non-oxidising acids. Pure copper and the high copper alloys can be considered to exhibit similar resistance to most corrosive environments. They possess excellent resistance to atmospheric environments. (corossion is a spontaneous process for which free energy change must be negative.

117. (c) : K_{sp} of AgCl > K_{sp} of AgBr.
For the precipitation to occur, its ionic product should exceed solubility product.

118. (b) : Zeolites are shape-selective porous solid acid catalysts, their catalytic activity originates from the presence of highly acidic Al – O(H) – Si hydroxyl in the framework.

119. (c) : Due to greater lone pair - bond pair repulsions than bond pair - bond pair repulsions, the F – S – F bond angle decreases from 180°.

120. (c) : Molecular size decreases from left to right while it increases in a group from top to bottom. Thus molecular size of nitrogen is greater than oxygen.

BIOLOGY

121. (d) : Cotton and other monocultured crops require an intensive use of pesticides as various types of pests attack these crops causing extensive damage.
So far, the only successful approach to engineering crops for insect tolerence has been the addition of Bt toxin, a family of toxins originally derived from soil bacteria. The Bt toxin contained by the Bt crops is no different from other chemical pesticides, but causes much less damage to the environment. These toxins are effective against a variety of economically important crops pests but pose no hazard to non-target organisms like mammals and fish. The Bt gene was isolated and transferred from a bacterium *Bacillus thuringiensis* to American cotton. The American cotton was subsequently crossed with Indian cotton to introduce the gene into native varieties. Bt toxin protects the cotton plants from ballworm (*A. lepidoptera*), a major pest of cotton. The worm feeding on the leaves of a Bt cotton plant becomes lethargic and sleepy, thereby causing less damage to the plant.

122. (b) : The ventral nerve cord, as its name suggests, is a cord of nervous tissue that runs the length of the animal in the lower part of its body. It is the characteristic of lower chordates like leech, cockroach and scorpion.

123. (d) : A synapse occurs where the axon of one neurone (the pre-synaptic neurone) meets either the dendrite or the cell body of another (the post-synaptic neurone). At the tip of the pre-synaptic axon is a button shaped swelling called a synaptic knob, inside which are numerous mitochondria and vesicles packed with a substance called a neurotransmitter is present.
This neurotransmitters at the time of nerve impulse diffuse across the space and bind to receptors in the membrane of the post-synaptic cell. This opens ion channels in the post-synaptic membrane of the post-synaptic cell resulting in a change in the post-synaptic cell's membrane potential and (if the cell is sufficiently excited) in the consequent generation of a nerve impulse.

124. (d) : The two DNA strands are held together by weak (hydrogen) bonds between the bases on each strand, forming base pairs. Genome size is usually stated as the total number of base pairs; the human genome contains roughly 3 billion base pairs.

125. (c) : The great Barrier Reef - the largest system of coral reefs in the world - is more than 2,000 km in length and comprises 2,900 separate reefs and 940 islands. Its high species diversity includes more than 400 species of coral, 4,000 species of molluscs, 1,500 species of fish, 6 species of turtles, 35 species of seabirds and 23 species of sea mammals. The Great Barrier Reef is one of the richest and most complex natural systems in the world. The Reef's diverse range of habitats all connect and support each other, which means they are all vital to the life of the Great Barrier Reef.

126. (d) : The species or taxa, which are in dangers of extinction and which may not survive if the adverse factors continue to operate or the species whose numbers have been reduced to a critical level or their habitats have been drastically reduced in such a way that they are in instant danger of extinction are called endangered species. In India, aconite and horn bill are endangered species.

127. (a) : Amphetamines are powerful drugs (stimulant), they 'speed' up the whole body, increasing the heart rate, blood pressure and breathing. Amphetamines make the user feel excited, confident and energetic. Some people use amphetamines to suppress their appetite, so they can go for a long time without eating. There are many health risks from taking this type of drug. Long-term use can cause mental illness and will put a strain on the heart, due to increased blood pressure.

128. (b) : SA node or sino-atrial node is known as the pacemaker of heart because the cells in the SA node contract the most number of times per minute and because each wave of excitation begins here and acts as the stimulus for the next wave of excitation.

129. (b) : The photosynthetic bacteria (e.g. purple non-sulphur bacteria) photosynthesise using bacterio-chlorophylls *a* and *b* in anoxic environments, such as the bottom mud of ponds and other stagnant water, although they are able to survive in air. The reducing agent involved is hydrogen rather than water, so oxygen is not produced. These bacteria efficiently use infrared light for photosynthesis.

130. (c) : There are some rare cases in medical literation which could be interpreted as atavisms, that is the reappearance of our ancestor's organs, in which more prolonged traits, already lost by human beings throughout evolution, are expressed again. Such is the case of supranumerary mammary glands, sacral tail etc.

131. (a) : The Virus Research Centre (VRC), Pune came to existance in 1952 under the joint auspices of the ICMR and the Rockefeller Foundation, as a part of the global programme of investigations on the arthropod - borne group of viruses. In view of its expanded scope and activities, the VRC was undesignated as the National Institute of Virology (NIV) in 1978. The NIV is identified today as the WHO collaborating centre for arbovirus reference and research. NIV also acts as the National Monitoring Centre for Influenza and Hepatitis.

132. (c) : Electron Beam Therapy or radiation therapy involves the use of radioactive waves to treat certain types of cancer. The therapy can be given with external beams of radiation. Electron beams are of low energy. They are often used in skin conditions and cancers. The procedure to deliver external beam radiation is somewhat similar to giving an X-ray. The person is put into position, and the machine delivers the radiation to the desired area. This beam therapy involves iodine, cobalt, protons and electrons. This therapy is used in cancer of cervix, cancer of larynx, germ cell cancer, Hodgkin's lymphoma, prostate cancer, breast cancer, lung cancer etc.

133. (b) : SARS (severe acute respiratory syndrome) has now affected 30 countries on five continents, with more than 8,000 cases and more than 900 deaths. The disease is due to infection with the SARS coronavirus (SARS-CoV). The genome of this virus has been completely sequenced. When viruses resembling SARS-CoV were isolated from Himalayan palm civets found in a live animal market in the Guangdong Province of China; it implicated these animals as the reservoir of the virus.

134. (c) : A better understanding of the mode of action of vitamin K is made possible by the use of an anti-coagulant. One such naturally occurring antagonist of vitamin K is known as Dicumarol. The discovery of the anti-coagulating property of Dicumarol took place when it was established that consumption of improperly cured sweet clover hay caused cattle to develop the so-called "sweet clover disease" which is attributable to a serious alternation in the coagulability of the blood that, in turn, often result in fatal haemorrhage.

135. (c)

136. (b) : Sulfur and nitrogen oxides emitted into the atmosphere react to form compounds that are transported long distances and are subsequently deposited to the Earth's surface in wet and dry forms. Although the term "acid rain" is widely recognized, the dry deposition portion ranges from 20 to 60 percent of total pollutant deposition, and represents the particulate and gaseous forms. A more accurate description of the overall process is acid deposition rather than acid rain.

Dry deposition occurs when sulfur dioxide and nitrogen oxides react, but not with water. It settles out of the atmosphere as particle or gases.

The effects of acid deposition include acidification of lakes and streams, nutrient enrichment of coastal waters and large river basins, soil nutrient depletion and decline of sensitive forests, agricultural crop damage, and impacts on ecosystem biodiversity. Toxic pollutants and metals also can be transported and deposited through atmospheric processes. Both local and long-range emission sources contribute to atmospheric deposition.

137. (c) : Domestic sewage rich in organic waste will exert a very high demand of oxygen in order to get biodegraded. Thus depleting the dissolved oxygen below critical level necessary to support aquatic life. Especially fish, which is very sensitive to the dissolved oxygen available in water, starts dying if the level goes below 4 mg/L.

138. (b) : The Minamata disease got its name from Minamata Bay in Southwestern Japan where it was first observed in nearby communities. It was officially discovered in 1956, and a few years later it was known to be caused by ingestion of fish that had been contaminated by mercury left off from a chemical manufacturing plant. Levels of methylmercury chloride were very high: upto 50 ppm in fish and 85 ppm in shellfish from the contaminated areas. 121 people were poisoned from eating the contaminated fish, 46 of which died. Dogs, cats, pigs, rats and birds that were living around the bay also showed the signs of mercury poisoning, and many died.

The initial symptoms were numbness of the limbs and the area around the mouth, sensory disturbance, and difficulty with everyday hand movements. Also there occurred a lack of coordination, weakness and tremor, slowed and slurred speech, and altered vision and hearing. These symptoms worsened and led to general paralysis, involuntary movements, difficulty in swallowing, convulsions, brain damage and death.

139. (c) : A pacemaker (or "artificial pacemaker"), is a medical device designed to regulate the beating of the heart. The purpose of an artificial pacemaker is to stimulate the heart when either the heart's native pacemaker is not fast enough or if there are blocks in the heart's electrical conduction system preventing the propagation of electrical impulses from the native pacemaker to the lower chambers of the heart, known as the ventricles. Generally, pacemakers do not treat fast rhythms of the heart.

140. (c) : On September 14, 1990 researchers at the U.S. National Institutes of Health performed the first (approved) gene therapy procedure on four-year old Ashanti DeSilva. Born with a rare genetic disease called severe combined immune deficiency (SCID), she lacked a healthy immune system, and was vulnerable to every passing germ. Children with this illness usually develop overwhelming infections and rarely survive to adulthood. In this gene therapy procedure, doctors removed white blood cells from the child's body, let the cells grow in the lab, inserted the missing gene into the cells, and then infused the genetically modified blood cells back into the patient's blood stream. Laboratory test have shown that the therapy strengthened her immune system.

141. (a) : After entering the wall of the embryo sac the pollen tube during its entry into the embryo sac passes through the nucellar cells and the synergids, e.g. *Fagopyrum*. The pollen tubes passes between the egg and one synergid. In *Cardiospermum*, it passes between embryo sac wall and synergid. In *Oxalis*, it passes directly through a synergid. In *Viola* it enters a synergid and makes its way through the base of the synergid. In normal cases only one synergid destroys by the impact of the pollen tube and the other remains intact until sometimes afterwards.

142. (d) : Southern blotting was named after Edward M. Southern who developed this procedure in Edinburgh University in the 1970's. Southern blotting is designed to locate a particular sequence of DNA within a complex mixture. For example, Southern Blotting could be used to locate a particular gene within an entire genome. The amount of DNA needed for this technique is dependent on the size and specific activity of the probe. Before, starting the procedure, the desired DNA should be isolated from a specific nucleated cell.

143. (d) : Even a single dose of thalidomide can cause severe birth defects or fetal death, thalomid (a form of thalidomide) must not be used during pregnancy. Pregnancy must be ruled out 24 hours before starting therapy with thalidomide. Women must be monitored for pregnancy while using thalomid because it can give rise to underdeveloped limbs in fetus.

144. (d)

145. (c) : During inversion a segment of chromosome gets inverted in the process of reattachment. Thus a chromosome having the genes A B C D E F G H I in linear order may get the segment D E F inverted. The new arrangement will be A B C F E D G H I. It is a chromosome aberration entailing two breaks in a chromosome followed by a reversal of the segment and consequently of the gene sequence in the segment.

Pericentric inversion includes the centromere in the inverted segment, whereas paracentric inversions do not.

146. (b)

147. (b) : Passive immunity may be artificially acquired, particularly when antiserum or antibodies produced by one individual are transfused into a second individual. In all cases, passive immunity represents the passive acquisition of an immune response that was actively acquired by another individual. Passive immunity can last for at most months since antibodies have a finite life span within the body.

148. (b) : *Pseudomonas aeruginosa* is a Gram-negative, aerobic rod belonging to the bacterial family *Pseudomonadaceae*. These bacteria are common inhabitants of soil water. They occur regularly on the surfaces of plants and occassionally on the surfaces of animals.

- The bacterium will grow in the absence of O_2 if NO_3 is available as a respiratory electron acceptor.
- *P. aeruginosa* possesses the metabolic versatility. Organic growth factors are not required, and it can use more than thirty organic compounds for growth.
- *Pseudomonas aeruginosa* is often observed growing in "distilled water" which is evidence of its minimal nutritional requirements.
- It is able to grow at temperatures as high as 42 degrees.
- Its tolerance to a wide variety of physical conditions, including temperature, contributes to its ecological success and makes it suitable for decomposing a variety of organic compounds in varied environmental conditions.

149. (c) : DNA is present both in mitochondria and chloroplast. The DNA molecules are circular, relatively small, double stranded (except for the DNA of some algae and protozoans). The mitochondrial DNA varies in size starting from 5 μm to 30 μm. Average length of chloroplast DNA is 45 μm.

150. (c) : Cytokinins are a group of phenyl urea derivatives of adenine, one of the molecules in DNA during pruning axillary bud, which is under repression due to effect of auxin, get sensitized to cytokinin, which releases it from apical dominance.

Cytokinin functions

- Cytokinins promote cytokinesis. They are found primarily in root meristems, embryos and fruits, and migrate from roots to the shoot systems of plants in xylem tissue.
- Cytokinins can promote axillary bud growth by over-riding the apparent inhibiting effect of auxin. This is one of the ways in which plants balance root and shoot growth. Shoot tip auxins inhibit lateral bud activation. Cytokinins produced in root meristems travel upward in xylem and if in higher concentration counter the inhibition of auxins to activate lateral buds.
- Cytokinins also retard leaf senescence, probably by stimulating RNA and protein synthesis and delaying degradation of chlorophyll.

151. (a) : Guard cells are semilunar or kidney shaped cells which surrounds the minute apertures of epidermis called stomata. Guard cells are living and have chloroplast. In sugarcane and in some other monocots like doob, maize guard cells are dumb bell shaped.

152. (b) : Analogous organs are those organs, which are different in origin but similar in function. Potato and sweet potato are absolutely different in their origin as potato is modified underground stem (tuber), while sweet potato is tuberous root. It means both have edible parts, which are different organs.

153. (c) : In *Ulothrix* sexual reproduction is of isogamous type. Two isogametes of + and – strain come together and fuse as a result a quadriflagellate zygospore is formed which floats on water after sometime it rests on the bottom of the pond at this time its four flagella disintegrate and a wall is formed surrounding it from all sides. After taking rest for a long period this zygote divides meiotically and gives rise to 16 zoospores. These zoospores come out of sac and give rise to the new plants of *Ulothrix*.

154. (d) : Due to continued formation of secondary tissues in the older stem and roots however the epidermis gets stressed and ultimately tends to rupture and followed by death of epidermal cells and outer tissues, and a new protective layer is developed called periderm. Structurally it consists of three parts Phellogen or Cork cambium, phellem or cork and phelloderm.

Usually in the periderm of most plants, certain areas with loosely arranged cells have been found, which possess more or less raised and corky spots where the underneath tissues break through the epidermis. Such areas are universally found in the stems of woody plants. These broken areas are called lenticels, which perform the function of exchange of gases in the absence of stomata.

155. (c) : Somaclonal variation refers to all types of variation occur in plants regenerated from cultured cells or tissues. Genetic changes take place in plant tissue culture and these changes are passed to their progenies. This technology can be used for disease resistance, improvement of quality and yield in plants.

156. (d)

157. (c) : The companion cells occur only in angiosperms where they accompany most sieve tube elements. Companion cell is a speciliased type of parenchyma cell which is closely associated in origin, position and function with sieve tube elements. These cells are living having abundant granular cytoplasm and a prominent elongated nucleus. Usually, the nuclei of the companion cell serve for the nuclei of the sieve tubes as they lack them. The companion cells do not contain starch. They live only so long as the sieve tube element with which they are associated and they are crushed with those cells. Longitudinal division of the mother cell of the sieve tube element forms the companion cells. One daughter cell becomes a companion cell and other sieve tube element.

158. (a) : During fertilization ventral canal cell and the neck canal cell, along with tip of the neck disintegrate and the neck forms a canal like passage full of mucilage and some chemicals like malic acids. These chemicals attract antherozoids (chemotactic movement of antherozoids) and one of the male gametes fuses with the oospore forming a diploid oospore. Water is essential for this process.

159. (b) : Corkcambium is a secondary lateral meristem that may arise from permanent living cells of hypodermis or outer cortex. It is composed of a single layer of meristematic cells. Its cells divide tangentially and periclinally toward the outer face and produce cork cells. These cells are compactly arranged and have thin cellulose walls in the beginning. As they mature there is a gradual loss of living matter and cells get elongated radially, vertically or tangentially. The cell walls become thick because of development of fatty substance called Suberin, which is impervious to water.

160. (b) :

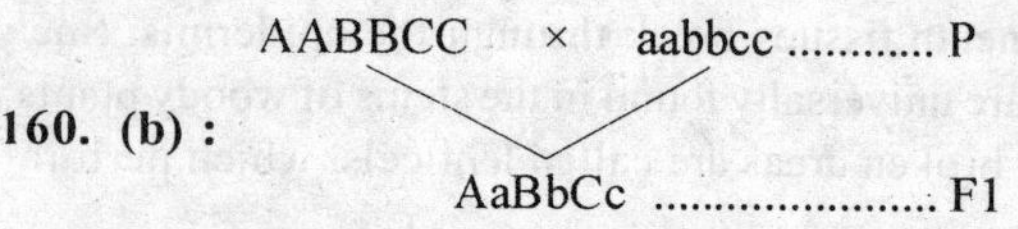

∴ Number of heterozygote is 3

∴ Number of progenies in F_1 will be 2^n or $2^3 = 8$.

161. (a) : DDT or dichloro-diphenyl trichloroethane was the first important synthetic pesticide (organo chlorine) discovered in 1939 by a Swiss chemist Paul Muller. It was toxic to wide range of insect pests ("broad spectrum") yet appeared to have low toxicity to mammals. It was persistent *i.e.* didn't break down rapidly in the environment, so that it didn't have to be reapplied often. DDT was so effective at killing pests and thus boosting crop yields and was so inexpensive to make that its use quickly spread over the globe. Farmers used more and more DDT throughout the 1950s and 1960s to get an increased yield of crop.

162. (b) : Antidiuretic hormone (ADH) or vasopressin is secreted from posterior pituitary gland. It is released in response to a fall in the water content of blood plasma and lead to an increase in the permeability to water of the distal and collecting tubules of the nephron. Deficiency or hyposecretion of ADH results in diabetes insipidus. Diabetes insipidus is characterised by micturating dilute urine several times a day which results in excessive thirst (polydipsia) and dehydration.

163. (c) : Oparin and Sydney Fox held that large organic molecules synthesised abiotically on primitive earth and formed large colloidal aggregates due to intermolecular attraction. These colloidal particles were called coacervates. In coacervates, lipid molecules are joined end to end forming a layer around each aggregate. This represents a single lipid membrane. Coacervates divide by budding like bacteria.

164. (c) : Tapeworm belonging to phylum platyhelminthes, pinworms and roundworm belonging to phylum nematoda, are all endoparasites. They all are intestinal parasites. In case of *Taenia solium* man gets infection by uncooked or improperly cooked measly pork. Cysticercus becomes active on reaching the intestine. Proscolex everts or evaginates in the intestinal wall. *Ascaris,* being an endoparasite inhabits the small intestine of man, more frequently of children than of adults. Man gets infection through skin contact. *Enterobius vermicularis* or pinworm live in caecum, appendix and at the junction of large and small intestine. They are transmitted by the improper sanitary condition.

165. (c) : The fish meal is prepared from the wastes of fish oil or canning industry or from the whole fish of non-oil type. The protein content of this meal is highly digestable, nutritive and of biological importance. Fish meal is also used for domestic animals like pigs, poultry, cattle etc.

166. (b) : Adaptation is the most basic and rather self-evident concept. It is the morphological or physiological modification in an organism to adjust itself in a particular environment. In some animals, it is known as mimicry as for example praying mantis or stick insect. The stick insect or praying mantis having green body colour exhibits close resemblance with twigs and foliages. It is a type of protective mimicry. They exhibit close resemblances also with the twigs in having slender body, attenuated limbs, sympathetic colouration and slow movement.

167. (a) : Carolus Linnaeus called humans as *Homo sapiens* or wise men and placed them along with apes and monkeys. There are certain similarities between human and chimpanzee. These are -
(i) RNA content of diploid cells is similar
(ii) DNA matching shows that human similarity is 100 % with chimpanzee and
(iii) banding pattern of chromosomes shows very little difference in chromosomes 3 and 6 between humans and chimpanzee.
Thus it can be concluded that among the primates, chimpanzee is the closest relative of the present day humans.

168. (d) : Dope test is an official test to discover whether a person or animal taking part in a competition has been given any drugs (such as anabolic steroids, erythropoietin etc.) to make their performance better or worse. It is a type of blood test. Alcohol is not used in this purpose. Alcohol has an effect on cerebellum and it results into imbalanced muscular activities, posture etc.

169. (b) : Queen is the only fertile female in beehive, having immensely developed ovaries. She lives for several successive years laying about 2000 or more eggs a day and upto about 1,500000 eggs during her life time. The queen has a remarkable capacity of controlling the fertilization of its eggs. A fertilized egg is laid in a worker or queen cell or honey comb, while an unfertilized egg in a drone cell, the latter develops parthogenetically. The queen mates only once in a life time. The sperms stored in her spermatheca fertilize her eggs as long as she lives.

170. (d) : Assertion is false as the humans would require more gestation period (should have been 21 months as compared to 9 months and will increase). Similarly the head size is increasing (especially the frontal brain) hence growth rate needs to increase but surprisingly most of the brain growth occurs after birth till 2 years (when the arterior fontanellae close at 18 months) and some more till 30 years when finally the cranial sutures close. Thus an increase in brain/skull size would required increase in gestation period, hence both assertion and reason are false.

171. (a) : The Darwin Wallace theory of Natural Selection can be generalised as the change in species by the survival of an organismal type exhibiting a natural variation that gives it an adaptive advantage in an environment. Thus leading to a new environmental equilibrium. The idea of the survival of the fittest explain the above evolution by natural selection. According to survival of fittest, some of the variations exhibited by living things make it easier for them to survive and reproduce thus more adaptive forms increase. Those which are not fit (or less adaptive) become eliminated.

172. (b) : Rhizome is normally a prostrate, thickened stem, creeping horizontally under the surface of the soil. The common example is ginger. It is provided with distinct node and long or short internode. It bears some scaly leaves at the nodes, possesses a bud in the axil of the scaly leaf and ends in a terminal bud.
The response of plant to gravity is called **geotropism.** The roots are *positively geotropic* and grow downwards, while the shoot is *negatively geotropic* and grows away from the gravitational pull from the centre of earth. Parts which show no effect of gravity are called **ageotropic**.

173. (c) : Flowering is a phytochrome regulated process. Phytotchrome is a blue protein pigment with a molecular mass of about 125 k Da (kilodaltons). Phytochrome occurs in two interconvertible form P_R (which absorbs red light) and P_{FR} (which absorbs far red light). The studies with mutants of *Arabidopsis* support and prove that the P_{FR} is the active form of phytochrome. When P_R molecules are exposed to red light, most of them absorb it and converted to P_{FR}. This causes floral induction in the shoot. A night interruption inhibits flowering of short-day plants and promotes flowering of long-day plants. Red light is more effective with short-day plants and a mixture of red and far-red with long-day plants.

174. (b) : Cyclic pathway of photosynthesis is appeared first in some eubacterial species. It is supposed to be the first evidence of production of ATP in the presence of light. During non-cyclic photophosphorylation photolysis of water takes place. Under the influence of light energy and the catalytic action of chlorophyll, water, a substance of low energy value, is split up into oxygen and hydrogen. Oxygen is used in the chloroplast. Non-cyclic photophosphorylation is the only natural process which adds molecular oxygen to the atmosphere.

175. (d) : Symbiotic nitrogen fixation occurs in legume plants. It takes place in the *Rhizobium* bacteroids which are located within root nodules cells. Rhizobium is an aerobic bacteria and hence it survive in presence of oxygen. But the important enzyme *Nitrogenase* (synthesise by *Rhizobium*) that reduces N_2, is oxygen sensitive. It can only function at low oxygen concentration. This low oxygen concentration in bacteriod is provided by leghaemoglobin. Leghaemoglobin (pink in colour) is a form of haemoglobin found in the nitrogen fixing root nodules of legume. They bound oxygen and thus protect the nitrogen fixing enzyme, nitrogenase (that is oxygen sensitive). It regulates oxygen diffusion to bacteroids and nitrogenase.

176. (a) : In some species of red algae called coralline algae, the cell walls become hardened with calcium carbonate. These algae hence important for the formation of coral reefs.

Coral reefs are formed through the accumulation of calcareous exoskeletons of coral animals, calcareous red algae and molluscs. They form the foundation of reefs by secreting a calcium carbonate skeleton that provides protection for the coral polyps. Calcium carbonate is secreted continuously by the coral colony.

177. (d) : Insect visit flowers to get nectar. Nectar is contained in a special gland called nectary and sometimes in a special structure called spur.

The attraction of flower in plants is not to diverge the insect from damaging other part, but to bring about pollination (*i.e.* transfer of pollen to the stigma). The pollen grains in insect pollinated flowers are either sticky or provided with spinous outgrowths. The stigma is also sticky. Insect often visit these flower for nectar and inevidently bring about pollination.

178. (b) : Coconut require the hot and wet climate hence it is grown in coastal areas. It is widely grown in coastal and deltic regions of tropical and subtropical countries.

Coconut fruit show hydrochory *i.e.* the dispersal takes place through water medium. Being the habitant of coastal area the fruit is so adapted that it can float and dispersed over thousand of kilometers before losing viability.

179. (c) : Sulphur is not a constituent of chlorophyll but it helps in chlorophyll formation. Due to the deficiency of sulphur, chlorosis often appears first in the young leaves. Mineral constituent of chlorophyll is magnesium which is situated in the centre of the porphyrin ring.

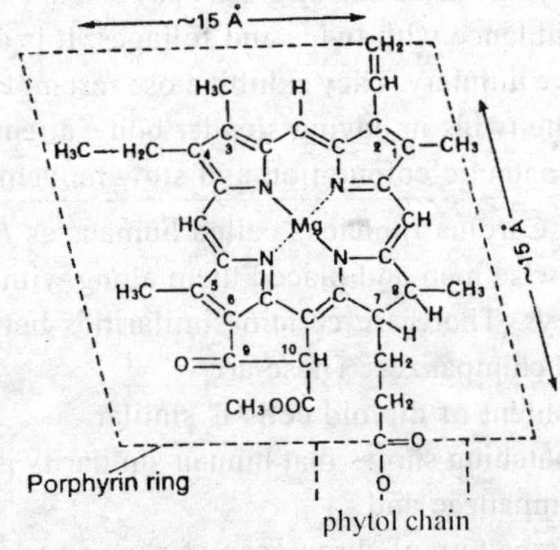

180. (b) : Superovulation is an effort to increase the fertility of cattle breeds. Inducing an animal to ovulate multiple oocytes can translate into producing more offsprings from selected females. Superovulation and embryo transfer involves the following steps.

- Donor cows of particularly fine pedigree are treated with hormones (mainly FSH and LH) to increase the number of eggs released at ovulation - multiple ovulation (MO)
- The cows are artificially inseminated using semen from a proven bull
- After 6 - 7 days the embryos are flushed out non-surgically, using a catheter placed into the uterus. This is possible because, in cattle, there is delay in embryos becoming implanted in the uterine wall. On average, 4-7 embryos are collected.
- The embryos may then be implanted into recipient cows whose oestrous cycle is at the correct receptive stage - usually as the result of hormonal manipulation.
- Embryos may be frozen and stored, using techniques similar to those applied to semen, (though precise control of the regime is somewhat more critical).

Farmers may, of course, buy-in embryos from sources anywhere in the world to transfer to their own recipient cows.

Embryo transfer has the potential to bring about genetic improvement twice as fast as AI (Artificial Insemination) alone.

GENERAL KNOWLEDGE

181.	(d)	**182.**	(a)
183.	(b)	**184.**	(c)
185.	(a)	**186.**	(a)
187.	(a)	**188.**	(b)
189.	(d)	**190.**	(b)
191.	(b)	**192.**	(a)
193.	(c)	**194.**	(d)
195.	(b)	**196.**	(a)
197.	(b)	**198.**	(d)
199.	(a)	**200.**	(c)

SOLVED PAPER
AIIMS - 2005

Time : 3½ Hours

Max. Marks : 200

PHYSICS

1. For skywave propagation of a 10 MHz signal, what should be the minimum electron density in ionosphere?
(a) $\sim 1.2 \times 10^{12}$ m^{-3} (b) $\sim 10^6$ m^{-3}
(c) $\sim 10^{14}$ m^{-3} (d) $\sim 10^{22}$ m^{-3}.

2. Which of the following logic gates is an universal gate?
(a) OR (b) NOT
(c) AND (d) NAND.

3. What should be the maximum acceptance angle at the air-core interface of an optical fibre if n_1 and n_2 are the refractive indices of the core and the cladding, respectively?
(a) $\sin^{-1}(n_2/n_1)$ (b) $\sin^{-1}\sqrt{n_1^2 - n_2^2}$
(c) $\left[\tan^{-1}\frac{n_2}{n_1}\right]$ (d) $\left[\tan^{-1}\frac{n_1}{n_2}\right]$

4. A conducting ring of radius 1 meter is placed in an uniform magnetic field B of 0.01 tesla oscillating with frequency 100 Hz with its plane at right angle to B. What will be the induced electric field?
(a) π volts/m (b) 2 volts/m
(c) 10 volts/m (d) 62 volts/m.

5. Consider an *n-p-n* transistor amplifier in common-emitter configuration. The current gain of the transistor is 100. If the collector current changes by 1 mA, what will be the change in emitter current?
(a) 1.1 mA (b) 1.01 mA
(c) 0.01 mA (d) 10 mA.

6. A telescope has an objective lens of focal length 200 cm and an eye piece with focal length 2 cm. If this telescope is used to see a 50 meter tall building at a distance of 2 km, what is the height of the image of the building formed by the objective lens?
(a) 5 cm (b) 10 cm
(c) 1 cm (d) 2 cm.

7. The ground state energy of hydrogen atom is -13.6 eV. What is the potential energy of the electron in this state?
(a) 0 eV (b) -27.2 eV
(c) 1 eV (d) 2 eV.

8. Solid targets of different elements are bombarded by highly energetic electron beams. The frequency (f) of the characteristic X-rays emitted from different targets varies with atomic number Z as
(a) $f \propto \sqrt{Z}$ (b) $f \propto Z^2$
(c) $f \propto Z$ (d) $f \propto Z^{3/2}$.

9. Two infinitely long parallel conducting plates having surface charge densities $+\sigma$ and $-\sigma$ respectively, are separated by a small distance. The medium between the plates is vacuum. If ε_0 is the dielectric permittivity of vacuum, then the electric field in the region between the plates is
(a) 0 volt/meter (b) $\sigma/2\varepsilon_0$ volt/meter
(c) σ/ε_0 volt/meter (d) $2\sigma/\varepsilon_0$ volt/meter.

10. In a semiconducting material the mobilities of electrons and holes are μ_e and μ_n respectively. Which of the following is true?
(a) $\mu_e > \mu_n$ (b) $\mu_e < \mu_n$
(c) $\mu_e = \mu_n$ (d) $\mu_e < 0$; $\mu_n > 0$.

11. The magnetic moment (μ) of a revolving electron around the nucleus varies with principal quantum number n as
(a) $\mu \propto n$ (b) $\mu \propto 1/n$
(c) $\mu \propto n^2$ (d) $\mu \propto 1/n^2$.

12. A radioactive material has a half-life of 10 days. What fraction of the material would remain after 30 days?
(a) 0.5 (b) 0.25
(c) 0.125 (d) 0.33

13. According to Hubble's law, the redshift (Z) of a receding galaxy and its distance r from earth are related as
(a) $Z \propto r$ (b) $Z \propto 1/r$
(c) $Z \propto 1/r^2$ (d) $Z \propto r^{3/2}$.

14. When exposed to sunlight, thin films of oil on water often exhibit brilliant colours due to the phenomenon of
(a) interference (b) diffraction
(c) dispersion (d) polarisation.

15. "Parsec" is the unit of
(a) time (b) distance
(c) frequency (d) angular acceleration.

16. The voltage gain of the following amplifier is

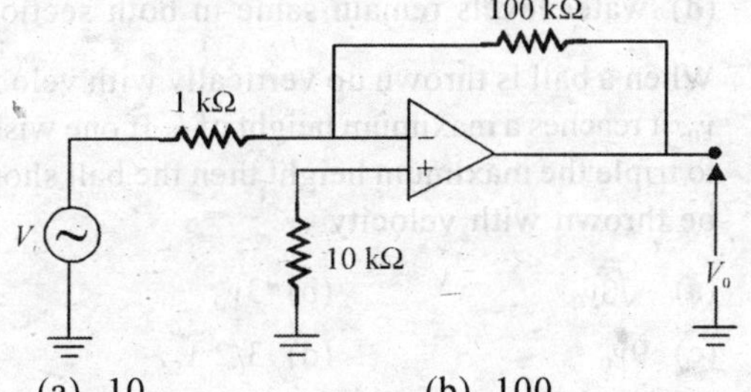

(a) 10 (b) 100
(c) 1000 (d) 9.9

17. A 50 Hz a.c. source of 20 volts is connected across R and C as shown in figure. The voltage across R is 12 volt. The voltage across C is

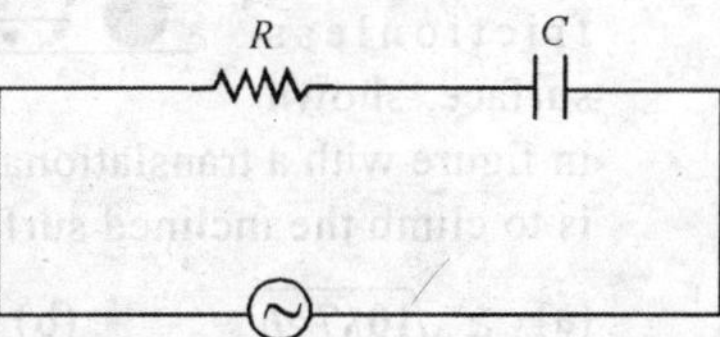

(a) 8 V (b) 16 V
(c) 10 V
(d) not possible to determine unless values of R and C are given.

18. In the figure given, the position-time graph of a particle of mass 0.1 kg is shown.

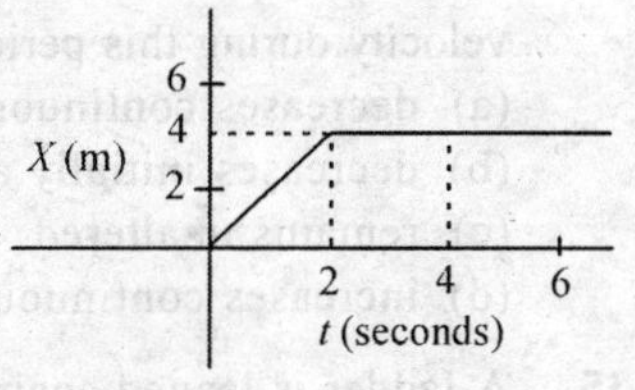

The impulse at $t = 2$ sec is
(a) 0.2 kg m sec^{-1} (b) – 0.2 kg m sec^{-1}
(c) 0.1 kg m sec^{-1} (d) – 0.4 kg m sec^{-1}.

19. The pressure exerted by an electromagnetic wave of intensity I (watt/m^2) on a nonreflecting surface is [c is the velocity of light]
(a) Ic (b) Ic^2
(c) I/c (d) I/c^2.

20. A block of mass 10 kg is moving in x-direction with a constant speed of 10 m/sec. It is subjected to a retarding force $F = -0.1x$ joule/meter during its travel from $x = 20$ meter to $x = 30$ meter. Its final kinetic energy will be
(a) 475 joule (b) 450 joule
(c) 275 joule (d) 250 joule.

21. Energy required to break one bond in DNA is approximately
(a) ~ 1 eV (b) ~ 0.1 eV
(c) ~ 0.01 eV (d) ~ 2.1 eV.

22. The condition for a uniform spherical mass m of radius r to be a black hole is [G = gravitational constant and g = acceleration due to gravity]
(a) $\left(\frac{2Gm}{r}\right)^{1/2} \le c$ (b) $\left(\frac{2gm}{r}\right)^{1/2} = c$
(c) $\left(\frac{2Gm}{r}\right)^{1/2} \ge c$ (d) $\left(\frac{gm}{r}\right)^{1/2} \ge c$

23. Which of the following is an amorphous solid?
(a) glass (b) diamond
(c) salt (d) sugar.

24. For a constant hydraulic stress on an object, the fractional change in the object's volume ($\Delta V/V$) and its bulk modulus (B) are related as
(a) $\frac{\Delta V}{V} \propto B$ (b) $\frac{\Delta V}{V} \propto \frac{1}{B}$
(c) $\frac{\Delta V}{V} \propto B^2$ (d) $\frac{\Delta V}{V} \propto B^{-2}$

25. Which of the following functions represents a simple harmonic oscillation?
(a) $\sin\omega t - \cos\omega t$ (b) $\sin^2\omega t$
(c) $\sin\omega t + \sin 2\omega t$ (d) $\sin\omega t - \sin 2\omega t$.

26. In case of linearly polarised light, the magnitude of the electric field vector
(a) does not change with time
(b) varies periodically with time
(c) increases and decreases linearly with time
(d) is parallel to the direction of propagation.

27. The circuit shown below acts as

(a) tuned filter
(b) low pass filter
(c) high pass filter (d) rectifier.

28. For ensuring dissipation of same energy in all three resistors (R_1, R_2, R_3) connected as shown in figure, their values must be related as

(a) $R_1 = R_2 = R_3$ (b) $R_2 = R_3$ and $R_1 = 4R_2$
(c) $R_2 = R_3$ and $R_1 = 1/4R_2$
(d) $R_1 = R_2 + R_3$.

29. The apparent depth of water in cylindrical water tank of diameter $2R$ cm is reducing at the rate of x cm/minute when water is being drained out at a constant rate. The amount of water drained in c.c. per minute is (n_1 = refractive index of air, n_2 = refractive index of water).

(a) $\dfrac{x\pi R^2 n_1}{n_2}$ (b) $\dfrac{x\pi R^2 n_2}{n_1}$

(c) $\dfrac{2\pi R n_1}{n_2}$ (d) $\pi R^2 x$.

30. A candle of diameter d is floating on a liquid in a cylindrical container of diameter D ($D >> d$) as shown in figure. If it is burning at the rate of 2 cm/hour then the top of the candle will

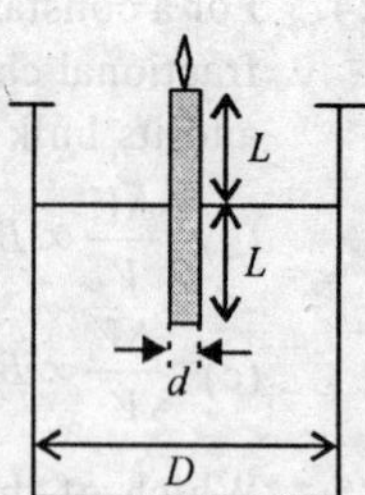

(a) remain at the same height
(b) fall at the rate of 1 cm/hour
(c) fall at the rate of 2 cm/hour
(d) go up at the rate of 1 cm/hour.

31. A given shaped glass tube having uniform cross section is filled with water and is mounted on a rotatable shaft as shown in figure. If the tube is rotated with a constant angular velocity ω when

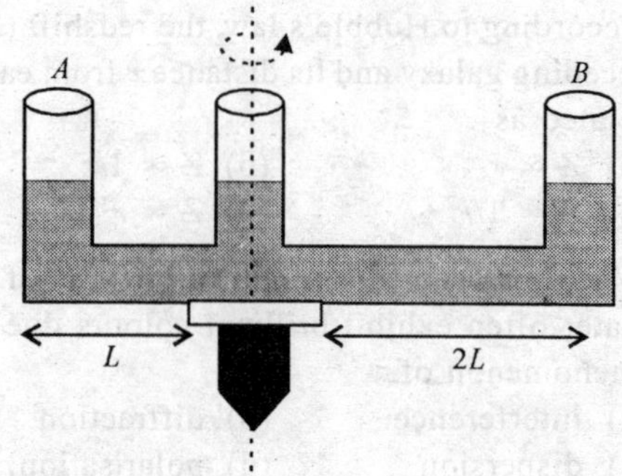

(a) water levels in both sections A and B go up
(b) water level in section A goes up and that in B comes down
(c) water level in section A comes down and that in B it goes up
(d) water levels remain same in both sections.

32. When a ball is thrown up vertically with velocity v_0, it reaches a maximum height of h. If one wishes to triple the maximum height then the ball should be thrown with velocity

(a) $\sqrt{3}v_0$ (b) $3v_0$
(c) $9v_0$ (d) $3/2\ v_0$.

33. A solid sphere is rolling on a frictionless surface, shown in figure with a translational velocity v m/s. If it is to climb the inclined surface then v should be

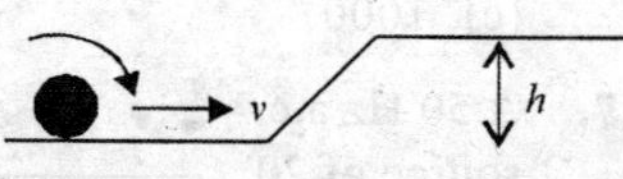

(a) $\geq \sqrt{10/7gh}$ (b) $\geq \sqrt{2gh}$
(c) $2gh$ (d) $10/7gh$.

34. A horizontal platform is rotating with uniform angular velocity around the vertical axis passing through its centre. At some instant of time a viscous fluid of mass m is dropped at the centre and is allowed to spread out and finally fall. The angular velocity during this period

(a) decreases continuously
(b) decreases initially and increases again
(c) remains unaltered
(d) increases continuously.

35. A ladder is leaned against a smooth wall and it is allowed to slip on a frictionless floor. Which figure represents trace of its centre of mass.

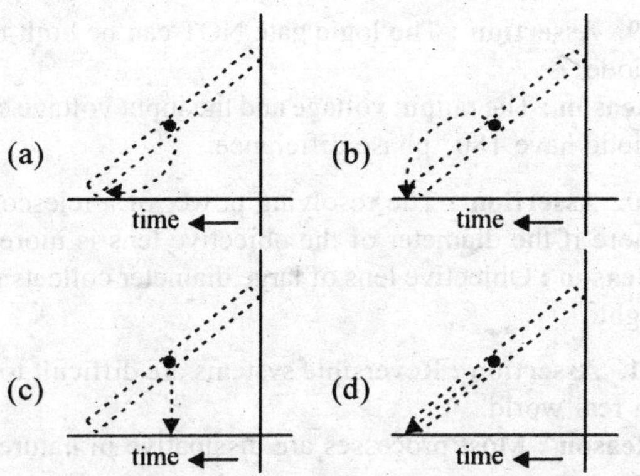

36. A person is standing in an elevator. In which situation he finds his weight less?

(a) when the elevator moves upward with constant acceleration.
(b) when the elevator moves downward with constant acceleration.
(c) when the elevator moves upward with uniform velocity
(d) when the elevator moves downward with uniform velocity.

37. A magnet is made to oscillate with a particular frequency, passing through a coil as shown in figure. The time variation of the magnitude of e.m.f. generated across the coil during one cycle is

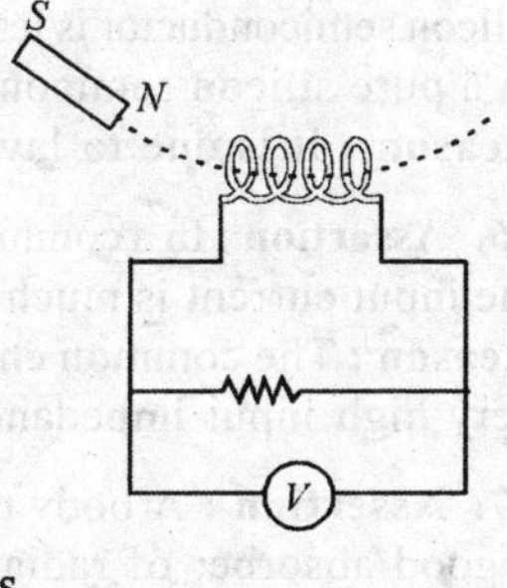

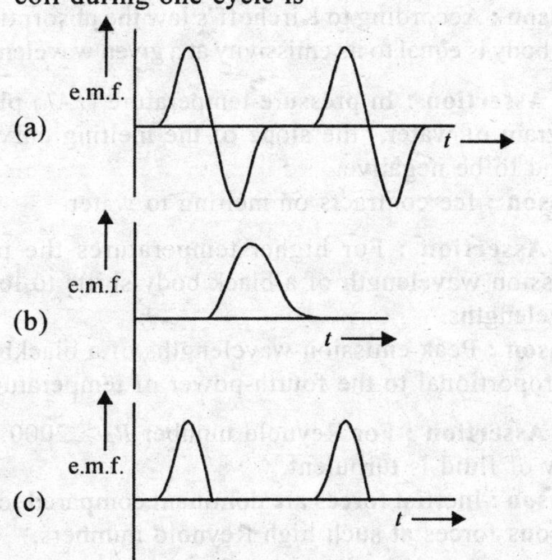

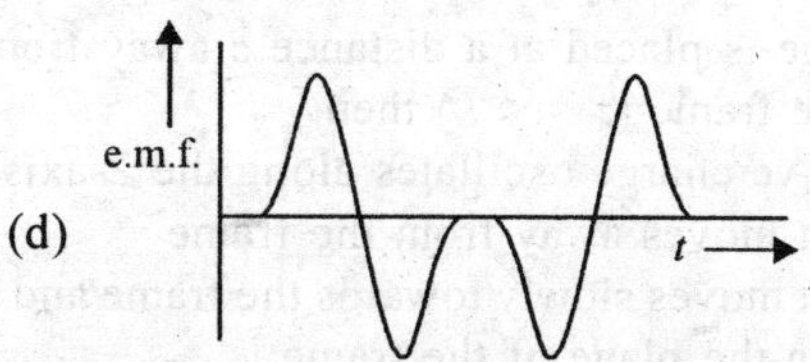

38. Two concentric conducting thin spherical shells A and B having radii r_A and r_B ($r_B > r_A$) are charged to Q_A and $-Q_B$ ($|Q_B| > |Q_A|$). The electrical field along a line, (passing through the centre is)

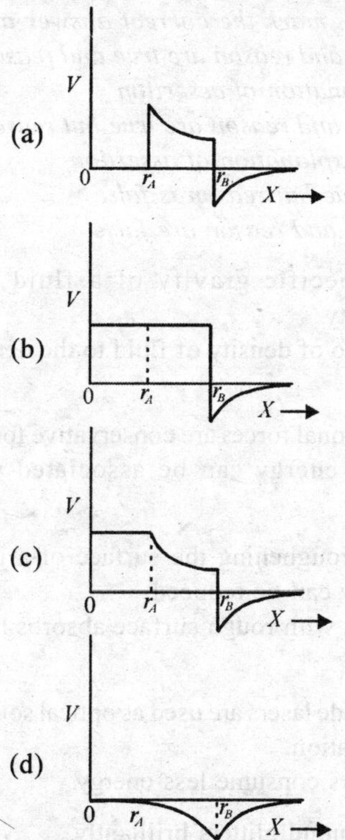

39. Dimension of electrical resistance is

(a) $ML^2T^{-3}A^{-1}$ (b) $ML^2T^{-3}A^{-2}$
(c) $ML^3T^{-3}A^{-2}$ (d) $ML^{-1}L^3T^3A^2$.

40. Four point +ve charges of same magnitude (Q) are placed at four corners of a rigid square frame as shown in figure. The plane of the frame is perpendicular to Z-axis. If a –ve point

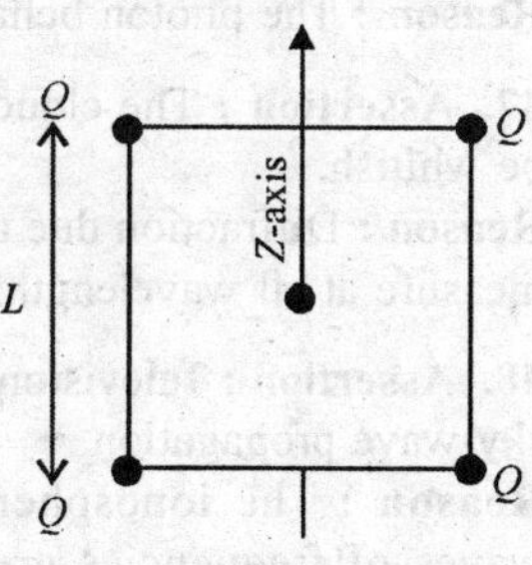

charge is placed at a distance z away from the above frame ($z << L$) then
(a) –ve charge oscillates along the Z-axis
(b) it moves away from the frame
(c) it moves slowly towards the frame and stays in the plane of the frame
(d) it passes through the frame only once.

Directions for questions 41-60 : *In each of the following questions, a statement of Assertion (A) is given followed by a corresponding statement of Reason (R) just below it. Of the statements, mark the correct answer as*
(a) If both assertion and reason are true and reason is the correct explanation of assertion
(b) If both assertion and reason are true but reason is not the correct explanation of assertion
(c) If assertion is true but reason is false
(d) If both assertion and reason are false.

41. Assertion : Specific gravity of a fluid is a dimensionless quantity.
Reason : It is the ratio of density of fluid to the density of water.

42. Assertion : Frictional forces are conservative forces.
Reason : Potential energy can be associated with frictional forces.

43. Assertion : By roughening the surface of a glass sheet its transparency can be reduced.
Reason : Glass sheet with rough surface absorbs more light.

44. Assertion : A diode lasers are used as optical sources in optical communication.
Reason : Diode lasers consume less energy.

45. Assertion : Diamond glitters brilliantly.
Reason : Diamond does not absorb sunlight.

46. Assertion : The energy (E) and momentum (p) of a photon are related by $p = E/c$.
Reason : The photon behaves like a particle.

47. Assertion : The clouds in sky generally appear to be whitish.
Reason : Diffraction due to clouds is efficient in equal measure at all wavelengths.

48. Assertion : Television signals are received through sky-wave propagation.
Reason : The ionosphere reflects electromagnetic waves of frequencies greater than a certain critical frequency.

49. Assertion : The logic gate NOT can be built using diode.
Reason : The output voltage and the input voltage of the diode have 180° phase difference.

50. Assertion : The resolving power of a telescope is more if the diameter of the objective lens is more.
Reason : Objective lens of large diameter collects more light.

51. Assertion : Reversible systems are difficult to find in real world.
Reason : Most processes are dissipative in nature.

52. Assertion : For a system of particles under central force field, the total angular momentum is conserved.
Reason : The torque acting on such a system is zero.

53. Assertion : Air quickly leaking out of a balloon becomes cooler.
Reason : The leaking air undergoes adiabatic expansion.

54. Assertion : It is not possible to use ^{35}Cl as the fuel for fusion energy.
Reason : The binding energy of ^{35}Cl is too small.

55. Assertion : The number of electrons in a p-type silicon semiconductor is less than the number of electrons in a pure silicon semiconductor at room temperature.
Reason : It is due to law of mass action.

56. Assertion : In a common emitter transistor amplifier the input current is much less than the output current.
Reason : The common emitter transistor amplifier has very high input impedance.

57. Assertion : A body that is a good radiator is also a good absorber of radiation at a given wavelength.
Reason : According to Kirchoff's law the absorptivity of a body is equal to its emissivity at a given wavelength.

58. Assertion : In pressure-temperature (P-T) phase diagram of water, the slope of the melting curve is found to be negative.
Reason : Ice contracts on melting to water.

59. Assertion : For higher temperatures the peak emission wavelength of a black body shifts to lower wavelengths.
Reason : Peak emission wavelengths of a blackbody is proportional to the fourth-power of temperature.

60. Assertion : For Reynold number $R_e > 2000$, the flow of fluid is turbulent.
Reason : Inertial forces are dominant compared to the viscous forces at such high Reynold numbers.

CHEMISTRY

61. Among the following molecules

(i) $\ddot{X}eO_3$ (ii) $\ddot{X}eOF_4$ (iii) $\ddot{X}eF_6$

Those having same number of lone pairs on Xe are

(a) (i) and (ii) only
(b) (i) and (iii) only
(c) (ii) and (iii) only
(d) (i), (ii) and (iii).

62. An aqueous solution of $CoCl_2$ on addition of excess of concentrated HCl turns blue due to formation of

(a) $[Co(H_2O)_4Cl_2]$ (b) $[Co(H_2O)_2Cl_4]^{2-}$
(c) $[CoCl_4]^{2-}$ (d) $[Co(H_2O)_2Cl_2]$

63. In which of the following pairs both the complex's show optical isomerism?

(a) *cis*-$[Cr(C_2O_4)_2Cl_2]^{3-}$, *cis*-$[Co(NH_3)_4Cl_2]$
(b) $[Co(en)_3]Cl_3$, *cis*-$[Co(en)_2Cl_2]Cl$
(c) $[PtCl(dien)]Cl$, $[NiCl_2Br_2]^{2-}$
(d) $[Co(NO_3)_3(NH_3)_3]$, *cis*-$[Pt(en)_2Cl_2]$.

64. The diamagnetic species is

(a) $[Ni(CN)_4]^{2-}$ (b) $[NiCl_4]^{2-}$
(c) $[CoCl_4]^{2-}$ (d) $[CoF_6]^{2-}$.

65. In the balanced chemical reaction

$IO_3^- + aI^- + bH^+ \rightarrow cH_2O + dI_2$

a, b, c and d respectively corresponds to

(a) 5, 6, 3, 3 (b) 5, 3, 6, 3
(c) 3, 5, 3, 6 (d) 5, 6, 5, 5

66. Among the following pairs of ions, the lower oxidation state in aqueous solution is more stable than the other, in

(a) Tl^+, Tl^{3+} (b) Cu^+, Cu^{2+}
(c) Cr^{2+}, Cr^{3+} (d) V^{2+}, VO^{2+}.

67. The number of P – O – P bridges in the structure of phosphorus pentoxide and phosphorus trioxide are respectively

(a) 6, 6 (b) 5, 5
(c) 5, 6 (d) 6, 5.

68. In diborane, the two H – B – H angles are nearly

(a) 60°, 120° (b) 95°, 120°
(c) 95°, 150° (d) 120°, 180°.

69. Which of the following gives propyne on hydrolysis?

(a) Al_4C_3 (b) Mg_2C_3
(c) B_4C (d) La_4C_3.

70. The pair of amphoteric hydroxides is

(a) $Al(OH)_3$, LiOH
(b) $Be(OH)_2$, $Mg(OH)_2$
(c) $B(OH)_3$, $Be(OH)_2$
(d) $Be(OH)_2$, $Zn(OH)_2$.

71. Which of the following is a carbonate ore?

(a) pyrolusite (b) malachite
(c) diaspore (d) cassiterite.

72. $^{238}_{92}U$ emits 8 α-particles and 6 β-particles. The neutron/proton ratio in the product nucleus is

(a) 60/41 (b) 61/40
(c) 62/41 (d) 61/42.

73. The correct order for the wavelength of absorption in the visible region is

(a) $[Ni(NO_2)_6]^{4-} < [Ni(NH_3)_6]^{2+} < [Ni(H_2O)_6]^{2+}$
(b) $[Ni(NO_2)_6]^{4-} < [Ni(H_2O)_6]^{2+} < [Ni(NH_3)_6]^{2+}$
(c) $[Ni(H_2O)_6]^{2+} < [Ni(NH_3)_6]^{2+} < [Ni(NO_2)_6]^{4-}$
(d) $[Ni(NH_3)_6]^{2+} < [Ni(H_2O)_6]^{2+} < [Ni(NO_2)_6]^{4-}$

74. F_2 formed by reacting K_2MnF_6 with

(a) SbF_5 (b) MnF_3
(c) $KSbF_6$ (d) MnF_4.

75. The isoelectronic pair is

(a) Cl_2O, ICl_2^- (b) ICl_2^-, ClO_2
(c) IF_2^+, I_3^- (d) ClO_2^-, ClF_2^+.

76. Which of the following chemicals are used to manufacture methyl isocyanate that caused "Bhopal Tragedy"?

(i) methylamine (ii) phosgene
(iii) phosphine (iv) dimethylamine.

(a) (i) and (iii) (b) (iii) and (iv)
(c) (i) and (ii) (d) (ii) and (iv).

77. α-Particles can be detected using

(a) thin aluminium sheet
(b) barium sulphate
(c) zinc sulphide screen
(d) gold foil.

78. Which of the following molecules is most suitable to disperse benzene in water?

(a) 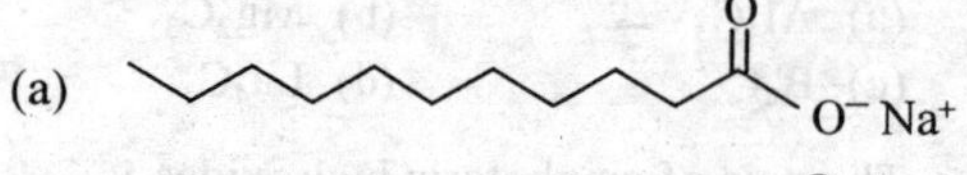

(b) 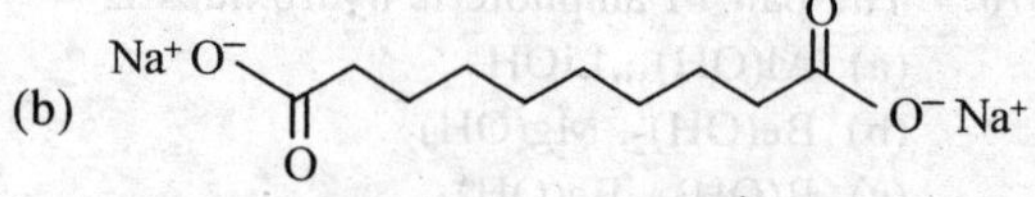

(c) CH_3

(d) 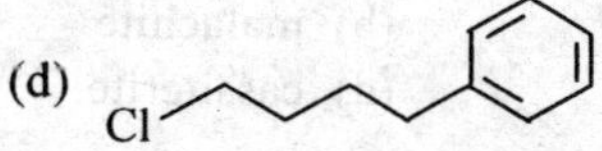

79. The chemical reaction,

$$2AgCl_{(s)} + H_{2\,(g)} \rightarrow 2HCl_{(aq)} + 2Ag_{(s)}$$

taking place in a galvanic cell is represented by the notation

(a) $Pt_{(s)} \mid H_{2\,(g)}$, 1 bar $\mid$ 1M $KCl_{(aq)} \mid AgCl_{(s)} \mid Ag_{(s)}$

(b) $Pt_{(s)} \mid H_{2(g)}$, 1 bar $\mid$ 1M $HCl_{(aq)} \mid$ 1M$Ag^+_{(aq)} \mid Ag_{(s)}$

(c) $Pt_{(s)} \mid H_{2\,(g)}$, 1 bar $\mid$ 1M $HCl_{(aq)} \mid AgCl_{(s)} \mid Ag_{(s)}$

(d) $Pt_{(s)} \mid H_{2\,(g)}$, 1 bar $\mid$ 1M $HCl_{(aq)} \mid Ag_{(s)} \mid AgCl_{(s)}$

80. If Z is the number of atoms in the unit cell that represents the closest packing sequence ... $A\ B\ C\ A\ B\ C$ ..., the number of tetrahedral voids in the unit cell is equal to

(a) Z (b) $2Z$
(c) $Z/2$ (d) $Z/4$.

81. ΔH_f° (298 K) of methanol is given by the chemical equation

(a) $CH_{4\,(g)} + \frac{1}{2}O_{2\,(g)} \rightarrow CH_3OH_{(g)}$

(b) $C\ (\text{graphite}) + \frac{1}{2}O_{2\,(g)} + 2H_{2\,(g)} \rightarrow CH_3OH_{(l)}$

(c) $C\ (\text{diamond}) + \frac{1}{2}O_{2\,(g)} + 2H_{2\,(g)} \rightarrow CH_3OH_{(l)}$

(d) $CO_{(g)} + 2H_{2\,(g)} \rightarrow CH_3OH_{(l)}$.

82. An endothermic reaction with high activation energy for the forward reaction is given by the diagram

(a) 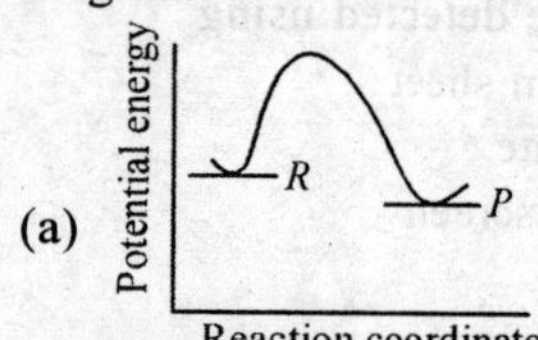

(b) 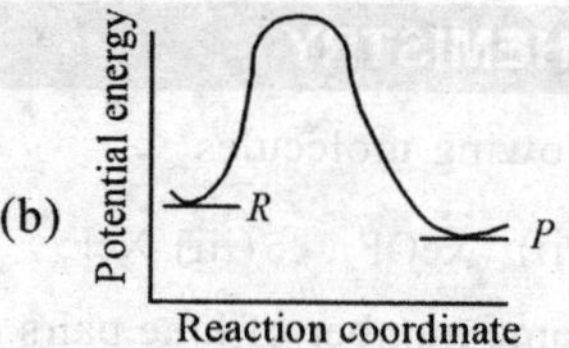

(c) 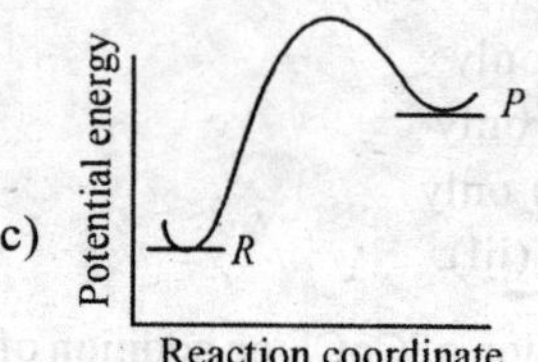

(d) 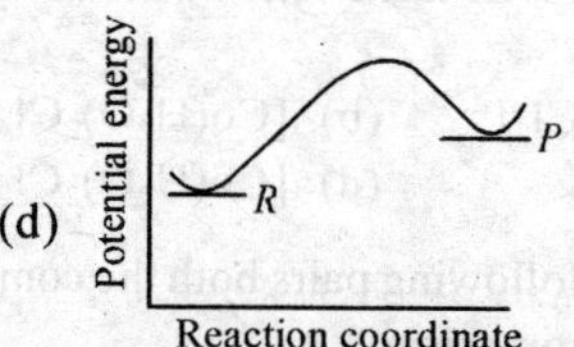

83. When 10 ml of 0.1 M acetic acid ($pK_a = 5.0$) is titrated against 10 ml of 0.1 M ammonia solution ($pK_b = 5.0$), the equivalence point occurs at pH

(a) 5.0 (b) 6.0
(c) 7.0 (d) 9.0

84. The most probable radius (in pm) for finding the electron in He^+ is

(a) 0.0 (b) 52.9
(c) 26.5 (d) 105.8

85. For the reaction of one mole of zinc dust with one mole of sulphuric acid in a bomb calorimeter, ΔU and w corresponds to

(a) $\Delta U < 0,\ w = 0$ (b) $\Delta U < 0,\ w < 0$
(c) $\Delta U > 0,\ w = 0$ (d) $\Delta U > 0,\ w > 0$.

86. For reaction $aA \rightarrow xP$, when $[A] = 2.2$ mM, the rate was found to be 2.4 mM s^{-1}. On reducing concentration of A to half, the rate changes to 0.6 mM s^{-1}. The order of reaction with respect to A is

(a) 1.5 (b) 2.0
(c) 2.5 (d) 3.0

87. For reaction, $2NOCl_{(g)} = 2NO_{(g)} + Cl_{2\,(g)}$, K_C at 427°C is 3×10^{-6} L. mol^{-1}. The value of K_p is nearly

(a) 7.50×10^{-5} (b) 2.50×10^{-5}
(c) 2.50×10^{-4} (d) 1.75×10^{-4}.

88. For the chemical equilibrium,

$$CaCO_{3\,(s)} \rightleftharpoons CaO_{\,(s)} + CO_{2\,(g)},$$

$\Delta H_r°$ can be determined from which one of the following plots?

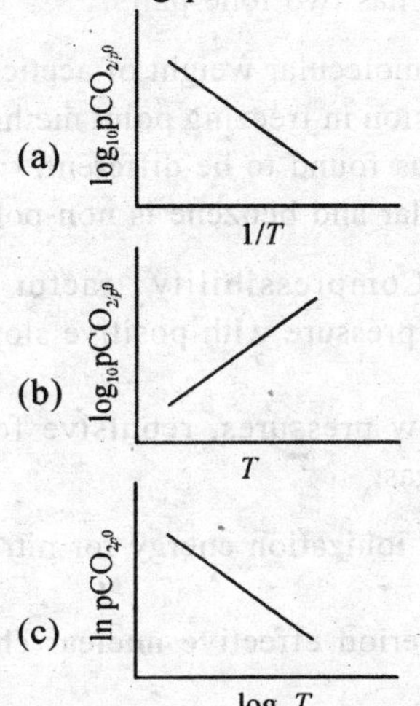

89. Among the following the strongest nucleophile is

(a) C_2H_5SH (b) CH_3COO^-

(c) CH_3NH_2 (d) $NCCH_2^-$

90. The major product formed in the following reaction is

$$CH_3-\overset{\overset{\large CH_3}{|}}{\underset{\underset{\large H}{|}}{C}}-CH_2Br \xrightarrow[CH_3OH]{CH_3O^-}$$

(a) $CH_3-\overset{\overset{\large CH_3}{|}}{\underset{\underset{\large H}{|}}{C}}-CH_2OCH_3$

(b) $CH_3-\underset{\underset{\large OCH_3}{|}}{CH}-CH_2CH_3$

(c) $CH_3-\overset{\overset{\large CH_3}{|}}{C}=CH_2$ (d) $CH_3-\overset{\overset{\large CH_3}{|}}{\underset{\underset{\large OCH_3}{|}}{C}}-CH_3$

91. The major product obtained on treatment of $CH_3CH_2CH(F)CH_3$ with CH_3O^-/CH_3OH is

(a) $CH_3CH_2CH(OCH_3)CH_3$

(b) $CH_3CH=CHCH_3$

(c) $CH_3CH_2CH=CH_2$

(d) $CH_3CH_2CH_2CH_2OCH_3$.

92. Among the following the most stable compound is

(a) *cis*-1,2-cyclohexanediol

(b) *trans*-1,2-cyclohexanediol

(c) *cis*-1,3-cyclohexenediol

(d) *trans*-1,3-cyclohexanediol.

93. 3-Phenylpropene on reaction with HBr gives (as a major product)

(a) $C_6H_5CH_2CH(Br)CH_3$

(b) $C_6H_5CH(Br)CH_2CH_3$

(c) $C_6H_5CH_2CH_2CH_2Br$

(d) $C_6H_5CH(Br)CH=CH_2$.

94. $CH_3CO_2C_2H_5$ on reaction with sodium ethoxide in ethanol gives A, which on heating in the presence of acid gives B. Compound B is

(a) CH_3COCH_2COOH (b) CH_3COCH_3

(c) $CH_2=$ (four-membered ring containing O) $=O$ (d) $CH_2=C(OC_2H_5)_2$

95. Among the following which one does not act as an intermediate in Hofmann rearrangement?

(a) RNCO (b) $RCO\ddot{N}$

(c) $RCO\ddot{N}HBr$ (d) RNC

96. Pyridine is less basic than triethylamine because

(a) pyridine has aromatic character

(b) nitrogen in pyridine is sp^2 hybridised

(c) pyridine is a cyclic system

(d) in pyridine, lone pair of nitrogen is delocalised.

97. Which one of the following biomolecules is insoluble in water?

(a) α-keratin (b) haemoglobin

(c) ribonuclease (d) adenine.

98. Correct configuration of the following is

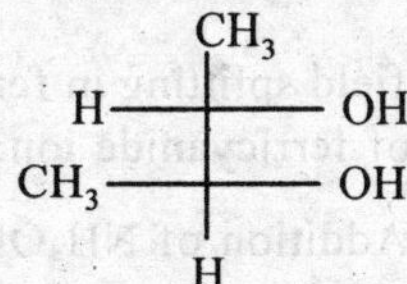

(a) 1S, 2S (b) 1S, 2R

(c) 1R, 2S (d) 1R, 2R.

99. Which one of the following statements is true for protein synthesis (translation)?
(a) amino acids are directly recognized by *m*-RNA
(b) the third base of the codon is less specific
(c) only one codon codes for an amino acid
(d) every *t*-RNA molecule has more than one amino acid attachment.

100. $C_6H_5CONHCH_3$ can be converted into $C_6H_5CH_2NHCH_3$ by
(a) $NaBH_4$ (b) H_2 - Pd/C
(c) $LiAl_4$ (d) Zn-Hg/HCl.

Directions for questions 101-120 : *In each of the following questions, a statement of Assertion (A) is given followed by a corresponding statement of Reason (R) just below it. Of the statements, mark the correct answer as*
(a) If both assertion and reason are true and reason is the correct explanation of assertion
(b) If both assertion and reason are true but reason is not the correct explanation of assertion
(c) If assertion is true but reason is false
(d) If both assertion and reason are false.

101. Assertion : Reaction of SO_2 and H_2S in the presence of Fe_2O_3 catalyst gives elemental sulphur.
Reason : SO_2 is a reducing agent.

102. Assertion : SiF_6^{2-} is known but $SiCl_6^{2-}$ is not.
Reason : Size of fluorine is small and its lone pair of electrons interacts with *d*-orbitals of Si strongly.

103 Assertion : Borax bead test is not suitable for Al(III).
Reason : Al_2O_3 is insoluble in water.

104. Assertion : Ozone is a powerful oxidising agent in comparison to O_2.
Reason : Ozone is diamagnetic but O_2 is paramagnetic.

105. Assertion : Potassium ferrocyanide is diamagnetic whereas potassium ferricyanide is paramagnetic.
Reason : Crystal field splitting in ferrocyanide ion is greater than that of ferricyanide ion.

106. Assertion : Addition of NH_4OH to an aqueous solution of $BaCl_2$ in the presence of NH_4Cl (excess) precipitates $Ba(OH)_2$.
Reason : $Ba(OH)_2$ is insoluble in water.

107. Assertion : $SeCl_4$ does not have a tetrahedral structure.
Reason : Se in $SeCl_4$ has two lone pairs.

108. Assertion : The molecular weight of acetic acid determined by depression in freezing point method in benzene and water was found to be different.
Reason : Water is polar and benzene is non-polar.

109. Assertion : Compressibility factor for hydrogen varies with pressure with positive slope at all pressures.
Reason : Even at low pressures, repulsive forces dominate hydrogen gas.

110. Assertion : First ionization energy for nitrogen is lower than oxygen.
Reason : Across a period effective nuclear charge decreases.

111. Assertion : B_2 molecule is diamagnetic.
Reason : The highest occupied molecular orbital is of σ type.

112. Assertion : Rate of hydrolysis of methyl chloride to methanol is higher in DMF than in water.
Reason : Hydrolysis of methyl chloride follows second order kinetics.

113. Assertion : Galvanised iron does not rust.
Reason : Zinc has a more negative electrode potential than iron.

114. Assertion : Extraction of iron metal from iron oxide ore is carried out by heating with coke.
Reason : The reaction $Fe_2O_{3\,(s)} \rightarrow Fe_{(s)} + 3/2\ O_{2\,(g)}$ is a spontaneous process.

115. Assertion : Rates of nitration of benzene and hexadeuterobenzene are different.
Reason : C – H bond is stronger than C – D bond.

116. Assertion : *t*-Butyl methyl ether is not prepared by the reaction of *t*-butyl bromide with sodium methoxide.
Reason : Sodium methoxide is a strong nucleophile.

117. Assertion : Maltose is a reducing sugar which gives two moles of D-glucose on hydrolysis.
Reason : Maltose has a 1,4-β-glycosidic linkage.

118. Assertion : $p\text{-}O_2N - C_6H_5COCH_3$ is prepared by Friedel Crafts acylation of nitrobenzene.

Reason : Nitrobenzene easily undergoes electrophilic substitution reaction.

119. Assertion : Alkyl isocyanides in acidified water give alkyl formamides.

Reason : In isocyanides, carbon first acts as a nucleophile and then as an electrophile.

120. Assertion : Cyclopentadienyl anion is much more stable than allyl anion.

Reason : Cyclopentadienyl anion is aromatic in character.

BIOLOGY

121. Based on cellular mechanisms there are two major types of regeneration found in the animals. Which one of the following is the correct example of the type mentioned?

(a) Morphallaxis – Regeneration of two transversely cut equal pieces of a Hydra into two small Hydras.

(b) Epimorphosis - Replacement of old and dead erythrocytes by the new ones.

(c) Morphallaxis - Healing up of a wound in the skin.

(d) Epimorphosis - Regeneration of crushed and filtered out pieces of a *Planaria* into as many new Planarians.

122. Which one of the following four secretions is correctly matched with its source, target and nature of action?

	Secretion	Source	Target	Action
(a)	Gastrin	Stomach lining	Oxyntic cells	Production of HCl
(b)	Inhibin	Sertoli cells	Hypoth-alamus	Inhibition of secretion of gonadotropin releasing hormone
(c)	Enterokinase	Duodenum	Gall bladder	Release of bile juice
(d)	Atrial Natriuretic Factor (ANF)	Sinu atrial node(SAN) M-cells of Atria	Juxta-glomerular apparatus (JGA)	Inhibition of release of renin

123. Which one of the following four glands is correctly matched with the accompanying description ?

(a) Thyroid - hyperactivity in young children causes cretinism

(b) Thymus - starts undergoing atrophy after puberty

(c) Parathyroid - secretes parathormone which promotes movement of calcium ions from blood into bones during calcification

(d) Pancreas - Delta cells of the Islets of Langerhans secrete a hormone which stimulates glycolysis in liver.

124. Given below is a pedigree chart showing the inheritance of a certain sex-linked trait in humans.

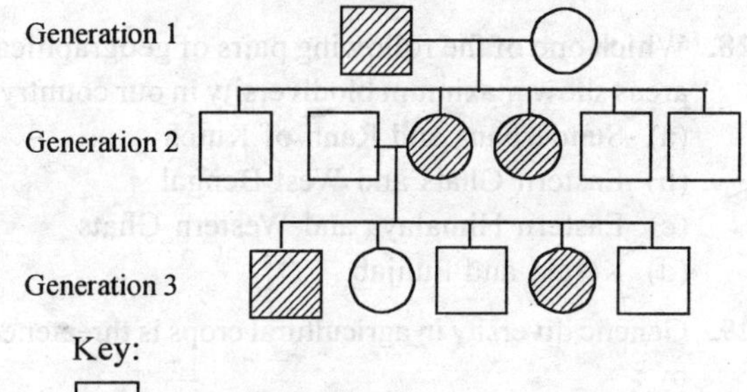

Key:

Unaffected male

Affected male

Unaffected female

Affected female

The trait traced in the above pedigree chart is

(a) dominant X-linked

(b) recessive X-linked

(c) dominant Y-linked

(d) recessive Y-linked.

125. A cross section at the midpoint of the middle piece of a human sperm will show

(a) centriole, mitochondria and 9 + 2 arrangement of microtubules

(b) centriole and mitochondria

(c) mitochondria and 9 + 2 arrangement of microtubules

(d) 9 + 2 arrangement of microtubules only.

126. Which one of the following is a correct statement?

(a) "Bt" in "Bt-cotton" indicates that it is a genetically modified organism produced through biotechnology.

(b) Somatic hybridization involves fusion of two complete plant cells carrying desired genes.
(c) The anticoagulant hirudin is being produced from transgenic *Brassica napus* seeds.
(d) "Flavr Savr" variety of tomato has enhanced the production of ethylene which improves its taste.

127. An insect bite may result in inflammation of that spot. This is triggered by the alarm chemicals such as:
(a) histamine and dopamine
(b) histamine and kinins
(c) interferons and opsonin
(d) interferons and histones.

128. Which one of the following pairs of geographical areas show maximum biodiversity in our country?
(a) Sunderbans and Rann of Kutch
(b) Eastern Ghats and West Bengal
(c) Eastern Himalaya and Western Ghats
(d) Kerala and Punjab.

129. Genetic diversity in agricultural crops is threatened by :
(a) introduction of high yielding varieties
(b) intensive use of fertilizers
(c) extensive intercropping
(d) intensive use of biopesticides.

130. One of the *ex situ* conservation methods for endangered species is
(a) wildlife sanctuaries
(b) biosphere reserves
(c) cryopreservation (d) national parks.

131. Formation of non-functional methaemoglobin causes blue-baby syndrome. This is due to
(a) excess of arsenic concentration in drinking water
(b) excess of nitrates in drinking water
(c) deficiency of iron in food
(d) increased methane content in the atmosphere.

132. Two of the body parts which do not appear in MRI may be:
(a) molar teeth and eye lens
(b) scapula and canines
(c) ligaments and ribs
(d) tendons and premolars.

133. A young drug addict used to show symptoms of depressed brain activity, feeling of calmness, relaxation and drowsiness. Possibly he was taking
(a) amphetamine (b) marijuna
(c) pethidine (d) valium.

134. Antigen binding site in an antibody is found between
(a) two light chains
(b) two heavy chains
(c) one heavy and one light chain
(d) either between two light chains or between one heavy and one light chain depending upon the nature of antigen.

135. Which one of the following events is correctly matched with the time period in a normal menstrual cycle?
(a) release of egg : 5th day
(b) endometrium regenerates : 5 - 10 days
(c) endometrium secretes nutrients for implantation : 11-18 days
(d) rise in progesterone level : 1 - 15 days.

136. A tumor inducing plasmid widely used in the production of transgenic plants is that of
(a) *Escherichia coli*
(b) *Bacillus thuringiensis*
(c) *Staphylococcus aureus*
(d) *Agrobacterium tumefaciens*.

137. Which one of the following statement pertaining to pollutants is correct?
(a) DDT is a non-biodegradable pollutant
(b) excess fluoride in drinking water causes osteoporosis
(c) excess cadmium in drinking water causes black foot disease
(d) methylmercury in water may cause "Itai Itai" disease.

138. Which one of the following statements is correct with respect to salt water balance inside the body of living organisms?
(a) when water is not available camels do not produce urine but store urea in tissues
(b) Salmon fish excretes lot of stored salt through gill membrane when in fresh water.
(c) *Paramecium* discharges concentrated salt solution by contractile vacuoles

(d) The body fluids of fresh water animals are generally hypotonic to surrounding water.

139. The "cri-du-chat" syndrome is caused by change in chromosome structure involving
(a) deletion (b) duplication
(c) inversion (d) translocation.

140. The family containing mustard and its main characters are
(a) Brassicaceae – Tetramerous flowers, six stamens, bicarpellary gynoecium, siliqua type fruit
(b) Brassicaceae – Pentamerous flowers, many stamens, pentacarpellary gynoecium, capsule type fruit
(c) Solanaceae - Pentamerous flowers, five stamens, bicarpellary gynoecium, berry type fruit
(d) Poaceae – Trimerous flowers, three stamens, monocarpellary gynoecium, caryopsis type of fruit.

141. Grain colour in wheat is determined by three pairs of polygenes. Following the cross AABBCC (dark colour) x aabbcc (light colour), in F_2 generation what proportion of the progeny is likely to resemble either parent?
(a) none (b) less than 5 percent
(c) one third (d) half.

142. Which one of the following statements pertaining to plant structure is correct?
(a) cork lacks stomata, but lenticels carry out transpiration
(b) passage cells help in transfer of food from cortex to phloem
(c) sieve tube elements possess cytoplasm but no nuclei
(d) the shoot apical meristem has a quiescent centre.

143. When synapsis is complete all along the chromosome, the cell is said to have entered a stage called
(a) zygotene (b) pachytene
(c) diplotene (d) diakinesis.

144. Primary source of allelic variation is
(a) independent assortment
(b) recombination
(c) mutation (d) polyploidy

145. Many cells function properly and divide mitotically even though they do not have
(a) plasma membrane (b) cytoskeleton
(c) mitochondria (d) plastids.

146. Three of the following statements regarding cell organelles are correct while one is wrong. Which one is wrong?
(a) Lysosomes are double membraned vesicles budded off from Golgi apparatus and contain digestive enzymes.
(b) Endoplasmic reticulum consists of a network of membranous tubules and helps in transport, synthesis and secretion.
(c) Leucoplasts are bound by two membranes, lack pigment but contain their own DNA and protein synthesizing machinery.
(d) Sphaerosomes are single membrane bound and are associated with synthesis and storage of lipids.

147. In which one of the following would you expect to find glyoxysomes?
(a) endosperm of wheat
(b) endosperm of castor
(c) palisade cells in leaf
(d) root hairs.

148. Which one of the following correctly represents an organism and its ecological niche?
(a) *Vallisneria* and pond
(b) desert locust (*Scistocerca*) and desert
(c) plant lice (aphids) and leaf
(d) vultures and dense forest.

149. Given below is one of the types of ecological pyramids.
This type represents
(a) pyramid of numbers in a grassland
(b) pyramid of biomass in a fallow land
(c) pyramid of biomass in a lake
(d) energy pyramid in a spring.

150. The given graph shows the effect of substrate concentration on the rate of reaction of the enzyme green-gram-phosphatase
What does the graph indicate?

(a) The rate of enzyme reaction is directly proportional to the substrate concentration
(b) Presence of an enzyme inhibitor in the reaction mixture
(c) Formation of an enzyme-substrate complex
(d) at higher substrate concentration the pH increases.

151. Which one of the following groups of structures/organs have similar function?
(a) Typhlosole in earthworm, intestinal villi in rat and contractile vacuole in *Amoeba.*
(b) Nephridia in earthworm, Malpighian tubules in cockroach and urinary tubules in rat.
(c) Antennae of cockroach, tympanum of frog and clitellum of earthworm.
(d) Incisors of rat, gizzard (proventriculus) of cockroach and tube feet of starfish.

152. Given diagram shows bone of the left human hindlimb as seen from front. It has certain mistakes in labeling. Two of the wrongly labelled bones are:

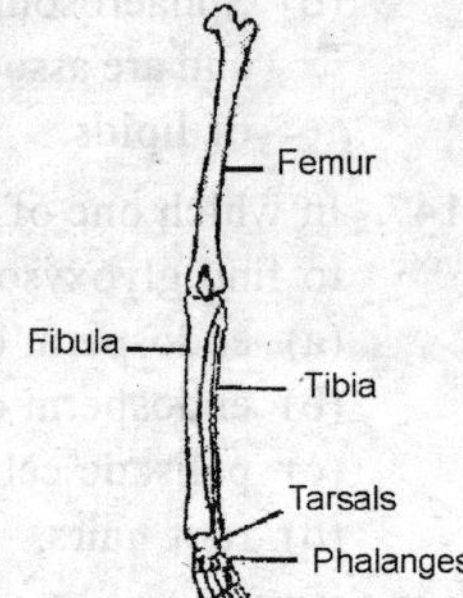

(a) tibia and tarsals
(b) femur and fibula
(c) fibula and phalanges
(d) tarsals and femur.

153. Electroporation procedure involves :
(a) fast passage of food through sieve pores in phloem elements with the help of electric stimulation
(b) opening of stomatal pores during night by artificial light
(c) making transient pores in the cell membrane to introduce gene constructs
(d) purification of saline water with the help of a membrane system.

154. Somaclonal variation appears in
(a) organisms produced through somatic hybridization
(b) plants growing in highly polluted conditions
(c) apomictic plants
(d) tissue culture raised plants.

155. In an experiment freshly hatched larvae of an insect (Khapra beetle) were reared on a basal diet (complete diet without cholesterol) with increasing amounts of cholesterol. Results obtained are shown in the graph given in the table :
The graph indicates that

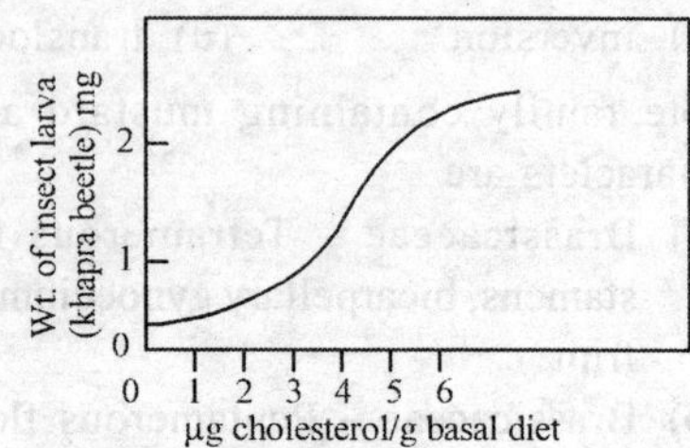

(a) cholesterol is an essential dietary requirement of khapra beetle
(b) growth of khapra beetle is directly proportional to cholesterol concentration
(c) cholesterol concentration of 2 μg/g diet is the optimum level
(d) growth of khapra beetle is inhibited when cholesterol concentration exceeds 5 μg/g diet.

156. Which one of the following is correct matching of a plant, its habit and the forest type where it normally occurs?
(a) *Prosopis*, tree, scrub
(b) *Saccharum*, grass, forest
(c) *Shorea robusta*, herb, tropical rain forest
(d) *Acacia catechu*, tree, coniferous forest.

157. cDNA probes are copied from the messenger RNA molecules with the help of
(a) restriction enzymes
(b) reverse transcriptase
(c) DNA polymerase
(d) adenosine deaminase.

158. Gibberellins can promote seed germination because of their influence on
(a) rate of cell division
(b) production of hydrolyzing enzymes
(c) synthesis of abscisic acid
(d) absorption of water through hard seed coat.

159. Which one of the following features is common in silverfish, scorpion, dragonfly and prawn?
(a) Three pairs of legs and segmented body
(b) Chitinous cuticle and two pairs of antennae
(c) Jointed appendages and chitinous exoskeleton
(d) Cephalothorax and tracheae.

160. Double fertilization involves
(a) fertilization of the egg by two male gametes
(b) fertilization of two eggs in the same embryo sac by two sperms brought by one pollen tube
(c) fertilization of the egg and the central cell by two sperms brought by different pollen tubes
(d) fertilization of the egg and the central cell by two sperms brought by the same pollen tube.

In the following questions (161-180), a statement of assertion (A) is followed by a statement of reason (R).

(a) If both Assertion & Reason are true and the reason is the correct explanation of the assertion, then mark *a*
(b) If both Assertion & Reason are true but the reason is not the correct explanation of the assertion, then mark *b*
(c) If Assertion is true statement but Reason is false, then mark *c*
(d) If both Assertion and Reason are false statements, then mark *d*.

161. *Assertion :* Senescence is the time when age associated defects are manifested.
Reason : Certain genes may be undergoing sequential switching on and off during one's life.

162. *Assertion :* In recombinant DNA technology, human genes are often transferred into bacteria (prokaryotes) or yeast (eukaryote).
Reason : Both bacteria and yeast multiply very fast to form huge populations which express the desired gene.

163. *Assertion :* A suspended particulate matter (SPM) is an important pollutant released by diesel vehicles.
Reason : Catalytic converters greatly reduce pollution caused by automobiles.

164. *Assertion :* Methane component of green house gases contributing to global warming is about 20 percent.
Reason : Introduction of multi-point fuel injection engines in automobiles has decreased methane content in the exhausts.

165. *Assertion :* Interferons are a type of antibodies produced by body cells infected by bacteria.
Reason : Interferons stimulate inflammation at the site of injury.

166. *Assertion :* Organ transplantation patients are given immunosuppressive drugs.
Reason : Transplanted tissue has antigens which stimulate the specific immune response of the recipient.

167. *Assertion :* Persons suffering from haemophilia fail to produce blood clotting factor VIII.
Reason : Prothrombin producing platelets in such persons are found in very low concentration.

168. *Assertion :* In humans, the gamete contributed by the male determines whether the child produced will be male or female.
Reason : Sex in humans is a polygenic trait depending upon a cumulative effect of some genes on X-chromosome and some on Y-chromosome.

169. *Assertion :* Mitochondria and chloroplasts are semi-autonomous organelles.
Reason : They are formed by division of pre-existing organelles as well as contain DNA but lack protein synthesizing machinery.

170. *Assertion :* Replication and transcription occur in the nucleus but translation occurs in the cytoplasm.
Reason : *m*RNA is transferred from the nucleus into the cytoplasm where ribosomes and amino acids are available for protein synthesis.

171. *Assertion :* The fungi are widespread in distribution and they even live on or inside other plants and animals.
Reason : Fungi are able to grow anywhere on land, water or on other organisms because they have a variety of pigments, including chlorophyll, carotenoids, fucooxanthin and phycoerythrin.

172. *Assertion :* C_4 photosynthetic pathway is more efficient than the C_3 pathway.
Reason : Photorespiration is suppressed in C_4 plants.

173. *Assertion :* Human ancestors never used their tails and so the tail expressing gene has disappeared in them.
Reason : Lamarck's theory of evolution is popularly called theory continuity of germ plasm.

174. *Assertion :* Presently, the global atmosphere is warming up.
Reason : The depletion of stratospheric ozone layer has resulted in increase in ultraviolet radiations reaching the earth.

175. *Assertion :* Comparative biochemistry provides a strong evidence in favour of common ancestry of living beings.
Reason : Genetic code is universal.

176. *Assertion :* Darwin's finches show a variety of beaks suited for eating large seeds, flying insects and cactus seeds.
Reason : Ancestral seed-eating stock of Darwin's finches radiated out from South American mainland to different geographical areas of the Galapagos Islands, where they found competitor-free new habitats.

177. *Assertion :* The atmospheric concentration of CO_2 at which photosynthesis just compensates for respiration is referred to as CO_2 compensation point.
Reason : The CO_2 compensation point is reached when the amount of CO_2 uptake is less than that generated through respiration because the level of CO_2 in the atmosphere is more than that required for achieving CO_2 compensation point.

178. *Assertion :* The age-sex structure of human population in countries like France and Germany gives a steep pyramid.
Reason : In countries like Sudan and India the population is increasing at a rapid rate.

179. *Assertion :* The duck-billed *Platypus* and the spiny ant-eater, both are egg-laying animals yet they are grouped under mammals.
Reason : Both of them have seven cervical vertebrae and 12 pairs of cranial nerves.

180. *Assertion : Agrobacterium tumefaciens* is popular in genetic engineering because this bacterium is associated with the roots of all cereal and pulse crops.
Reason : A gene incorporated in the bacterial chromosomal genome gets automatically transferred to the crop with which the bacterium is associated.

GENERAL KNOWLEDGE

181. Metaphysics refers to :
(a) A branch of philosophy concerned with the rational query of reality.
(b) A branch of physics concerned with investigation of reality.
(c) Meta-analysis of physics for the purpose of theory of relativity.
(d) Analysis of human body at atomic level.

182. Who is called as numismatist?
(a) an expert on numerology
(b) a numerator
(c) an expert on mathematics
(d) a person who studies coins.

183. Anjali Bhagwat is related to which field:
(a) Lawn tennis (b) Badminton
(c) Shooting (d) Athletics.

184. Who received Stains International award for religion harmony?
(a) Teesta Setalvad
(b) Kuldeep Nayar
(c) Bharatiya Vidya Bhawan
(d) Pope John Paul.

185. A 'dirty' nuclear bomb means :
(a) it has small amount of cobalt 60
(b) it involves low grade fusion reaction
(c) it involves low grade fission reaction
(d) it involves small Ce-137.

186. National Inland Navigation Institute (NINI) is situated in:
(a) Patna
(b) Kolkata
(c) Goa
(d) Gomukh, Uttaranchal.

187. 'Blogs' means:
(a) On line journals where cyber-diarists unreveal their stories.
(b) Black spots in somebody's life.
(c) Big logs used to cross the river in hills.
(d) Big blocks of land used for grazing animals.

188. What is the colour of Black Box, that is found in aircraft?
(a) Orange (b) Red
(c) Blue (d) Black.

189. Which author was a Bengali writer and an Oscar-winning film director?
(a) Bankimchandra Chatterjee
(b) Satyajit Ray
(c) Chhabi Biswas
(d) Rabindranath Tagore.

190. What is the symbol of Laloo Prasad Yadav's RJD party?
(a) Lantern (b) Tea Leaves
(c) Elephant (d) Palm.

191. Where is the Tibetan government-in-exile based?
(a) Delhi (b) Dharamsala
(c) Phomphenh (d) London.

192. What is true of Leonardo da Vinci's Mona Lisa?
(a) he painted without a model
(b) the model was the wife of a client
(c) he dreampt her in the night
(d) the model was an unmarried women.

193. Which is the annual pilgrimage that every Muslim should make once in the lifetime?
(a) Haj (b) Sharjah
(c) Jihad (d) Zakat.

194. What is the term used in e-mail and online conversations to convey mood along with the words?
(a) smiley (b) pictures
(c) emoticon (d) flames.

195. Whose quote is "I hear and I forget. I see and I remember. I do and I understand"?
(a) Caskie Stinnet (b) Mickey Mantle
(c) Confucious
(d) Arthur Schopenhauer.

196. Whose autobiography is "Sunny Days"?
(a) Sunil Gavaskar (b) Geofrey Boycott
(c) Sunny Deol (d) Sunil Shetty.

197. Which age in Indian history is referred to as the "Golden Age"?
(a) Maurya (b) Gupta
(c) Mughal (d) Ancient.

198. Which novel of Amitav Ghosh is called *Esteremi Orienti* in its Italian version?
(a) In An Antique Land
(b) Dancing in Cambodia
(c) The Circle of Reason
(d) The Shadow Lines.

199. Which of the following is President A.P.J. Abdul Kalam's autobiography?
(a) Wings of Fire (b) Crossroads
(c) Ignited Minds: Unleashing the Power Within India
(d) My experiment with truth.

200. Which of the following units of measurement is not named after a person?
(a) Hertz (b) Curie
(c) Barleycorn (d) Apgar.

SOLUTIONS

PHYSICS

1. (a) : The critical frequency of a sky wave for reflection from a layer of atmosphere is given by

$$f_c = 9\,(N_{max})^{1/2}$$

where N is the density of electron/m^3.

$$10 \times 10^6 = 9\,(N_{max})^{1/2}$$

$$N_{max} = \left(\frac{10\times10^6}{9}\right)^2 \simeq 1.2\times10^{12}\ \text{m}^{-3}.$$

2. (d) : NAND and NOR gate are used as universal gate.

3. (b) : Core of acceptance angle $\theta = \sin^{-1}\sqrt{n_1^2 - n_2^2}$.

4. (b) : As a constant magnetic field conducting ring oscillates with a frequency of 100 Hz.

i.e. $T = \frac{1}{100}$ s, for $\frac{T}{2}$, it goes up to B

$\therefore$ The corresponding frequency is 200 Hz.

Induced emf $= \frac{\text{change in flux}}{\text{time}}$

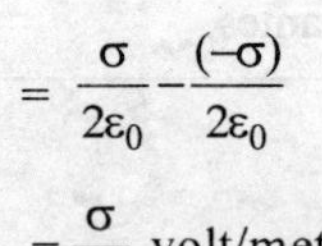

$= \frac{2BA\cos\theta}{T} = 2BA\,f\cos\theta$

$= \pi r^2 \times 2 \times 0.01 \times 200$ as $r = 1$ m

$= \pi r^2 \times 2 \times 0.01 \times 200 = 4\pi$ V.

Non-electrostatic induced electric field along the circle,

$$E = \frac{1}{2\pi r}\times\left(\pi r^2 \times \frac{dB}{dt}\right) = \frac{e}{2\pi r} = \frac{4\pi}{2\pi r} = 2\ \text{V/m}.$$

5. (b) : Current gain $= \frac{\Delta I_C}{\Delta I_B}$

$\therefore\quad \Delta I_B = \frac{1\ \text{mA}}{100} = 10^{-2}$ mA.

As $\Delta I_E = \Delta I_B + \Delta I_C = (0.01 + 1)$ mA $= 1.01$ mA.

6. (a) : From the formula for convex lens,

$$\frac{1}{v} - \frac{1}{u} = \frac{1}{f}$$

$$\therefore\quad v = \frac{f\times u}{u-f} = \frac{200\times200\times10^3}{[200\times10^3 - 200]} = \frac{200\times10^3}{999}.$$

Also, magnification,

$$m = \left|\frac{v}{u}\right| = \left|\frac{I}{O}\right|$$

$$= \frac{200\times10^3}{999\times200\times10^3} = \frac{I}{50\times100}$$

$$I = \frac{5000}{999} \simeq 5\ \text{cm}.$$

7. (b) : Total energy = kinetic energy + potential energy

Potential energy = 2 total energy

$= -2 \times 13.6 = -27.2$ eV.

8. (b) : According to Moseley's law

$$(Z-\sigma) \propto \sqrt{f} \quad\text{or,}\quad f \propto (Z-\sigma)^2.$$

Note : The correct answer should have been $f \propto (Z-\sigma)^2$ where σ is the screening constant. Many authors use at this level, $\sigma = 1$ approximately.

9. (c) : Electric field between the plates is

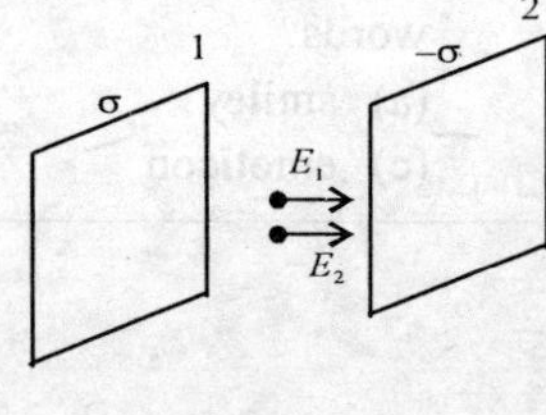

$$= \frac{\sigma}{2\varepsilon_0} - \frac{(-\sigma)}{2\varepsilon_0}$$

$$= \frac{\sigma}{\varepsilon_0}\ \text{volt/meter}.$$

10. (a) : $\mu_e > \mu_n$ because electron is lighter than hole.

11. (a) : $\vec{L} = n\cdot\frac{h}{2\pi}$,

$$\mu_n = \frac{e}{2m}\cdot n\frac{h}{2\pi}\quad\text{i.e. } \mu \propto n.$$

12. (c) : $T_{1/2} = 10$ days, $T = 30$ days

$$T = n \times T_{1/2}.\quad n = \frac{T}{T_{1/2}} = \frac{30}{10} = 3$$

$$\frac{N}{N_0} = \left(\frac{1}{2}\right)^n = \left(\frac{1}{2}\right)^3 = \frac{1}{8} = 0.125.$$

13. (a) : Hubble's law is a statement of a direct correlation between the distance (r) to a galaxy and its recessional velocity as determined by the red shift (Z). It is stated as $Z = H_0 r$,
where Z = recessional velocity
H_0 = Hubble constant and r = distance.

14. (a) : The colour in the oil film is formed due to interference of sunlight where the colour of the film will depend upon the thickness and the angle of inclination.

15. (b) : Parsec (pc) is an astronomical unit of length equal to the distance at which a baseline of one astronomical unit subtends an angle of one second of arc.
1 parsec = 3.085677×10^{16} m = 3.26 light years.

16. (b) : This is an example of operational amplifier in this voltage gain.

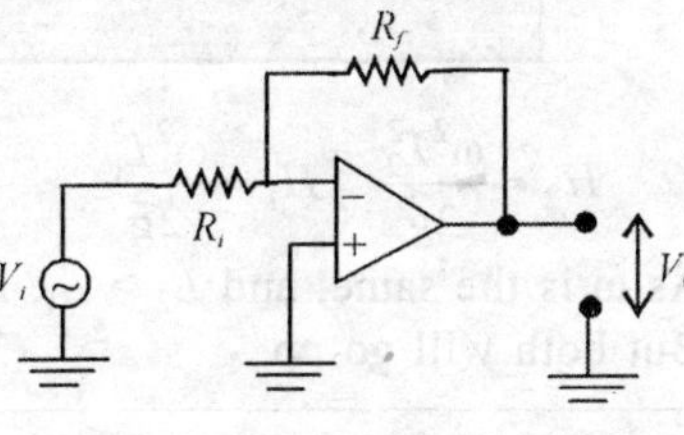

$$A = \frac{V_0}{V_i} = \frac{R_f}{R_i}$$

$$= \frac{100\ \text{k}\Omega}{1\ \text{k}\Omega} = 100.$$

17. (b) : $\upsilon = 50$ Hz, $V = 20$ V, $V_R = 12$ V

In case of RC circuit, $V = \sqrt{V_R^2 + V_C^2}$

$\Rightarrow (20)^2 = (12)^2 + (V_C)^2$

$\Rightarrow (V_C)^2 = 400 - 144 = 256 \quad \Rightarrow \quad V_C = 16$ V.

18. (a) : Impulse = change in momentum

$$= m\Delta V = \frac{m\Delta x}{\Delta t} = 0.1 \times \frac{4-0}{2-0} = 0.2\ \text{kgmsec}^{-1}.$$

19. (c) : Pressure = Force/area

$$I = \frac{\text{Energy}}{\text{area-time}} = \frac{F \cdot S}{At} = \frac{Fc}{A}. \quad I/c = P.$$

20. (a) : According to work energy theorem,

$$W = \Delta\text{K.E.} \quad \Rightarrow \quad W = \frac{1}{2}mv_2^2 - \frac{1}{2}mv_1^2$$

$$\Rightarrow F \cdot dx = \text{K.E.}_F - \frac{1}{2} \times 10 \times 100$$

$$\Rightarrow F \cdot dx = \text{K.E.}_F - 500$$

$$\Rightarrow \int_{20}^{30} -0.1x\, dx = \text{K.E.}_F - 500$$

$$\Rightarrow -0.1\left[\frac{x^2}{2}\right]_{20}^{30} = \text{K.E.}_F - 500$$

$$\Rightarrow -0.1\left[\frac{900-400}{2}\right] = \text{K.E.}_F - 500$$

$\Rightarrow$ K.E.$_F$ = 500 − 25 = 475 J.

21. (a)

22. (c) : The criterion for a star to be black hole is

$$\frac{GM}{c^2 R} \geq \frac{1}{2} \quad \text{or,} \quad \sqrt{\frac{2GM}{R}} \geq c.$$

23. (a) : Amorphous solids are the solids in which atoms are arranged in a completely irregular manner. They are also known as glassy solids.

24. (b) : Bulk modulus $\propto \dfrac{1}{\Delta V/V}$

25. (a) : $y = \sin\omega t - \cos\omega t$

$$\frac{dy}{dt} = \omega\cos\omega t + \omega\sin\omega t$$

$$\frac{dy}{dt} = -\omega^2\sin\omega t + \omega^2\cos\omega t$$

$$= -\omega^2(\sin\omega t - \cos\omega t).$$

$a = -\omega^2 y. \quad \therefore \quad a \propto -y.$

which is the condition of simple harmonic motion.

26. (b) : The magnitude of electric field vector varies periodically with time because it is the form of electromagnetic wave.

27. (a)

28. (c) : As the voltage in R_2 and R_3 is same therefore, according to,

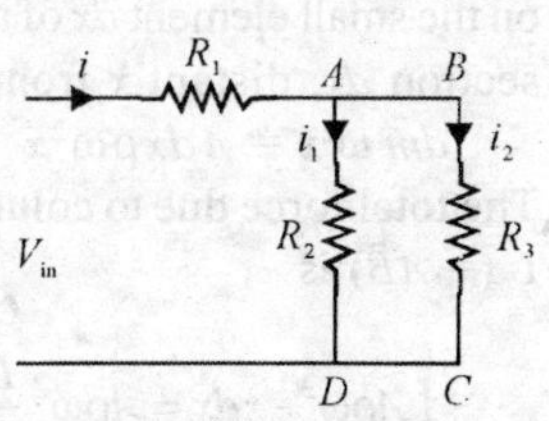

$$H = \frac{V^2}{R} \cdot t, \quad R_2 = R_3$$

Also the energy in all resistance is same.

$\therefore \quad i^2 R_1 t = i_1^2 R_2 t$

Using $i_1 = \frac{R_3}{R_2+R_3}i = \frac{R_3}{R_3+R_3}i = \frac{1}{2}i$

Thus $i^2 R_1 t = \frac{i^2}{4}R_2 t$ or, $R_1 = \frac{R_2}{4}$.

29. (b) : $\frac{n_2}{n_1} = \frac{\text{real depth}}{\text{apparent depth}}$ or, $\frac{n_2}{n_1} = \frac{h}{x}$

Differentiating with respect to time,

$$\frac{n_2}{n_1} = \frac{dh/dt}{dx/dt}$$

Change in real depth $= \frac{n_2}{n_1} \times$ change in apparent depth

$\frac{dh}{dt} = \frac{n_2}{n_1}x$ cm/min.

The amount of water drained in c.c. per minute

$= \frac{dh}{dt} \times \pi R^2 = x\,\pi R^2 \frac{n_2}{n_1}$.

30. (b) : Initial weight of the candle = weight of liquid displaced

$\rho_C V_C g = \rho_L$ (volume displaced) g

$\Rightarrow \rho_C \pi \left(\frac{d}{2}\right)^2 2L = \rho_L \pi \frac{d^2}{2} Lg \Rightarrow \frac{\rho_C}{\rho_L} = \frac{1}{2}$ ... (i)

When 2 cm has been burnt, total length $= 2L - 2$

But $\rho_C(2L-2) = \rho_L(L-x)$

$\rho_C 2(L-1) = 2\rho_C(L-x)$ [Using eqn. (i)]

$\therefore$ $x = 1$ cm.

Outside also it has decreased 1 cm as the total decrease is 2 cm. The level of the candle comes down at half the rate of burning.

31. (a) : Due to rotation about the axis OO', a force is acting on the liquid column AB outwards, pushing up the liquid column on the right. This centrifugal force acting on the small element dx of area of cross-section dx, distant x from the axis is

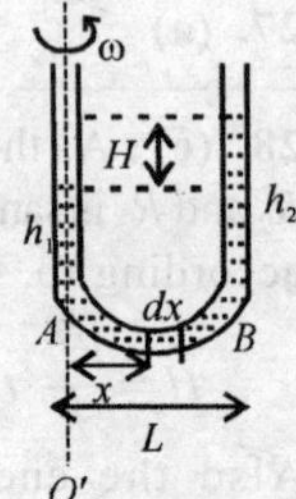

$dm\,\omega^2 x = A\,dx\,\rho\omega^2 x$

The total force due to column of length L (= AB) is

$$\int_0^L A\rho\omega^2 \cdot x\,dx = A\rho\omega^2 \frac{L^2}{2}$$

Pressure at B = atmospheric pressure + $h_1\rho g + \frac{A\rho\omega^2}{A}\frac{L^2}{2}$

Pressure at B due to liquid column on the right hand side = atmospheric pressure + $h_2\rho g$

Net pressure due to the left hand side = pressure at B due to liquid column

atm. pressure $+ h_1\rho g + \rho\omega^2 \frac{L^2}{2}$ = atm. pressure $+ h_2\rho g$

$\therefore$ $h_2 - h_1 = H_0 = \frac{\omega^2 L^2}{2g}$.

Here one has

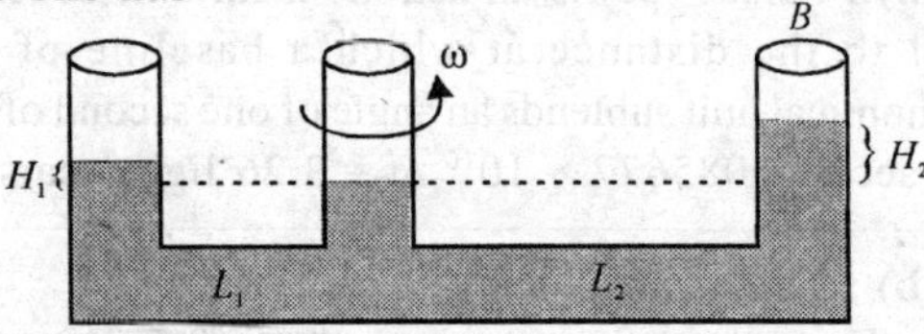

$H_2 = \frac{\omega^2 L_2^2}{2g}$, $H_1 = \frac{\omega^2 L_1^2}{2g}$

As ω is the same, and $L_2 > L_1$, $H_2 > H_1$.

But both will go up.

32. (a) : As $v^2 = u^2 + 2as$

$\therefore$ $u^2 \propto s$ ... (i)

For given condition, $u'^2 \propto 3s$ ... (ii)

From eqn. (i) and (ii),

$\frac{u'^2}{u^2} = 3 \Rightarrow u' = \sqrt{3}v_0$.

33. (a) : From conservation of energy

Potential energy = translational kinetic energy + rotational kinetic energy

$$mgh = \frac{1}{2}mv^2 + \frac{1}{2}\left(\frac{2}{5}\right)mR^2 \cdot \frac{v^2}{R^2}$$

$$\Rightarrow \frac{7}{10}mv^2 = mgh \Rightarrow v \geq \sqrt{\frac{10}{7}gh}.$$

34. (b) : According to law of conservation of momentum,

$I\omega$ = constant.

When viscous fluid of mass m is dropped and start spreading out then its moment of inertia increases and angular velocity decreases. But when it start falling then its moment of inertia again starts decreasing and angular velocity increases.

35. (c) :

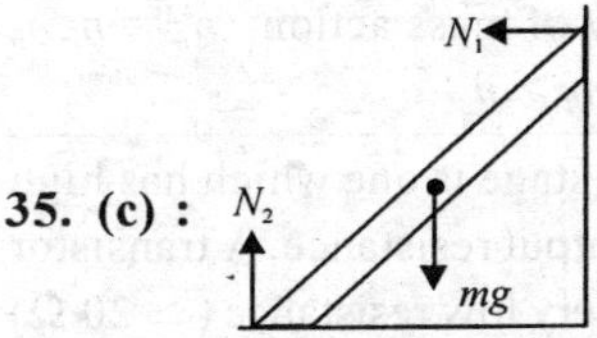

36. (b) : When elevator moves downward with constant acceleration, $a = g$. Then person standing in an elevator find himself weightless.
(g' with respect to the lift is $(g - a)$).

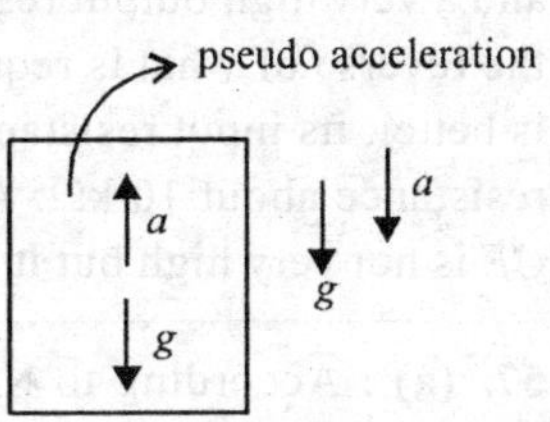

37. (a) : As the north pole approaches, a north pole is developed at that face *i.e.* the current flows anticlockwise. Finally when it completes the oscillation, when it is ready, no emf is present. Now south pole approaches the other side R.H.S. the current flows clockwise to repel the south pole. This means the current is anticlockwise at the L.H.S. as before. This is possible in (a). The breaks show when the pendulum is at the extreme and momentarily stationary.

38. (c) : $|Q_B| > |Q_A|$ (given). Inside the shell B, the potential is a constant and negative.
But V_A inside r_A is positive and greater than that of B because $r_A < r_B$. Upto r_B, one as hence positive potential. Beyond r_A, $V_A \propto (1/r)$, this is $> V_B$, one gets the course $\propto 1/r$. At B, the negative potential is more therefore the potential line is still negative. (c) explains all these factors.
Note : ***However the question asked is the field and the diagrams given are for the potential. This is an error.***

39. (b) : Resistance $= \dfrac{\text{potential difference}}{\text{current}}$

$$= \frac{ML^2T^{-3}A^{-1}}{A} = ML^2T^{-3}A^{-2}.$$

40. (a) : The negative charge oscillates, the resultant force acts as a restoring force and is cosθ component, proportional to displacement. When it reaches the plane XY, the resultant force is zero and the mass moves down due to inertia. Thus oscillation is set.

[This problem is similar to Q^+ —— q —— Q^+]

41. (a) : Specific gravity is former name of relative density and relative density is the density of a substance divided by the density of water.
∴ Specific gravity = relative density

$$= \frac{\text{density of substance}}{\text{density of water}} = \text{dimensionless.}$$

42. (d) : Frictional work is not completely recoverable. When the force of friction is the total mechanical energy is not conserved. The friction force is therefore called a nonconservative or a dissipative force.

43. (c) : When glass surface is made rough then the light falling on it is scattered in different direction due to which its transparency decreases.

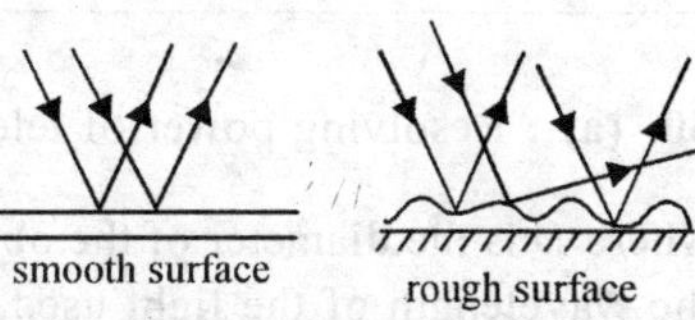

44. (b) : In optical communication, a semiconductor bases laser (diode laser) is used to generate analog signals or digital pulses for transmission through optical fibres. The advantages of diode lasers are their small size and low power input.

45. (b) : Diamond glitters brilliantly because light enters in diamond suffers total internal reflection. All the light entering in it comes out of diamond after number of reflections and no light is absorb by it.

46. (a) : Momentum of a platform is given by
$p = h/\lambda$ (by de Broglie hypothesis) ... (i)
Also the photon is a form of energy packet behave as a particle and having energy
$E = hc/\lambda$ ... (ii)
From (i) and (ii), $p = \dfrac{E}{c}$ or, $\dfrac{h\upsilon}{c}$.

47. (c) : The clouds consists of dust particles and water droplets. Their size is very large as compared to the wavelength of the incident light from the sun. So there is very little scattering of light. Hence the light which we receive through the clouds has all the colours of light. As a result of this, we receive almost white light. Therefore, the cloud are generally white.

48. (d) : In sky wave propagation, the radio waves having frequency range 2 MHz to 30 MHz are reflected back by the ionosphere. Radio waves having frequency

nearly greater than 30 MHz penetrates the ionosphere and is not reflected back by the ionosphere. The TV signal having frequency greater than 30 MHz therefore cannot be propagated through sky wave propagation. In case of sky wave propagation, critical frequency is defined as the highest frequency that is returned to the earth by the considered layer of the ionosphere after having sent straight to it. Above this frequency, a wave will penetrate the ionosphere and is not reflected by it.

49. (d) : In diode the output is in same phase with the input therefore it cannot be used to built NOT gate.

50. (a) : Resolving power of telescope $= \frac{D}{1.22\lambda}$

where D is the diameter of the objective lens and λ is the wavelength of the light used.
With increase in D, resolving power of telescope increases. A telescope will have large light gathering power if the diameter of the objective lens is large. Hence a bright image will be formed by the telescope.

51. (a) : In a perfectly reversible system, there is no loss of energy. Losses can be minimised, friction can be reduced, the resistance in L-C oscillating system can also be negligible. But one cannot completely eliminate energy losses. This makes a perfectly reversible system, an ideal.

52. (a) : When external torque acting on the system is zero then only the total angular momentum of system is considered to be conserved.
If $\vec{L} = I\omega = \text{constant}$, $\tau = I\alpha = 0$.

$$\because \alpha = \frac{d\omega}{dt} = 0 \text{ for constant } \omega.$$

53. (a) : Adiabatic expansion produces cooling.

54. (c) : The process of nuclear fusion can be explained with the help of concept of binding energy per nucleon of very light nuclei and the intermediate nuclei. Binding energy per nucleon of very light nuclei is less than that of intermediate nuclei. It means light nuclei are less stable than that of intermediate nuclei. As ^{35}Cl has a large binding energy therefore it cannot be used as fuel for fusion energy.

55. (a) : According to law of mass action, $n_i^2 = n_e n_h$
In p-type semiconductor $n_h > n_e$

56. (c) : A good amplifier stage is one which has high input resistance and low output resistance. A transistor in CB configuration has a very low resistance ($\simeq 20\ \Omega$) and a very high output resistance ($\simeq 1\ M\Omega$). It is just the reverse of what is required. The CE configuration is better, its input resistance is about 1 kΩ and output resistance about 10 kΩ. Although input resistance of CE is not very high but it still prefers better amplifier.

57. (a) : According to Kirchhoff's law, $a = e$.
or the absorptivity of a body equals its emissivity. A good absorber is a good emitter. As a good absorber is poor reflector, emitting (or radiating) ability of body is oppositely related to its ability to reflect. Therefore good emitter (or radiator) is a poor reflector.

58. (a) : The negative slope is because of change of

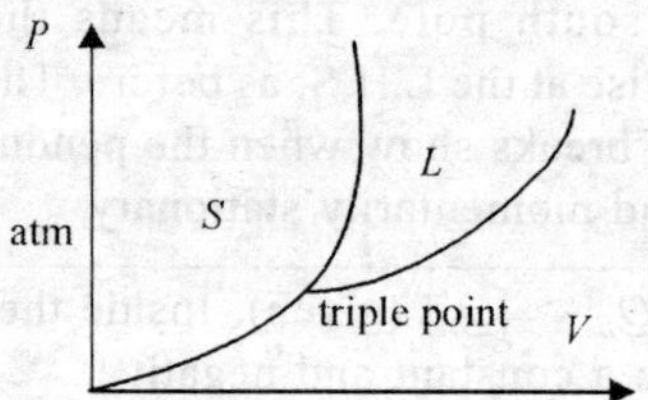

phase. This happens to liquids which contract on melting.

59. (b) : Wien's relation gives λ at maximum intensity, $\lambda_m \cdot T = \text{constant}$.

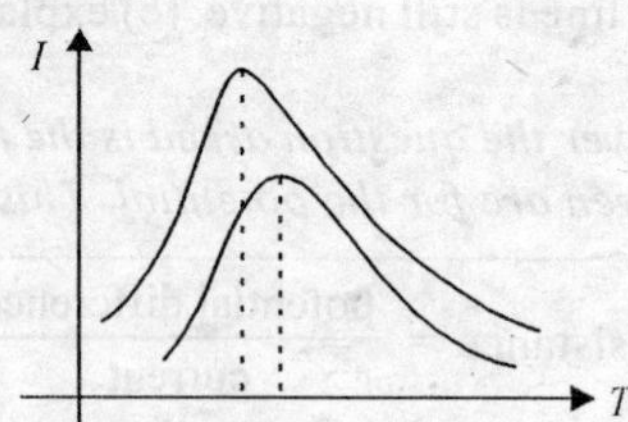

Stefan's law,
σT^4 = intensity of emission of a particular wavelength does not explains the shift of λ_m with absolute temperature.

60. (a) : Reynold's number represents the ratio of the inertial force is refer as inertia (mass of moving fluid) per unit area to the viscous force per unit area. When $R_e > 2000$, the flow is often turbulent in that case internal force dominate viscous force.

CHEMISTRY

61. (d) : XeO_3 :

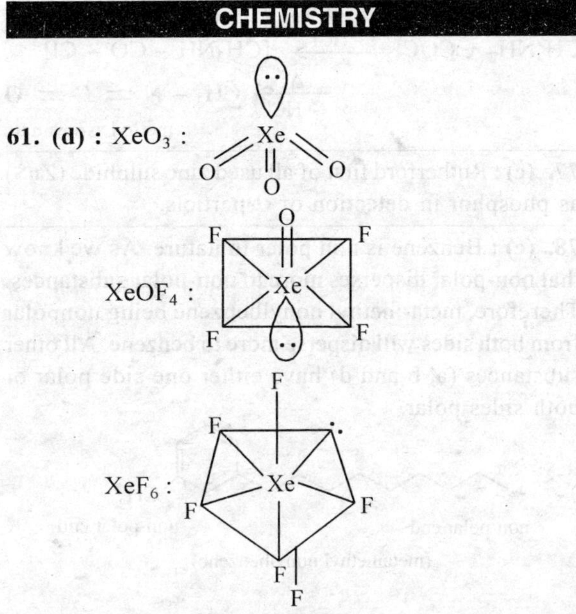

62. (c) : $CoCl_2$ is a weak Lewis acid, reacting with chloride ion to produce salt containing the tetrahedral $[CoCl_4]^{2-}$ ion. $CoCl_2$ is blue when anhydrous, and a deep magneta colour when hydrated, for this reason it is widely used as an indicator for water.

63. (b) : $[Co(en)_3]Cl_3$

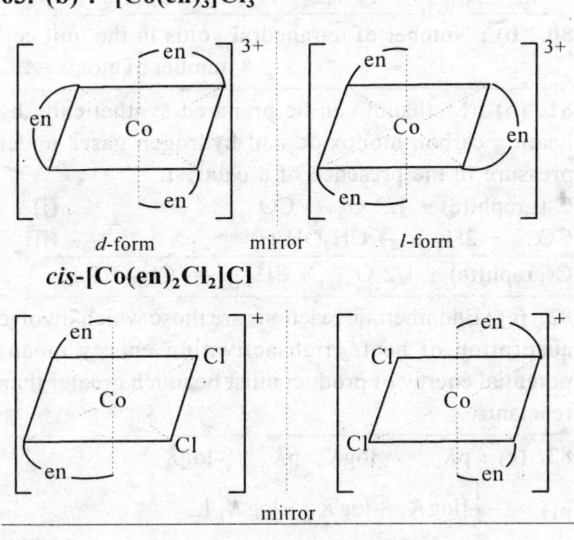

64. (a) :

$[Ni(CN)_4]^{2-}$ ⥮ ⥮ ⥮ ⥮ ×× | ×× | ×× ××

diamagnetic

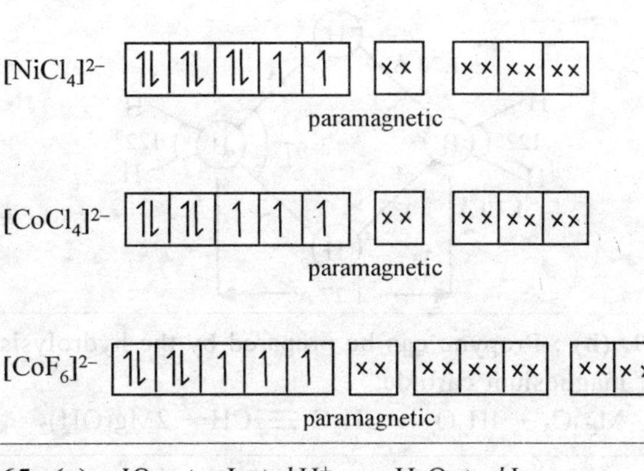

65. (a) : $IO_3^- + aI^- + bH^+ \rightarrow cH_2O + dI_2$

Step 1 : $I^- \rightarrow I_2$ (oxidation)

$IO_3^- \rightarrow I_2$ (reduction)

Step 2 : $2IO_3^- + 12H^+ \rightarrow I_2 + 6H_2O$

Step 3 : $2IO_3^- + 12H^+ + 10e \rightarrow I_2 + 6H_2O$

$2I^- \rightarrow I_2 + 2e$

Step 4 : $2IO_3^- + 12H^+ + 10e^- \rightarrow I_2 + 6H_2O$

$[2I^- \rightarrow I_2 + 2e]5$

Step 5 : $2IO_3^- + 10I^- + 12H^+ \rightarrow 6I_2 + 6H_2O$

$IO_3^- + 5I^- + 6H^+ \rightarrow 3I_2 + 3H_2O$

On comparing, $a = 5$, $b = 6$, $c = 3$, $d = 3$.

66. (a) : Tl^+ ions are more stable than Tl^{3+} and thus, Tl^{3+} ions change to Tl^+ ions thereby acting as oxidising agents.

Tl^{3+} compounds + $2e \rightarrow Tl^+$ compounds
(less stable oxidising agent) (more stable reducing agent)

67. (a) :

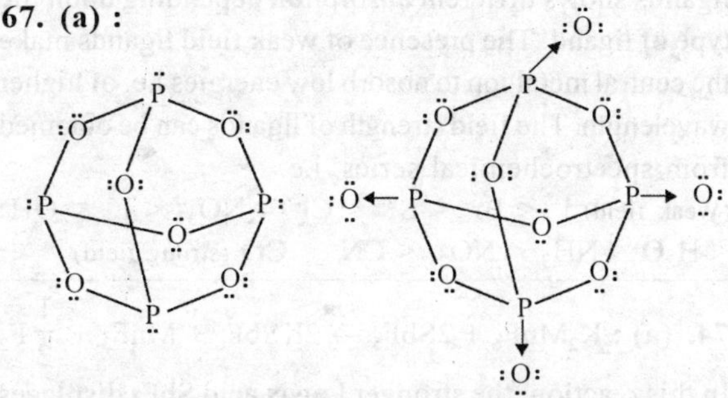

68. (b) : Dilthey in 1921 proposed a bridge structure for diborane. Four hydrogen atoms, two on the left and two on the right, known as terminal hydrogens and two boron atoms lie in the same plane. Two hydrogen atoms forming bridges, one above and other below, lie in a plane perpendicular to the rest of molecule.

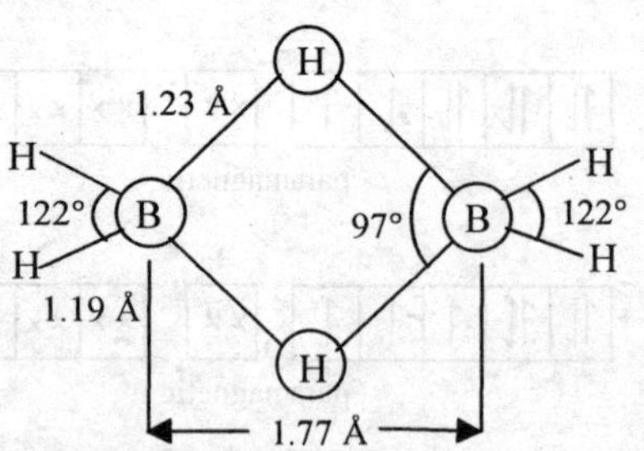

69. (b) : Propyne can be prepared by the hydrolysis of magnesium carbide.

$Mg_2C_3 + 4H_2O \rightarrow CH_3C \equiv CH + 2Mg(OH)_2$

70. (d) : Both $Be(OH)_2$ and $Zn(OH)_2$ are amphoteric in nature.

71. (b) : Pyrolusite = MnO_2

Malachite - $CuCO_3{\cdot}Cu(OH)_2$

Diaspore - $Al_2O_3{\cdot}H_2O$

Cassiterite - SnO_2

72. (c) : ${}_{92}U^{238} \xrightarrow[-6\beta]{-8\alpha} {}_{82}X^{206}$

Number of protons = 82

Number of neutrons = 124

Neutron/proton ratio in the product nucleus = $\frac{124}{82} = \frac{62}{41}$.

73. (a) : The absorption of energy or the observation of colour in a complex transition compound depends on the charge of the metal ion and the nature of the ligands attached. The same metal ion with different ligands shows different absorption depending upon the type of ligand. The presence of weak field ligands make the central metal ion to absorb low energies i.e. of higher wavelength. The field strength of ligands can be obtained from spectrochemical series. i.e.

(Weak field) $I^- < Br^- < S^{2-} < Cl^- < NO_3^- < F^- < OH^- < H_2O < NH_3 < NO_2^- < CN^- < CO$ (strong field)

74. (a) : $K_2MnF_6 + 2SbF_5 \rightarrow 2KSbF_6 + MnF_3 + \frac{1}{2}F_2$

In this reaction, the stronger Lewis acid SbF_5 displaces the weaker one, MnF_4 from its salt. MnF_4 is unstable and readily decomposes to give MnF_3 and fluorine.

75. (d) : Number of electrons in ClO_2^-

= 7 + 6 + 6 + 1 = 20

Number of electrons in ClF_2^+ = 7 + 7 + 7 − 1 = 20.

76. (c) : Methyl isocyanate is industrially prepared by the action of methyl amine with phosgene.

$CH_3NH_2 + COCl_2 \xrightarrow{-HCl} [CH_3NH - CO - Cl]$

$\xrightarrow[-HCl]{\Delta} CH_3 - N = C = O$

methyl isocyanate

77. (c) : Rutherford first of all used zinc sulphide (ZnS) as phosphor in detection of α-particls.

78. (c) : Benzene is non polar in nature. As we know that non-polar disperses more to non-polar substances. Therefore, meta-methyl nonylbenzene being nonpolar from both sides will disperse more to benzene. All other substances (a, b and d) have either one side polar or both sides polar.

CH_3

non-polar end   non-polar end

(metamethyl nonylbenzene)

$\equiv \quad H_{19}C_9 - C_6H_4 - CH_3$

79. (b) : $2AgCl_{(s)} + H_{2\,(g)} \rightarrow 2HCl_{(aq)} + 2Ag_{(s)}$

The activities of solids and liquids are taken as unity and at low concentrations, the activity of a solute is approximated to its molarity.

The cell reaction will be

$Pt_{(s)} | H_{2\,(g)}$, 1 bar $| H^+_{(aq)}$ 1 M $| AgCl_{(aq)}$ 1 M $| Ag_{(s)}$

80. (b) : Number of tetrahedral voids in the unit cell = 2 × number of atoms = 2Z.

81. (b) : Methanol can be prepared synthetically by heating carbon monoxide and hydrogen gases under pressure in the presence of a catalyst.

C (graphite) + 1/2 $O_2 \rightarrow CO_{(g)}$ ... (i)

$CO_{(g)} + 2H_{2\,(g)} \rightarrow CH_3OH\ (l)$ ... (ii)

C(graphite) + 1/2 $O_{2\,(g)} + 2H_{2\,(g)} \rightarrow CH_3OH_{(l)}$

82. (c) : Endothermic reactions are those which involve absorption of heat. High activation energy means potential energy of product must be much greater than reactants.

83. (c) : $pK_a = -\log K_a$, $pK_b = -\log K_b$

$$pH = -\frac{1}{2}[\log K_a + \log K_w - \log K_b]$$

$$= -\frac{1}{2}[-5 + \log(1\times10^{-14}) - (-5)]$$

$$= -\frac{1}{2}[-5 - 14 + 5] = -\frac{1}{2}(-14) = 7.$$

84. (c) : Most probable radius = a_0/Z
where a_0 = 52.9 pm. For helium ion, Z = 2.

$$r_{mp} = \frac{52.9}{2} = 26.45 \text{ pm}.$$

85. (a) : Bomb calorimeter is commonly used to find the heat of combustion of organic substances which consists of a sealed combustion chamber, called a bomb. If a process is run in a sealed container then no expansion or compression is allowed, so $w = 0$ and $\Delta U = q$.
$\Delta U < 0$, $w = 0$.

86. (b) : $aA \rightarrow xP$
Rate of reaction = $[A]^a$
Order of reaction = a.
$[A]_1 = 2.2$ mM, $r_1 = 2.4$ m M s^{-1} ... (i)
$[A]_2 = \frac{2.2}{2}$ mM, $r_2 = 0.6$ mM s^{-1} or, $\frac{2.4}{4}$ ... (ii)
On reducing the concentration of A to half, the rate of reaction is decreased by four times.
Rate of reaction = $[A]^2$
Order of reaction = 2.

87. (d) : $2NOCl_{(g)} = 2NO_{(g)} + Cl_{2(g)}$
$K_p = K_C (RT)^{\Delta n}$
$K_p = 3 \times 10^{-6} (0.0821 \times 700) = 172.41 \times 10^{-6}$
$= 1.72 \times 10^{-4}$.

88. (a) : For the reaction,
$CaCO_{3(s)} \rightleftharpoons CaO_{(s)} + CO_{2(g)}$
$K_p = p_{CO_2}$ and $K_C = [CO_2]$
($\because$ $[CaCO_3] = 1$ and $[CaO] = 1$ for solids)
According to Arrhenius equation we have
$K = Ae^{-\Delta H^\circ_r/RT}$
Taking logarithm, we have

$$\log K_p = \log A - \frac{\Delta H^\circ_r}{RT(2.303)}$$

This is an equation of straight line. When $\log K_p$ is plotted against $1/T$. we get a straight line.
The intercept of this line = $\log A$, slope = $-\Delta H^\circ_r/2.303R$
Knowing the value of slope from the plot and universal gas constant R, ΔH_r° can be calculated.
(Equation of straight line : $Y = mx + C$. Here,

$$\underset{Y}{\log K_p} = \underset{m}{-\frac{\Delta H^\circ_r}{2.303R}}\underset{x}{\left(\frac{1}{T}\right)} + \underset{C}{\log A}\,)$$

89. (a) : Nucleophiles are those substances which can donate a pair of electrons. These can be neutral or negative. The nucleophilic power depends on the tendency of species to donate electrons. This is more, when an electron pushing group (+I group) is present. Among the alkyl groups, those have higher number of C-atoms will push more, hence ethyl > methyl.

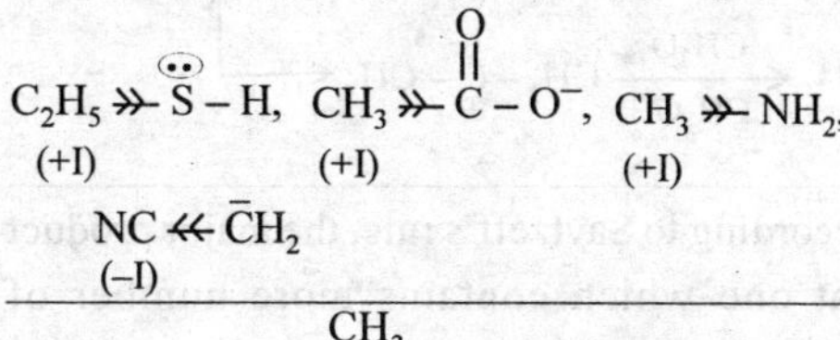

$C_2H_5 \ggg \ddot{S}-H$ (+I), $CH_3 \ggg C(=O)-O^-$ (+I), $CH_3 \ggg NH_2$ (+I),
$NC \lll \bar{C}H_2$ (–I)

90. (d) : $H_3C-C(CH_3)(H)-CH_2-Br \xrightarrow[CH_3OH]{CH_3O^-} A$?

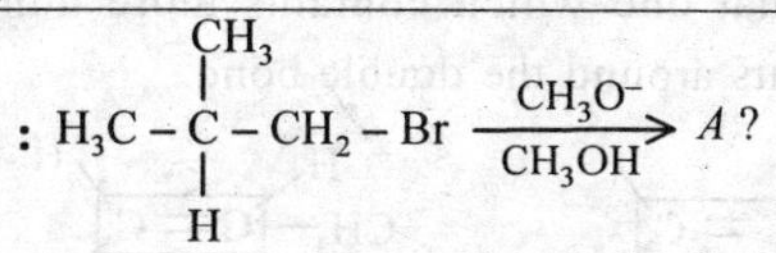

Alkyl halide is 1°.
Keep in mind 1° halide give product by S_N2/E-2 mechanism and 1° halide always gives substitution reaction except when strongly hindered base is used.

ex.: With $CH_3-C(CH_3)_2-O^{\ominus}$ it gives mainly elimination.

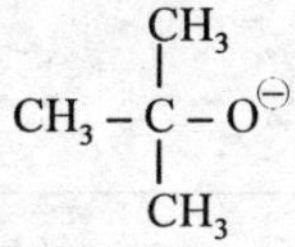

The reaction involves carbocation intermediate.

i.e. $CH_3-C(CH_3)(H)-\overset{\oplus}{C}H_2$
(primary carbocation)

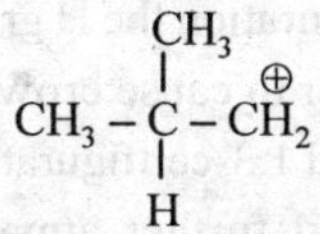

but as it is a primary carbocation it will rearrange to give a tertiary carbocation, which completes the reaction

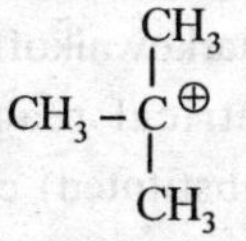

$CH_3-\overset{\oplus}{C}(CH_3)-CH_3$
(tertiary carbocation)

Stability of carbocation : 3° > 2° > 1° > $\overset{\oplus}{C}H_3$
It is because the stability of a charged system is increased by dispersal of the charge. The more stable the carbocation, the faster it is formed.
N.B. - Rearrangement can be done in two ways.

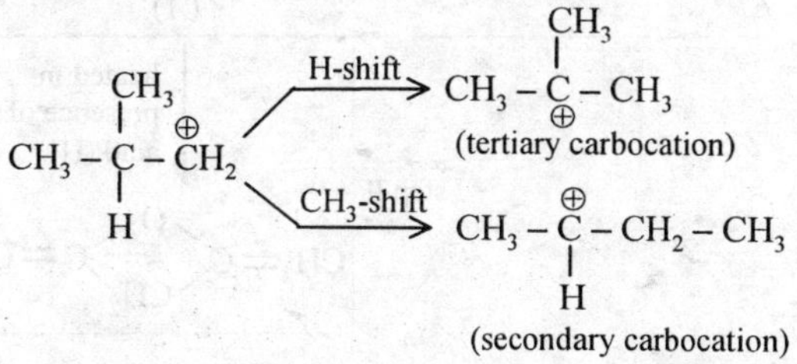

$CH_3-C(CH_3)(H)-\overset{\oplus}{C}H_2 \xrightarrow{\text{H-shift}} CH_3-\overset{\oplus}{C}(CH_3)-CH_3$ (tertiary carbocation)

$CH_3-C(CH_3)(H)-\overset{\oplus}{C}H_2 \xrightarrow{CH_3\text{-shift}} CH_3-\overset{\oplus}{C}(H)-CH_2-CH_3$ (secondary carbocation)

Therefore,

$$CH_3-\overset{CH_3}{\underset{H}{C}}-CH_2-Br = CH_3-\overset{CH_3}{\underset{H}{C}}-\overset{\oplus}{C}H_2+Br^-$$

$$CH_3-\overset{CH_3}{\underset{OCH_3}{C}}-CH_3 \xleftarrow[CH_3OH]{CH_3O^-} CH_3-\overset{CH_3}{\underset{\oplus}{C}}-CH_3$$

91. (b) : According to Saytzeff's rule, the major product will be that one which contains more number of substituents around the double bond.

>C=C<

CH_3-(H)C=C(H)$-CH_3$ 2-substituents (major)

(H)(H)C=C(H)(H) with CH_3CH_2 — one substituent (minor)

92. (d) : *Trans* configuration is more stable than *cis* configuration because in *cis*-configuration the H groups are thrown closely enough together to cause crowding or repulsion. Again between 1,2-and 1,3-configurations, in 1-3, the OH groups are placed further appart to minimise the repulsion. Hence, more stable is 1,3-configuration.

93. (b) : According to Markownikoff's rule, the negative part of the unsymmetrical reagent adds to less hydrogenated (more substituted) carbon atom of the double bond.

$$C_6H_5CH=CH-CH_3+HBr \rightarrow C_6H_5\overset{Br}{C}HCH_2CH_3$$

94. (c) : ***Claisen condensation***

step I $CH_3CO_2C_2H_5 \xrightarrow[C_2H_5OH]{NaOC_2H_5} CH_3COCH_2COOC_2H_5$ (*A*)

step II — heated in presence of acid (H^+) → $CH_2=C\langle{}^{O}_{CH_2}\rangle C=O$

Step II :

$$CH_3-\overset{O}{\overset{\|}{C}}-\underset{H}{\overset{H}{C}}-\overset{O}{\overset{\|}{C}}-OC_2H_5 \xrightarrow[heat]{H^+} CH_3-\overset{O}{\overset{\|}{C}}-\overset{H}{C}=\overset{O}{\overset{\|}{C}}$$

$$\rightarrow CH_2=C\langle{}^{O}_{CH_2}\rangle C=O$$

$$\overset{\ominus}{C}H_2-\overset{O^{\ominus}}{\overset{\|}{C}}-CH=\overset{O}{\overset{\|}{C^+}} \;(H) \equiv CH_2=C\langle{}^{O}_{CH_2}\rangle C=O$$

95. (d) : (i) $R\overset{O}{\overset{\|}{C}}NH_2+Br_2+KOH \longrightarrow RCONHBr + KBr + H_2O$

(ii) $RCONHBr+KOH \rightarrow RNCO+KBr+H_2O$

(iii) $RNCO+2KOH \rightarrow RNH_2+K_2CO_3$

$RCONH_2+Br_2+4KOH \rightarrow RNH_2+2KBr + K_2CO_3+2H_2O$

96. (d) : Basicity of amines is due to availability of an unshared pair (lone pair) of electrons on nitrogen. This lone pair of electrons is available for the formation of a new bond with a proton or Lewis acid.

Pyridine is less basic than triethylamine because lone pair of nitrogen in pyridine is delocalised.

97. (a) : α-Keratin is a water insoluble fibrous protein, serves as the major constituent of hair, nails and skin.

98. (a) :

	CH_3	
H	—	OH
CH_3	—	OH
	H	

Following the procedure outlined under 'Golden Rule' the absolute configuration is 1S, 2S.

99. (b) : Genetic code shows degeneracy i.e. occurrence of more than 1 codon per amino acid. All the amino acid except methionine and tryptophan are coded by more than 1 codon.

For example, valine is specified by GUU, GUC, GUA, GUG.

This shows that first two bases are common in all the four codons coding for valine. But the third base can be changed.

100. (d) : $C_6H_5CONHCH_3 \xrightarrow[HCl]{Zn-Hg} C_6H_5CH_2NHCH_3$
This reaction is known as Clemmenson reduction.

101. (b) : SO_2 shows both oxidising as well as reducing nature.
The reaction given in assertion is due to oxidising nature of SO_2.

$$2H_2S + SO_2 \rightarrow 2H_2O + 3S$$

102. (a) : (i) Due to smaller size of F; steric repulsions will be less in SiF_6^{2-}.
(ii) Interaction of F lone pair electrons with Si is stronger than that of chlorine lone pairs.

103. (b) : Borax bead test is not suitable for Al(III) because its oxidising as well as reducing flame is colourless in both hot as well as cold.
Alumina is insoluble in water as they exist in hydrated form like $Al_2O_3 \cdot 2H_2O$, $Al_2O_3 \cdot H_2O$ etc.

104. (b) : Due to the ease with which it can liberate nascent oxygen, O_3 acts as a powerful oxidising agent.

$$O_3 \rightarrow O_2 + O$$

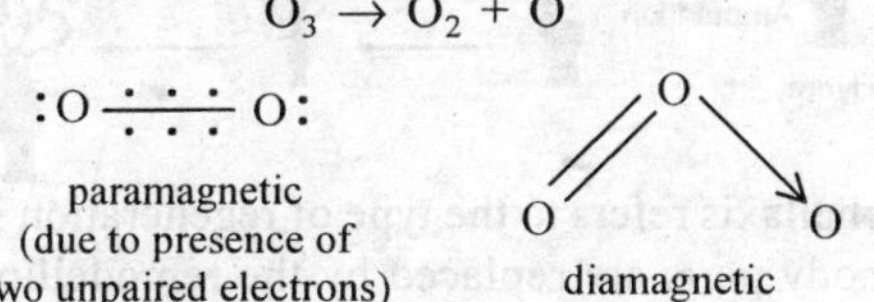

105. (c) : Ferrocyanide ion

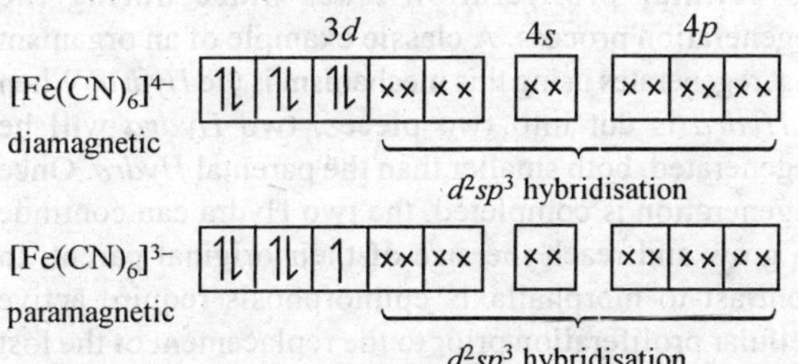

In ferrocyanide ion, the oxidation state of Fe is +2 however in ferricyanide ion, the oxidation number of Fe is +3.
Generally, the higher the oxidation state of the metal, the greater the crystal field splitting. It means crystal field splitting in ferrocyanide ion is lower than that of ferricyanide ion.

106. (d) : $Ba(OH)_2$ is soluble in water.

107. (c) : $SeCl_4$ possess see saw geometry, which can be regarded as a distorted trigonal bipyramidal structure, having one lone pair (lp) of electrons in the basal position of the trigonal bipyramidal. See-saw geometry of $SeCl_4$ molecules arises due to the sp^3d hybridisation of the central atom. The distortion in shape is due to the presence of one lone pair of electrons.

108. (a) : Depression in freezing point is a colligative property which depends upon the number of particles. The number of particles are different in case of benzene and water that is why molecular weight of acetic acid determined by depression in freezing point method is also different.

109. (a) : In case of H_2, compressibility factor increases with the pressure. At 273 K, $Z > 1$ which shows that it is difficult to compress the gas as compared to ideal gas. In this case repulsive forces dominate.

110. (d) : First ionization energy for nitrogen is greater than oxygen.

	N	O
eV	14.5	13.6

This is due to stable configuration of nitrogen (half-filled 2p-orbital).
Due to screening effect the valency electron experiences less attraction towards the nucleus. This brings decrease in the nuclear charge (Z) actually present on the nucleus. The reduced nuclear charge is termed effective nuclear charge and its magnitude increases in a period when we move from left to right.

111. (d) : In B_2, total number of electrons = 10
$B_2 \rightarrow \sigma(1s)^2\ \sigma^*(1s^2)\ \sigma(2s)^2\ \sigma^*(2s)^2\ \sigma(2p_x)^1\ \pi(2p_y)^1$
Presence of unpaired electron shows the paramagnetic nature.
The highest occupied molecular orbital is of π-type.

112. (a) : Hydrolysis of methyl chloride to methanol follows S_N2 reaction. The rates of many S_N2 reactions are affected by the solvent. Protic solvents – those that contain – OH or – NH group are generally the worst solvents for S_N2. Polar protic solvents, (like water, alcohols and carboxylic acids), which have strong dipoles but don't have – OH or – NH groups are the best. In contrast to protic solvents, which decrease the rates of S_N2 reactants by lowering the ground state energy of nucleophile, polar aprotic solvents (DMF) increase the rates of S_N2 reactions by raising the ground state energy of nucleophile.

113. (a) : Zinc metal which has a more negative electrode potential than iron will provide electrons in preference to the iron, and therefore corrode first. Only when all the zinc has been oxidised does the iron start to rust.

114. (d) : Extraction of iron metal from iron oxide ore is carried out by heating with coke and flux (calcium carbonate). Flux is a slag forming substance. It converts infusible impurities into fusible slag.
The reaction : $Fe_2O_{3\,(s)} \rightarrow Fe_{\,(s)} + 3/2\ O_{2\,(g)}$ is not a spontaneous process. Fe_2O_3 is converted to FeO at about 400°C. FeO is converted to Fe at about 800°C-1000°C.

115. (d) : Rates of nitration of benzene and hexadeutero benzene are same because nitration depends upon availability of electrophile.

116. (b) : In Williamson's synthesis, if a tertiary alkyl halide is used, an alkene is the only reaction product and no ether is formed.

$$CH_3-\underset{CH_3}{\overset{CH_3}{\underset{|}{\overset{|}{C}}}}-Br + NaOCH_3 \longrightarrow CH_3-\underset{CH_3}{\underset{|}{C}}{=}CH_2 + NaBr$$

2-methyl propene

It is because alkoxides are not only nucleophiles but also strong bases as well. They react with alkyl halides leading to elimination reaction.

117. (c) : On hydrolysis one mole of maltose yields two moles of D-glucose. It is a reducing sugar. The two glucose units are linked through α-glucosidic linkage between C - 1 of one unit and the C-4 of another.

118. (d) : The nitro group strongly deactivates the benzene ring towards electrophilic substitution. Nitrobenzene does not undergo Friedel-Craft acylation reaction.

119. (a) : In an isocyanide, first an electrophile and then a nucleophile add at the carbon to form a species which usually undergoes further transformations.

$$R\overset{+}{N}\equiv\bar{C} + E^+ \longrightarrow R\overset{+}{N}\equiv CE \xrightarrow{Nu} RN\equiv C(Nu)E$$

$$R\overset{+}{N}\equiv\bar{C} + H_2O \longrightarrow RN{=}CHOH \longrightarrow RNHCHO$$

alkylformamide

120. (a) :

cyclopentadienyl anion

$$\bar{C}H_2CH{=}CH_2 \longleftrightarrow CH_2{=}CH\bar{C}H_2$$

allyl anion

Here the resonance approach is a poor predictor of stability. The Huckel rule, based on molecular orbital theory, is a much better predictor of stability for these aromatic and antiaromatic system.

121. (a) : Based on cellular mechanisms, regeneration can be divided into two broad categories : morphallaxis and epimorphosis.

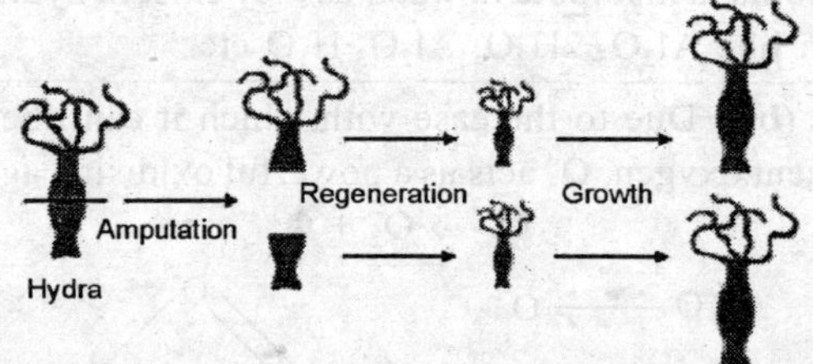

Morphallaxis refers to the type of regeneration in which lost body parts are replaced by the remodelling of the remaining tissue. In this type of regeneration, little or no cellular proliferation takes place during the regeneration process. A classic example of an organism that regenerates using this mechanism is the *Hydra*. When a *Hydra* is cut into two pieces, two *Hydra* will be regenerated, both smaller than the parental *Hydra*. Once regeneration is completed, the two Hydra can continue to grow and reach the size of their original parent. In contrast to morphallaxis epimorphosis require active cellular proliferation prior to the replacement of the lost body part. For eg. *Planarian*, which are flatworms, regenerate using a mechanism in which pre-existing stem cells, known as neoblasts, begin to proliferate and migrate to the injured site in response to injury. These cells then form a mass of proliferating cells, known as regeneration blastema, that will later differentiate into the specialized cells that comprise the regenerated structure. Most tissue regeneration in mammals also belongs to the epimorphosis. For example, mammals can regenerate their muscle, bone epithelia of the skin and gut, blood, and some neurons by activating pre-existing stem cells or progenitor cells.

122. (d) : Gastrin is a polypeptide hormone produced by the enteroendocrine cells of the stomach after exposure to mechanical stimuli or stimulation of vagus nerve and of the duodenum, after the exposure of chyme that contains undigested proteins. It plays an important role in the control of gastric acid secretion. Inhibin hormone is secreted from corpus luteum, placenta and testes. It supplements the effect of excess sex hormones for depressing gonadotrophic activity (FSH, LH, ICSH). The target of inhibin is anterior lobe of pituitary. Duodenal enterokinase converts trypsinogen to activate trypsin which, in turn, activates the other pancreatic enzymes. Atrial natriuretic factor (ANF) is released by walls of the cardiac atrium in response to high sodium concentration, high extracellular fluid volume, or high blood volume. It then acts *via* various mechanisms to excrete Na, and to cause vasodilation in the circulatory system. It dilates the afferent glomerular arteriole, constricts the efferent glomerular arteriole, and relaxes the mesangial cells. The increases the glomerular filtration rate, resulting in greater excretion of Na^+ and water. It also decreases Na resorption in the renal distal convoluted tubule and cortical collecting duct. It also inhibits renin secretion.

123. (b) : Cretinism is a type of mental retardation and bodily malformation caused by severe, uncorrected thyroid deficiency in infancy and early childhood .Delta cells is a type of cell in the pancreas (the organ of the digestive system located behind the stomach). Within the pancreas, the delta cells are located in areas called the islets of Langerhans. The delta cells make somatostatin, a hormone that inhibits the release of numerous hormones in the body. Somatostatin has a variety of functions. Taken together, they work to reduce the rate at which food is absorbed from the contents of the intestine. Somatostatin is also secreted by the hypothalamus and by the intestine.Beta cells in the pancreatic islets secrete the hormone insulin in response to a high concentration of glucose in the blood. Parathyroid hormone is a hormone secreted by the parathyroid glands that regulates the metabolism of calcium and phosphate in the body. Parathyroid hormone acts to raise the extracellular calcium concentration, that is, the concentration of calcium ions in the spaces between the cells of the body and in the blood plasma; it promotes the absorption of calcium by the intestine, mobilizes calcium salts from the bones, and increases the tendency of the kidney to recover calcium from the urine. The hormone also enhances both the excretion of phosphate by the kidneys and its uptake by the cells.

124. (a) : In the given chart the disease is inherited by female child from his father and none of the male child is affected hence it shows that the disease is X linked. Moreover, in the progeny the disease is expressed phenotypically by female child even if it is carrier, so the disease is dominant. Hence the pattern of disease is X linked dominant.

125. (c) : The cross section of the sperm midpiece shows the axial bundle of microtubules or axoneme surrounded by a microtubular sheath in which the mitochondria of the spermatid have become arranged in a helical manner. The microtubular structure provide the ability of the sperm to swim through the reproductive tract of the female. The microtubules are in 9 + 2 arrangement.

126. (c) : Bt in "Bt Cotton" stands for *Bacillus thurengiensis.* This is naturally occurring soil bacterium. Somatic hybridization involves fusion of protoplast of two cells. "Flavr savr" is genetically engineered tomatoes which express delayed softening by insertion of an additional copy of PG endociding gene. PG is poly galacturonase enzyme which is responsible for the breakdown of cell wall pectin. Transgenic *Brassica napus* seeds are being used to produce the anticoagulant hirudin.

127. (b) : Inflammation is common to almost all diseases that involve microbiologic, chemical, or physical injury to living tissues. Acute inflammation may be defined as the microcirculation response to injury; the cardinal signs are heat, redness, pain, swelling, and loss of function. The accompanying microcirculatory changes comprise arteriolar vasodilation, increased small vein permeability, formation of edema fluid, and WBC migration to the site of injury. Histamine is stored in mast cell granules and basophils and is released by inflammatory and immunologic stimuli. It plays an important role in acute inflammation, exerting a dilator action on arterioles, increasing the permeability of small venules to plasma proteins and causing pain by stimulating nociceptors. However, the generally poor clinical efficacy of antihistamines suggests that their role in nonimmune inflammation is limited. Plasma kinins such as bradykinin are not stored but are released by the action of kininogenase on plasma $á_2$-globulin. Bradykinin is a potent vasodilator, increasing small vein permeability and causing pain by stimulating peripheral nociceptors, but it has a short half-life.

128. (c) : Eastern Himalayas and Western Ghats are the geographical areas in India which shows the maximum diversity.

129. (a) : Introduction of high yield varieties is the major threat to the genetic diversity in agricultural crops. This would eliminate other crop type/variety from the pool.

130. (c) : *Ex situ* conservation is the preservation of components of biological diversity outside their natural habitats: in zoos, aquaria, botanic gardens and gene banks, for example. Zoos, botanical gardens and arboretums are the most conventional methods of ex-situ conservation, all of which house whole, protected specimens for breeding and reintroduction into the wild when necessary and possible. These facilities provide not only housing and care for specimens of endangered species, but also have an educational value.
Rest of the given options are example of *insitu* conservation.

131. (b) : Blue baby syndrome is blood related condition found in babies due to nitrate poisoning (poisoning limits blood's ability to carry oxygen thereby causing baby to look blue); known as metheamoglobanemia. This is a serious illness in infants which is caused when nitrate is converted into nitrite in the infant's body. Nitrite interferes with the oxygen carrying capacity of the child's blood (It replaces the oxygen on the red blood cells). This is an acute disease in that symptoms can develop rapidly in infants. However, in most cases, health deteriorates over a period of days. Clearly, expert medical advice should be sought immediately if these symptoms occur.

132. (b) : MRI is a non-invasive technique which uses strong magnetic field for generating resonance and low radio frequency in protons present in body. Most common protons are H nuclei of H_2O molecules. Scapula and canine are osteocytic structures with negligible H_2O content.

133. (d) : Valium (diazepam) is in a class of drugs called benzodiazepines. Valium (diazepam) affects chemicals in the brain that may become unbalanced and cause anxiety, seizures, and muscle spasms. Valium (diazepam) is used to relieve anxiety, nervousness, and tension associated with anxiety disorders. It is also used to treat certain types of seizure disorders and muscle spasms.

134. (c)

135. (b) : Menstruation is a part of the female reproductive cycle that starts when girls become sexually mature at the time of puberty. The parts of the body involved in the menstrual cycle include the brain, pituitary gland, uterus and cervix, ovaries, fallopian tubes and vagina. The following events given in the options occur in a normal menstrual cycle.
(i) Release of egg called ovulation usually takes place roughly 14 days after the first day of the start of a period for fertilization.
(ii) Following menstruation endometrium regenerates about 8 days during the proliferative phase.
(iii) Implantation occurs after 7 days of fertilization.
(iv) Progesterone level rises after ovulation which occurs after 14 days.

136. (d) : T_1 plasmid is found extragenomically in *Agarobacterium tumefaciens* which possess T-DNA that is responsible for causing tumor in host plant.

137. (a) : Non-biodegradable pollutant: a pollutant which retains its toxicity for extremely long periods of time. Some lead and mercury compounds, certain chlorinated hydrocarbon pesticides (e.g., DDT)and radioactive substances are nonbiodegradable pollutants. Osteoporosis is a condition that is characterized by a decrease in bone mass and density, causing bones to become fragile. Blackfoot disease (BFD) is a severe form of peripheral vascular disease (PVD), in which the blood vessels in the lower limbs are severely damaged, resulting eventually in progressive gangrene. It has been observed in Taiwan. Itai-itai disease is a chronic cadmium poisoning with renal tubular dysfunction followed by osteomalacia.

138. (a) : Camel excrete a highly concentrated urine to conserve water. They do not sweat till body temperature rises about 55°C-60°C. Camel can also tolerate desiccation upto 40% cellular content.

139. (a) : Cri du chat a rare syndrome (1 in 50,000 live births) caused by a deletion on the short arm of chromosome 5, is a rare genetic disorder due to a missing portion of chromosome 5. It was first described by Lejeune in 1963. The name of this syndrome is French for "cry of the cat," referring to the distinctive cry of children with this disorder. The cry is caused by abnormal larynx development, which becomes normal within a few weeks of birth. Infants with cri du chat have low birth weight and may have respiratory problems.

140. (a) : Brassica (mustard) belongs to family Brassicaceae. Family brassicaceae is characterised by polypetalous 4 petals, polysepalous 4 sepals, six stamens (which are in tetradynamous condition *i.e.* 4 + 2 or in two whorls, 4 inner long and 2 outer short). Gynoecium is bicarpellary, syncarpous unilocular with parietal placentation. Fruit is usually siliqua (Dry dehiscent fruit formed by bicarpellary syncarpous gynoecium with replum) and rarely lomentum.

141. (b) : Polygene results in quantitative inheritance. Quantitative inheritance is characterised by occurrence of intermediate forms between the parental type. There will be 7 (1 : 6 : 15 : 20 : 15 : 6 : 1) phenotypes when three polygene pairs are involved. The total number of progeny would be 64. Out of these sixty four only two will be likely to resemble either parents. Hence their proportion in F_2 generation would be 3·12 *i.e.* less than five per cent.

142. (c) : Mature cork cells are plant cells that form the protective water resistant tissue in the outer covering of stems and trunks. Cork cells are genetically programmed not to divide, but instead to remain as they are dead cells. Cork cells possess lenticels. A lenticel is produced beneath a former stomata or stoma of the epidermis. They encloses intercellular space for gaseous exchange. Passage cells help in transfer of water from cortex. Quiscent centre is present in root apical meristem.

143. (b): The synapsis, pairing of homologous chromosomes takes place during zygotene. Synapsis results in the formation of bivalents during zygotene. The formation of special proteinaceous structure called synaptonemal complex occur. After zygotene stage cell entered in pachytene stage in which the bivalents become spiralled, shortened and thickened.

144. (b) : Recombination is the natural process of breaking and rejoining DNA strands to produce new combinations of genes and, thus, generate genetic variation. This is the phenomenon occur during meiosis I.

145. (d) : The presence of plastid is a feature of plant cells but animal cells are devoid of them. Even then they function properly and divide mitotically similar to plant cells.

146. (a) : Lysosomes are roughly spherical bodies bounded by a single membrane. They are manufactured by the Golgi apparatus. Lysosomes are small membrane bound vesicles in the cytoplasm of cells which contain toxic enzymes. When a cell dies, these membranes rupture and the enzymes are released. They break down the cells structure, and the debris is removed. The lysosome also contains cytokines which summon inflammatory cells and stimulate inflammation. The contents of lysosomes can be released by macrophages and neutrophils both to kill bacteria and viruses, and to stimulate inflammation.

147. (b) : Glyoxysomes are enzymes which play a critical role in lipid metabolism in seedlings. Hence they are supposed to be present in endosperm of castor as endosperm of wheat will posses starch.

148. (c) : Ecological niche is the term used to describe the status of a plant or animal in its community.

149. (c) : Pyramid of energy is always upright as only 10% energy is transferred from one trophic level to another. Pyramid of number in a grassland is also upright as the producers are always maximum in number than herbivores and carnivores. Pyramid of biomass in a lake shows spindle shaped pyramid.

150. (b)

151. (b) : Nephridia in earthworm, malpighian tubules in cockroach and urinary tubules in rat are all excretory in function.

152. (c) : According to the correct labelling shown the pair fibula and phalanges is wrongly marked.

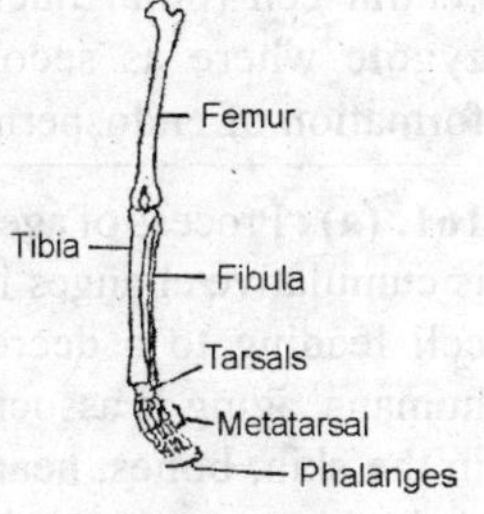

153. (c) : Electroporation is the process used for the transformation of bacteria or plant protoplasts. Electroporation occurs as a result of the reconcentration of lipid molecules of the bilayer membrane to form hydrophilic pores in the membrane. The distribution of such pores, both in terms of size and number, determine the electrical properties of the cell membrane.

154. (d) : Somaclonal variations is the term used to

describe the variation seen in plants that have been produced by plant tissue culture. Chromosomal rearrangements are an important source of this variation.

155. (a) : According to the graph the growth of the insect takes place as the amount of the cholesterol increase and at 6 μg cholesterol/g the growth get static. If the growth rate would have been directly proportional to the cholesterol concentration then the graph would have been straight line. (3) is wrong as the optimum level is 6 μg/g cholesterol concentration.

156. (b) : Prosopis are tree found in scrub. *Saccharum* is grass which is cultivated. *Shorea robusta* (Sal) is tree found in moist tropical forest. *Acacia catechu* is tree found in dry deciduous forests.

157. (b) : Reverse transcriptase is an enzyme used by retroviruses to from complementary DNA (cDNA) from their RNA. The resulting DNA is then inserted into the chromosome of the host cell.

158. (b) : Gibberellins induces the hydrolyzing enzymes in the endosperm of germinating seeds. It stimulates the production of digestive enzymes like proteases, amylase, lipase which help to mobilise stored nutrients.

159. (c) : Silverfish, scorpion, dragonfly and prawn all fall in phylum arthropods which have jointed appendages and chitinous exoskeleton as the characteristic feature.

160. (d) : Double fertilization is the characteristic feature of angiosperms. Here one male nucleus fertilizes the egg nucleus and the other male nucleus fertilizes the central cell (polar nuclei). First fertilization result in zygote where as second fertilization results in the formation of endosperm.

161. (a) : Process of ageing is called senescence. Ageing, is cumulative changes in an organism, organ, tissue, or cell leading to a decrease in functional capacity. In humans, aging is associated with degenerative changes in the skin, bones, heart, blood vessels, lungs, nerves, and other organs and tissues.

It is genetically controlled programme regulated by regulatory genes. This view is suggested by the great range of lifespans among different animal species—from a few days in the fruit fly to more than 100 years in some tortoises. Scientists have recently learned how to double the lifespans of such laboratory organisms as roundworms and fruit flies through genetic manipulation, and mutant genes in mice have been observed to have a comparable effect in postponing ageing.

Genes which have a deleterious effect on individual's fitness are selected against by natural selection. Mutations in these genes which postponed the deleterious effect of the gene to a later time in individual's life history reduce the effect of natural selection to the gene, because the selection has less time to act on it. If the gene doesn't have a negative effect until after the individual has reproduced, the gene may escape natural selection altogether, because when selection starts to affect the gene, it has already propagated to the next generation. In a related fashion, some genes may help to ensure reproduction at the cost of diseases later in life. For instance, our immune system generally helps to keep us healthy during reproductive age, but many adults acquire autoimmune diseases such as rhemuatoid arthritis as they age.

162. (a) : In recombinant DNA technology widely used host for replication and amplification of recombinant DNA are prokaryotic *E. coli* and the eukaryotic yeast. They replicate very fast to form a large population which expressed desired gene. Yeast artificial chromosome (YAC) are important cloning tools for the analysis of complex genome such as that of humans. They allow the maintenance, propagation and analysis of such genome in an experimentally tractable system, the yeast.

163. (b) : SPM (Suspended Particulate Matter) is defined as particles floating in the air with a diameter below 10 μ m. Studies have shown that high SPM concentrations in the air can have a detrimental impact on respiratory organs. SPM is generated from natural sources (e.g., volcanoes or dust storms) and human activities (vehicles, incinerators and industrial plants).

SPM	Other aerosols
Less than 10 μm	Less than 100 μm
Tend to float longer in air due to small size.	Tend to settle fairly quickly due to comparative heaviness

Catalytic converter is a device designed to reduce the amount of emissions from automobiles. The current (so-called three-way) systems use a heated metal catalyst to reduce the emissions of carbon monoxide (CO), hydrocarbons, and nitric oxide (NO), all of which contribute to the formation of photochemical smog. In an automobile's exhaust system, a catalytic converter provides an environment for a chemical reaction where unburnt hydrocarbons completely combust. Hence the combustion process continues but outside the engine combustion chamber where no useful energy is extracted. Toxic car gases such as unburnt hydrocarbon (UHC) and carbon monoxide (CO) would not exist if the fuel to energy conversion in the engine were perfect.

164. (b) : Methane is largely a product of incomplete decomposition and is produced by a group of bacteria called methanogens under anaerobic conditions. The major sources of methane include freshwater wetlands, enteric fermentation in cattle and flooded rice fields. Biomass burning also produces methane. Major gases contributing in greenhouse effect with their percentage contribution are given in the given pie chart.

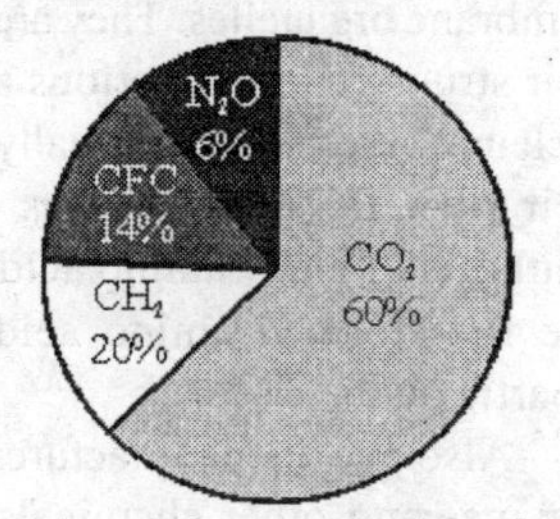

The relative contribution of different gases to global warming

Efficient engine (for example, multi point fuel injection engine) can reduce the unburnt carbons (like methane etc.) in auto emission.

165. (d) : Interferons are not antibodies. These are natural proteins produced by the cells of the immune systems of most animals in response to challenges by foreign agents such as viruses, bacteria, parasites and tumor cells. Interferons belong to the large class of glycoproteins known as cytokines. In human body there are three types of interferon – α, β and γ. Interferon alpha and beta are produced by many cell types, including T-cells and B-cells and are important component of the antiviral response. They stimulate both macrophages and NK (Natural Killer) cells. They both are also active against tumors. Interferon gamma is involved in the regulation of the immune and inflammatory response. Interferon gamma has had some antiviral and antitumor effect but these are generally weak, however, it potentiates the effect of interferon alpha and interferon beta.

Inflammation is the first response to infection and injury and is critical to body defence. Basically, the inflammatory response is an attempt by the body to restore and maintain homeostasis after injury. Inflammation is the influx of fluid and cells that results in redness, swelling, heat, and pain at the infection site.

166. (a) : An organ transplant is the transplantation of an organ (or part of one) from one body to another, for the purpose of replacing the recipient's damaged or failing organ with a working one from the donor. Organ donors can be living, or cadaveric (dead). Immunosuppressive drug are any of a variety of substances used to prevent production of *antibodies*. They are clinically used to

- prevent rejection by a recipient's body of an organ (e.g. *bone marrow, heart, kidney, liver*) transplanted from a donor. A transplant is rejected when the recipient's immune system acts against it.
- treatment of autoimmune diseases or diseases that are most likely of autoimmune origin (e.g. rheumatoid arthritis). The *steroids*, such as *cortisone*, which suppress the antibody-forming lymphocyte cells, have been used to prolong human organ transplants. Steroids may also prevent antigens from entering cells and thereby prevent local allergic inflammation reactions. In another immunosuppressive method, human lymphocytes are injected into horses, stimulating the animals to produce antilymphocyte serum. The serum, administered to humans with transplanted organs, in some way inactivates lymphocyte cells. Another group of immunosuppressive drugs act by interfering with the synthesis of *nucleic acids* and are especially effective against proliferating cells such as stimulated lymphocytes. Some of these are analogs of purines and pyrimidines, substances that are nucleic acid subunits; the purine analog azothioprine has been used to suppress rejection of transplanted human kidneys. Most substances that inhibit nucleic acid synthesis, such as nitrogen mustard, cyclophosphamide (Cytoxan), chloramphenicol, actinomycin, and colchicine, are not widely used clinically because they are too toxic.

167. (c) : Haemophilia is a blood disorder where the blood does not clot normally. Haemophilia A is the most common form, caused by a deficiency of blood clotting factor VIII. Haemophilia B is due to a deficiency of blood clotting factor IX. Haemophilia is an hereditary disorder. In almost all cases, it is males that suffer the condition, although it is passed on by both females and males carrying the gene. Queen Victoria was a carrier of haemophilia A. It is also known as classical haemophilia and factor VIII deficiency haemophilia. Haemophilia B is also known as Factor IX haemophilia, and Christmas disease after the first patient diagnosed with it. Prothrombin producing platelets in such persons are not found in very low concentration.

168. (c) : In most animal species, chromosomes can be categorized as two types: autosomes and sex chromosomes. Autosomes are non-sex chromosomes that are the same number and kind between sexes. Sex chromosomes determine if the individual is male or female. Sex chromosomes in the human female are XX; those of the male are XY. Males produce X-containing and Y-containing gametes; therefore males determine the sex of offspring. Besides genes that determine sex, sex chromosomes carry many genes for traits unrelated to sex. X-linked gene is any gene located on X chromosome; used to describe genes on X chromosome that are missing on the Y chromosome.

When the female ovum is fertilized by the male, there is initiated an incredibly complex chain of events which culminate nine months later in the birth of a child. During the very early stages of this gestation period the development of the embryo is predisposed in certain directions by the possession of the sex chromosomes which are composed of two elements, one contributed by the mother and the other by the father. The mother can contribute only what is termed as an X chromosome which predisposes towards the development of female structural, functional and temperamental characteristics, but the father can contribute either an X or a Y chromosome predisposing in the first instance to female, or in the second to male structural and functional and temperamental characteristics. In short, the sex of the child to be born is initially governed by the chromosomal contribution of the father. All chromosomes are paired, and the Y is dominant over the X chromosome when combined with it. A child conceived will therefore be subject during development thereafter to a predisposition towards femaleness if receiving an X chromosome from the mother and an X chromosome from the father (XX), or towards maleness if receiving an X chromosome from the mother but a Y chromosome from the father (XY). Therefore sex in human is a monogenic not polygenic.

Polygenic traits or continuous traits are those traits that are determined by the combined effect of more than one pair of genes. An example of this is human stature. The combined size of all of the body parts from head to foot determines the height of an individual.There is an additive effect. The sizes of all of these body parts are, in turn, determined by numerous genes. Human skin, hair, and eye colour are also polygenic traits because they are influenced by more than one allele at different loci. The result is the perception of continuous gradation in the expression of these traits.

169. (c) : Mitochondria and chloroplasts both are double membrane organelles. They are semi autonomous as both their structure and functions are partially controlled by nucleus of the cell and partially themselves. Both possess their own DNA and arises from pre-existing cells. Synthesis of many amino acids occurs in mitochondria. The first formed amino acids are glutamic acid and aspartic acid.

Also plastid manufactures some of its own proteins, enzymes and other chemicals because of the presence of 70s ribosomes which can help translate the coded information contained in *m*RNAs transcribed over chloroplast DNA.

170. (a) : DNA replication is the process of forming carbon copy of DNA. Whereas transcription is the formation of RNA over DNA template.

DNA replication and transcription takes place in nucleus as the required material DNA and RNA are present in the nucleus.

During transcription *m*RNA take the coded information from DNA to the cytoplasm where translation takes place. Translation is the process of protein synthesis. It is separated from transcription in both space and time. It prevents the intermixing of raw materials, protect DNA from respiratory enzymes and ribosomal machinery from nuclease.

171. (c) : Fungi are considered ubiquitous *i.e.* they occur in a variety of habitats. Most of them are moisture loving and terrestrial and few (eg. *Monoblepharis*) are aquatic. Fungi may be **epiphytic** (*i.e.* live on plants eg. *Armillaria*), **saprophytic** (*i.e.* grow in dead organic matter eg. *Mucor*), **symbiotic** (*i.e.* live with association with other plants eg. lichen, mycorrhiza) and **predacious** (eg. *Dactyldela*) and parasitic (eg *Erysipi*) fungi are achlorophyllus *i.e.* devoid of chlorophyll hence cannot prepare their own food. They are heterotrophic and show absorptive type of nutrition.

172. (a) : C_4 photosynthetic pathway is more efficient than C_3 pathway as C_4 plants can pick up CO_2 even when it is found in low concentration. PEP enzymes shows high affinity for CO_2. C_4 plants contain two types of chloroplast (Kranz anatomy) : bundle sheath chloroplast and mesophyll chloroplast. Bundle sheath cells contain Calvin cycle enzymes. Due to high concentration of CO_2 in bundle sheath cells, RuBP carboxylase works only for Calvin cycle and not for photorespiration.

Photorespiration is a wasteful process as it works to undo the act of photosynthesis in C_3 plants. No energy rich compound is produced in this process. When temperature increase more and more photosynthetically fixed carbon is lost by photorespiration thus reducing the efficiency of C_3 plants.

173. (d) : If humans share ancestry with other primates, then we should expect to see remnants of that common ancestry in our genes. For example, tails; this characteristic is still exhibited occssionally in atavism. According to current evolutionary theory, the ancestors of humans lost their tails about 25 million years ago, when apes (tail-less primates) diverged from monkeys (tailed primates). Theory of the continuity of the germplasm was given by Weismann. The German biologist Weismann recognized that animals are made up of: body cells (somaplasm), which contain gamete-producing cells (germplasm). At each generation, the embryo that develops from the zygote not only sets aside some germplasm for the next generation but also produces the cells that will develop into the body, the soma, of the organism. Jean-Baptise Lamarck (1744-1829), presented the first widely discussed theory of Evolution, the idea that organisms are connected through time by ancestor-descendent relationships and that they change through time. Lamarck's theory of evolution had four main components. (1) Spontaneous generation of organisms from inanimate matter occurs continuously throughout Earth history (2) Extinction does not occur. (3) Traits developed by parents are passed on directly to offspring (The Inheritance of Aquired Characteristics). (4) Use or disuse of parts causes them to transformation (*i.e.,* it drove evolutionary change).

174. (b) : The warming up of global atmosphere present day is due to the increase in green house effect.

Green house effect (GHE) describe the roles of water vapour, CO_2 and other trace gases in keeping the Earth's surface warmer than it would be otherwise. These radiatively active gases are relatively transparent to incoming shortwave radiation (visible spectrum), but are relatively opaque to outgoing reradiating (infrared rays) longwave radiation. The latter radiation, which would otherwise escape to space, is trapped by these gases within the lower levels of the atmosphere. The subsequent reradiation of some of the energy back to the surface maintains surface temperature higher than they would be if the gases were absent (without the green house effect the Earth's average global temperature would be –18 degree celsius rather than the present 15 degree celsius). There is concern that increasing concentration of the green house gases including CO_2, CH_4, and man made chlorofluorocarbons (CFCS), may enhance the green house effect and cause global warming.

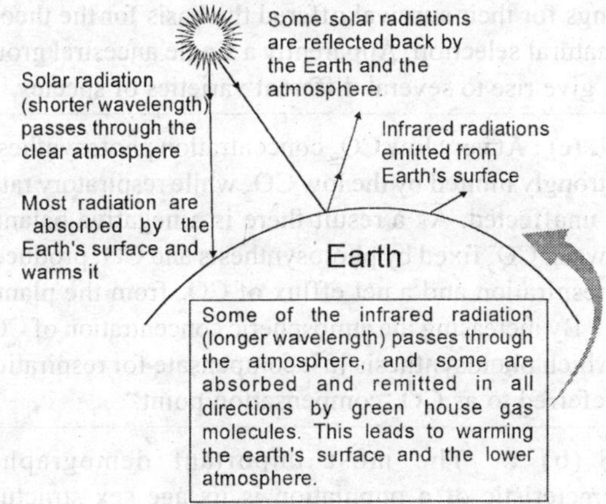

Ozone layer present in the stratosphere is depleted by the aerosols and chloroflurocarbons. Ozone protects the earth from high energy ultra violet radiation.

175. (b) : Convincing evidence of common ancestry comes from the similarities in the biochemical composition, reactions and physiological activities of living beings, like metabolic process, enzymes, cytochrome C, insulin, haemoglobin, blood and lymph etc. Genetic code is the sequence of DNA nucleotides that determines the amino acid sequence of the translated protein. The genetic code is read in triplets of bases called codons.

Genetic code is applicable universally *i.e.* a codon specifies the same amino acid from a virus to a tree or human beings. The *m*RNA from chick oviduct introduced in *E.coli* produces an ovalbumen in the bacterium exactly similar to one formed in chick.

176. (a) : Darwin finches are an excellent example of the way in which the species gene pools have adapted in order for long term survival via their offspring. Finches were formed due to divergent evolution (adaptive radiation) to avoid interspecific competition.

The common birds of Galapagos islands, the finches were markedly different from the finches of main land. The closely related species of finches had beak of different shapes and sizes, and adapted for feeding on completely different diets. Darwin also found that fossils of Galapagos islands are most similar to living species of South America. The food supply increases in arithmetic ratio but the population increases in geometric ratio. With the study of this theory it struck to Darwin that there is struggle for existence among plants and animals. This concept of competition among the living beings for their survival offered the basis for the theory of natural selection. Apparently a single ancestral group can give rise to several different varieties of species.

177. (c) : At very low CO_2 concentration photosynthesis is strongly limited by the low CO_2 while respiratory rates are unaffected. As a result there is a negative balance between CO_2 fixed by photosynthesis and CO_2 produced by respiration and a net efflux of CO_2 from the plant.

By increasing the atmospheric concentration of CO_2 at which photosynthesis just compensate for respiration is referred to as CO_2 compensation point.

178. (b) : The most important demographic characteristic of a population is its age sex structure which is also known as population pyramids. Age sex pyramids display the percentage or actual amount of a population broken down by gender and age. Developed countries with stable population gives a steep pyramid.

The population of Sudan and India are increasing at a rapid rate. The population growth rate for Sudan is 2.60% and for India it is 1.40%.

179. (a) : To be a mammal the presence of hair and milk or mammary gland is must, but presence of 7 cervical vertebrae and 12 pairs of cranial nerves are also additional mammalian characteristics.The monotremes make up by far the smallest subclass of mammals, with just three species, found in Australia, Tasmania, and New Guinea. One of these is the duck-billed platypus, and the remaining two are the echidnas, or spiny anteaters.The duck-billed platypus and the spiny anteater are mammals that lay eggs rather than give live birth to young ones. The platypus has a bill like a duck, fur like a mammal and webbed feet. It lays eggs that look like reptile eggs. Its young feed from the mother's mammary glands.The spiny anteater's covering looks like that of the porcupine. It has a long tongue to catch insects and a bill. It lays several eggs which it keeps in a pouch on its side.

180. (d) : *Agrobacterium tumefacines* is a gram negative non sporing, motile, rod shaped bacterium, closely related to *Rhizobium*. It is found commonly on and around root surfaces. The region termed rhizosphere where it seems to survive by using nutrients that leak from the root tissues. But it infects only through the wound-site either naturally occurring or caused by transplanting of seedling and nursery stock. It is harmful to plants and useful to scientists for the same reason *i.e.* it transfers DNA into plant genomes found in soil worldwide. *A. tumefaciens* cause crown gall disease of a wide range of dicot (broad leaved) plants especially members of rose family by transferring its own DNA into plant cells. But in laboratory, the ability to move all sorts of genes into plants has made the microbe the standard tool for investigating plant genetics and modifying crops.

181. (a)	**182.** (d)	**183.** (c)	**184.** (a)
185. (d)	**186.** (a)	**187.** (a)	**188.** (a)
189. (b)	**190.** (a)	**191.** (b)	**192.** (b)
193. (a)	**194.** (c)	**195.** (c)	**196.** (a)
197. (b)	**198.** (b)	**199.** (a)	**200.** (c)

☺☺☺

SOLVED PAPER
AIMS - 2006

Time : 3½ Hours Max. Marks : 200

PHYSICS

1. In refraction, light waves are bent on passing from one medium to the second medium, because in the second medium
(a) the frequency is different
(b) the coefficient of elasticity is different
(c) the speed is different
(d) the amplitude is smaller.

2. Two spheres of same size, one of mass 2 kg and another of mass 4 kg are dropped simultaneously from the top of Qutab Minar (height ≈ 72 m). When they are 1 m above the ground the two spheres have the same
(a) momentum (b) kinetic energy
(c) potential energy (d) acceleration.

3. The moment of inertia of a rod about an axis through its centre and perpendicular to it is $\frac{1}{12}ML^2$ (where M is the mass and L, the length of the rod). The rod is bent in the middle so that the two halves make an angle of 60°. The moment of inertia of the bent rod about the same axis would be
(a) $\frac{1}{48}ML^2$ (b) $\frac{1}{12}ML^2$
(c) $\frac{1}{24}ML^2$ (d) $\frac{ML^2}{8\sqrt{3}}$.

4. A boat at anchor is rocked by waves whose crests are 100 m apart and velocity is 25 m/sec. The boat bounces up once in every
(a) 2500 s (b) 75 s
(c) 4 s (d) 0.25 s.

5. By sucking through a straw, a student can reduce the pressure in his lungs to 750 mm of Hg (density = 13.6 g/cm^3). Using the straw, he can drink water from a glass upto a maximum depth of
(a) 10 cm (b) 75 cm
(c) 13.6 cm (d) 1.36 cm.

6. Two parallel large thin metal sheets have equal surface charge densities ($\sigma = 26.4 \times 10^{-12}$ C/m^2) of opposite signs. The electric field between these sheets is
(a) 1.5 N/C (b) 1.5×10^{-10} N/C
(c) 3 N/C (d) 3×10^{-10} N/C.

7. The magnetic moment has dimensions of
(a) [LA] (b) [L^2A]
(c) [$LT^{-1}A$] (d) [$L^2T^{-1}A$].

8. A wire mesh consisting of very small squares is viewed at a distance of 8 cm through a magnifying converging lens of focal length 10 cm, kept close to the eye. The magnification produced by the lens is
(a) 5 (b) 8
(c) 10 (d) 20.

9. Hard X-rays for the study of fractures in bones should have a minimum wavelength of 10^{-11} m. The accelerating voltage for electrons in X-ray machine should be
(a) < 124.2 kV (b) > 124.2 kV
(c) between 60 kV and 70 kV
(d) = 100 kV.

10. In photoelectric effect, the electrons are ejected from metals if the incident light has a certain minimum
(a) wavelength (b) frequency
(c) amplitude (d) angle of incidence.

11. A lens is made of flint glass (refractive index = 1.5). When the lens is immersed in a liquid of refractive index 1.25, the focal length
(a) increases by a factor of 1.25
(b) increases by a factor of 2.5
(c) increases by a factor of 1.2
(d) decreases by a factor of 1.2

12. The voltage of clouds is 4×10^6 volt with respect to ground. In a lightening strike lasting 100 msec, a charge of 4 coulombs is delivered to the ground.

The power of the lightening strike is
(a) 160 MW (b) 80 MW
(c) 20 MW (d) 500 MW.

13. Five capacitors, each of capacitance value C are connected as shown in the figure. The ratio of capacitance between P and R, and the capacitance between P and Q is

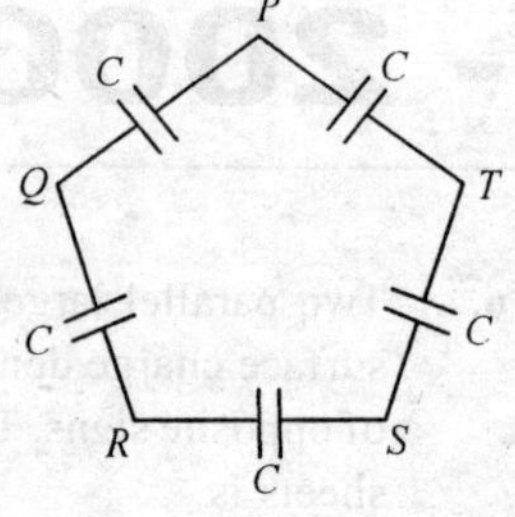

(a) 3 : 1 (b) 5 : 2
(c) 2 : 3 (d) 1 : 1.

14. A stone thrown into still water, creates a circular wave pattern moving radially outwards. If r is the distance measured from the centre of the pattern, the amplitude of the wave varies as
(a) $r^{-1/2}$ (b) r^{-1}
(c) r^{-2} (d) $r^{-3/2}$.

15. For inelastic collision between two spherical rigid bodies
(a) the total kinetic energy is conserved
(b) the total potential energy is conserved
(c) the linear momentum is not conserved
(d) the linear momentum is conserved.

16. When a p-n diode is reverse biased, then
(a) no current flows
(b) the depletion region is increased
(c) the depletion region is reduced
(d) the height of the potential barrier is reduced.

17. Which of the following diagrams represents the variation of electric field vector with time for a circularly polarized light?

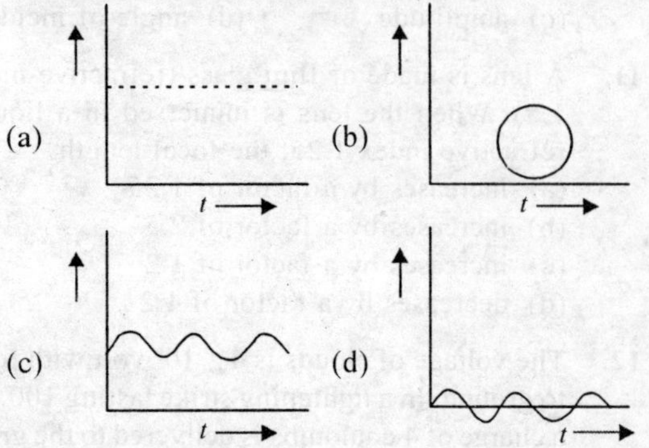

18. The operation of a nuclear reactor is said to be critical, if the multiplication factor (κ) has a value
(a) 1 (b) 1.5
(c) 2.1 (d) 2.5

19. The circuit given below represents which of logic operations?

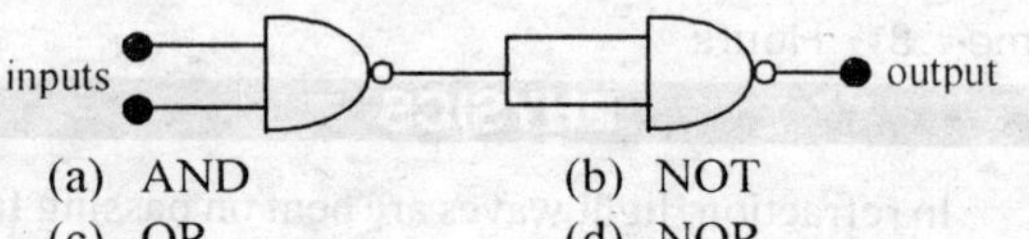

(a) AND (b) NOT
(c) OR (d) NOR.

20. A person used force (F), shown in figure to move a load with constant velocity on surface. Identify the correct surface profile.

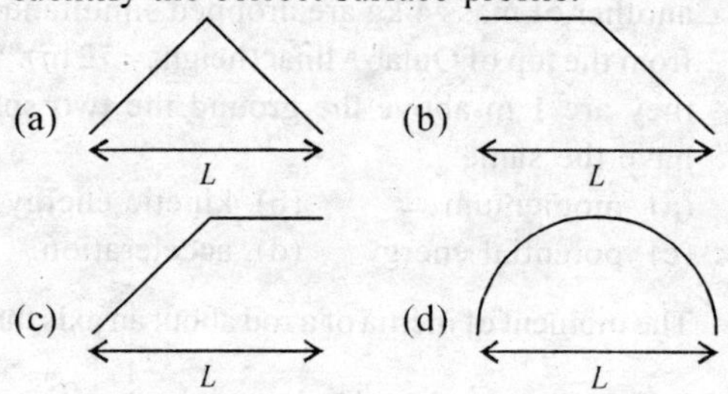

(a) (b) (c) (d)

21. Three objects coloured black, gray and white can withstand hostile conditions upto 2800°C. These objects are thrown into a furnace where each of them attains a temperature of 2000°C. Which object will glow brightest?
(a) the white object (b) the black object
(c) all glow with equal brightness
(d) gray object.

22. Two balloons are filled, on with pure He gas and other by air, respectively. If the pressure and temperature of these balloons are same then the number of molecules per unit volume is
(a) more in the He filled balloon
(b) same in both balloons
(c) more in air filled balloon
(d) in the ratio of 1 : 4.

23. Flash light equipped with a new set of batteries, produces bright white light. As the batteries wear out,

(a) the light intensity gets reduced with no change in its colour
(b) light colour changes first to yellow and then red with no change in intensity
(c) it stops working suddenly while giving white light
(d) colour changes to red and also intensity gets reduced.

24. The spatial distribution of the electric field due to two charges (A, B) is shown in figure. Which one of the following statements is correct?

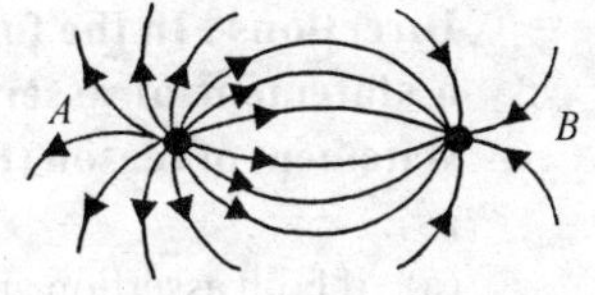

(a) A is +ve and B –ve and $|A| > |B|$
(b) A is –ve and B +ve; $|A| = |B|$
(c) both are +ve but $A > B$
(d) both are –ve but $A > B$.

25. Circular loop of a wire and a long straight wire carry currents I_c and I_e respectively as shown in figure. Assuming that these are placed in the same plane, the magnetic fields will be zero at the centre of the loop when separation H is

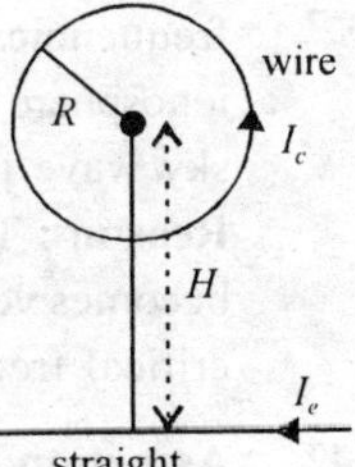

(a) $\dfrac{I_e R}{I_c \pi}$ (b) $\dfrac{I_c R}{I_e \pi}$
(c) $\dfrac{\pi I_c}{I_e R}$ (d) $\dfrac{I_e \pi}{I_c R}$.

26. If a street light of mass M is suspended from the end of a uniform rod of length L in different possible patterns as shown in figure, then

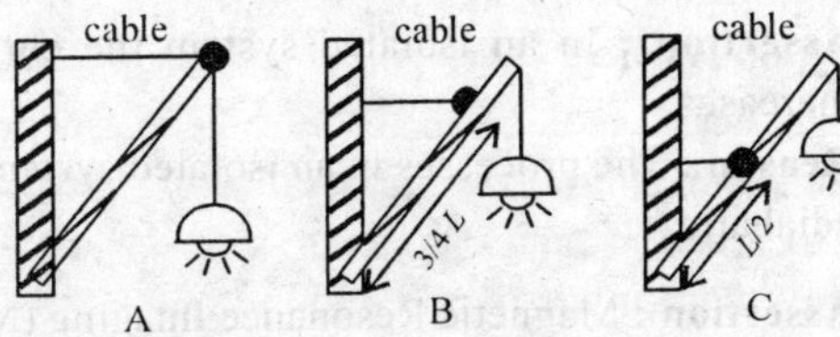

(a) pattern A is more sturdy
(b) pattern B is more sturdy
(c) pattern C is more sturdy
(d) all will have same sturdiness.

27. $^{238}_{92}U$ has 92 protons and 238 nucleons. It decays by emitting an alpha particle and becomes
(a) $^{234}_{92}U$ (b) $^{234}_{90}Th$
(c) $^{235}_{92}U$ (d) $^{237}_{93}Np$.

28. The fossil bone has a ^{14}C : ^{12}C ratio, which is [1/16] of that in a living animal bone. If the half-life time of ^{14}C is 5730 years, then the age of the fossil bone is
(a) 11460 years (b) 17190 years
(c) 22920 years (d) 45840 years.

29. Which one of the following is a possible nuclear reaction?
(a) $^{10}_{5}B + ^{4}_{2}He \rightarrow ^{13}_{7}N + ^{1}_{1}H$
(b) $^{23}_{11}Na + ^{1}_{1}H \rightarrow ^{20}_{10}Ne + ^{4}_{2}He$
(c) $^{239}_{93}Np \rightarrow ^{239}_{94}Pu + \beta^- + \bar{\nu}$
(d) $^{11}_{7}N + ^{1}_{1}H \rightarrow ^{12}_{6}C + \beta^- + \bar{\nu}$.

30. When a guitar string is sounded with a 440 Hz tuning fork, a beat frequency of 5 Hz is heard. If the experiment is repeated with a tuning fork of 437 Hz, the beat frequency is 8 Hz. The string frequency (Hz) is
(a) 445 (b) 435
(c) 429 (d) 448.

31. A metallic ring is dropped down, keeping its plane perpendicular to a constant and horizontal magnetic field. The ring enters the region of magnetic field at $t = 0$ and completely emerges out at $t = T$ sec. The current in the ring varies as

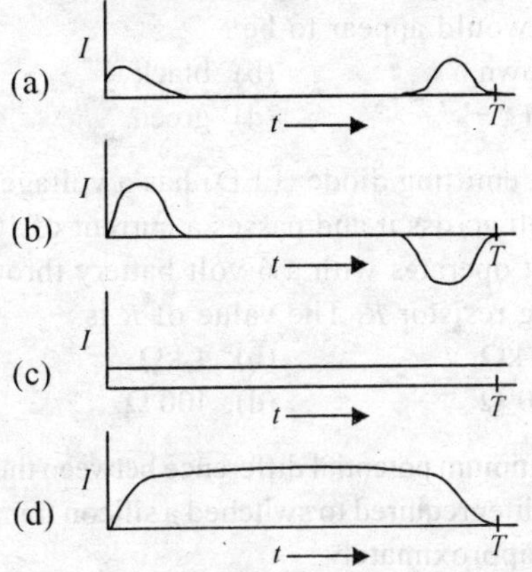

32. If alpha, beta and gamma rays carry same momentum, which has the longest wavelength

(a) alpha rays (b) beta rays
(c) gamma rays
(d) none, all have same wavelength.

33. An amplifier has a voltage gain $A_V = 1000$. The voltage gain in dB is
(a) 30 dB (b) 60 dB
(c) 3 dB (d) 20 dB.

34. When you make ice cubes, the entropy of water
(a) does not change (b) increases
(c) decreases
(d) may either increase or decrease depending on the process used.

35. A bimetallic strip consists of metals X and Y. It is mounted rigidly at the base as shown. The metal X has a higher coefficient of expansion compared to that for metal Y. When the bimetallic strip is placed in a cold bath

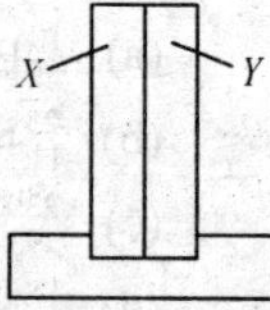

(a) it will bend towards the right
(b) it will bend towards the left
(c) it will not bend but shrink
(d) it will neither bend or shrink.

36. For a wave propagating in a medium, identify the property that is independent of the others.
(a) velocity (b) wavelength
(c) frequency
(d) all these depend on each other.

37. A leaf which contains only green pigments is illuminated by a laser light of wavelength 0.6328 μm. It would appear to be
(a) brown (b) black
(c) red (d) green.

38. A light emitting diode (LED) has a voltage drop of 2 volt across it and passes a current of 10 mA when it operates with a 6 volt battery through a limiting resistor R. The value of R is
(a) 40 kΩ (b) 4 kΩ
(c) 200 Ω (d) 400 Ω.

39. The minimum potential difference between the base and emitter required to switched a silicon transistor ON is approximately
(a) 1 V (b) 3 V
(c) 5 V (d) 4.2 V.

40. Given below is the circuit diagram of an AM demodulator. For good demodulation of AM signal of carrier frequency f, the value of RC should be

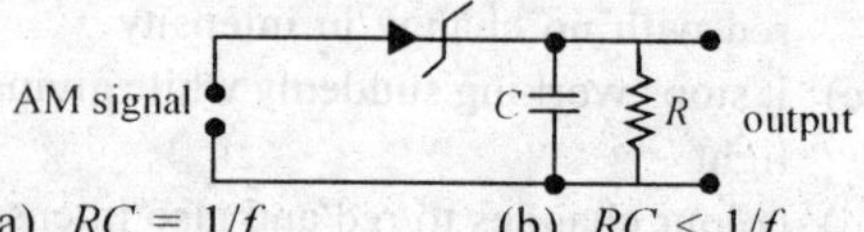

(a) $RC = 1/f$ (b) $RC < 1/f$
(c) $RC \geq 1/f$ (d) $RC >> 1/f$.

Directions : In the following questions (41-60), a statement of assertion (A) is followed by a statement of reason (R). Mark the correct choice as :
(a) if both assertion and reason are true and reason is the correct explanation of the assertion
(b) if both assertion and reason are true but reason is not the correct explanation of the assertion
(c) if assertion is true, but reason is false
(d) both assertion and reason are false statements.

41. **Assertion :** Electromagnetic waves with frequencies smaller than the critical frequency of ionosphere cannot be used for communication using sky wave propagation.
Reason : The refractive index of the ionosphere becomes very high for frequencies higher than the critical frequency.

42. **Assertion :** The binding energy per nucleon, for nuclei with atomic mass number $A > 100$ decreases with A.
Reason : The nuclear forces are weak for heavier nuclei.

43. **Assertion :** In common base configuration, the current gain of the transistor is less than unity.
Reason : The collector terminal is reverse biased for amplification.

44. **Assertion :** In an isolated system the entropy increases.
Reason : The processes in an isolated system are adiabatic.

45. **Assertion :** Magnetic Resonance Imaging (MRI) is a useful diagnostic tool for producing images of various parts of human body.
Reason : Protons of various tissues of human body play a role in MRI.

46. **Assertion :** A judo fighter in order to throw his opponent on to the mat tries to initially bend his opponent and then rotate him around his hip.
Reason : As the mass of the opponent is brought closer to the fighter's hip, the force required to throw the opponent is reduced.

47. **Assertion :** The root mean square and most probable speeds of the molecules in a gas are the same.
Reason : The Maxwell distribution for the speed of molecules in a gas is symmetrical.

48. **Assertion :** Use of ball bearings between two moving parts of a machine is a common practice.
Reason : Ball bearings reduce vibrations and provide good stability.

49. **Assertion :** Standard optical diffraction gratings cannot be used for discriminating between different X-ray wavelengths.
Reason : The grating spacing is not of the order of X-ray wavelengths.

50. **Assertion :** Diamagnetic materials can exhibit magnetism.
Reason : Diamagnetic materials have permanent magnetic dipole moment.

51. **Assertion :** A man in a closed cabin which is falling freely does not experience gravity.
Reason : Inertial and gravitational mass have equivalence.

52. **Assertion:** The photoelectrons produced by a monochromatic light beam incident on a metal surface, have a spread in their kinetic energies.
Reason : The work function of the metal varies as a function of depth from the surface.

53. **Assertion :** The Carnot cycle is useful in understanding the performance of heat engines.
Reason : The Carnot cycle provides a way of determining the maximum possible efficiency achievable with reservoirs of given temperatures.

54. **Assertion :** A *p-n* junction with reverse bias can be used as a photo-diode to measure light intensity.
Reason : In a reverse bias condition the current is small but is more sensitive to changes in incident light intensity.

55. **Assertion :** Perspiration from human body helps in cooling the body.
Reason : A thin layer of water on the skin enhances its emissivity.

56. **Assertion :** When a glass of hot milk is placed in a room and allowed to cool, its entropy decreases.
Reason : Allowing hot object to cool does not violate the second law of thermodynamics.

57. **Assertion :** Cobalt-60 is useful in cancer therapy.
Reason : Cobalt-60 is a source of γ-radiations capable of killing cancerous cells.

58. **Assertion :** A thin stainless steel needle can lay floating on a still water surface.
Reason : Any object floats when the buoyancy force balances the weight of the object.

59. **Assertion :** An emf $\vec{E}$ is induced in a closed loop where magnetic flux is varied. The induced $\vec{E}$ is not a conservative field.
Reason : The line integral $\vec{E} \cdot d\vec{l}$ around the closed loop is non-zero.

60. **Assertion :** In optical fibre, the diameter of the core is kept small.
Reason : This smaller diameter of the core ensures that the fibre should have incident angle more than the critical angle required for total internal reflection.

CHEMISTRY

61. The pair in which both species have same magnetic moment (spin only value) is
(a) $[Cr(H_2O)_6]^{2+}$, $[CoCl_4]^{2-}$
(b) $[Cr(H_2O)_6]^{2+}$, $[Fe(H_2O)_6]^{2+}$
(c) $[Mn(H_2O)_6]^{2+}$, $[Cr(H_2O)_6]^{2+}$
(d) $[CoCl_4]^{2-}$, $[Fe(H_2O)_6]^{2+}$.

62. The pair in which both species have iron is
(a) nitrogenase, cytochromes
(b) carboxypeptidase, haemoglobin
(c) haemocyanin, nitrogenase
(d) haemoglobin, cytochromes.

63. Borax is used as a cleansing agent because on dissolving in water it gives
(a) alkaline solution (b) acidic solution
(c) bleaching solution (d) basic solution.

64. The incorrect statement among the following is
(a) C_{60} is an allotropic form of carbon

(b) O_3 is an allotropic form of oxygen
(c) S_8 is only allotropic form of sulphur
(d) red phosphorus is more stable in air than white phosphorus.

65. The pair whose both species are used in anti-acid medicinal preparation is
(a) $NaHCO_3$ and $Mg(OH)_2$
(b) Na_2CO_3 and $Ca(HCO_3)_2$
(c) $Ca(HCO_3)_2$ and $Mg(OH)_2$
(d) $Ca(OH)_2$ and $NaHCO_3$.

66. The colour imparted by Co(II) compounds to glass is
(a) green (b) deep-blue
(c) yellow (d) red.

67. The number of possible isomers of an octahedral complex $[Co(C_2O_4)_2(NH_3)_2]^-$ is
(a) 1 (b) 2
(c) 3 (d) 4.

68. The ligands in anti-cancer drug cisplatin are
(a) NH_3, Cl (b) NH_3, H_2O
(c) Cl, H_2O (d) NO, Cl.

69. Given below, catalyst and corresponding process/reaction are matched. The mismatch is
(a) $[RhCl(PPh_3)_2]$: hydrogenation
(b) $TiCl_4 + Al(C_2H_5)_3$: polymerization
(c) V_2O_5 : Haber-Bosch process
(d) nickel : hydrogenation.

70. Among the following, the species having square planar geometry for central atom are
(i) XeF_4, (ii) SF_4, (iii) $[NiCl_4]^{2-}$, (iv) $[PdCl_4]^{2-}$
(a) (i) and (iv) (b) (i) and (ii)
(c) (ii) and (iii) (d) (iii) and (iv).

71. Tincture iodine is
(a) aqueous solution of I_2
(b) solution of I_2 in aqueous KI
(c) alcoholic solution of I_2
(d) aqueous solution of KI.

72. In $[Ag(CN)_2]^-$, the number of π bonds is
(a) 2 (b) 3
(c) 4 (d) 6.

73. The compound molecular in nature in gas phase but ionic in solid state is
(a) PCl_5 (b) CCl_4
(c) PCl_3 (d) $POCl_3$.

74. Which two of the following salts are used for preparing iodized salt?
(i) KIO_3, (ii) KI, (iii) I_2, (iv) HI
(a) (i) and (ii) (b) (i) and (iii)
(c) (ii) and (iv) (d) (iii) and (iv).

75. The compound used in enrichment of uranium for nuclear power plant is
(a) U_3O_8 (b) UF_6
(c) $UO_2(NO_3)_2$ (d) UCl_4.

76. The de Broglie wavelength associated with a ball of mass 1 kg having kinetic energy 0.5 J is
(a) 6.626×10^{-34} m (b) 13.20×10^{-34} m
(c) 10.38×10^{-21} m (d) 6.626×10^{-34} Å.

77. Dominance of strong repulsive forces among the molecules of the gas (Z = compressibility factor)
(a) depends on Z and indicated by $Z = 1$
(b) depends on Z and indicated by $Z > 1$
(c) depends on Z and indicated by $Z < 1$
(d) is independent of Z.

78. 40 ml of 0.1 M ammonia solution is mixed with 20 ml of 0.1 M HCl. What is the pH of the mixture? (pK_b of ammonia solution is 4.74)
(a) 4.74 (b) 2.26
(c) 9.26 (d) 5.00

79. For a spontaneous process the correct statement is
(a) entropy of the system always increases
(b) free energy of the system always increases
(c) total entropy change is always negative
(d) total entropy change is always positive.

80. The Ca^{2+} and F^- are located in CaF_2 crystal, respectively at face centred cubic lattice points and in
(a) tetrahedral voids
(b) half of tetrahedral voids
(c) octahedral voids
(d) half of octahedral voids.

81. The charge required for the reduction of 1 mol of MnO_4^- to MnO_2 is
(a) 1 F (b) 3 F
(c) 5 F (d) 6 F.

82. For the reaction, $2N_2O_5 \rightarrow 4NO_2 + O_2$

rate of reaction is

(a) $\frac{1}{2}\frac{d}{dt}[N_2O_5]$ (b) $2\frac{d}{dt}[N_2O_5]$

(c) $\frac{1}{4}\frac{d}{dt}[NO_2]$ (d) $4\frac{d}{dt}[NO_2]$

83. For a phase change

$$H_2O_{(l)} \xrightleftharpoons[0°C,\ 1\ bar]{} H_2O_{(s)}$$

(a) $\Delta G = 0$ (b) $\Delta S = 0$

(c) $\Delta H = 0$ (d) $\Delta U = 0$.

84. A 5% solution (by mass) of cane sugar in water has freezing point of 271 K and freezing point of pure water is 273.15 K. The freezing point of a 5% solution (by mass) of glucose in water is

(a) 271 K (b) 273.15 K

(c) 269.07 K (d) 277.23 K.

85. The energy gaps (E_g) between valence band and conduction band for diamond, silicon and germanium are in the order

(a) E_g (diamond) > E_g (silicon) > E_g (germanium)

(b) E_g (diamond) < E_g (silicon) < E_g (germanium)

(c) E_g (diamond) = E_g (silicon) = E_g (germanium)

(d) E_g (diamond) > E_g (germanium) > E_g (silicon).

86. The enthalpy change (ΔH) for the reaction,

$$N_{2\,(g)} + 3H_{2\,(g)} \rightarrow 2NH_{3\,(g)}$$

is –92.38 kJ at 298 K. The internal energy change ΔU at 298 K is

(a) –92.38 kJ (b) –87.42 kJ

(c) –97.34 kJ (d) –89.9 kJ.

87. The products formed when an aqueous solution of NaBr is electrolysed in a cell having inert electrodes are

(a) Na and Br_2 (b) Na and O_2

(c) H_2, Br_2 and NaOH (d) H_2 and O_2.

88. Among the following L-serine is

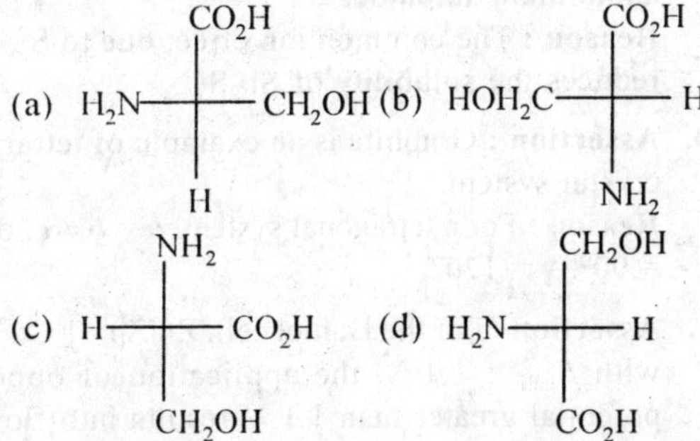

89. Among the following which one can have a meso form?

(a) $CH_3CH(OH)CH(Cl)C_2H_5$

(b) $CH_3CH(OH)CH(OH)CH_3$

(c) $C_2H_5CH(OH)CH(OH)CH_3$

(d) $HOCH_2CH(Cl)CH_3$.

90. Which of the following sequence of reactions (reagents) can be used for the conversion of $C_6H_5CH_2CH_3$ into $C_6H_5CH = CH_2$?

(a) $SOCl_2$; H_2O (b) SO_2Cl_2; alc. KOH

(c) $Cl_2/h\upsilon$; H_2O (d) $SOCl_2$; alc. KOH.

91. Isopropyl benzene on air oxidation in the presence of dilute acid gives

(a) C_6H_5COOH (b) $C_6H_5COCH_3$

(c) C_6H_5CHO (d) C_6H_5OH.

92. The major product obtained on the monobromination (with $Br_2/FeBr_3$) of the following compound *A* is

OCH_3, CH_3 (compound *A*)

(a) OCH_3, Br, CH_3 (b) OCH_3, CH_3, Br

(c) OCH_3, Br, CH_3 (d) OCH_3, Br, CH_3

93. The following sequence of reactions on *A* gives

A (CH_2CONH_2, $COOCH_3$) $\xrightarrow[2.\ heat]{1.\ Br_2/NaOH}$

(a) 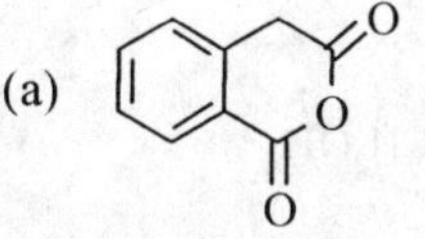 (b) 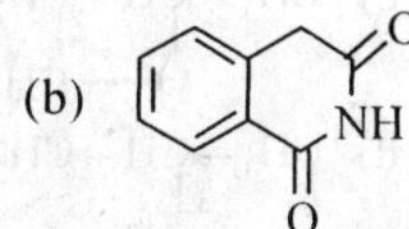

(c) 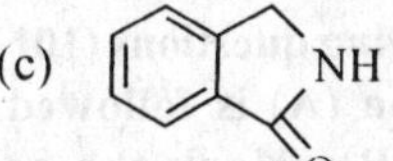 (d) 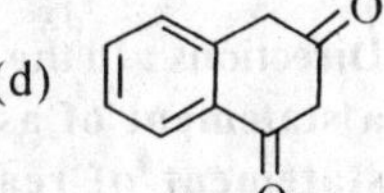

94. Nitrobenzene on treatment with zinc dust and aqueous ammonium chloride gives
(a) $C_6H_5N = N - C_6H_5$
(b) $C_6H_5NH_2$
(c) C_6H_5NO (d) C_6H_5NHOH.

95. Thymine is
(a) 5-methyluracil (b) 4-methyluracil
(c) 3-methyluracil (d) 1-methyluracil.

96. Lysine is least soluble in water in the pH range
(a) 3 to 4 (b) 5 to 6
(c) 6 to 7 (d) 8 to 9.

97. Methyl-α-D-glucoside and methyl-β-D-glucoside are
(a) epimers (b) anomers
(c) enantiomers
(d) conformational diastereomers.

98. Which of the following compounds has the highest boiling point?
(a) $CH_3CH_2CH_2Cl$ (b) $CH_3CH_2CH_2CH_2Cl$
(c) $CH_3CH(CH_3)CH_2Cl$ (d) $(CH_3)_3CCl$.

99. The correct increasing order of the reactivity of halides for S_N1 reaction is
(a) $CH_3 - CH_2 - X < (CH_3)_2CH - X < CH_2 = CH - CH_2 - X < PhCH_2 - X$
(b) $(CH_3)_2CH - X < CH_3 - CH_2 - X < CH_2 = CH - CH_2 - X < PhCH_2 - X$
(c) $PhCH_2 - X < (CH_3)_2CH - X < CH_3 - CH_2 - X < CH_2 = CH - CH_2 - X$
(d) $CH_2 = CH - CH_2 - X < Ph - CH_2 - X < (CH_3)_2CH - X < CH_3 - CH_2 - X$.

100. The major product formed in the following reaction is
$$CH_3CH(Cl)CH_2 - CH_2OH \xrightarrow{\text{aq. KOH}}$$
(a) $CH_3CH = CH - CH_2OH$
(b) $CH_2 = CH - CH_2 - CH_2OH$
(c) $CH_3 - CH - CH_2$ (with the CH and CH_2 linked through O — CH_2, a ring)
(d) $CH_3 - CH(OH) - CH_2 - CH_2OH$

Directions : In the following questions (101-120), a statement of assertion (A) is followed by a statement of reason (R). Mark the correct choice as :
(a) if both assertion and reason are true and reason is the correct explanation of the assertion
(b) if both assertion and reason are true but reason is not the correct explanation of the assertion
(c) if assertion is true, but reason is false
(d) both assertion and reason are false statements.

101. Assertion : In the iodometric titration starch is used as an indicator.
Reason : Starch is a polysaccharide.

102. Assertion : Molecular nitrogen is less reactive than molecular oxygen.
Reason : The bond length of N_2 is shorter than that of oxygen.

103. Assertion : $[Co(NO_2)_3(NH_3)_3]$ does not show optical isomerism.
Reason : It has a plane of symmetry.

104. Assertion : $E°$ for Mn^{3+}/Mn^{2+} is more positive than Cr^{3+}/Cr^{2+}.
Reason : The third ionization energy of Mn is larger than that of Cr.

105. Assertion : $K_2Cr_2O_7$ is used as primary standard in volumetric analysis.
Reason : It has a good solubility in water.

106. Assertion : Silicones are hydrophobic in nature.
Reason : Si – O – Si linkages are moisture sensitive.

107. Assertion : According to transition state theory, for the formation of an activated complex, one of the vibrational degrees of freedom is converted into a translational degree of freedom.
Reason : Energy of the activated complex is higher than the energy of reactant molecules.

108. Assertion : Water in liquid state is more stable than ice at room temperature.
Reason : Water in liquid form has higher entropy than ice.

109. Assertion : Sb_2S_3 is not soluble in yellow ammonium sulphide.
Reason : The common ion effect due to S^{2-} ions reduces the solubility of Sb_2S_3.

110. Assertion : Graphite is an example of tetragonal crystal system.
Reason : For a tetragonal system, $a = b \neq c$, $\alpha = \beta = 90°$, $\gamma = 120°$.

111. Assertion : For the Daniel cell, $Zn|Zn^{2+} || Cu^{2+}|Cu$ with $E_{cell} = 1.1$ V, the application of opposite potential greater than 1.1 V results into flow of

electron from cathode to anode.
Reason : Zn is deposited at anode and Cu is dissolved at cathode.

112. **Assertion :** Fe^{3+} can be used for coagulation of As_2S_3 sol.
Reason : Fe^{3+} reacts with As_2S_3 to give Fe_2S_3.

113. **Assertion :** If red blood cells were removed from the body and placed in pure water, pressure inside the cells increases.
Reason : The concentration of salt content in the cells increases.

114. **Assertion :** Change in colour of acidic solution of potassium dichromate by breath is used to test drunk drivers.
Reason : Change in colour is due to the complexation of alcohol with potassium dichromate.

115. **Assertion :** Anilinium chloride is more acidic than ammonium chloride.
Reason : Anilinium ion is resonance-stabilised.

116. **Assertion :** Diastereomers have different physical properties.
Reason : They are non-superimposable mirror images.

117. **Assertion :** The presence of nitro group facilitates nucleophilic substitution reactions in aryl halides.
Reason : The intermediate carbanion is stabilised due to the presence of nitro group.

118. **Assertion :** 1,3-butadiene is the monomer for natural rubber.
Reason : Natural rubber is formed through anionic addition polymerization.

119. **Assertion :** Addition of HBr on 2-butene gives two isomeric products.
Reason : Addition of HBr on 2-butene follows Markovnikov's rule.

120. **Assertion :** The water pouch of instant cold pack for treating athletic injuries breaks when squeezed and NH_4NO_3 dissolves lowering the temperature.
Reason : Addition of non-volatile solute into solvent results into depression of freezing point of solvent.

BIOLOGY

121. Given below is a table comparing the effects of sympathetic and parasympathetic nervous system for four feature (1–4). Which one feature is correctly described ?

Feature	Sympathetic nervous system	Parasympathetic nervous system
(a) salivary glands	stimulates secretion	inhibits secretion
(b) pupil of the eye	dilate	constricts
(c) heart rate	decreases	increases
(d) intestinal peristalsis	stimulates	inhibits

122. Which one of the following animals is correctly, matched with its one characteristic and the taxon ?

Animal	Characteristic	Taxon
(a) millipede	ventral nerve cord	arachnida
(b) duckbill platypus	oviparous	mammalia
(c) silverfish	pectoral & pelvic fins	chordata
(d) sea anemone	triploblastic	cnidaria

123. All mammals without any exception are characterized by
(a) viviparity and biconcave red blood cells
(b) extra-abdominal testes and a four chambered heart
(c) heterodont teeth and 12 pairs of cranial nerves
(d) a muscular diaphragm and milk producing glands

124. Which one of the following pairs of the kind of cells and their secretion is correctly matched ?
(a) oxyntic cells — a secretion with pH between 2.0 and 3.0
(b) alpha cells of islets of Langerhans — secretion that decreases blood sugar level
(c) Kupffer cells — a digestive enzyme that hydrolyses nucleic acids
(d) sebaceous glands — a secretion that evaporates for cooling

125. Examine the diagram of the two cell types A and B given below and select the correct option

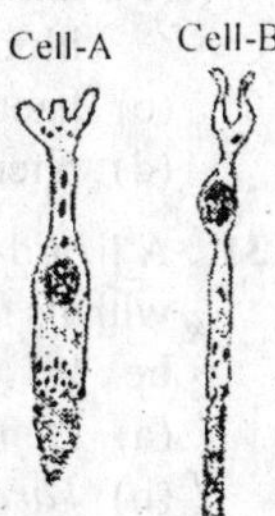

(a) cell A is the rod cell found evenly all over retina
(b) cell A is the cone cell more concentrated in the fovea centralis

(c) cell B is concerned with colour vision in bright light
(d) cell A is sensitive to low light intensities

126. Which one of the following pairs of features is a good example of polygenic inheritance ?
(a) human height and skin colour
(b) ABO blood group in humans and flower colour of *Mirabilis jalapa*
(c) hair pigment of mouse and tongue rolling in humans
(d) human eye colour and sickle cell anaemia

127. Mating of an organism to a double recessive in order to determine whether it is homozygous or heterozygous for a character under consideration is called
(a) reciprocal cross (b) test cross
(c) dihybrid cross (d) back cross

128. In which one of the following sets of three items each belong to the category mentioned against them?
(a) lysine, glycine, thiamine — amino acids
(b) myosin, oxytocin and gastrin — hormones
(c) rennin, helicase and hyaluronidase — enzymes
(d) optic nerve, oculomotor, vagus — sensory nerves

129. A cricket player is fast chasing a ball in the field. Which one of the following groups of bones are **directly** contributing in this movement ?
(a) femur, malleus, tibia, metatarsals
(b) pelvis, ulna, patella, tarsals
(c) sternum, femur, tibia, fibula
(d) tarsals, femur, metatarsals, tibia

130. Given below is a highly simplified representation of the human sex chromosomes from a karyotype.
Gene *a*
Gene *b*
The gene *a* and *b* could be of
(a) colour blindness and body height
(b) attached ear lobe and Rhesus blood group
(c) haemophilia and red-green colour blindness
(d) phenylketonuria and haemophilia

131. A lizard-like member of reptilia is sitting on a tree with its tail coiled around a twig. This animal could be
(a) *Hemidactylus* showing sexual dimorphism
(b) *Varanus* showing mimicry
(c) garden lizard (*Calotes*) showing camouflage
(d) *Chamaeleon* showing protective colouration

132. The figure given below shows three velocity-substrate concentration curves for an enzyme reaction. What do the curves a, b, and c depict respectively ?

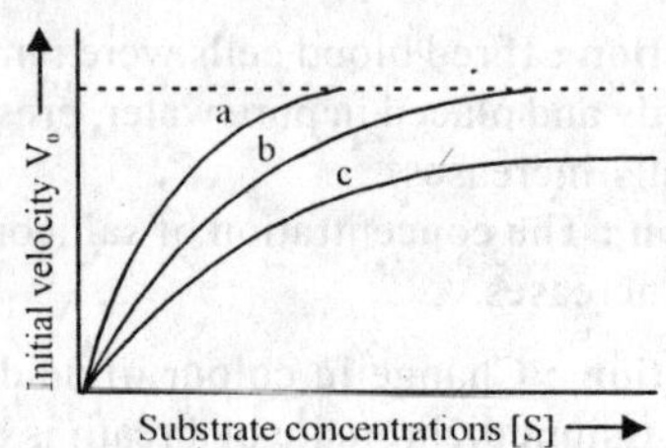

(a) a-normal enzyme reaction, b-competitive inhibition, c-non-competitive inhibition
(b) a-enzyme with an allosteric modulator added, b-normal enzyme activity, c-competitive inhibition
(c) a-enzyme with an allosteric stimulator, b-competitive inhibition added c-normal enzyme reaction
(d) a-normal enzyme reaction, b-non-competitive inhibitor added c-allosteric inhibitor added

133. Pollution from animal excreta and organic waste from kitchen can be most profitably minimized by
(a) storing them in underground storage tanks
(b) using them for producing biogas
(c) vermiculture
(d) using them directly as biofertilizers

134. A person who shows unpredictable moods, outbursts of emotion, quarrelsome behaviour and conflicts with others is suffering from
(a) borderline personality disorder (BPD)
(b) mood disorder
(c) addictive disorder (d) schizophrenia

135. Genes present in the cytoplasm of eukaryotic cells are found in
(a) mitochondria and inherited *via* egg cytoplasm
(b) lysosomes and peroxisomes
(c) golgi bodies and smooth endoplasmic reticulum
(d) plastids and inherited *via* male gamete

136. The type of epithelial cells which line the inner surface of fallopian tubes, bronchioles and small bronchi are known as

(a) squamous epithelium
(b) columnar epithelium
(c) ciliated epithelium
(d) cubical epithelium

137. Tadpoles of frog can be made to grow as giant sized tadpoles, if they are
(a) administered antithyroid substance like thiourea
(b) administered large amounts of thyroxine
(c) reared on a diet rich in egg yolk
(d) reared on a diet rich in both egg yolk and glucose

138. When children play bare footed in pools of dirty water and flood water, they may suffer from disease like
(a) leptospirosis and bilharzia
(b) malaria, amoebic dysentery and leptospirosis
(c) bilharzia, infective hepatitis and diarrhoea
(d) guinea worm infection, elephantiasis and amoebic dysentery

139. Which one of the following is an environment-related disorder with the correct main cause ?
(a) black lung disease (pneumoconiosis) found mainly in workers in stone quarries and crushers
(b) blue baby disease (methaemoglobinaemia) due to heavy use of nitrogenous fertilizers in the area
(c) Non-hodgkin's lymphoma found mainly in workers involved in manufacture of neem based pesticides
(d) skin cancer mainly in people exposed to benzene and methane

140. The given figure shows an angiogram of the coronary blood vessel. Which one of the following statements correctly describes, what is being done ?

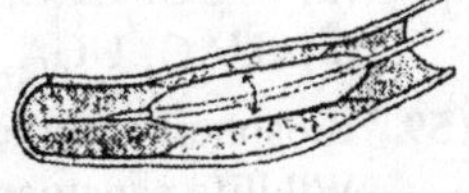

(a) it is coronary artery which has a cancerous growth that is being removed
(b) it is coronary artery which is blocked by a plaque and the same is being cracked
(c) it is coronary vein in which the defective valves are being opened
(d) it is coronary vein blocked by a parasite (blood fluke) that is being removed

141. In the following table identify the correct matching of the crop, its disease and the corresponding pathogen.

	Crop	Disease	Pathogen
(a)	citrus	canker	*Pseudomonas rubrilineans*
(b)	potato	late blight	*Fusarium udum*
(c)	brinjal	root-knot	*Meloidogyne incognita*
(d)	pigeon pea	seed gall	*Phytophthora infestans*

142. In which one of the following combinations (a-d) of the number of chromosomes is the present day hexaploid wheat correctly represented ?

Combination	Monosomic	Haploid	Nullisomic	Trisomic
(a)	21	28	42	43
(b)	7	28	40	42
(c)	21	7	42	43
(d)	41	21	40	43

143. Grafting is successful in dicots but not in monocots because the dicots have
(a) vascular bundles arranged in a ring
(b) cambium for secondary growth
(c) vessels with elements arranged end to end
(d) cork cambium

144. In the sieve elements, which one of the following is the most likely function of P-proteins ?
(a) deposition of callose on sieve plates
(b) providing energy for active translocation
(c) autolytic enzymes
(d) sealing mechanism on wounding

145. Myxomycetes are
(a) saprobes or parasites, having mycelia, asexual reproduction by fragmentation, sexual reproduction by fusion of gametes
(b) slimy mass of multinucleate protoplasm, having pseudopodia-like structures for engulfing food, reproduction through fragmentation or zoospores
(c) prokaryotic organisms, cellular or acellular, saprobes or autotrophic, reproduce by binary fission
(d) eukaryotic, single-celled or filamentous, saprobes or autotrophic, asexual reproduction by fusion of two cells or their nuclei

146. "Ordines Anomali" of Bentham and Hooker includes

(a) seed plants showing abnormal forms of growth and development
(b) plants described only in fossil state
(c) plants described in the literature but which Bentham and Hooker did not see in original
(d) a few orders which could not be placed satisfactorily in the classification

147. Hirudin is
(a) a protein produced by *Hordeum vulgare*, which is rich in lysine
(b) a toxic molecule isolated from *Gossypium hirsutum*, which reduces human fertility
(c) a protein produced from transgenic *Brassica napus*, which prevents blood clotting
(d) an antibiotic produced by a genetically engineered bacterium, *Escherichia coli*

148. A scion is grafted to a stock. The quality of fruits produced will be determined by the genotype of
a) stock
(b) scion
(c) both stock and scion
(d) neither stock nor scion

149. In prokaryotes, chromatophores are
(a) specialized granules responsible for colouration of cells
(b) structures responsbile for organizing the shape of the organism
(c) inclusion bodies lying free inside the cells for carrying out various metabolic activities
(d) internal membrane systems that may become extensive and complex in photosynthetic bacteria

150. Among rust, smut and mushroom all the three
(a) are pathogens (b) are saprobes
(c) bear ascocarps (d) bear basidiocarps

151. The function of leghaemoglobin during biological nitrogen fixation in root nodules of legumes is to
(a) convert atmospheric N_2 to NH_3
(b) convert ammonia to nitrite
(c) transport oxygen for activity of nitrogenase
(d) protect nitrogenase from oxygen

152. *Avena* curvature test is a bioassay for examining the activity of
(a) auxins (b) gibberellins
(c) cytokinins (d) ethylene

153. What is common between chloroplasts, chromoplasts and leucoplasts ?
(a) presence of pigments
(b) possession of thylakoids and grana
(c) storage of starch, proteins and lipids
(d) ability to multiply by a fission-like process

154. Plants of which one of the following groups of genera are pollinated by the same agency ?
(a) *Triticum, Cocos, Mangifera*
(b) *Ficus, Kigelia, Casuarina*
(c) *Salvia, Morus, Euphorbia*
(d) *Bombax, Butea, Bauhinia*

155. The Montreal Protocol refers to
(a) persistent organic pollutants
(b) global warming and climate change
(c) substances that deplete the ozone layer
(d) biosafety of genetically modified organisms

156. Keystone species deserve protection because these
(a) are capable of surviving in harsh environmental conditions
(b) indicate presence of certain minerals in the soil
(c) have become rare due to overexploitation
(d) play an important role in supporting other species

157. In India, we find mangoes with different flavours, colours, fibre content, sugar content and even shelf-life. The large variation is on account of
(a) species diversity (b) induced mutations
(c) genetic diversity (d) hybridization

158. During protein synthesis in an organism at one point the process comes to a halt. Select the group of the three codons from the following, from which any one of the three could bring about this halt.
(a) UUU, UCC, UAU (b) UUC, UUA, UAC
(c) UAG, UGA, UAA (d) UUG, UCA, UCG

159. Biosphere reserves differ from National Parks and Wildlife sanctuaries because in the former
(a) human beings are not allowed to enter
(b) people are an integral part of the system
(c) plants are paid greater attention than the animals
(d) living organisms are brought from all over the world and preserved for posterity

160. Somaclonal variation is seen in
(a) tissue culture grown plants
(b) apomicts (c) polyploids
(d) vegetatively propagated plants

Direction : In the following questions (161–180), a statement of assertion is given and a corresponding statement of reason is given just below it. Of the statements, mark the correct answer as -

(a) *If both Assertion & Reason are true and the reason is the correct explanation of the assertion.*

(b) *It both Assertion & Reason are true but the reason is not the correct explanation of the assertion.*

(c) *If Assertion is true statement but Reason is false.*

(d) *It both Assertion and Reason are false statements.*

161. Assertion : A person who has received a cut and is bleeding needs to be given anti-tetanus treatment.
Reason : Anti-tetanus injection provides immunity by producing antibodies for tetanus.

162. Assertion : Cancer cells are virtually immortal until the body in which they reside dies.
Reason : Cancer is caused by damage to genes regulating the cell division cycle.

163. Assertion : A network of food chains existing together in an ecosystem is known as a food web.
Reason : An animal like kite cannot be a part of a food web.

164. Assertion : Inflammation of a skeletal joint may immobilize the movements of the joint.
Reason : Uric acid crystals in the joint cavity and ossification of articular cartilage lead to this.

165. Assertion : The earliest organisms that appeared on the Earth were non-green and presumably anaerobes.
Reason : The first autotrophic organisms were the chemoautotrophs that never released oxygen.

166. Assertion : *Escherichia coli, Shigella* sp. and *Salmonella* sp. are all responsible for diarrhoeal disease.
Reason : Dehydration is common to all types of diarrhoeal diseases and adequate supply of fluids electrolytes should be ensured.

167. Assertion : Deforestation is one main factor contributing to global warming.
Reason : Besides CO_2, two other gases methane and CFCs are also included under green house gases.

168. Assertion : LSD and marijuana are clinically used as analgesics.
Reason : Both these drugs suppress brain function.

169. Assertion : An organism with lethal mutation may not even develop beyond the zygote stage.
Reason : All types of gene mutations are lethal.

170. Assertion : Our body secretes adrenaline in intense cold.
Reason : Adrenaline raises metabolic rate.

171. Assertion : When the ambient temperature is high and soil contains excess of water, the plants tend to lose water in the form of droplets from lenticels.
Reason : Root pressure regulates the rate of loss of water form lenticels.

172. Assertion : In angiosperms the conduction of water is more efficient because their xylem has vessels.
Reason : Conduction of water by vessel elements is an active process with energy supplied by xylem parenchyma rich in mitochondria.

173. Assertion : Polytene chromosomes have a high amount of DNA.
Reason : Polytene chromosomes are formed by repeated replication of chromosomal DNA without separation of chromatids.

174. Assertion : UV radiation causes photodissociation of ozone into O_2 and O, thus causing damage to the stratospheric ozone layer.
Reason : Ozone hole is resulting in global warming and climate change.

175. Assertion : The concentration of methane in the atmosphere has more than doubled in the last 250 years.
Reason : Wetlands and rice fields are the major sources of methane.

176. Assertion : In tropical rain forests, O-horizon and A-horizon of soil profile are shallow and nutrient-poor.
Reason : Excessive growth of micro-organisms in the soil depletes its organic content.

177. Assertion : Gram-negative bacteria do not retain the stain when washed with alcohol.
Reason : The outer face of the outer membrane of Gram-negative bacteria contains lipopolysaccharides, a part of which is integrated into the membrane lipids.

178. Assertion : Under conditions of high light intensity and limited CO_2 supply, photorespiration has a useful role in protecting the plants from photo-oxidative damage.

Reason : If enough CO_2 is not available to utilize light energy for carboxylation to proceed, the excess energy may not cause damage to plants.

179. Assertion : Photosynthetically C_4 plants are less efficient than C_3 plants.

Reason : The operation of C_4 pathway requires the involvement of only bundle-sheath cells.

180. Assertion : Eukaryotic cells have the ability to adopt a variety of shapes and carry out directed movements.

Reason : There are three principal types of protein filaments - microfilaments, microtubules and intermediate filaments, which constitute the cytoskeleton.

GENERAL KNOWLEDGE

181. The term 'CPR' often used in first aid stands for
(a) Clinic for Pulmonary Rehabilitation
(b) Chemical Prevention of Rhinitis
(c) Chemo-Prophylaxis response
(d) Cardio-Pulmonary resuscitation

182. Alzheimer's disease affects
(a) childhood (b) adolescent
(c) young people (d) elderly people

183. Central Council for Research in Yoga and Naturopathy (CCRYN) is an organization that funds research in the given field in our country. It is located in
(a) New Delhi (b) Rishikesh
(c) Bangalore (d) Hyderabad

184. The vaccination for which one of the following diseases is not covered in the immunization schedule so far ?
(a) tuberculosis (b) diphtheria
(c) measles (d) pneumonia

185. Which one of the following is true and is not a misconception ?
(a) cutting the top of a bitter cucumber and rubbing it with the corresponding surface removes bitterness
(b) pearl is produced from a drop of rain water falling into the oyster in Swati Nakshatra
(c) while dreaming during sleep at night the eyes move rapidly
(d) peahen gets conceived from the tears that drop from the peacock's eye and she drinks them

186. A drug called reserpine was discovered by
(a) Jal Vakil (b) Paul Ehrlish
(c) Hansen (d) Alexander Wood

187. Biometry refers to
(a) identification of humans by scanning face and fingerprints
(b) measurement of mechanical displacement in humans
(c) a method of lie detection
(d) body length relationships across the evolutionary scale

188. Which one of the following is one of the two days when the sun rises exactly in the east ?
(a) 14th January (b) 21st March
(c) 21st June (d) 23nd December

189. X-rays were discovered by
(a) Wilhelm K. Roentgen
(b) H. Kissinger
(c) Sir C.V. Raman (d) Meghnad Saha

190. Which one of the following literary titles is correctly matched with its author ?
(a) Ramayana - Tulsidas
(b) Mahabharat - Vedvyas
(c) Kumarsambhav - Ravidas
(d) Shakuntala - Bhushan

191. A very much publicized treatment method "DOTS" is being adopted for the cure of
(a) dementia (b) tetanus
(c) tuberculosis
(d) sexually transmitted disease

192. Which of the following Indian cricket player after India-Pakistan ODI (One-day International) at Abudhabi became no.1 ODI batsman in the ICC (International Cricket Club) ranking
(a) Rahul Dravid (b) Yuvraj
(c) Sachin Tendulkar (d) M.S. Dhoni

193. The Jungle in Rudyard Kipplling's Jungle book, describes which part of Indian forest ?
(a) central Indian forest near Satpura range
(b) Uttaranchal thick forest
(c) Himalayan forest in Himachal
(d) Niligiri jungles

194. Sardar Sarovar Dam is built on the river
(a) Jhelam (b) Narmada
(c) Tapti (d) Vyas

195. One ream of paper equals to
(a) 100-110 sheets (b) 256 sheets
(c) 480-500 sheets (d) 1000 sheets

196. Which of the following honour is given by UNESCO ?
(a) the Kalinga prize
(b) Magasay award
(c) Pulitzer prize
(d) order of the Golden Ark award

197. 'Body line' in cricket refers to
(a) bowling that hits the body
(b) the line of body close to wicket line
(c) the white line on ground within which the player stands
(d) the line of moving ball

198. 'Hindu view of life' is written by
(a) S. Radhakrishnan (b) R.K. Narayan
(c) V.D. Savarkar (d) John Ruskin

199. Lagoon refers to
(a) a full moon
(b) the sea breaking into the land and then separated by sand dunes
(c) a spot in a desert made fertile by presence of water
(d) horse shoe shaped coral reef

200. Ecology deals with
(a) the earth and planets
(b) the relationship between organism and their environments
(c) the life under the sea
(d) economical growth of poor people

SOLUTIONS

PHYSICS

1. (c)

2. (d) : Acceleration is independent of mass in kinematics.

3. (b) : Moment of inertia of uniform rod about one end $= \frac{ML^2}{3}$

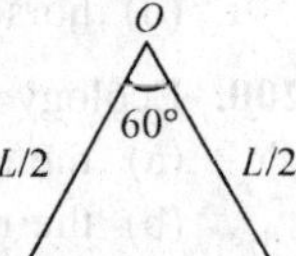

$\therefore$ Moment of inertia of a rod about an axis passing through O and perpendicular to the plane of the rod will be

$= 2\left(\frac{M}{2}\right)\frac{(L/2)^2}{3} = \frac{ML^2}{4\times 3} = \frac{ML^2}{12}$.

4. (c) : $\lambda = 100$ m, $v = 25$ m/s

$\therefore \quad \upsilon = \frac{25}{100} = 0.25$ Hz. $\quad \therefore \quad T = 4$ s.

5. (c) : Pressure difference between lungs and atmosphere = 760 mm – 750 mm = 10 mm = 1 cm of Hg.
Pressure difference $= 1 \times 13.6 \times g = l \times 1 \times g$ of water
i.e., one can draw from a depth of 13.6 cm of water.

6. (c) : Electric field between the sheets is

$$E = \frac{\sigma}{\varepsilon_0} = \frac{26.4\times 10^{-12}}{8.85\times 10^{-12}} \approx 3 \text{ N/C.}$$

7. (b) : The S.I. unit of magnetic moment is Am^2. Therefore its dimensions is $[\text{L}^2\text{A}]$.

8. (a) : $u = -8$ cm, $f = 10$ cm

As, $\frac{1}{v} - \frac{1}{u} = \frac{1}{f}$,

$\therefore \quad \frac{1}{v} = \frac{1}{f} + \frac{1}{u} = \frac{1}{10} + \frac{1}{-8} = \frac{1}{10} - \frac{1}{8} = \frac{4-5}{40} = \frac{-1}{40}$

or, $\quad v = -40$ cm.

Magnification produced by the lens,

$m = \frac{v}{u} = \frac{-40}{-8} = 5.$

This is a virtual image, erect and on the same side as the object.

9. (b) : $\lambda_{min} = \frac{hc}{eV} = \frac{1.242\times 10^{-6}}{V}$

$V = \frac{1.242\times 10^{-6}}{10^{-11}} = 124.2$ kV

The accelerating voltage for electrons in X-ray machine should be greater than 124.2 kV.

10. (b) : Minimum energy *i.e.* minimum frequency is needed.

11. (b) : Let f be focal length of lens.

$\frac{1}{f} = ({}^a\mu_g - 1)\left(\frac{1}{R_1} - \frac{1}{R_2}\right) = (1.5-1)\left(\frac{1}{R_1} - \frac{1}{R_2}\right)$

or, $\quad \frac{1}{f} = 0.5\left(\frac{1}{R_1} - \frac{1}{R_2}\right)$ or, $\frac{1}{R_1} - \frac{1}{R_2} = \frac{1}{0.5f}$ .. (i)

Let f' be focal length of the lens when immersed in a liquid.

$\frac{1}{f'} = ({}^L\mu_g - 1)\left(\frac{1}{R_1} - \frac{1}{R_2}\right) = \left(\frac{1.5}{1.25} - 1\right)\left(\frac{1}{R_1} - \frac{1}{R_2}\right)$

$= \left(\frac{0.25}{1.25}\right)\left(\frac{1}{R_1} - \frac{1}{R_2}\right) = \frac{0.25}{1.25} \times \frac{1}{0.5f}$ (using (i))

$\frac{1}{f'} = \frac{1}{2.5f}$ or, $f' = 2.5f$.

i.e. focal length of lens when immersed in a liquid is increased by a factor of 2.5.

12. (a) : Work done = charge × potential difference
$W = 4 \times (4 \times 10^6 - 0) = 16 \times 10^6$ J.

Power of the lightening strike, $P = \frac{W}{t}$

$= \frac{16\times 10^6}{100\times 10^{-3}} = 160$ MW.

13. (c) : Between the points P and Q, a capacitor C_1 and series combination of C_2, C_3, C_4, C_5 are connected in parallel.

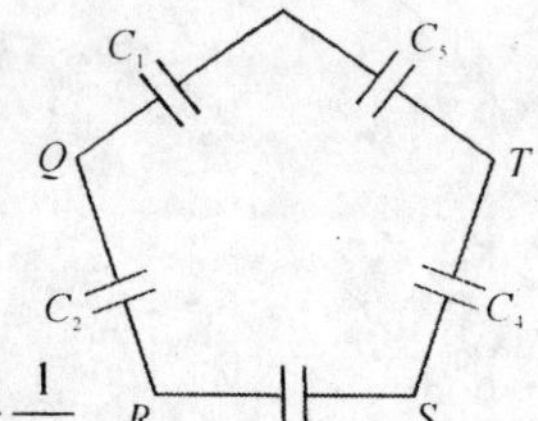

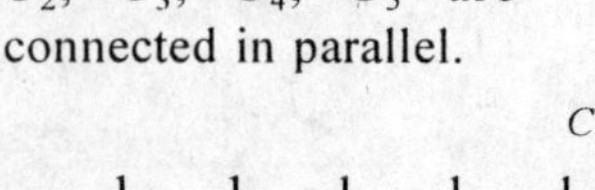

$\therefore \quad \frac{1}{C_s} = \frac{1}{C_2} + \frac{1}{C_3} + \frac{1}{C_4} + \frac{1}{C_5}$

$$=\frac{1}{C}+\frac{1}{C}+\frac{1}{C}+\frac{1}{C}=\frac{4}{C}$$

or, $C_s = C/4$.

The equivalent capacitance between P and Q is

$$C' = C_1 + C_s = C + \frac{C}{4} = \frac{5C}{4}$$

Between the points P and R a series combination of C_1, C_2 and a series combination of C_3, C_4, C_5 are connected in parallel.

$$\therefore \frac{1}{C_s'} = \frac{1}{C_1} + \frac{1}{C_2} = \frac{1}{C} + \frac{1}{C} = \frac{2}{C} \text{ or, } C' = \frac{C}{2}$$

$$\frac{1}{C_s''} = \frac{1}{C_3} + \frac{1}{C_4} + \frac{1}{C_5} = \frac{1}{C} + \frac{1}{C} + \frac{1}{C} = \frac{3}{C} \text{ or, } C'' = \frac{C}{3}$$

The equivalent capacitance between P and R is

$$C'' = C_s' + C_s'' = \frac{C}{2} + \frac{C}{3} = \frac{5C}{6}$$

$$\therefore \frac{C''}{C'} = \frac{(5C/6)}{(5C/4)} = \frac{4}{6} = \frac{2}{3}.$$

14. (a) : For circular wave, intensity $I \propto \frac{1}{r}$.

Amplitude, $A \propto \sqrt{I}$, $A \propto \sqrt{\frac{1}{r}}$ or, $A \propto r^{-1/2}$.

15. (d) : In inelastic collision linear momentum is conserved, but total kinetic energy is not conserved.

16. (b) : In reverse biased, the depletion region of *p-n* diode is increased.

17. (b) : By superposition of two perpendicular waves polarised and having a phase difference of $\pi/2$ will result in circular polarisation of light.

18. (a) : If it is less than one, reaction can be sustained and if the multiplication factor is more than one, the reaction becomes uncontrolled. It is an explosion.

19. (a) : $Y = \overline{\overline{A \cdot B}} = A \cdot B$

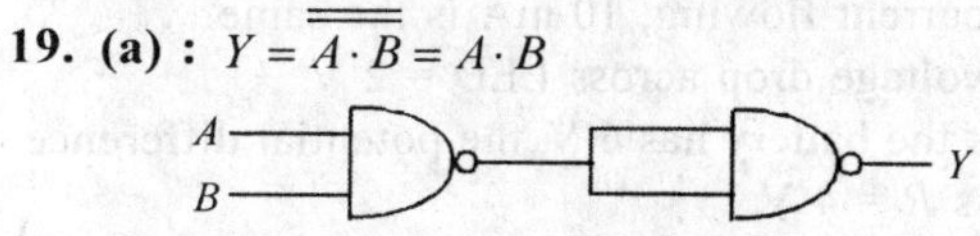

The given circuit is AND gate.

20. (c) : First a force is used to move the body when it has to be more than the static friction. Then the body starts moving and is getting accelerated. Then suddenly the force is decreased to match the kinetic friction. The body then moves with a constant velocity.

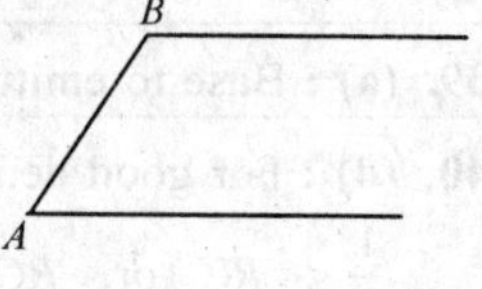

Force > $\mu_s \cdot N$.

Constant acceleration, velocity increases proportionately with time. Then suddenly force applied is just equal to $\mu_K N$. It is just sufficient to cancel friction. Whatever be the earlier maximum velocity attained will be continued.

21. (b) : Black object. That which can absorb maximum can also emit maximum. (Kirchhoff's law).

22. (b) : Assuming the balloons have the same volume, as $PV = nRT$, if P, V and T are the same, n, the number of moles present will be the same, whether it is He or air *i.e.* nitrogen will be the same.

23. (d) : If the voltage is not sufficient to heat it to white hot temperature, the filament will become red. But the intensity will be very much reduced because of low voltage. But if the voltage is only reduced a little only intensity will be reduced. It can be (a) also.

24. (a) : The lines proceed from the positive and lines will reach B, if B is negative.

The number of lines/unit area *i.e.* the density of lines is greater for the greater charge.

A is +ve, B is –ve and $|A| > |B|$.

25. (a) : Magnetic field due to a circular loop at the centre of the loop is $B_1 = \frac{\mu_0}{4\pi}\frac{2\pi I_c}{R}$.

Magnetic field due to a straight line at the centre of the loop is $B_2 = \frac{\mu_0 2I_e}{4\pi H}$

Both these fields act in opposite direction hence total magnetic field at the centre of the loop is

$$B = B_1 - B_2 = \frac{\mu_0 2\pi I_c}{4\pi R} - \frac{\mu_0 2I_e}{4\pi H}$$

$B = 0$ (given).

$$\therefore \frac{\mu_0 2\pi I_c}{4\pi R} = \frac{\mu_0 2I_e}{4\pi H} \text{ or, } H = \frac{I_e R}{\pi I_c}.$$

26. (a) : Pattern A is more sturdy because the moment of the tension about the fulcrum is maximum in A to counterbalance the moment of mg acting from the centre of mass of the rod.

27. (b) : Emission of alpha particle, decrease the mass

number by 4 and charge number by 2.

$\therefore$ Decrease in mass number = 238 – 4 = 234

Decrease in charge number = 92 – 2 = 90

${}^{234}_{90}Th$ is emitted.

28. (c) : After 5730 years, the number of C^{14} remaining is $\frac{1}{2}^{th}$ original. To have (1/16) original value, it takes $(1/2)^4$, 4 half lives.

Therefore, the bone is 4 × 5730 years = 22920 years old.

29. (c) : According to conservation of mass number

10 + 4 = 13 + 1

According to conservation of charge number,

5 + 2 ≠ 7 + 1

Hence (a) is not possible.

According to conservation of charge number,

93 = 94 – 1

According to conservation of mass number,

239 = 239

Hence (c) is possible.

According to conservation of mass number,

11 + 1 = 12

According to conservation of charge number,

7 + 1 ≠ 6 – 1

Hence (d) is not possible.

${}^{23}_{11}Na + {}^{1}_{1}H$ also satisfies both the conservation of mass number and charge. However, ^{23}Na is a very stable isotope and nuclear reaction will be very difficult. The formation of Pu from Np is well known. It satisfies the conditions of conservations and Np is also very unstable. Therefore (c) is the only correct answer.

30. (a) : υ – 5 = 440 Hz

υ – 8 = 437 Hz

(υ; 5; 440 Hz; 3; 437 Hz)

$\therefore$ υ = 445 Hz by both the methods.

It could have been 435 Hz. It would have satisfied 440 – υ = 5. But this would not have satisfied 437 Hz.

31. (b) :

1. When the ring is just entering the magnetic field, emf is induced and the current flows in one direction.

2. When the whole ring is surrounding the flux inside, there is no change in the flux.

Induced emf = 0, current is zero.

3. When the ring just goes out of the region of flux, a pulse of current is produced which is opposite to that of 1 given above.

(b) is the only figure that describes this.

32. (d) : If the momentum of α and β particles are p, if this is also equal to $h\upsilon/c$ of the photon - γ-rays,

$\lambda_{\text{de Broglie}} = h/p$

As p is the same, the wavelength will be the same. For α and β particles, they are de Broglie waves and in the case of photons (γ-rays), it is the wavelength of the associated electromagnetic wave.

33. (b) : Voltage gain in dB = $20 \log_{10} A_V$

$= 20 \log_{10}(1000) = 60$ B.

34. (c) : Entropy is a measure of disorder.

When water is converted to ice, disorder decreases, entropy decreases.

35. (b) : When the bimetallic strip is kept in a cold bath, the length of X decreases faster and therefore the strip binds towards the left.

36. (c) : As $v = \upsilon\lambda$, the velocity = frequency × wavelength. When light is travelling in a medium, υ is assumed to be the same and the velocity of light in the medium is less. λ gets adjusted so that $\frac{c'}{\lambda'} = \upsilon$. Here υ is independent.

It is frequency of light *i.e.* energy that is a constant. Wavelength and velocity change. $\therefore c/\lambda$ = constant.

37. (b)

38. (d) : As LED is connected to a battery through a resistance in series.

The current flowing, 10 mA is the same.

The voltage drop across LED = 2 V

$\therefore$ As the battery has 6 V, the potential difference across R = 4 V.

$\therefore iR = 4\text{ V} \Rightarrow R = \frac{4\text{ V}}{10 \times 10^{-3}\text{ A}} = 400\ \Omega.$

39. (a) : Base to emitter in Si transistor is 1 V.

40. (d) : For good demodulation,

$\frac{1}{f} << RC$ or, $RC >> \frac{1}{f}$.

41. If the frequencies of the waves are less than that of the critical frequency. They will be reflected back as the ionosphere has refractive index less than free space. This is the principle of sky wave propagation. Therefore the assertion is wrong.
The statement given in the reason that the refractive index becomes high is correct. But the reason given is not true for the assertion.
Assertion is wrong. Reason-statement is correct. But not the reason. We have to put (e) as this is a rare case where the assertion itself is wrong.

42. (b) : The decrease in binding energy per nucleon for heavy nuclei ($A > 100$) due to increase in coulomb repulsion between the protons inside the nucleus.

43. (c) : The common base configuration of *npn* transistor is used for voltage amplification. The current amplification is very small. Assertion is true.
The collector is reverse biased for voltage amplification. The reason given has not mentioned that it is voltage amplification. The reason is therefore incomplete by itself. It is wrong.

44. (b) : In an isolated system the entropy increases in accordance with the second law of thermodynamics.

45. (a) : Magnetic Resonance Imaging is based on the nuclear magnetic resonance of protons.
Therefore both assertion and reason are correct.

46. (a) : Rotation of the opponent makes it difficult for the person rotated to resist. Any torque given by a force by pushing the person about an axis will be resisted but not the torque by rotation. By bringing him close to the hip, the opponents moment of inertia is reduced.

47. (d) : $v_{r.m.s} = \sqrt{\frac{3kT}{m}}$ or, $\sqrt{\frac{3RT}{M}}$

$v_{probable} = \sqrt{\frac{2kT}{m}}$ or, $\sqrt{\frac{2RT}{M}}$

$\therefore$ Assertion is wrong.

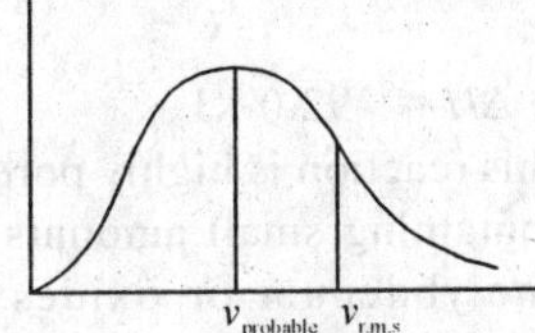

This is asymmetric. Therefore reason is also wrong.

48. (c) : Assertion is correct. But ball bearing is used for reducing friction.

49. (a)

50. (d) : Diamagnetic materials have $L = 0, S = 0, J = 0$. They have no magnetic moment. Reason given is wrong.

51. (b) : If a man inside a lift which is falling freely *i.e.* with acceleration *g*, the relative acceleration of the man with respect to the lift
= acceleration of man with respect to earth (g)
– acceleration of lift with respect to earth, g
$= g - g = 0$. Assertion is correct.
The statement given by the reason is correct but not what is given is the reason for the assertion.

52. (c) : Statement is correct, but the work function only depends on the photoelectric metal.

53. (a) **54. (a)** **55. (c)** **56. (b)** **57. (a)**

58. (b) : A thin stainless steel needle on a still water may floats due to surface tension as upward force due to surface tension balances the weight of the needle.

59. (a)

60. (a) : Total internal reflection will be for rays incident at an angle greater than *C*. If the fibres are thin, only rays almost parallel will pass, further for non-paraxial rays, the angle of incidence is large and therefore they also will be totally internally reflected. Both are right.

CHEMISTRY

61. (b) : Spin only magnetic moment, $\mu_s = \sqrt{n(n+2)}$
where n = number of unpaired electrons.
Number of unpaired electrons in Cr^{2+} ([Ar] $3d^4$) is 4, in Co^{2+} ([Ar] $3d^7$) is 3, in Fe^{2+} ([Ar] $3d^6$) is 4, in Mn^{2+} ([Ar] $3d^5$) is 5.
As the number of unpaired electrons in Cr^{2+} and Fe^{2+} are same, hence $[Cr(H_2O)_6]^{2+}$ and $[Fe(H_2O)_6]^{2+}$ will have same magnetic moment.

62. (d) : Cytochromes are conjugated proteins consisting of an apoprotein and a prosthetic group (heme). The heme consists of a porphyrin with a central iron atom.
The name haemoglobin is the concatenation of heme and globin, reflecting the fact that each subunit of haemoglobin is a globular protein with an embedded

heme (or haem) group; each heme group contains an iron atom, and this is responsible for the binding of oxygen. The most common types of haemoglobin contains four such subunits, each with one heme group.

63. **(a) :** Borax dissolves in water to give alkaline solutions.

$Na_2B_4O_7 + 2H_2O \rightarrow \underset{\text{strong base}}{2NaOH} + \underset{\text{weak acid}}{H_3BO_3}$

Borax is therefore used as a water softener and cleansing agent.

64. **(c) :** The different allotropic forms of sulphur arises partly from the extent to which S has polymerised and partly from the crystal structures adopted. The two common crystalline forms are α or rhombic sulphur and β or monoclinic sulphur. A third modification is γ-monoclinic sulphur. All three forms contain puckered S_8 rings with a crown conformation.
Engel's sulphur (ε-sulphur) contains S_6 rings.
S_7, S_9, S_{10}, S_{11}, S_{12}, S_{18} and S_{20} rings have been made by Schmidt and his group.
Plastic or γ-sulphur contains spiral chains and sometimes S_8 and other rings.
The other allotropic forms of sulphur are milk of sulphur and colloidal or δ-sulphur.

65. **(a) :** Intestine is acidic due to formation of HCl during digestion. Excessive acidity in the intestine creates problem of intestinal ulcer, gastric reflux and oesophagitis. The compound which reduced or neutralise acidity are called antacids.

$NaHCO_3 + HCl \rightarrow NaCl + H_2O + CO_2$

$Mg(OH)_2 + 2HCl \rightarrow MgCl_2 + 2H_2O$

66. **(b) :** Glass is an amorphous and transparent or translucent solid obtained by solidification of a mixture of silicates of different metals, one of which is always an alkali metal. Addition of small amounts of transition metal salts to the glass mixture imparts colour to the glass. For example, addition of small amounts of Fe^{3+}, Fe^{2+}, Co^{2+}, Cr^{3+} and Mn^{4+} salts imparts yellow-brown, light blue, deep blue, green or violet colour respectively.

67. **(c) :** $[Co(C_2O_4)_2(NH_3)_2]^-$

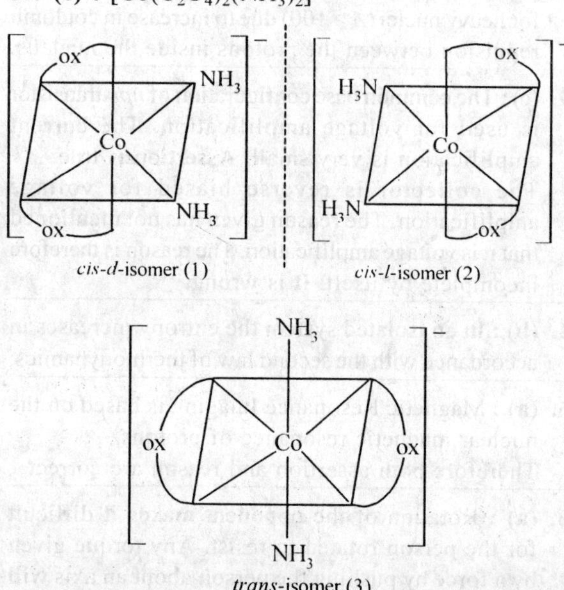

cis-d-isomer (1) *cis-l*-isomer (2)

trans-isomer (3)

68. **(a) :** *Cis*-diamminedichloroplatinum(II) (cisplatin) is a widely used anticancer drug. Ligands in cisplatin are NH_3 and Cl.

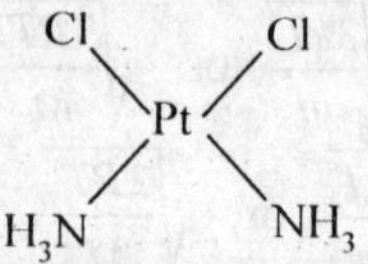

69. **(c) :** Haber-Bosch process is used for the synthesis of ammonia.

$N_2 + 3H_2 \rightleftharpoons 2NH_3$; $\Delta H = -92.0$ kJ

The best catalyst for this reaction is highly porous finely divided iron containing small amounts of promoters usually molybdenum or oxides of potassium and aluminium.

70. **(a) :** XeF_4 : sp^3d^2 hybridisation, shape is square

planar instead of octahedral due to presence of two lone pair of electrons on Xe atom.

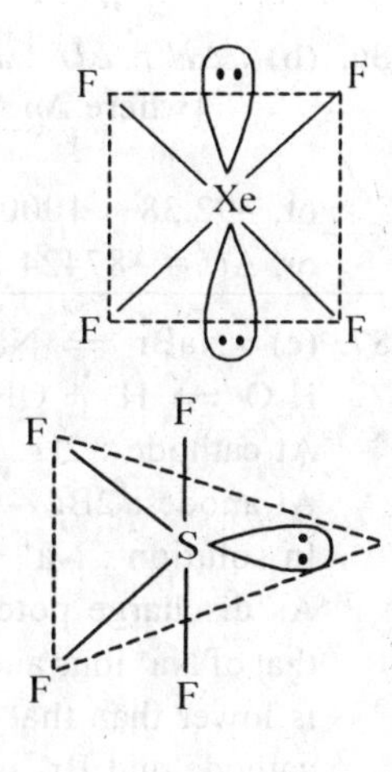

SF_4 : SF_4 molecule shows sp^3d hybridisation but its expected trigonal bipyramidal geometry gets distorted due to presence of a lone pair of electrons and it becomes distorted tetrahedral or see-saw with the bond angles equal to 89° and 177° instead of the expected angles of 90° and 180° respectively.

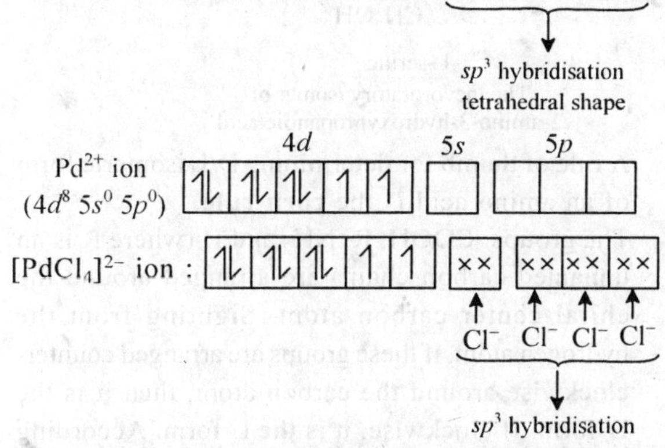

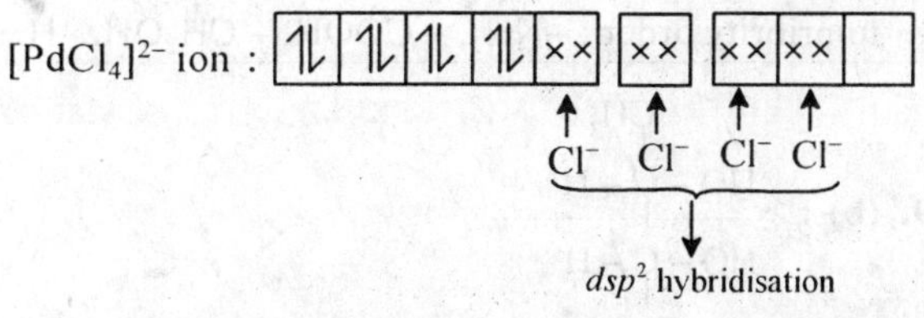

Experiments have, however, shown that 4-coordinated complexes of Pd(II) are diamagnetic (n = 0). Thus it is dsp^2 hybridisation which is involved in the formation of $[PdCl_4]^{2-}$ ion *i.e.* 4-coordinated complexes of Pd(II) have square planar geometry with n = 0 (diamagnetic).

71. (b) : Tincture of iodine is an aqueous solution of I_2 in KI, and French iodine is a solution in alcohol.

72. (c) : Cyanide is considered, in a broad sense, to be the most potent ligand for many transition metals. The very high affinities of metals for cyanide can be attributed to its negative charge, compactness and ability to engage in π-bonding.

The dicyanides $[M(CN)_2]^-$ (M = Cu, Ag, Au) are linear in geometry.

$-C \overset{1\sigma}{\underset{2\pi}{\equiv}} N-$ Thus two cyanide ions have 4π-bonds.

73. (a) : PCl_5 is molecular in the gas phase but exists as $[PCl_4]^+[PCl_6]^-$ in the crystalline solid.

74. (a) : When traces of iodide in the form of KIO_3/KI is added to the salt, iodised salt is obtained.

75. (a) : The fuel used in nuclear power plant is enriched uranium-235 in the form of U_3O_8.

76. (a) : Kinetic energy $= \frac{1}{2}mv^2$

[m = mass, v = velocity]

or, $0.5 = \frac{1}{2}\times 1\times v^2$ or, $v = 1\ ms^{-1}$

de Broglie wavelength, $\lambda = \frac{h}{mv}$

or, $\lambda = \frac{6.626\times10^{-34}\ \text{Js}}{1\ \text{kg}\times 1\ \text{ms}^{-1}} = 6.626\times10^{-34}$ m.

77. (b) : When the value of $Z < 1$, it is due to attractive forces between molecules. At high pressure, when $Z > 1$, it is due to repulsive forces between electron clouds of the molecules of gases.

78. (c) : 40 ml of 0.1 M ammonia solution = 40 × 0.1

= 4 milli equivalent ammonia solution

20 ml of 0.1 M HCl = 20 × 0.1

= 2 milli equivalent of HCl

$NH_4OH + HCl \rightarrow NH_4Cl + H_2O$

	NH_4OH	HCl	NH_4Cl
Initial milli-eqv.	4	2	0
Milli-eqv. after reaction	4 2 = 2	0	2

$\therefore pOH = pK_b + \log\frac{[NH_4Cl]}{[NH_4OH]} = 4.74 + \log\frac{2}{2}$

$= 4.74 + \log 1 = 4.74$

$\therefore pH = 14 - 4.74 = 9.26$

79. (d) : $\Delta S_{total} = \Delta S_{system} + \Delta S_{surroundings}$

For a spontaneous process ΔS_{total} must be positive.

i.e. $\Delta S_{total} > 0$.

80. (a) : In CaF_2 crystal, the Ca^{2+} ions are present at all corners and at the centre of each face of the cube and the F^- ions occupy all the tetrahedral sites.

81. (b) : $MnO_4^- + 2H_2O + 3e^- \rightarrow MnO_2 + 4OH^-$
Charge required for the reduction of 1 mol of MnO_4^- to MnO_2 = 3 F.

82. (c) : In general for a reaction,

$$x_1A + x_2B \rightarrow y_1C + y_2D$$

The rate expression may be expressed as

$$-\frac{1}{x_1}\frac{d[A]}{dt} = -\frac{1}{x_2}\frac{d[B]}{dt} = \frac{1}{y_1}\frac{d[C]}{dt} = \frac{1}{y_2}\frac{d[D]}{dt}.$$

For $2N_2O_5 \rightarrow 4NO_2 + O_2$

$$-\frac{1}{2}\frac{d[N_2O_5]}{dt} = \frac{1}{4}\frac{d[NO_2]}{dt} = \frac{d[O_2]}{dt}$$

83. (a) : $\Delta G^\circ = -RT\ln K$
[ΔG° = standard free energy change, K = equilibrium constant]
If a substance is in equilibrium between two phases at constant temperature and pressure, its chemical potential must have the same value in both the phases.
$\therefore \Delta G^\circ = 0$.

84. (c) : K_f for water $= \frac{\Delta T_f \times W \times m}{1000 \times w}$
(where W = wt. of water, w = wt. of cane sugar, m = molecular wt. of cane sugar)

$$= \frac{2.15 \times 100 \times 342}{1000 \times 5} = 14.7$$

Now, for 5% glucose,

$$\Delta T_f = \frac{K_f \times 1000 \times w'}{W \times m'}$$ (where w' = wt. of glucose, m' = molecular wt. of glucose)

$$= \frac{14.7 \times 1000 \times 5}{100 \times 180} = 4.08$$

$\therefore$ Freezing point of glucose solution
= 273.15 – 4.08 = 269.07 K.

85. (a) : Semiconductors are solids where there is only a small difference in energy, called a 'band gap', between the filled valence band of electrons and a conduction band.

Compound	**Energy gap (kJ mol^{-1})**
Diamond	579
Silicon	106
Germanium	68

86. (b) : $\Delta H = \Delta U + \Delta nRT$
[where Δn = no. of molecules of products – no. of molecules of reactants]
or, $-92.38 \times 1000 = \Delta U - 2 \times 8.314 \times 298$
or, $\Delta U = -87424$ J = –87.424 kJ.

87. (c) : $NaBr \rightleftharpoons Na^+ + Br^-$
$H_2O \rightleftharpoons H^+ + OH^-$
At cathode : $2H^+ + 2e^- \rightarrow H_2$
At anode : $2Br^- - 2e \rightarrow Br_2$
In solution : $Na^+ + OH^- \rightarrow NaOH$
As discharge potential of H^+ ions is lower than that of Na^+ ions and discharge potential of Br^- ions is lower than that of OH^- ions, H_2 is liberated at cathode and Br_2 is liberated at anode.

88. (c) :

NH$_2$
H—+—CO$_2$H
CH$_2$OH

L-serine
The laevorotatory isomer of 2-amino-3-hydroxypropanoic acid

A rule of thumb for determining D/L isomeric form of an amino acid is the **corn rule**.
The groups: COOH, R, NH_2 and H (where R is an unnamed carbon chain) are arranged around the chiral center carbon atom. Sighting from the hydrogen atom, if these groups are arranged counter-clockwise around the carbon atom, then it is the D-form. If clockwise, it is the L-form. According to priority order : $-NH_2$, – COOH, – CH_2OH, –H.

89. (b) :

CH$_3$
HO – C – H
HO – C – H
CH$_3$
meso form

90. (b) : $C_6H_5CH_2CH_3 \xrightarrow{SO_2Cl_2} C_6H_5CH(Cl)CH_3 \xrightarrow{\text{KOH alc.}} C_6H_5CH{=}CH_2$

91. (d) : Isopropyl benzene or cumene on air oxidation in presence of dilute acid gives phenol.

$$\underset{\text{cumene}}{C_6H_5-CH(CH_3)_2} \xrightarrow[\Delta]{O_2} \underset{\text{cumene hydroperoxide}}{C_6H_5-C(CH_3)_2-O-OH} \xrightarrow{H_2O/H^+} \underset{\text{phenol}}{C_6H_5OH} + CH_3\overset{O}{\overset{\|}{C}}CH_3$$

92. (b) : The position taken up by a third group entering the ring depends on the nature of the two groups already present.

When both groups show *o*- and *p*-directing nature, the directive power of each group is generally in the following order :

$O^- > NH_2 > NR_2 > OH > OMe, NHAc > Me > X$

In case of compound *A* (3-methylanisole, $C_6H_4(OCH_3)(CH_3)$), the arrows are used to indicate the possible positions that may be taken up by an incoming group.

(with respect to $-OCH_3$ group) (with respect to both $-CH_3$ group and $-OCH_3$ group)

Due to presence of bulky group, steric effect works, and the favourable product will be this.

$$\text{3-methylanisole} \xrightarrow{Br_2/FeBr_3} \text{4-bromo-3-methylanisole}$$

93. (c) : $o\text{-}C_6H_4(CH_2CONH_2)(COOCH_3) \xrightarrow{Br_2/NaOH} o\text{-}C_6H_4(CH_2NH_2)(COOCH_3) \xrightarrow[\Delta]{-CH_3OH}$ cyclic amide (C_6H_4 fused ring with CH_2–NH–C(=O))

94. (d) : When reduced with a neutral reducing agent like zinc dust and aqueous ammonium chloride, nitrobenzene gives phenyl hydroxyl amine.

$$\underset{\text{nitrobenzene}}{C_6H_5NO_2} + Zn + H_2O \xrightarrow[\text{warm}]{NH_4Cl} \underset{\text{phenyl hydroxyl amine}}{C_6H_5\overset{H}{N}-OH} + ZnO$$

95. (a) : Thymine, also known as 5-methyluracil, is a pyrimidine nucleobase. As the name implies, thymine may be derived by methylation of uracil at the 5th carbon.

(Structure of thymine: pyrimidine ring with H_3C at C-5, C=O at C-4 and C-2, NH at N-3 and N-1.)

96. (d) : Any amino acid has its lowest solubility on its isoelectronic point and the isoelectric point is the pH at which the amino acid carries no charge.

97. (b) : Methyl-α-D-glucoside and methyl-β-D glucoside differs at C-1, hence are called anomers.

methyl α-D-glucoside: $H-C(OCH_3)-(CHOH)_3-CH(-O-)-CH_2OH$ methyl-β-D-glucoside: $OCH_3-C(H)-(CHOH)_3-CH(-O-)-CH_2OH$

98. (b) : For the same halogen, boiling point of alkyl halide decreases as the size of the alkyl group decreases.

For isomeric alkyl halides, boiling point decreases as branching increases. So the decreasing order of boiling point is

$CH_3CH_2CH_2CH_2Cl > CH_3CH_2CH_2Cl > CH_3CH(CH_3)CH_2Cl > (CH_3)_3CCl$.

99. (a) : Reactivity of halides towards S_N1 mechanism is

benzyl > allyl > 3° > 2° > 1°.

100. (d) : Halogenated compounds on treatment with aq. KOH form alcohols. The halogen atom is substituted by – OH group.

$$CH_3CH(Cl)CH_2 - CH_2OH \xrightarrow{\text{aq. KOH}} CH_3CH(OH)CH_2 - CH_2OH$$

Here OH^- acts as a nucleophile.

101. (b) : Starch $(C_6H_{10}O_5)_n$ is a polysaccharide. It consists of two fractions - one is known as α-amylose and the other is β-amylose or amylopectin. In iodimetric and iodometric titrations, starch solution is used as an indicator. It gives blue or violet colour with free iodine. At the end point the blue or violet colour disappears when iodine is completely changed to iodide.

102. (a) : Bond order of $N_2 = 3$, bond order of $O_2 = 2$. Higher the bond order, higher is the bond dissociation energy. *i.e.* higher stability or less reactivity. Thus N_2 is less reactive than O_2. Higher the bond order, shorter is the bond length. Shorter bond length of N_2 shows its higher bond order.

103. (a) : The essential requirement for a substance to be optically active is that the substance should not have a plane of symmetry in its structure.

104. (b) : It is known that the value of $E°$ becomes more negative down the series. As the chromium is present below in electrochemical series than Mn, so Mn has more positive $E°$ value than Cr.

$Mn \rightarrow 3d^5\ 4s^2$, $\quad Mn^{2+} \rightarrow 3d^5\ 4s^0$

$Cr \rightarrow 3d^5\ 4s^1$, $\quad Cr^{2+} \rightarrow 3d^4\ 4s^0$

For elimination of one electron from Mn^{2+}, more energy is required due to its stable configuration. That is why third ionization energy of Mn is larger than Cr.

105. (c) : $K_2Cr_2O_7$ is less soluble in water. $K_2Cr_2O_7$ can be found in pure state and can be accurately weighed. It is not hygroscopic in nature. So $K_2Cr_2O_7$ is used as a primary standard solution.

106. (c) : Silicones are strongly water repellent. Their water repellency arises because a silicone chain is surrounded by organic side groups and looks like an alkane from the outside.

107. (a) : $A + B \rightleftharpoons (AB)^{\#} \rightarrow$ products.

The activated complex can also be treated as a distinct chemical species in equilibrium with the reactants which then decompose into products. It is, however, a special molecule in which one vibrational degree of freedom has been converted to a translational degree of freedom along the reaction coordinate. It must be remembered that the activated complex is not merely an intermediate in process of breaking or forming of chemical bonds. It is unstable because it is situated at the maximum of the potential energy barrier separating the produts from the reactants. The difference between the energy of the activated complex (E_1) and the energy of the reactants (E_2) is the activation energy, E_a.

$$E_1 - E_2 = E_a, \quad E_1 >> E_2.$$

108. (a) : Fusion of ice is a spontaneous process, because the process again proceeds in the direction of more random state, *i.e.* liquid state is more random (higher entropy) in comparison to solid state. *i.e.* ice.

109. (d) : Sb_2S_3 is soluble in yellow ammonium sulphide.

$$Sb_2S_3 + 3(NH_4)_2S \rightarrow 2(NH_4)_3SbS_3$$

The stability of sulphides increases with increase in atomic number of the element.

110. (d) : Graphite has a two dimensional sheet structure. Each C-atom is in sp^2 hybridised state and is linked to three other carbon atoms in a hexagonal planar structure.

For a tetragonal system, $a = b \neq c$, $\alpha = \beta = \gamma = 90°$.

For a hexagonal system, $a = b \neq c$, $\alpha = \beta = 90°$, $\gamma = 120°$.

111. (b) : If the opposing potential becomes slightly larger than that of the cell, the direction of current flow is reversed, and so is the cell reaction. Now zinc ions are converted to zinc at one electrode and Cu is converted into copper ion and the overall cell reaction becomes

$$Zn^{++} + Cu \rightarrow Zn + Cu^{++}$$

112. (c) : When oppositely charged sols are mixed in almost equal proportions, their charges are neutralised. Both sols may be partially or completely precipitated. When negatively charged As_2S_3 sol is added to positively charged $Fe(OH)_3$ sol, in suitable amounts, precipitation of both the sols take place simultaneously.

113. (c) : If the red blood cells are placed in pure water, pressure inside the cells increases as the water is drawn in and the cell swells.

114. (c) : Change in colour is due to the oxidation of alcohol with potassium dichromate. Oxidation of alcohols with $K_2Cr_2O_7$ in dilute H_2SO_4 (orange solution):

Primary — RCH_2OH (alcohol) $\xrightarrow[K_2Cr_2O_7 + H_2SO_4]{[O]}$ $RCHO$ (aldehyde) $\xrightarrow[K_2Cr_2O_7 + H_2SO_4]{[O]}$ $RCOOH$ (acid) (orange solution becomes green)

Secondary — $RR'CHOH$ $\xrightarrow[K_2Cr_2O_7 + H_2SO_4]{[O]}$ $RR'C=O$ (ketone) (orange solution becomes green)

Tertiary — $RR'R''C-OH$ $\xrightarrow[K_2Cr_2O_7 + H_2SO_4]{[O]}$ no reaction (solution remains orange)

$K_2Cr_2O_7$ in presence of dilute H_2SO_4 acts as an oxidising agent. It is converted into chromic sulphate which is green in colour.

$$\underset{\text{(orange)}}{K_2Cr_2O_7} + 4H_2SO_4 \rightarrow K_2SO_4 + \underset{\text{(green)}}{Cr_2(SO_4)_3} + 4H_2O + 3O$$

115. (c) : $\underset{\substack{\text{anilinium ion} \\ \text{stronger acid}}}{C_6H_5\overset{+}{N}H_3} \longrightarrow \underset{\substack{\text{aniline} \\ \text{weaker conjugated base}}}{C_6H_5NH_2} + H^+$

Aniline is weaker base than ammonium chloride. In NH_4Cl or aliphatic amines, the non-bonding electron pair of N is localized and is fully available for coordination with a proton. On the other hand, in aniline or other aromatic amines, the non-bonding electron pair is delocalised into benzene ring by resonance.

[Resonance structures of aniline]

But anilinium ion is less resonance stabilised than aniline.

[Anilinium ion Kekulé structures] ⟷ no other resonating structure possible

116. (c) : Stereoisomers which are not mirror images of each other are called diastereomers.

Diastereomers have different physical properties.

Note : Diastereomers have similar chemical properties because they belong to the same family, but they do not have identical chemical properties because of difference in their relative configurations.

117. (a) : The C-atom of C – Cl in chloronitrobenzene carries a small +ve charge.

[Resonance structures of o-chloronitrobenzene]

Because of the positive charge, attack at this carbon atom by the nucleophile is facilitated.

[Mechanism: Nu^- + o-chloronitrobenzene → intermediate → o-Nu-nitrobenzene + Cl^-]

118. (d) : Isoprene (2-methyl-1,3-butadiene) is the monomer for natural rubber.

Natural rubber is formed through cationic addition polymerisation. Cationic addition polymerisation is catalysed by acids and Lewis acids. Alkenes containing electron-donating groups usually undergoes cationic addition polymerisation.

$$n\,CH_2=\underset{|}{\overset{CH_3}{C}}-CH=CH_2 \xrightarrow{\text{polymerisation}} \left(CH_2-\overset{CH_3}{\overset{|}{C}}=CH-CH_2\right)_n$$

119. (d) : Addition of HBr on 2-butene gives only one product, 2-bromobutane.

$$\underset{\text{2-butene}}{CH_3-CH=CH-CH_3} \xrightarrow{HBr} \underset{\text{2-bromobutane}}{CH_3-\underset{Br}{\underset{|}{CH}}-CH_2-CH_3}$$

As 2-butene is a symmetrical alkene, it does not follow Markownikoff's rule.

120. (a) : Freezing point of a substance is defined as the temperature at which the vapour pressure of its liquid is equal to the vapour pressure of the corresponding solid. Since the addition of a non-volatile solute always lowers the vapour pressure of solvent, therefore it will be in equilibrium with solid phase at a lower pressure and hence at a lower temperature.

BIOLOGY

121. (b) : Sympathetic and parasympathetic nervous system are the parts of autonomic nervous system. Autonomic nervous system is a part of peripheral nervous system that supplies stimulation *via* motor nerves to the smooth and cardiac muscles (the involuntary muscles) and to the glands of the body. The activity of the ANS is controlled principally by the medulla oblongata and hypothalamus of brain. Sympathetic and parasympathetic nervous system tend to work antagonistically on the same organ.

Feature	Sympathetic nervous system	Parasympathetic nervous system
(i) salivary glands	inhibit secretion	stimulate secretion
(ii) pupil of the eye	dilate	constricts
(iii) heart rate	increase strength & rate of heart beat	decrease strength & rate of heart beat
(iv) intestinal peristalsis	inhibits	stimulates

122. (b) : Millipede - Millipedes belongs to order or class diplopoda of myriapoda. Millipedes are called thousand leggers because of possession of numerous legs. Inspite of this they move very slowly.

Silver fish - *Lepisma* is commonly known as silver fish because of its glistening silvery white fish like body. It belongs to the insect order thysanura.

Sea anemone - Sea anemone (*Admasia*), belongs to coelenterates, shows commensalism. It is found attached to the empty shell of gastropods occupied by hermit crab. Its body wall is two layered *i.e.*, outer epidermis and inner gastrodermis. In between these two layers is present mesogloea.

123. (d) : All mammals without any exception are characterized by a muscular diaphragm and milk producing glands.

124. (d) : Oxyntic (or parietal) cell is present in the wall of the stomach that produce HCl which forms the part of gastric juice. Oxyntic cell also produce intrinsic factor which is involved in the absorption of vitamin B_{12} in the small intestine. The pH of gastric acid is 2-3 in the stomach of the lumen. The acidity being maintained by the proton pump, a H^+/K^+ ATPase.

Alpha cell of islets of langerhans secrete glucagon hormone which raises blood glucose level by stimulating liver to convert glycogen to glucose and by stimulating the conservation of fatty acids and amino acids to glucose. **Kupffer cells** are specialized macrophages that disposes of old blood cells and particulate matter. Kupffer cells, named after Karl Wilhem Von Kupffer, are found in the bloodstreams and in the liver, attached to the walls of the sinusoids.

Sebaceous gland is a simple or branched glands in the skin that secrete an oily substance, sebum which is fatty mildly antiseptic material that protects, lubricates, and waterproofs the skin and hair & help prevent dessication.

125. (b) : Cone cell is one of two types (other is rod) of light sensitive cells in the retina of the eye. The human retina contains 6-7 million cones which function best in bright light and are essential for active vision (receiving a sharp accurate image). The area of retina called the fovea contains the greatest concentration of cone. Cones can also distinguish colours. There are 3 types of cone, each sensitive to the wavelength of a different primary colour - red, green or blue.

126. (a) : Polygenic inheritance is the inheritance pattern of a trait controlled by two or more genes. Genes may be on the same or different chromosomes and each gene may have two or more alleles. The gene expression is influenced by a variety of factors including gender, nutrition, breed, rate of growth, and amount of exercise. These traits are quantitative traits - that is, there is a wide range within the population. Such traits include height, weight, character, working abilities, and some genetic defects.

One example is height in humans - there are a larger number of phenotypes, each differing slightly from the next and forming a graduated series. Some variation in height in humans is due to environmental factors such as diet, exercise and disease. However, if the environmental factors were constant, there would still be continuous variation in height due to such things as formation and hormone levels. The more genes that control a characteristic, the more possible gene combinations exist and the more phenotypes.

Other examples of polygenic inheritance include : skin colour in humans, colour in wheat kernels, egg weight in poultry, fleece weight in sheep. Kernal colour in wheat is determined by two gene pairs, so called polygenes that produce a range of colors from white to dark red depending on the combinations of alleles. Dark red plants are homozygous *AABB* and white plants are homozygous *aabb*. When these homozygotes are crossed the F_1 offspring are all double heterozygotes *AaBb*. Thus crossing individuals with the phenotype extremes yield offspring that are a 'blend' of the two parents.

127. (b) : Test cross is a cross made to identify hidden recessive alleles in an individual of unknown genotype. This individual is crossed with one that is homozygous for the allele being investigated (*i.e.*, a homozygous recessive). The homozygous recessive individual may be the parent of the individual being investigated.

128. (c) : Rennin, helicase and hyaluronidase are all enzymes. Rennin (chymosin), secreted by the stomach is responsible for clotting milk. It acts on a soluble milk protein (caseinogen) to converts it into the insoluble form casein. Helicase unwinds double stranded helical DNA during replication. Hyaluronidase is able to digest hyaluronic acid (major glycosaminoglycan) & is therefore important in modulating the removal of cell matrix in order to facilitate cell movement or tissue organization.

Thiamine is **not an amino acid**, it is vitamin B_1, which is active in the form of thiamin pyrophosphate, a coenzyme in decarboxylation reactions in carbohydrate metabolism. A deficiency of vitamin B_1 leads to beri beri.

Myosin is a **contractile protein** that interacts with actin to bring about contraction of muscle or cell movement.

Among optic, oculomotor and vagus, which are cranial nerves, optic is sensory in nature, oculomotor is motor and vagus is mixed sensory nerves.

129. (d)

130. (c) : The figure shows, human sex chromosome with genes 'a' and 'b'. So, 'a' and 'b' are sexlinked genes, that are inherited through sex chromosomes. The most important character of sex linked inheritance are colourblindness and haemophilia. Both the disorders are due to recessive sex linked genes. The gene for red green colour blindness is located on X chromosomes. The person suffering from this disease is unable to distinguish red and green colours. Haemophilia, also called bleeder's disease, is due to presence of recessive gene on X-chromosome. The person suffering from this disease have blood which does not clot properly *i.e*, lacking a factor (plasma thromboplastin) which is responsible for clotting of blood.

131. (d) : *Chamaeleon* (or girgit) is a lizard like member of reptilia which is famous for changing its colour according to its surroundings. The phenomenon is called metachrosis. *Chamaeleon* lives on trees in south India and is insectivorous and can catch an insects about 20 cm away by eversible tongue. Its tails is long cylindrical & prehensile (means able to grasp or grab by wrapping around).

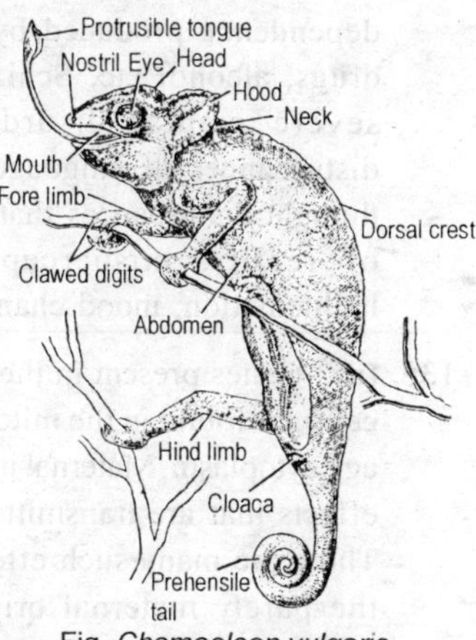

Fig. *Chamaeleon vulgaris*.

132. (a) : Enzymes or biocatalysts are proteinaceous substance that are capable of catalysing chemical reactions of biological systems without themselves undergoing any change. In the graph *a* shows normal enzyme reaction, graph *b* shows competitive inhibition and graph *c* shows non competitive inhibition. In competitive inhibition the inhibitor, which is a substrate analogue, combines reversibly to the free enzyme at the active site. In non competitive inhibition, the inhibitor binds to enzyme at a place other than substrate binding site. It results in destruction of enzyme activity.

133. (b) : Pollution from animal excreta and organic waste from kitchen can be most profitable minimized using them in the generation of biogas. Biogas is a mixture of methane and carbon dioxide resulting from the anaerobic decomposition of such waste materials as domestic, industrial and agricultural sewage.

134. (a) : Borderline personality disorder (BPD) is a serious mental illness. Borderline describing a personality disorder characterized by unstable and intense relationships, exploiting and manipulating other people, rapidly changing moods, recurrent suicidal or self injuring acts & a prevasive inner feelings of emptiness & boredom.

A mood disorder is a condition where the prevailing emotional moods is distorted or inappropriate to the circumstances. Addiction is a state of dependence produced by the habitual taking of drugs, alcohol etc. Schizophrenia is a group of severe mental disorders characterized by disturbances of languages and communications, thought disturbances that may involve distortion of reality, misperceptions, delusions and hallucination, mood changes & withdrawn etc.

135. (a) : Genes present in the cytoplasm of eukaryotic cells are found in the mitochondria & inherited *via* egg cytoplasm. Maternal inheritances are the genetic effects that are transmitted *via* the maternal line. There are many such effects some resulting from the purely maternal origin of mitochondria or chloroplasts, others from effects on the phenotype of the embryo by easily development within the female, such as maternal influence on coiling of snails.

136. (c) : Ciliated epithelium is a region of epithelium consisting of columnar or cuboidal cells bearing hairlike appendages that are capable of beating rapidly. Ciliated epithelium performs the functions of moving particles of fluids over the epithelial surface. Cubical ciliated epithelium occurs in certain parts of uriniferous tubules whereas columnar ciliated epithelium occurs in fallopian tubules, nasal passages, bronchioles, small bronchi and buccopharyngeal cavity of frog. It often occurs in the vicinity of mucus secreting goblet cells.

Squamous epithelium are found in linning of alveoli in the lungs and Bowman's capsule in the kidney. Columnar epithelium are found in the lining layer of gastrointestinal tract, gall bladder, uterus etc. and cubical or cuboidal epithelium lines the salivary ducts, pancreated ducts, gastric glands, thyroid follicles, germinal epithelium of ovary, proximal part of uriniferous tubules etc.

137. (a) : Thyroxine, the principal hormone, of thyroid gland, is required for tissue differentiation and metamorphosis (the rapid transformation from the larval to the adult form) in amphibians. So in its absence of presence of antithyoid substance, eg. thiourea, tadpoles or axolotl remain in the larval stage indefinitely. Thiourea is an organic compound of carbon, nitrogen, sulphur and hydrogen, with the formula CSN_2H_4 or $(NH_2)_2CS$. It is similar to urea, except that oxygen atom is replaced by a sulphur atom.

Antithyroid agents and the thiouracils and mercaptoglyoxalines owe their activity to the presence of the potentially free thiol group, which by its ready reduction of elementary iodine to iodide ion,

2R-S + 12 -+ R-S-S-R + 2I

interferes with the iodination of tyrosine in the thyroid protein and hence inhibits the synthesis of the thyroid hormone.

138. (a) : Leptospirosis (also known as Weil's disease, canicola fever, canefield fever, nanukayami fever or 7-day fever) is a bacterial zoonotic disease caused by spirochaetes of the genus Leptospira that affects humans and a wide range of animals, including mammals, birds, amphibians, and reptiles. It was first described by Adolf Weil in 1886 when he reported an "acute infectious disease with enlargement of spleen, jaundice and nephritis.Humans become infected through contact with water, food, or soil containing urine from these infected animals. This may happen by swallowing contaminated food or water or through skin contact. Leptospirosis is common among watersport enthusiasts in certain areas as prolonged immersion in water is known to promote the entry of the bacteria.

Schistosomiasis or bilharzia is also called snail fever or swimmer's itch. Schistosomiasis is a life-threatening parasitic disease caused by a worm that lives in a host snail. Humans can become infected when they come in contact with water in ponds and rivers where the snail lives. The pathology is mostly caused by the large number of eggs becoming stuck in various body parts, in particular the liver (causing liver enlargement and malfunction) and the kidneys (causing kidney damage, detectable by blood in the urine).

139. (b) : Blue baby syndrome is a pathological condition, called methemoglobinemia, in which blood's capacity for oxygen transport is reduced, resulting in bluish skin discoloration in infants. Blue baby syndrome begins when large amounts of nitrates in water are ingested by an infant and converted to nitrite by the digestive system. The nitrite then reacts with oxyhaemoglobin (the oxygen-carrying blood protein) to form metheglobin, which cannot carry oxygen.
Pneumoconiosis is a man-made, occupational lung diseases that are contracted by prolonged breathing of coal mine dust *i.e.* caused by the inhalation of dust, characterized by formation of nodular fibrotic changes in lungs. Non-Hodgkin lymphoma (or NHL) is a cancer of lymphoid tissue, a part of the lymphatic system. NHL is a heterogenous disease. Skin cancer is a malignant tumor that grows in the skin cells. It is commonly caused by exposure to the sun's UV rays.

140. (b) : Angiogram is an X-ray diagnostic procedure used to visualize the blood vessels following injection of a contrast substance into an artery. It is used to image arteries in the brain, heart, kidneys, gastrointestinal tract, aorta, neck (carotids), chest, limbs and pulmonary circuit.
Coronary angiography is performed to detect obstruction in the coronary arteries, which can lead to heart attack. It may be performed if you have unstable angina, atypical chest pain, aortic stenosis, or unexplained heart failure.

141. (c) : The root knot disease of brinjal is quite common in all vegetative growing areas especially when the climate is warm, with short winters. The disease is caused by root knot nematode *Meloidogyne incognita*. It devitalizes root tips, develop swelling over roots and reduces flow of water and minerals to the aerial parts. As a result yield and quality of fruits are affected.
Citrus canker is a common bacterial diseases of citrus tree, caused by *Xanthomonas citri*. Late blight is a disease of potato caused by fungus *Phytophthora infestans* having blight type symptoms. Wilt of pigeon pea is caused by *Fusarium udum* (fungi) where wilting of seedlings and adult plants occur.

142. (d) : The present day wheat is hexaploid, known as triticale (2n = 42) with 3 genomes A, B and D *i.e*, AABBDD. The 3 genomes are obtained from 3 different diploid species.
(i) *Triticum aegilopoides* -AA (2n = 14)
(ii) *Aegilops speltoides* - BB (2n = 14)
(iii) *Aegilops squarossa* - DD (2n = 14)
By crossing of first two diploids sps *Triticum dicoccoides* (2n = 28) *i.e.*, tetraploid is produced AABB which on crossing with third species gives rise to *Triticum aestivum* (2n = 42) hexaploid (AABBDD).
So its haploid set will have 21 chromosomes, monosomic (2n - 1) will have 41 chromosomes, nullisomics (2n - 2) will have 40 chromosomes, and trisomic (2n + 1) will have 43 chromosomes.

143. (b) : Grafting is the technique of joining parts of two plants so as to form a composite plant. Grafting is carried out during period of active growth and rapid healing between two related plants having vascular cambium. One plant has strong root system and the other plant possesses better flower or fruit yield. The former is called stock and the latter is known as scion or graft. Vascular cambium are the lateral meristem found in those vascular plants that exhibit secondary growth. It forms secondary xylem and secondary phloem mostly by periclinal division.

144. (d) : Sieve elements are a component of phloem tissue and are responsible for conduction of food in plants. A sieve tube element has peripheral layer of cytoplasm without any nucleus. The central part is occupied by a network of canals which contain fibrils of *p*-protein. The protein is vibratite and is believed to actively participate in the transport of nutrients. One general property of its ability to form a gel and it functions as a puncture repair substance forming a plug at any site of damage in sieve element, thus preventing loss of food materials being translocated by the phloem. Thus it is believed to have sealing function on wounding.

145. (b) : Myxomycetes are generally placed under fungi but are also placed under protista. They are known as slime mould and are surrounded by plasma membrane only. They are multinucleate, showing amoeboid like nature (pseudopodia for engulfing food). Both sexual and asexual mode of reproduction is found. They produce spores within sporangia. Asexual reproduction is by fragmentation and sexual reproduction by spores.

146. (d) : The system of classification of seed plants presented by Bentham and Hooker, represented the most well developed classification of natural system. The classification was published in 3 volume work '*Genera plantarum*'. The system divided phanerogams or seed plants into 3 classes - dicotyledons, gymnospermae and monocotyledons. Dicotyledons were further subdivided into 3 subclasses – polypetalae, gamopetalae and monochlamydae based on the presence or absence of petals and their fusion. They were further divided into series, orders and families. No orders were recognised within monochlamydae and monocotyledons, the series being directly divided into families. But the system had a lot of demerits within it. He did not know the affinities of the families placed under 'Ordines anomate' and the families were tentativily grouped together. So, a few orders were not placed satisfactorily in the classification. Monochlamydae is an unnatural assemblage of taxa, which belongs elsewhere. The creation of this group has resulted in the separation of many closely related families.

147. (c) : Transgenic plants are those plants in which a foreign gene has been introduced and stably integrated into the host DNA. A gene that is transferred using the tools of molecular biology is called transgene. *Brassica napas* is one of the transgenic plant species. Recently transgenic plants have been explored for production of biologically active peptides and proteins having pharmaceutical applications including use as blood proteins, enzymes, growth, hormones etc. The protein hirudin present in leech, prevents blood clotting. The gene was chemically synthesized and introduced in *Brassica napas* and later on the seeds contained the protein.

148. (b) : Grafting is the technique of joining parts of two plants so as to form a composite plant. One plant has a strong root system called the stock, and the other plant having better flower or fruit yield is known as scion. When a scion is grafted to a stock the root system of the plant has the genotype of stock and fruits produced show genotypes of the scion.

149. (d) : Chromatophores are internal membrane systems present in photosynthetic prokaryotes. These develop as membrane lined sacs or thylakoids from plasma membrane. Thylakoid membranes contain photosynthetic pigments in cyanobacteria and purple bacteria. Small sacs or granules containing pigments phycobilin are attached to these membranes. In green bacteria chromatophores are covered by non unit non lipid protein membrane. They are sometimes called chlorosomes.

150. (a) : Rust, smut and mushroom all belong to the group of pathogenic fungi. These fungi belong to the class basidiomycetes, and produce basidiospores. Mushroom are placed in the order agaricales. *Amanita* and *Marasmius* are pathogenic or disease causing fungi. *Marasmius ordeades* causes fairy rings on turf grasses. Rusts and smuts are included in the subclass teliomycetidae. Rust fungi comes under order uredinales, eg. *Puccinia graminis* causes black rust of wheat, *P. recondita* causes leaf rust of wheat. Smut fungi comes under order ustilaginales which produce teliotospores, eg. *Ustilago tritici* causes loose smut of wheat.

151. (d) : *Rhizobium* is the nitrogen fixing bacteria present in root nodules of legumes. Roots of a legume secrete chemical attractants flavonoids and betaines. Bacteria collect over the root hairs, release nod factors that causes curling of root hairs around the bacteria, degradations of cell wall and formation of an infection thread enclosing bacteria. The infected cortical cells differentiate and start dividing. It produces swelling of nodules and the infected cells enlarge. Bacteria stop dividing and form irregular polyhedral structures called bacteroids. The host cells develops a pinkish coloured pigment called leg haemoglobin. It is an oxygen scavenger and protects nitrogenase from oxygen. Symbiotic nitrogen fixation requires co-operations of 'Nod' genes of legumes, 'nod' 'nif' and 'fix' genes of bacteria.

152. (a) : Bioassay is a testing of biological activity like growth response of a substance by employing plant part. *Avena* curvature test is a bioassay for examining the activity of auxins. It is based upon experiments of Went. 10° curvature is produced by auxin concentration of 150 μg/lit at 25°C and 90% relative humidity. It can measure auxin upto 300 μg/lit. Auxin from shoot tip or any other plant organ is allowed to diffuse in a standard size agar block. 15 - 30 mm long oat coleoptile grown in dark is held vertically over water. 1mm tip of coleoptile is removed without injuring the primary leaf. After 3 hrs a second decapitation is carried out for 4mm distance. Primary leaf is now pulled loose and agar block supported against it - at the tip of decapitated coleoptile. After 90 - 110 mm the coleoptile is found to have bent. The curvature is measured.

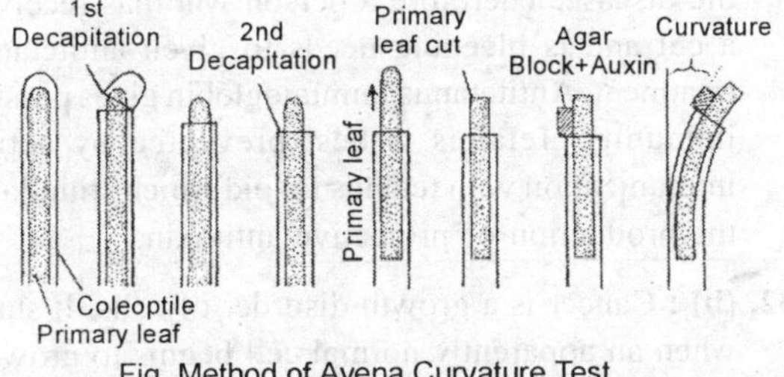

Fig. Method of Avena Curvature Test.

153. (d) : Chloroplast, chromoplast and leucoplast are all types of plastids which are classified on the basis of pigments they contain. Plastids are semiautonomous cell organelles bounded by two membranes and are found in only plant cells & some unicellular organisms (*Euglena*) of uncertain affinity. The common among all the three organelles are that they have ability to multiply by a fission like process because these organelles contain there own genetic material and protein synthesizing machinery, *i.e.*, DNA, RNA and ribosomes. Plastids are thought to have arisen as a result of an endosymbiotic event in which an early photosynthetic prokaryotic invaded a primitive eukaryotic host. All plastids are derived initially from small undifferentiated plastids termed proplastids which are found in the dividing cells in meristems. During cell differentiation, proplastids differentiate into particular plastids types according to the type of cell in which they reside.

Chloroplasts are the organelles in which photosynthesis takes place. Photosynthesis is an important process by which autotrophic cells manufacture their own food. Chloroplasts contain the green pigment chlorophyll (this is why plant leaves are green) which absorbs light to provide the energy necessary to complete photosynthesis. Chromoplasts are very similar to chloroplasts, but they do not contain the green pigment chlorophyll. Instead, they contain other pigments which give colour to flowers and to leaves during the fall. These other pigments absorb colours of light than chlorophyll. Leucoplasts are non-pigmented colourless plastids. Lacking pigments, leucoplasts are not green, so they are predictably located in roots and non-photosynthetic tissues of plants. They may become specialized for bulk storage of starch, lipid or protein and are then known as amyloplasts, elaioplasts, or proteinoplasts. These materials are released from the leucoplast when the cell requires them.

154. (d) : Pollination by birds is called ornithophily, eg. humming birds, honey eaters, sunbirds etc. are sensitive to colours and have powerful vision. Plants like *Bombax, Butea,* etc are ornithophilous plants. There flowers are characterised by tubular, cup shaped corolla, bright colour to attract insect, excess of nectar and pollens. They are generally odourless. *Bauhinia* is mostly visited by hummingbirds and their propagules are dispersed by birds.

155. (c) : The montreal protocol on substances that deplete the ozone layer was signed in Montreal, Canada, by over 150 countries at a convention in 1987 to cut use of CFCs (chlorofluorocarbons). The aim of the Protocol was to protect the ozone layer in the stratosphere by decreasing and eventually eliminating the use of ozone-depleting substances like CFCs. It is regarded as one of the most successful international treaties in modern history.

156. (d) : Keystone species is a species which has significant and disproportionately large influence on the community removal or decrease in number of keystone species causes disruption in structure and function of community. For example in intertidal regions star fish feeds on mussels. Removal of star fish leads to dominance of mussels that excludes algae and browsing species. In tropical rain forests fig functions as keystone species as they provide fruit to a number of animals during the period of food scarcity.

157. (c) : Genetic diversity is the diversity in the number and types of genes as well as chromosomes present in different species and the variations in the genes and their alleles in the same species. Variations in the genes of a species increase with the increase in size and environmental parameters of the habitat. It helps in speciation and evolution of new species.

158. (c) : Nonsense codon is a set of three nucleotides for which there is no corresponding tRNA molecule to insert an amino acid into the polypeptide chain. Protein synthesis is hence terminated and the completed polypeptide released from the ribosome. Three stop codons are UAA (ochre), UAG (amber) and UGA (opal). Mutations which generate any of these three codons in a position which normally contains a codon specifying an amino acid are known as nonsense mutations.

159. (b) : Biosphere reserves, National Park and wild life sanctuaries are all protected areas but differ from each other in some ways. National parks are reserved for betterment of wild life. Cultivation, grazing forestry and habitat manipulations are not allowed. Sanctuaries are tracts of land with or with out lake where wild life can take refuge. Harvesting of timber, collection of forest products, tilling of land, private ownership of land etc., are allowed. Biosphere reserves are multipurpose protected area which are meant for preserving genetic diversity in representative ecosystems of various national biomass and unique biological communities by protecting wild life, traditional life style of tribals and domesticated plant/animal genetic resources. Each biosphere reserve has 3 zones – (i) Natural zone - where no human activity is allowed, (ii) Buffer zone - limited human activity is allowed like education, research, (iii) Transition zone - has different parts like agriculture, tourism, and restoration regions.

160. (a) : Genetic variation present among plants cells of a culture is called somaclonal variation. The term is also used for the genetic variation present in plants regenerated from a single culture. This variation has been used to develop sexual/useful variations.

161. (a) : Tetanus is a serious and often fatal disease caused by the neurotoxin tetanospasmin which is produced by the gram positive obligate anaerobic bacterium *Clostridium tetani*. Infections begins when the bacteria are introduced into an open injury or wound where they produce tetanospasmin toxin which blocks messages from the spinal cord to the muscles, forcing muscles to go into severe spasm. Deep puncture wound or those with devitalized (dead) tissue are particularly prone to tetanus infection because the bacillus thrives in an anaerobic environment. Tetanus often begins with mild spasm in the jaw muscles (hence called **lock jaw** or **trismus**), neck muscles and facial muscles. Stiffness rapidly develops in the chest, back and abdominal muscles. Immunization against tetanus can prevent the disease. Therefore a person who has received a cut and is bleeding needs to given antitetanus treatment. Antitetanus immunoglobin gives passive immunity. Tetanus is best prevented by active immunization with tetanus toxoid which stimulates the production of protective antitoxin.

162. (b) : Cancer is a growth disorder of cells. It starts when an apparently normal cell begins to grow in an uncontrolled and invasive way. The result is a cluster of cells, called a tumor, that constantly expands in size. Cells that leave the tumor and spread throughout the body, forming new tumors at distant sites, are called metastases. Cancer is a gene disorder of somatic tissue, in which damaged genes fail to properly control cell proliferation. The cell division cycle is regulated by a sophisticated group of proteins. Cancer results from the mutation of the genes encoding these proteins. More than one mutation is necessary for carcinogenesis. In fact, a series of several mutations to certain classes of genes is usually required before a normal cell will transform into a cancer cell. Only mutations in those certain types of genes which play vital roles in cell division, cell death, and DNA repair will cause a cell to lose control of its proliferation. Cancer can be caused by chemicals that mutate DNA or in some instances by viruses that circumvent the cell's normal proliferation controls. Whatever the immediate cause, however, all cancers are characterized by unrestrained growth and division. Cell division never stops in a cancerous line of cells. Cancer cells are virtually immortal—until the body in which they reside dies.

163. (c) : The process of transfer of energy from producers through a series of organisms *i.e.* from primary consumers to secondary consumers to tertiary consumers by process of eating and being eaten constitute a food chain, eg. grassland ecosystem. Food chains can never occur independently in ecosystem but various food chains are inter-connected with each other forming an interlocked system known as food web. In grassland ecosystem food chains may be–

(i) Grass → Rabbit → Hawk/kite
(ii) Grass → Mouse → Snake → Kite/Hawk
(iii) Grass → Grasshopper → Lizard → Kite/Hawk

So, the food web will always include kite.

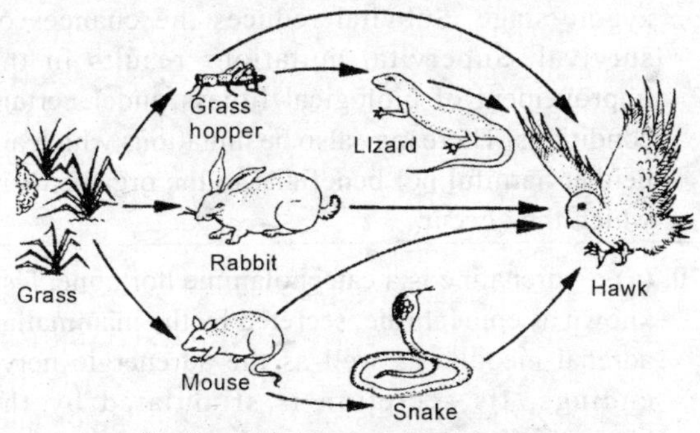

Fig. Food web in a grassland ecosystem

164. (a) : Inflammation is a process in which the body's WBCs and the chemicals released into the blood or the affected tissue to protect us from infection and foreign substances such as bacteria and viruses. This releases of chemicals increases the blood flow to the area of injury or infection. Inflammation is characterized by redness, swollen joint that's warm to touch, joint pain, joint stiffness & loss of joint function.

The increase number of cells and inflammatory substances within the joint causes irritation, wearing down of cartilage (cushions at the end of bones) and swelling of the joint lining. Inflammation of one or more joint results in arthritis. When there is a deposition of uric acid and crystals of sodium urates in the joints it will lead to gout arthritis. Uric acids is the end metabolism products of nitrogen containing purine nucleic acid. Gout generally affects one or two joints only. It is very painful particularly at night, and makes movement difficult. Gout generally affects great toe.

165. (b) : The first living organisms originated among organic molecules and in oxygen free atmosphere. They presumably obtained energy by fermentation of some of these organic molecules. They were non-green and anaerobes, capable of respiring in absence of oxygen. They depended on the existing organic molecules for their nutrition, hence they were heterotrophs. Then came autotrophs when the supply of existing organic molecules were exhausted. These organisms were capable of producing their own organic molecules by chemosynthesis. They synthesized food from inorganic molecules. Photoautotrophs were also anaerobic at first but later on oxygen releasing photosynthetic organism developed.

166. (b) : *E.coli*, *Shigella sp.* and *Salmonella* species are all bacteria which are responsible for the diarrhoea diseases. Diarrhoea is a frequent bowel evacuation or the passage of abnormally soft or liquid faeces. It may be caused by intestinal infections, other form of intestinal inflammation (such as Colitis or Crohn's disease), malabsorption, anxiety and the irritable bowel syndrome. Severe or prolonged diarrhoea may lead to excess losses of fluid, salts and nutrients in the faeces. Dehydration (whose symptoms includes great thirst, nausea and exhaustion) is common to all types of diarrhoeal diseases. The condition is treated by drinking plenty of water, severe cases require oral rehydration therapy or intravenous administration of water and salts. One litre of ORS (Oral rehydration solution) contains 1.5 gm glucose, 3.5 gm NaCl, 2.9 gm KCl & 2.9 gm trisodium citrate.

167. (b) : Deforestation increases atmospheric CO_2 content by releasing carbon stored in organic matter and reduced primary productivity. So deforestation is one of the main factors contributing to global warming other than green house gases. The various green house gases are CO_2 (60% effect), CH_4 (20% effect) CFC_s (14% effect) and nitrogen oxide

(N_2O, 6% effect). Due to increase of CO_2 concentration, the absorption of heat radiation also increase thus increasing the temperature. This increase in temperature may causes melting of glacier and polar ice caps, which is called global warming. This melting of glaciers and polar ice results in raising the sea level. Actually these green house gases absorbs infra red radiations (heat) of the sun like glass and thus traps the heat and does not allow it to radiate back to the space. They instead radiate the heat back to earth, thus causing increase in temperature.

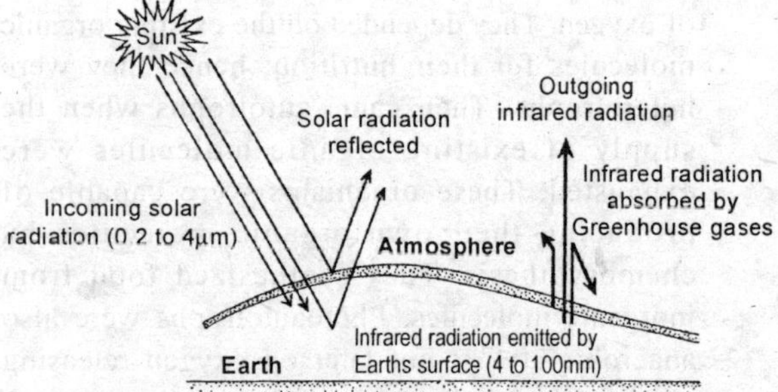

Fig. Greenhouse effect in keeping the earth warm.

168. (d) : An analgesic is any member of the diverse group of drugs used to relieve pain and to achieve analgesia. Analgesic drugs act in various ways on the peripheral and central nervous system; they include paracetamol (acetaminophen), the nonsteroidal anti-inflammatory drugs (NSAIDs) such as the salicylates, narcotic drugs such as morphine, synthetic drugs with narcotic properties such as tramadol, and various others.

LSD and marijuana are used as hallucinogens. Hallucinogens are natural and synthetic (synthesized) substances that, when ingested (taken into the body), significantly alter one's state of consciousness. Hallucinogenic compounds often cause people to see (or think they see) random colours, patterns, events, and objects that do not exist. These substances are sometimes called "pyschedelic," or "mind-expanding" drugs.

Marijuana and hashish, two substances derived from the hemp plant (*Cannabis sativa*), are also considered natural hallucinogens. Marijuana (also called grass, pot, tea, weed, or reefer), a green herb from the flower of the hemp plant, is considered a mild hallucinogen. Hashish is marijuana in a more potent, concentrated form. Both drugs are usually smoked. Their effects include a feeling of relaxation, faster heart rate, the sensation that time is passing more slowly, and a greater sense of hearing, taste, touch, and smell. LSD (Lysergic Acid Diethylamide) is the most common hallucinogen and one of the most potent mood-changing chemicals. It is manufactured from lysergic acid, found in a fungus that grows on rye and other grains. LSD users may experience flashbacks of visions they had when on the drug. Some LSD users suffer organic brain damage, which results in impaired memory and attention span, confusion, and difficulty in thinking.

169. (c) : Mutations are sudden and abruptive qualitative or quantitative change in the genetic material of an organism. According to their effects on the phenotype mutations may be classified as lethals, subvitals and supervitals. Lethal mutations results in death of the cells or organism in which they occur. The organism may not even develop beyond the zygote stage. Subvital reduces the chances of survival. Supervital mutations results in the improvement of biological fitness under certain conditions. There may also be mutations which are neither harmful nor beneficial to the organisms in which they occur.

170. (a) : Adrenaline is a catecholamine hormone, also known as epinephrine, secreted by the mammalian adrenal medulla as well as the adrenergic nerve endings. Its secretion is stimulated by the sympathetic nervous system under conditions of stress. Adrenaline stimulates blood flow to skeletal muscles and increases blood glucose levels. It also raises metabolic rate.

171. (d) : When the ambient temperature is high and soil contains excess water, the rate of transpiration is increased *i.e.,* loss of water takes place from leaves through stomata. Lenticular transpiration is only 0.1% of the total transpiration. It however continues day and night because lenticels have no mechanism of closure. The lenticels connect the atmospheric air with the cortical tissue of stem through intercellular spaces present amongst the complementary cells. Root pressure regulates the rate of loss of water from the stomata in some plants.

Root pressure is a positive pressure that develops in the xylem sap of the roots of some plants.

172. (c) : Xylem is the main conducting tissue in plants. It consists of 4 different components – tracheids, trachea or vessels, xylem fibre and xylem parenchyma. Tracheids are elongated cells with tapering end. They are generally present in ferns and gymnosperms for conduction of water. In angiosperms, vessels are composite structure as these are formed by dissolution of end walls of row of cells *i.e.*, vessels elements. So angiosperms, have more efficient system of conduction due to presence of vessels. Conduction of water by vessel elements is also known as ascent of sap. Water absorbed by roots, goes upward to replace the water loss by transpiration. The most accepted theory for ascent of sap is transpiration pull theory *i.e.,* when water is lost by transpiration from the leaves, a tension is created in the xylem and due to this water absorbed by roots hair is passed through vessels to the leaves. The xylem parenchyma are mainly for storage function but sometimes help in conduction.

173. (a) : Polytene chromosomes are quite common in salivary glands of insects and so are called salivary chromosomes. These chromosomes have high amount of DNA of almost 1000 times in *Drosophila* as compared to ordinary somatic chromosomes. These chromosomes are multistranded. They are in permanent prophase stage. These chromosomese are formed by somatic pairing between homologous chromosomes and repeated replication of their chromonemata without separation of chromatids. All the chromosomes may remain attached to one another at a common point called chromocentre.

174. (a) : Stratosphere zone of earth's atmosphere contains a layer of ozone (O_3) which prevents the earth surface from about 99% of incoming solar ultra violet radiations. The primary chemicals responsible for ozone depletion are a group of chlorine containing compounds called chloroflourocarbons (CFCs) used as coolants in refrigerators and air conditioners and propellants for aerosol cans and foam blowing agents for insulation and packaging and also as solvents. After their release into troposphere CFCs go to stratosphere when these are broken down by ultraviolet radiations releasing chlorine or bromine which break O_3 molecules into O_2 and O. Due to depletion of O_3 layer, higher levels of ultra violet rays reach earth surface. Depletion in the concentration of ozone over a restricted area is called ozone hole. Ozone depletions results in problems like skin cancer, cataract animals becoming blind, mutations, inhibiting photosynthesis, decreases in productivity. Decreased photosynthetic activity will increase O_2 concentration of the atmosphere resulting in global warming.

175. (a) : Hydrocarbon are major air pollutants. Methane is produced naturally during decomposition of organic matter, incomplete biomass combustion. Its concentration was 700 ppb in pre industrial times and 1750 ppb in 2000. So the concentration has more than doubled in the last 250 years. Flooded paddy fields, marshes, cattles etc. are the major sources of this gas.

176. (b) : A cross section of well developed soil shows more or less distinct layers called horizons. O-horizon is the topmost layer of soil and A-horizon comes below O horizon. In the topmost layer, vegetation grows and various biological activities takes place. Tropical rain forests are found in tropical zone of the world and are characterized by very high temperature and abundance of rainfall. Soil in these area are red latosols and are exceedingly thick. Leaching of minerals from the top soil occurs rapidly but cycling of nutrients also occur here. The laterite soils are generally infertile because of intensive leaching and not due to growth of micro-organism.

177. (a) : The technique of staining bacteria was given by a Dutch microbiologist Christian Gram and this technique is known as Gram staining. In the cell wall of gram +ve bacteria both horizontal and vertical peptide linkages are present due to which mesh is dense and stain does not come out. Futher outer layer of cell wall of Gram +ve bacteria is made up of techoic acid. In the cell wall of gram –ve bacteria, either horizontal or vertical peptide linkages are present, due to which mesh is loose and hence stain comes out when washed with alcohol. Further outermost layer of cell wall of Gram –ve bacteria is made up lipopolysaccharides.

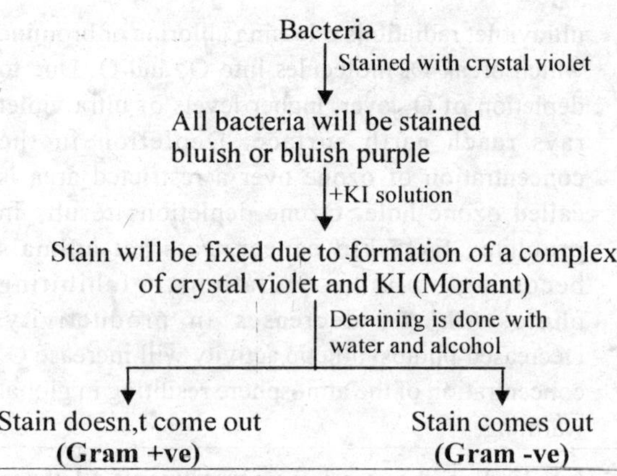

178. (c) : Photorespiration protects the plants from photoxidative damage by dissipating excess of excitation energy. When the CO_2 supply is limited and under high light intensity photorespiration takes place thus protecting the plants. If enough CO_2 is not available to utilize light energy for carboxylation to proceed, the excess energy will cause photoxidative damage to the plants. The energy liberated should be used in photophosphorylation in presence of CO_2. If CO_2 is less then in C_3 plants O_2 combines with RuBP to form phosphoglycollate thus utilizing the excess energy.

179. (d) : C_4 plants are those plants that produce C_4 compound like malic acid or aspartic acid as the first stable compound of CO_2 fixation cycle, eg. maize, sugar cane etc. These plants can grow in dense tropical, forests where there is poor supply of CO_2 because there is internal supply of CO_2. Also photorespiration is negligible or absent in these plants. So, they are photosynthetically more efficient than C_3 plants. These plants show a special type of leaf anatomy called Kranz anatomy. The C_4 pathway shows 2 carboxylation reactions one in mesophyll chloroplast and the other in bundle sheath. Chloroplasts - CO_2 acceptor is PEP and not RuBP and PEP carboxylase is the key enzyme.

180. (a) : The cytoskeleton is a fibrous network made of proteins that contributes to the structure and internal organization of eukaryotic cells within the cytoplasm. It is a dynamic structure that maintains cell shape, enables some cell motion (using structures such as flagella and cilia), and plays important roles in both intra-cellular transport (the movement of vesicles and organelles, for example) and cellular division. The cytoskeleton has three major fibre types: microfilaments made of actin protein, intermediate filaments made of various kinds of proteins (eg keratin), and microtubules made of tubulin.

GENERAL KINOWLEDGE

181. (d)	**182. (d)**	**183. (a)**	**184. (d)**
185. (c)	**186. (a)**	**187. (d)**	**188. (b)**
189. (a)	**190. (b)**	**191. (c)**	**192. (d)**
193. (a)	**194. (b)**	**195. (c)**	**196. (a)**
197. (a)	**198. (a)**	**199. (b)**	**200. (b)**

☺☺☺

SOLVED PAPER
AIIMS - 2007

Time : 3½ Hours

Max. Marks : 200

PHYSICS

1. The camera lens has an aperture of f and the exposure time is (1/60) s. What will be the new exposure time if the aperture become $1.4f$?
(a) $\frac{1}{42}$ (b) $\frac{1}{56}$
(c) $\frac{1}{72}$ (d) $\frac{1}{31}$

2. A point source is kept at a distance of 1000 m has an illumination I. To change the illumination to $16I$ the new distance should become
(a) 250 m (b) 500 m
(c) 750 m (d) 800 m

3. If collector current is 120 mA and base current is 2 mA and resistance gain is 3, what is power gain?
(a) 180 (b) 10800
(c) 1.8 (d) 18

4. With the decrease of current in the primary coil from 2 amperes to zero value in 0.01s the emf generated in the secondary coil is 1000 volts. The mutual inductance of the two coils is
(a) 1.25 H (b) 2.50 H
(c) 5.00 H (d) 10.00 H

5. In case of infinite long wire electric field is proportional to
(a) $\frac{1}{r}$ (b) $\frac{1}{r^2}$
(c) $\frac{1}{r^3}$ (d) r^0

6. What is the magnetic field at a distance R from a coil of radius r carrying current I?
(a) $\frac{\mu_0 IR^2}{2(R^2+r^2)^{\frac{3}{2}}}$ (b) $\frac{\mu_0 Ir^2}{2(R^2+r^2)^{\frac{3}{2}}}$
(c) $\frac{\mu_0 I}{2r}$ (d) $\frac{\mu_0 I}{2R}$

7. In the following diagram, which particle has highest e/m value?

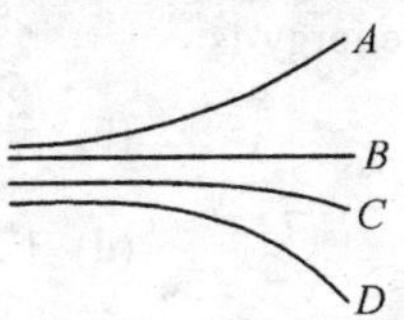

(a) A (b) B
(c) C (d) D

8. What is the energy of He^+ electron in first orbit?
(a) 40.8 eV (b) –27.2 eV
(c) –54.4 eV (d) –13.6 eV

9. What is the dimensions of impedance ?
(a) $ML^2T^{-3}I^{-2}$ (b) $M^{-1}L^{-2}T^3I^2$
(c) $ML^3T^{-3}I^{-2}$ (d) $M^{-1}L^{-3}T^3I^2$

10. If the highest modulating frequency of the wave is 5 kHz, the number of stations that can be accomodated in a 150 kHz bandwidth ?
(a) 15 (b) 10
(c) 5 (d) None of these

11. Zener diode acts as a/an
(a) oscillator (b) regulator
(c) rectifier (d) filter

12. In communication with help of antenna if height is doubled then the range covered which was initially r would become
(a) $\sqrt{2}r$ (b) $3r$
(c) $4r$ (d) $5r$

13. Which wavelength of sun is used finally as electric energy?
(a) Radio waves (b) Infra red waves
(c) Visible light (d) Micro waves

14. CO_2 laser uses
(a) microwaves (b) infra red
(c) ultra violet (d) visible light

15. Shear modulus is zero for
(a) solids (b) liquids
(c) gases (d) liquids and gases

16. Height of geostationary satellite is
(a) 16000 km (b) 22000 km
(c) 28000 km (d) 36000 km

17. If a solid sphere of mass 1 kg and radius 0.1 m rolls without slipping at a uniform velocity of 1 m/s along a straight line on a horizontal floor, the kinetic energy is
(a) $\frac{7}{5}$ J (b) $\frac{2}{5}$ J
(c) $\frac{7}{10}$ J (d) 1 J

18. In the diagram shown below all three rods are of equal length L and equal mass M. The system is rotated such that rod B is the axis. What is the moment of inertia of the system?

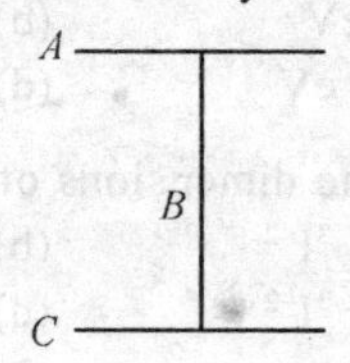

(a) $\frac{ML^2}{6}$ (b) $\frac{4}{3}ML^2$
(c) $\frac{ML^2}{3}$ (d) $\frac{2}{3}ML^2$

19. In the half wave rectifier circuit operating from 50 Hz mains frequency, the fundamental frequency in the ripple would be
(a) 25 Hz (b) 50 Hz
(c) 70.7 Hz (d) 100 Hz

20. In an AC circuit the potential differences across an inductance and resistance joined in series are respectively 16 V and 20 V. The total potential difference of the source is
(a) 20.0 V (b) 25.6 V
(c) 31.9 V (d) 53.5 V

21. The focal length of the objective and eye lenses of a microscope are 1.6 cm and 2.5 cm respectively. The distance between the two lenses is 21.7 cm. If the final image is formed at infinity. What is the linear magnification?
(a) 11 (b) 110
(c) 1.1 (d) 44

22. If the temperature of a black body increases from 7°C to 287°C then the rate of energy radiation increases by
(a) $\left(\frac{287}{7}\right)^4$ (b) 16
(c) 4 (d) 2

23. Faraday law of electrolysis indirectly shows
(a) quantisation of charge
(b) quantisation of angular momentum
(c) quantisation of current
(d) quantisation of viscosity

24. What is the amount of energy released by deuterium and tritum fusion?
(a) 60.6 eV (b) 12.6 eV
(c) 17.6 eV (d) 28.3 eV

25. What is the energy of photon whose wavelength is 6840 Å ?
(a) 1.81 eV (b) 3.6 eV
(c) −13.6 eV (d) 12.1 eV

26. Calculate power output of ${}^{235}_{92}U$ reactor, if it takes 30 days to use up 2 kg of fuel, and if each fission gives 185 MeV of useable energy. Avogadro's number = 6×10^{23}/mol?
(a) 56.3 MW (b) 60.3 MW
(c) 58.3 MW (d) 54.3 MW

27. A transistor is a/an
(a) chip (b) insulator
(c) semiconductor (d) metal

28. The number 0 (zero) is required for
(a) transistor (b) abacus
(c) computer (d) calculator

29. The magnetic susceptibility of an ideal diamagnetic substance is
(a) −1 (b) 0
(c) + 1 (d) ∞

30. The direction of the angular velocity vector is along
(a) the tangent to the circular path
(b) the inward radius
(c) the outward radius (d) the axis of rotation

31. A man of mass 60 kg records his wt. on a weighing machine placed inside a lift. The ratio of wts. of man recorded when lift is ascending up with a

uniform speed of 2 m/s to when it is descending down with a uniform speed of 4 m/s will be
(a) 0.5 (b) 1
(c) 2 (d) none of these

32. The force of gravitation is
(a) repulsive (b) conservative
(c) electrostatic
(d) non-conservative

33. In old age arteries carrying blood in the human body become narrow resulting in an increase in the blood pressure. This follows from
(a) Pascal's law
(b) Stoke's law
(c) Bernoulli's principle
(d) Archimede's principle

34. In an adiabatic change, the pressure and temperature of a monoatomic gas are related as $P \propto T^C$, where C equals
(a) $\frac{2}{5}$ (b) $\frac{5}{2}$
(c) $\frac{3}{5}$ (d) $\frac{5}{3}$

35. A large horizontal surface moves up and down in S.H.M. with an amplitude of 1 cm. If a mass of 10 kg (which is placed on the surface) is to remain continuously in contact with it, the maximum frequency of S.H.M. will be
(a) 5 Hz (b) 0.5 Hz
(c) 1.5 Hz (d) 10 Hz

36. A siren emitting sound of frequency 800 Hz is going away from a static listener with a speed of 30 m/s. The frequency of sound heard by listener is (velocity of sound = 300 m/s)
(a) 727.3 Hz (b) 481.2 Hz
(c) 644.8 Hz (d) 286.5 Hz

37. Which of the following physical quantities do not have same dimensions?
(a) pressure and stress
(b) tension and surface tension
(c) strain and angle
(d) energy and work.

38. Which of the following velocity-time graphs shows a realistic situation for a body in motion?

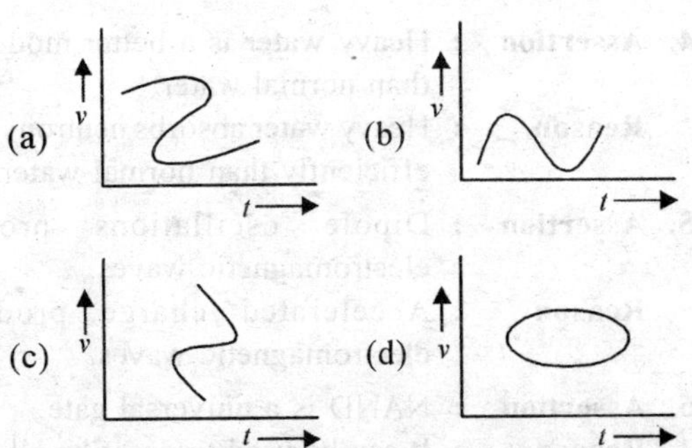

39. Work of 3.0×10^{-4} joule is required to be done in increasing the size of a soap film from 10 cm × 6 cm to 10 cm × 11 cm. The surface tension of the film is
(a) 5×10^{-2} N/m (b) 3×10^{-2} N/m
(c) 1.5×10^{-2} N/m (d) 1.2×10^{-2} N/m

40. If the water falls from a dam into a turbine wheel 19.6 m below, then the velocity of water at the turbines, is (Take $g = 9.8$ m/s^2)
(a) 9.8 m/s (b) 19.6 m/s
(c) 39.2 m/s (d) 98.0 m/s

Directions : In the following questions (41-60), a statement of assertion (A) is followed by a statement of reason (R). Mark the correct choice as :

[a] If both assertion and reason are true and reason is the correct explanation of assertion
[b] If both assertion and reason are true but reason is not the correct explanation of assertion
[c] If assertion is true but reason is false
[d] If both assertion and reason are false.

41. Assertion : Goggles have zero power.
Reason : Radius of curvature of both sides of lens is same

42. Assertion : A white source of light during interference forms only white and black fringes.
Reason : Width of fringe is inversely proportional to the wavelength of the light used.

43. Assertion : A current continues to follow in superconducting coil even after switch is off.
Reason : Superconducting coils show Meissner effect.

44. **Assertion** : Heavy water is a better moderator than normal water.
Reason : Heavy water absorbs neutrons more efficiently than normal water.

45. **Assertion** : Dipole oscillations produce electromagnetic waves.
Reason : Accelerated charge produces electromagnetic waves.

46. **Assertion** : NAND is a universal gate.
Reason : It can be used to describe all other logic gates.

47. **Assertion** : Ferro magnetic substances become paramagnetic above Curie temp.
Reason : Domains are destroyed at high temp.

48. **Assertion** : In a cavity within a conductor, the electric field is zero.
Reason : Charges in a conductor reside only at its surface.

49. **Assertion** : Voltmeter is connected in parallel with the circuit
Reason : Resistance of a voltmeter is very large.

50. **Assertion** : Ohm's law is applicable for all conducting elements.
Reason : Ohm's law is a fundamental law.

51. **Assertion** : No power loss associated with pure capacitor in ac circuit.
Reason : No current is flowing in this circuit.

52. **Assertion** : In a metal all the free electrons have same energy.
Reason : Electrons do not obey Pauli's exclusion principle.

53. **Assertion** : Optical fibres are used for telecommunication
Reason : Optical fibres are based on the phenomenon of total internal reflection.

54. **Assertion** : A hollow metallic closed container maintained at a uniform temperature can act as a source of black body radiation.
Reason : All metals act as black bodies.

55. **Assertion** : Machine parts are jammed in winter.
Reason : The viscosity of lubricant used in machine parts increase at low temperatures.

56. **Assertion** : An astronaut experience weightlessness in a space satellite.
Reason : When a body falls freely it does not experience gravity.

57 **Assertion** : A brass tumbler feels much colder than a wooden tray on a chilly day.
Reason : The thermal conductivity of brass is more than the thermal conductivity of wood.

58. **Assertion** : In free expansion of an ideal gas, the entropy increases.
Reason : Entropy increases in all natural processes.

59. **Assertion** : ^{94}Sr from the radioactive fall out from a nuclear bomb ends up in the bones of human beings through the milk consumed by them. It causes impairment of the production of red blood cells.
Reason : The energetics β-particles emitted in the decay of ^{94}Sr damage the bone marrow.

60. **Assertion** : Sound waves cannot travel in vacuum but light can travel in vacuum.
Reason : Sound waves are longitudinal waves and they cannot be polarised but electromagnetic waves are transverse and they can be polarised.

CHEMISTRY

61. In the following sequence of the reactions, what is *D* ?

$$C_6H_5CH_3 \xrightarrow{[O]} A \xrightarrow{SOCl_2} B \xrightarrow{NaN_3} C \xrightarrow{Heat} D$$

(a) Primary amine (b) An amide
(c) Phenyl isocyanate
(d) A chain lengthed hydrocarbon

62. The coordination number in *hcp* is
(a) 6 (b) 12
(c) 18 (d) 24.

63. Cyanogen gas is obtained in the reaction
(a) $CuSO_{4(aq)} + KCN \longrightarrow$
(b) $K_4[Fe(CN)_6] \xrightarrow{heat}$
(c) $CH_3CN + H_2O \xrightarrow{\Delta}$
(d) $CH_3CONH_2 + P_2O_5 \xrightarrow{\Delta}$

64. The pH of the solution obtained on neutralisation of 40 mL 0.1 M NaOH with 40 ml 0.1 M CH_3COOH is

(a) 7 (b) 8
(c) 6 (d) 3.

65. Inert gases are mixed in iodine vapours. Then there are _____ between them.

(a) H-bonding
(b) van der Waals forces
(c) Electrostatic forces
(d) Metallic bonds.

66. Bond length order is

(a) $O_2 < O_3 < O_2^{2-}$ (b) $O_2 < O_2^{2-} < O_3$
(c) $O_2^{2-} < O_3 < O_2$ (d) $O_2 = O_2^{2-} > O_3$.

67. Largest difference in radii is found in case of the pair

(a) Li, Na (b) Na, K
(c) K, Rb (d) Rb, Cs.

68. 1 mol each of the following compounds is dissolved in 1L of solution. Which will have the largest ΔT_b value?

(a) HF (b) HCl
(c) HBr (d) HI.

69. $CH_3OC_2H_5$ and $(CH_3)_3C - OCH_3$ are treated with hydroiodic acid. The fragments after reactions obtained are

(a) $CH_3I + HOC_2H_5$; $(CH_3)_3C - I + HOCH_3$
(b) $CH_3OH + C_2H_5I$; $(CH_3)_3Cl + HOCH_3$
(c) $CH_3OH + C_2H_5$; $(CH_3)_3C - OH + CH_3I$
(d) $CH_3I + HOC_2H_5$; $CH_3I + (CH_3)_3 - C - OH$.

70. Carbon and CO gas are used to reduce which of the following pairs of metal oxides for extraction of metals?

(a) FeO, SnO (b) SnO, ZnO
(c) BaO, Na_2O_2 (d) FeO, ZnO

71. Which of the following amines will not give N_2 gas on treatment with nitrous acid ($NaNO_2$ + HCl) ?

(a) $C_2H_5NH_2$ (b) CH_3NH_2
(c) $(CH_3)_2CH - NH_2$ (d) All will give N_2.

72. X-rays are emitted during

(a) α, *n* reaction (b) *K*-capture
(c) *n*, α reaction (d) β-emission.

73. In *P* versus *V* graph, the horizontal line is found in which _____ exists.

(a) Gas (b) Liquid
(c) Equilibrium between gas and liquid
(d) Super critical temperature.

74. During estimation of nickel, we prepare nickel dimethylglyoxime, a scarlet red solid. This compound is _____.

(a) ionic (b) covalent
(c) metallic
(d) non-ionic complex.

75. Critical temperatures for *A*, *B*, *C* and *D* gases are 25°C, 10°C, –80°C and 15°C respectively. Which gas will be liquefied more easily ?

(a) *A* (b) *B*
(c) *C* (d) *D*.

76. Which of the following metal ions will form complexes with the same magnetic moment and geometry irrespective of the nature of ligands?

(a) Ni^{2+} (b) Fe^{2+}
(c) Cu^{2+} (d) Co^{2+}

77. During titration of acetic acid with aq. NaOH solution, the neutralisation graph has a vertical line. This line indicates

pH —V→

(a) alkaline nature of equivalence
(b) acidic nature of equivalence
(c) neutral nature of equivalence
(d) depends on experimental proceeding.

78. Which of the following radioisotopes is used as anticancerous?

(a) Na-24 (b) C-14
(c) U-235 (d) Co-60.

79. XeF_6 on complete hydrolysis produces

(a) $XeOF_4$ (b) XeO_2F_2
(c) XeO_3 (d) XeO_2.

80. Calculate change in internal energy if $\Delta H = -92.2$ kJ, $P = 40$ atm and $\Delta V = -1$L.

(a) –42 kJ (b) –88 kJ
(c) +88 kJ (d) +42 kJ.

81. ΔH_{fusion} of a substance is '*x*' and ΔH_{vap} is '*y*', then $\Delta H_{sublimation}$ will be

(a) $x + y$ (b) $x - y$
(c) x/y (d) y/x.

82. Decay constant of a radioactive substance is 69.3 sec^{-1}, find $t_{1/16}$ of the same substance.
(a) 4×10^{-2} sec (b) 2×10^{-2} sec
(c) 1×10^{-2} sec (d) none of these.

83. The repeating unit in silicone is

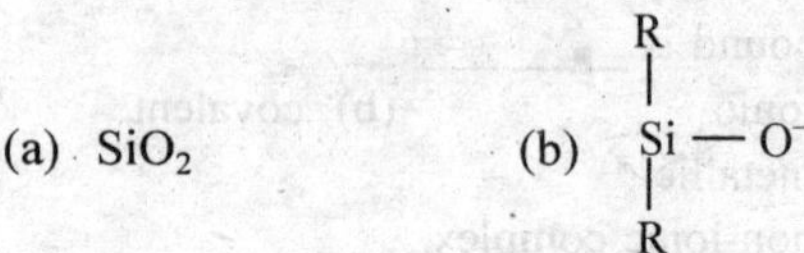

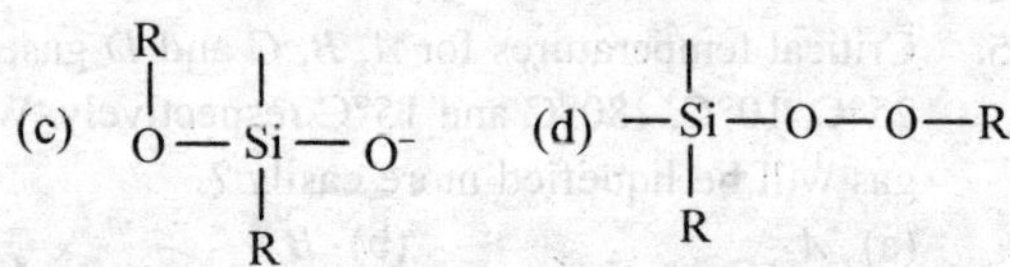

84. Propene on hydroboration and oxidation produces
(a) $CH_3CH_2CH_2OH$ (b) $CH_3CHOHCH_3$
(c) $CH_3CHOHCH_2OH$ (d) CH_3CH_2CHO.

85. $C_6H_5-CH_2CH=CH_2$ on mercuration and demercuration produces
(a) $C_6H_5-CH_2CHOHCH_3$
(b) $C_6H_5-CH_2CH_2CH_2OH$
(c) $C_6H_5-CH_2CHOHCH_2OH$
(d) none of these.

86. $C_6H_5-O-COCH_3 \xrightarrow[\Delta]{AlCl_3}$
The product obtained is/are
(a) *o*-product (b) *m*-product
(c) *o*- and *p*-products
(d) *o*-, *m*- and *p*-products.

87. The element which is the most abundant in the earth crust is
(a) O (b) S
(c) Al (d) H.

88. Wavelength of red light is absorbed by the complex
(a) $[Cu(CN)_4]^{2-}$ (b) $[Cu(NH_3)_4]^{2+}$
(c) $CuSO_4$ (d) $Cu(CN)_2$.

89. In the change $[Cu(H_2O)_6]^{2+} \xrightarrow{HCl} [CuCl(H_2O)_5]^{+}$, the colour changes from
(a) blue to green (b) blue to pink
(c) pink to green (d) pink to blue.

90. Benzoic acid is treated with lithium aluminium hydride. The compound obtained is
(a) benzaldehyde (b) benzyl alcohol
(c) toluene (d) benzene.

91. Chain transfer reagent is
(a) CCl_4 (b) CH_4
(c) O_2 (d) H_2.

92. Among the following components of cement which is present in highest amount?
(a) Ca_2SiO_4 (b) Ca_3SiO_5
(c) Al_2O_3 (d) $Ca_3Al_2O_6$.

93. A catalyst
(a) changes the equilibrium constant
(b) lowers the activation energy
(c) increases the forward and backward reactions at different speeds
(d) follows same mechanism for the reaction.

94. Which of the following does not contain any coordinate bond?
(a) H_3O^+ (b) BF_4^-
(c) HF_2^- (d) NH_4^+

95. Which of the following species participate in sulphonation of benzene ring ?
(a) H_2SO_4 (b) SO_3
(c) HSO_3^- (d) SO_2^-

96. Which of the following statement is true ?
(a) Trimethyl amines form a soluble compound with Hinsberg reagent and KOH.
(b) Dimethylamines react with KOH and phenol to form an azo dye.
(c) Methylamine reacts with nitrous acid and liberates N_2 from aq. soln.
(d) None of these.

97. ΔS_{surr} for an exothermic reaction is
(a) always positive (b) always negative
(c) zero
(d) may be positive or negative.

98. The vapour pressure of pure benzene at a certain temperature is 0.850 bar. A non-volatile, non-electrolyte solid weighing 0.5g is added to 39.0 g of benzene (molar mass 78 g/mol). The vapour pressure of the solution then is 0.845 bar. What is the molecular mass of the solid substance?
(a) 58 (b) 180
(c) 170 (d) 145.

99. Which of the following is optically inactive?

(a) Fischer projection: top H; H_3C—C—Cl; Cl—C—CH_3; bottom H

(b) Fischer projection: top H; Cl—C—CH_3; H_3C—C—Cl; bottom H

(c) Fischer projection: top H; H_3C—C—Cl; H_3C—C—Cl; bottom H

(d) none of these.

100. Which statement is true for ferrocene?

(a) All Fe-C are of equal length

(b) C are sp^3 hybridized

(c) It was the first discovered organometallic compound

(d) All of these.

Directions : In the following questions (101-120), a statement of assertion (A) is followed by a statement of reason (R). Mark the correct choice as :

[a] If both assertion and reason are true and reason is the correct explanation of assertion.

[b] If both assertion and reason are true but reason is not the correct explanation of assertion.

[c] If assertion is true but reason is false.

[d] If both assertion and reason are false.

101. ***Assertion*** : Copper sulphate solution is not stored in zinc vessel.
Reason : Zinc forms complex with $CuSO_4$.

102. ***Assertion*** : Benzene diazonium salt on boiling with water forms phenol.
Reason : C – N bond is polar.

103. ***Assertion*** : *trans*-butene on reaction with bromine forms racemic mixture.
Reason : *trans*-compound in *trans* addition forms two types of stereoisomers.

104. ***Assertion*** : Ozone is an allotrope of oxygen.
Reason : Oxygen is bluish colour liquid and in singlet state it is more paramagnetic.

105. ***Assertion*** : SnI_4 is an orange solid.
Reason : The colour arises due to charge transfer.

106. ***Assertion*** : Acetamide has more polar $>C=O$ group than in ethyl acetoacetate.
Reason : $\ddot{N}H_2$ is more electron donating than $\ddot{O}C_2H_5$.

107. ***Assertion*** : Magnetic moment of Dy is the highest among the lanthanoids.
Reason : Orbital motion contributes magnetic moment.

108. ***Assertion*** : C – O bond in metal carbonyl is long.
Reason : There is delocalisation of electrons from filled *d* orbitals into the empty orbitals on the CO ligands.

109. ***Assertion*** : Chloral reacts with phenyl chloride to form DDT.
Reason : It is an electrophilic substitution reaction.

110. ***Assertion*** : Mixture of CH_3COOH and CH_3COONH_4 is an example of acidic buffer.
Reason : Acidic buffer contains equimolar mixture of weak acid and its salt with weak base.

111. ***Assertion*** : Alkyl iodide can be prepared by treating alkyl chloride/bromide with NaI in acetone.
Reason : NaCl/NaBr are soluble in acetone while NaI is not.

112. ***Assertion*** : F is more electronegative than Cl.
Reason : F has high electron affinity than Cl.

113. ***Assertion*** : Acetylene on reacting with sodamide gives sodium acetylide and ammonia.
Reason : *sp* hybridised carbon atoms of acetylene are considerably electronegative.

114. ***Assertion*** : As a salt such as NaCl dissolves, the Na^+ and Cl^- ions leaving the crystal lattice acquire far greater freedom.
Reason : In thermodyanamic terms, the formation of solution occurs with a favourable change in free energy, *i.e.*, ΔH has a high positive value and $T\Delta S$ a low negative value.

115. ***Assertion*** : Alpha (α)-amino acids exist as internal salt in solution as they have amino and carboxylic acid groups in near vicinity.
Reason : H^+ ion given by carboxylic group (–COOH) is captured by amino group ($-NH_2$) having lone pair of electrons.

116. ***Assertion*** : The kinetics of the reaction –

$$mA + nB + pC \rightarrow m'X + n'Y + p'Z$$

obeys the rate expression as –

$$\frac{dx}{dt} = k[A]^m[B]^n$$

Reason : The rate of reaction does not depend upon the concentration of *C*.

117. ***Assertion*** : Molecular nitrogen is less reactive than molecular oxygen.
Reason : The bond length of N_2 is shorter than that of oxygen.

118. ***Assertion*** **:** The lactic acid shows the geometrical isomerism.
Reason **:** Lactic acid has carbon-carbon double bond.

119. ***Assertion*** **:** The equilibrium constant is fixed and a characteristic for any given chemical reaction at a specified temperature.
Reason **:** The composition of the final equilibrium mixture at a particular temperature depends upon the starting amount of reactants.

120. ***Assertion*** **:** The position of an element in periodic table after emission of one α and two β-particles remains unchanged.
Reason **:** Emission of one α and two β-particles give isotope of the element which acquires same position in periodic table.

BIOLOGY

121. Which of the following is an eye disease?
(a) hepatitis (b) measles
(c) glaucoma (d) bronchitis

122. Which match is true?

	Vitamin deficiency disease	Vitamin	Source
(a)	Severe bleeding	Tocopherol	Milk, egg
(b)	Anaemia	Ascorbic acid	Lemon, orange
(c)	Night blindness	Retinol	Carrot, milk
(d)	Sterility	Calciferol	Milk, butter

123. A child took sugar cane and sucked its juice. Regarding this which of the following match is correct?

	Substrate	Enzyme	Site of secretion of enzyme	Products formed
(a)	Proteins	Pepsin	Duodenum	Polypeptides
(b)	Starch	Amylase	Salivary glands	Glucose
(c)	Lipids	Lipase	Pancreas	Fat globules
(d)	Sucrose	Invertase	Duodenum	Glucose + Fructose

124. Which of the following does not come under the class mammals?
(a) flying fox (b) hedgehog
(c) manatee (d) lamprey

125. The black pigment in the eye which reduces the internal reflection is located in
(a) retina (b) iris
(c) cornea (d) sclerotic

126. Which of the following match is correct?

	Hormone	Effect
(a)	Oxytocin	Milk ejection hormone
(b)	Glucagon	Decreases blood sugar level
(c)	Adrenaline	Decreases heart rate
(d)	Thyroxine	Decreases BMR

127. Which of the following statements regarding glucagon is false?
(a) it is secreted by α-cells of Langerhans
(b) it acts antagonistically to insulin
(c) it decreases blood sugar level
(d) the gland responsible for its secretion is heterocrine gland

128. Which of the following is true regarding sperm?
(a) fertilizin : for penetrating egg membrane
(b) hyalurodinase : for penetrating egg membrane
(c) acrosin : dissolves corona radiata
(d) capacitation : takes place in penis

129. Which form of reproduction is correctly matched?
(a) *Euglena* → transverse binary fission
(b) *Paramecium* → longitudinal binary fission
(c) *Amoeba* → multiple fission
(d) *Plasmodium* → binary fission

130. Hearing impairment affects which part of brain?
(a) frontal lobe (b) parietal lobe
(c) temporal lobe (d) cerebellum

131. Which of the following match is correct?
(a) Emphysema : reduction of surface area of alveoli and bronchi
(b) Pneumonia : occupational disease with asbestos
(c) Silicosis : inflammation of alveoli
(d) Asthma : excessive secretion of bronchial mucus

132. The shoulder blade is made of
(a) clavicle (b) humerus
(c) ilium (d) scapula

133. "*Homo sapiens*" implies
(a) human race (b) human beings
(c) modern man (d) none of these

134. "*Omnis-cellula-e-cellula*" was given by
(a) Virchow (b) Hooke
(c) Leeuwenhoek (d) Brown

135. XO-chromosomal abnormality in human beings causes
(a) Turner's syndrome (b) Down's syndrome
(c) Klinefelter's syndrome
(d) none of these.

136. The component of blood which prevents its coagulation in the blood vessels is
(a) haemoglobin (b) plasma
(c) thrombin (d) heparin.

137. Wings of pigeon, mosquito and bat show
(a) divergent evolution
(b) atavism
(c) convergent evolution
(d) all of these.

138. Which of the following is responsible for the mechanical support, protein synthesis and enzyme transport?
(a) cell membrane (b) mitochondria
(c) dictyosome
(d) endoplasmic reticulum.

139. Thickening of arteries due to cholesterol deposition is
(a) arteriosclerosis (b) rheumatic heart
(c) blood pressure (d) cardiac arrest.

140. An example of competitive inhibition of an enzyme is the inhibition of
(a) succinic dehydrogenase by malonic acid
(b) cytochrome oxidase by cyanide
(c) hexokinase by glucose-6-phosphate
(d) carbonic anhydrase by carbon dioxide.

141. Which of the following is the connecting link between glycolysis and Krebs cycle?
(a) acetyl Co-A (b) oxalosuccinic acid
(c) pyruvic acid (d) citric acid

142. Which of the following contain β-1, 4 linkage?
(a) maltose (b) sucrose
(c) lactose (d) fructose

143. What is PAR range?
(a) 200 nm - 800 nm (b) 400 nm - 700 nm
(c) 350 nm - 550 nm (d) 600 nm - 100 nm

144. Which statement is true?
(a) adenine has 4 nitrogen atoms
(b) cytosine has 3 nitrogen atoms
(c) guanosine has 3 nitrogen atoms
(d) uracil has 5 nitrogen atoms

145. Beta diversity is diversity
(a) in a community
(b) between communities
(c) in a mountain gradient
(d) on a plain

146. Which of the following is correct match?

	Disease	Pathogen
(a)	Wilt disease	*Synchytrium*
(b)	Citrus canker	*Xanthomonas*
(c)	Red rot of sugarane	*Ustilago*
(d)	Powdery mildew	*Fusarium*

147. Which of the following helps in ascent of sap?
(a) root pressure (b) transpiration
(c) capillarity (d) all of these

148. Which of the following is correct set of micronutrient for plants?
(a) Mg, Si Fe, Cu Ca (b) Cu, Fe, Zn, B, Mn
(c) Mg, Fe, Zn, B, Mn (d) Mo, Zn, Cl, Mg, Ca

149. Velamen present in orchids help in
(a) absorbing water from support
(b) respiration
(c) absorption of moisture from air
(d) synthesising food

150. Hydroponics is
(a) nutrient less culture
(b) water less culture
(c) soilless culture
(d) none of these

151. Leghaemoglobin helps in
(a) nitrogen fixation
(b) protecting nitrogenase from O_2
(c) destroys bacteria
(d) transport of food in plants

152. Which among the following is a rootless plant?
(a) *Nymphaea* (b) *Sagittaria*
(c) *Ceratophyllum* (d) *Vallisneria*

153. Composite fruit develops from
(a) single ovary (b) inflorescence
(c) apocaropous ovary (d) pericarp

154. Ozone in stratosphere extends
(a) 10-20 km (b) 20-25 km
(c) 15-30 km (d) 25-40 km

155. Apomixis is
(a) formation of seeds by fusion of gametes
(b) formation of seeds without syngamy and meiosis
(c) formation of seeds with syngamy but no meiosis
(d) none of the above

156. Cocoa is the plant from which chocolate is made. Which part is used to extract it?
(a) flower (b) fruit
(c) seeds (d) bark

157. If a homozygous red-flowered plant is crossed with a homozygous white-flowered plant, the offsprings will be
(a) half-white flowered
(b) half red-flowered
(c) all white-flowered (d) all red-flowered

158. Gene which suppresses other gene's activity but does not lie on the same locus is called as
(a) epistatic (b) supplementary
(c) hypostatic (d) codominant

159. Pure line breed refers to
(a) heterozygosity only
(b) heterozygosity and linkage
(c) homozygosity only
(d) homozygosity and self assortment

160. Which part of the world has a high density of organism?
(a) deciduous forests
(b) grasslands
(c) tropical rain forests
(d) savannahs

Directions : In the following questions (161-180), a statement of assertion (A) is followed by a statement of reason (R). Mark the correct choice as :

[a] If both assertion and reason are true and reason is the correct explanation of assertion
[b] If both assertion and reason are true but reason is not the correct explanation of assertion
[c] If assertion is true but reason is false
[d] If both assertion and reason are false.

161. Assertion (A) : Haemophilia is a recessive sex linked disease.
Reason (R) : Haemophilia occurs due to mutation of a structural gene on chromosome 15.

162. Assertion (A) : Astigmatism is due to uneven curvature of lens.
Reason (R) : It is treated with cylindrical lenses.

163. Assertion (A) : Antigen can be easily recognized because it has antigenic determinants.
Reason (R) : The recognition ability is innate.

164. Assertion (A) : Blood coagulate in uninjured blood vessels.
Reason (R) : Uninjured blood vessels release an anticoagulant heparin.

165. Assertion (A) : Smaller the organism higher is the rate of metabolism per gram weight.
Reason (R) : The heart rate of a six month old baby is much lower than that of an old person.

166. Assertion (A) : Torison can be seen in ctendium.
Reason (R) : Ctenidium acts as the respiratory organ.

167. Assertion (A) : The earliest fossil form in the phylogeny of horse is eohippus.
Reason (R) : Eohippus lived during the early pliocene epoch.

168. Assertion (A) : Secreting hypotonic urine is effective in reducing urinary loss of water.
Reason (R) : Hypotonic urine is more concentrated and higher in osmotic pressure than the blood.

169. Assertion (A) : Aldosterone is a steroid hormone and is important in the control of sodium and potassium ion concentration in mammals.
Reason (R) : It upgrades sodium ion concentration in the ECF by promoting reabsorption of sodium ions from renal tubules and excretion of potassium ions in urine.

170. Assertion (A) : Pollution is always caused by human activities.
Reason (R) : Pollution is not different from contamination.

171. **Assertion (A) :** Algae and fungi are classified as thallophytes.

Reason (R) : They both are autotrophs.

172. **Assertion (A) :** Conifer trees produce a large quantity of wind borne pollen grains.

Reason (R) : The pollen grains have wings.

173. **Assertion (A) :** *Neurospora* is commonly called water mould.

Reason (R) : It belongs to basidomycetes fungi.

174. **Assertion (A) :** In woody stems, the amount of heart wood continues to increase year after year.

Reason (R) : The cambial activity continues uninterrupted.

175. **Assertion (A) :** Vernalization is acceleration of subsquent flowering by low temperature treatment.

Reason (R) : Site of vernalization is apical meristem.

176. **Assertion (A) :** Plants absorb sulphur in the form of sulphate ions.

Reason (R) : Sulphur bacteria are required for the formation of sulphate.

177. **Assertion (A) :** Chlorofluorocarbons are responsible for ozone depletion.

Reason (R) : Ozone level decreases by as much as 67% every year.

178. **Assertion (A) :** Dark reaction is purely enzymatic reaction.

Reason (R) : It occurs only in absence of light.

179. **Assertion (A) :** Vegetable oils are fats which are present in plant cells in soluble form.

Reason (R) : Vegetable oils occur only in cells of embryo.

180. **Assertion (A) :** Petroplants produce large amount of latex.

Reason (R) : The latex contains łong chain hydrocarbons.

GENERAL KNOWLEDGE

181. Only zero and one are used for operating
(a) Calculator (b) Computer
(c) Abacus (d) Type writer

182. Transistor is
(a) semi conductor (b) inductor
(c) modulator (d) demodulator

183. Computer cannot
(a) send message (b) abstract thought
(c) read files (d) play music

184. Which of the following is not a carbohydrate
(a) wax (b) starch
(c) sucrose (d) maltose

185. Which of the following is an eye disease?
(a) hepatitis (b) measles
(c) glaucoma (d) bronchitis

186. Which of the following is the vaccine for tuberculosis?
(a) DPT (b) BCG
(c) salk vaccine (d) rubella vaccine

187. Horns, nails and hair are
(a) soluble fats
(b) insoluble carbohydrates
(c) keratin proteins (d) complex lipids

188. Who conducts the State assembly elections?
(a) Chief Justice of the High Court concerned
(b) Chief Justice of the Supreme Court
(c) Chief Election Commission
(d) Governor of the state concerned

189. Which is an ore of aluminium?
(a) chromite (b) cuprite
(c) bauxite (d) siderite

190. Kalidas was
(a) A poet during the Gupta period
(b) A dramatist during Harshvardhana's reign
(c) An astronomer during Gupta period
(d) None of these

191. Which mirror is used as a rear view mirror in vehicles?
(a) plain (b) convex
(c) concave (d) spherical

192. The compilation "Meri Ekyawan Kavitayen's is by
(a) A.B. Vajpayee
(b) Harivanshrai Bachchan
(c) Dharam Vir Bharti
(d) Shiv Mangal Singh Suman

193. 'Equinox' means
(a) days are longer than nights
(b) days and nights are equal
(c) days are shorter than nights
(d) none of these

194. Who was known as "Nightingale of India"?
(a) Vijaylaxmi Pandit (b) Sarojini Naidu
(c) Suraiya (d) None of these

195. Gaya is associated with Lord buddha, where he
(a) was born
(b) attained enlightenment
(c) died
(d) delivered his first sermon

196. Chemical change does not take place in
(a) souring of milk into curd
(b) rusting of iron in atmosphere
(c) burning of magnesium ribbon in air
(d) emitting of light by a red hot platinum wire

197. Who is the highest wicket taker in Indian Cricket team?
(a) Javagal Srinath (b) Anil Kumble
(c) Maninder Singh (d) Kapil Dev

198. Which country leads in production of aluminium and aluminium goods
(a) Australia (b) U.S.
(c) Russia (d) Japan

199. Which of the following places was known as a centre of learning in ancient India?
(a) Nalanda (b) Ujjain
(c) Allahabad (d) none of these

200. The process of transfer of heat by matter but without actual movement of the particles themselves is called
(a) conduction (b) convection
(c) radiation
(d) none of the above

SOLUTIONS

PHYSICS

1. **(d) :** Time of exposure $\propto f^2$

$\frac{1}{60}\times\frac{1}{1}=\frac{t}{1.4^2} \Rightarrow t = 0.3266$ s

$t=\frac{1}{31}$ s.

2. **(a) :** For a point source, illuminance at a distance r is given by

Illuminance $I = \frac{\text{luminous flux} \times \phi}{4\pi r^2}$

$\therefore \quad \frac{I}{I'}=\left(\frac{r'}{r}\right)^2$

$\frac{I}{16I}=\frac{r'^2}{(1000\text{ m})^2}$

or $r'^2=\frac{(1000\text{ m})^2}{16}$ or $r'=\frac{(1000\text{ m})}{4}$

$r' = 250$ m

3. **(b) :** Current gain $\beta=\frac{I_C}{I_B}=\frac{(120\text{ mA})}{(2\text{ mA})}=60$

Power gain = Resistance gain × β^2
= (3) × $(60)^2$ = 10800

4. **(c) :** Induced emf $\varepsilon=\frac{-MdI_P}{dt}$

where M is the mutual inductance of two coils and $\frac{dI_P}{dt}$ is the rate of change of current in the primary.

$\therefore \quad 1000\text{ V}=\frac{-M(O\text{A}-2\text{ A})}{0.01\text{ s}}$

or $M=\frac{(1000\text{ V})(0.01\text{ s})}{(2\text{A})}=5$ H.

5. **(a) :** Electric field due to a infinite long wire of linear charge density λ is given by

$E=\frac{1\lambda}{2\pi\varepsilon_0 r}$

6. **(b) :** A coil of radius r carrying current I, magnetic field at a point at a distance R from the centre of the coil is given by

$B=\frac{\mu_0 Ir^2}{2[R^2+r^2]^{3/2}}$

At the centre of a coil, $R = 0$

$\therefore \quad B=\frac{\mu_0 Ir^2}{2r^3}=\frac{\mu_0 I}{2r}$

7. **(d) :** $evB=\frac{mv^2}{r}$

$\frac{e}{m}\propto\frac{1}{r}$, if B and v are the same. The radius of curvature of D is minimum. Therefore $\frac{e}{m}$ is maximum.

8. **(c) :** For hydrogen like atoms like He^+, Li^{++} etc, the energy in an nth orbit is given by

$E_n=\frac{-Z^2\,13.6}{n^2}$ eV

For He^+, $Z = 2$

$\therefore \quad E_1=\frac{-(2)^2\,13.6}{(1)^2}$ eV $= -54.4$ eV

9. **(a) :** Impedance has the same dimensions as that of a resistance

$\therefore$ Resistance $R=\frac{\text{Voltage } V}{\text{current } I}$

$=\frac{[\text{ML}^2\text{T}^{-3}\text{I}^{-1}]}{[\text{I}]}=[\text{ML}^2\text{T}^{-3}\text{I}^{-2}]$

10. **(a) :** Number of stations $=\frac{\text{Band width}}{\text{Band width/stations}}$;

Bandwidth per station = 2 × 5 kHz

Total bandwidth = 150 kHz.

Number of stations $=\frac{150}{10}=15$

11. **(b) :** Zener diode acts as an a voltage regulator.

12. **(a) :** Range $r=\sqrt{2Rh}$

where R is the radius of the earth and h is the height of a antenna

$\therefore \quad r'=\sqrt{2R(2h)}=\sqrt{2}(\sqrt{2Rh})=\sqrt{2}\,r$

13. **(b) :** Infrared rays or heat rays used for heating thermocouples to produce electricity.

14. **(c) :** One has to use higher energy to produce radiation in the visible region. In CO_2 laser two electrodes produce discharge which is used. Therefore ultraviolet rays are used to produce light in any lower energy region.

15. **(c) :** Even viscosity is due to shearing when flow takes place in stream lined motion. In gases, there is no shearing and therefore no shear modulus.

16. **(d) :** The principle of the geostationary satellite is its period of rotation is the same as that of the earth.

$$\frac{-GMm}{r^2} + m\omega^2 r = 0$$

i.e. $\frac{GM}{(R+h)^2} = \left(\frac{2\pi}{T}\right)^2 (R+h)$

h works out to 36000 km.

17. **(c) :** K.E of rolling $= \left(\frac{1}{2}mv^2 + \frac{1}{2}I.\frac{v^2}{R^2}\right)$

$$\Rightarrow \quad \text{K.E} = \frac{1}{2}mv^2 + \frac{1}{2}\cdot\frac{2}{5}\cdot\frac{mr^2.v^2}{r^2}$$

$$\text{K.E} = \frac{1}{2}mv^2 \times \frac{7}{5}$$

m = 1 kg , v = 1 m/s

$$\text{K.E} = \frac{1}{2}\times 1\times 1\times\frac{7}{5} = \frac{7}{10}\text{ J}$$

18. **(a) :** Since the width negligible, the moment of inertia of B is zero along its length.

$$I_A + I_C = \frac{mL^2}{12} + \frac{mL^2}{12} = \frac{mL^2}{6}$$

19. (b) :

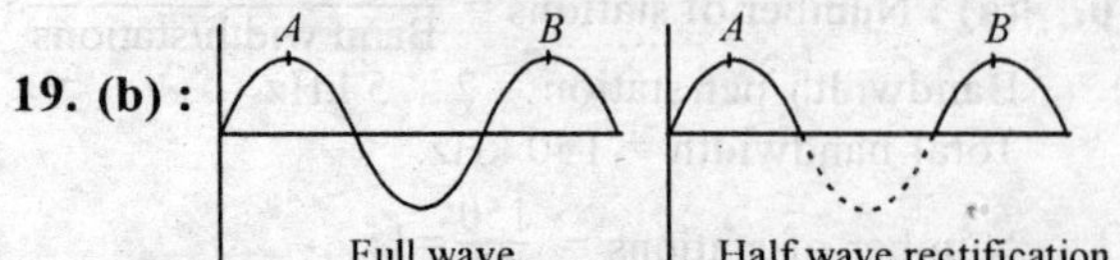

Full wave Half wave rectification

In full wave a.c. or half rectified, the time interval between two peaks are the same. But in half wave rectification, the negative wave part is cut off. But as for frequency or the period, they will be the same as seen from the figures. Therefore, this also will be 50 cycles/second.

20. **(b) :** V_L = 16 V, V_R = 20 V.

In the inductor the current lags by $\frac{\pi}{2}$.

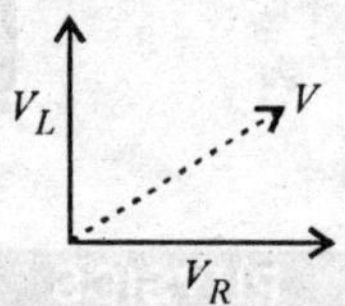

$$\therefore \quad V = \sqrt{V_L^2 + V_R^2} = \sqrt{256+400}$$

$\therefore V_{total} = 25.6$ V.

21. **(b) :**

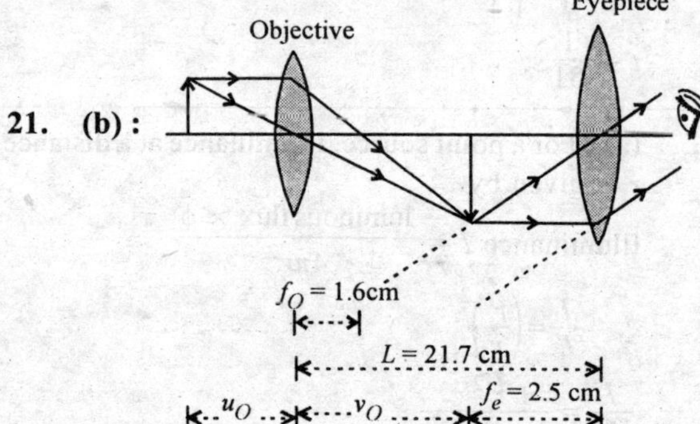

Here $v_O = L - f_e = 21.7$ cm $- 2.5$ cm $= +19.2$ cm

+ve sign show that image is real.

For a objective lens $\frac{1}{u_O} + \frac{1}{v_O} = \frac{1}{f_O}$

[using real-virtual sign convention]

$$\therefore \quad \frac{1}{u_O} = \frac{1}{f_O} - \frac{1}{v_O} \quad \therefore \quad \frac{1}{u_O} = \frac{1}{(+1.6)} - \frac{1}{(+19.2)}$$

$$\frac{1}{u_O} = \frac{19.2-1.6}{(1.6)(19.2)} \quad \text{or} \quad u_O = +1.745 \text{ cm}$$

+ve sign show that object is real

When the image is formed at infinity, the magnification is given by

$$m = \left(\frac{v_O}{u_O}\right)\left(\frac{D}{f_e}\right)$$

where D is the distance of distinct vision.

$$\therefore \quad m = \left(\frac{19.2\text{ cm}}{1.745\text{ cm}}\right)\left(\frac{25\text{ cm}}{2.5\text{ cm}}\right) = 110.$$

22. **(b) :** The energy radiated per unit time by a black body at absolute temperature T is given by $H = A\sigma T^4$.

where A is the area of a black body

$$\text{or} \quad \frac{H'}{H} = \frac{[(287+273)\text{K}]^4}{[(7+273)\text{K}]^4} = \left[\frac{560}{280}\right]^4 = 16$$

23. **(a)**

24. **(c) :** $^{2}_{1}H + ^{3}_{1}H \rightarrow ^{4}_{2}He + ^{1}_{0}n + Q$
Deuterium Tritium Helium neutron

The energy released in the process is given by

$$Q = \left[M_{^{2}_{1}H} + M_{^{3}_{1}H} - M_{^{4}_{2}He} - M_{^{1}_{0}n}\right]c^2$$

$= [2.014102 + 3.016050 - 4.002603 - 1.008665]uc^2$

$= (0.018884\text{ u})\left[931.5\frac{\text{MeV}}{\text{u}}\right] = 17.6\text{ MeV}.$

25. **(a) :** $\lambda = 6840$ Å

$\therefore \quad \upsilon = \frac{c}{\lambda} \Rightarrow h\upsilon = \frac{hc}{\lambda}$; $hc = 12400$ eVÅ

Energy of the photon $= \frac{12400\text{ eVÅ}}{6840\text{ Å}} = 1.81$Å

26. **(c) :** Mass of $^{235}_{92}U$ per second in the reactor is

$$m = \frac{2\times10^3}{30\times24\times60\times60} = 7.72\times10^{-4}\text{ g/sec}$$

$\therefore$ Number of fissions reaction per second

$= \frac{6\times10^{23}}{235}\times m = \frac{6\times10^{23}\times7.72\times10^{-4}}{235}$

$= 1.97\times10^{18}$/sec

Power of nuclear reactor $= 1.97\times10^{18}\times185$ MeV/s

$= 1.97\times10^{18}\times185\times10^{6}\times1.6\times10^{-19}$ J/s.

$= 58.3$ MW.

27. **(c) :** A transistor is an semiconductor.

28. **(c) :** A computer is working on a binary system of calculations based on zero and 1.

29. **(a) :** For dimagnetic substance, magnetic susceptibility is $-1 \le \chi < 0$

For ideal or perfect diamagnetic substances magnetic susceptibility is –1.

Type 1- superconductors are perfect diamgnetic.

30. **(d) :** $v = r \times \omega$.

v is the tangential. If r is in the XY plane and v is also in this plane, ω is in the Z direction. + or – is decided by whether the particle is rotating in the anticlockwise direction or clockwise direction.

31. **(b) :** Uniform speed will not affect his weight.

The ratio is $\frac{60\times g}{60\times g} = 1$

32. **(b) :** Conservative force

The work done is independent of the path.

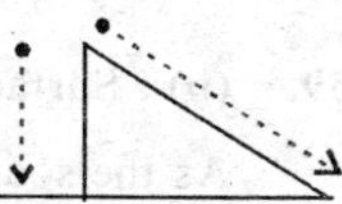

33. **(c) :** Bernoulli's principle,

If one has water flowing in a horizontal tube, the pressure will be the same.

But the velocity will be more. If there is any obstruction, then pressure will also build up. Bernoulli's law is valid for luminous flow.

In old age arteries get thicker and narrow.

34. **(b) :** $\gamma = 1 + \frac{2}{f}$

$\Rightarrow \gamma$ for mono atomic gas $= 1 + \frac{2}{3} = \frac{5}{3}$

For adiabatic relation $\frac{P^{\gamma-1}}{T^{\gamma}} = $ const;

$P \propto T^{\frac{\gamma}{\gamma-1}} \Rightarrow P \propto T^{\frac{5}{3}\times\frac{3}{2}}$

$\therefore \quad T^C = T^{\frac{5}{2}} \Rightarrow C = \frac{5}{2}$.

35. **(a) :** Here, $a = 1$ cm $= 0.01$ m; The mass will remain in contact with surface, if

$mg = m\omega^2 a$ or $\omega = \sqrt{g/a}$

or $2\pi\upsilon = \sqrt{g/a}$ or $\upsilon = \frac{1}{2\pi}\sqrt{\frac{g}{a}}$

$\upsilon = \frac{7}{2\times22}\sqrt{\frac{980}{1}} = 4.9\text{ s}^{-1} = 5\text{ Hz}$

36. **(a) :** Here, $\upsilon = 800$ Hz, $v_s = 30$ m/s, $v = 300$ m/s.

As the source is going away from the stationary observer, therefore,

$\upsilon' = \frac{v\times\upsilon}{v+v_s} = \frac{300\times800}{300+30} = \frac{300\times800}{330} = 727.3$ Hz .

37. **(b) :** Pressure and stress both have the dimensions of force/area. Strain and angle are both dimensionless. Energy and work have the same dimensions force × distance.

Tension and surface tension refer to two different physical quantities and their dimensions are different. Tension is a force and surface tension is force per unit length.

38. **(b) :** In the other graphs, at a particular time more than one velocity is shown which is not possible in realistic situation.

39. **(b) :** Surface tension, $S = \frac{\text{work done}}{\text{increase in area}}$

As the soap film has two surfaces.

$$S = \frac{3.0\times10^{-4}\text{ J}}{2\times(10\times11-10\times6)\times10^{-4}\text{ m}^2}$$

$= 3 \times 10^{-2}$ N/m.

40. **(b) :** $v=\sqrt{2gh}=\sqrt{2\times9.8\times19.6}=19.6$ m/s.

41. **(a) :** *Both assertion and reason are true and reason is the correct explanation of assertion.*

Assertion : Goggles have zero power. True

The focal length is given by $\frac{1}{f}=(\mu-1)\left(\frac{1}{R_1}-\frac{1}{R_2}\right)$.

For goggle lenses, both sides are curved the same way. R_1 and R_2 are positive. If they are the same, $\frac{1}{f}=0$ *i.e.* power is zero. Reason is also true and it is the explanation for the assertion.

42. **(d) :** *Both the assertion and reason are false.*

Fringe width $\beta=\frac{\lambda D}{d}$. This depends on the wavelength. Diffraction depends on the wavelength of light. Therefore if a white source of light is used, only the central fringe will be white. All the rest have different wavelengths and some orders will also overlap for different colours. Both the assertion and the reason are false because the fringe width is not independent of wavelength.

43. **(b) :** *Both assertion and reason are true but reason is not the correct explanation of assertion.*

The assertion is true. Even when the *emf* is switched off, the current continues to flow because its resistance becomes zero.

The Meissner effect is another property of the superconductor and not the reason for the assertion. Meissner effect repels the magnetic field lines from the interior of the superconductor. (b)

44. **(c) :** *Assertion is true but reason is false.*

The assertion is true because heavy - water is a better moderator than ordinary water. This is because heavy water absorbs fewer neutrons than normal water. The assertion is right. The reason is false.

45. **(a) :** *Both assertion and reason are true and reason is the correct explanation of assertion.*

Assertion is true. The reason is also true according to the classical theory of Maxwell. The dipole oscillation gives radiation because the charges are accelerated. (Any oscillation has acceleration).

46. **(a) :** *Both assertion and reason are true and reason is the correct explanation of assertion.*

NAND and NOR gates are treated as universal gates because all other basic gates AND gate OR gate and NOT gate can be constructed using only NAND gate (or NOR gate).

47. **(a) :** *Both assertion and reason are true and reason is the correct explanation of assertion.*

The assertion is true. From Curie Weiss law where the susceptibility $\chi=\frac{C}{(T-\theta_C)}$. If the temperature rises above the Curie temperature θ_C, ferromagnetic materials become paramagnetic materials because the domains get destroyed as stated.

48. **(a) :** *Both assertion and reason are true and reason is the correct explanation of assertion.*

Both the assertion and reason are true and the reason is the correct explanation. It is because the charges are only at the surface of a conductor; the charge enclosed in the Gaussian surface in the cavity is zero. The field is therefore zero.

49. **(a) :** *Both assertion and reason are true and reason is the correct explanation of assertion.*

A voltmeter is always connected in parallel. This has of course a large resistance. The assertion and reason are correct and it is the correct explanation.

50. **(d) :** *Both the assertion and reason are false.*

Both the assertion and reason are false. Ohms law is obeyed by metals for a certain range of temperature, not obeyed by superconductors, valves, diodes and semiconductors. It is not a universal law but it is purely empirical.

51. **(c) :** *Assertion is true but reason is false.*

Assertion is true. When a capacitor is connected to an a.c. circuit, $\varepsilon_{rms}=i_{rms}\left(\frac{1}{C\omega}\right)$ where $\frac{1}{C\omega}$ is the impedance due to capacitative resistance. The power consumed in this circuit is zero because the phase difference ϕ between *emf* and current in a pure capacitance a.c. circuit is $\frac{\pi}{2}$. Power factor $\cos\phi = 0$. It is only for d.c. that a current does not flow. Reason is false.

52. **(c) :** *Assertion is true but reason is false.*
Assertion is correct in the sense that the free electrons occupy a single energy band. But a band has a distribution of energy. One can treat assertion as correct. But the reason is false because electrons in a metal follow Pauli's exclusion principle. It is because of this, one has different bands. Therefore the answer is (c).

53. **(a) :** *Both assertion and reason are true and reason is the correct explanation of assertion.*
Optical fibers are used in communication and it is because the phenomenon of total internal reflection, taking place inside the fiber for the signal incident. Both the statements are correct and the reason given is the right explanation.

54. **(d) :** *Both the assertion and reason are false.*
A hollow metallic container with a small orifice and coated with lamp black inside is taken as a source of black-body radiation when it is heated. A closed container cannot act as a source of blackbody because it cannot absorb all radiations. All metals are not black bodies. A black body is described above. It is the hole that absorbs and emits the radiation, which is treated as a black body and not even the whole container.
Assertion is only partially correct. The statement given in the reason is wrong.

55. **(a) :** *Both assertion and reason are true and reason is the correct explanation of assertion.*
Both the assertion and the reason are correct. Special lubricants have to be used at low temperature.

56. **(b) :** *Both assertion and reason are true but reason is not the correct explanation of assertion*
Both the statements of assertion and the reason are correct. They are independent statements. The statement given in the reason is not the reason for the weightlessness of the astronaut. The centripetal and centrifugal forces cancel out. In the case of free fall, the pseudo acceleration, *g* acts upwards. The body does not feel it. But all the same it will fall down to the earth. His mind which feels, is riding the lift of his body. The body is falling down with acceleration *g*. In the first case, the force of acceleration due to gravity is cancelled by the centrifugal force acting outwards. Both the statements are correct but the reason given is not the reason for the assertion.

57. **(a) :** *Both assertion and reason are true and reason is the correct explanation of assertion.*
Both the assertion and reason are correct because the conducting brass tumbler absorbs heat from the body. The hand feels cold when the tumbler is touched.

58. **(a) :** *Both assertion and reason are true and reason is the correct explanation of assertion.*

59. **(a) :** *Both assertion and reason are true and reason is the correct explanation of assertion.*

^{94}Sr from ^{235}U fission is absorbed through milk. Their emission of β^- particles will damage the bone-marrow as Sr is absorbed in bones.

60. **(b) :** *Both assertion and reason are true but reason is not the correct explanation of assertion.*
Both the assertion and reason are correct statements but the reason given is not the explanation for the assertion.

CHEMISTRY

61. **(c) :**

$$C_6H_5CH_3 \xrightarrow{[O]} \underset{(A)}{C_6H_5COOH} \xrightarrow[-SO_2,\,-HCl]{SOCl_2} \underset{(B)}{C_6H_5COCl}$$

$$\xrightarrow[-NaCl]{NaN_3} \underset{(C)}{C_6H_5CON_3} \xrightarrow[-N_2,\ \text{rearrangement}]{\Delta} \underset{(D)}{C_6H_5NCO}$$

62. (b) : The number of nearest neighbour with which a given sphere is in contact is called coordination number. The C.N. in *hcp* and *ccp* arrangement is 12.

63. (a) : $2CuSO_4 + 4KCN \rightarrow (CN)_2 + 2CuCN + 2K_2SO_4$
On combining solution of copper (II) salts and cyanides, an unstable copper (III) cyanide is formed which rapidly decomposes into copper (I) cyanide and cyanogen.

64. (b) : $NaOH + CH_3COOH$ forms CH_3COONa which gives basic solution with pH > 7.

65. (b) : There are several types of van der Waals attraction : dipole/dipole, dipole/induced-dipole and spontaneous-dipole/induced-dipole. The spontaneous-dipole/induced-dipole attractions are also known as *London dispersion forces*. LDF are surprisingly strong but are only short range forces *e.g.* surface of neutral molecules or inert gases. All molecules have LDF and strength increases with the size/surface area of the molecule. In case of halogens, LDF increases as $F_2 < Cl_2 < Br_2 < I_2$.

66. (a) : Ozone molecule is V-shaped with O – O bond length 1.278 Å.

(O–O bonds 1.278 Å, 1.278 Å; angle 116.8°)

The bond length is intermediate between that for a single bond (1.48 Å as in H_2O_2) and for a double bond (1.21 Å as in O_2).

Also, bond order $\propto \frac{1}{\text{bond length}}$

Hence, $O_2 < O_2^{2-}$.

67. (b) : Atomic as well as ionic radii increases from Li to Fr due to the presence of one extra shell of electron.

	Li	Na	K	Rb	Cs
Metallic radii (pm)	152	186	227	248	265

68. (d) : Bond dissociation energy increases in the order.

HI < HBr < HCl < HF

HF is most stable halogen acid and HI is the least. Higher the bond dissociation energy, lower is the degree of ionisation.

As we know $\Delta T_b = ik_bm$.
Hence ΔT_b value is largest in HI. All colligative properties depend on number of particles.

69. (a) : When mixed ethers are used, the alkyl iodide produced depends on the nature of alkyl groups. If one group is Me and the other a pri- or sec-alkyl group, then methyl iodide is produced. Here reaction occurs via S_N2 mechanism and because of the steric effect of the larger group, I^- attacks the smaller (Me) group.

$$CH_3OC_2H_5 + HI \rightarrow CH_3I + C_2H_5OH$$

When the substrate is a methyl *t*-alkyl ether, the products are *t*-*R*I and MeOH. Here reaction occurs by S_N1 mechanism and formation of products is controlled by the stability of carbocation. Since carbocation stability order is $3^o > 2^o > 1^o > \overset{\oplus}{C}H_3$.

$\therefore$ Alkyl halide is always derived from *tert*-alkyl group.

$$CH_3-\underset{CH_3}{\overset{CH_3}{|}}{C}-O-CH_3 + HI \xrightarrow[S_N1]{373\text{ K}} CH_3-\underset{CH_3}{\overset{CH_3}{|}}{C}-O-I + CH_3OH$$

tert - Butyl methyl ether   *tert* - Butyl iodide

70. (d) : $Fe^{+2}O + C \rightarrow Fe^0 + CO$ (reduction)

$$FeO + C \rightarrow Fe + CO_2$$

Similarly, $Zn^{+2}O + C \rightarrow Zn^0 + CO$ (reduction)

$$ZnO + C \rightarrow Zn + CO_2$$

71. (d) : All aliphatic primary amines liberate N_2 gas on treatment with HNO_2.

$$R-NH_2 + HONO \xrightarrow{273-278\text{ K}} R-OH + N_2 + H_2O$$

Since no other class of amines liberate N_2 gas on treatment with HNO_2, this reaction is used as a test for aliphatic primary amines.

72. (c) : In certain nucleus, the nucleus captures an electron from the *K*-shell (being nearest to the nucleus). The vacancy created is filled up with the electron from the higher shells thereby emitting X-rays. As a result of *K*-electron capture, a proton in the nucleus is converted into a neutron ($P^+ + e^- \rightarrow n$).

73. (c) :

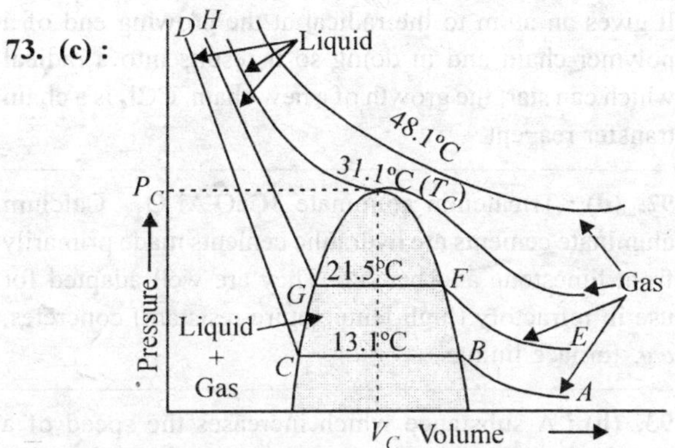

From the graph, at point A, CO_2 exists as a gas, As pressure is increased, the volume of the gas decreases along the curve AB. At B liquefaction of the gas starts. Hence, volume decreases rapidly along BC because liquid has much less volume than the gas. At point C, liquefaction is complete.

Amount of gas decreased = Amount of liquid formed or increased.

Because along horizontal line, gas converts into liquid.

74. (d) :

$$\begin{matrix} & O^- \\ & | \\ H_3C-C{=}N: \\ | \\ H_3C-C{=}N: \\ & | \\ & O-H \end{matrix} + Ni^{2+} + \begin{matrix} H-O \\ | \\ :N{=}C-CH_3 \\ | \\ :N{=}C-CH_3 \\ | \\ O^- \end{matrix}$$

$$\longrightarrow \begin{matrix} {}^-O \cdots H - O \\ | \qquad\qquad | \\ H_3C-C{=}N \rightarrow Ni^{2+} \leftarrow N{=}C-CH_3 \\ H_3C-C{=}N \rightarrow \qquad \leftarrow N{=}C-CH_3 \\ | \qquad\qquad | \\ O - H \cdots O^- \end{matrix}$$

Bis-(dimethylglyoximato) nickel (II) chelated complex (red ppt)

This planar complex is very poorly soluble and is used for the gravimetric determination of nickel *e.g.* ores.

75. (a) : Critical temperature of gas may be defined as that temperature above which it cannot be liquefied how so ever high pressure may be applied on the gas.

As we know, $T_C = \dfrac{8a}{27Rb}$

where a = van der Waal's constant which is a measure of intermolecular forces of attraction. Greater the value of a more easily the gas can be liquefied and hence larger T_C mean larger the value of a.

76. (c) : In presence of either strong field or weak field, the number of unpaired electron remains the same in case of Cu^{2+} ion.

$$Cu \longrightarrow 3d^{10}4s^1$$
$$Cu^{2+} \longrightarrow 3d^9$$

↑↓	↑↓	↑↓	↑↓	↑

77. (a) : In any type of acid-base titration, there is a sudden change in the pH value at the end point. During the titration of a weak acid with a strong base, beyond the equivalent point, the solution will contain the salt and excess of free base.

$$CH_3COOH + NaOH \longrightarrow \underset{\text{Sodium acetate}}{CH_3COONa} + H_2O$$

Due to the presence of free base, solution becomes alkaline in nature.

78. (d) : Radiation (γ-rays) emitted by the radioactive substances ($_{27}Co^{60}$) destroys the cells. Hence, it is used in treatment of cancer in which the malignant cells are wiped out.

79. (c) : $XeF_{6(s)} + 3H_2O_{(l)} \longrightarrow \underset{\substack{\text{highly} \\ \text{explosive}}}{XeO_{3(s)}} + 6HF_{(aq)}$

80. (b) : $\Delta H = \Delta E + P\Delta V$

$$\Delta E = \Delta H - P\Delta V = -92.2 - 40 \times (-1) \times 101 \times 10^{-3}$$
$$= -92.2 + 4.04 = -88.16 \text{ kJ} \approx -88 \text{ kJ}.$$

81. (a) : Solid $\xrightarrow{\text{fusion}}$ Liquid $\quad \Delta H_{\text{fusion}} = x$

Liquid $\xrightarrow{\text{vaporisation}}$ Gas $\quad \Delta H_{\text{vap}} = y$

Solid $\xrightarrow{\text{sublimation}}$ Gas $\quad \Delta H_{\text{sub}}$

So, $\Delta H_{\text{sub}} = \Delta H_{\text{fusion}} + \Delta H_{\text{vap.}}$, $\Delta H_{\text{sub}} = x + y$.

82. (a) : $1 \xrightarrow{t_{1/2}} \frac{1}{2} \xrightarrow{t_{1/2}} \frac{1}{4} \xrightarrow{t_{1/2}} \frac{1}{8} \xrightarrow{t_{1/2}} \frac{1}{16}$

So, $t_{1/16} = 4t_{1/2}$

$$= 4 \times \frac{0.693}{\lambda} = 4 \times \frac{0.693}{69.3} = 4 \times 10^{-2} \text{ sec.}$$

83. (b) : R_2SiO^- is the repeating unit in silicone.

$$HO-\underset{R}{\overset{R}{\underset{|}{\overset{|}{Si}}}}-O-\underset{R}{\overset{R}{\underset{|}{\overset{|}{Si}}}}-O-\underset{R}{\overset{R}{\underset{|}{\overset{|}{Si}}}}-O-$$

84. (a) : $3CH_3-CH=CH_2 \xrightarrow[THF]{BH_3} (CH_3CH_2CH_2)_3B \xrightarrow[OH^-]{H_2O_2} 3CH_3CH_2CH_2OH$

85. (a) :

$C_6H_5CH_2CH=CH_2 + Hg(OCOCH_3)_2 \longrightarrow C_6H_5CH_2-\overset{+}{CH}\cdots CH_2 \cdots Hg(OCOCH_3) \xrightarrow{H_2\ddot{O}:}$

$C_6H_5CH_2-CH(OH)-CH_2-Hg(OCOCH_3) \xrightarrow{NaBH_4} C_6H_5CH_2CH(OH)CH_3$

86. (c) : This reaction is Fries rearrangement -

$C_6H_5OCOCH_3 \xrightarrow[\Delta]{AlCl_3}$ o-hydroxy acetophenone + p-hydroxy acetophenone

o-hydroxy acetophenone

p-hydroxy acetophenone

87. (a) : Oxygen is the most abundant element in the earth's crust. (above 45.5 wt %)

88. (b) : When NH_4OH is added to the solution containing Cu^{2+} ions, deep blue solution is obtained.

$$Cu^{2+} + 4NH_4OH \rightarrow \underset{\text{deep blue solution}}{[Cu(NH_3)_4]^{2+}} + 4H_2O$$

Hydrated cupric compounds absorb radiations corresponding to red light and the transmitted colour is greenish blue (which is complementary to red colour). Thus, cupric compounds give greenish-blue colour.

89. (b)

90. (b) : $C_6H_5COOH \xrightarrow[\text{reduction}]{LiAlH_4} C_6H_5CH_2OH$

benzyl alcohol

91. (a) : A substance that is able to cause a chain transfer in a chain polymerisation is called a chain transfer agent. It gives an atom to the radical at the growing end of a polymer chain and in doing so it results into a radical which can start the growth of a new chain. CCl_4 is a chain transfer reagent.

92. (d) : Tricalcium aluminate $3CaO.Al_2O_3$ - Calcium aluminate cements are hydraulic cements made primarily from limestone and bauxite. They are well adapted for use in refractory (high temperature resistant) concretes. *e.g.* furnace linings.

93. (b) : A substance which increases the speed of a reaction without being consumed in the reaction is called a catalyst. Catalyst reduces the height of barrier by providing an alternative path for the reaction and lowers the activation energy.

94. (c) : Only HF_2^- has H-bonding $[F–H.....F]^-$ rest all the molecules have coordinate bonds.

95. (b) : Most electrophilic substitution reactions are irreversible but sulphonation is an exception. Treatment of benzene with "oleum" (a solution of SO_3 in conc. sulphuric acid) will give the sulphonic acid, the electrophile is sulphur trioxide (SO_3).

$C_6H_6 + SO_3 \longrightarrow [C_6H_6^{\oplus}(H)SO_3^{\ominus}] \longrightarrow C_6H_5SO_3H$

96. (c) : Aliphatic 1° amines react with cold nitrous acid to give alcohols with quantitative evolution of N_2 gas.

$$\underset{\text{Methylamine}}{CH_3NH_2} + HONO \xrightarrow{273\text{ - }278K} CH_3OH + N_2 + H_2O$$

This reaction is used as a test for aliphatic primary amines.

97. (d) : In exothermic processes, heat released by the reaction increases the entropy of the surrounding. The overall entropy change is certainly positive when the entropy of the system is positive. In some exothermic reactions, entropy of the system may decrease. If reaction is highly exothermic and increase in entropy of the surroundings is very high, the total entropy change will be positive and the reaction will be spontaneous.

98. (c) : $P^o_A = 0.850$ bar, $P_S = 0.845$ bar

$w = 0.5$ g, $m = ?$

weight of solvent (benzene) = 39.0 g

and molecular weight of benzene = 78 g

As we know, $\frac{P_A^\circ - P_S}{P_A^\circ} = x_B = \frac{n_B}{n_A}$

$$\frac{0.850 - 0.845}{0.850} = \frac{\frac{w_B}{M_B}}{\frac{w_A}{M_A}} = \frac{\frac{0.5}{m}}{\frac{39}{78}}$$

On solving, we get
molecular mass of solid structure (m) = 170 g.

99. (c) : Due to internal compensation, this compound is strictly inactive.

$$\begin{array}{c} H \\ H_3C - \overset{|}{\underset{|}{C_1}} - Cl \\ H_3C - \overset{|}{\underset{|}{C_2}} - Cl \\ H \end{array}$$ (*meso*)

C – 1 = *R* - configuration
C – 2 = *S* - configuration

100.(d) : Ferrocene (structure: two cyclopentadienyl rings bonded to Fe)

Ferrocene

101.(a) : Electropositive elements like zinc precipitate copper from a solution of copper sulphate and finally forms a complex.

$$CuSO_4 + Zn \rightarrow Cu + ZnSO_{4(aq)} \rightarrow [Zn(H_2O)_4]SO_4$$

102.(b) : This is the substitution or replacement reaction of benzene diazonium salt, where nitrogen is lost as N_2 and different groups are introduced in its place.

$$C_6H_5N^+{\equiv}N \xrightarrow{H_2O} C_6H_5O^+H_2 + N_2 \xrightarrow{H_2O} C_6H_5OH + H_3O^+$$

Phenol

103.(d) : With *trans*-but-2-ene, the product of Br_2 addition is optically inactive due to the formation of symmetric *meso* compounds.

$$H{-}C{-}CH_3 \;\Vert\; CH_3{-}C{-}H + Br_2 \longrightarrow$$

$$\begin{array}{c} CH_3 \\ H - | - Br \\ H - | - Br \\ CH_3 \end{array} + \begin{array}{c} CH_3 \\ Br - | - H \\ Br - | - H \\ CH_3 \end{array}$$

Meso

In general, for symmetrical alkenes and symmetrical reagents, the addition takes place as :

cis-alkene + syn-addition → meso
trans-alkene + syn-addition → racemic
cis-alkene + anti-addition → racemic
trans-alkene + anti-addition → meso

104.(c) : Oxygen is a colourless, odourless and tasteless gas. It is paramagnetic in gaseous, liquid and solid states. It can be liquefied to a pale blue liquid by compressing the gas at a very low temperature. Its allotropic modification is ozone.

105.(a) : The orange colour of SnI_4 is caused by the absorption of blue light, the reflected light thus containing a higher proportion of red and orange. The energy absorbed in this way causes the transfer of an electron from I to Sn. Since transferring an electron to another atom is transferring a charge, such spectra are called charge transfer spectra.

106.(a) : Weaker bases are good leaving groups. Hence, the acyl derivatives with weaker bases as leaving groups can easily rupture the bond and are more reactive. Cl^- is the weakest base while NH_2^- is the strongest base. The correct order of basicity of the leaving group and their tendency to leave is $H_2N^-: > RO^-: > RCOO^-: > :Cl^-$

107.(a) : The magnetic moment of transition elements may be calculated from the equation :

$$\mu_{S+L} = \sqrt{4S(S+1) + L(L+1)}$$

S = resultant spin quantum number
L = resultant orbital momentum quantum number

$$\mu = g\sqrt{J(J+1)}$$

where $g = \frac{3}{2} + \frac{S(S+1) - L(L+1)}{2J(J+1)}$

we know, $J = L - S$ when the shell is less than half full.
$J = L + S$ when it is more than half full.

Electronic configuration of Dy = $[Xe]4f^{10}6s^2$

$Dy^{3+} = [Xe]4f^9$

−3	−2	−1	0	+1	+2	+3
↑↓	↑↓	↑	↑	↑	↑	↑

Here $S = 5/2$ (since there are five unpaired electron)

$L = -1 \times 1 + 0 \times 1 + 1 \times 1 + 2 \times 1 + 3 \times 1 = 5$

So, $J = L + S = 15/2$

Now, $g = \frac{3}{2} + \frac{35/4 - 30}{2 \times \frac{15}{2} \times \frac{17}{2}} = 1.334$

$$\mu = g\sqrt{J + (J+1)} = 10.65 \text{ BM}$$

Thus calculated value of magnetic moment of Dy is the highest among the lanthanoid.

108.(a) : C – O bond in metal carbonyl is long as ligated CO has lower bond order. The lower B.O. is due to the transfer of metal $d\pi$ electrons into the π^* orbitals of ligated CO.

109.(c) : When chlorobenzene is heated with chloral in the presence of conc. H_2SO_4, a powerful insecticide, DDT is formed with the elimination of water molecule.

$$CCl_3CHO + 2\,H\text{–}C_6H_4\text{–}Cl \xrightarrow[\Delta,\,-H_2O]{H_2SO_4} CCl_3CH(C_6H_4\text{–}Cl)_2$$

DDT

110.(d) : CH_3COOH/CH_3COONH_4 is not an example of acidic buffer. Acidic buffer contains equimolar mixture of weak acid and its salt with strong base.
e.g. CH_3COOH/CH_3COONa.

111.(c) : This is Finkelstein reaction which involves the conversion of an alkyl chloride/bromide to an alkyl iodide by the addition of sodium iodide in acetone. Because sodium iodide is soluble in acetone and NaCl and NaBr are not, the equilibrium is shifted by the precipitation of insoluble salt.

$$R\text{—}X \underset{MX}{\overset{MX'}{\rightleftharpoons}} R\text{—}X'$$

The equilibrium position of the reaction depends on the nucleophilicity of the anion, whether a good leaving group is present and whether one anion is better stabilised than the other in a given solvent.

112.(c) : Chlorine has high electron affinity than fluorine. The less negative electron gain enthalpy of fluorine as compared to chlorine is due to very small size of the fluorine atom.

113.(a) : $HC\equiv CH + NaNH_2 \xrightarrow{\text{Ether}} HC\equiv C^-Na^+ + NH_3$

C–H bond is strongly polar due to high electronegativity of carbon atom. Hence it gives H^+ ion on reacting with a base or acetylene behaves as an acid.

114.(c) : In thermodynamic terms, formation of solution occurs with a favourable change in free energy

$$\Delta G = \Delta H - T\Delta S$$

where ΔH has a small positive value and $T\Delta S$ a large positive value; thus ΔG is negative.

115.(a) : $NH_2\text{—}CH_2\text{—}COOH$ is a typical α-amino acid. In solution it exists as, internal salt or Zwitter ion,

$$(^+NH_3\text{—}CH_2\text{—}COO^-)$$

because the proton (H^+) of COOH group is captured by $-NH_2$ group as NH_2 has a lone pair of electrons on N atom.

116.(a) : Rate expression $\frac{dx}{dt} = k[A]^m[B]^n$ shows that the total order of reactions is $m + n + 0 = m + n$ as the rate of reaction is independent of concentration of C, *i.e*, the order with respect to C is zero. This is the reason that C does not figure in the rate expression.

117.(b) : Bond order of N_2 = 3, bond order of O_2 = 2. Higher the bond order, higher is the bond dissociation energy *i.e.* higher stability or less reactivity. Thus N_2 is less reactive than O_2.
Higher the bond order, shorter is the bond length. Higher bond order of N_2 shows its shorter bond length.

118.(d) : 2-Hydroxy propanoic acid is known as lactic acid. It has following structure–

$$CH_3\text{—}\overset{H}{\underset{OH}{C^*}}\text{—}\overset{O}{\overset{\|}{C}}\text{—}OH$$

It has no carbon-carbon double bond and hence cannot show geometrical isomerism. However, it shows optical isomerism due to the presence of a chiral carbon atom.

119.(c) : The equilibrium constant is always fixed and is a characteristic of a reaction at specified temperature. It defines the composition of the final equilibrium mixture of that reaction, regardless of the starting amount of reactants and products.

120.(a) : The loss of one α-particle will reduce the mass number by four and atomic number by two. Subsequent two β-emissions will increase the atomic number by two without affecting the mass number. Hence, the new element will be only an isotope of the parent nucleide and hence its position in the periodic table remains unchanged.

BIOLOGY

121.(c) : Glaucoma is a condition in which loss of vision occurs because of an abnormally high pressure in the eye. In most cases there is no other ocular disease. This is known as primary glaucoma and there are two pathologically distinct types- acute and chronic simple. In acute (or angle-closure) glaucoma, there is an abrupt rise in pressure due to sudden closure of the angle between the cornea and iris where aqueous humour

usually drains from the eye. This is accompanied by pain and marked blurring of vision associated with inflammation of the anterior segment. In the more common chronic simple (or open-angle) glaucoma, the pressure increases gradually, usually without producing, pain, and the visual loss is insidious. The same type of visual loss may rarely occur in eyes with a normal pressure, this is called low-tension glaucoma.
Hepatitis is an inflammation of the liver caused by viruses, toxic substances or immunological abnormalities. Measles (Rubeola disease) is an acute infectious eruptive viral disease of childhood (3-5 years old) caused by specific virus of the group myxoviruses. Basically it is caused by an RNA containing *Rubeola virus*/*Polynosa morbillorum*. Measles is the infection of respiratory tract and conjunctiva which is transmitted by contact, fomite and droplet methods. Bronchitis is the inflammation of the bronchi.

122.(c) : Night blindness is the inability to see in dim light or at night. It is due to disorder of the cells in the retina that are responsible for vision in dim light and can result from dietary deficiency of vitamin A (retinol).

Name	Sources	Effect of deficiency
Vit. C (Ascorbic acid)	Lemon, orange and other citrus fruits, tomatoes, green vegetables, potatoes, carrots, pepper etc.	**Scurvy** (also called *sailor's disease*) is characterised by wound - healing and growth retardation etc.
Vit. D (Ergocal-ciferol and Cholecal-ciferol)	Synthesized in skin cells in sunlight from 7-dehydrocholesterol (*i.e.* provitamin D_3), also found in butter, liver, kidneys, egg yolk, fish, oil, etc.	**Rickets**, a disorder of children of 6 months to 2 years, and **osteomalacia,** a disorder of adults.
Vit. E (Tocoph-erol)	Green vegetables, oils, egg yolk, wheat, animal tissues	Reversible sterility in female. In male causes atrophy of spermatogenic tubules of testes.

123.(d) : Sucrose (cane sugar; beet sugar; saccharose) is a sugar comprising one molecule of glucose linked to a fructose molecule. It occurs widely in plants and is particularly abundant in sugar cane and sugar beet (15-20%), from which it is extracted and refined for table sugar. If heated to 200°C, sucrose becomes caramel. Sucrose is broken down into the monosaccharides glucose and fructose with the help of carbohydrate digesting enzyme, invertase, produced in the small intestine (duodenum).

124.(d) : Lamprey (or *Petromyzon*) belongs to class cyclostomata. The lamprey has about 1 m. long greenish brown, cylindrical body with smooth, scaleless, slimy skin; anterior circular, jawless mouth; a single dorsal naris; seven pairs of circular gill slits; 2 dorsal fins and a tail fin. Its life cycle includes two quite different phases. The larval phase (called ammocoete) is a fresh water sedentary, filter feeding and microphagus creature reminiscent of the lancet. The fish like adult lives in the sea and is parasitic on fishes.

125.(a) : The black pigment in the eye, which reduces the internal reflection is known as retina. It is the inner most coat of the eyeball and it is a thin, light sensitive nervous layer. The external coat of the eyeball is known as sclerotic but in front of the sclerotic, there is a transparent connective tissue called cornea. Iris is the pigmented part present in front of choroid.

126.(a) : Oxytocin is a hormone that causes both contraction of smooth muscle in the uterus during birth and expulsion of milk from the mammary glands during suckling. Oxytocin is produced in the neurosecretory cells of the hypothalamus but is stored and secreted by the posterior pituitary gland. Glucagon is a hormone, secreted by the α (or A) cells of the islets of Langerhans in the pancreas, that increases the concentration of glucose in the blood by stimulating the metabolic breakdown of glycogen. It thus antagonizes the effects of insulin. Adrenaline (epinephrine) is a hormone produced by the medulla of the adrenal glands, that increases heart activity, improves the power and prolongs the action of muscles, and increases the rate and depth of breathing to prepare the body for 'fright, flight, or fight'. At the same time it inhibits digestion and excretion. Thyroxine is secreted by thyroid gland. It controls the rate of all metabolic processes in the body and influence physical development and activity of the nervous system.

127.(c) : *Refer answer 126*

128.(b) : Hyaluronidase is a hydrolytic enzyme present in the acrosome of sperm. It lyses the glycosaminoglycans in the extracellular matrix holding the cell of the corona radiata together. As the coronal cells become more loosely associated, sperm cells can propel themselves inward, toward the zona pellucida by making a receptive cone or fertilization cone through the cytoplasm of the egg. Hyaluronidase may also be involved in breaking down the zona pellucida.

Fertilizin is a chemical substance secreted from the cortical region of egg cytoplasm to attract the sperm towards the egg. Acrosin is released from the acrosome of a spermatozoa as a consequence of the acrosome reaction. Capacitation is the final stage in the maturation process of spermatozoa. This takes place inside the genital tract as the sperm penetrates the ovum.

129.(c) : Reproduction is an essential feature of all living organisms. It is the process by which an individual multiplies in number by producing more individuals of its own type. It maintains the continuity of race by replacing old dying members and helps in increasing the total number of individuals. *Amoeba proteus* does not reproduce sexually. The reproduction is essentially asexually and takes place by various methods such as binary fission, multiple fission and sporulation. Binary fission is the most common mode of reproduction. It results in the division of the parent *Amoeba* into two daughter amoebea. *Amoeba* reproduces by multiple fission during adverse environmental conditions. The animals secretes a three-layered protective, chitinous cyst around it and becomes inactive. Inside the cyst, the nucleus repeatedly divides to form several daughter nuclei, which arrange themselves near the periphery. When favourable conditions arrive, the cyst breaks off liberating the young pseudopodiospores, each with fine pseudopodia. They feed and grow rapidly to become adults and lead an independent life.

Form of reproduction present in the following animals are –

Euglena – Longitudinal binary fission
Paramecium – Transverse binary fission
Plasmodium – Multiple fission

130.(c) : Temporal lobe is one of the main divisions of the cerebral cortex in each hemisphere of the brain, lying at the side within the temple of the skull and separated from the frontal lobe by a cleft, the lateral sulcus. Areas of the cortex in this lobe are concerned with the appreciation of sound and spoken language.

131.(a) : Emphysema means air in the tissues. In pulmonary emphysema the air sacs (alveoli) of the lungs are enlarged and damaged, which reduces the surface area for the exchange of oxygen and carbon dioxide. Severe emphysema causes breath-lessness, which is made worse by infections. Pneumonia is inflammation of the lung caused by bacteria, in which the air sacs (alveoli) become filled with inflammatory cells and the lung becomes solid. The symptoms include those of any infection (fever, malaise, headaches, etc.), together with cough and chest pain. Silicosis, a lung disease, is a form of pneumoconiosis produced by inhaling silica dust particles. It affects workers in hard-rock mining and tunnelling, quarrying, stone dressing, sand blasting, and boiler scaling. Silica stimulates fibrosis of lung tissue, which produces progressive breathlessness and considerebly increased susceptibility to tuberculosis. Asthma is the condition of subjects with widespread narrowing of the bronchial airways, which changes in severity over short periods of time (either spontaneously or under treatment) and leads to cough, wheezing, and difficulty in breathing.

132.(d) : Scapula (shoulder blade) is the largest of the bones that make up each half of the pectoral (shoulder) girdle. It is a flat triangular bone, providing anchorage for the muscles of the forelimb and an articulation for the humerus at the glenoid cavity. It is joined to the clavicle (collar bone) in front. Clavicle is a bone that forms part of the pectoral (shoulder) girdle, linking the scapula (shoulder blade) to the sternum (breast bone). In humans it forms the collar bone and serves as a brace for the shoulders. Humerus is the long bone of the upper arm which articulates with the scapula (shoulder blade) at the glenoid cavity and with the ulna and radius (*via* a condyle) at the elbow. Ilium is the largest of the three bones that make up each half of the pelvic girdle. The ilium bears a flattened wing of bone that is attached by ligaments to the sacrum.

133.(a) : Humans, or human beings, are bipedal primates belonging to the mammalian species *Homo sapiens* (Latin "wise man" or "knowing man") in the family Hominidae (the great apes). It includes both archaric and modern humans, as well as the subspecies *Homo sapeins neanderthalensis*, also known as the Neanderthals. *Homo sapiens* first started appearing about 500,000 or fewer years ago.

134.(a) : Rudolf Virchow was the first to suggest that new cells are formed from the division of the pre-existing cells - *omnis-cellula-e-cellula* (every cell is derived from a cell). Robert Hooke was the first to coin the term "cell" for small structures in a piece of cork under a microscope. His observations were published in a book named *micrographia*. Leeuwenhoek was the first person to observe and describe microscopic organisms and living cell. He observed nucleus in RBC of salmon fish and used simple lens and observed nuclei and unicellular organisms including bacteria. In 1676, he described the bacteria and gave the term *animalcules*. His observations laid the foundations for the science of bacteriology and microbiology. Robert Brown (1831) described and named nucleus.

135.(a) : Turner's syndrome is characterised by the monosomy of XO type. It is characterized by a lack of ovaries and menstrual cycle. Affected women are sterile and lack secondary sexual characteristics, although the external genitalia are present. The syndrome is named after the US endocrinologist H. H. Turner (1892–1970), who first described it.

Down's syndrome is a congential form of mental retardation due to a chromosome defect in which there are three copies of chromosome no. 21 instead of the usual two. The affected individual has a short broad face and slanted eyes (as in the Mongolian races), short fingers, and weak muscles. Down's syndrome can be detected before birth by amniocentesis. It is named after the British physician John Down (1828-96), who first studied the incidence of the disorder. Klinefelter's syndrome is characterised by trisomy (XXY). These are male individuals, who are phenotypically fairly normal but have a fairly low sperm count and therefore sterile.

136.(d) : Heparin prevents blood coagulation in the blood vessels. It is secreted by mast cells. It is an anticoagulant, blocking conversion of prothrombin to thrombin. Haemoglobin is the blood pigment necessary for oxygen transport. Plasma is the component of blood. Thrombin is the product of blood clotting.

137.(a) : Wings of pigeon, mosquito and bat show divergent evolution. It is the evolutionary process resulting in dissimilarity in structural features of organisms that occupy similar habitat.

Atavism is the regaining of same structures after a certain gap of few generations. Convergent evolution is the development of superficially similar structures in unrelated organisms, usually because the organisms live in the same kind of environment. Examples are the wings of insects and birds and the streamlined bodies of whales and fish.

138.(d) : Endoplasmic reticulum functions as cytoskeleton or intracellular and ultrastructural skeletal framework by providing mechanical support to colloidal cytoplasmic matrix. Proteins and enzymes synthesized by ribosomes enter the channels of rough endoplasmic reticulum both for intracellular use as well as extracellular transport.

139.(a) : Thickening of arteries due to cholesterol deposition is arteriosclerosis. This is extremely widespread disease predisposes to myocardial infarction, cerebral thrombosis, and other serious illness. It is characterized by infiltration of cholesterol and appearance of foam cells in certain lesions of the arterial wall, distorting the vessels and making them rigid.

140.(a) : An example of competitive inhibition of an enzyme is the inhibition of succinic dehydrogenase by malonic acid. It is the simple type of competitive inhibition. A competitive inhibitor resembles the substrate and binds to the active site of the enzyme. The substrate is then prevented from binding to the same active site.

141.(a) : During glycolysis 1 molecule of glucose is converted to 2 molecules of pyruvic acid in the cytoplasm. These two molecules of pyruvic acid is then converted to acetyl CoA by decarboxylation. This acetyl CoA is the connecting link between glycolysis and Krebs cycle. Acetyl CoA thus formed participates in Krebs cycle and combines with oxalo acetic acid to form citric acid.

142.(c) : Lactose or milk sugar (carbohydrate) is reducing sugar formed through β-1-4 condensation between galactose and glucose. Lactose does not occur in nature except as a product of the mammary gland. It is highest in human milk as compared to that of cow, buffalo and goat.

143.(b) : Light is the visible part of electromagnetic radiations. Sunlight or solar radiations reaching the earth have wavelength between 300 nm to 2600 nm. Part of the spectrum used in photosynthesis has a wavelength between 400-700 nm. It is called photosynthetically active radiations (PAR).

144.(a) : Nitrogen containing organic ring compounds are present in the nucleotides of nucleic acid. They are of two types two ringed nitrogenous compounds *eg.*, adenine and guanine. Purines are 9-membered double rings and each has four N-atoms at 1', 3', 7' and 9' positions. Pyrimidines are single ringed nitrogenous compounds *eg.*, cytosine and thymine. A pyrimidine has two N-atoms at 1' and 3' positions.

145.(b) : Community and ecosystem diversity is of three types α, β and γ. β-diversity (β index diversity between community diversity) is a biodiversity which appears in a range of communities due to replacement of species with the change in community habitat due to presence of different microhabitats, niches and difference in environmental conditions.

146.(b) : Citrus canker is a bacterial disease. It is caused by bacteria *Xanthomonas citri* which is aerobic, rod shaped and monotrichous. It is a world wide disease of most *Citrus* plants but the most susceptible are grape fruits, sweet orange, lime and lemon. The symtoms first appear on the undersurface of leaves as small watery slightly raised, round light green spots that finally rupture to form corky crater like lesions or canker. Twigs, fruits, also develop lesions. The disease reduces the quantity and quality of fruits.

Powdery mildew is caused by *Erysiphe* sp, red rot of sugarcane by *Colletotrichum falcatum* and wilt disease by *Fusarium* sp. Thus, they are all fungal diseases.

147.(d) : Water is mainly absorbed by roots which goes upwards so as to replace water loss in transpiration and to be used in photosynthesis. This upward movement of water from roots to leaves through stem against force of gravity is called ascent of sap. Different theories have been put forward in support of ascent of sap. They include root pressure theory, capillary theory and transpiration pull theory. Root pressure is developed when rate of absorption is more than rate of transpiration and so water is pushed up in the tracheary elements. Capillary force theory was given by Boehm according to which xylem vessels act as minute capillaries and water rises in these capillaries due to capillary action or surface tension. According to transpiration pull theory by Dixon and Jolly, due to water loss by transpiration suction pressure is increased and water is absorbed from adjacent xylem vessels of leaves and thus sap in under tension.

148.(b) : Plants require nutrients for proper growth and development. 16 elements are necessary for plants and are called essential elements as C, H, O, N, P, S, K, Mg, Ca, Fe, Cu, B, Zn, Mn, Mo and Cl. These essential elements are categorised into 2 groups as macro elements and micro elements. Marco elements are required by plants in larger amounts *eg.*, C, H, O, N, S, P, K, Ca, Mg. Microelements or trace elements are required by plants in very small amounts *ie* in traces *eg.*, Fe, Cu, B, Mn, Mo and Cl.

149.(c) : Some epiphytes *eg.*, orchids have aerial roots. In these roots, the outer covering is made up of a spongy tissue called velamen which absorbs moisture from the air. Thus, the aerial plant can prepare food by photosynthesis.

150.(c) : Solution culturc is being used for raising flowers and vegetables at home. This soilless production of plants is called hydroponics (Gk. *hydor* – water, *ponas* – excretion) Plans are raised in small tanks of concrete or metal; The tanks are covered over by wire netting or gauze. They are filled up with a water solution containing appropriate quantities of all mineral elements. The solution is changed from time to time. There is a mechanism for aeration and circulation. *p*H is checked and corrections are made regularly. Iron is added as Fe-EDTA otherwise it gets precipitated, especially in alkaline *p*H. The agent which keeps metals in the soluble state is called chelating agent or ligand. EDTA (Ethylene diamine tetra-acetic acid) is one such agent. Fe-EDTA complex is called chelate. As soon as the plant enlarge they are tied to the roof of the chambers by means of strings. Hydroponics is useful in areas having thin, infertile and dry soils. They conserve water. Additionally hydroponics can regulate *p*H optimum for a particular crop, control soil borne pathogens, avoid problems of weeding and obtain consistently better yield.

151.(b) : Leghaemoglobin is a pinkish pigment present inside the root nodules of nitrogen fixing plants like legumes. It is an oxygen scavenger and is related to blood pigment haemoglobin. It protects nitrogen fixing enzyme nitrogenase from oxygen. The most important bacteria present inside the nodules is *Rhizobium*.

152.(c) : All the given options are hydrophytes in nature which grow in extremely wet or watery conditions. But among them only in *Ceratophyllum* roots are completely absent even in embryonic stage. They remain under water completely. *Nymphaea* is a rooted hydrophyte with floating leaves, *Vallisneria* is rooted submerged hydrophyte and *Sagittaria* is rooted emergent hydrophyte.

153.(b) : Composite fruits are multiple fruits which are developed from the complete inflorescence and are also called as infructescence. They are of two types sorosis and syconus. Spike, spadix and catkin type of inflorescence gives rise to this type of fruit eg *Ananas*, *Artocarpus*. Syconus develops from a hypanthodium inflorescence eg *Ficus*.

154.(b) : Stratosphere zone of earth's atmosphere contains a layer of ozone (O_3) which prevents the earth surface from about 99% of incoming solar UV radiations. Ozone layer is present in the stratosphere which is also called ozonosphere. It lies at an altitude of 23-25 km over equator and its concentration is 300 dobsons.

155.(b) : Amphimixis is normal type of sexual reproduction having both meiosis and fertilization. But in some plants, the normal sexual reproduction is replaced by some abnormal type of sexual reproduction where there is no meiosis and syngamy. It is of two types vegetative reproduction and agamospermy. In vegetative reproduction plants develop from parts other than seeds. In agamospermy, plants produce seeds as means of propagation by abnormal method.

156.(c) : Cocoa or *Theobroma* belongs to family sterculiaceae, and is a native of tropical America for preparation of cocoa and chocolates, the seeds are used.

157.(d) : The red colour of flower dominates upon white colour of flower. In the present varieties both parents are of pure variety, therefore, the offsprings will be all heterozygous red flowered as shown below :

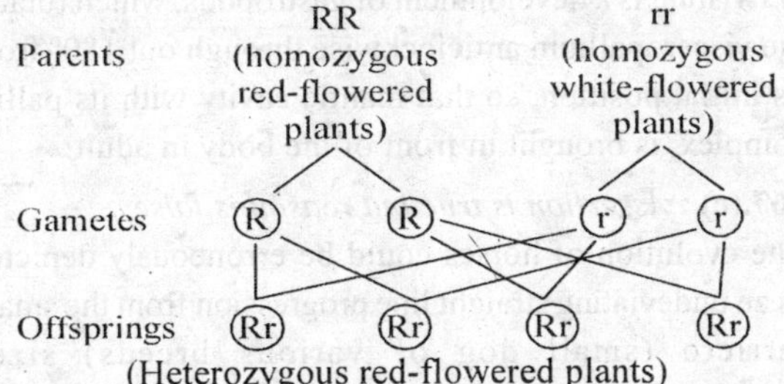

158.(a) : The phenomenon by which a gene suppresses the phenotypic expression of a nonallelic gene is called epistasis. The ratio for epistatic gene is 12 : 3 : 1in F_2 generation. The alleles which do not show dominant recessive relationship and are able to express themselves independently when present together are called codominant alleles. Supplementary genes are a pair of nonallelic genes, one of which produces its effect independently in the dominant state while the dominant allele of the second gene is without any independent effect but is able to modify the effect of the former to produce a new trait.

159.(c) : Pure line is true breeding genotypes, a line that has been rendered homozygous for all genes under consideration in successive generations, a line in which homozygous individuals produce only homozygous offspring like parents. Thus, pure line breed refers to homozygosity only.

160.(c) : Tropical rain forests are mainly found in central America, along Amazon and Orinoco rivers, South America, Congo river basin of Africa, Malagasy Republic and South east Asia including India. Diversity of life is so high that a hectare of the forest may have as many as 200 species of trees, 70% - 80% of all insects and 80 - 85% of all birds are known from tropical forests. Productivity of this biome is also very high and life is abundant. It has different varieties and number of plants and animals.

161.(c) : *Assertion is true but reason is false.*
Haemophilia (also known as bleeder disease) is an popular example of sex linked inheritance in human beings. Haemophilia is either of two hereditary disorders in which the blood clots very slowly, due to a deficiency of either of two coagulation factors – haemophilia A, due to deficiency of factor VIII (antihaemophilic factor); or haemophilia B, due to deficiency of factor IX (Christmas factor). The patient may experience prolonged bleeding following any injury or wound, and in severe cases there is spontaneous bleeding into muscles and joints. Haemophilia is controlled by a sex-linked gene, which means that it is almost exclusively restricted to males; women can carry the disease – and pass it on to their sons – without being affected themselves. The genes encoding factors VIII and IX have been used in gene therapy trials for haemophilia.
Mutation of a structural gene on chromosome 15 is the molecular basis of Marfan syndrome. This disease is due to domiant mutation resulting in the production of abnormal form of connective tissues and characteristic extreme looseness of joints.

162.(b) : *Both assertion and reason are true but reason is not the correct explanation of assertion.*
Astigmatism is a defect of vision in which the image of an object is distorted, usually in either the vertical or the horizontal axis, because not all the light rays come of a focus on the retina. Some parts of the object may be in

focus but light from other parts may be focused in front of or behind the retina. This is usually due to abnormal curvature of the cornea and/or lens whose surface resembles part of sphere. The defect can be corrected by wearing cylindrical lenses, which produce exactly the opposite degree of distortion and thus cancel out the distortion caused by the eye itself.

163.(b) : *Both assertion and reason are true but reason is not the correct explanation of assertion.*

Antigen is any substance that may be specifically bound by an antibody molecule. The antigens are mostly protcins, but can be polysaccharides, glycoproteins or other types of conjugated proteins, nucleic acid or such chemicals. Each antigen has many antigenic determinants (called epitopes) of the antigen. As each antibody binds with 2 or more such determinants, the one antigen can bind with many antibodies. In order to generate antibodies specific for small molecules, the latter are attached to a larger molecule before immunization. The number of different antigens recognized by lymphocytes in the body is extremely large. The recognition ability is innate and develops without exposure to the antigen. Stem cells differentiate into many million different T and B lymphocytes, each with the ability to respond to a particular antigen. When the antigen first enters the body, it can bind directly to the appropriate receptors on B cells. However, a full antibody response requires that the B cells contact helper T cells. In the case of T cells, the antigen is taken up by an antigen-presenting cells and partially digested. A peptide fragment of it is presented to the appropriate receptors on T cells. In either case, the cells are stimulated to divide, forming clones of cells that respond to this antigen.

164.(d) : *Both the assertion and reason are false.*

When a blood vessel gets injured, blood platelets get clumped at the injured spot and release certain chemicals called platelet factors, which promote blood coagulation. Injured tissues or platelets also release coagulation promoting substances called thromboplastins which help in the formation of an enzyme prothrombinase. This enzyme activates inactive protein prothrombin to active thrombin which further promotes the coagulation process. Blood normally contains an anticoagulant heparin which is released from mast cell granules that prevents the activation of prothrombin in uninjured blood vessels. Blood also contains antithrombin which inhibits any thrombin formed accidentally. Moreover, uninjured tissues do not release thromboplastins, hence blood does not coagulate in uninjured blood vessels.

165.(b) : *Both assertion and reason are true but reason is not the correct explanation of assertion.*

The basal metabolic rate is defined as the energy requirement of the human body at rest and reflects the caloric needs of the body. BMR can be determined by total body weight and the amount of muscle mass. BMR is inversely related with the weight or volume of an organism, *i.e.* smaller the organism, higher is the basal metabolic rate and *vice versa*.

Heart rate of six month old baby is 110-112 beats/min. Though it is higher than normal adult person, but it is lower than the old person. At the age of 60, a man may have maximum heart rate of 160 beats/min (avg 120 beats/min).

166.(b) : *Both assertion and reason are true but reason is not the correct explanation of assertion.*

Ctenidium is a monopectinate gill situated on the right side of the branchial chamber. Ctenidium helps in respiration by beating of cilia, thus creating water current. Ctenidium is innervated by nerves from the left pleural and supra-intestinal ganglia. This nerve supply indicates that it is actually an organ of the left side but has shifted to the right side during development (torsion). Torsion or twisting is a development of gastropods, which rotates the visceropallium anticlockwise through out 180° from its initial position, so that mantle cavity with its pallial complex, is brought in front of the body in adult.

167.(c) : *Assertion is true but reason is false.*

The evolution of horses could be erroneously depicted as an undeviating straight line progression from the small, terriero (small dog of various breeds) sized *Hydracotherium eohippus* to the large modern horse, *Equus eohippus* originated from Eocene period. Eohippus (meaning "dawn horse") was the earliest-known horse. It was the size of a tiny dog. Another name for this genus is Hyracotherium (meaning "mole beast"). Eohippus was only 2 feet (60 cm) long and 8 to 9 inches (20 cm) high at the shoulder. This primitive horse had 4 hoofed toes on the front feet and 3 hoofed ant on each hind foot. It had a long skull with 44 long-crowned teeth. Eohippus was a grazing herbivore that ate soft leaves and plant shoots. Eohippus lived during the early Eocene Epoch, about 50 million years ago. The major stages in evolution of horse are : (i) eohippus, (ii) mesohippus, (iii) merychippus, (iv) pliohippus, and (v) equus.

168.(d) : *Both the assertion and reason are false.*

When there is a threat of excessive water loss from the body of the animal, then the urine excreted needs to be hypertonic and not hypotonic because excessive water loss from the body posses the threat of a rise in osmoconcentration of the blood. Since hypertonic urine is more concentrated and higher in osmotic pressure than the blood, therefore it helps in reducing the loss of water with urine. Mammals and birds can excrete hypertonic urine which is more concentrated than their blood. For this, an isotonic glomerular filtrate is first filtered into the Bowman's capsules of nephrons in kidneys. The tubules of nephrons then reabsorb a large volume of water from the glomerular filtrate not accompanied by the reabsorption of proportionate amounts of solutes. This leaves the urine more concentrated than the blood which is very effective in reducing the urinary loss of water.

169.(a) : *Both assertion and reason are true and reason is the correct explanation of assertion.*

Aldosterone is a steroid hormone (mineralocorticoid) produced by the outer-section (zona glomerulosa) of the adrenal cortex in the adrenal gland to regulate sodium and potassium balance in the blood. At the late distal tubule & collecting duct,, aldosterone has two main actions:

- Acting on mineralocorticoid receptors (MR) on principal cells in the distal tubule of the kidney nephron, it increases the permeability of their apical (luminal) membrane to potassium and sodium and activates their basolateral Na^+/K^+ pumps, stimulating ATP hydrolysis leading to phosphorylation of the pump and a conformational change in the pump exposes the Na^+ ions to the outside. The phosphorylated form of the pump has a low affinity for Na^+ ions, hence reabsorbing sodium (Na^+) ions and water into the blood, and secreting potassium (K^+) ions into the urine. (Chlorine anions are also reabsorbed in conjunction with sodium cations to maintain the system's electrochemical balance.)
- Aldosterone stimulates H^+ secretion by intercalated cells, in the collecting duct, regulating plasma bicarbonate (HCO_3^-) levels and its acid/base balance.

Aldosterone may act on the central nervous system *via* the posterior pituitary gland to release vasopressin (ADH) which serves to conserve water by direct actions on renal tubular resorption.

Aldosterone is responsible for the reabsorption of about 2% of filtered sodium in the kidneys, which is nearly equal to the entire sodium content in human blood under normal GFR (glomerular filtration rate).

170.(d) : *Both the assertion and reason are false.*

Pollution may be defined as an undesirable change in the physical, chemical or biological characteristics of our air, water and land that may or will harmfully affect human lives or other organism. Pollution can be natural or man made. Natural pollution comes from volcanic eruptions, emission of natural gas, soil erosion, ultraviolet rays, etc. Most of the pollution is man-made. Contamination occurs due to the presence of harmful organisms or their products or undersirable products in a desirable product causing disease or discomfort, for the organism who consume it. Therefore pollution and contamination are two different things.

171.(c) : *Assertion is true but reason is false.*

According to Eichler's classification, plant kingdom is divided into two subdivisions cryptogamae and phanerogamae. Cryptogamae has 3 divisions thallophyta, bryophyta and pteridophyta. Thallophyta in turn is divided into 2 classes, algae and fungi. As both these groups have generally undifferentiated plant body (not differentiated into true root, stem and leaves) they are called thallophyta. Also they are non vascular plants. But algae are chlorophyllous and hence show autotrophic mode of nutrition *ie* can prepare their own food. But fungi are non-chlorophyllous and cannot prepare their own food. So they are heterotrophic in nature.

172.(a) : *Both assertion and reason are true and reason is the correct explanation of assertion.*

Conifer or *Pinus* is a heterosporous plant producing mega and microspores inside megasporangium and micro-sporangium respectively. Each micro-sporangium is a small, sessile and elongated sac like structure having two layered wall. Inside the wall lie tapetum which is a nourishing layer. Inside the cavity are large number of dusty and two winged micro-spores present. On maturity the microsporangium wall bursts from the upper side forming a longitudinal slit. A large number of yellow pollen grains are liberated which are carried by wind due to the presence of wings.

173.(d) : *Both assertion and reason are false.*
Neurospora is commonly called pink /red bread mould or pink mould. It belongs to class ascomycetes fungi or sac fungi. It is used in experimental genetics as it can be grown easily in a definite medium in laboratory. It is a haploid fungus. It is a heterothallic fungus having + ve and – ve mycelia and somatic fusion of two halpoid nuclei produce a diploid zygote. The zygote by one meiotic and another mitotic divisions forms 8-nuclei and hence ascospores, a characteristic structure of ascomycetes are produced.

174.(a) : *Both assertion and reason are true and reason is the correct explanation of assertion.*
As a result of continued secondary growth for several years, the older parts of the stem and its old branches have a part of its secondary xylem rendered non - functional. Such a modified and non - functional secondary xylem is called the heart wood or duramen, the functional outer younger rings of secondary xylem constitute the sap wood or alburnum. With the passage of time and addition of new outer rings of secondary xylem due to cambial activity more rings of the sap wood are changed into heart wood. This leads to the increase in the thickness of heart wood, whereas the sap wood remains of about the same thickness.

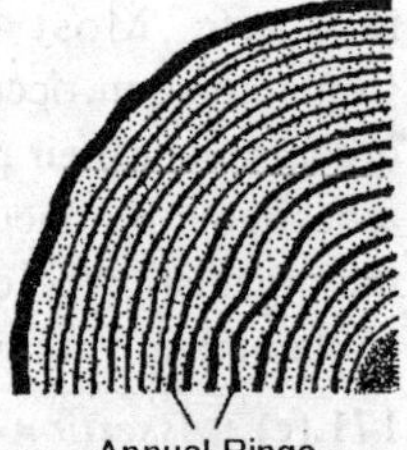

175.(b) : *Both assertion and reason are true but reason is not the correct explanation of assertion.*
Term vernalization was first given by T.D. Lysenko (1928). In colder countries, there are cereals of 2 physiological types, *i.e.*, winter cereals and spring cereals. Winter cereals are sown in winter and flower in following summer whereas spring cereals are sown in spring and flower in summer. If winter cereal is sown in spring, it shows vegetative growth but does not flower unless it receives low temperature of winter. But winter cereal can be converted into spring cereal by providing artificial low temperature treatment, (*i.e.*, springification.) Some plants requiring low temperature requirement (vernalization) for flowering are *Secale cereale* (European rye), *Triticum vulgare, Brassica oleracea, Beta vulgaris, Apium and Lolium perenne,* etc. Site of vernalization is apical meristem or all the meristematic cells. As a result of vernalization, a flowering hormone called "vernalin" is formed (reported by Melchers), but venalin has never been isolated. Once a plant is vernalized, it can be devernalized by exposing the plant to temperature of 30°C or above. For establishing vernalization, plant should be kept at 20°Cfor 4–5 days.

176.(a) : *Both assertion and reason are true and reason is the correct explanation of assertion.*
Organic sulphur is made available to the plant through biological oxidation through the activity of certain microorganisms. Sulphur is transformed from the organic form to the sulfate ion, the form of sulphur that higher plants absorb. Soil microorganisms oxidize not only organic sulphur but also sulphide minerals such as ferrous sulphide. The elemental sulphur is then oxidized to sulphate by sulphur bacteria.

177.(b) : *Both assertion and reason are true but reason is not the correct explanation of assertion.*
A slight thinning of ozone layer occurs naturally for a few months every year over Antarctica. It decreases by 67% every year. The primary chemicals responsible for ozone depletion are a group of chlorine containing compounds called chloroflurocarbons (CFCs), used as coolants in air conditioners and refrigerators (freon) and propellants for aerosol cans and form blowing agents for insulation and packaging and also as solvents. Besides halons, methyl bromide, methyl chloroform, carbon tetrachloride and nitrous oxide are also responsible for O_3 loss. After their release into troposphere, CFCs and other chlorine containing compounds go to stratosphere where these are broken down by UV-radiations releasing chlorine. Similarly bromine is released by breakdown of halons and methyl bromide. The sunlight catalyzes the chemical reaction by which chlorine or bromine break O_3 molecules and convert them into O_2 molecules. This chemical reaction does not change chlorine or bromine and thus single chlorine or bromine atom can breakdown many thousands of O_3 molecules.

178.(c) : *Assertion is true but reason is false.*
Photosynthesis is actually oxidation reduction process in which water is oxidised and CO_2 is reduced to carbohydrates. Assimilatory power ATP and $NADPH_2$ are required for reduction of CO_2. But this reduction is independent of light *i.e* occurs in presence or absence of light but production of assimilatory power is light dependent. This reaction is called light reaction or Hill's

reaction and the light independent phase is an enzymatic reaction called dark reaction. It occurs is stroma of chloroplast and is enzyme radiated one. It was first of all established by F.F. Blackman and so is also called Blackman's reaction. During this process CO_2 is fixed to carbohydrate.

179.(d) : *Both assertion and reason are false.*

Vegetable oils and fats are located in the form of small insoluble droplets within the plant cells. They occur predominantly in seeds most commonly in the endosperm and cotyledons. In most of the cereals, however, the fat occurs almost exclusively in the embryo. Olive and palm oils are two important examples that are obtained from the fleshy pericarp of the fruit. Less frequently, oils and fats are extracted from the roots, stems and foliage.

180.(a) : *Both assertion and reason are true and reason is the correct explanation of assertion.*

Latex of some plants containing long chain hydrocarbons is considered to be a good substitute for liquid fuels or petroleum. Such plants having large amount of latex with long chain hydrocarbons are called petroplants. Cultivation of petroplants is also a part of energy-cropping. Cultivation of these petrocrops was first of all done by Italians in Ethiopia about fifty years back, although actual credit for identifying the petrocrops goes to Dr. Calvin. The most common petroplants belong to families of euphorbiaceae, asclepiadaceae, apocynaceae, compositae, labiatae, sapotaceae, urticaceae, etc., which have property of converting large amounts of their photosynthates into latex with hydrocarbons. Their hydrocarbon contents can be increased by genetic manipulations (genetic engineering). But commercial production of petroleum or liquid fuel alternative (through petroplants) is in early stage. The use of these petroplants may reduce the pressure on liquid fuel or petroleum.

GENERAL KNOWLEDGE

181. (c)	**182. (a)**	**183. (b)**	**184. (a)**	**185. (c)**
186. (b)	**187. (c)**	**188. (c)**	**189. (c)**	**190. (a)**
191. (b)	**192. (a)**	**193. (b)**	**194. (b)**	**195. (b)**
196. (d)	**197. (b)**	**198. (b)**	**199. (a)**	**200. (a)**

Chapterwise Index - '08

Physics • Chemistry • Biology

Use the index for topicwise analysis of last year's AIIMS paper and refer to these questions when you are practising MCQs chapterwise.

PHYSICS

Chapter's Name	Question No.	Total
Units and Dimensions	1	1
Motion in One Dimension	2	1
Motion in Two Dimensions	3, 42	2
Laws of Motion and Friction	6	1
Work, Power and Energy	4	1
Centre of Mass and Rotational Motion	5	1
Gravitation	7, 19	2
Properties of Matter	21, 40, 43	3
Oscillations	52	1
Waves	16, 41	2
Heat and Thermodynamics	9, 17	2
Electrostatics	14, 20, 28	3
Current Electricity	22, 37, 57	3
Thermal and chemical effects of current	25, 30, 58	3
Magnetic Effects of Current	26, 46, 56, 59	4
Magnetism	23, 51	2
Electromagnetic Induction and Alternating Current	15, 24, 29, 45, 53, 55	6
Electromagnetic Waves	13	1
Ray Optics	12, 27, 33, 38, 39, 44, 43	7
Wave Optics	10, 35	2
Modern Physics	11, 18, 31, 47, 48, 54, 60	7
Solids and Semiconductor Devices	8, 32, 34	3
Universe	36	1
Principle of Communication	50	1

CHEMISTRY

Chapter's Name	Question No.	Total
Basic Concepts	85	1
Atomic Structure	104	1
Periodic Properties		0
Chemical Bonding	88, 118	2
Nuclear Chemistry		0
Gaseous and Liquid States	89, 103	2
Solid State	76, 94	2
Mole Concept & Solutions	114	1
Colloids, Surface Chemistry & Catalysis	71, 91	2
Equilibrium	65, 84, 105	3
Kinetics	62, 80	2
Energetics	108	1
Electrochemistry	70, 90, 92, 93	4
Redox Reactions		0
Metallurgy		0
Hydrogen and its Compounds		0
s-Block Elements		0
p-Block Elements	63, 86, 97, 98, 110, 119	6
d and *f*-Block Elements	113	1
Complex Compounds	66, 112	2
Purification and Analysis of Compound		0
General Organic Chemistry	68, 72, 73, 102	4
Aliphatic Hydrocarbons	67, 75	2
Aromatic Hydrocarbons	64, 69, 77, 78, 83, 99, 100	7
Halogen Derivatives		0
Alcohols, Phenols and Ethers	61, 87, 107, 117, 120	5
Aldehydes and Ketones	81, 101, 106, 109	4
Carboxylic acids & their derivatives	79	1
Nitrogen Containing Compounds	95, 96, 115, 116	4
Biochemistry		0
Chemistry in Action	82, 111	2
Environmental Chemistry	74	1

BIOLOGY		
Chapter's Name	**Question No.**	**Total**
General Biology		0
Biological Classification		0
Kingdom Monera	154	1
Kingdom Fungi	161	1
Plant Kingdom	140, 162	2
Cell and its Structural Component		0
Cell Reproduction		0
Cell Respiration	149	1
Enzymes	165	1
Biomolecules	148	1
Mendelian Genetics		0
Hereditary Material		0
Anatomy of Flowering Plants	153, 155, 156	3
Morphology of Flowering Plants	168	1
Physiology of Flowering Plants	152, 170, 171, 172	4
Embryology of Flowering Plants	132, 138, 144, 176, 177	5
Growth and Development in Flowering Plants	136, 150	2
Angiosperm Families		0
Ecology and Pollution	123, 133, 134, 143, 179, 180	6

Chapter's Name	Question No.	Total
Applied Botany	124, 158	2
Animal Kingdom	147, 163, 164, 173	4
Gene and Chromosome	157, 159	2
Gene regulation and Applied Genetics		0
Human Genetics & Genetic Disorder	166	1
Animal Tissue	125	1
Musculo-skeletal system		0
Digestive System and Nutrition		0
Respiration	145, 169	2
Circulatory system and Immunity	129, 142	2
Excretion and Osmoregulation		0
Reproduction and Embryonic Development	122, 135, 137, 178	4
Nervous system and sense organ	139, 141	2
Endocrine system	146, 174	2
Common Human Diseases	128, 175	2
Growth and Regeneration	160	1
Evolution		0
Drug and Addiction	126, 151	2
Applied Zoology	127, 130, 131, 167	4
Wild Life and Conservation		0
Human Population & Growth	121	1

Solved Paper
AIIMS - 2008

Time : 3½ Hours | Max. Marks : 200

PHYSICS

1. In an electrical circuit containing L, C and R which of the following does not denote the dimensions of frequency?
(a) LC (b) $\frac{1}{\sqrt{LC}}$
(c) $\frac{1}{RC}$ (d) $\frac{R}{L}$

2. The displacement time graph of a particle moving along a straight line is drawn below.

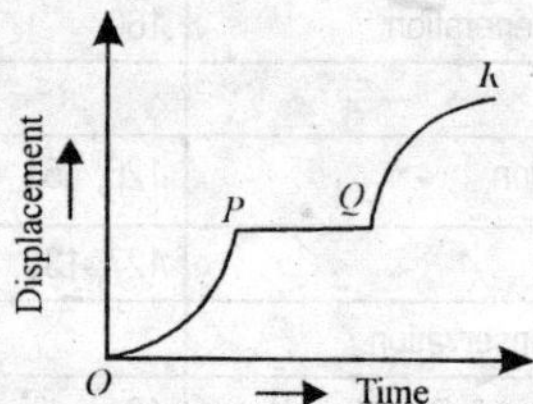

The accelerations of the particle during the regions OP, PQ and QR are

	OP	PQ	QR
(a)	–	0	+
(b)	+	0	+
(c)	+	0	–
(d)	–	0	–

3. A particle of mass m moves with constant speed along a circular path of radius r under the action of force F. Its speed is
(a) $\sqrt{\frac{Fr}{m}}$ (b) $\sqrt{\frac{F}{r}}$
(c) $\sqrt{Fmr}$ (d) $\sqrt{\frac{F}{mr}}$

4. A bullet is fired from a rifle and the rifle recoils. Kinetic energy of rifle is
(a) less than K.E. of bullet
(b) greater than K.E. of bullet
(c) equal to K.E. of bullet
(d) none of the above

5. Side of an equilateral triangle is l. Three point masses, each of magnitude m, are placed at the three vertices of the triangle. Moment of inertia of this system about one side of the triangle as axis is given by
(a) $\frac{3ml^2}{4}$ (b) $\frac{4}{3}ml^2$
(c) $\frac{3}{2}ml^2$ (d) $\frac{2}{3}ml^2$

6. P, Q and R are three coplanar forces acting at a point and are in equilibium.

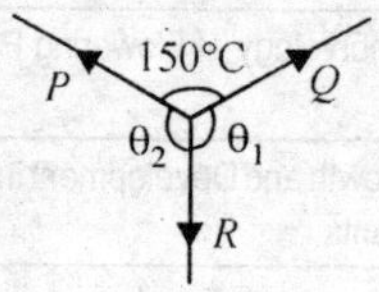

Given $P = 1.9318$ kg wt [$\sin\theta_1 = 0.9659$], the value of R (in kg wt) is
(a) 0.9659 (b) 2
(c) 1 (d) 1/2.

7. Suppose the gravitational force varies inversely as the nth power of distance. Then the time period of a planet in circular orbit of radius R around the sun will be proportional to
(a) $R^{\left(\frac{n+1}{2}\right)}$ (b) $R^{\left(\frac{n-1}{2}\right)}$
(c) R^n (d) $R^{\left(\frac{n-2}{2}\right)}$

8. A Ge specimen is doped with Al. The concentration of acceptor atoms is ~ 10^{21} atoms/m³. Given that the intrinsic concentration of electron hole pairs is $10^{19}/m^3$, the concentration of electrons in the specimen is
(a) $10^{17}/m^3$ (b) $10^{15}/m^3$
(c) $10^4/m^3$ (d) $10^2/m^3$.

9. A slab consists of two layers of different materials of the same thickness and having thermal conductivities K_1 and K_2 are connected in series.

The equivalent thermal conductivity of the slab is

(a) $\frac{2K_1K_2}{K_1+K_2}$ (b) $\sqrt{K_1K_2}$

(c) $\frac{K_1K_2}{K_1+K_2}$ (d) $K_1 + K_2$.

10. In Young's double slit experiment, the distance between two slits is made three times then the fringe width will become

(a) 9 times (b) 1/9 times

(c) 3 times (d) 1/3 times.

11. A laser beam is used for carrying out surgery because, it

(a) is highly monochromatic

(b) is highly coherent

(c) is highly directional

(d) can be sharply focussed.

12. A converging lens forms a real image I of an object on its principal axis. A rectangular slab of refractive index μ and thickness x is introduced between I and the lens, I will move

(a) towards the lens $(\mu - 1)x$

(b) towards the lens by $\left(1-\frac{1}{\mu}\right)x$

(c) away from the lens by $(\mu - 1)x$

(d) away from the lens by $\left(1-\frac{1}{\mu}\right)x$.

13. The velocity of electromagnetic radiation in a medium of permittivity ε_0 and permeability μ_0 is given by

(a) $\frac{1}{\sqrt{\mu_0\varepsilon_0}}$ (b) $\sqrt{\frac{\mu_0}{\varepsilon_0}}$

(c) $\sqrt{\frac{\varepsilon_0}{\mu_0}}$ (d) $\sqrt{\mu_0\varepsilon_0}$

14. Electric field at centre of a uniformly charged semicircle of radius a is

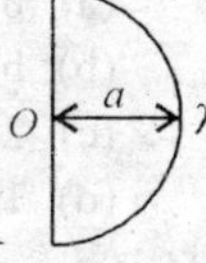

(a) $\frac{\lambda}{2\pi\varepsilon_0 a^2}$ (b) $\frac{\lambda}{4\pi^2\varepsilon_0 a^2}$

(c) $\frac{\lambda^2}{2\pi\varepsilon_0 a}$ (d) $\frac{\lambda}{2\pi\varepsilon_0 a}$

15. If frequency of $R - L$ circuit is f then impedence will be

(a) $\sqrt{R^2+(2\pi fL)^2}$ (b) $R^2 + (2\pi f^2)^2$

(c) $\sqrt{(R^2+L\pi f^2)}$ (d) $R^2 + (2\pi f)^2$.

16. Two closed organ pipes of length 100 cm and 101 cm produces 16 beats in 20 sec. When each pipe is sounded in its fundamental mode calculate the velocity of sound.

(a) 303 ms^{-1} (b) 332 ms^{-1}

(c) 323.2 ms^{-1} (d) 300 ms^{-1}.

17. A certain gas is taken to the five states represented by dots in the graph. The plotted lines are isotherms. Order of the most probable speed v_p of the molecules at these five states is

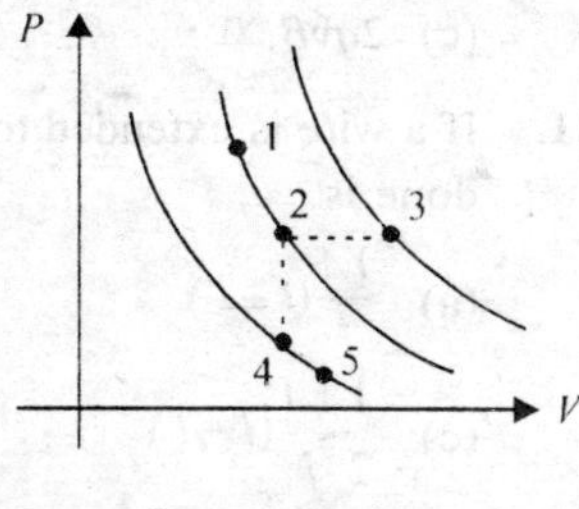

(a) $v_{p\text{ at }3} > v_{p\text{ at }1} = v_{p\text{ at }2} > v_{p\text{ at }4} = v_{p\text{ at }5}$

(b) $v_{p\text{ at }1} > v_{p\text{ at }2} = v_{p\text{ at }3} > v_{p\text{ at }4} = v_{p\text{ at }5}$

(c) $v_{p\text{ at }3} > v_{p\text{ at }2} = v_{p\text{ at }4} > v_{p\text{ at }1} = v_{p\text{ at }5}$

(d) insufficient information to predict the result.

18. N_1 atoms of a radioactive element emit N_2 beta particles per second. The decay constant of the element is (in s^{-1})

(a) N_1/N_2 (b) N_2/N_1

(c) N_1 (ln 2) (d) N_2 (ln 2)

19. Figure shows the variation of energy with the orbit radius r of a satellite in a circular motion. Mark the correct statement.

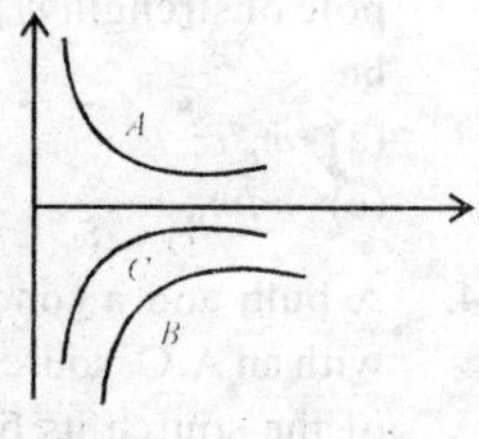

(a) C is total energy, B kinetic energy and A is potential energy

(b) A is kinetic energy, B total energy and C potential energy

(c) A and B are the kinetic and potential energies and C the total energy of the satellite.

(d) C and A are kinetic and potential energy respectively and B the total energy of the satellite.

20. Two changes $+q$ and $-q$ are attached to the two ends of a light rod of length L, as shown in figure. The system is given a velocity v perpendicular to magnetic field $\vec{B}$. The magnetic force on the system of charges and magnitude of force on one charge by the rod, are respectively

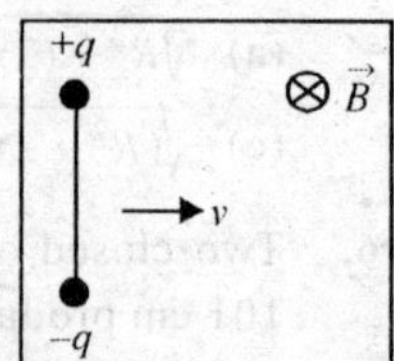

(a) zero, zero (b) zero, qvB
(c) $2qvB$, 0 (d) $2qvB$, qvB

21. If a wire is extended to a new length l, the work done is

(a) $\frac{YA}{l}(l-l')$ (b) $\frac{YA}{l}(l-l')^2$
(c) $\frac{1}{2}\frac{YA}{l}(l-l')^2$ (d) $2\cdot\frac{YA}{l}(l-l')^2$.

22. The equivalent resistance between the points X and Y in the following circuit diagram will be

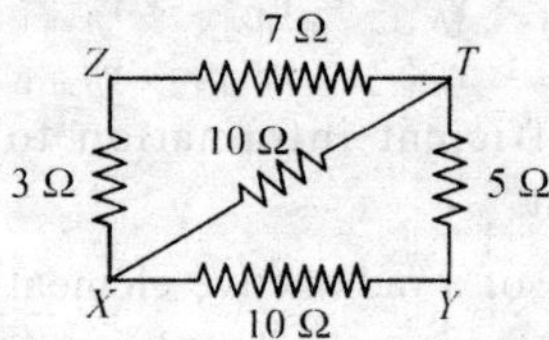

(a) 10 Ω (b) 5 Ω
(c) 7 Ω (d) 3 Ω.

23. The intensity of magnetic field due to an isolated pole of strength m_p at a point distant r from it will be

(a) m_p/r^2 (b) $m_p r^2$
(c) r^2/m_p (d) m_p/r.

24. A bulb and a condenser are connected in series with an A.C. source. On increasing the frequency of the source its brightness will

(a) increase (b) decrease
(c) sometimes increase and sometimes decrease
(d) neither increase nor decrease.

25. Two heater wires, made of the same material and having the same length and the same radius, are first connected in series and then in parallel to a constant potential difference. If the rates of heat produced in the two cases are H_s and H_p respectively, then H_s/H_p will be

(a) 1/2 (b) 2
(c) 1/4 (d) 4.

26. The ratio of magnetic fields on the axis of a circular current carrying coil of radius a to the magnetic field at its centre will be

(a) $\frac{1}{\left(1+\frac{x^2}{a^2}\right)^{3/2}}$ (b) $\frac{1}{\left(1+\frac{a^2}{x^2}\right)^{1/2}}$

(c) $\frac{1}{\left(1+\frac{a^2}{x^2}\right)^{2}}$ (d) $\frac{1}{\left(1+\frac{a^2}{x^2}\right)^{3}}$

27. Lumen is the unit of

(a) luminous flux (b) luminosity
(c) illumination (d) quantity of light.

28. A charge q is uniformly distributed on a ring of radius r. A sphere of an equal radius is constructed with its centre lying on the periphery of the ring. The flux of electric field through the surface of the sphere will be

(a) $\frac{q}{\varepsilon_0}$ (b) $\frac{q}{2\varepsilon_0}$

(c) $\frac{q}{3\varepsilon_0}$ (d) $\frac{q}{4\varepsilon_0}$

29. When 100 V d.c. is applied across a coil, a current of 1 A flows through it. When 100 V a.c. of 50 Hz is applied to the same coil only 0.5 A flows. The inductance of the coil is

(a) 0.55 H (b) 5.5 mH
(c) 0.55 mH (d) 55 mH.

30. A bulb of 25 W, 200 V and another bulb of 100 W, 200 V are connected in series with a supply line of 220 V. Then

(a) both bulbs will glow with same brightness
(b) both bulbs will get fused
(c) 25 W bulb will glow more brightly
(d) 100 W bulb will glow more brightly.

31. Which of the following is matched wrongly?

(a) oil drop experiment → Millikan
(b) dual nature of light → de Brogile
(c) uncertainty principle → Heisenberg
(d) none of these

32. The forbidden gap in the energy bands of silicon is
(a) 2.6 eV (b) 1.1 eV
(c) 0.1 eV (d) 6 eV

33. When white light passes through a prism, the deviation is maximum for
(a) violet light (b) green light
(c) red light (d) yellow light

34. Which of the following gates correspond to the truth table given below?

A	B	Y
0	0	1
0	1	0
1	0	0
1	1	0

(a) NAND (b) OR
(c) XOR (d) NOR

35. Light is incident normally on a diffraction grating through which the first diffraction is seen at 32°. In this case the second order diffraction will be
(a) at 80° (b) at 64°
(c) at 48°
(d) there is no second order diffraction

36. If there were no atmosphere, the average temperature on earth surface would be
(a) lower (b) higher
(c) same (d) 0°C.

37. The current curve between $\log_e \frac{J}{T^2}$ and $\frac{1}{T}$ is

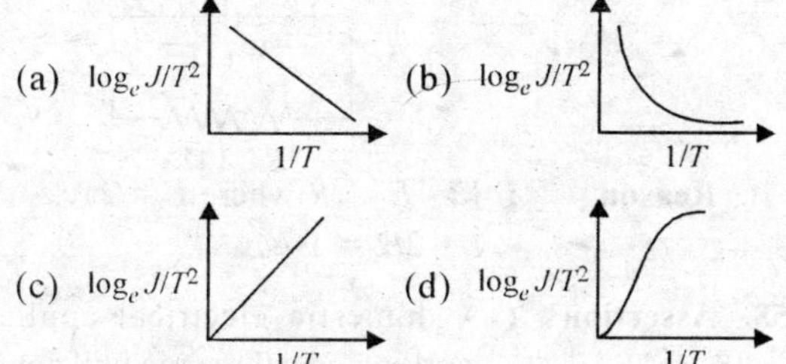

38. An object 5 cm tall is placed 1 m from a concave spherical mirror which has a radius of curvature of 20 cm. The size of the image is
(a) 0.11 cm (b) 0.50 cm
(c) 0.55 cm (d) 0.60 cm.

39. The magnifying power of a compound microscope increase with
(a) the focal length of objective lens is increased and that of eye lens is decreased
(b) the focal length of eye lens is increased and that of objective lens is decreased
(c) focal lengths of both objects and eye-piece are increased
(d) focal lengths of both objects and eye-piece are decreased.

40. A thread is tied slightly loose to a wire frame as in figure and the frame is dropped into a soap solution and taken out. The frame is completely covered with the film. When the portion A is punctured with a pin, the thread

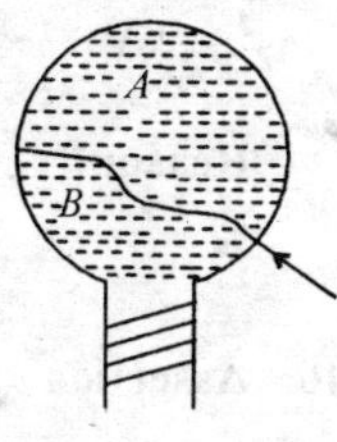

(a) becomes concave towards A
(b) becomes convex towards A
(c) either (a) or (b) depending on the size of A with respect to B
(d) remains in the initial position.

Directions : In the following questions (41-60), a statement of assertion (A) is followed by a statement of reason (R). Mark the correct choice as :
(a) If both assertion and reason are true and reason is the correct explanation of assertion
(b) If both assertion and reason are true but reason is not the correct explanation of assertion
(c) If assertion is true but reason is false
(d) If both assertion and reason are false.

41. **Assertion** : In the relation $f = \frac{1}{2l}\sqrt{\frac{T}{\mu}}$, where symbols have standard meaning, m represent linear mass density.
Reason : The frequency has the dimensions of inverse of time.

42. **Assertion** : When the velocity of projection of a body is made n times, its time of flight becomes n times.
Reason : Range of projectile does not depend on the initial velocity of a body.

43. **Assertion** : A needle placed carefully on the

surface of water may float, whereas a ball of the same material will always sink.

Reason : The buoyancy of an object depends both on the material and shape of the object.

44. Assertion : The colour of the green flower seen through red glass appears to be dark.

Reason : Red glass transmits only red light.

45. Assertion : The alternating current lags behind the e.m.f. by a phase angle of $\pi/2$, when AC flows through an inductor.

Reason : The inductive reactance increases as the frequency of AC source decreases.

46. Assertion : A spark occur between the poles of a switch when the switch is opened.

Reason : Current flowing in the conductor produces magnetic field.

47. Assertion : X-rays can penetrate through the flesh but not through the bones.

Reason : The penetrating power of X-rays depends on voltage.

48. Assertion : It is essential that all the lines available in the emission spectrum will also be available in the absorption spectrum.

Reason : The spectrum of hydrogen atom is only absorption spectrum.

49. Assertion : A double convex lens (μ = 1.5) has focal length 10 cm. When the lens is immersed in water (μ = 4/3) its focal length becomes 77 cm.

Reason : $\frac{1}{f}=\frac{\mu_v-\mu_m}{\mu_m}\left(\frac{1}{R_1}-\frac{1}{R_2}\right)$

50. Assertion : Diode lasers are used as optical sources in optical communication.

Reason : Diode lasers consume less energy.

51. Assertion : We cannot think of magnetic field configuration with three poles.

Reason : A bar magnet does exert a torque on itself due to its own field.

52. Assertion : In a SHM, kinetic and potential energies become equal when the displacement is $1/\sqrt{2}$ times the amplitude.

Reason : In SHM, kinetic energy is zero when potential energy is maximum.

53. Assertion : A bird perches on a high power line and nothing happens to the bird.

Reason : The level of bird is very high from the ground.

54. Assertion : Stopping potential depends upon the frequency of incident light but is independent of the intensity of the light.

Reason : The maximum kinetic energy of the photoelectrons is proportional to stopping potential.

55. Assertion : Inductance coils are usually made of thick copper wire.

Reason : Induced current is more in wire having less resistance.

56. Assertion : When radius of circular loop carrying current is doubled, its magnetic moment becomes four times.

Reason : Magnetic moment depends on area of the loop.

57. Assertion : In the following circuit, emf is 2 V and internal resistance of the cell is 1 Ω and R = 1 Ω, then reading of the voltmeter is 1 V.

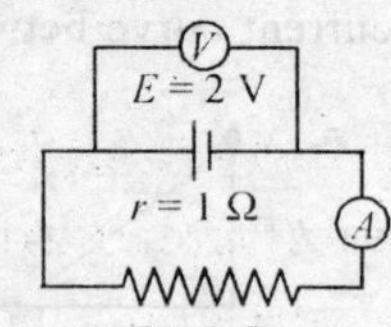

Reason : $V = E - IR$ where E = 2 V, I = 2/2 = 1 A.

58. Assertion : A domestic electrical appliance, working on a three pin will continue working even if the top pin is removed.

Reason : The third pin is used only as a safety device.

59. Assertion : The energy of charged particle

moving in a uniform magnetic field does not change.

Reason : Work done by magnetic field on the charge is zero.

60. Assertion : ^{90}Sr from the radioactive fall out from a nuclear bomb ends up in the bones of human beings through the milk consumed by them. It causes impairment of production of red blood cells.

Reason : The energies β-particles emitted in the decay of ^{90}Sr damage the bone marrow.

CHEMISTRY

61. Identify Z in the reaction.

$$C_6H_5OH \xrightarrow{CHCl_3 + NaOH} X \xrightarrow[conc]{NaOH} Z$$

(a) o-HOC$_6$H$_4$–CH(OH)–C$_6$H$_4$OH-o

(b) o-HOC$_6$H$_4$CH$_2$OH + o-HOC$_6$H$_4$COONa

(c) o-HOC$_6$H$_4$–C(=O)–C$_6$H$_4$OH-o

(d) o-HOC$_6$H$_4$–C(=O)–CH(OH)–C$_6$H$_4$OH-o

62. For the reaction, $2NO_2 + F_2 \rightarrow 2NO_2F$, following mechanism has been provided.

$$NO_2 + F_2 \xrightarrow{Slow} NO_2F + F$$

$$NO_2 + F \xrightarrow{Fast} NO_2F$$

Thus, rate expression of the above reaction can be written as

(a) $r = K[NO_2]_2[F_2]$ (b) $r = K[NO_2][F_2]$

(c) $r = K[NO_2]$ (d) $r = K[F_2]$.

63. What is the correct relationship between the pHs of isomolar solutions of sodium oxide (pH_1), sodium sulphide (pH_2), sodium selenide (pH_3) and sodium telluride (pH_4)?

(a) $pH_1 > pH_2 = pH_3 = pH_4$

(b) $pH_1 < pH_2 < pH_3 < pH_4$

(c) $pH_1 < pH_2 > pH_3 < pH_4$

(d) $pH_1 > pH_2 > pH_3 > pH_4$.

64. Toluene is nitrated and the resulting product is reduced with tin and hydrochloric acid. The product so obtained is diazotised and then heated with cuprous bromide. The reaction mixture so formed contains

(a) mixture of *o*- and *m*-bromotoluenes

(b) mixture of *o*- and *p*-bromotoluenes

(c) mixture of *o*- and *p*-dibromobenzenes

(d) mixture of *o*- and *p*-bromo anilines.

65. The dissociation equilibrium of a gas AB_2 can be represented as

$$2AB_{2\,(g)} \rightleftharpoons 2AB_{(g)} + B_{2\,(g)}$$

The degree of dissociation is x and is small compared to 1. The expression relating the degree of dissociation (x) with equilibrium constant K_p and total pressure p is

(a) $(2K_p/p)^{1/2}$ (b) K_p/p

(c) $2K_p/p$ (d) $(2K_p/p)^{1/3}$.

66. Which of the following is considered as an anticancer species?

(a) $[Pt(H_3N)_2Cl_2]$ (cis: H_3N, H_3N / Cl, Cl)

(b) $[Pt(H_3N)Cl(Cl)(NH_3)]$ (trans: H_3N, Cl / Cl, NH_3)

(c) $[PtCl_3(CH_2{=}CH_2)]$

(d) $[PtCl_4]$

67. $CH_3CH = CHCH_3 + CHCl_3 + t\text{-BuOK} \rightarrow A$. A is

(a) $CH_3CH-CHCH_3$ bridged by CH_2 (cyclopropane)

(b) $CH_3CH-CHCH_3$ bridged by CCl_2 (C with Cl, Cl)

(c) $CH_3CH(OBu) - CH(Cl)CH_3$

(d) $CH_3CH-CHCH_3$ bridged by O (epoxide)

68. In which of the following preparations of ether,

the configuration about chiral centre is not retained?

(a) $CH_3-C(H)(D)-OH + Na \xrightarrow{CH_3Br}$

(b) $CH_3-C(H)(D)-OH + TsCl \xrightarrow{CH_3ONa}$

(c) $CH_3-C(H)(D)-CH{=}CH_2 + Hg(OAc)_2 \xrightarrow{NaBH_4} + CH_3OH$

(d) $CH_3-C(H)(D)-CH{=}CH_2 + CF_3CO_3H \longrightarrow$

69. Toluene on treatment with CrO_3 and $(CH_3CO)_2O$ followed by hydrolysis with dil. HCl gives
(a) benzaldehyde (b) benzoic acid
(c) phenol
(d) phenylacetaldehyde.

70. The time period to coat a metal surface of 80 cm^2 with 5×10^{-3} cm thick layer of silver (density 1.05 g cm^{-3}) with the passage of 3 A current through a silver nitrate solution is
(a) 115 sec (b) 125 sec
(c) 135 sec (d) 145 sec.

71. Correct equation of Freundlich isotherm is
(a) $\log\left(\frac{m}{x}\right) = \log k + \frac{1}{n}\log c$
(b) $\log\left(\frac{x}{m}\right) = \log c + \frac{1}{n}\log k$
(c) $\log\left(\frac{x}{m}\right) = \log c + \frac{1}{k}\log c$
(d) $\log\left(\frac{x}{m}\right) = \log k + \frac{1}{k}\log c$

72. Which of the following compounds is not chiral?
(a) 1-Chloropentane
(b) 2-Chloropentane
(c) 1-Chloro-2-methyl pentane
(d) 3-Chloro-2-methyl pentane.

73. Which of the following molecules will not show optical activity?
(a) HOOC, COOH; H, H; HO, H (structure)
(b) $H_3C-CH(OH)-CD$
(c) HO, H, CH_3, OH, H, CH_3 (structure)
(d) Br, H, H, Br (cyclopropane structure)

74. Green chemistry means such reactions which
(a) are related to the depletion of ozone layer
(b) study the reactions in plants
(c) produce colour during reactions
(d) reduce the use and production of hazardous chemicals.

75. Identify the final product.
$H_3C-CH{=}CH-CH_2-CO-CH_3 \xrightarrow[\text{(ii) } H_3O^+]{\text{(i) } m\text{-CPBA}}$
(a) H_3C, H, HO; OH, H, CH_2COCH_3 (structure)
(b) H_3C, H, HO; H, OH, CH_2COCH_3 (structure)
(c) H_3C, H, HO; OH, CH_2COCH_3, H (structure)
(d) none of these.

76. The flame colours of metal ions are due to
(a) Frenkel defect (b) Schottky defect
(c) metal deficiency defect
(d) metal excess defect.

77. The reaction of an organic compound with ammonia followed by nitration of the product gives a powerful explosive called RDX. The organic compound is
(a) phenol (b) toluene
(c) glycerine (d) formaldehyde.

78. Cumene process is the most important commercial method for the manufacture of phenol. Cumene is
(a) *iso*-propyl benzene (b) ethyl benzene
(c) vinyl benzene (d) propyl benzene.

79. Prolonged exposure of fat or oil in moist air and light causes bad smell (rancidity). It is due to
(a) formation of $C_6 - C_{12}$ fatty acids
(b) formation of ketone and aldehyde
(c) both of these causes
(d) formation of glycerol.

80. Acid hydrolysis of sucrose is a
(a) pseudo first order reaction
(b) zero order reaction
(c) second order reaction
(d) unimolecular reaction.

81. Which of these compounds is synthesised by chloral?
(a) DDT (b) BHC
(c) chloroform (d) Michlers ketone.

82. When phenol reacts with phthalic anhydride in presence of H_2SO_4 and heated and hot reaction mixture is poured in NaOH solution, then product formed is
(a) alizarin (b) methyl orange
(c) fluorescein (d) phenolphthalein.

83. The function of $AlCl_3$ in Friedel-Craft's reaction is to
(a) absorb HCl (b) absorb water
(c) produce nucleophile
(d) produce electrophile.

84. The correct order of increasing $[H_3O^+]$ in the following aqueous solutions is
(a) 0.01 M H_2S < 0.01 M H_2SO_4 < 0.01 M NaCl < 0.01 M $NaNO_2$
(b) 0.01 M NaCl < 0.01 M $NaNO_2$ < 0.01 M H_2S < 0.01 M H_2SO_4
(c) 0.01 M $NaNO_2$ < 0.01 M NaCl < 0.01 M H_2S < 0.01 M H_2SO_4
(d) 0.01 M H_2S < 0.01 M $NaNO_2$ < 0.01 M NaCl < 0.01 M H_2SO_4.

85. Percentage of Se (at. mass = 78.4) in peroxidase anhydrase enzyme is 0.5% by weight, then minimum molecular mass of peroxidase anhydrase enzyme is
(a) 1.576×10^4 (b) 1.576×10^3
(c) 15.76 (d) 2.136×10^4.

86. The number of S – S bonds in sulphur trioxide trimer (S_3O_9) is
(a) three (b) two
(c) one (d) zero.

87. Oxidation product 1,2-cyclopentanediol with HIO_4 gives
(a) $HC(=O) - CH_2 - CH_2 - CH_2 - C(=O) - H$
(b) 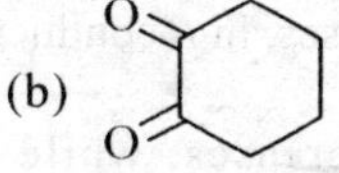
(c) $O{=}C(OH) - CH - CH_2 - CH_2 - C(OH){=}O$
(d) none of these.

88. The correct order of dipole moment is
(a) $CH_4 < NF_3 < NH_3 < H_2O$
(b) $NF_3 < CH_4 < NH_3 < H_2O$
(c) $NH_3 < NF_3 < CH_4 < H_2O$
(d) $H_2O < NH_3 < NF_3 < CH_4$.

89. The root mean square speed of the molecules of diatomic gas is u. When the temperature is doubled, the molecules dissociate into two atoms. The new rms speed of the atom is
(a) $\sqrt{2}u$ (b) u
(c) $2u$ (d) $4u$.

90. For the following concentration cell, to be spontaneous $Pt(H_2)P_1$ atm. |HCl|$Pt(H_2)P_2$ atm. Which of the following is correct?
(a) $P_1 = P_2$ (b) $P_1 < P_2$
(c) $P_1 > P_2$ (d) can't be predicted.

91. Which one of the following is not a surfactant?
(a) $CH_3 - (CH_2)_{15} - \overset{\oplus}{N}(CH_3)_2 - CH_3Br$
(b) $CH_3 - (CH_2)_{14} - CH_2 - NH_2$
(c) $CH_3 - (CH_2)_{16} - CH_2OSO_2^- Na^+$
(d) $OHC - (CH_2)_{14} - CH_2 - COO^- Na^+$.

92. The standard oxidation potential $E°$ for the half cell reaction are
$Zn \rightarrow Zn^{2+} + 2e^-$; $E° = + 0.76V$
$Fe \rightarrow Fe^{2+} + 2e^-$; $E° = + 0.41V$

EMF of the cell reaction is
$Zn + Fe^{2+} \rightarrow Zn^{2+} + Fe$
(a) – 0.35 V (b) + 0.35 V
(c) 0.17 V (d) 1.17 V.

93. To observe the effect of concentration on the conductivity electrolytes of different nature were taken in two vessels *A* and *B*. *A* contains weak electrolyte NH_4OH and *B* contains strong electrolyte NaCl. In both containers, concentration of respective electrolyte was increased and conductivity observed.
(a) in *A* conductivity increases, in *B* conductivity decreases
(b) in *A* conductivity decreases, while in *B* conductivity increases
(c) in both *A* and *B* conductivity increase
(d) in both *A* and *B* conductivity decreases.

94. A unit cell of sodium chloride has four formula units. The edge length of the unit cell is 0.0564 nm. What is the density of sodium chloride?
(a) 1.2 g/cm³ (b) 2.165 g/cm³
(c) 3.64 g/cm³ (d) 4.56 g/cm³.

95. The reaction

$$R-\underset{\underset{O}{||}}{C}-R \xrightarrow[H_2SO_4]{N_3H} RCONHR + N_2$$

is called
(a) Claisen-Schmidt reaction
(b) Kolbe-Schmidt reaction
(c) Schmidt reaction
(d) Kolbe's reaction.

96. Which of the following amines, can give N-nitrosoamine on treatment with HNO_2?
(a) $C_6H_5-NH_2$ (b) $CH_3-\underset{\underset{NH_2}{|}}{CH}-CH_3$
(c) C_6H_5-NH-R (d) $C_6H_5-NR_2$

97. The purification of alumina is called
(a) Baeyer's process (b) Bosch process
(c) Castuer process (d) Hoop's process.

98. Which acid has P – P linkage?
(a) Hypophosphoric acid
(b) Pyrophosphoric acid
(c) Metaphosphoric acid
(d) Orthophosphoric acid.

99. $C_6H_6 \xrightarrow[H_2SO_4]{HNO_3} X \xrightarrow[FeCl_3]{Cl_2} Y$. In the above sequence *Y* can be
(a) 3-nitrochlorobenzene
(b) 1-nitrochlorobenzene
(c) 4-nitrochlorobenzene
(d) none of these.

100. Which of the following is aromatic?

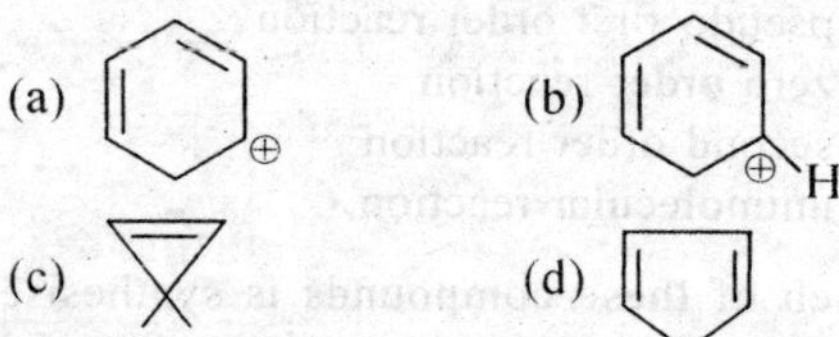

Directions : In the following questions (101-120), a statement of assertion (A) is followed by a statement of reason (R). Mark the correct choice as :
(a) If both assertion and reason are true and reason is the correct explanation of assertion
(b) If both assertion and reason are true but reason is not the correct explanation of assertion
(c) If assertion is true but reason is false
(d) If both assertion and reason are false.

101. Assertion : $(CH_3)_3CCOC(CH_3)_3$ and acetone can be distinguished by the reaction with $NaHSO_3$.
Reason : HSO_3^- is the nucleophile in bisulphite addition.

102. Assertion : Tertiary carbonium ions are generally formed more easily than primary carbonium ions.
Reason : Hyperconjugation as well as inductive effect due to additional alkyl groups stabilize tertiary carbonium ions.

103. Assertion : If H_2 and Cl_2 enclosed separately in the same vessel exert pressure of 100 and 200 mm respectively, their mixture in the same vessel at the same temperature will exert a pressure of 300 mm.

Reason : Dalton's law of partial pressures states that total pressure is the sum of partial pressures.

104. Assertion : The quantized energy of an electron is largely determined by its principal quantum number.

Reason : The principal quantum number n is a measure of the most probable distance of finding the electron around the nucleus.

105. Assertion : According to Le-Chatelier's principle addition of heat to an equilibrium solid $\rightleftharpoons$ liquid results in decrease in the amount of solid.

Reason : Reaction is endothermic, so on heating forward reaction is favoured.

106. Assertion : Cyclohexanone exhibits keto-enol tautomerism.

Reason : In cyclohexanone, one form contains the keto group (C═O) while other contains enolic group (– C═C – OH).

107. Assertion : Phenol is more reactive than benzene towards electrophilic substitution reaction.

Reason : In the case of phenol, the intermediate carbocation is more resonance stabilised.

108. Assertion : Many endothermic reactions that are not spontaneous at room temperature become spontaneous at high temperature.

Reason : Entropy of the system increases with increase in temperature.

109. Assertion : Benzaldehyde is more reactive than ethanal towards nucleophilic attack.

Reason : The overall effect of $-I$ and $+R$ effect of phenyl group decreases the electron density on the carbon atom of $>C=O$ group in benzaldehyde.

110. Assertion : Bleaching powder reacts with dilute acids to evolve chlorine.

Reason : The chlorine liberated by the action of dilute acids on bleaching powder is called available chlorine.

111. Assertion : Teflon has high thermal stability and chemical inertness.

Reason : Teflon is a thermoplastic.

112. Assertion : In high spin situation, configuration of d^5 ions will be $t^3_{2g}\ e^2_g$.

Reason : In high spin situation, pairing energy is less than crystal field energy.

113. Assertion : Copper metal gets readily corroded in acidic aqueous solution.

Reason : Free energy change for this process is negative.

114. Assertion : When a concentrated solution is diluted by adding more water, molarity of the solution remains unchanged.

Reason : Product of moles of a solute and volume is equal to the molarity.

115. Assertion : Anilinium chloride is more acidic than ammonium chloride.

Reason : Anilinium chloride is resonance stabilised.

116. Assertion : Pyrrole is an aromatic heterocyclic compound.

Reason : It has cyclic delocalised 6π electrons.

117. Assertion : 2-Butanol on heating with H_2SO_4 gives 1-butene and 2-butene.

Reason : Dehydration of 2-butanol follows Saytzeff's rule.

118. Assertion : $SeCl_4$ does not have a tetrahedral structure.

Reason : Se in $SeCl_4$ has two lone pairs.

119. Assertion : Liquid NH_3 is used for refrigeration.

Reason : Liquid NH_3 quickly vapourises.

120. Assertion : Ethers behave as bases in the presence of mineral acids.

Reason : It is due to the presence of lone pair of electrons on the oxygen.

BIOLOGY

121. Two opposite forces operate in the growth and development of every population. One of them is related to the ability to reproduce at a given rate. The force opposite to it is called

(a) fecundity
(b) environmental resistances
(c) biotic control (d) mortality.

122. Acrosome reaction in sperm is triggered by

(a) capacitation (b) release of lysin
(c) influx of Na^+ (d) release of fertilizin.

123. What is a keystone species?

(a) a species which makes up only a small proportion of the total biomass of a community, yet has a huge impact on the community's organization and survival
(b) a common species that has plenty of biomass, yet has a fairly low impact on the community's organization
(c) a rare species that has minimal impact on the biomass and on other species in the community
(d) a dominant species that constitutes a large proportion of the biomass and which affects many other species.

124. Which one of the following pairs is not correctly matched?

(a) *Streptomyces* - Antibiotic
(b) *Serratia* - Drug addiction
(c) *Spirulina* - Single cell protein
(d) *Rhizobium* - Biofertilizer.

125. You are required to draw blood from a patient and to keep it in a test tube for analysis of blood corpuscles and plasma. You are also provided with the following four types of test tubes. Which of these will you not use for the purpose?

(a) test tube containing calcium bicarbonate
(b) chilled test tube
(c) test tube containing heparin
(d) test tube containing sodium oxalate.

126. Smoking addiction is harmful because it produces polycyclic aromatic hydrocarbons, which cause

(a) reduction in oxygen transport
(b) increase in blood pressure
(c) cancer
(d) retardation of growth of foetus.

127. The main reason why antibiotics could not solve all the problems of bacteria mediated diseases is

(a) insensitivity of the individual following prolonged exposure to antibiotics
(b) inactivation of antibiotics by bacterial enzymes
(c) decreased efficiency of the immune system
(d) the development of mutant strains resistant to antibiotics.

128. Which of the following sets includes the bacterial disease?

(a) cholera, typhoid, mumps
(b) tetanus, tuberculosis, measles
(c) malaria, mumps, poliomyelitis
(d) diphtheria, leprosy, plague.

129. The binding of antibodies to the antigens to produce a large insoluble complex is known as

(a) antibody-antigen complex
(b) agglutination (c) immunization
(d) suppressor cell reaction.

130. One of the major difficulties in the biological control of insect pest is that

(a) the predator develops a preference to other diets and may itself become a pest
(b) the predator does not always survive when transferred to a new environment
(c) the method is less effective as compared with the use of insecticides
(d) the practical difficulty of introducing the predator to specific areas.

131. Cattle fed with spoilt hay of sweet clover which contains dicumarol

(a) are healthier due to a good diet
(b) catch infections easily
(c) may suffer vitamin K deficiency and prolonged bleeding
(d) may suffer from beri-beri due to deficiency of vitamin B_1.

132. Which one of the following methods is commonly used to maintain the genetic traits of a given plant?

(a) by propagating through seed germination
(b) by propagating through vegetative multiplication
(c) by generating hybrids through intergeneric pollination
(d) by treating the seeds with gamma radiations.

133. The bacteria which attack dead animals are
(a) first link of the food chain and are known as primary producers
(b) second link of the food chain and are herbivorous
(c) third link of the food chain and are tertiary consumers
(d) the end of food chain and are decomposers.

134. Which of the following statements is incorrect?
(a) lichen, an association of fungus and algae is an example of mutualism.
(b) those epiphytes which use other plants for support only and not for water or food supply and are examples of commensalism.
(c) sea-anemone on hermit-crab is an example of protocooperation.
(d) mutualism, protocøoperation, commensalism cannot be included under symbiosis.

135. How many sperms are formed from a secondary spermatocyte?
(a) 4 (b) 8
(c) 2 (d) 1.

136. Phytohormones are
(a) hormones regulating growth from seed to adulthood
(b) growth regulators synthesised by plants and influencing physiological process
(c) hormones regulating flowering
(d) hormones regulating secondary growth.

137. Grey crescent is the area
(a) at the point of entry of sperm into ovum
(b) just opposite to the site of entry of sperm into ovum
(c) at the animal pole (d) at the vegetal pole.

138. Even after killing the generative cell with a laser beam, the pollen grain of a flowering plant germinates and produces normal pollen tube because
(a) laser beam stimulates pollen germination and pollen tube growth
(b) the laser beam does not damage the region from which pollen tube emerges
(c) the contents of killed generative cell permits germination and pollen tube growth
(d) the vegetative cell has not been damaged.

139. One common example of simple reflex is
(a) tying your shoe laces while talking to another person and not looking at them
(b) watering of mouth at the sight of a favourite food
(c) climbing up a stairs in dark without stumbling
(d) closing of eyes when strong light is flashed across them.

140. Select one of the following pairs of important features distinguishing *Gnetum* from *Cycas* and *Pinus* and showing affinities with angiosperms.
(a) Perianth and two integuments.
(b) Embryo development and apical meristem.
(c) Absence of resin duct and leaf venation.
(d) Presence of vessel elements and absence of archegonia.

141. Injury to vagus nerve in humans is not likely to affect
(a) tongue movements
(b) gastrointestinal movements
(c) pancreatic secretion
(d) cardiac movements.

142. Which one of the following is a matching pair?
(a) Lubb-Sharp closure of AV valves at the beginning of ventricular systole.
(b) Dup-Sudden opening of semilunar valves at the beginning of ventricular diastole.
(c) Pulsation of the radial artery-Valves in the blood vessels.
(d) Initiation of the heart beat - Purkinje fibres.

143. A lake near a village suffered heavy mortality of fishes within a few days. Consider the following reasons for this?
(a) lots of urea and phosphate fertilizer were used in the vicinity.
(b) the area was sprayed with DDT by an aircraft.
(c) the lake water turned green and stinky.
(d) phytoplankton polulations in the lake declined initially thereby greatly reducing photosynthesis.

144. Which one of the following pairs of plant structures has haploid number of chromosomes?

(a) nucellus and antipodal cells.
(b) egg nucleus and secondary nucleus.
(c) megaspore mother cell and antipodal cells.
(d) egg cell and antipodal cells.

145. When a man inhales air containing normal concentration of O_2 as well as CO he suffers from suffocation because
(a) CO reacts with O_2 reducing its percentage in air
(b) haemoglobin combines with CO instead of O_2 and forms carboxyhaemoglobin
(c) CO affects diaphragm and intercostal muscles
(d) CO affects the nerves of the lungs.

146. A patient of diabetes mellitus excretes glucose in urine even when he is kept in a carbohydrate free diet. It is because
(a) fats are catabolised in adipose tissues to form glucose
(b) amino acids are catabolised in kidney to form glucose
(c) amino acids are discharged in blood stream from liver
(d) glycogen from muscles is released in blood stream.

147. During the life-cycle, *Fasciola hepatica* (liver fluke) infects its intermediate host and primary host at the following larval stages respectively
(a) redia and miracidium
(b) cercaria and redia
(c) metacercaria and cercaria
(d) miracidium and metacercaria

148. Enzymes, vitamins and hormones can be classified into a single category of biological chemicals because of all of these
(a) enhance oxidative metabolism
(b) are conjugated proteins
(c) are exclusively synthesised in the body of a living organism as at present
(d) help in regulating metabolism.

149. Cut surfaces of fruit and vegetables often become dark because
(a) dirty knife makes it dark
(b) oxidation of tannic acid in the presence of trace of iron from the knife makes it dark
(c) dust of the air makes it dark
(d) none of the above.

150. *Nicotiana sylvestris* flowers only during long days and *N.tabacum* flowers only during short days. If raised in the laboratory under different photoperiods, they can be induced to flower at the same time and can be cross-fertilized to produce self-fertile offspring. What is the best reason for considering *N.sylvestris* and *N.tabacum* to be separate species ?
(a) they cannot interbreed in nature
(b) they are reproductively distinct
(c) they are physiologically distinct
(d) they are morphologically distinct

151. Which one of the following is the correct statement regarding the particular psychotropic drug specified?
(a) morphine leads to delusions and disturbed emotions.
(b) barbiturates cause relaxation and temporary euphoria.
(c) hashish causes alteration of thoughts, perceptions and hallucinations.
(d) opium stimulates nervous system and causes hallucinations.

152. In succulent plants the stomata open in night and close in day. Which among the following would be best hypothesis to explain the mechanism of stomatal action in night only?
(a) CO_2 accumulates, reduces pH, stimulate enzymes resulting in accumulation of sugars.
(b) increase in CO_2 concentration, conversion of organic acids into starch resulting in the increased conversion into sugars resulting in K^+ transport.
(c) low CO_2 concentration accumulates organic acids resulting in the increased concentration of cell sap.
(d) CO_2 used up, increase pH results in accumulation of sugars.

153. The cells of the quiescent centre are characterised by
(a) having dense cytoplasm and prominent nuclei
(b) having light cytoplasm and small nuclei

(c) dividing regularly to add to the corpus
(d) dividing regularly to add to tunica

154. *Thermococcus*, *Methanococcus* and *Methanobacterium* exemplify
(a) bacteria whose DNA is relaxed or positively supercoiled but which have a cytoskeleton as well as mitochondria
(b) bacteria that contain a cytoskeleton and ribosomes
(c) archaebacteria that contains protein homologous to eukaryotic core histones
(d) archaebacteria that lack any histones resembling those found in eukaryotes but whose DNA is negatively supercoiled.

155. Ectophloic siphonostele is found in
(a) *Osmunda* and *Equisetum*
(b) *Marsilea* and *Botrychium*
(c) *Adiantum* and *Cucurbitaceae*
(d) *Dicksonia* and *Maidenhair fern*.

156. Chlorenchyma is known to develop in the
(a) cytoplasm of *Chlorella*
(b) mycelium of a green mould such as *Aspergillus*
(c) spore capsule of a moss
(d) pollen tube of *Pinus*

157. The distance between two genes in a chromosome is measured in cross-over units which represent
(a) ratio of crossing over between them
(b) percentage of crossing over between them
(c) number of crossing over between them
(d) none of these.

158. In transgenics, expression of transgene in target tissue is determined by
(a) enhancer (b) transgene
(c) promoter (d) reporter.

159. How many genome types are present in a typical green plants cell?
(a) more than five (b) more than ten
(c) two (d) three.

160. The growth curve of bacterial population in lab is plotted against time. What will be the shape of graph?
(a) sigmoid (b) hyperbolic
(c) ascending straight line
(d) descending straight line.

Directions : In the following questions (161-180), a statement of assertion (A) is followed by a statement of reason (R). Mark the correct choice as :
(a) If both assertion and reason are true and reason is the correct explanation of assertion
(b) If both assertion and reason are true but reason is not the correct explanation of assertion
(c) If assertion is true but reason is false
(d) If both assertion and reason are false.

161. Assertion : Protoplasmic continuity is maintained in perforated septum.
Reason : Usually a small pore remains in the centre of the septum.

162. Assertion : The primary protenema of moss by death and decay of cells may break into fragments.
Reason : Each fragment gives rise to leafy gametophyte.

163. Assertion : Cephalization is advantageous to an animal.
Reason : It improves the appearance of the animal.

164. Assertion : Koel does not build nest for egg laying.
Reason : Koel lays its eggs in the nest of tailor bird.

165. Assertion : Competitive inhibitor is also called as substrate analogue.
Reason : It resembles the enzymes in structure.

166. Assertion : Persons suffering from haemophilia fail to produce blood clotting factor VIII.
Reason : Prothrombin producing platelets in such persons are found in very low concentration.

167. Assertion : Hybridoma cells are shifted to a medium deficient in nutrient which cannot be synthesized by myeloma cells.
Reason : This medium allows selection of hybridoma cells.

168. Assertion : Maize is an albuminous seed.

Reason : Endosperm is completely absorbed by its growing embryo.

169. Assertion : Ciliated epithelium is present in the inner lining of trachea and large bronchi.

Reason : Ciliary movement propel the mucus and foreign particle towards the larynx.

170. Assertion : Light is one of the important factor in transpiration.

Reason : It induces stomatal opening and closing. Therefore, transpiration increases in light and decreases in dark.

171. Assertion : The higher concentration of O_2 in the atmosphere is inhibitory to photosynthesis.

Reason : CO_2 is the main substrate of photosynthesis.

172. Assertion : F_1 particles are present in the inner mitochondrial membrane.

Reason : An electron gradient formed on the inner mitochondrial membrane, forms ATP.

173. Assertion : Rhabdome is present in *Palaemon.*

Reason : Rhabdome has an important role in digestion.

174. Assertion : Pituitary is attached to hypothalamus by a vein.

Reason : This attachment is done through a hypophysial portal vein.

175. Assertion : Rabies is acute infectious disease of warm blooded mammals characterised by involvement of central nervous system resulting in paralysis and finally death.

Reason : This is caused due to neurotropic filterable bacteria in saliva of rabid animals.

176. Assertion : Many plants are propagated vegetatively even though they bear seeds.

Reason : Potatoes multiply by tubers and apple by cutting.

177. Assertion : Nuclear endosperm is formed by subsequent nuclear division without wall formation.

Reason : Coconut is an example of such endosperm, where the endosperm remains nuclear throughout the development of the fruit.

178. Assertion : In mammals the female secondary sexual characters are developed by gonadotropins.

Reason : Gonadotropins are secreted by graafian follicle.

179. Assertion : The plant biomass which serves as the food of herbivores and decomposers is said to result from the gross primary productivity.

Reason : Gross primary productivity is the rate of net production of organic material (biomass).

180. Assertion : Methyl mercury is a highly persistent pollutant that accumulates in food chains.

Reason : Mercury pollution is responsible for minamata.

GENERAL KNOWLEDGE

181. The first of the GAEL (Global Alliance for the elimination of Leprosy) was held in
(a) New Delhi (b) Bombay
(c) Culcutta (d) Paris.

182. Megger is an instrument to measure
(a) very low resistance
(b) insulation resistance
(c) inductance of a coil
(d) all of the above.

183. Terminator technology promotes sale of which of the following that is/are generated by it?
(a) gransgenic fertile seed.
(b) gene modified plants.
(c) genetically engineered seeds fertilized in next generation.
(d) all of these.

184. Which among the following has become the third

tiger reserve of Assam?
(a) Manas Wildlife Sanctury
(b) Kaziranga National Park
(c) Nameri National Park
(d) none of these.

185. To make the acidic soil suitable for agricultural, one of the following material is used.
(a) lime (b) gypsum
(c) calcium superphosphate
(d) vegetable compost.

186. The landform which is not associated with wind erosion is
(a) sand dune (b) inselberg
(c) drumlin (d) mushroom rock.

187. BCG vaccination is to be given to a new born child
(a) immediately after child birth
(b) within 48 hours
(c) within seven days
(d) within six months.

188. For reproducing sound, CD (compact disc) audioplayer uses a
(a) quartz crystal (b) titanium needle
(c) laser beam
(d) barium titanate ceramic

189. In a three pin electrical plug, longest pin should be connected to
(a) ground terminal (b) live terminal
(c) neutral terminal (d) any terminal.

190. The new addition to the commonwealth games 2010 is
(a) shooting (b) hockey
(c) wrestling (d) football.

191. The name of the player who established record in World Cup Cricket 2007 of making six sixes is
(a) Sanath Jaisurya (b) Virendra Sehwag
(c) Adam Gilchrist (d) Hershelle Gibbs.

192. The lateral meaning of the word Arya is
(a) superior (b) learned
(c) priest (d) warrior.

193. When T.V. is switched on
(a) audio and video both start simultaneously
(b) audio is heard immediately but video starts later because video needs some warm up time
(c) video starts immediately but audio is heard later because sound travels at a lesser speed than light
(d) it depends on the T.V. stand.

194. The instrument of music in which Ustad Amjad Ali Khan has distinguished himself is
(a) sarod (b) violin
(c) sitar (d) shehnai.

195. A deep and narrow river valley with steep bank is called
(a) geyser (b) bluff
(c) delta (d) canyon.

196. A 'breath test' used by traffic police to check drunken drivers uses -
(a) potassium dichormate-sulphuric acid
(b) potassium permanganate sulphuric acid
(c) turmeric on filter paper
(d) silica gel coated with silver nitrate

197. In which of the following books is 'Knowledge is Power' written?
(a) Essay on Man (b) Paradise Lost
(c) Leviathan (d) Das Capital.

198. Who said "where weather accumulates, men decay"?
(a) Abraham Lincoln (b) Mao Tsetung
(c) Karl Marx (d) Goldsmith.

199. Which of the following computer viruses is named aftc: cherry and caffein soft drink popular with programmers ?
(a) sircam (b) code pink
(c) code red (d) malisa

200. The fourth Buddist council was held during the reign of
(a) Ashoka
(b) Chandragupta
(c) Kanishka
(d) Chandragupta Vikramaditya

SOLUTIONS

PHYSICS

1. (d)

2. (c): Acceleration = $\frac{d^2x}{dt^2}$

For part OP, the acceleration is positive as the velocity is increasing. Slope is increasing. For part PQ, the acceleration is zero. Horizontal straight line shows that the velocity is zero. For part QR, acceleration is negative. It is retarded motion. Velocity is decreasing as the slope decreases with time. Hence option (c) is correct.

3. (a): Centripetal force $(F) = \frac{mv^2}{r}$ $\therefore v = \sqrt{\frac{Fr}{m}}$

4. (b): Momentum of rifle = Momentum of bullet

$m_1v_1 = m_2v_2$, Also $m_1 > m_2$

$$\frac{\text{K.E. of rifle}}{\text{K.E. of bullet}} = \frac{\frac{1}{2}m_1v_1^2}{\frac{1}{2}m_2v_2^2}$$

$$= \frac{m_1^2v_1^2}{m_1} \cdot \frac{m_2}{m_2^2v_2^2} = \frac{m_2}{m_1}$$

K.E. of rifle is less than K.E. of bullet.

5. (a): Distance of corner mass from opposite side = r

$$r^2 = l^2 - \left(\frac{l}{2}\right)^2 = \frac{3l^2}{4}$$

$$I = mr^2 = \frac{3}{4}ml^2$$

6. (c) : Using Lami's theorem, we have

$$\frac{P}{\sin\theta_1} = \frac{R}{\sin 150°} \Rightarrow \frac{P}{\sin\theta_1} = \frac{R}{\sin(180° - 30°)}$$

$$\Rightarrow \frac{1.9318 \text{ kgwt}}{0.9659} = \frac{R}{1/2}$$

$$\Rightarrow R = \frac{1.9318}{0.9659} \times \frac{1}{2} \text{ kgwt} = 1 \text{ kgwt.}$$

7. (a) : Gravitational force, $F \propto \frac{1}{r^n}$

$F = \frac{k}{r^n}$ where k is a constant.

For a planet, moving in a circular orbit of radius R, $F = \frac{k}{R^n}$

But, $F = m\omega^2R$

$$\Rightarrow \frac{k}{R^n} = mR \cdot \left(\frac{2\pi}{T}\right)^2 \Rightarrow \frac{k}{R^{n+1}} = \frac{m(2\pi)^2}{T^2}$$

$$\Rightarrow T^2 \propto R^{n+1}$$

$$\therefore T \propto R^{\frac{n+1}{2}}$$

8. (a) : $n_h = 10^{21}$ atoms/m^3

$n_i = 10^{19}$ atoms/m^3, n_e = ?

$n_en_h = n_i^2$

$$n_e = \frac{n_i^2}{n_h} = \frac{(10^{19})^2}{10^{21}} = \frac{10^{38}}{10^{21}} = 10^{17} \text{ atoms/m}^3.$$

9. (a) : In series combination, $\frac{t}{K_1} + \frac{t}{K_2} = \frac{2t}{K}$

$$\Rightarrow \frac{1}{K_1} + \frac{1}{K_2} = \frac{2}{K} \Rightarrow k = \frac{2K_1K_2}{K_1+K_2}.$$

10. (d) : Fringe width, $\beta = \frac{\lambda D}{d}$

From question, $d' = 3d$

$\therefore$ New fringe width, $\beta' = \frac{\lambda D}{d'}$

$$\therefore \beta' = \frac{\lambda D}{3d} = \frac{\beta}{3}.$$

11. (a)

12. (d) : Due to insertion of slab, the optical path increases by x/μ, where x is thickness of slab. Therefore the converging point will shift away by $\left[x - \frac{x}{\mu}\right] = x\left(1 - \frac{1}{\mu}\right)$.

13. (a) : Velocity of electromagnetic wave is

$$c = \frac{1}{\sqrt{\mu_0\varepsilon_0}}.$$

14. (d) :

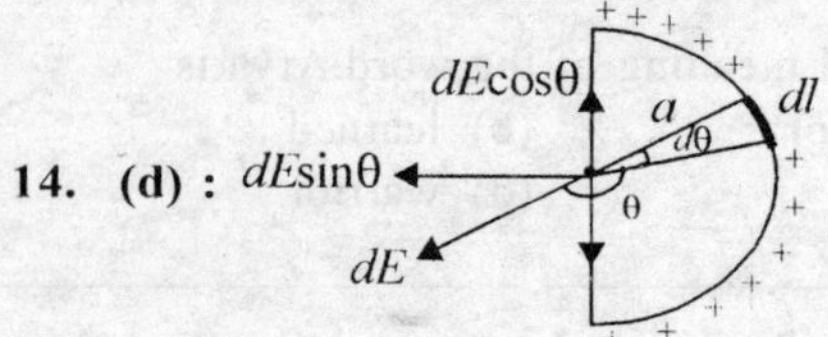

Electric field intensity at O due to small elemental length dl of charged ring,

$$dE = \frac{1}{4\pi\varepsilon_0}\cdot\frac{\lambda dl}{a^2} = \frac{1}{4\pi\varepsilon_0}\cdot\frac{\lambda a d\theta}{a^2}$$

$$dE = \frac{1}{4\pi\varepsilon_0}\cdot\frac{\lambda}{a}d\theta$$

$\therefore$ Net electric field at centre O is

$$E = \int dE\sin\theta = \int_0^{\pi}\frac{1}{4\pi\varepsilon_0}\frac{\lambda}{a}\sin\theta d\theta$$

$$= \frac{\lambda}{4\pi\varepsilon_0 a}\left[-\cos\theta\right]_0^{\pi}$$

$\therefore$ $E = \dfrac{\lambda}{2\pi\varepsilon_0 a}$.

15. (a) : Impedance of RL circuit is

$$Z = \sqrt{R^2 + X_L^2}$$

where $X_L = \omega L = 2\pi f L$

$\therefore$ $Z = \sqrt{R^2 + (2f L)^2}$.

16. (c) : Frequency of fundamental mode of vibrations of 1st closed organ pipe,

$$\upsilon_1 = \frac{v}{4l_1} = \frac{v}{4\times 100} \quad \ldots \text{(i)}$$

Frequency of fundamental mode of vibrations of 2nd closed organ pipe,

$$\upsilon_2 = \frac{v}{4l_2} = \frac{v}{4\times 101} \quad \ldots \text{(ii)}$$

From question, $\upsilon_1 - \upsilon_2 = \dfrac{16}{20}$

$$\Rightarrow \frac{v}{4\times 100} - \frac{v}{4\times 101} = \frac{16}{20}$$

$$\Rightarrow \frac{v}{4}\cdot\left[\frac{1}{100} - \frac{1}{101}\right] = \frac{16}{20}$$

$$\Rightarrow \frac{v}{4}\left[\frac{101-100}{101}\right] = \frac{16}{20} \Rightarrow \frac{v}{4}\times\frac{1}{101} = \frac{16}{20}$$

$$\Rightarrow v = \frac{16\times 101\times 4}{20} = 323.2 \text{ m/s.}$$

17. (a) : Stages 1 and 2 are at the same temperature. Also stages 4 and 5 are at same temperature. As V_p is more at higher temperature and same at all stages at equal temperature.

$\therefore$ $V_{P_3} > V_{P_1} = V_{P_2} > V_{P_4} = V_{P_5}$.

18. (b) : $-\dfrac{dN}{dt} = \lambda N \Rightarrow N_2 = \lambda N_1$

19. (c) : Kinetic energy is +ve (A)

|total energy| < |P.E.|

$\therefore$ $C \rightarrow$ total energy, B the P.E.

20. (b) : Net charge on system = 0

$\therefore$ Net force on system = 0.

Now consider one charge : $T = qvB$.

21. (c) : $Y = \dfrac{F/A}{\dfrac{\Delta l}{l}}$

$\therefore$ $F = \dfrac{YA}{l}\cdot\Delta l = k\cdot\Delta l$

Force $\propto$ extension

If the extension is x, work done in extending by dx

$dW = kx\, dx \qquad \therefore W = \dfrac{1}{2}k\cdot x^2$

If x is $l' - l$, $W = \dfrac{1}{2}k(l'-l)^2$

i.e. work done is $\dfrac{1}{2}\dfrac{YA}{l}(l-l')^2$.

22. (b) :

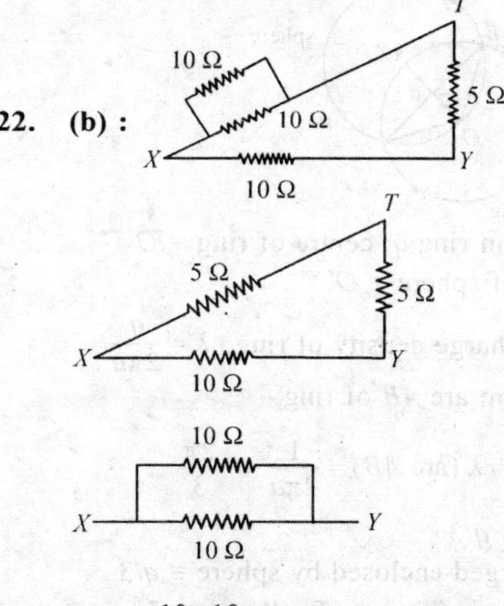

$$R_{XY} = \frac{10\times 10}{10+10} = 5\ \Omega.$$

23. (a) : The magnetic intensity due to an isolated pole of strength m_p at a distance $(r) = \dfrac{m_p}{r^2}$

24. (a) : With increase in frequency, reactance of LC circuit will increase. As a result, voltage increases. So, brightness will increase.

25. (c) : When heater wires are connected in series, then equivalent resistance,

$$R_s = R_1 + R_2 = 2R \qquad (\because R_1 = R_2)$$

Rate of heat produced, $H_s = \frac{V^2}{R_s}$

$$H_s = \frac{V_2}{2R} \quad \text{... (i)}$$

In second case, $R_p = \frac{R_1 R_2}{R_1 + R_2} = \frac{R \cdot R}{2R}$

or $R_p = \frac{R}{2}$

$\therefore$ Rate of heat produced, $H_p = \frac{V^2}{R_p}$

$$H_p = \frac{2V^2}{R} \quad \text{... (ii)}$$

Dividing (i) by (ii), we get

$$\frac{H_s}{H_p} = \frac{(V^2/2R)}{(2V^2/R)} = \frac{v^2}{2R} \times \frac{R}{2V^2} = \frac{1}{4}.$$

26. **(a)**

27. **(a)** : Lumen is the S.I. unit of luminous flux.

28. **(c)** :

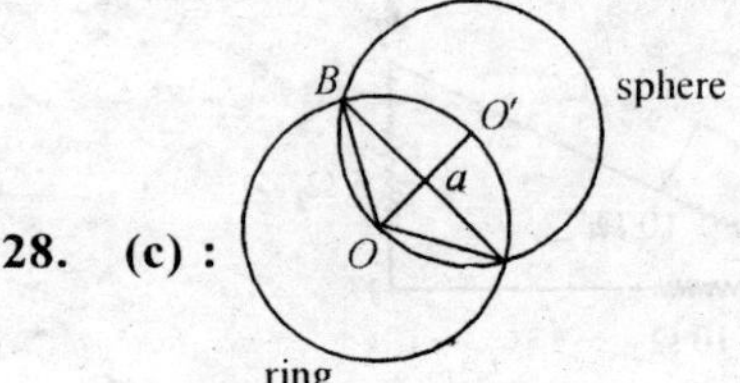

Charge on ring q, centre of ring = O

Centre of sphere = O'

Linear charge density of ring, $\lambda = \frac{q}{2\pi a}$

Charge on arc AB of ring,

$$q_{AB} = \lambda\,(\text{arc } AB) = \frac{1}{2\pi a} \cdot a \cdot \frac{2\pi}{3}$$

$$q_{AB} = q/3$$

i.e., charged enclosed by sphere = $q/3$

$\therefore$ Flux coming out of sphere = $q/3\varepsilon_0$.

29. **(a)** : For dc, $V = IR$ (R is resistance of inductor)

$100 = 1 \times R \quad \Rightarrow \quad R = 100\ \Omega.$

For ac, $Z = \sqrt{R^2 + X_L^2}$

$\because V = IZ$

$$\Rightarrow 100 = 0.5\sqrt{R^2 + X_L^2}$$

$$\Rightarrow 100 = 0.5\sqrt{(100)^2 + X_L^2}$$

$$\Rightarrow 100 = \frac{5}{10}\sqrt{(100)^2 + X_L^2}$$

$$X_L^2 = (200)^2 - (100)^2 = 300 \times 100$$

$$\Rightarrow X_L = \sqrt{3 \times (100)^2} = 100\sqrt{3}$$

$$\Rightarrow \omega L = 100\sqrt{3} \quad \Rightarrow \quad 2\pi\upsilon L = 100\sqrt{3}$$

$$\Rightarrow 2 \times \pi \times 50 \times L = 100\sqrt{3}$$

$$\Rightarrow 100 \times \pi L = 100\sqrt{3}$$

$$\therefore \quad L = \frac{\sqrt{3}}{\pi} = \frac{\sqrt{3}}{3.14} \quad \Rightarrow \quad L = 0.55\text{ H}.$$

30. **(c)** : Resistance of 25 W, 200 V bulb

$$R_1 = \frac{(200)^2}{25}\ \Omega.$$

Resistance of 100 W, 200 V bulb

$$R_2 = \frac{(200)^2}{100}\ \Omega.$$

Clearly, $R_1 > R_2$. $\quad \therefore \quad H_1 > H_2$.

$\therefore$ 25 W bulb will glow more brightly.

31. **(d)**

32. **(b)** : The forbidden gap in the energy band of Si = 1.1 eV.

33. **(a)** : Since the wavelength of violet light is the smallest, therefore maximum deviation will occur for violet light.

34. **(d)** : By truth table, $Y = \overline{A + B}$. Therefore it is a NOR gate operation.

35. **(d)** : Angle of first order diffraction $(\theta_1) = 32°$. We know that the angle of diffraction for the nth order (θ_n) is given by $d \sin\theta_n = n\lambda$.

For first order diffraction we get

$d \sin 32° = 1 \times \lambda$ or, $\lambda = d \sin 32°$.

Now for second order diffraction,

$d \sin\theta_2 = 2 \times \lambda$ or, $d \sin\theta_2 = 2 \times d \sin 32°$

or $\sin\theta_2 = 2 \times \sin 32° = 2 \times 0.529 = 1.06$.

Since the sine of any angle cannot be greater than 1, therefore there is no second order diffraction.

36. **(a)**

37. **(a)** : We know that $J = AT^2 e^{-b/T}$

$$\frac{J}{T^2} = Ae^{-b/T}$$

Taking log both side, we get

$$\log_e \frac{J}{T^2} = \log_e(A \cdot e^{-b/T})$$

$$\log_e \frac{J}{T^2} = \log_e A - \frac{b}{T}$$

Comparing with $y = mx + C$ we get correct option (a).

38. (c) : $h_0 = 5$ cm, $h_i = ?$

$u = -100$ cm, $R = -20$ cm. $\therefore f = -10$ cm

Using mirror formula,

$$\frac{1}{v}+\frac{1}{u}=\frac{1}{f} \Rightarrow \frac{1}{v}-\frac{1}{100}=-\frac{1}{10}$$

$$\frac{1}{v}=\frac{1}{100}-\frac{1}{10}=\frac{1-10}{100}=-\frac{9}{100}$$

$$\therefore v=-\frac{100}{9} \text{ cm.}$$

$$\frac{h_i}{h_0}=\frac{v}{u} \Rightarrow \frac{h_i}{5 \text{ cm}}=\frac{(100/9)}{100}=\frac{1}{9}$$

$\therefore h_i = 5/9 = 0.55$ cm.

39. (b) : Magnifying power of compound microscope

$$M=-\frac{v_o}{u_o}\left(1+\frac{D}{f_e}\right)=-\frac{L}{f_o}\left(1+\frac{D}{f_e}\right)$$

40. (c)

41. (b) : From, $f=\frac{1}{2l}\sqrt{\frac{T}{\mu}}, f^2=\frac{T}{4l^2\mu}$

or, $\mu=\frac{T}{4l^2f^2}=\frac{[\text{MLT}^{-2}]}{\text{L}^2\text{T}^{-2}}=\frac{\text{M}}{\text{L}}$

$=\frac{\text{Mass}}{\text{length}}$ = linear mass density.

42. (c) : As time of flight,

$$T=\frac{2u\sin\theta}{g} \quad \therefore T'=\frac{2(nu)\sin\theta}{g}=nT$$

But range

$$R=\frac{u^2\sin 2\theta}{g} \therefore R'=\frac{n^2u^2\sin 2\theta}{g}=n^2R.$$

43. (c) : A needle placed carefully on the surface of water may float due to surface tension as upward force due to surface tension balances the weight of the needle. But these upward force due to surface tension are very small as compared to weight of ball. Also the weight of liquid displaced by the ball immersed in liquid is less than the weight of the ball, hence ball sinks into the liquid.

44. (a) : Green flower emit all folour except green and the emitted colours are dominated by red colour. So flower appear black.

45. (c) : Assertion is correct but reason is false because inductance reactance $X_L = 2\pi fL$. So, higher frequency greater inductance reactance.

46. (b)

47. (b) : Hardness penetrating power of X-ray depends upon accelerating voltage applied across X-ray tube. Characteristic X-ray relate to the material of target. X-ray can't pass through matter of heavier element like bones (which contain phosphorus and calcium) but can pass through matter of lighter element as flesh (which contain oxygen, hydrogen and carbon)

48. (d) : Emission transitions can take place between any higher energy level and any energy level below it while absorption transitions start from the lowest energy level only and may end at any higher energy level. Hence number of absorptions transitions between two given energy level. Hence number of absorptions transitions between two given energy levels is always less than the number of emission transitions between the same two levels.

49. (a) : $\frac{1}{f}=({}^a\mu_g-1)\left[\frac{1}{R_1}-\frac{1}{R_2}\right]$

$$=\left(\frac{\mu_g}{\mu_W}-1\right)\left(\frac{1}{R_1}-\frac{1}{R_2}\right)$$

$$\frac{1}{f}=\left(\frac{\mu_g-\mu_w}{\mu_w}\right)\cdot\left[\frac{1}{R_1}-\frac{1}{R_2}\right]$$

$$=\left(\frac{1.5-1.33}{1.33}\right)\cdot\left[\frac{1}{20}+\frac{1}{20}\right]$$

$$\frac{1}{f}=\frac{0.13\times 2}{20} \Rightarrow f=\frac{20}{0.26}$$

$\therefore f = 76.92$ cm.

50. (b)

51. (d) : It is quite clear that magnetic poles always exists in pairs. Since, one can imagine magnetic field configuration with three poles. When north poles or south poles of two mangets are glued together. They provide a three pole field configuration. It is also know that a bar magnet does not exert a torque on itself due to own its field.

52. (b) : When the displacement of a particle executing SHM is y, then its

$$K.E.=\frac{1}{2}m\omega^2(a^2-y^2) \text{ and}$$

$$P.E.=\frac{1}{2}m\omega^2y^2.$$

For $K.E. = P.E.$ or $2y^2 = a^2$ or, $y = a/\sqrt{2}$. Since total energy remains constant through out the motion, which is $E = K.E. + P.E.$ So, when $P.E.$ is maximum then $K.E.$ is zero and vice versa.

53. (c) : Electric shock is due to the electric current flowing through a living body. When the bird perches on a single high power line, no current passes through its body because its body is at equipotential surface i.e., there is no potential difference. While when man touches the same line, standing bare foot on ground the electrical circuit is completed through the ground. The hands of man are at high potential and his feets are at low potential. Hence large amount of current flows through the body of the man and person therefore gets a fatal shock.

54. (b) : Stopping potential is a measure of maximum kinetic energy of emitted photoelectron ($eV_0 = K_{max}$) and K_{max} depends upon the frequency of incident light but is independent of intensity.

55. (a)

56. (a) : Magnetic moment, $M = nIA$

57. (a) : $V = E - I(R + r)$

58. (a)

59. (d) : The force on a charged particle moving in a uniform magnetic field always acts in direction perpendicular to the direction of motion of the charge. As work done by magnetic field on the charge is zero. [$W = FS\cos\theta$], so the energy of the charged particle does not change.

60. (a)

CHEMISTRY

61. (b) : X is [benzene ring with OH and CHO] ; which undergoes Cannizzaro's reaction to give Z.

62. (b) : Slowest step of mechanism decides the rate expression. Thus rate $= K[NO_2][F_2]$.

63. (d) :

I $Na_2O + H_2O \rightarrow 2NaOH$

II $Na_2S + H_2O \rightarrow 2NaOH + H_2S$

III $Na_2Se + H_2O \rightarrow 2NaOH + H_2Se$

IV $Na_2Te + H_2O \rightarrow 2NaOH + H_2Te$

I will have the highest pH. Among H_2S, H_2Se, H_2Te acidity goes on increasing on going down the group as bond length increases on increasing size of central atom. So, $pH_4 < pH_3 < pH_2$

Overall order is $pH_1 > pH_2 > pH_3 > pH_4$

64. (b) :

Toluene (CH_3) $\xrightarrow[H_2SO_4]{HNO_3}$ o-nitrotoluene (CH_3, NO_2) + p-nitrotoluene (CH_3, NO_2)

$\downarrow$ Sn/HCl

o-toluidine (CH_3, NH_2) + p-toluidine (CH_3, NH_2)

$\downarrow$ $NaNO_2$/HCl

(CH_3, $\overset{+}{N}\equiv N\overset{-}{Cl}$) + ($CH_3$, $\overset{+}{N}\equiv N\overset{-}{Cl}$)

$\downarrow$ CuBr

(CH_3, Br) + (CH_3, Br)

65. (d) :

	$2AB_{2\,(g)}$	$\rightleftharpoons 2AB_{(g)}$	$+ B_{2\,(g)}$
Initial	2	0	0
Equilibrium	$2(1-x)$	$2x$	x

Moles at equilibrium $= 2(1-x) + 2x + x$

$= 2 - 2x + 2x + x = x + 2.$

$$K_p = \frac{[P_{AB}]^2[P_{B_2}]}{[P_{AB_2}]} = \frac{\left(\frac{2x}{x+2}\times p\right)^2\left(\frac{x}{2+x}\times p\right)}{\left[\frac{2(1-x)}{x+2}\times p\right]^2}$$

$$= \frac{\frac{4x^3}{x+2}\times p}{4(1-x)^2} = \frac{4x^2\times p}{2}\times\frac{1}{4}$$

$$x=\left(\frac{2K_p}{p}\right)^{1/3} \qquad \text{(as } 1-x\approx 1,\ 2+x\approx 2)$$

66. **(a)** : Cisplatin is effective in curing cancer

$$\begin{matrix} H_3N & & Cl \\ & Pt & \\ H_3N & & Cl \end{matrix}$$

67. **(b)** :It is a method of preparation of cycloalkanes.

$$CH_3-CH=CH-CH_3+CHCl_3 \xrightarrow{(CH_3)_3C-OK}$$

$$CH_3-\underset{\underset{Cl\quad Cl}{\diagdown C \diagup}}{CH-CH}-CH_3+CH_3-\underset{CH_3}{\overset{CH_3}{\underset{|}{\overset{|}{C}}}}-OH+KCl$$

68. **(b)**

$$H_3C-\underset{D}{\overset{H}{C}}-OH+Na\longrightarrow H_3C-\underset{D}{\overset{H}{C}}-O^-$$

$$\xrightarrow[-Br^-]{CH_3Br} H_3C-\underset{D}{\overset{H}{C}}-OCH_3$$

retention of configuration

$$H_3C-\underset{D}{\overset{H}{C}}-OH+TsCl\longrightarrow H_3C-\underset{D}{\overset{H}{C}}-OTs$$

$$\xrightarrow[S_N2]{CH_3ONa} H_3CO-\underset{D}{\overset{H}{C}}-CH_3$$

inversion

$$H_3C-\underset{D}{\overset{H}{C}}-CH=CH_2+Hg(OAc)_2+CH_3OH$$

$$\xrightarrow[\text{Markownikoff's addition}]{NaBH_4} H_3C-\underset{D}{\overset{H}{C}}-\underset{H}{\overset{OCH_3}{C}}-CH_3$$

retention

$$H_3C-\underset{D}{\overset{H}{C}}-CH=CH_2 \xrightarrow{CF_3CO_3H} H_3C-\underset{D}{\overset{H}{C}}-\text{(epoxide)}$$

retention

69. **(a)** : $C_6H_5CH_3 \xrightarrow[(CH_3CO)_2O]{CrO_3} C_6H_5CH(OAc)_2 \longrightarrow C_6H_5CHO$

70. **(b)** : Weight of Ag required = $V \times d$

$= 80 \times 5 \times 10^{-3} \times 1.05 = 0.42$

$$\because \quad W=\frac{Eit}{96500}$$

$$\therefore \quad 0.42=\frac{108\times 3\times t}{96500} \Rightarrow t=125 \text{ sec.}$$

71. **(a)** : The empirical relation, *viz.*, $\frac{x}{m}=kc^{1/n}$, put forward by Freundlich is known as Freundlich's adsorption isotherm. Taking log on both sides

$$\log\left(\frac{x}{m}\right)=\log k+\frac{1}{n}\log c$$

72. **(a)** : $CH_3-CH_2-CH_2-CH_2-\underset{Cl}{\overset{H}{C}}-H$

1-chloropentane

$\Rightarrow$ absence of asymmetric carbon atom.

73. **(c)** : As it has plane of symetry

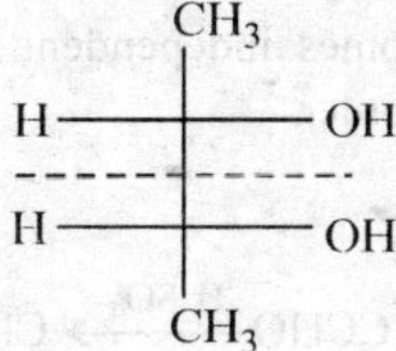

74. **(d)**

75. **(b)** :

$$\text{(CH}_3\text{)(H)C=C(CH}_3\text{)-CH}_2\text{-C(=O)- ...} \xrightarrow{m\text{-CPBA}} \text{epoxide} \xrightarrow{H_3O^+}$$

(product: CH$_3$, H, H, OH, OH, CH$_2$CH$_3$ substituted diol)

76. **(d)** : This defect arises when a compound has excess metal ion. If a negative ion is absent from its lattice site leaving a hole occupied by electron. The holes occupied by electrons are called F- centres. Greater the number of F-centres greater is the intensity of colour.

77. **(b) :** Trinitrotoluene (TNT) with ammonium nitrate is extensively employed as blasting explosive.

78. **(a) :**

$$\text{Cumene (C}_6\text{H}_5\text{CH(CH}_3)_2) \xrightarrow[\text{Catalyst}]{O_2} C_6H_5-C(CH_3)_2-O-OH \xrightarrow{H_2O/H^+} \text{Phenol} + (CH_3)_2CO$$

79. **(c) :** On long storage in contact with air and moisture, oils and fats develop unpleasant smell. This process is known as ranicidification. It is due to

(a) Enzymatic hydrolysis - producing bad smelling lower fatty acids.

(b) Oxidation of unsaturated acids - producing aldehydes and ketones.

80. **(a) :** It is an example of pseudo unimolecular reaction where molecularity ≥ 2 but order of reaction is one.

Rate = k[Sugar] [H_2O]

In the reaction, water is present in excess and its concentration is taken to be constant, thus the reaction becomes independent of [H_2O] and is pseudo first order.

81. **(a) :**

$$2C_6H_5Cl + Cl_3CCHO \xrightarrow{H_2SO_4} Cl_3C-H(C_6H_4Cl)_2$$

D.D.T.

82. **(d) :** Phenol couples with phthalic anhydride in presence of conc. H_2SO_4 to form phenolphthalein which is used as an indicator :

$$\text{Phthalic anhydride} + 2\,C_6H_5OH \xrightarrow[(-H_2O)]{H_2SO_4\text{ (conc)}} \text{Phenolphthalein}$$

83. **(d) :**

$$H_3C-C(CH_3)_2-Cl + AlCl_3 \longrightarrow H_3C-C^{\oplus}(CH_3)_2 + AlCl_4^-$$

$$C_6H_6 + {}^{\oplus}C(CH_3)_3 \longrightarrow [C_6H_6C(CH_3)_3]^+ \xrightarrow{AlCl_4^-} C_6H_5C(CH_3)_3 + AlCl_3 + HCl$$

84. **(c) :** H_2SO_4 is strong acid having pH < 7. $NaNO_2$ on hydrolysis gives alkaline solution of pH > 7. NaCl is neutral and H_2S is weak acid.

85. **(a) :** The enzyme must contain at least one atom of Se.

∵ 0.5 g of Se is present in 100 g of enzyme

∴ 78.4 g of Se will be present in $= \dfrac{100 \times 78.4}{0.5}$

$= 1.576 \times 10^4$ g of enzymes

86. **(d) :** Cyclic. trimer (S_3O_9: ring of three SO_2 units linked by O atoms)

87. **(a) :** Cyclopentane-1,2-diol $\xrightarrow{-H_2O}$ cyclopentene oxide

$\xrightarrow{-HIO_4}$ OH$(CH_2)_3$CHO

To cuase oxidative cleavage of bonds carrying groups prone to undergo oxidation. One mole of reagent is required to cleave one bond.

88. **(a) :** In H_2O, electronegativity difference is highest. So, dipole moment is highest in this. CH_4 is a symmetrical tetrahedral structure and its dipole moment is zero.

99. **(c) :** $u = \sqrt{\dfrac{3RT}{M}}$

If $T = 2T$ and $M = M/2$, then $u_1 = \sqrt{\frac{3R\times 2T}{M/2}}$

$\therefore \quad \frac{u_1}{u} = \sqrt{4} = 2.$

90. **(c) :** Pt (H_2) P_1 atm. | Pt(H_2) P_2 atm.
For spontaneous reaction, E_{cell} should be positive so $P_1 > P_2$

$$E_{cell} = \frac{0.059}{2}\log\frac{P_1}{P_2}$$

Also, if $P_1 > P_2$ oxidation occurs at L.H.S. electrode and reduction occurs at R.H.S. electrode.

91. **(b) :** Molecule is simply amine in nature.

92. **(b) :** $E^\circ_{cell} = 0.76 - 0.41 = 0.35$ V.

93. **(d) :** Solution which contains large number of ions compared to another solution of same concentration at the same temperature has more conductance and is said to be stronger electrolyte. The one which has relatively small number of ions is called weak electrolyte. If concentration of respective electrolyte was increased, the equivalent conductance decreased in each case, but rapid decrease in equivalent conductance is seen in weak electrolyte.

94. **(b):** Density $= \frac{nM}{N_A \times a^3}$

$$= \frac{4\times 58.5}{6.023\times 10^{23}\times(5.64\times 10^{-8})^3} = 2.17 \text{ g/cm}^3.$$

95. **(c) :**

$$R-\overset{O}{\overset{\|}{C}}-R \xrightarrow{H^+} R-\overset{OH}{\overset{|}{\underset{+}{C}}}-R \xrightarrow{H-\overset{-}{N}-\overset{+}{N}\equiv N} R-\overset{OH}{\overset{|}{C}}-R \text{ (with } H-N-\overset{\oplus}{N}\equiv N)$$

$$\xrightarrow{-H_2O} R_2C=N-\overset{+}{N}\equiv N \xrightarrow{-N_2} R-\overset{+}{C}=N-R \xrightarrow{H_2O} R-C(\overset{+}{O}H_2)=NR \xrightarrow{-H^+} R-C(OH)=NR \rightarrow R-\underset{\underset{O}{\|}}{C}-NHR$$

96. **(c) :** Secondary amines form nitrosoamines which are yellow oily liquids insoluble in water.

$$R_2NH + HONO \rightarrow R_2NNO + H_2O$$

Dialkyl nitrosoamine

97. **(a) :** Baeyer's process = Bauxite ore is roasted as to convert FeO into Fe_2O_3

$$\text{Roasted ore} + NaOH \xrightarrow[80\text{ atm}]{150°C} NaAlO_2 \xrightarrow{\text{Hydrolysis}} Al(OH)_3 + NaOH$$

(NaOH recycled)

98. **(a) :** Hypophosphoric acid is

$$HO-\overset{O}{\overset{\|}{\underset{HO}{\underset{|}{P}}}}-\overset{O}{\overset{\|}{\underset{OH}{\underset{|}{P}}}}-OH$$

Pyrophosphoric acid

$$O\leftarrow\overset{OH}{\overset{|}{\underset{OH}{\underset{|}{P}}}}-O-\overset{OH}{\overset{|}{\underset{OH}{\underset{|}{P}}}}\rightarrow O$$

Metasphoric acid

(cyclic structure: HO, O, OH; P, P; O, O, O)

Orthophosphoric acid

$$HO-\overset{O}{\overset{\uparrow}{\underset{OH}{\underset{|}{P}}}}-OH$$

99. **(a) :** $(HNO_3 + H_2SO_4)$ will generate $\overset{+}{N}O_2$ (nitronium ion) which will give nitrobenzene, as $-NO_2$ is deactivating and *meta* directing so, product formed will be 3-nitrochlorobenzene.

100. **(c) :** It follows Huckel's rule of $(4n + 2)\pi$ electrons. If we keep $n = 0$ the total number of π electrons will be 2.

So, (cyclopropenyl cation) follows the aromaticity rule whereas options (a), (b), (d) have 4π electrons.

101. **(b) :** HSO_3^- is a bulky nucleophile, hence, cannot attack on sterically hindered ketones.

102. **(a) :** Greater the number of H-atoms present on the carbon atoms α to unsaturation the more resonating forms are possible due to hyperconjugation and thus greater is the stability of carbonium ion.

$$H_3C-\overset{CH_3}{\underset{CH_3}{C^{\oplus}}} \longleftrightarrow H_3C-\overset{CH_2H^+}{\underset{CH_3}{C}}$$

(9-equivalent forms)

103. (d) : H_2 and Cl_2 react chemically. Hence Dalton's law is not applicable. Dalton's law states that "at a given temperature, the total pressure exerted by two or more non-reacting gases occupying a definite volume is equal to the sum of the partial pressures of the component gases."

104. (a) : $E = -\dfrac{2\pi^2 k^2 m_e{}^4}{n^2 h^2}$

where n = principal quantum number which has only integral value, it follows that total energy is quantized.

105. (a) : Solid + heat $\rightleftharpoons$ liquid. So on heating forward reaction is favoured and amount of solid will decrease.

106. (a) : Cyclohexanone exists in two readily interconvertible different structures leading to dynamic equilibrium known as tautomerism.

keto $\rightleftharpoons$ enol

107. (c) : – OH group shows + M effect and is an activating group, moreover the arenium ion of phenolic substitution is more stable.

108. (b) : The factor $T\Delta S$ increases with increase in temperature.

109. (a) :

110. (b) : The reaction involved is

$CaOCl_2 + H_2SO_4 \rightarrow CaSO_4 + H_2O + Cl_2$

The available chlorine may be defined as the % of chlorine liberated when one mole of bleaching powder (127 g) is treated with excess of dilute H_2SO_4.

111. (b) : Due to presence of strong C-F bonds teflon has high thermal stability and chemical intertness. As, it softens on heating and can be remoulded. So, it is a thermoplastic.

112. (c) :

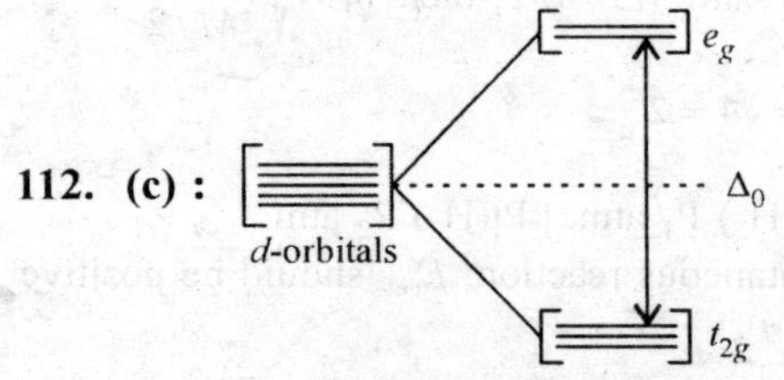

d-orbital splitting in an octahedral crystal field

$\therefore$ In high spin situation, $\Delta_0 < P$, in d^5 configuration, 4th and 5th electron are added to e_g rather than t_{2g}. So configuration of d^5 ion will be $t_{2g}^3\, e_g^2$.

113. (d) : Non-oxidising acids (HCl and dil. H_2SO_4) do not have any effect on copper. However they dissolve the metal in presence of air. As it is a non-spontaneous process so, ΔG can not be –ve.

114. (d) : Molarity equation is written as $M_1V_1 = M_2V_2$ thus if the V_2 changes M_2 also changes.

$$\text{Molarity} = \frac{\text{moles of solute}}{\text{volume of solution in litre}}$$

115. (c) : Aniline is weaker base than ammonium chlordie. In NH_4Cl or aliphatic amines, then non-bonding electron pair of N is localised and is fully available for coordination with a proton.

$$\underset{\text{(stronger acid)}}{C_6H_5NH_3^{\oplus}} \longrightarrow \underset{\text{(weaker-conjugate base)}}{C_6H_5NH_2 + H^+}$$

On the other hand, in aniline and other aromatic amines, the non-bonding electron pair is delocalised into benzene ring by resonance.

But anilinium ion is less resonance stabilised than aniline

$\longleftrightarrow$ no other resonating structure possible.

116. (a)

117. (a) : Saytzeff's rule : The alkene formed in greatest amount is the one that corresponds to removal of the hydrogen from the β-carbon having the fewest hydrogen substituent.

In case of 2° and 3° alc. Saytzeff's rule is followed

$$H_3C-CH_2-\underset{\large OH}{\underset{|}{CH}}-CH_3 \xrightarrow[(1:1)]{H_2SO_4} H_3C\ CH{=}CH-CH_3 + H_2O$$

118. (c) : $SeCl_4$ possesses see-saw geometry, which can be regarded as a distorted trigonal bipyramidal structure, having one lone pair of electrons in the basal position of the trigonal bipyramid. See-saw geometry of $SeCl_4$ molecules arises due to the sp^3d hybridisation of the central atom. The distortion in shape is due to the presence of one lone pair of electrons.

119. (a) : Liq. NH_3 has high heat of vaporisation (327 cal/g). So, it takes up lots of heat and helps in cooling. So, it is used in ice-plants.

120. (a) : Due to the presence of lone pair of electrons on oxygen atom, ethers behave as base and form stable oxonium salts with mineral acids.

$$C_2H_5-\ddot{O}-C_2H_5 + HCl \rightarrow C_2H_5-\underset{H}{\overset{\oplus}{O}}-C_2H_5\ \overset{\ominus}{Cl}$$

Diethyl oxonium chloride

BIOLOGY

121. (b) : The environmental factors which can check the growth of population size constitute the environmental resistance. These include predators, food, water, nesting sites, similar competitors, etc. All living things tend to reproduce until the point at which their environment becomes a limiting factor. No population, human or otherwise, can grow indefinitely; eventually, some biotic or abiotic variable will begin to limit population growth.

122 (c) : The activated spermatozoan on reaching the egg plasma membrane, undergoes a number of changes in its acrosomal region. All these changes are collectively described under acrosome reaction. Acrosome reaction is calcium-dependent involving massive uptake of calcium and sodium with an efflux of hydrogen generating high pH and osmotic pressure, producing negative surface charge, and partial or total release of the acrosomal enzymes. Calcium influx may activate phospholipase resulting in accumulation of unsaturated fatty acids and fusiogenic lysophospholipids contributing to acrosome reaction.

123. (a) : Keystone species are those species which has significant and disproportionately large influence on the community structure and characteristics. It has often considerably low abundance and biomass as compared to dominant species. Removal of such species causes serious disruption in structure and function of community.

124. (b) : *Serratia marcescens* is considered a harmful human pathogen which has been known to cause urinary tract infections, wound infections, and pneumonia. *Serratia* bacteria also have many antibiotic resistance properties which may become important if the incidence of *Serratia* infections dramatically increases.

125. (c) : Clotting of collected blood can be prevented by -

– coating test tubes with silicon (which produce non wettable surface similar in its smoothness to endothelial lining of blood vessels).

– adding chelating agents (includes trisodium citrate, sodium oxalate and sodium EDTA) which remove calcium which is important for blood coagulation, and prevent blood clotting.

– adding Heparin, most powerful anticoagulant which acts indirectly by activating plasma antithrombin III. Heparin is effective both *in vivo* and *in vitro*. Whereas the option a, b and d are effective *in vitro*.

Heparinized blood is not suitable for blood counts (as it alters the shape of RBC's and WBC's which affects blood testing), Fragility testing and complement fixation tests. Hence (c) is the correct answer.

126. (c) : Cancer is caused by cells dividing repeatedly out of control. They cease to respond to the normal signals around them and form unspecialised masses of cells called tumours. Lung cancer usually starts in the epithelium of the bronchioles, so-called bronchial carcinoma. It then usually spreads throughout the lungs. It is caused almost exclusively by smoking. Tobacco smoke contains chemicals responsible for lung cancer. The most important of

these are polycyclic hydrocarbons which are converted in the body to carcinogens.
Besides, carbon monoxide combines with haemoglobin and reduces oxygen transport by about 15% in smokers and nicotine increases blood pressure, heart rate and constriction of blood vessels.

127. **(d) :** A major problem in the treatment of bacterial mediated diseases is that many bacteria have been found to show resistance to antibiotics. The emergence of antibiotic-resistant bacteria is closely linked to the extent that antibiotics are used in humans and items of human diet. Resistant strains may appear rapidly or slowly, according to the amount or type of antibiotic used. Bacteria occur in such large numbers that there is a high chance of a mutant individual eventually appearing in the population. As soon as it does, use of the antibiotic to which it is resistant will give it a selective advantage over non-resistant types and it will multiply and eventually become the dominant type. Antibiotics may also be destroyed by enzymes inside the cells being targetted. A well-known and important example is the group of enzymes known as penicillinases which hydrolyses and destroys penicillins and cephalosporins.

128. **(d) :** Diptheria, leprosy and plague are the bacterial diseases of humans. Diptheria is a serious air-borne contagious disease. It is caused by *Cornybacterium diptheriae* which is a Gram-positive bacterium. It is inhaled through droplets and reaches to respiratory tract and infects it. Leprosy or Hansen's disease is a contact disease, caused by bacterium *Mycobacterium leprae*. It degenerates the tissues and deforms the body organs. Plague is a disease caused by bacterium *Yersinia pestis* or *Pasteurella pestis*.

129. **(b) :** Binding of antibodies to the antigens produces a large insoluble complex known as agglutination. It is a specific reaction, *i.e.*, a particular antigen will only clump in the presence of its specific antibody. Each antibody has two antigen binding sites. It combines with two antigens, causing them to agglutinate.

130. **(a) :** The predator develops a preference to other diets and can give unforeseen negative results that could outweigh all benefits. For example, when the mongoose was introduced in Hawaii in order to control the rat population, it preyed on the endemic birds of Hawaii, especially their eggs, more often than it ate the rats. As most of the birds feed on insect and keep insect population low. The mangoose who destroy birds acts as secondary pest.

131. **(c) :** Dicumarol is an anticoagulant found in spoilts sweet clover causes hemorrhage and other symptoms of bleeding disorder by disrupting vitamin K metabolism and preventing the activation of prothrombin and certain other clotting factors by the liver.

132. **(b) :** The propagation through vegetative multiplication is used to maintain the genetic traits of a given plant. It gives rise to genetically uniform population or clone. In case of plants propagated through seeds, variations creep in due to chance segregation of genes during meiosis and their chance combination during fertilization.

133. **(d) :** Bacteria attacking the dead animals represent the end of the food chain and are decomposers. These are the organisms that obtain energy from chemical breakdown of organisms. They secrete enzymes onto dead matter and then absorb the breakdown products. Bacteria are specialised to breakdown organic materials that are difficult for other organisms to digest. They also fulfil a vital role in the ecosystem, returning the constituents of organic matter to the environment in inorganic forms so that they can again be assimilated by producers.

134. **(d) :** Symbiosis means "living together". It is a beneficial coaction between two (or more) different species in which one or both the species are benefited and neither species is harmed. Symbiotic relationships are manifested through commensalism, protocooperation and mutualism and are widespread in nature. Commensalism is an association or relationship between two different organisms in which one is always benefited while the other is neither benefited nor harmed. This relationship may be permanent or temporary and the benefit derived from the other organism may consist of protection, transportation,

living space and food. Protocooperation is a relationship between two species, which is favourable but not obligatory to both. Mutualism is a relationship between two or more individuals of different species in which all are benefited by one another.

135. (c) : At sexual maturity, the undifferentiated primordial germ cells divide several times by mitosis to produce a large number of spermatogonia. Each spermatogonium actively grows to a larger primary spermatocyte. Each primary spermatocyte undergoes two successive divisions, called maturation divisions. The first maturation division is reductional or meiotic. Hence, the primary spermatocyte divides into two haploid daughter cells called secondary spermatocytes. Both secondary spermatocytes now undergo second maturation division which is an ordinary mitotic division to form, four haploid spermatids. Thus each secondary spermatocyte gives rise to two spermatids that undergo transformation to form two sperms. Overall, both secondary spermatocytes give rise to four sperms.

136. (b) : Growth regulators are organic substances, other than nutrients, which in low concentration regulate growth, differentiation and development by promoting or inhibiting the same. Phytohormones are growth regulators produced naturally in plants and translocated to another region for regulating one or more physiological reactions when present in low concentration. Phytohormone can have a promoting or inhibiting effect on a process.

137. (b) : Grey crescent is the area just opposite to the site of entry of sperm into ovum. It marks the future dorsal side of the embryo.

138. (d) : During the post-pollination development, germination of pollen grain takes place. The pollen grain absorbs water and nutrients on the stigma from the stigmatic secretion through its germ pores. The tube or vegetative cell enlarges and comes out of the pollen grain through one of the germ pores or germinal furrows to form a pollen tube. Generative cell does not produces pollen tube instead it passes into the pollen tube and divides into 2 male gametes. Thus even after killing the generative cell with a laser beam, the pollen grain produces normal pollen tube because the vegetative cell has not been damaged.

139. (d) : Simple or unconditional reflexes are present in an individual right from birth. They are specific, predictable, purposeful and have survival value, *e.g.* breast feeding and swallowing in newly born babies and blinking of eyes are examples of unconditioned reflexes. (a), (b) and (c) are the examples of conditional reflexes and are not present at birth but develop later in life through learning habit.

140. (d) : Unlike *Cycas* and *Pinus*, *Gnetum* shows the occurrence of vessel elements and the absence of archegonia. Archegonia are altogether absent in the female gametophyte and vessels occur in the xylem along with the tracheids in the secondary wood. Thus *Gnetum* shows affinities with angiosperms. Besides it resembles angiosperms in several other aspects like presence of tetrasporic embryo sac, free nuclear divisions in the embryo sac, two cotyledonous embryo etc.

141. (a) : Vagus nerve arises from the side of medulla oblongata. It innervates the larynx, trachea, oesophagus, stomach, lungs, heart and intestines. It is a mixed nerve. It controls the visceral sensations and visceral movements, *i.e.*, heart beat, respiratory movements, peristalsis, sound production, etc. Movement of the tongue is controlled by hypoglossal nerve as it innervates the muscles of the tongue.

142. (a) : Lubb (first sound, systolic sound) is the first heart sound which is low pitched, not very loud, of long duration (about 0.15 seconds) and is produced partly due to closure of atrio-ventricular valves (tricuspid and bicuspid) and partly by the contraction of the muscles in the ventricles.

143. (a) : Part of fertilizers added to crop fields are passed down to water bodies during rains through surface run-off. Presence of extra nutrients brings about dense growth of plant and animal life. The phenomenon is called eutrophication. Eutrophication leads to organic loading, depletion of oxygen, death of animals and fouling of water.

144. **(d) :** The egg cell is one of the haploid cell of egg apparatus present in the micropylar end of embryo sac in seeded plants. It is also called oosphere and represents the single female gamete of the embryo sac. Antipodal cells are the haploid cells, usually three in number, present in embryo sac at the opposite end of micropyle. Their function is unknown and at fertilization, they may disintegrate or multiply and enlarge.

145. **(b) :** Affinity of carbon monoxide for haemoglobin is 200 times more than oxygen. At 0.5 partial pressure, CO combines with 50% of haemoglobin. It produces a relatively stable compound called carboxy-haemoglobin. This causes low supply of oxygen to the body which is characterised by headache, dizziness, nausea, etc.

146. **(a) :** A patient of diabetes mellitus is unable to produce or fail to utilize insulin hormone. Thus, he is unable to store glucose in the form of glycogen. Hence, he started to excrete glucose in the urine. A patient is kept in carbohydrate free diet yet he excretes glocose in urine becuase high level of glucose not only depends on dietary carbohydrates but also on glycogenolysis (degradation of glycogen in liver) and gluconeogenesis (breakdown of fats into glucose in adipose tissues and coversion of muscle lactate into glucose *via* cori cycle).

147. **(d) :** Life cycle of *F.hepatica* is complete and completed in two hosts. Primary host, in which the adult fluke lives, is sheep. While the intermediate host, in which numerous larval stages are passed, is a snail (*Lymnaea*, *Planorbis*, etc.). This type of life cycle, involving two different kinds of hosts, is termed digenetic.

Miracidium larva is the larval stage involved in life cycle. When suitable conditions become available, the encapsulated embryo, in 4-15 days, differentiates into a miracidium larva. It hatches out and swims in water. Metacercaria develops into adult fluke only inside its definitive host or sheep. The latter gets infection by grazing on leaves and grass blades to which the cysts are attached. Metacercaria survives action of host's gastric juice as its cyst is insoluble in it. Cyst wall finally dissolves in proximal part of intestine and liberates the larva.

148. **(d) :** Enzymes are protein that, in small amounts, speed up the rate of a biological reactions and help in regulating metabolism.

Hormones are also metabolic regulator and help in stimulation or inhibition of one or more physiological processes.

Vitamines are accessory food factors which are required in small quantity for controlling metabolism and body functioning.

149. **(b)**

150. **(a) :** The process by which N_2 is reduced to NH_4^+ is called nitrogen fixation. Nitrogenase enzyme catalyzes this reduction. It is only carried out by prokaryotic microorganisms. Principal N_2-fixers include certain free living cyanobacteria in symbiotic associations with fungi in lichens or with ferns, mosses, and liverworts, and by bacteria or other microbes associated symbiotically with roots, especially those of legumes. About 15 percent of the nearly 20,000 species in the fabaceae (Leguminosae) family have been examined for N_2 fixation, and approximately 90 percent of these have root nodules in which fixation occurs. So without active nitrogenase enzyme there will be no N_2 fixation in legumes.

151. **(c) :** Hallucination means apparent perception of external objects or sounds not actually present. It is caused by psychedelic drugs or hallicinogens. The hallucinogens act mainly on CNS (central nervous system) and greatly alter one's thoughts, feelings and perceptions. Hashish is the example of hallucinogen.

152. **(b) :** In CAM plants stomata open at night. In these plants night acidification occurs. *i.e.*, malic acid is synthesised during night due to incomplete oxidation of carbohydrates.

In night, $2C_6H_{12}O_6 + 3O_2 \rightarrow 3C_4H_6O_5 + 3H_2O$
(malic acid)
↓
leads to opening of stomata

At night malic acid formed in guard cells dissociates into H^+ and malate ions. K^+ ion exchange from subsidiary cells with H^+ ions. Thus due to accumulation of K^+ ions osmotic pressure of guard cells increases, endosmosis occurs and guard cells become turgid due to which stomata opens. The malic acid at day time breaks into CO_2 and pyruvic acid thus increasing the concentration of CO_2 in mesophyll cells. This is utilised in Calvin cycle to form sugar which is finally converted into starch.

153. **(b) :** In the apices of some roots, (e.g., *Zea mays*, maize), there is a central region of cells which normally does not divide. This central inactive region was called quiescent centre by F.A.L. Clowes (1959, 1961). The cells of this region have lesser amounts of RNA and DNA so they have small nuclei. These cells also have a lower rate of protein synthesis. Mitochondria and endoplasmic reticulum are less developed. The cells of the quiescent centre are usually inactive. However, if already existing meristematic cells are injured or become inactive due to any other reason, the cells of quiescent centre become active.

154. **(d) :** *Thermococcus*, *Methanococcus* and *Methanobacterium* exemplify archaebacteria that lack any histones resembling those found in eukaryotes but whose DNA is negatively supercoiled. Archaebacteria do not have a nucleus, the genetic material floats freely in the cytoplasm. They consist of ribosomal RNA. DNA contains a single, circular molecule, which is compact and tightly wound. No protein is associated with DNA. The archaebacterial cell may contain plasmids, which are small, circular pieces of DNA and have a highly negatively supercoiled DNA.

155. **(a) :** Stele is a column containing vascular tissues which is surrounded by pericycle and separated from ground tissue by endodermis.

Siphonostele is medullated protostele or protostele with a central non-vascular pith. Leaf gaps are absent. Siphonostele is of two types :

In Ectophloic siphonostele, central pith is surrounded successively by xylem, phloem, pericycle and endodermis. In amphiphloic siphonostele there is a central pith and xylem is surrounded on either side by phloem, pericycle and endodermis. It is found in *Osmunda* and *Equisetum*.

156. **(c) :** Chlorenchyma or assimilatory parenchyma are parenchymatous cells that possess abundant chloroplasts in them. They are capable of photosynthesis. A spore capsule of moss can perform photosynthesis because of the presence of chlorenchyma cells in them.

157. **(b) :** The physical distance between two genes determines both the strength of the linkage and the frequency of the crossing over between two genes. The strength of the linkage increases with the closeness of the two genes. On the other hand the frequency of crossing over increases with the increase in the physical distance between the two genes.

158. **(d) :** The plants, in which a functional foreign gene has been incorporated by any biotechnological methods that generally is not present in plant, are called transgenic plants. When plant cell are transformed by any of the transformation methods it is necessary to isolate the transformed cells/tissue. There are certain selectable marker genes present in vectors that facilitate the selection process. In transformed cells the selectable marker genes or are introduced through vector. There is a number of marker genes which are commonly described as reporter genes screenable genes. Some of the reporter genes which are most commonly used in plant transformation are : cat, gus, lux, nptII., etc.

159. **(c) :** Since a typical green plant is diploid, therefore it has two sets of chromosomes. So the number of genome will be two, because genome is the entire set of gene carried by a gamete or present in the haploid cell of a particular organism.

160. **(b) :** Under continuous supply of food and space in the laboratory conditions the bacterial population grows exponentially and shows a J-shaped curve, thus the curve would be hyperbolic.

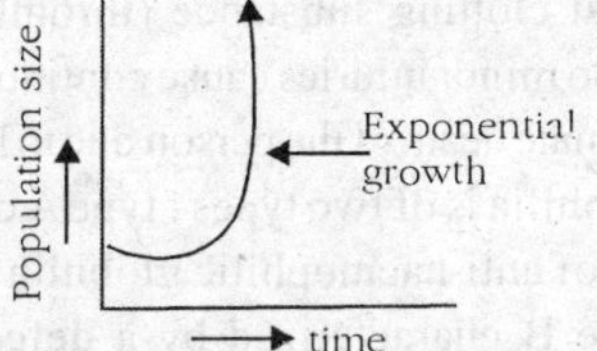

Such populations ultimately crash when the population size grows beyond carrying capacity.

161. **(a) :** In all the septate fungi except basidiomycetes (dolipore septum), the septa are seldom complete. They are perforated and contain plasmodesmata or small central pores. Septal pores allow protoplasmic continuity between adjacent cells. This is useful for quick translocation of nutrients to all part of the body, mobilisation of reserve materials from older parts to younger parts and from vegetative hyphae to reproductive hyphae.

162. **(a) :** The haploid spores on germination gives rise to alga-like filamentous branched portion called primary protonema. This protonema develops buds, from which leafy gametophyte arises. Sometimes this primary protonema breaks up into small fragments accidentally and these fragments give rise to leafy gametophores.

163. **(c) :** Cephalization is the concentration of nervous tissues and sense organs in or towards the anterior end forming a distinct head. It provides greater prominence and domination of the head over the rest of the body. It does not improve the appearance of the animal.

164. **(c) :** Koel is a nest parasite and does not build a nest of its own. It simply lays its eggs in a crow's nest so that the eggs and young ones, are looked after by the foster parents.

165. **(c) :** Competitive inhibition is the inhibition of enzyme activity by the presence of a chemical that competes with the substrate for binding to the active site of the enzyme. The inhibitor chemical is called substrate analogue or competitive inhibitor. It resembles the substrate in structure and gets bound up to the active site of the enzyme without getting transformed by the latter.

166. **(c) :** Haemophilia, also called bleeder's disease is a X-linked recessive disorder. The person which contains the recessive gene for haemophilia lacks a normal clotting substance (thromboplastin) in blood. So minor injuries cause continuous bleeding and ultimate death of the person due to hemorrhages. Haemophilia is of two types : type A characterized by lack of anti-haemophilic globulin (factor VIII) and type B characterized by a defect in plasma thromboplastic component (factor IX).
Prothrombin is an inactive plasma protein and is produced by liver. It helps in blood clotting. It is not produced by platelets.

167. **(a) :** The hybridoma cells are shifted to a medium deficient in nutrient which cannot be synthesized by myeloma cells so that myleoma cells could be removed or hybridoma cells could be purified. The unfused myleoma cells *die* while hybridoma cells survive. The hybridoma cells are allowed to multiply separately.

168. **(c) :** Any seed which contains endosperm or perisperm at maturity is called albuminous or endospermic seed *i.e.*, food reserve of the seed is stored in endosperm or perisperm, *e.g.* rubber, coconut, castor bean, maize and other cereals. Seed that does not have endosperm at maturity and in which cotyledons absorb food reserve from endosperm during development and act as storage organs is called exalbuminous or non-endospermic seed, *e.g.*, mustard, groundnut, bean, pea etc.

169. **(b) :** Trachea and large bronchi are lined by pseudostratified ciliated columnar epithelium bearing glandular cells (mucous gland). The secretion of mucous glands keeps the walls of trachea and large bronchi moist and traps dust particles which enter with the air. The vibratile cilia of the epithelium then carry the mucous containing dust particles upto the larynx where they can be spitted out.

170. **(a) :** Light has got no direct effect on the rate of transpiration but indirectly it affects the rate in two ways firstly by controlling the stomatal opening and secondly by affecting the temperature. With the increase in the light intensity the rate of transpiration increases because the stomata get opened and the temperature increases. The rate of transpiration increases markedly in light and decreases in dark. There is a close relationship between the opening of stomata and presence of light.

171. **(b) :** Oxygen accumulation causes substantial inhibition of photosynthesis. Both oxygen evolution and CO_2 assimilation were reduced in the presence of atmospheric oxygen. Oxygen causes a direct and indeed competitive inhibition of Ribulose diphosphate carboxylase. As a result glycolate synthesis is enhanced and leads to begin photorespiration. Carbon dioxide being one of the raw materials for photosynthesis, its concentration affects the rate of photosynthesis markedly. Because of its very low concentration in atmosphere (0.03 per cent only) it acts as a limiting factor in natural photosynthesis.

172. (c) : Oxysomes or $F_0 - F_1$ particles are present on the inner mitochondrial membrane. The F_1 head-piece of oxysome functions as ATP-synthetase which synthesises ATP from ADP and ip (inorganic phosphate) using energy from proton gradient or ATP synthetase becomes active in ATP formation only when there is a proton gradient having high concentration of protons on F_0 side (base) as compared to F_1 side (head piece) of $F_0 - F_1$ particles or oxysomes.

173. (c) : Inner ends of cone cells lie upon an elongated, spindle shaped rod, the rhabdome. Rhabdome is secreted and surrounded by a group of seven elongated retinal cells. Rhabdome and retinal cells together form the receptor region of eye.

174. (d) : Pituitary gland or hypophysis is situated in a depression, the sella turcica of sphenoid bone of the skull. It is directly attached to the hypothalamus by a stalk, the infundibulum. Hypophysial portal veins carry blood containing neurohormones (releasing factors) from the hypothalamus to the anterior pituitary.

175. (c) : Rabies (hydrophobia) is an acute viral disease of the central nervous system that affects all warm-blooded animals and is usually transmitted to humans by a bite from an infected dog. Symptoms appear after an incubation period ranging from 10 days to over a year and include malaise, fever, difficulty in breathing, salivation, periods of intense excitement, and painful muscle spasms of the throat induced by swallowing. In the later stages of the disease the mere sight of water induces convulsions and paralysis, death occurs within 4-5 days.

176. (a) : The most common form of asexual reproduction in plants is called vegetative propagation. It is the formation of new plants from vegetative units (propagules) such as buds, tubers, rhizomes, roots, stem, leaf etc. Besides the natural methods of vegetative propagation, there are a number of techniques for artificial vegetative propagation of economically and aesthetically important plants. Potatoes are produced by tubers and not by seeds. Stem tubers are found in potato and artichoke. They have buds in the region of nodes or eyes for vegetative multiplication. Root cuttings are used in propagation of lemon, apple, orange, blackberry etc.

177. (c) : In nuclear endosperm, first and further divisions of primary endosperm nucleus are not followed by cytokinesis or wall formation and thus these free nuclear divisions lead to formation of a large number of free nuclei in embryo sac. At maturity, centripetal wall formation may occur to make the tissue partly cellular. Endosperm of coconut is unique in sense that it is both nuclear and cellular. Here the primary endosperm nucleus undergoes a number of free nuclear divisions. When the fruit is about 50 mm long the embryo sac remains filled with a watery fluid or milk containing free nuclei and fine cytoplasmic particles. At a later stage when the fruit becomes about 100 mm in length the liquid shows in addition to free nuclei, several cells each enclosing variable number of nuclei. Thus coconut has multicellular endosperm (called coconut meat) in the outer part and free nuclear as well as vacuolate endosperm (called coconut milk) in the centre.

178. (d) : The female secondary sexual characters are developed by estrogens. Estrogens are steroid hormones secreted by growing ovarian follicles. It includes estradiol, estriol and estrone. This hormone is responsible for the development of female secondary sexual and accessory characters. In humans it is also formed in the adrenal cortex, testis and foetoplacental unit.

Gonadotrophic hormones (LH and FSH) are secreted by the anterior lobe of pituitary gland. LH is responsible for ovulation and transforms graafian follicle into corpus luteum and FSH stimulates spermatogenesis and maturation of graafian follicle and secretion of estrogen in ovaries.

179. (d) : Net primary productivity is the available biomass for the consumption to heterotrophs (herbivores and decomposers). The rate of biomass production is called productivity. It has two aspects, gross primary productivity and net primary productivity. The rate of total production of organic matter during photosynthesis is known as gross primary productivity. Its considerable amount is utilised by plants in respiration. The organic matter synthesised by plants (GPP) minus the rate of respiration and other loss represents the net primary productivity.

180. (b) : Mercury is an important toxic pollutant. It is changed to water soluble dimethyl mercury which undergoes biomagnification, *i.e.*, accumulates in the body of organisms inhabiting in the water. Eating poisoned animals causes deformity known as minamata disease which is characterized by diarrhoea, impairment of various senses, numbness of lips, blurring of vision, mental dearrangement and death.

GENERAL KNOWLEDGE

181. (a)	**182. (b)**	**183. (c)**	**184. (b)**	**185. (c)**
186. (c)	**187. (d)**	**188. (c)**	**189. (a)**	**190. (c)**
191. (d)	**192. (a)**	**193. (b)**	**194. (a)**	**195. (d)**
196. (a)	**197. (a)**	**198. (d)**	**199. (c)**	**200. (c)**

Chapterwise Index - '09

Physics • Chemistry • Biology

Use the index for topicwise analysis of this year's AIIMS paper and refer to these questions when you are practising MCQs chapterwise.

PHYSICS

Chapter's Name	Question No.	Total
Units and Dimensions	5, 15, 60	3
Motion in One Dimension		0
Motion in Two Dimensions	16, 56	2
Laws of Motion and Friction	17, 59	2
Work, Power and Energy	10, 11, 12, 13, 18	5
Centre of Mass and Rotational Motion	58	1
Gravitation	38, 57	2
Properties of Matter	21, 41	2
Oscillations	22, 36, 42	3
Waves		0
Heat and Thermodynamics	20, 54, 55	3
Electrostatics	8, 19, 23, 43, 44	5
Current Electricity	35	1
Thermal and chemical effects of current	24, 25	2
Magnetic Effects of Current	26, 27	2
Magnetism	45	1
Electromagnetic Induction and Alternating Current	6, 28, 29, 46	4
Electromagnetic Waves	30	1
Ray Optics	1, 14, 47, 48	4
Wave Optics	31, 32, 39, 40	4
Modern Physics	2, 4, 7, 9, 33, 34, 37, 49, 51	9
Solids and Semiconductor Devices	3, 50, 52, 53	4
Universe		0
Principles of Communication		0

CHEMISTRY

Chapter's Name	Question No.	Total
Basic Concepts	63, 80, 87	3
Atomic Structure		0
Periodic Properties		0
Chemical Bonding	83	1
Nuclear Chemistry		0
Gaseous and Liquid States	82, 109	2
Solid State	85	1
Mole Concept & Solutions	62, 69, 81	3
Colloids, Surface Chemistry & Catalysis		0
Equilibrium	65, 68, 92, 114	4
Kinetics	66, 67, 106	3
Energetics	98, 103, 108	3
Electrochemistry	73, 95	2
Redox Reactions		0
Metallurgy		0
Hydrogen and its Compounds		0
s-Block Elements	79, 84, 89, 90, 102	5
p-Block Elements	61, 64, 70, 71, 72, 94, 97, 111, 116	9
d- and *f*-Block Elements	78	1
Complex Compounds	120	1
Purification and Analysis of Compound		0
General Organic Chemistry	74, 86, 88,91, 93, 101	6
Aliphatic Hydrocarbons	104, 107	2
Aromatic Hydrocarbons	75, 76, 77	3
Halogen Derivatives		0
Alcohols, Phenols and Ethers	96, 105	2
Aldehydes and Ketones	99, 100, 110	3
Carboxylic acids & their derivatives	112, 117	2
Nitrogen Containing Compounds	113	1
Biochemistry	119	1
Chemistry in Action	115, 118	2
Environmental Chemistry		0

BIOLOGY		
Chapter's Name	**Question No.**	**Total**
General Biology	153	1
Biological Classification		0
Kingdom Monera	142, 156	2
Kingdom Fungi		0
Plant Kingdom	143	1
Cell and its Structural Components	173	1
Cell Reproduction		0
Cell Respiration	150, 168	2
Enzymes		0
Biomolecules	144, 157	2
Mendelian Genetics	158, 180	2
Hereditary Material		0
Anatomy of Flowering Plants	140, 149	2
Morphology of Flowering Plants	147	1
Physiology of Flowering Plants	139, 151, 152, 175, 178	5
Embryology of Flowering Plants	160, 166, 172	3
Growth and Development in Flowering Plants	164	1
Angiosperm Families		0
Ecology and Pollution	154, 161, 170	3
Applied Botany	141, 148, 159, 169	4
Animal Kingdom	124, 128, 167	3
Genes and Chromosomes	136, 138, 146	3
Gene regulation and Applied Genetics	145	1
Human Genetics & Genetic Disorder	137	1
Animal Tissue	129, 162, 163	3
Musculo-Skeletal System	133	1
Digestive System and Nutrition	135	1
Respiration	134	1
Circulatory System and Immunity	121, 155, 165	3
Excretion and Osmoregulation		0
Reproduction and Embryonic Development	131, 132, 171, 179	4
Nervous System and Sense Organs	123	1
Endocrine System	174	1
Common Human Disease	127	1
Growth and Regeneration		0
Evolution	125, 126, 176, 177	4
Drug Addiction	122, 130	2
Applied Zoology		0
Wild Life and Conservation		0
Human Population & Growth		0

SOLVED PAPER
AIIMS - 2009

Time : 3½ hours | Max. Marks : 200

PHYSICS

1. A convex lens of refractive index $\frac{3}{2}$ has a power of 2.5 D in air. If it is placed in a liquid of refractive index 2, then the new power of the lens is
(a) – 1.25 D (b) – 1.5 D
(c) 1.25 D (d) 1.5 D

2. What is ratio of Bohr magneton to the nuclear magneton?
(a) m_p/m_e (b) m_p^2/m_e^2
(c) 1 (d) $\frac{m_e}{m_p}$

3. When the inputs of a two input logic gate are 0 and 0, the output is 1. When the inputs are 1 and 0, the output is zero. The type of logic gate is
(a) XOR (b) NAND
(c) NOR (d) OR

4. de Broglie wavelength λ associated with neutrons is related with absolute temperature T as
(a) $\lambda \propto T$ (b) $\lambda \propto \frac{1}{T}$
(c) $\lambda \propto \frac{1}{\sqrt{T}}$ (d) $\lambda \propto T^2$

5. The dimensions of specific resistance are
(a) $[M L^2T^{-2}A^{-1}]$ (b) $[M L^3T^{-3}A^{-2}]$
(c) $[M L^3T^{-2}A^{-1}]$ (d) $[M L^2T^{-2}A^{-2}]$

6. Reciprocal of impedance is
(a) susceptance (b) conductance
(c) admittance (d) transconductance

7. A nucleus of mass number 220 decays by α decay. The energy released in the reaction is 5 MeV. The kinetic energy of an α- particle is
(a) $\frac{1}{54}$ MeV (b) $\frac{27}{11}$ MeV
(c) $\frac{54}{11}$ MeV (d) $\frac{55}{54}$ MeV

8. Four charges are arranged at the corners of a square as shown in the figure. The direction of electric field at the centre of the square is along

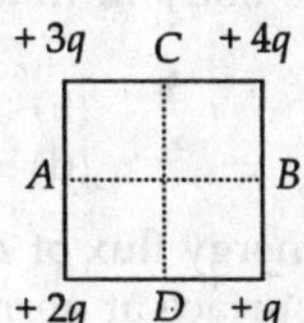

(a) DC (b) BC
(c) AB (d) AD

9. The wavelengths of K_α X-rays for lead isotopes Pb^{208}, Pb^{206} and Pb^{204} are λ_1, λ_2 and λ_3 respectively. Then
(a) $\lambda_2 = \sqrt{\lambda_1\lambda_3}$ (b) $\lambda_2 = \lambda_1 + \lambda_3$
(c) $\lambda_2 = \lambda_1\lambda_3$ (d) $\lambda_2 = \frac{\lambda_1}{\lambda_3}$

10. A force F acting on an object varies with distance x as shown in the figure. The force is in N and x in m. The work done by the force in moving the object from $x = 0$ to $x = 6$ m is

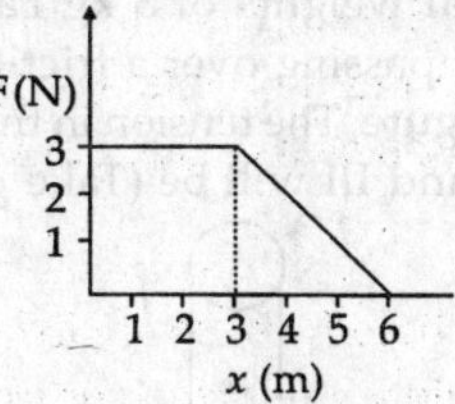

(a) 13.5 J (b) 10 J
(c) 15 J (d) 20 J

11. Which of the following graph depicts spring constant k versus length l of the spring correctly?

(a) (b)

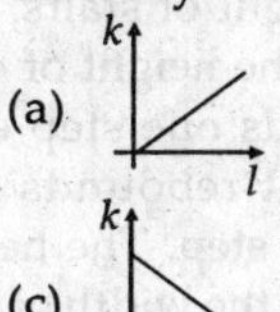

(c) (d)

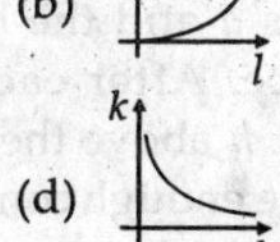

12. A body of mass 5 kg moving with a speed of 1.5 m/s on a horizontal smooth surface collides with a nearly weightless spring of force constant k = 5 N/m. The maximum compression of the spring would be

1.5 m/s

(a) 0.5 m (b) 0.15 m
(c) 1.5 m (d) 0.12 m

13. A body is moved along a straight line by a machine delivering constant power. The distance travelled by the body in time t is proportional to

(a) $t^{1/2}$ (b) t
(c) $t^{3/2}$ (d) t^2

14. Light with an energy flux of 18 W/cm^2 falls on a non-reflecting surface at normal incidence. The pressure exerted on the surface is

(a) 2 N/m^2 (b) 2×10^{-4} N/m^2
(c) 6 N/m^2 (d) 6×10^{-4} N/m^2

15. The dimensional formula of Planck's constant is

(a) $[ML^2T^{-1}]$ (b) $[ML^2T^{-2}]$
(c) $[ML^0T^2]$ (d) $[MLT^2]$

16. A body is projected horizontally with a velocity of $4\sqrt{2}$ m/sec. The velocity of the body after 0.7 seconds will be nearly (Take g = 10 m/sec^2)

(a) 10 m/sec (b) 9 m/sec
(c) 19 m/sec (d) 11 m/sec

17. Three equal weights of 3 kg each are hanging on a string passing over a frictionless pulley as shown in figure. The tension in the string between masses II and III will be (Take g = 10 m/sec^2)

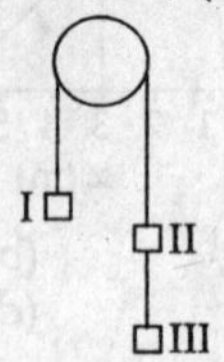

(a) 5 N (b) 6 N
(c) 10 N (d) 20 N

18. A ball is bouncing down a flight of stairs. The coefficient of restitution is e. The height of each step is d and the ball descends one step each bounce. After each bounce it rebounds to a height h above the next lower step. The height is large enough compared with the width of step so that the impacts are effectively head-on. Find the relationship between h and d.

(a) $h = \frac{d}{1-e^2}$ (b) $h = \frac{d}{1+e^2}$
(c) $h = \frac{d}{1+e}$ (d) $h = \sqrt{\frac{d}{1-e^2}}$

19. A conducting sphere of radius R carrying charge Q lies inside an uncharged conducting shell of radius $2R$. If they are joined by a metal wire, the amount of heat that will be produced is

(a) $\frac{1}{4\pi\varepsilon_0} \cdot \frac{Q^2}{4R}$ (b) $\frac{1}{4\pi\varepsilon_0} \cdot \frac{Q^2}{2R}$
(c) $\frac{1}{4\pi\varepsilon_0} \cdot \frac{Q^2}{R}$ (d) $\frac{2}{4\pi\varepsilon_0} \cdot \frac{Q^2}{3R}$

20. Black holes in orbit around a normal star are detected from the earth due to the frictional heating of infalling gas into the black hole, which can reach temperatures greater than 10^6 K. Assuming that the infalling gas can be modelled as a blackbody radiator, then the wavelength of maximum power lies

(a) in the visible region
(b) in the X-ray region
(c) in the the microwave region
(d) in the gamma-ray region of electromagnetic spectrum

21. Neglecting the density of air, the terminal velocity obtained by a raindrop of radius 0.3 mm falling through air of viscosity 1.8×10^{-5} N s m^{-2} will be

(a) 10.9 m s^{-1} (b) 7.48 m s^{-1}
(c) 3.7 m s^{-1} (d) 12.8 m s^{-1}

22. A particle executes simple harmonic motion of period T and amplitude l along a rod AB of length $2l$. The rod AB itself executes simple harmonic motion of the same period and amplitude in a direction perpendicular to its length. Initially, both the particle and the rod are in their mean positions. The path traced out by the particle will be

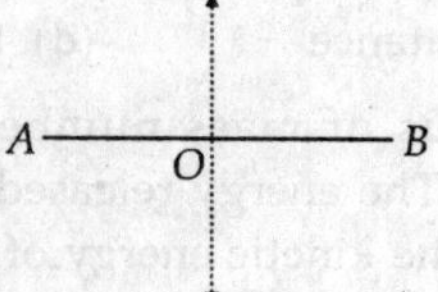

(a) a circle of radius l
(b) a straight line inclined at $\frac{\pi}{4}$ to the rod
(c) an ellipse

(d) a figure of eight

23. What is the energy stored in the capacitor between terminals *a* and *b* of the network shown in the figure? (Capacitance of each capacitance $C = 1\ \mu F$)

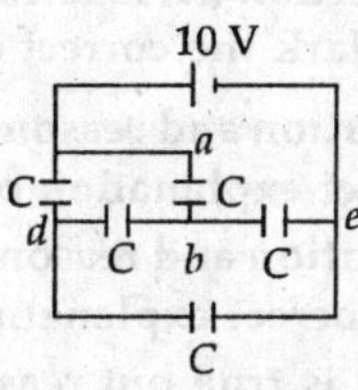

(a) 12.5 μJ (b) Zero
(c) 25 μJ (d) 50 μJ

24. When a current is passed in a conductor, 3°C rise in temperature is observed. If the strength of current is made thrice, then rise in temperature will approximately be
(a) 36°C (b) 27°C
(c) 18°C (d) 9°C

25. In a metal with positive Thomson coefficient, current is passed from the lower temperature to higher temperature side. Then heat will be
(a) absorbed (b) constant
(c) evolved (d) either 'b' or 'c'

26. A moving coil galvanometer has a resistance of 900 Ω. In order to send only 10% of the main current through this galvanometer, the resistance of the required shunt is
(a) 0.9 Ω (b) 100 Ω
(c) 405 Ω (d) 90 Ω

27. A current I_1 carrying wire *AB* is placed near another long wire *CD* carrying current I_2. If wire *AB* is free to move, it will have

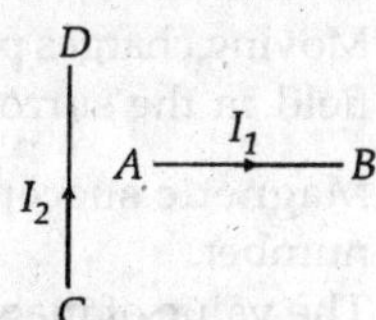

(a) rotational motion only
(b) translational motion only
(c) rotational as well as translational motion
(d) neither rotational nor translational motion

28. A coil of wire of a certain radius has 100 turns and a self inductance of 15 mH. The self inductance of a second similar coil of 500 turns will be
(a) 75 mH (b) 375 mH
(c) 15 mH (d) none of these

29. In a series *LCR* circuit, the voltage across the resistance, capacitance and inductance is 10 V each. If the capacitance is short circuited the voltage across the inductance will be
(a) 10 V (b) $10\sqrt{2}$ V
(c) $10/\sqrt{2}$ V (d) 20 V

30. If v_s, v_x and v_m are the speeds of gamma rays, X-rays and microwaves respectively in vacuum, then.
(a) $v_s > v_x > v_m$ (b) $v_s < v_x < v_m$
(c) $v_s > v_x > v_m$ (d) $v_s = v_x = v_m$

31. Which out of following, cannot produce two coherent sources?
(a) Lloyd's mirror (b) Fresnel biprism
(c) Young's double slit (d) Prism

32. In Young's double slit experiment, the two slits act as coherent sources of equal amplitude *a* and of wavelength λ. In another experiment with the same set up, the two slits are sources of equal amplitude *a* and wavelength λ, but are incoherent. The ratio of intensities of light at the mid point of the screen in the first case to that in the second case is
(a) 2 : 1 (b) 1 : 2
(c) 3 : 4 (d) 4 : 3

33. If the kinetic energy of a particle is increased by 16 times, the percentage change in the de Broglie wavelength of the particle is
(a) 25% (b) 75%
(c) 60% (d) 50%

34. If the half lives of a radioactive element for α and β decay are 4 years and 12 years respectively, the ratio of its inital activity and that after 12 years will be
(a) 6.25% (b) 12.5%
(c) 25% (d) 50%

35. In the given circuit, the potential difference between *A* and *B* is

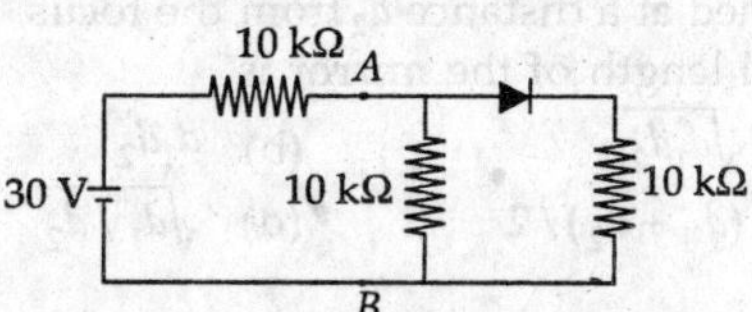

(a) 0 (b) 5 volt
(c) 10 volt (d) 15 volt.

36. A ball is suspended by a thread of length *L* at the point *O* on a wall which is inclined to the vertical by α. The thread with the ball is displaced by a small angle β away from the vertical and also away from the wall. If the ball is released, the period of oscillation of the pendulum when $\beta > \alpha$ will be

(a) $\sqrt{\frac{L}{g}}\left[\pi+2\sin^{-1}\frac{\alpha}{\beta}\right]$ (b) $\sqrt{\frac{L}{g}}\left[\pi-2\sin^{-1}\frac{\beta}{\alpha}\right]$

(c) $\sqrt{\frac{L}{g}}\left[2\sin^{-1}\frac{\beta}{\alpha}-\pi\right]$ (d) $\sqrt{\frac{L}{g}}\left[2\sin^{-1}\frac{\alpha}{\beta}+\pi\right]$

37. A radioactive nucleus is being produced at a constant rate α per second. Its decay constant is λ. If N_0 are the number of nuclei at time $t = 0$, then the maximum number of nuclei possible are

(a) $N_0+\frac{\alpha}{\lambda}$ (b) N_0

(c) $\frac{\lambda}{\alpha}+N_0$ (d) $\frac{\alpha}{\lambda}$

38. A wire of length l and mass m is bent in the form of a semicircle. The gravitational field intensity at the centre of semicircle is

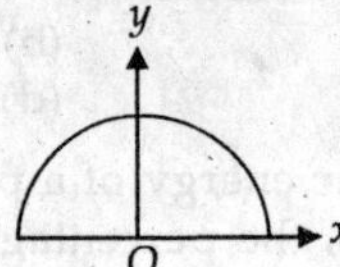

(a) $\frac{Gm}{\pi l}$ along x-axis

(b) $\frac{Gm}{\pi l}$ along y-axis

(c) $\frac{2\pi Gm}{l^2}$ along y-axis

(d) $\frac{2\pi Gm}{l^2}$ along x-axis

39. In a concave mirror, an object is placed at a distance d_1 from the focus and the image is formed at a distance d_2 from the focus. Then the focal length of the mirror is

(a) $\sqrt{d_1 d_2}$ (b) $d_1 d_2$

(c) $(d_1+d_2)/2$ (d) $\sqrt{d_1/d_2}$

40. A short linear object, of length l, lies along the axis of a concave mirror, of focal length f, at a distance d from the pole of the mirror. The size of the image is then (nearly)

(a) $\frac{lf}{d-f}$ (b) $\frac{d-f}{lf}$

(c) $l\frac{f^2}{(d-f)^2}$ (d) $\frac{(d-f)^2}{f^2}l$

Directions : In the following questions (41-60), a statement of assertion (A) is followed by a statement of reason (R). Mark the correct choice as :

(a) If both assertion and reason are true and reason is the correct explanation of assertion

(b) If both assertion and reason are true but reason is not the correct explanation of assertion

(c) If assertion is true but reason is false

(d) If both assertion and reason are false.

41. Assertion : Liquid molecules have greater potential energy at the melting point.

Reason : Intermolecular spacing between molecules increases at melting point.

42. Assertion : The bob of a simple pendulum is a ball full of water, if a fine hole is made in the bottom of the ball, the time period first increases and then decreases.

Reason : As water flows out of the bob the weight of bob decreases.

43. Assertion : Electric potential of earth is taken zero.

Reason : No electric field exists on earth surface.

44. Assertion : A charge, whether stationary or in motion produces a magnetic field around it.

Reason : Moving charges produce only electric field in the surrounding space.

45. Assertion : Magnetic susceptibillity is a pure number.

Reason : The value of magnetic susceptibility for vacuum is one.

46. Assertion : Transformers are used only in alternating current source not in direct current.

Reason : Only a.c. can be stepped up or down by means of transformers.

47. Assertion : A total reflecting prism is used to erect the inverted image without deviation.

Reason : Rays of light incident parallel to base of prism emerge out as parallel rays.

48. **Assertion :** The edges of the images of white object formed by a concave mirror on the screen appear white.

Reason : Concave mirror does not suffer chromatic aberration.

49. **Assertion :** A photon has no rest mass, yet it carries definite momentum.

Reason : Momemtum of photon is due to its energy and hence its equivalent mass.

50. **Assertion :** A photocell is called an electric eye.

Reason : When light is incident on some semiconductor its electrical resistance is reduced.

51. **Assertion :** Nuclei having number about 60 are most stable.

Reason : When two or more light nuclei are combined into a heavier nucleus, then the binding energy per nucleon will increase.

52. **Assertion :** In a common-emitter amplfier, the load resistance of the output circuit is 1000 times the load resistance of the input circuit. If $\alpha = 0.98$, then voltage gain is 49×10^3.

Reason : $\alpha = \dfrac{\beta}{1-\beta}$ (symbols have their usual meaning).

53. **Assertion :** Most amplifiers use common emitter circuit configuration.

Reason : Its input resistance is comparatively higher.

54. **Assertion :** For an isothermal process in an ideal gas, the heat obsorbed by the gas is entirely used in the work done by the gas.

Reason : During a process taking place in a system, the temperature remains constant then the process is isothermal.

55. **Assertion :** When hot water is poured in a beaker of thick glass, the beaker cracks.

Reason : Outer surface of the beaker expands suddenly.

56. **Assertion :** Generally the path of a projectile from the earth is parabolic but it is elliptical for projectiles going to a very great height.

Reason : Up to ordinary height the projectile moves under a uniform gravitational force, but for great heights, projectile moves under a variable force.

57. **Assertion :** Angular speed of a planet around the sun increases, when it is closer to the sun.

Reason : Total angular momentum of the system remains constant.

58. **Assertion :** The size and shape of the rigid body remains unaffected under the effect of external forces.

Reason : The distance between two particles remains constant in a rigid body.

59. **Assertion :** Impulsive force is large and acts for a short time.

Reason : Finite change in momentum should be produced by the force.

60. **Assertion :** The dimensional formula for product of resistance and conductance is same as for dielectric constant.

Reason : Both have dimensions of time constant.

CHEMISTRY

61. KF combines with HF to form KHF_2. This compound contains the species
(a) K^+, F^- and H^+ (b) K^+, F^- and HF
(c) K^+ and $[HF_2]^-$ (d) $[KHF]^+$ and F_2

62. For a dilute solution, Raoult's law states that
(a) The relative lowering of vapour pressure is proportional to the amount of solute in solution
(b) The relative lowering of vapour pressure is equal to the mole fraction of solute
(c) The lowering of vapour pressure is equal to the mole fraction of the solute
(d) The vapour pressure of the solution is equal to the mole fraction of the solvent.

63. To a 25 ml H_2O_2 solution, excess of acidified solution of KI was added. The iodine liberated required 20 ml of 0.3 N $Na_2S_2O_3$ solution.

The volume strength of H_2O_2 solution is
(a) 1.344 g/L (b) 3.244 g/L
(c) 5.4 g/L (d) 4.08 g/L

64. Which of the following shows bond in silicone?
(a) Si-C-Si-C-Si (b) Si-Si-Si-Si
(c) -Si-O-Si-O-Si- (d) Si-C-Si-O-Si.

65. pH of a 0.01 M solution ($K_a = 6.6 \times 10^{-4}$)
(a) 7.6 (b) 8
(c) 2.6 (d) 5

66. In a homogenous reaction $A \longrightarrow B + C + D$ the initial pressure was P_0 and after time t it was P. Expression for rate constant k in terms of P_0, P and t will be

(a) $k = \frac{2.303}{t} \log \frac{2P_0}{3P_0 - P}$

(b) $k = \frac{2.303}{t} \log \frac{2P_0}{P_0 - P}$

(c) $k = \frac{2.303}{t} \log \frac{3P_0 - P}{2P_0}$

(d) $k = \frac{2.303}{t} \log \frac{2P_0}{3P_0 - 2P}$

67. Which curve corresponds to the temperature dependance of the rate R of a simple one step reaction ?

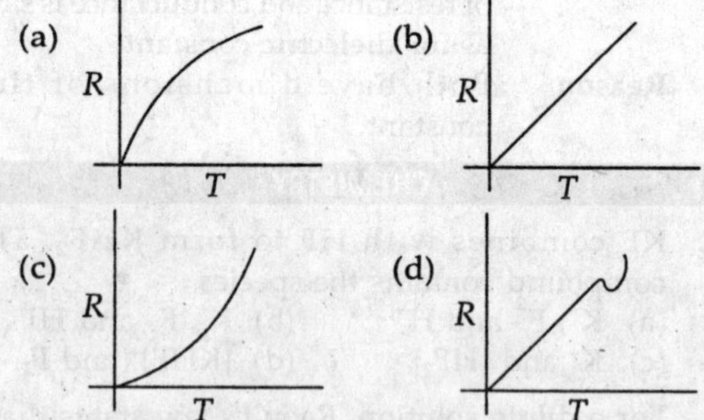

68. A vessel of one litre capacity containing 1 mole of SO_3 is heated till a state of equilibrium is attained.
$2SO_{3(g)} \rightleftharpoons 2SO_{2(g)} + O_{2(g)}$.
At equilibrium, 0.6 moles of SO_2 had formed. The value of equilibrium constant is
(a) 0.18 (b) 0.36
(c) 0.45 (d) 0.68.

69. A 0.1 molal solution of an acid is 4.5% ionized. Calculate freezing point. (molecular weight of the acid is 300). $K_f = 1.86$ K mol^{-1} kg.
(a) – 0.199°C (b) 2.00°C
(c) 0°C (d) – 0.269°C

70. Which of the following is an example of chain silicates ?
(a) Kaolinite (b) Zircon
(c) Benitonite (d) Diopside

71. Which of the element shows +4 oxidation state?
(a) Sn (b) Ra
(d) Fr (d) Sc

72. Tincture of iodine is
(a) aqueous solution of I_2
(b) solution of I_2 in aqueous KI
(c) alcoholic solution of I_2
(d) aqueous solution of KI.

73. The specific conductance of a N/10 KCl at 25°C is 0.0112 ohm^{-1} cm^{-1}. The resistance of cell containing solution at the same temperature was found to be 55 ohm. The cell constant will be
(a) 6.16 cm^{-1} (b) 0.616 cm^{-1}
(c) 0.0616 cm^{-1} (d) 616 cm^{-1}

74. Decreasing order of stability of ions is
(i) $CH_3 - \overset{+}{C}H - CH_3$
(ii) $CH_3 - \overset{+}{C}H - OCH_3$
(iii) $CH_3 - \overset{+}{C}H - COCH_3$
(a) (i) > (ii) > (iii) (b) (ii) > (i) > (iii)
(c) (ii) > (iii) > (i) (d) (iii) > (i) > (ii)

75. $C_6H_4(CH_3)_2 \xrightarrow{O_3} A$, what is A ?
(a) $CH_3-C(=O)-C(=O)H$ + 2 $CHO-CHO$
(b) 3 $CHO-CHO$
(c) 2 $CH_3-C(=O)-C(=O)H$ + $CHO-CHO$
(d) 2 $CH_3-C(=O)-CH_3$ + $CHO-CHO$

76. $C_6H_5-CH(CH_3)-CH_3$ ($H_3C-CH-CH_3$ on benzene) $\xrightarrow{KMnO_4} A \xrightarrow[630°C]{\text{sodalime}} B$
What is B ?

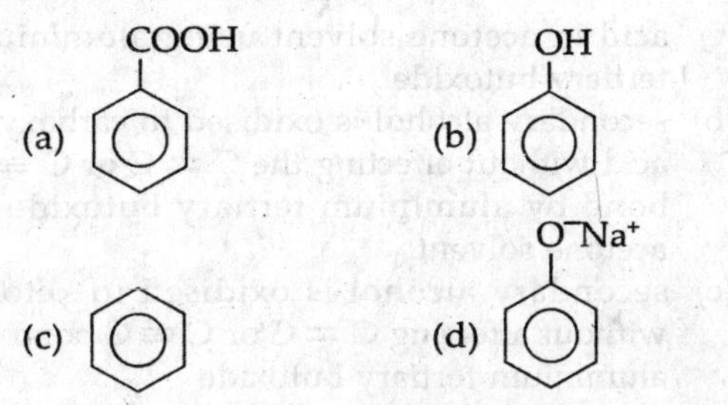

77. $CH_3(CH_2)_4CH_3 \xrightarrow[773\text{ K, }10-20\text{ atm}]{Cr_2O_3/Al_2O_3} A \xrightarrow{Br_2/Fe} B \xrightarrow[\text{ether}]{Mg} C \xrightarrow{H_2O} D$

What is D ?

(a) benzene (b) phenol (OH)

(c) bromobenzene (Br) (d) benzoic acid (COOH)

78. Mercurous chloride exists in the form of

(a) Hg^+ (b) Hg_2^{2+}

(c) Hg^{2+} (d) Hg_3^{2+}

79. Formula of microcosmic salt is

(a) Na_2HPO_4 (b) $Na(NH_4)HPO_4$

(c) K_2HPO_4 (d) $Na_2PO_4{\cdot}K_2PO_4$

80. What is the molarity of H_2SO_4 solution that has a density of 1.84 g/cc at 35°C and contains 98% by weight ?

(a) 4.18 M (b) 8.14 M

(c) 18.4 M (d) 18 M.

81. A mixture of two miscible liquids A and B is distilled under equilibrium conditions at 1 atm pressure. The mole fraction of A in solution and vapour phase are 0.30 and 0.60 respectively. Assuming ideal behaviour of the solution and the vapour, calculate the ratio of the vapour pressure of pure A to that of pure B.

(a) 4.0 (b) 3.5

(c) 2.5 (d) 1.85

82. The variation of volume V, with temperature T, keeping pressure constant is called the coefficient of thermal expansion (α) of a gas. *i.e.*, $\alpha = \frac{1}{V}\left(\frac{\partial V}{\partial T}\right)_P$.

For an ideal gas α is equal to

(a) T (b) $1/T$

(c) P (d) $1/P$.

83. The molecules having the same hybridization, shape and number of lone pairs of electrons are

(a) SeF_4, XeO_2F_2 (b) SF_4, XeF_2

(c) $XeOF_4$, TeF_4 (d) $SeCl_4$, XeF_4

84. The correct order of stability of the superoxides is

(a) $KO_2 > RbO_2 > CsO_2$

(b) $KO_2 > CsO_2 > RbO_2$

(c) $CsO_2 > RbO_2 > KO_2$

(d) $RbO_2 > CsO_2 > KO_2$

85. Schottky defect in crystals is observed when

(a) unequal number cations and anions are missing from the lattice

(b) equal number of cations and anions are missing from the lattice

(c) an ion leaves its normal site and occupies an interstitial site

(d) density of the crystal is increased

86. Consider the reaction

$C_6H_5-CH_2-CH(OTs)-CH(CH_3)-CH_3 \xrightarrow[t\text{-BuOH}]{(CH_3)_3CO^-} C_6H_5-CH{=}CH-CH(CH_3)-CH_3$ (major product)

The correct explanation is

(a) The product is formed due to nucleophilic substitution

(b) The product is formed according to Saytzeff's rule

(c) Conjugated double bond product is formed due to higher stability because of resonance stabilization

(d) $(CH_3)_3CO^-$ is a better leaving group

87. 2.5 g of the carbonate of a metal was treated with 100 ml of 1N H_2SO_4. After the completion of the reaction, the solution was boiled off to expel CO_2 and was then titrated against 1N NaOH solution. The volume of alkali that would be consumed, if the equivalent weight of the metal is 20

(a) 50 (b) 25

(c) 75 (d) 100.

88. In solvents like DMSO, acetonitrile, F^- ion of dissolved NaF is more reactive than in methyl alcohol. Explain

(a) CH_3OH is more polar than DMSO and CH_3CN
(b) CH_3OH is less polar than DMSO and CH_3CN
(c) unsolvated F^- ion is DMSO or CH_3CN acts more efficiently as nucleophile
(d) –OH group is a better leaving group than F^- ion

89. Which of the following fluorides has the lowest melting point ?
(a) BaF_2 (b) SrF_2
(c) CaF_2 (d) BeF_2

90. Which of the following has the highest tendency to give the reaction,
$M^+_{(g)} \xrightarrow[\text{medium}]{\text{aqueous}} M^+_{(aq)}$?
(a) Na (b) Li
(c) K (d) Rb

91. How many geometrical isomers are possible in the following two alkenes ?
(i) $CH_3-CH=CH-CH=CH-CH_3$
(ii) $CH_3-CH=CH-CH=CH-Cl$
(a) 4 and 4 (b) 4 and 3
(c) 3 and 3 (d) 3 and 4.

92. The equilibrium constant for mutarotation α-D Glucose $\rightleftharpoons$ β-D Glucose 1.8. What percentage of α form remains at equilibrium?
(a) 35.7 (b) 64.3
(c) 55.6 (d) 44.4

93. 2-phenylethylbromide when heated with NaOEt, elimination takes place. No deuterium exchange takes place when the reaction is carried out in C_2H_5OD solvent. The mechanism will be
(a) E1 elimination (b) E2 elimination
(c) E1cB elimination (d) E2 or E1cB

94. The $M-O-M$ bond angles in M_2O (where M is halogen) is in the order
(a) $Br_2O > Cl_2O > F_2O$
(b) $F_2O > Br_2O > Cl_2O$
(c) $F_2O > Cl_2O > Br_2O$
(d) $Cl_2O > F_2O > Br_2O$

95. Hydrofluoric acid is a weak acid. At 25°C, the molar conductivity of 0.002 M HF is 176.2 Ω^{-1} cm^2 mol^{-1}. If its Λ°_m = 405.2 Ω^{-1} cm^2 mol^{-1}. Equilibrium constant at the given concentration is
(a) 6.7×10^{-4} M (b) 3.2×10^{-4} M
(c) 6.7×10^{-5} M (d) 3.2×10^{-5} M

96. In Oppenauer's oxidation,
(a) secondary alcohol is oxidised to carboxylic acid in acetone solvent using aluminium tertiary butoxide
(b) secondary alcohol is oxidised to carboxylic acid without affecting the $C=C$ or $C\equiv C$ bond by aluminium tertiary butoxide in acetone solvent
(c) secondary alcohol is oxidised to ketone without affecting $C=C$ or $C\equiv C$ bond by aluminium tertiary butoxide
(d) secondary alcohol is oxidised to ketone by chromic acid - pyridine complex.

97. Incorrect statement about Ge is
(a) GeO_2 is weakly acidic
(b) $Ge(OH)_2$ is amphoteric
(c) $GeCl_2$ is more stable than $GeCl_4$
(d) Ge–Ge bond energy is lesser than that of Si – Si

98. In an isobaric process, when temperature changes from T_1 to T_2, ΔS is equal to
(a) 2.303 $C_P \log (T_2/T_1)$ (b) 2.303 $C_P \ln (T_2/T_1)$
(c) $C_P \ln (T_1/T_2)$ (d) $C_V \ln (T_2/T_1)$

99. In one reaction,
(cyclohexyl)–Mg–Br is treated with CH_3CN and then hydrolysed. In another reaction (cyclohexyl)–Mg–Br is treated with ethyl acetate and then hydrolysed.

$$\text{C}_6\text{H}_{11}\text{-MgBr} \xrightarrow[\text{(ii) } H_3O^+]{\text{(i) } CH_3CN} A$$

$$\text{C}_6\text{H}_{11}\text{-MgBr} \xrightarrow[\text{(ii) } H_3O^+]{\text{(i) } CH_3-\overset{O}{\overset{\|}{C}}-OC_2H_5} B$$

A and B are
(a) (cyclohexyl)–CHO and (cyclohexyl)–CO–CH_3
(b) (cyclohexyl)–CO–CH_3 and (cyclohexyl)–CO–CH_3
(c) (cyclohexyl)–CO–CH_3 and (cyclohexyl)–CO–OC_2H_5
(d) (cyclohexyl)–CO–CH_3 and (cyclohexyl)–$O-\overset{O}{\overset{\|}{C}}-CH_2-CH_3$

100. In the following sequence of the reactions, identify the final product.

$$CH_3-Mg-Br + \text{(cyclohexanone)} \xrightarrow{H_3O^{\oplus}} A \xrightarrow{HBr} B \xrightarrow{\text{Mg, ether}} C \xrightarrow[H_3O^{\oplus}]{CH_3CHO} D$$

(a) 1-methylcyclohexyl with CH_3 and $-CHOH-CH_3$ (ring carbon bearing CH_3 and CHOH(CH_3))

(b) 1-methylcyclohexyl with CH_3 and $-C(=O)-CH_3$

(c) 2-methylcyclohexyl $-CHOH-CH_3$

(d) 2-methylcyclohexyl $-CH_2OH$

Directions : In the following questions (101-120), a statement of assertion (A) is followed by a statement of reason (R). Mark the correct choice as :

(a) If both assertion and reason are true and reason is the correct explanation of assertion

(b) If both assertion and reason are true but reason is not the correct explanation of assertion

(c) If assertion is true but reason is false

(d) If both assertion and reason are false.

101. Assertion : Electromeric effect is brought into play only at the requirement of the reagent.

Reason : It is a temporary effect in which bond pair is shifted to one of the constituent atoms.

102. Assertion : In fused state, calcium chloride cannot be used to dry alcohol or NH_3.

Reason : $CaCl_2$ is not a good dessicant.

103. Assertion : Heat of neutralisation of nitric acid with NaOH is same to that of HCl and NaOH.

Reason : In both cases strong acid and strong bases are neutralised.
$H^+ + OH^- \rightarrow H_2O$.

104. Assertion : *Cis*-2-butene gives *meso*-2, 3-butanediol with dilute alkaline $KMnO_4$ solution.

Reason : Dilute alkaline $KMnO_4$ solution gives *trans* addition with alkenes.

105. Assertion : Ethers can be dried by using sodium wire.

Reason : Ethers do not react with sodium.

106. Assertion : In rate law, unlike in the expression for equilibrium constants, the exponents for concentrations do not necessarily match the stoichiometric coefficients.

Reason : It is the mechanism and not the balanced chemical equation for the overall change that governs the reaction rate.

107. Assertion : The presence of Ag^+ enhances the solubility of alkenes in water.

Reason : Alkenes are weakly polar in nature.

108. Assertion : A reaction which is spontaneous and accompanied by decrease of randomness must be exothermic.

Reason : All exothermic reactions are accompanied by decrease of randomness.

109. Assertion : Compressibility factor for hydrogen varies with pressure with positive slope at all pressure.

Reason : Even at low pressure, repulsive forces dominate for hydrogen gas

110. Assertion : *p*-N,N-dimethylaminobenzaldehyde undergoes benzoin condensation.

Reason : The aldehydic (–CHO) group is meta directing.

111. Assertion : The S-S-S bond angle in S_8 molecule is 105º.

Reason : S_8 has a V-shape.

112. Assertion : Sodium formate has both the C – O bonds have same value 1.27 Å.

Reason : Equal bond length is due to the phenomenon of resonance.

113. Assertion : C_2H_5Br reacts with alcoholic solution of $AgNO_2$ to form nitroethane as the major product.

Reason : NO_2^- is an ambidient ion.

114. Assertion : Ice $\rightleftharpoons$ water, if pressure is applied water will evaporate.
Reason : Increases of pressure pushes the equilibrium towards the side in which number of gaseous molecule increases.

115. Assertion : Ebonite is highly vulcanised rubber.
Reason : Perlon is used in the manufacture of fibres.

116. Assertion : Al forms $[AlF_6]^{3-}$ but B does not form $[BF_6]^{3-}$.
Reason : B does not react with fluorine.

117. Assertion : Esters which contain α-hydrogens undergo Claisen condensation.
Reason : $LiAlH_4$ reduction of esters gives acids.

118. Assertion : In an acid-base titration involving strong base and a weak acid, methyl orange can be used as an indicator.
Reason : Methyl orange changes its colour in pH range of 7 to 9.

119. Assertion : Millon's test is a test for identification of proteins.
Reason : Millon's reagent is a solution of mercurous nitrate and mercuric nitrate in nitric acid containing little nitrous acid.

120. Assertion : $Cu(OH)_2$ is soluble in NH_4OH but not in NaOH.
Reason : $Cu(OH)_2$ forms a soluble complex with NH_3.

BIOLOGY

121. What is diapedesis?
(a) a kind of amoeboid movement
(b) the process of filtration of urea in kidney
(c) a type of locomotion found in *Hydra*
(d) migration of WBCs into the tissue spaces from blood capillaries

122. Which one of the following depresses brain activity and produces feelings of calmness, relaxation and drowsiness?
(a) morphine (b) valium
(c) amphetamines (d) hashish.

123. Which of the following nerves arises from organ of Corti?
(a) olfactory nerve (b) cochlear nerve
(c) abducens nerve (d) none of these

124. Delicate hair-like feathers which remain sparsely distributed over the body are
(a) coverts (b) filoplumes
(c) plumules (d) remiges

125. *Homo erectus* evolved during
(a) pleistocene (b) miocene
(c) pliocene (d) holocene

126. Which of the following postulates is related with Neo-Darwinism?
(a) mutations are believed to help form new species
(b) it incorporates isolation as an essential component of evolution
(c) it can explain the occurrence of unchanged forms over millions of years
(d) all of the above

127. Intermediate host is absent in the infection of
(a) *Plasmodium* (b) *Trypanosoma*
(c) *Entamoeba* (d) filarial worm.

128. Which one feature is common to leech, cockroach and scorpion?
(a) nephridia
(b) ventral nerve cord
(c) cephalization (d) antennae.

129. The type of epithelial cells which line the inner surface of Fallopian tubes, bronchioles and small bronchi are known as
(a) squamous epithelium
(b) columnar epithelium
(c) ciliated epithelium
(d) cuboidal epithelium

130. A person who shows unpredictable moods, outbursts of emotions, quarrelsome behaviour and conflicts with others is suffering from
(a) borderline personality disorder (BPD)
(b) mood disorder
(c) addictive disorder
(d) schizophrenia

131. In humans at the end of first meiotic division, the male germ cells differentiate into the
(a) primary spermatocytes
(b) secondary spermatocytes
(c) spermatids
(d) spermatogonia

132. Contraceptive oral pills help in birth control by
(a) killing the sperms in uterus

(b) preventing implantation
(c) preventing ovulation
(d) both (b) and (c).

133. Which one of the following is a sesamoid bone?
(a) pelvis (b) patella
(c) pterygoid (d) pectoral girdle.

134. Respiration is controlled by
(a) medulla oblongata
(b) cerebellum
(c) hypothalamus (d) cerebrum

135. Duodenum has characteristic Brunner's gland which secretes two hormones called
(a) prolactin, parathormone
(b) secretin, cholecystokinin
(c) enterocrinin, duocrinin
(d) gastrin, euterogastrone.

136. Which of the following species has the chromosome complement similar to that of *Triticum aestivum*?
(a) *Zea mays*
(b) *Secale cereale*
(c) *Gossypium*
(d) *Aegilops*

137. Eugenics is the branch concerned with
(a) improving the quality of human race by symptomatic treatment of genetic diseases
(b) improving the quality of human populations by the application of genetic principles
(c) improving the quality of human race by providing best suitable environment
(d) none of the above.

138. What is incorrect about the following figure representing DNA replication?

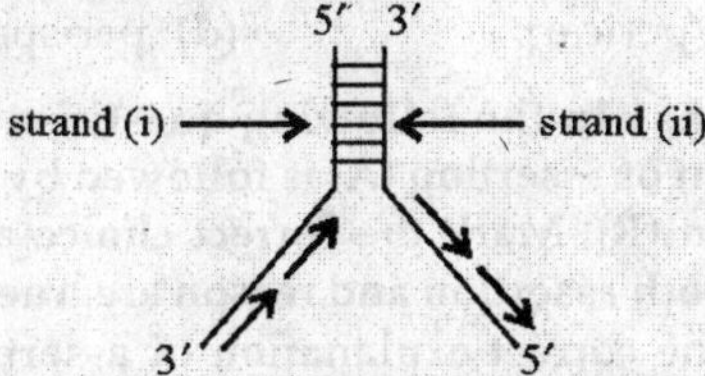

(a) the direction of DNA replication in strand (i)
(b) the direction of DNA replication in strand (ii)
(c) discontinuous replication of strand (i)
(d) discontinuous replication of strand (ii)

139. Which of the following is the characteristic of PS-I.
(a) it is active only upto 680 nm of light
(b) the reaction centre of PS-I is P_{680}
(c) PS-I is reduced by the electrons released in photolysis of water
(d) PS-I is involved in non-cyclic photophosphorylation.

140. Bark refers to
(a) phellem + phellogen + phelloderm
(b) periderm + cortex
(c) phellem + phelloderm + secondary phloem
(d) periderm + cortex + pericycle + secondary phloem

141. Cotton fibres mainly contains
(a) cellulose (b) glycogen
(c) protein (d) lipid

142. The outermost limiting layer of mycoplasma is made up of
(a) cell wall (b) cell membrane
(c) mucilaginous sheath
(d) slime layer

143. Which of the following statements about *Spirogyra* is correct?
(a) lateral conjugation takes place in homothallic species
(b) scalariform conjugation takes place in homothallic species
(c) lateral conjugation takes place in heterothallic species
(d) the type of conjugation is unrelated to homothallic & heterothallic species

144. Which of the following sugars is not found in plants ?
(a) sucrose (b) glucose
(c) lactose (d) fructose

145. The binding site of *t*RNA with *m*RNA & amino acids respectively are
(a) *m*RNA with DHU loop & amino acid with CCA end
(b) *m*RNA with CCA end & amino acid with anticodon loop
(c) *m*RNA with anticodon loop & amino acid with DHU loop
(d) *m*RNA with anticodon loop & amino acid with CCA end

146. Percentage of recombination between A and B is 9%, A and C is 17%, B and C is 26% , then the arrangement of genes is
(a) ABC (b) ACB
(c) BCA (d) BAC

147. Which of the following is true?
(a) umbel is a racemose inflorescence where all stalked flower aggregate on the flat receptacle
(b) raceme is a racemose inflorescence having main axis shortened & flower born acropetally
(c) spadix is a racemose inflorescence having pendulous spike with main axis much flattened
(d) spike is a racemose inflorescence having sessile flowers

148. Jute fibres deteriorate quickly because
(a) cellulose content is high
(b) lignin content is high
(c) cellulose content is low
(d) lignin content is low

149. The branched sclereids present in hydrophytes are
(a) osteosclereids (b) trichosclereids
(c) macrosclereids (d) astrosclereids.

150. The enzyme decarboxylase catalyses the following step
(a) conversion of citric acid to *cis* aconitic acid
(b) fumaric acid to malic acid
(c) oxalosuccinic acid to α-ketoglutaric acid
(d) malic acid to oxaloacetic acid

151. Which of the following is true regarding the given electron transport chain?
CoQ → Cyt c → Cyt aa_3 → O_2
(a) CoQ → Cyt c is H^+ absorbing site
(b) $aa_3 \rightarrow O_2$, H^+ yielding site
(c) CoQ → Cyt c is H^+ yielding site and $aa_3 \rightarrow O_2$ is H^+ absorbing site
(d) no H^+ is absorbed or released

152. Which one of the following is not a microelement for plants?
(a) Cu (b) B
(c) Zn (d) Cr

153. National bird of India is
(a) *Psittacula* (b) *Passer domesticus*
(c) *Pavo cristatus* (d) *Parakeet*.

154. Rain is called acid-rain when its pH is below
(a) 7 (b) 6.5
(c) 6 (d) 5.6

155. Cytokines that provide non specific immunity against virus are
(a) interleukin (b) tumour necrosis
(c) colony stimulating
(d) interferon.

156. By all of the following ways bacteria become resistant to antibiotic except
(a) making enzymes that inactivate the drug
(b) becoming impermeable to the drug
(c) modifying the target of the drug
(d) moving away from the drug.

157. Specific proteins responsible for the flow of materials and information into the cell are called
(a) membrane receptors
(b) carrier proteins
(c) integral proteins (d) none of these

158. Which of the following conditions represents a case of co-dominant genes?
(a) a gene expresses itself, suppressing the phenotypic effect of its alleles
(b) genes that are similar in phenotypic effect when present separately, but when together interact to produce a different trait
(c) alleles, both of which interact to produce a trait, which may or may not resemble either of the parental types
(d) alleles, each of which produces an independent effect in a heterozygous condition

159. The first bioherbicide developed in 1981 was based on
(a) *Phytophthora palmivora*
(b) *Phytophthora infestans*
(c) *Bacillus thuringiensis*
(d) *Azadirachta indica*

160. Upon fertilization, what structure develops from carpel?
(a) testa (b) tegmen
(c) pericarp (d) perisperm

Directions : In the following questions (161-180), a statement of assertion (A) is followed by a statement of reason (R). Mark the correct choice as :
(a) If both assertion and reason are true and reason is the correct explanation of assertion
(b) If both assertion and reason are true but reason is not the correct explanation of assertion
(c) If assertion is true but reason is false
(d) If both assertion and reason are false.

161. Assertion : Secondary succession takes place in recently denuded area.
Reason : It is caused due to baring of an area.

162. Assertion : Connective tissue inside the brain is essential for conduction of nerve impulse.

Reason : Connective tissue hold together the nerve cells of brain.

163. Assertion : Mammary glands are apocrine glands.

Reason : The distal part containing secretory granules break down and leaves as a secretion.

164. Assertion : Cytokinins increases shelf life of fruits and vegetables.

Reason : Cytokinins induce cell division.

165. Assertion : Angina pectoris means "pain in the chest".

Reason : It results due to carrying of extra blood to the heart muscle.

166. Assertion : Protandry and protogyny ensures cross fertilization.

Reason : Cross fertilization introduces variation in progeny.

167. Assertion : Bursa fabricii lies on the ventral side of the cloaca in birds.

Reason : Bursa fabricii is related with flight adaptation.

168. Assertion : Glycolysis is the first step of respiration in which glucose completely breaks into CO_2 and H_2O.

Reason : In this process, there is net gain of twenty four molecules of ATP.

169. Assertion : Restriction enzymes cut the strand of DNA to produce sticky ends.

Reason : Stickiness of the ends facilitates the action of the enzyme DNA polymerase.

170. Assertion : Excess of nitrates in drinking water are harmful for infants.

Reason : Nitrates are responsible for blue baby syndrome.

171. Assertion : Amniocentesis is a process of foetal sex determination.

Reason : Metabolic errors and other diseases can be diagnosed prenatally by this process.

172. Assertion : Pollen mother cells (PMCs) are the first male gametophytic cells.

Reason : Each PMC gives rise to two pollens.

173. Assertion : Nucleus is the controlling centre of a cell.

Reason : Pores in the nuclear envelop regulate the flow of materials in and out of the nucleus.

174. Assertion : Hormone calcitonin has antagonistic effect to that of parathormone.

Reason : Calcitonin decreases blood calcium level while parathormone increases blood calcium level.

175. Assertion : Dark reaction occurs only at night in the stroma of chloroplast.

Reason : CO_2 fixation occurs only during C_3 cycle.

176. Assertion : The primitive atmosphere was reducing one *i.e.* without oxygen.

Reason : In the primitive atmosphere, oxygen was involved in forming ozone layer.

177. Assertion : Jave Ape-man, Peking man and Heidelberg man are the fossils of *Homo erectus*.

Reason : *Homo erectus* evolved from *Homo habilis*.

178. Assertion : Loss of water produces a negative hydrostatic pressure.

Reason : Positive hydrostatic pressure is developed due to osmotic entry of water into it.

179. Assertion : Mammalian ova produces hyaluronidase.

Reason : The eggs of mammal are microlecithal and telolecithal.

180. Assertion : A gamete may carry either of the traits but not both.

Reason : This is Mendel's second law or law of independent assortment.

GENERAL KNOWLEDGE

181. A pendulum clock is set to give correct time at the sea level. The clock is moved to a hill station at an altitude h above sea level. In order to keep correct time on the hill station which one of the following adjustments is required?
(a) the length of the pendulum has to be reduced
(b) the length of the pendulum has to be increased
(c) the mass of the pendulum has to be increased
(d) the mass of the pendulum has to be reduced.

182. Match List I with List II and select the correct answer using the codes given below the lists:

List I (Date)	List II (Events)
(A) 24th October	(1) Human Rights Day
(B) 10th December	(2) Common wealth Day
(C) 24th May	(3) United Nations Day
(D) 21st September	(4) International Day of Peace.

Codes :

	A	B	C	D
(a)	4	1	2	3
(b)	3	1	2	4
(c)	3	2	1	4
(d)	4	2	1	3

183. The President of India is elected by
(a) members of both Houses of Parliament
(b) members of both Houses of Parliament and of State Legislatures
(c) members of both Houses of Parliament and of State Legislative Assemblies
(d) elected members of both Houses of Parliament and elected members of state Legislative Assemblies.

184. Who wrote the book 'India Wins Freedom'?
(a) Maulana Abul Kalam Azad
(b) Mahatma Gandhi
(c) Sir Mohammad Iqbal
(d) Abdul Ghaffar Khan.

185. Consider the following statements about the National Anthem:
1. It was first sung on December 27, 1911 at the Calcutta session of the Indian National Congress.
2. It was adopted by the Constituent Assembly on January 26, 1950
3. Playing time of the full version of the National Anthem is approximately 52 seconds.

Which of the statements given above is/are correct?
(a) 1 only (b) 1 and 2
(c) 1 and 3 (d) 2 and 3.

186. Match List I with List II and select the correct answer using the codes given below the lists.

List I (Vitamin)	List II (Function)
(A) Vitamin A	(1) Assists in normal reproductive function
(B) Vitamin C	(2) Assists in absorption and metabolism of calcium
(C) Vitamin D	(3) Essential for healthy skin and normal vision.
(D) Vitamin B_{12}	(4) Essential for formation of collagen.
	(5) Essential for red blood cell formation.

Codes :

	A	B	C	D
(a)	2	1	5	4
(b)	3	4	2	5
(c)	3	2	4	1
(d)	2	1	3	5.

187. The metal compound commonly found in Sindhoor or Kumkum is based on
(a) tin (b) lead
(c) copper (d) zinc.

188. Which among the following thermometers is preferred for measuring temperature around 1250°C?
(a) mercury thermometer
(b) constant volume gas thermometer
(c) optical pyrometer
(d) platinum resistance thermometer.

189. The term stagflation refers to a situation where
(a) growth has no relation with the change in prices
(b) rate of growth and prices both are decreasing
(c) rate of growth is faster than the rate of price increase
(d) rate of growth is slower than the rate of price increase.

190. Which event brought about a profound change

in Ashoka's administrative policy?
(a) the third Buddhist council
(b) the Kalinga war
(c) his embracing of buddhism
(d) his sending of missionary to Ceylon.

191. The plant dye *Henna* imparts orange-red colour to skin and hair due to its reaction with which of the following?
(a) proteins and amino acids
(b) lipids
(c) carbohydrates
(d) nucleic acids.

192. Match the List I with List II and select the correct answer using the codes given below the lists.

List I (Islands)	List II (Ocean)
(A) Hawaiian Islands	(1) Indian Ocean
(B) Solomon Islands	(2) North Pacific Ocean
(C) St. Helena	(3) South Pacific Ocean
(D) Seychelles	(4) South Atlantic Ocean

Codes :

	A	B	C	D
(a)	2	3	4	1
(b)	1	4	3	2
(c)	2	4	3	1
(d)	1	3	4	2

193. Delingha came recently in news? What is this?
(a) it is an endangered species of an Indian bird
(b) it is place in Europe which was struck by an earthquake
(c) China recently deployed missiles in the Delingha near Tibet sending alarming signals across political establishment in India
(d) none of the above.

194. Octopus is an anti-terror ageny of
(a) Kerala (b) Andhra Pradesh
(c) Karnataka (d) Gujarat.

195. Indira Gandhi Prize for peace, disarmament and development has recently been conferred on
(a) Bill Gates (b) Jacob Zuma
(c) Asma Jahangir
(d) none of the above.

196. India's Deep Joshi has recently been honoured with
(a) Magsaysay Award
(b) Whitely Prize
(c) Right to Livelihood Award
(d) none of these.

197. The runner up in 2009 Wimbledon Men's Singles was
(a) Roger Federer
(b) Rafael Nadal
(c) Andy Roddick
(d) none of the above.

198. Who amongst the following cricketers has been chosen for Rajiv Gandhi Khel Ratna Award, 2007?
(a) Rahul Dravid (b) M.S. Dhoni
(c) Sachin Tendulkar (d) Virender Sehwag.

199. Who amongst the following became the first woman pilot in the world to fly MIG-35 fighter plane?
(a) Suman Sharma
(b) Saudamini Deshmukh
(c) Kirsty Moore
(d) Nicole Malachowski.

200. Mr. Paul Krugman whose name was in news recently is a famous
(a) medical scientist
(b) economist
(c) author
(d) astrophysicist.

SOLUTIONS

PHYSICS

1. **(a) :** Focal length of a convex lens having power 2.5 D, $= \frac{1}{2.5}$ m

Also focal length of a lens in a medium of refractive index μ is given by

$$\frac{1}{f} = (\mu - 1)\left(\frac{1}{R_1} - \frac{1}{R_2}\right)$$

$$\Rightarrow 2.5 = \frac{1}{f} = \left(\frac{3}{2} - 1\right)\left(\frac{1}{R_1} - \frac{1}{R_2}\right) \quad \text{....(i)} \quad \text{(in air)}$$

$$\Rightarrow \frac{1}{f'} = \left(\frac{3}{4} - 1\right)\left(\frac{1}{R_1} - \frac{1}{R_2}\right) \quad \text{...(ii)} \quad [\because {}^{l}\mu_g = \tfrac{3}{4}] \text{ in liquid}$$

Dividing the two, $2.5f' = \frac{0.5}{-0.25}$

$$\Rightarrow \frac{1}{f'} = \frac{-5}{25 \times 0.25} = -1.25\,\text{D}$$

2. **(a) :** Magnetic moment associated with electrons orbitting around the nucleus is given in terms of Bohr magneton (μ_B)

$$\mu_B = \frac{e\hbar}{2m_e}$$

e = electronic charge, m_e = electronic mass.

In nuclear physics, magnetic moments associated with the spins of protons and neutrons are expressed in nuclear magnetons (μ_N)

$$\mu_N = \frac{e\hbar}{2m_p}$$

m_p = mass of a proton.

$$\Rightarrow \frac{\mu_B}{\mu_N} = \frac{m_p}{m_e}$$

3. **(c) :** If we make a truth table for the outputs given in the question. It matches with the truth table of an NOR gate.

$Y = \overline{A + B}$

A	B	Y (output)
1	0	0
0	1	0
0	0	1

4. **(c) :** $\lambda \propto \frac{1}{\sqrt{T}}$

5. **(b) :** Specific resistance $\rho = \frac{RA}{l}$

$= [ML^2T^{-3}A^{-2}]\,[L]$

$= [ML^3T^{-3}A^{-2}]$

6. **(c) :** The reciprocal of impedance is admittance.

7. **(c) :** Let the reaction be represented as

$$^{220}_{Z}X \longrightarrow {}^{216}_{Z-2}Y + {}^{4}_{2}He$$

$\because$ energy released in the reaction is 5 MeV

$$\Rightarrow \frac{1}{2}m_Y v^2{}_Y + \frac{1}{2}m_\alpha v_\alpha^2 = 5\,\text{MeV}$$

$$\Rightarrow \frac{1}{2}(216)v_Y^2 + \frac{1}{2}4(v_\alpha)^2 = 5\,\text{MeV} \quad \text{...(i)}$$

Also using conservation of linear momentum.

$$m_Y v_Y = -m_\alpha v_\alpha \Rightarrow v_Y = \frac{-m_\alpha}{m_Y}v_\alpha$$

$$v_Y = \frac{-4}{216}v_\alpha = \frac{-1}{54}v_\alpha$$

Putting in eqn. (i)

$$\frac{1}{2}(216)\left(\frac{v_\alpha}{54}\right)^2 + \frac{1}{2}4(v_\alpha)^2 = 5\,\text{MeV}$$

$$\frac{1}{2}(216)\left(\frac{v_\alpha}{54}\right)^2 + \text{K.E.}_\alpha = 5\,\text{MeV}$$

$$\Rightarrow \frac{1}{2} \times 4\,\frac{v_\alpha{}^2}{54} + \text{K.E.}_\alpha = 5\,\text{MeV}$$

$$\Rightarrow \frac{1}{54}(\text{K.E.}_\alpha) + \text{K.E.}_\alpha = 5\,\text{MeV}$$

$$\text{K.E.}_\alpha = \frac{5 \times 54}{55} = \frac{54}{11}\,\text{MeV}$$

8. **(a) :** The resultant electric fields due to diagonally opposite charges will act as shown below.

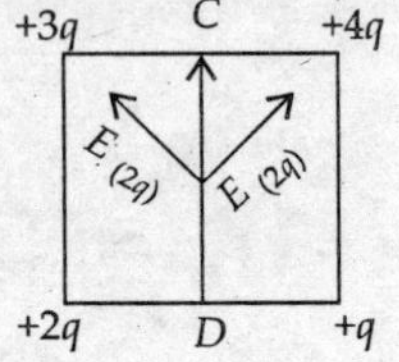

Hence the resultant field is along DC.

9. **(a) :** Wavelengths of the K_α lines for given isotopes of lead (Pb) can be given by a general expression

$$\frac{1}{\lambda} = R(Z-1)^2\left(\frac{1}{1^2} - \frac{1}{2^2}\right)$$

where R = Rydberg's constant, Z = atomic number of the isotopes. Though Pb^{208}, Pb^{206} and Pb^{204} have different atomic masses, Z will be same for them *i.e.* 82.

$$\therefore \frac{1}{\lambda_1} = R(82-1)^2\left(\frac{1}{1^2} - \frac{1}{2^2}\right) = \frac{3}{4}R(81)^2$$

$$\frac{1}{\lambda_2} = \frac{3}{4}R(81^2) \text{ and } \frac{1}{\lambda_3} = \frac{3}{4}R(81^2)$$

$$\Rightarrow \left(\frac{1}{\lambda_2}\right)^2 = \frac{1}{\lambda_1} \times \frac{1}{\lambda_3} \Rightarrow \lambda_2 = \sqrt{\lambda_1 \lambda_3}$$

10. **(a)** : Work done by force = Area under force-displacement graph.

$$= 3 \times 3 + \frac{1}{2} \times 3 \times 3 = 9 + 4.5 = 13.5 \text{ J}$$

11. **(d)** : Since $k \propto \frac{1}{l}$

12. **(c)** : At maximum compression the whole kinetic energy of ball = potential energy of spring.

$$\frac{1}{2}mv^2 = \frac{1}{2}kx^2 \Rightarrow x = v\sqrt{\frac{m}{k}}$$

$$x = 1.5 \times \sqrt{\frac{5}{5}} = 1.5 \text{ m}$$

13. **(c)**

14. **(d)** : Radiation pressure P_{rad} due to light falling on a non-reflecting surface at normal incidence is given by

$$P_{rad} = \frac{\text{Energy flux}}{\text{Speed of light}} = \frac{18 \text{ W/cm}^2}{3 \times 10^8 \text{ m/s}}$$

$$= \frac{18 \times 10^4 \text{ W/m}^2}{3 \times 10^8 \text{ m/s}} = 6 \times 10^{-4} \text{ N/m}^2$$

15. **(a)**

16. **(b)** : After 0.7 sec the horizontal velocity component of the body = $4\sqrt{2}$ m/sec since there is no change in velocity in horizontal direction.

The vertical velocity component after 0.7 seconds = 0 + gt = 0 + 0.7 × 10

= 7 m/sec

$\therefore$ resultant velocity of the body = $\sqrt{(4\sqrt{2})^2 + 7^2}$

= $\sqrt{32 + 49}$ = 9 m/sec

17. **(d)** : Three equal weights of 3 kg each are hanging on a string passing over a pulley as shown in figure.

If a is the common acceleration.

$T - 3g = 3a$ (For mass I)

$3g + T_1 - T = 3a$ (For mass II)

$3g - T_1 = 3a$ (For mass III)

Adding, above three equations

$3g = 9a$, $a = g/3$

$T_1 = 3g - 3a = 3g - g = 2g = 20$ N

18. **(a)** : The ball falls a distance h from its highest (rest) position and rebounds a distance $(h - d)$.

Thus the coefficient of restitution $e = \sqrt{\frac{h-d}{h}}$

$$e^2 = \frac{h-d}{h} \text{ or } h = \frac{d}{1-e^2}$$

19. **(a)** : The capacitances of two are $C_1 = 4\pi\varepsilon_0 R$ and $C_2 = 4\pi\varepsilon_0 (2R)$

Initial energy $= E_i = \frac{Q^2}{2C_1}$

Final energy $= E_f = \frac{Q^2}{2C_2}$

Heat produced = $E_i - E_f$

$$= \frac{Q^2}{2}\left[\frac{1}{4\pi\varepsilon_0 R} - \frac{1}{2 \times 4\pi\varepsilon_0 R}\right]$$

$$= \frac{1}{4\pi\varepsilon_0} \cdot \frac{Q^2}{2R}\left[1 - \frac{1}{2}\right]$$

$$= \frac{1}{4\pi\varepsilon_0} \cdot \frac{Q^2}{4R}$$

20. **(b)** : $\lambda_m T = 2.898 \times 10^{-3}$ mK

$\lambda_m = \frac{2.9 \times 10^{-3}}{10^6} = 2.9 \times 10^{-9}$ m = 2.9 nm. It lies in the X-ray region of the electromagnetic spectrum.

21. **(a)** : The terminal velocity of the spherical raindrop of radius r is given by

$v_t = \frac{2r^2 \rho g}{9\eta}$ where ρ is the density of water and η the viscosity of air. Substituting r = 0.3 mm = 0.3×10^{-3} m, $\rho = 10^3$ kg/m^3, g = 9.8 m/s^2 and $\eta = 1.8 \times 10^{-5}$ N s/m^2, we get

$$v_t = \frac{2\times(0.3)^2\times10^{-3}\times9.8}{9\times1.8\times10^{-5}}$$

$= 10.9$ m s^{-1}

22. **(b)** : Let the simple harmonic equation for the particle be $x = l\sin\omega t$ ... (i)

where ω is its angular velocity.

Since the S.H.M. of the rod has the same period and amplitude and its vibration is perpendicular to that of the particle, its equation is $y = l\cos(\omega t + \phi)$ where ϕ is the initial phase difference (phase angle for y). But both the particle as well as the rod pass through the mean position simultaneously. Hence $\phi = \pi/2$ since $x = y = 0$ at $t = 0$.

So, $y = l\cos(\omega t + \pi/2) = -l\sin\omega t$ ... (ii)

Eliminating t between (i) and (ii), we have

$y = -x$

which is the equation to a straight line at angle $\pi/4$ to the rod.

23. **(a)** : Network is redrawn as shown in figure.

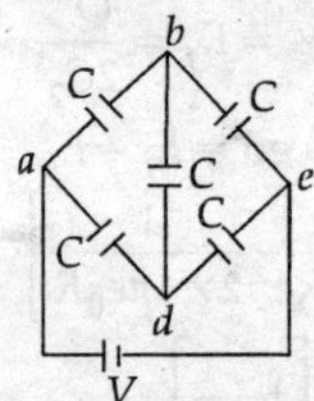

This is a balanced Wheatstone's network.

Equivalent capacitance $C_{eq} = C$

Charge on capacitor between the terminals a and b

$$\frac{Q}{2} = \frac{CV}{2}$$

Energy stored in that capacitor

$$= \frac{1}{2C}\left(\frac{Q}{2}\right)^2 = \frac{Q^2}{8C} = \frac{C^2V^2}{8C} = \frac{CV^2}{8}$$

Given: $C = 1$ μF, $V = 10$ V

$$= \frac{(1\times10^{-6})\times10^2}{8}$$

$$= \frac{100}{8}\times10^{-6} = 12.5\ \mu\text{J}$$

24. **(b)** : $H = I^2Rt = mc\Delta\theta$

$\therefore\ \Delta\theta \propto I^2$

Hence $\dfrac{\Delta\theta_2}{\Delta\theta_1} = \left(\dfrac{I_2}{I_1}\right)^2$ or $\dfrac{\Delta\theta_2}{3} = \left(\dfrac{3I}{I}\right)^2$

or $\Delta\theta_2 = 9\times3 = 27°C$

25. **(a)** : According to positive Thomson's effect the potential at a point of lower temperature is lower than at the point at higher temperature which is at higher potential. When current is passed from lower temperature to higher temperature of a metal, work is to be done, hence energy is absorbed.

26. **(b)** : $I_g = 0.1I$, $I_s = 0.9I$; $S = I_g G/I_s$

$= 0.1\times900/0.9 = 100\ \Omega$

27. **(c)** : Since the magnetic field, due to current through wire CD at various locations on wire AB is not uniform, therefore, the wire AB, carrying current I_1 is subjected to variable magnetic field due to which, neither the force nor the torque on the wire AB will be zero. As a result of which the wire AB will have both translational and rotational motions.

28. **(b)** : Inductance of a coil is given by

$$L = \frac{1}{2}\mu_0\pi N^2R \Rightarrow \frac{L_2}{L_1} = \frac{N_2^2}{N_1^2}$$

$$\therefore L_2 = L_1\frac{N_2^2}{N_1^2} = \left(\frac{500}{100}\right)^2 15\text{ mH} = 375\text{mH}$$

29. **(c)** : As $V_R = V_L = V_C$

$R = X_L = X_C$, $Z = R$

$V = IR = 10$ volt

When capacitor is short circuited,

$$Z = \sqrt{R^2 + X^2_L} = \sqrt{R^2+R^2} = R\sqrt{2}$$

New current $I' = V/Z = V/R\sqrt{2} = \dfrac{10}{R\sqrt{2}}$

Potential drop across inductance

$= I'X_L = I'R = \frac{10\times R}{R\sqrt{2}} = \frac{10}{\sqrt{2}}$ volt

30. **(d)**

31. **(d)**

32. **(a) :** When sources are coherent, intensity at mid point is

$I_{max} = (a + a)^2 = 4a^2$

When sources are incoherent, no interference occurs. Intensity at mid point is

$I = I_1 + I_2 = a^2 + a^2 = 2a^2$

$\therefore \frac{I_{max}}{I} = \frac{4a^2}{2a^2} = 2:1$

33. **(b) :** $\lambda = \frac{h}{mv} = \frac{h}{\sqrt{2mE}}$ or $\lambda \propto \frac{1}{\sqrt{E}}$

$\therefore \frac{\lambda'}{\lambda} = \sqrt{\frac{E}{E'}} = \sqrt{\frac{1}{16}} = \frac{1}{4}$

% change in wavelength $= \left(\frac{\lambda-\lambda'}{\lambda}\right)\times 100$

$= \left(1-\frac{\lambda'}{\lambda}\right)\times 100 = \left(1-\frac{1}{4}\right)\times 100 = 75\%$

34. **(a) :** $T = \frac{T_\alpha T_\beta}{T_\alpha + T_\beta} = \frac{4\times 12}{4+12}$

$n = \frac{t}{T} = \frac{12}{3} = 4$

$\frac{N}{N_0} = \left(\frac{1}{2}\right)^n = \left(\frac{1}{2}\right)^4 = \frac{1}{16} = 6.25\%$

35. **(c) :** Here *p-n* junction is forward biased. If *p-n* junction is ideal, its resistance is zero. The effective resistance across *A* and *B*

$= \frac{10\times 10}{10+10} = 5\ \text{K}\Omega$

Current in the circuit

$I = \frac{30}{(10+5)\times 10^3} = \frac{2}{10^3}$

$\therefore$ Current in each arm $= \frac{I}{2} = \frac{1}{10^3}$ A.

Pot. diff. across *A* and *B*

$= \frac{1}{10^3}\times 10\times 10^3 = 10$ V

36. **(a) :** $\theta = \theta_0 \sin\omega t \quad \omega = \sqrt{\frac{g}{L}}$

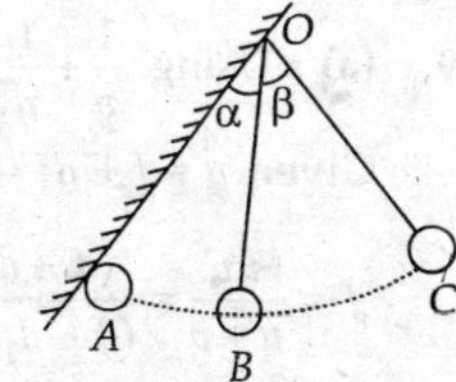

$\because T = 2\pi\sqrt{\frac{L}{g}}$

When $\beta > \alpha$, time taken by pendulum from B to C and C to *B*

$t_1 = \frac{T}{2} = \frac{1}{2}\times 2\pi\sqrt{\frac{L}{g}} = \pi\sqrt{\frac{L}{g}}$

Time taken by pendulum from *B* to *A* and *A* to *B*

$t_2 = 2t = \frac{2}{\omega}\sin^{-1}\left(\frac{\alpha}{\beta}\right)$ using $\theta = \theta_0 \sin\omega t$

$\alpha = \beta\sin\omega t$ or $t = \frac{1}{\omega}\sin^{-1}\left(\frac{\alpha}{\beta}\right)$

$\therefore$ Time period of motion

$T = t_1 + t_2 = \sqrt{\frac{L}{g}}\left[\pi + 2\sin^{-1}\frac{\alpha}{\beta}\right]$

37. **(d) :** Maximum number of nuclei will be present, when rate of decay = rate of formation

$\lambda\,.\,N = \alpha\,,\ N = \frac{\alpha}{\lambda}$

38. **(c) :** Consider two small elements each of length $dl = rd\theta$ symmetrically.

$\pi r = l$

Resolve the elemental field intensities

$\because |dE_1| = |dE_2|$

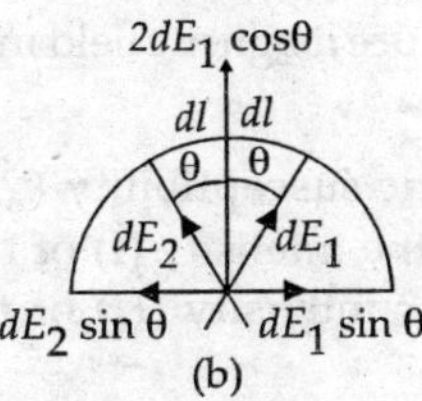

(b)

$dE = 2dE_1\cos\theta = \frac{2Grd\theta}{r^2}\cos\theta$

G = Gravitational constant

λ = Linear mass density $= \frac{m}{l}$

or $dE = \frac{2\lambda G}{r}\int_0^{90^\circ}\cos\theta\, d\theta = \frac{2\lambda G}{r} = \frac{2\pi Gm}{l^2}$

39. **(a)** : Using $\frac{1}{v}+\frac{1}{u}=\frac{1}{f}$

Given $u = f + d_1$ $\quad v = f + d_2$

$$f=\frac{uv}{u+v}=\frac{(f+d_1)(f+d_2)}{(f+d_1)+(f+d_2)}$$

On solving $f=\sqrt{d_1 d_2}$

40. **(c)** : Use $\frac{1}{v}+\frac{1}{u}=\frac{1}{f}$

Find v_1, when $u = d$ and v_2, when $u = d + l$

Size of image $= v_1 - v_2 = l\left(\frac{f}{d-f}\right)^2$

41. **(c)** : When a solid changes into a liquid, the work done against the attraction of molecules is stored in the form of potential energy.

42. **(b)** : When ball is completely filled with water, the centre of gravity of the pendulum is at the centre of the ball when water starts flowing out, the centre of gravity shifts below, thus increasing the length of pendulum, and increasing time period. When ball is more than half empty the centre of gravity again rises up so length of pendulum decreases and time period also decreases.

43. **(c)** : Electric potential of earth is taken as zero, because the capacitance of earth is taken infinite.

44. **(d)** : A charge, whether stationary or in motion, produces an electric field around it. If it is in motion, then in addition to the electric field, it also produces a magnetic field, because moving charges produce magnetic field in the surrounding space.

45. **(c)** : Magnetic susceptibility (χ_m) is defined as the ratio of the intensity (I) of magnetisation to the magnetic intensity (H) of the magnetising field, that is

$$\chi_m=\frac{I}{H}$$

It is a pure number, because I and H have the same unit. Its value for vacuum is zero as there can be no magnetisation in vacuum.

46. **(a)** : Transformers which convert low voltages into higher ones are called step-up transformers, while those which convert high voltages into lower ones are called step-down transformers. This is possible only for a.c. source and not for d.c. source.

47. **(a)** :

B, 90°, P, Q', Q, P', A, C

Beam of light incident on face AB, suffers refraction from air to glass and strikes the face AC suffering total internal reflection. The beam now strikes the face BC of the prism at an angle of incidence less than the critical angle hence it suffers refraction from glass to air and bends away from the normal. The beam emerges out parallel to the base. As a result of refraction, on emergence the rays are inverted.

48. **(a)** : The rays or all colours incident on a concave mirror at the same angle are reflected at the same angle. Hence image formed by reflection does not suffer chromatic aberration.

49. **(a)** : Equivalent mass of photon (m) is given from equation

$$E = mc^2 = h\upsilon \;\therefore\; m=\frac{h\upsilon}{c^2}$$

Where E is energy, m is mass, c is speed of light, h is Planck's constant, υ is frequency.

$\therefore$ Momentum of photon $= m\times\frac{h\upsilon}{c^2}\times c=\frac{h\upsilon}{c}$

50. **(b)** : Photo-conductive cell is based on the principle that when light is incident on some semiconductor, its electrical resistance is reduced. Such cells are used in solar batteries. Whereas photocell is used in electrolyte for giving theft warning in banks treasuries, etc., when the thief throws torch light on the cash box, the light is incident on a photocell placed there and a bell at some particular place rings.

51. **(b)** : The nuclei having mass number $A \approx 60$ have maximum binding energy per nuclean (about 8.7 MeV). So, these nuclei are most stable.

52. **(c)** : We know that

$$\alpha=\frac{\Delta i_C}{\Delta i_E} \text{ and } \beta=\frac{\Delta i_C}{\Delta i_B}$$

Also $\beta = \frac{\alpha}{1-\alpha} = \frac{0.98}{1-0.98} = 49$

$\therefore$ Voltage gain $= \beta = \frac{R_2}{R_1} = 49 \times 1000 = 49 \times 10^3$

53. (a) : Most amplifiers use the common emitter circuit configuration because the cricuit offers both current and voltage gains resulting in much higher power gain that can be obtained by a common-base amplifier. The other consideration for the use of the common-emitter amplifier is that its input resistance is higher and of the order of load resistance.

54. (b) : In case of an ideal gas internal energy depends only upon the temperature of the gas. Therefore, if an ideal gas undergoes an isothermal process, there will be no change in its internal energy

($\Delta U = 0$) Then $Q = W$.

55. (c) : When we pour hot water in beaker, the inner surface of the glass expands on heating. But heat from inside does not reach quickly the outer surface of the glass, because glass is a bad conductor of heat. Hence, the outer surface does not expand and the glass cracks.

56. (a) : Upto ordinary heights the change in the distance of a projectile from the centre of the earth is negligible compared to the radius of the earth. Hence projectile moves under a nearly uniform gravitational force and its path is parabolic. But for projectiles going to great heights, the gravitational force decreases in inverse poroportion to the square of the distance of the projectile from the centre of the earth. Under such a variable force the path of projectile is elliptical.

57. (a) : According to law of conservation of angular momentum, when sum of external torques acting on a system is zero, then the total angular momentum of the system remains constant.

$\tau = 0$, $L = I\omega$ = Constant

If I increases, ω decreases and vice versa.

58. (a)

59. (a) : Impulse = Force × time duration
= Change in momentum

A large force acting for a short time to produce a finite change in momentum is called an impulsive force.

60. (c) : Both the quantities are dimensionless. Resistance × conductance = $R \times 1/R = (M^0L^0T^0) = 1$ and Dielectric constant K is dimensionless.

CHEMISTRY

61. (c) : The fluoride ion, by a process of hydrogen bonding, forms the anion, HF_2^-. The compound is written as $K^+[HF_2]^-$.

62. (b)

63. (d) : $2KI + H_2SO_4 + H_2O_2 \longrightarrow K_2SO_4 + 2H_2O + I_2$

$2Na_2S_2O_3 + I_2 \longrightarrow Na_2S_4O_6 + 2NaI$

milli eq. of H_2O_2 in 50 ml = milli eq. of I_2
= milli eq. of $Na_2S_2O_3$

milli eq. of H_2O_2 in 25 ml = 20 × 0.3 = 6

milli eq. of H_2O_2 in 1000 ml $= \frac{6}{25} \times 1000 = 240$

Equivalent per litre $= \frac{240}{1000}$

Gram per litre of $H_2O_2 = \frac{240}{1000} \times 17 = 4.08$ g/L

(Equivalent weight of $H_2O_2 = \frac{34}{2} = 17$).

64. (c): Silicones are organic silicon polymers containing Si–O–Si linkages.

$$\begin{array}{ccccccc} & R & & R & & R & \\ -O- & Si & -O- & Si & -O- & Si & -O- \\ & O & & O & & O & \\ -O- & Si & -O- & Si & -O- & Si & -O- \\ & R & & R & & R & \end{array}$$ (cross linked silicone)

65. (c): $\alpha = \sqrt{\frac{K_a}{C}} = \sqrt{\frac{6.6 \times 10^{-4}}{0.01}} = \sqrt{6.6 \times 10^{-2}} = 0.257$

$[H^+] = C\alpha = 0.01 \times 0.257 = 2.57 \times 10^{-3}$

pH = 3 – log2.5 = 2.60

66. (a):

	$A \longrightarrow$	B +	C +	D
Initial	a	0	0	0
After time t	$a - x$	x	x	x

It is given that $a = P_0$ ...(i)

$a - x + x + x + x = P$

or $a + 2x = P$ ...(ii)

From (i),

$P_0 + 2x = P$ or $x = \frac{P - P_0}{2}$

From rate equation

$$k = \frac{2.303}{t} \log \frac{a}{a-x}$$

$$= \frac{2.303}{t} \log \frac{P_0}{P_0 - \left(\frac{P - P_0}{2}\right)} = \frac{2.303}{t} \log \frac{2P_0}{3P_0 - P}$$

67. **(b)**

68. **(d) :** $2SO_{3(g)} \rightleftharpoons 2SO_{2(g)} + O_{2(g)}$

Initial conc. 1.0 mole   0.0 mole   0.0 mole

Equilibrium 0.4 mole   0.6 mole   0.3 mole

$\Rightarrow$ Equilibrium constant is given by :

$$K = \frac{[SO_2]^2[O_2]}{[SO_3]^2} = \frac{(0.6)^2(0.3)}{(0.4)^2} = 0.675 \approx 0.68$$

69. **(d) :** If acid is 4.5% ionized then $\alpha = 0.45$.

ΔT_f = molality $\times K_f = 0.1 \times 1.86 = 0.186$

$\Delta T_{exp} = \Delta T_N(1 + \alpha) = 0.186(1 + 0.45) = 0.269°C$

70. **(d) :** Diopside $\rightarrow CaMg[(SiO_3)_2]$.

71. **(a)**

72. **(b) :** Tincture of iodine is an aqueous solution of I_2 in KI.

73. **(b) :** We know that

specific conductance = Cell constant × conductance

$\Rightarrow$ Cell constant = Resistance × sp. conductance

$= 55 \times 0.0112 = 0.616\ cm^{-1}$

74. **(b) :** The dispersal of the charge stabilizes the carbocation. More the number of electron donating groups are present, greater the dispersal of positive charge and therefore more the stability of carbocation can be observed.

So, the order is

$CH_3 - \overset{+}{C}H - OCH_3 > CH_3 - \overset{+}{C}H - CH_3 > CH_3 - \overset{+}{C}H - COCH_3$

75. **(c):** (m-xylene, with CH_3 and CH_3) $+ 3O_3 \longrightarrow$ (triozonide, with CH_3 and H_3C) $\xrightarrow{Zn/OH}$

$2CH_3-C=O$ (over $H-C=O$) + CHO (over CHO)

Methyl glyoxal   glyoxal

76. **(c):** $H_3C-CH-CH_3$ (attached to benzene) $\xrightarrow{KMnO_4}$ $COOH$ (attached to benzene) $\xrightarrow[\text{heat}]{\text{soda - lime}}$ (benzene)

77. **(a):** Benzene can be prepared by cyclization of long chain alkanes on heating at 500 - 550°C under high pressure in presence of catalyst Cr_2O_3 supported on alumina or $Pt - Al_2O_3$ (*i.e.*, catalytic reforming)

$$\underset{n\text{-hexane}}{C_6H_{14}} \xrightarrow[\text{773 K, at high pressure}]{Cr_2O_3/Al_2O_3} \underset{A}{C_6H_6} + 4H_2$$

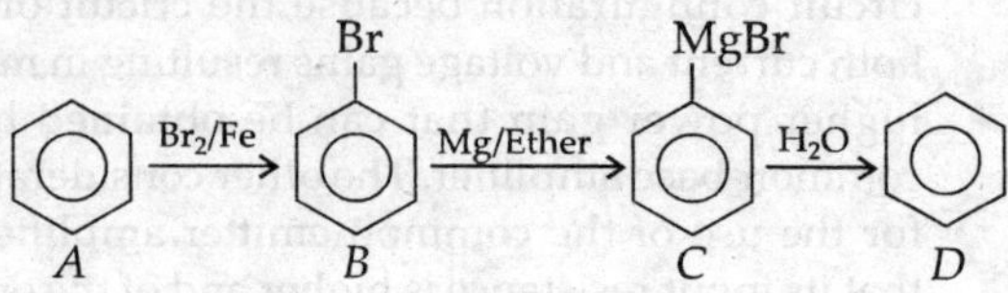

78. **(b)**

79. **(b)**

80. **(c):** Molarity

$$= \frac{\text{wt. of solute}}{\text{mol. wt.}} \times \frac{1000}{\text{vol. of solution (in ml.)}}$$

$$\left(\text{Volume of solution} = \frac{\text{mass}}{\text{density}} = \frac{100}{1.84} = 54.34\ \text{ml}\right)$$

$$\text{Now molarity} = \frac{98}{98} \times \frac{1000}{54.34} = 18.4\ \text{M}$$

81. **(b) :** In solution, $x_A = 0.30$; $x_B = 0.70$

In vapour phase, $x'_A = 0.60$; $x'_B = 0.40$

Using Dalton's law and Raoult's law

$$x'_A = 0.60 = \frac{p_A}{P} = \frac{p_A}{p_A + p_B} = \frac{0.30\ p_A^\circ}{0.30\ p_A^\circ + 0.70\ p_B^\circ}$$

$$x'_B = 0.40 = \frac{p_B}{P} = \frac{p_B}{p_A + p_B} = \frac{0.70\ p_B^\circ}{0.30\ p_A^\circ + 0.70\ p_B^\circ}$$

$$\frac{x'_A}{x'_B} = \frac{0.60}{0.40} = \frac{0.30\ p_A^\circ}{0.70\ p_B^\circ}$$

$$\frac{p_A^\circ}{p_B^\circ} = \frac{0.60 \times 0.70}{0.40 \times 0.30} = \frac{7}{2} = 3.5$$

82. **(b) :** For n moles of an ideal gas $PV = nRT$

or $V = n\dfrac{RT}{P}$

Differentiating with respect to T at constant P, we have

$$\left(\frac{\partial V}{\partial T}\right)_P = \frac{nR}{P} = \frac{V}{T}$$

$$\alpha = \frac{1}{V}\left(\frac{\partial V}{\partial T}\right)_P = \frac{1}{V} \times \frac{V}{T} = \frac{1}{T}$$

83. **(a):** SeF_4 and XeO_2F_2 are both sp^3d hybridized, trigonal bipyramidal and see-saw shaped with 1 lone pair of electrons each.

SF_4 has 1 lone pair, XeF_2 has 3 lone pairs. $XeOF_4$

is square pyramidal with 1 lone pair, TeF_4 is see-saw shaped with 1 lone pair, $SeCl_4$ has see-saw shape with 1 lone pair, XeF_4 has planar shape with 2 lone pairs.

84. **(c):** Stability of superoxides increases with increase in size and electropositivity of the metal. Hence the order $CsO_2 > RbO_2 > KO_2$.

85. **(b)**

86. **(c):** $(CH_3)_3CO^-$ is a better base than a nucleophile. Hence elimination occurs. The product formed is resonance stabilised.

87. **(a):** Equivalent weight of metal carbonate = 20 + 30 = 50

2.5 g of metal carbonate $= \frac{2.5}{50} = 0.05$ eq.

Number of equivalent of H_2SO_4 would have reacted = 0.05

Number of equivalent of H_2SO_4 taken

$= \frac{100 \times 1}{1000} = 0.1$

Number of equivalent of H_2SO_4 remains unreacted = 0.1 – 0.05 = 0.05 eq.

∴ Number of equivalent of alkali consumed = 0.05 eq.

milli eq. = Normality × Volume in mL

∴ $1.0 \times V = 0.05 \times 1000$

$V = \frac{0.05 \times 1000}{1.0} = 50$ ml

88. **(c):** In methyl alcohol, F^- ion is solvated but in DMSO or CH_3CN (aprotic solvent) F^- ion is not solvated. Unsolvated F^- ion acts more efficiently as a nucleophile.

89. **(d)** : Being covalent, BeF_2 has the lowest melting point (800°C) while other fluorides melt at around 1300°C.

90. **(b)** : Because of its smallest size, Li^+ has highest hydration energy and hence the highest stability of hydrated Li^+ ion.

91. **(d)** : When the ends of alkene containing n double bonds are different, the number of geometrical isomers is 2^n. Thus for

$CH_3-CH=CH-CH=CH-Cl$.

Number of geometrical isomers = $2^2 = 4$

When the ends of alkene containing n double bonds are same, then the number of geometrical isomers = $2^{n-1} + 2^{p-1}$

where $p = \frac{n}{2}$ for even n and $\frac{n+1}{2}$ for odd n, thus for

$CH_3-CH=CH-CH=CH-CH_3$

Number of geometrical isomers

$= 2^{2-1} + 2^{\frac{2}{2}-1} = 2^1 + 2^0 = 2 + 1 = 3.$

92. **(a)** :

	α-D glucose ⇌	β-D glucose
Initial	1	0
At equilibrium	1 – α	α

$K = \frac{\alpha}{1-\alpha} = 1.8$

Solving α = 0.642

1 – α = 0.358

Percent of α-D glucose remaining at equilibrium = 35.8%.

93. **(b)** : $C_6H_5-CH_2-CH_2-Br \xrightarrow[-HBr]{EtO^{\ominus}} C_6H_5-CH=CH_2$

2-phenyl ethyl bromide

It is a primary bromide. So it will undergo elimination either by E2 or E1cB. Since there is no deuterium exchange in C_2H_5OD solvent, C – H bond is not broken to form carbanion. Hence the actual mechanism is E2 only.

$$Ph-\underset{\underset{EtO-H}{}}{\overset{H}{C}}-\overset{Br}{C}-H \rightarrow Ph-CH=CH_2 + EtOH + Br^-$$

94. **(a):** Br_2O (116°), Cl_2O (111°), OF_2 (105°)

In OF_2 repulsion between lone pairs is greater than that between bond pair since electrons are away from O and nearer to F. In Cl_2O, bonding electrons are nearer to O than to Cl, so the bond angle is greater than 109°28′. In Br_2O, the bonding electrons are more closer to oxygen than in Cl_2O, so the bond angle is largest (116°).

95. **(a):** $\alpha = \frac{\Lambda_c}{\Lambda^\circ_m} = \frac{176.2\ \Omega^{-1}\ cm^2\ mol^{-1}}{405.2\ \Omega^{-1}\ cm^2\ mol^{-1}} = 0.435$

$K = \frac{[H^+][F^{-1}]}{[HF]} = \frac{C\alpha^2}{1-\alpha} = \frac{(0.002\ M)(0.435)^2}{1-0.435}$

96. (c): In Oppenauer's oxidation, secondary alcohol is oxidised to corresponding ketone in the presence of aluminium tertiary butoxide. Other oxidisable groups are not affected.

$$\begin{matrix}R_1\\R_2\end{matrix}\!\!>CHOH + [(CH_3)_3C-O]_3Al \xrightarrow{CH_3COCH_3} \begin{matrix}R_1\\R_2\end{matrix}\!\!>C=O + CH_3CHOH-CH_3$$

97. (c): $GeCl_4$ is more stable than $GeCl_2$. Ge has greater tendency to form +4 state than +2 state.

98. (a): The entropy change for a process, when T and P are the variables is given by

$$\Delta S = C_P \ln\frac{T_2}{T_1} - R\ln\frac{P_2}{P_1}$$

For an isobaric process $P_1 = P_2$. Hence the above equation reduces to

$$C_P \ln\frac{T_2}{T_1} = \Delta S.$$

or $\Delta S = 2.303 C_p \log\frac{T_2}{T_1}$.

99. (b): $C_6H_{11}-Mg-Br + CH_3-C\equiv N \longrightarrow CH_3-\underset{C_6H_{11}}{\underset{|}{C}}=N-MgBr \xrightarrow{H_3O^{\oplus}} CH_3-\underset{C_6H_{11}}{\underset{|}{C}}=O$ (A)

$C_6H_{11}-Mg-Br + CH_3-\overset{O}{\overset{||}{C}}-OC_2H_5 \longrightarrow CH_3-\overset{O-MgBr}{\overset{|}{\underset{C_6H_{11}}{\underset{|}{C}}}}-OC_2H_5 \xrightarrow{H_3O^{\oplus}} CH_3-\overset{OH}{\overset{|}{\underset{C_6H_{11}}{\underset{|}{C}}}}-OH \xrightarrow{-H_2O} CH_3-\underset{C_6H_{11}}{\underset{|}{C}}=O$ (B)

Thus in both cases, the same product, cyclohexyl methyl ketones is formed.

100. (a): Alkyl halides are starting materials for Grignard reagents which are used for preparing number of organic compounds.

$CH_3-Mg-Br$ + cyclohexanone $\longrightarrow$ 1-methylcyclohexyl-OMgBr (CH_3, OMgBr) $\xrightarrow{H_3O^+}$ 1-methylcyclohexanol (CH_3, OH) [A] $\xrightarrow[-H_2O]{HBr}$ 1-bromo-1-methylcyclohexane (CH_3, Br) [B] $\xrightarrow{Mg/Ether}$ (CH_3, Mg−Br) [C] $\xrightarrow{CH_3-\overset{H}{\overset{|}{C}}=O}$ (CH_3, $-\underset{CH_3}{\underset{|}{C}}(H)-OMgBr$) $\xrightarrow{H_3O^+}$ (CH_3, $\underset{CH_3}{\underset{|}{CHOH}}$) [D]

101. (a): It is a temporary effect. It comes into play instantaneously at the demand of the attacking reagent and as soon as the attacking reagent is removed the original condition is restored.

$$A{=}B \rightleftharpoons A^+ - B^-$$

This effect is applicable on a multiple bond.

102. (c): $CaCl_2$ forms addition products with alcohol and ammonia. ($CaCl_2.4NH_3$ or $CaCl_2.\ 4C_2H_5OH$).

103. (a)

104. (c):

$$\underset{cis\text{-2-butene}}{\begin{matrix}H_3C-C-H\\ \|\\ H_3C-C-H\end{matrix}} \xrightarrow[\text{(cold)}]{\text{Alk. }KMnO_4} \underset{\text{(Meso)}}{\begin{matrix}CH_3\\ |\\ H-C-OH\\ |\\ H-C-OH\\ |\\ CH_3\end{matrix}}$$

Alkaline $KMnO_4$ always gives *cis*-addition on olefins.

105. (a)

106. (a)

107. (b) : Ag^+ forms complex with the alkene by $p\pi$-$d\pi$ bonding giving an ion and the solubility increases.

$$Ag^+ \text{ bonded (dashed) to both C atoms of } C \text{---} C$$

108. (c): $\Delta G = \Delta H - T\Delta S$

$-ve = \Delta H - [T(-ve)]$ (as spontaneous)

Exothermic reactions may be accompanied by increase or decrease of randomness.

109. (a): In case of H_2, compressibility factor increases with the pressure. At 273 K, $Z > 1$ which shows that it is difficult to compress the gas as compared to ideal gas. In this case, repulsive force dominates.

110. (b) : $(CH_3)_2N-C_6H_4-CHO \xrightarrow{\text{alc. KCN}}$ $(CH_3)_2N-C_6H_4-\overset{O}{\overset{\|}{C}}-\underset{H}{\underset{|}{\overset{OH}{\overset{|}{C}}}}-C_6H_4-N(CH_3)_2$

111. (c): As atoms in S_8 molecule undergo sp^3 hybridisation and contain two lone pairs of electrons on each and exists as staggered 8 atoms-rings.

112. (a): Formate ion shows resonance and gives rise to identical bond lengths.

$$H-C(=O)-O-H \quad (C=O: 1.23\ \text{Å},\ C-O: 1.36\ \text{Å}) \qquad \left[H-C(\cdots O)_2\right]^- Na^+ \quad (\text{both } 1.27\ \text{Å})$$

Sodium formate

113. (b) : The lone pair electrons on N atom in $AgNO_2$ attacks C_2H_5Br to form nitroethane as the major product.

114. (d) : Increase in pressure favours melting of ice into water because at higher pressure melting point of ice is lowered.

According to Le-Chatelier's principle, if pressure is increased the equilibrium will shift in direction which produces smaller number of moles.

115. (b) : Ebonite is a very hard rubber contains 30-40% sulphur.

116. (c): B does not have vacant *d*-orbitals (sub-shell) as its valence shell.

117. (c): It is known that esters with α-hydrogens form carbanion when treated with base. It brings about nucleophilic substitution at the carbonyl group of the other molecule of the ester to yield β-keto ester. $LiAlH_4$ reduces esters to alcohols.

118. (d) : In a titration of strong base and weak acid phenolphthalein is used as indicator.

Methyl orange changes its colour in pH of range 3 to 5.

119. (b) : Millon's test is used for proteins. When Millon's reagent is added to the aqueous solution of a protein, a white precipitate is formed.

120. (a)

BIOLOGY

121. (d) : WBCs can change their shape like *Amoeba* and are thus, capable of amoeboid movement. This enables them to squeeze out of blood capillaries into the tissues. This process is called diapedesis.

122. (b) : Valium is a benzodiazephine (sedative) that gives a feeling of relaxation, calmness or drowsiness in the body. Morphine is the main opium alkaloid that depresses respiratory centre and contributes to the fall in blood pressure. Amphetamines are synthetic drugs and are stimulant in nature. Hashish is a hallucinogen.

123. (b) : The organ of Corti consists of outer hair cells, inner hair cells, inner pillar cells, outer pillar cells, tunnel of Corti, phalangeal cells (cells of Deiters), cells of Hensen and cells of Claudius. The sensory hairs project from the outer ends of the hair cells into the scala media, while from the inner end of the cells nerve fibres arise, which unite to form the cochlear nerve.

124. (b)

125. (a): *Homo erectus* appeared about 1.7 million years ago in middle pleistocene. *H. erectus* evolved from *Homo habilis*. He was about 1.5–1.8 metres tall.

126. (d)

127. (c): *Entamoeba histolytica* is a monogenetic parasite, *i.e.*, living in a single host, in the large intestine of humans. It causes amoebiasis or amoebic dysentery.

128. (b) : The ventral nerve cord, as its name suggests, is a cord of nervous tissue that runs the length of the animal in the lower part of its body. It is the characteristic of lower chordates like leech, cockroach and scorpion.

129. (c): Ciliated epithelium is a region of epithelium consisting of columnar or cuboidal cells bearing hairlike appendages that are capable of beating rapidly. Ciliated epithelium performs the functions of moving particles of fluids over the epithelial surface. Cuboidal ciliated epithelium occurs in certain parts of uriniferous tubules whereas columnar ciliated epithelium occurs in fallopian tubules, nasal passages, bronchioles, small bronchi and buccopharyngeal cavity of frog. It often occurs in the vicinity of mucus secreting goblet cells.

130. (a): Borderline personality disorder (BPD) is a serious mental illness. Borderline describing a personality disorder characterized by unstable and intense relationships, exploiting and manipulating other people, rapidly changing moods, recurrent suicidal or self injuring acts & a prevasive inner feelings of emptiness & boredom.

A mood disorder is a condition where the prevailing emotional moods are distorted or inappropriate to the circumstances. Addiction is a state of dependence produced by the habitual taking of drugs, alcohol etc. Schizophrenia is a group of severe mental disorders characterized by disturbances of languages and communications, thought disturbances that may involve distortion of reality, misperceptions, delusions and hallucination, mood changes etc.

131. (b) : At sexual maturity, the undifferentiated primordial germ cells divide several times by mitosis to produce a large number of spermatogonia. Each spermatogonium then actively grows to a larger primary spermatocyte. Each primary spermatocyte undergoes two successive divisions, called maturation divisions. The first maturation division is reductional or meiotic. Hence, the primary spermatocyte divides into the haploid daughter cells called secondary spermatocytes.

132. (d) : Oral contraceptive pills inhibit ovulation and implantation. They have to be taken daily for 21 days starting within the first five days of menstrual cycle. After a gap of 7 days, it has to be repeated.

133. (b) : Patella is a sesamoid bone. Sesamoid bones are small rounded masses of bones formed in tendons at the joints where they are subjected to great pressure.

134. (a)

135. (b) : Secretin and cholecystokinin are secreted by Brunner's gland located in duodenum. Secretin causes the pancreas to secrete alkaline pancreatic juice and stimulates bile production in the liver. Cholecystokinin induces the gall bladder to contract and eject bile into the intestine and stimulates the pancreas to secrete its digestive enzymes.

136. (c): The chromosome complement of *Triticum aestivum* (2n = 26) is similar to that of *Gossypium* whose ploidy level is also 2n = 26. *Zea mays* has ploidy level of 2n = 20. *Secale* and *Aegilops* both have the similar ploidy level of 2n = 14.

137. (b) : Eugenics is the study of methods of improving the quality of human populations by the application of genetic principles. Positive eugenics would seek to do this by selective breeding programmes. Negative eugenics aims to eliminate harmful genes (*e.g.*, those causing haemophilia and colour blindness) by counselling any prospective parents who are likely to be carriers.

138. (c): DNA polymerase can polymerize nucleotides only in $5' \rightarrow 3'$ direction on $3' \rightarrow 5'$ strand because it adds them at the $3'$ end. Since the two strands of DNA run in antiparallel directions, the two templates provide different ends for replication. Replication over the two templates thus proceeds in opposite directions. One strand with polarity $3' \rightarrow 5'$ forms its complementary strand continuously because $3'$ end of the latter is open for elongation. It is called leading strand. Replication is discontinuous on the other template with polarity $5' \rightarrow 3'$ because only a short segment of DNA strand can be built in $5' \rightarrow 3'$ direction due to exposure of a small stretch of template at one time. Short segments of replicated DNA are called Okazaki fragments.

139. (d) : Photosystem I is located in the nonappressed part of grana thylakoids as well as stroma thylakoids. In this photosystem chlorophyll :

carotenoid content is high. Its photocentre is P_{700}. Pigment molecules of PS I absorb at or below 700 nm wavelenth of light. It receives electrons from photosystem II. Photosystem I is involved in both cyclic and non cyclic photophosphorylation. It is not connected with photolysis of water. Usually it hands over its electron to $NADP^+$.

140. (d) : Bark is a loose term and is used to define all the tissues outside vascular cambium. It is differentiated into outer bark or rhytidome (consisting of dead cells) and inner bark (of living cells, *i.e.*, periderm, cortex, pericycle and secondary phloem). The outer layers of the bark are being constantly peeled off on account of the formation of new secondary vascular tissues in the interior. Bark is insect repellent, decay proof, fire-proof and acts as a heat screen.

141. (a): The cotton fibres represent epidermal prolongations of seed coat cells. A raw cotton fibre, on average, gives the following values on analysis : cellulose, 94%, protein - 1.3%, pectic substances - 0.9%, ash - 1.2%, wax - 0.6%, sugars - 0.3% and traces of pigments and mineral matter.

142. (b) : Mycoplasma are the smallest and simplest free living Gram negative prokaryotes or monerans. A cell wall is absent. Plasma membrane forms the outer boundary of the cell. A substantial amount of polysaccharides having acetyl glucosamine are associated with cell membrane.

143. (a): Sexual reproduction *in Spirogyra* takes place by the process of conjugation. In *Spirogyra*, the process of conjugation may be of two types – scalariform conjugation and lateral conjugation. Scalariform conjugation occurs in heterothallic species. Lateral conjugation occurs between the adjacent cells of the same filament of homothallic species of *Spirogyra*. Lateral conjugation are of two types. They are indirect lateral conjugation (chain type) and direct lateral conjugation.

144. (c): Sucrose, glucose and fructose, all the three sugars are found in plants. Sucrose is the commercial sugar which is obtained from sugarcane. Glucose is the main respiratory substrate in plants and animals. Fructose can also function similarly. Moreover fructose is also the common fruit sugar.
Lactose or milk sugar is found naturally in milk. It is reducing sugar which is formed in the mammary glands of mammal through condensation of two hexose molecules.

145. (d) : The binding site of *t*RNA with *m*RNA is anticodon loop and with amino acid is CCA end, as shown in the figure.

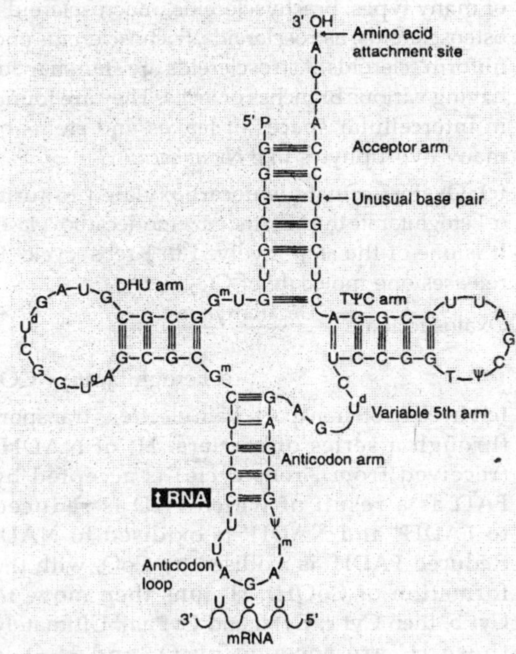

146. (d) : 1 map unit or centimorgan is equivalent to 1% recombination between two genes. The frequency of recombination can be used to depict the arrangement of the genes.
Recombination frequency between three genes is

A – B = 9%
A – C = 17% and
B – C = 26%

By manipulating the three possibilities of their arrangements A – B – C, A – C – B and B – A – C, it was found that the three gene must be arranged in the order B – A – C with distance between B – A being 9 cM and A – C being 17 cM and the distance between B – C being 26 cM.

147. (d) : Spike is a racemose inflorescence that bears sessile flowers in an acropetal fashion, *e.g.*, chaff flower (*Achyranthes*), bottle brush (*Callistemon*), *Adathoda vasica, Amaranthus.*

148. (b) : Lignin is a complex organic polymer that is deposited within the cellulose of plant cells. The lignin content is high in jute fibres which causes deterioration very quickly.

149. (d) : Sclereids are highly thickened dead sclerenchyma cells with very narrow cavities. They may also be branched. They provide stiffness to the parts in which they occur. Sclereids are of many types: brachysclereids, macrosclereids, osteosclereids, astrosclereids, trichosclereids and filiform sclereids. Astrosclereids are star-shaped, having various branches or arms. They are found in intercellular spaces of leaves and stems of many hydrophytes like *Nymphaea*.

150. (c): Oxalosuccinate is decarboxylated to form α-ketoglutarate through the enzyme decarboxylase. It is one of the step involved in Krebs' cycle. It releases one molecule of CO_2.

$$\text{Oxalosuccinate} \xrightarrow[Mg^{2+}]{\text{Decarboxylase}} \alpha\text{-ketoglutarate} + CO_2$$

151. (c): In electron transport chain electrons transport through a series of carriers. H^+ of $NADH^+$ (received from Krebs cycle) is accepted by FAD as a result of which FAD is reduced to $FADH^+$ and $NADH^+$ is oxidised to NAD. Reduced $FADH^+$ is oxidised by CoQ, with the formation of $CoQH^+$. H^+ ions then move to Cyt b, then Cyt c, Cyt a and Cyt aa_3. Ultimately these H^+ are acceped by O_2 and H_2O is formed.

152. (d) : Plants require many organic and inorganic nutrients to complete their life-cycle. It has been established that some elements are required by plants in relatively large amount and are called major elements or macronutrients, *e.g.*, C, H, O, N, S, P, K, Ca and Mg.
Microelements or minor elements or trace elements are required by plants in very small amount, less than 1ppm. *E.g.*, Fe, Cu, B, Zn, Mn, Mo, Cl. Thus Cr is not a microelement.

153. (c): The common peafowl or peacock, *Pavo cristatus*, called 'Mor' or Mayur' in hindi, is the national bird of India. It occurs throughout India upto 1650 meters in the himalayas. It displays a well-marked sexual dimorphism, the male having a gorgeous ocellated tail.

154. (d) : Acid rain is rainfall and other forms of precipitation with a pH less than 5. pH of normal rain is 5.6 – 6.5. It is caused by the large scale emission of acidic gases into the atmosphere from thermal power plants, industries and automobiles.

155. (d) : Interferon is a group of proteins that increases the resistance of cells to viral infection. Interferon also acts as cytokines and can enhance some immune responses. Three types of interferons have so far been discovered, alpha, beta and gamma, all of which have immune-modulating effects. Interferons are used in the treatment of cancer and autoimmune diseases.

156. (d) : Bacteria become resistant to antibiotic by either producing enzymes or forming impermeable capsule and modifying the target of the drug.

157. (b) : Active transport is the uphill movement of materials across the membrane where the solute particles move against their concentration gradient or electro-chemical gradient. It takes place through the agency of special organic molecules called carrier molecules, carrier particles or carrier proteins. There is a special carrier molecule for each solute particle (ion or molecule). The carrier has its binding site on two surfaces of the membrane. The solute particle (or substrate) combines with the carrier to form carrier solute complex. In the bound state the carrier undergoes a conformational change which transports the solute to the other side of the membrane. Here the solute is released. Energy is used in bringing about the conformational change in the carrier. It is provided by ATP.

158. (d) : Co-dominance is the phenomenon when the two genes neither show dominant-recessive relationship nor show intermediate condition, but both of them express themselves simultaneously. This has been reported in roan character of cattle (*i.e.*, patches of 2 different colours on the skin).

159. (a): The first bioherbicide is devine, which is a mycoherbicide, based on fungus *Phytophthora palmivora*. It is being used since 1981 to control *Morrenia odorata* (milkweed vines) in *Citrus* orchards.

160. (c): Ripened ovary or fertilized ovary is called fruit. The wall of the ovary forms fleshy or dry fruit wall known as pericarp. It means that the pericarp is developed from pistil or carpel.

161. (a) : Biotic or ecological succession is the formation of a series of biotic communities at the same site over a period of time one after the other, till a stable climax community develops over the area. It occurs generally in bare areas. Primary succession takes place on a biological sterile soilless primary barren area. Secondary succession takes place in a recently denuded area which still contains a lot of organic debris, remains and propagules of previous living organisms. The area has become bared due to destruction of the community previously present. The baring of an area can be caused due to forest fire, deforestation for wood, timber and habitat, overgrazing, landslides or earthquakes, excessive and repeated droughts, fallowing a cropland and repeated floods.

162. **(d)** : Connective tissue consists of variously shaped cells lying in an extracellular material called matrix. It joins one tissue to another in the organs. Connective tissue is absent inside the central nervous system i.e. brain and spinal cord and thus has no function in the conduction of nerve impulse.The nerve cells of the brain and spinal cord are held together by supporting cells called neuroglia cells.

163. **(a)**: Based on the mode of secretion, the glands are of three types : mesocrine, apocrine and holocrine. Mammary glands that are present in mammals to feed the young ones with milk are the example of apocrine glands. In apocrine glands, the secretion accumulates as secretory granules in the distal part of the cell. This part later breaks down and leaves as a secretion.

164. **(b)** : Application of cytokinins to marketed vegetables can keep them fresh for several days. Shelf life of cut shoots and flowers is prolonged by employing the hormone cytokinin. The reason is that the cytokinin increases retention of chlorophyll and delayed senescence in leaves. Cytokinin as the name suggests, is essential for cell division or cytokinesis. It promotes cell division along with auxin by controlling the activity of cyclin dependent kinases.

165. **(c)**: Angina pectoris literally means "pain in the chest". It results from arteriosclerosis of the arteries that supply the heart muscle itself, i.e., the coronary arteries. Arteriosclerosis is the hardening of arteries and arterioles due to thickening of the fibrous tissue, and the consequent loss of elasticity.
Due to the lack of required expansion, the arteries are unable to carry extra blood to the heart muscle at the time of stress when the heart is beating more vigorously. Deprived of oxygen the heart muscle experiences constricting pain.

166. **(b)** : Most of the animals have sex organs. They are either males or females. But in some lower animals, the organs of both the sexes are found in the same individual. These are called bisexual or monoecious animals or hermaphrodites. In these animals, testes and ovaries do not mature simultaneously. For example in earthworm, testes mature earlier, while in others, *e.g.*, sea-squirt, ovaries mature earlier. These conditions are respectively called protandry and protogyny. They ensure cross fertilization. Cross fertilization is a process in which gametes derived from different individuals are united to form zygote. It involves the mixing of two different genetic materials. This is better than self-fertilization as it introduces variation by combining traits of two individuals.

167. **(d)** : A small, glandular, blind pouch of lymphatic tissue, the bursa lies on the dorsal side of the cloaca. It is lined with endoderm, and opens into the proctodaeum. In a young bird, bursa fabricii forms lymphocytes, and probably it produces antibodies and protects against local infection, but it atrophies in the adult before sexual maturity. It is also called cloacal thymus, because like thymus, it secretes lymphocytes. Thus it is not related with flight adaptation, rather it helps in immunity.

168. **(d)** : Glycolysis is the process of breakdown of glucose or similar hexose sugar into two molecules of pyruvic acid through a series of enzyme mediated reactions, releasing energy (ATP) and reducing power ($NADH_2$). It is the first step of respiration, which occurs inside the cytoplasm and is independent of O_2. In glycolysis, two molecules of ATP are consumed during double phosphorylation of glucose to form fructose 1, 6 diphosphate. Four molecules of ATP are produced in the conversion of 1, 3-diphosphoglycerate to 3-phosphoglycerate and phosphenol pyruvate to pyruvate whereas, two molecules of $NADH_2$ are formed during oxidation of glyceraldehyde 3-phosphate to 1, 3-diphosphoglycerate. Since, each NADH is equivalent to 3 ATP, so net gain in glycolysis is 8 ATP.

169. **(c)**: Restriction enzyme, a type of endonuclease, functions by "inspecting" the length of a DNA sequence. Once it finds a recognition sequence,

it binds and cut each of the two strands of the double helix at specific point leaving single stranded portions at the ends. This results in overhanging stretches called sticky ends. These are named so because they form hydrogen bonds with their complementary counter parts *i.e.* they can join similar complementary ends of DNA fragment from some other source with the help of DNA ligase. This stickiness of the ends facilitates the action of the enzyme DNA ligase, not DNA polymerase.

170. (a): Excess of nitrates in drinking water are harmful for human health and may be fatal for infants. Excessive use of fertilizers often leads to accumulations of nitrates in water. In infants excess nitrate reacts with haemoglobin to form nonfunctional methaemoglobin that impairs oxygen transport. This condition is termed as methaemoglobinemia or blue baby syndrome. The disease can damage respiratory and vascular systems and even cause suffocation.

171. (b) : Amniocentesis is a foetal sex determination and disorder test based on the chromosomal pattern in the amniotic fluid surrounding the developing embryo. It is withdrawal of a sample of the amniotic fluid surrounding the embryo in the uterus by piercing the amniotic sac through the abdominal wall. Amniotic fluid drawn from the uterus contains cells from the embryo (mostly shed from the skin). Cell cultures enable chromosome patterns to be studied so that prenatal diagnosis of chromosomal abnormalities (such as Down's syndrome) can be made. Metabolic errors and other diseases such as spina bifida, can also be diagnosed prenatally from the biochemistry of the cells.

172. (d) : Primary sporogenous cell gives rise to microspore mother cells or pollen mother cells (PMCs). They are sporophytic in nature *i.e.*, diploid. These cells undergo meiosis (reduction division) which gives rise to 4 microspores or pollens and this formation of microspores or pollens is called microsporo-genesis. Microspores represent the beginning of the gametophytic phase and they are haploid in nature.

173. (b) : Nucleus is the controlling centre of a cell as it contains chromosomes and genes. Chromosomes contain the DNA which by transcription prepare RNA which in turn leads to the formation of proteins by translation. These proteins regulate the various metabolic processes going in the cell. Besides this, nucleus contains genetic information for reproduction, development & behaviour of an organism.

Nuclear membrane is double layered, semipermeable and is perforated by minute, circular nuclear pores. The pore controls the passage of macromolecules like tRNAs, mRNAs, ribosomal proteins, enzymes etc. during different processes of transcription, translation etc.

174. (a): Calcitonin or thyrocalcitonin is secreted by parafollicular cells of thyroid stroma. It retards bone dissolution and stimulates excretion of calcium in urine. Thus, it lowers calcium level in extra cellular fluid (ECF). Parathormone is secreted by chief cells of parathyroid gland and is also known as Collip's hormone. It maintains blood calcium level by increasing its absorption from food in intestine and its reabsorption from nephrons in the kidney. Maintenance of proper calcium level is in fact, a combined function of parathormone and calcitonin. When calcium level falls below normal then parathormone maintains it by promoting its absorption, reabsorption and also by demineralization of bones. When blood calcium level exceeds above normal then calcitonin hormone increases excretion of calcium in urine.

175. (d) : Dark reaction is also known as light-independent phase. Unlike, light reaction, it does not require light as an essential factor. Thus can takes place both in the presence or absence of light. The term dark reaction does not mean that it takes place only in dark period or at night. CO_2 fixation occurs in both C_3 and C_4 cycle. In C_3 cycle, CO_2 is added by the enzyme, RuBisco to a 5 carbon compound RuBP that is converted to 2 molecules of 3-carbon PGA. In C_4 cycle the first product of CO_2 fixation (takes place in mesophyll) is a 4-carbon compound, oxaloacetic acid. It is seen in some tropical plants.

176. (c): The lightest atoms of nitrogen, carbon etc. formed the primitive atmosphere. Hydrogen atoms were most numerous and most reactive in primitive atmosphere. Hydrogen atoms combined with all oxygen atoms to form water leaving no free oxygen. Thus primitive atmosphere was reducing atmosphere (without free oxygen) unlike the present oxidising atmosphere (with free oxygen).

Formation of ozone layer is the consequence of modern oxidizing atmosphere having plenty of free oxygen. As more oxygen accumulated in the atmosphere (due to photosynthesis) ozone began to appear in the top layers.

177. (b) : The fossil of Java Ape-man was discovered from pleistocene rocks in central Java. The fossil of Peking man was discovered from the lime stone caves of Choukoutien near Peking while that of Heidelberg man was discovered in mid pleistocene. All these three fossils come under the category of *Homo erectus*.

Homo erectus appeared about 1.7 million years ago in middle pleistocene. *H. erectus* evolved from *Homo habilis*. He was about 1.5–1.8 metres tall. He had erect posture. His skull was flatter than that of modern man. He had protruding jaws, projecting brow ridges, small canines and large molar teeth. He made more elaborate tools of stones and bones, hunted big game and perhaps knew use of fire.

178. (b) : Hydrostatic pressure is the pressure which develops in an osmotic system due to osmotic entry or exit of water from it.

Loss of water produces a negative hydrostatic pressure or tension. It develops in xylem due to loss of water in transpiration. This is very important in transport of sap over long distances in plants.

A positive pressure develops in a plant cell or system due to entry of water into it. Positive hydrostatic pressure is also called turgor pressure. Due to turgor pressure the protoplast of a plant cell wall press the cell wall to the outside. The cell wall, being elastic, presses the protoplast with an equal and opposite force. The force exerted by the cell wall over the protoplast is called wall pressure (WP). Normally wall pressure is equal and opposite to turgor pressure except when the cell becomes flaccid.

179. (d) : Hyaluronidase, a hydrolytic enzyme is an acrosomal content in mammalian sperm. It helps at the time of fertilization during the penetration of sperm into ovum. Based on the amount of yolk mammalian eggs are alecithal means egg without yolk. Microlecithal eggs are with very little yolk e.g., sea urchin, starfish. On the basis of distribution of yolk telolecithal eggs are those eggs in which the yolk is concentrated towards the vegetal pole and cytoplasm and nucleus lie near the animal pole e.g., birds and reptiles.

180. (c): The law of segregation states that the two alleles controlling each character maintain indentity in the organism but during the formation of gametes or spores by meiosis move apart due to separation of the homologous chromosomes which bear them, so that each gamete or spore receives only one allele of each character on random basis. Since the gametes or spores possess one allele of each character, they are always pure. The law of segregation is, therefore, also called the law of purity of gametes/spores. Mendel's second law or the law of independent assortment states that the alleles of different characters located in different pairs of homologous chromosomes are independent of one another in their segregation during gamete formation and in coming together into the offspring by fertilization, both processes occurring randomly.

GENERAL KNOWLEDGE

181. (a)	**182.** (b)	**183.** (d)	**184.** (a)	**185.** (c)
186. (b)	**187.** (d)	**188.** (d)	**189.** (d)	**190.** (b)
191. (a)	**192.** (a)	**193.** (c)	**194.** (b)	**195.** (a)
196. (a)	**197.** (c)	**198.** (b)	**199.** (a)	**200.** (b)

☺☺☺

Chapterwise Index - '10

Physics • Chemistry • Biology

Use the index for topicwise analysis of this year's AIIMS paper and refer to these questions when you are practising MCQs chapterwise.

PHYSICS

Chapter's Name	Question No.	Total
Units and Dimensions	28, 33	2
Motion in One Dimension		
Motion in Two Dimensions	5, 14, 41, 42	4
Laws of Motion and Friction	15, 16, 43, 45	4
Work, Power and Energy	31, 56	2
Centre of Mass and Rotational Motion	8, 29, 48	3
Gravitation	57	1
Properties of Matter	10, 30, 32, 49, 50	5
Oscillations	38	1
Waves	9, 36, 37	3
Heat and Thermodynamics	17, 18, 19, 20	4
Electrostatics	11, 21, 27, 44	4
Current Electricity	25	1
Thermal and chemical effects of current	1, 58	2
Magnetic Effects of Current	6, 22, 55	3
Magnetism	7, 46	2
Electromagnetic Induction and Alternating Current	23, 39, 40	3
Electromagnetic Waves	47	1
Ray Optics	4, 54	2
Wave Optics		
Modern Physics	2, 12, 13, 24, 25, 26, 34, 59, 60	9
Solids and Semiconductor Devices	3, 51, 52	3
Universe		
Principles of Communication	53	1

CHEMISTRY

Chapter's Name	Question No.	Total
Basic Concepts	113	1
Atomic Structure	77, 91	2
Periodic Properties	65, 80, 84, 106	4
Chemical Bonding	78, 79, 114	3
Nuclear Chemistry	107, 112	2
Gaseous and Liquid States	70, 81	2
Solid State	64, 108, 118	3
Mole Concept & Solutions	92, 98, 117	3
Colloids, Surface Chemistry & Catalysis	61	1
Equilibrium	83, 102	2
Kinetics	63, 68, 109	3
Energetics	82	1
Electrochemistry	69, 76, 95, 99, 104	5
Redox Reactions		
Metallurgy		
Hydrogen and its Compounds	85	1
s-Block Elements	86, 96, 101	3
p-Block Elements	74, 94, 103	3
d- and *f*-Block Elements	62, 71, 110, 115	4
Complex Compounds	75, 119	2
Purification and Analysis of Organic Compound		
General Organic Chemistry	66, 100, 105	3
Aliphatic Hydrocarbons	67, 87, 120	3
Aromatic Hydrocarbons	116	1
Halogen Derivatives		
Alcohols, Phenols and Ethers	93, 97	2
Aldehydes and Ketones	90, 111	2
Carboxylic acids & their derivatives	88	1
Organic Compounds Containing Nitrogen	72, 89	2
Biochemistry		
Chemistry in Action	73	1
Environmental Chemistry		

BIOLOGY

Chapter's Name	Question No.	Total
General Biology	158	1
Biological Classification	122, 141, 157	3
Kingdom Monera	153	1
Kingdom Fungi		
Plant Kingdom	127	1
Cell and its Structural Components	125, 138	2
Cell Reproduction		
Cell Respiration		
Enzymes		
Biomolecules		
Mendelian Genetics	170	1
Hereditary Material	135	1
Anatomy of Flowering Plants	124, 162	2
Morphology of Flowering Plants		
Physiology of Flowering Plants	126, 132, 137, 151, 160, 166, 176	7
Embryology of Flowering Plants	136, 169	2
Growth and Development in Flowering Plants		
Angiosperm Families		
Ecology and Pollution	129, 134, 171	3
Applied Botany	139, 155	2
Animal Kingdom	142, 149, 163, 179	4
Genes and Chromosomes		
Gene regulation and Applied Genetics	156, 174	2
Human Genetics & Genetic Disorder	131, 140	2
Animal Tissue	150	1
Musculo-Skeletal System	130	1
Digestive System and Nutrition	121, 128, 145, 172, 180	5
Respiration	147, 173	2
Circulatory System and Immunity	143, 144, 164	3
Excretion and Osmoregulation	165	1
Reproduction and Embryonic Development	148, 152, 168	3
Nervous System and Sense Organs	178	1
Endocrine System	146, 161, 177	3
Common Human Disease	123, 133, 159, 175	4
Growth and Regeneration		
Evolution	154	1
Drug Addiction		
Applied Zoology	167	1
Wild Life and Conservation		
Human Population & Growth		

SOLVED PAPER
AIIMS - 2010

Time : 3½ Hours

Max. Marks : 200

PHYSICS

1. Transmission lines transmit a voltage of V volt to our houses from power stations, then the power P supplied by them is proportional to

   (a) $\frac{1}{V}$ (b) V
   (c) V^2 (d) $\frac{1}{V^2}$

2. Whenever a stream of electrons collides with a stream of photons, in this collision, which of the following is not conserved?

   (a) Linear momentum
   (b) Total energy
   (c) No. of photons
   (d) No. of electrons

3. The logic gate represented in following figure is

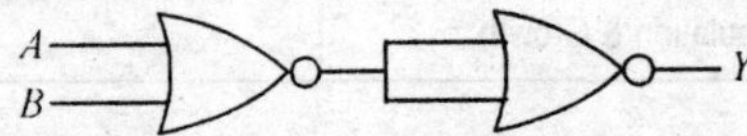

   (a) OR Gate (b) NOT Gate
   (c) NAND Gate (d) XOR Gate

4. For a person near point of vision is 100 cm. Then the power of lens he must wear so as to have normal vision, should be

   (a) +1 D (b) –1 D
   (c) +3 D (d) –3 D

5. Two projectiles of same mass have their maximum kinetic energies in ratio 4 : 1 and ratio of their maximum heights is also 4 : 1 then what is the ratio of their ranges ?

   (a) 2 : 1 (b) 4 : 1
   (c) 8 : 1 (d) 16 : 1

6. An uncharged particle is moving with a velocity of $\vec{v}$ in non-uniform magnetic field as shown.

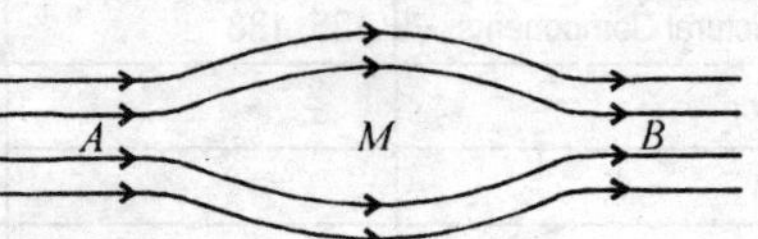

   Velocity $\vec{v}$ would be

   (a) Maximum at A & B
   (b) Minimum at A & B
   (c) Maximum at M (d) Same at all points

7. Which of the following is true regarding dimagnetic substances (symbols have their usual meaning)

   (a) $\mu_r > 1, \chi_m > 1$ (b) $\mu_r > 1, \chi_m < 1$
   (c) $\mu_r < 1, \chi_m < 0$ (d) $\mu_r < 1, \chi_m > 0$

8. What is moment of inertia of a cylinder of radius r, along its height ?

   (a) mr^2 (b) $\frac{mr^2}{2}$
   (c) $\frac{2mr^2}{5}$ (d) $\frac{mr^2}{5}$

9. A uniform string is vibrating with a fundamental frequency 'f'. The new frequency, if radius & length both are doubled would be

   (a) $2f$ (b) $3f$
   (c) $\frac{f}{4}$ (d) $\frac{f}{3}$

10. Two spherical soap bubbles of radii a and b in vacuum coaleasce under isothermal conditions. The resulting bubbles has a radius given by

    (a) $\frac{(a+b)}{2}$ (b) $\frac{ab}{a+b}$
    (c) $\sqrt{a^2+b^2}$ (d) $a + b$

11. What would be the voltage across C_3?

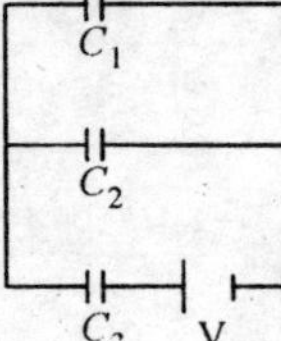

    (a) $\frac{(C_1+C_2)V}{C_1+C_2+C_3}$
    (b) $\frac{C_1V}{C_1+C_2+C_3}$

(c) $\dfrac{C_2V}{C_2+C_2+C_3}$

(d) $\dfrac{C_3V}{C_1+C_2+C_3}$

12. **What would be maximum wavelength for Brackett series of hydrogen-spectrum?**

(a) 74583 Å (b) 22790 Å
(c) 40519 Å (d) 18753 Å

13. **What would be the radius of second orbit of He^+ ion?**

(a) 1.058 Å (b) 3.023 Å
(c) 2.068 Å (d) 4.458 Å

14. **The position of a particle moving in the x-y plane at any time t is given by; $x = (3t^3 - 6t)$ metres; $y = (t^2 - 2t)$ metres. Select the correct statement.**

(a) acceleration is zero at $t = 0$
(b) velocity is zero at $t = 0$
(c) velocity is zero at $t = 1$ s
(d) velocity and acceleration of the particle are never zero.

15. **Two masses $M_1 = 5$ kg and $M_2 = 10$ kg are connected at the ends of an inextensible string passing over a frictionless pulley as shown. When the masses are released, then the acceleration of the masses will be**

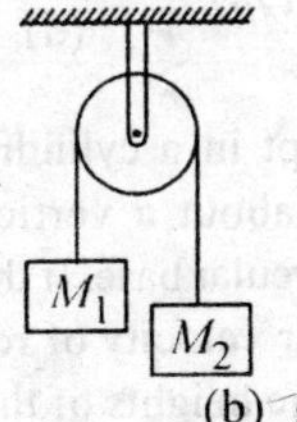

(a) g (b) $g/2$
(c) $g/3$ (d) $g/4$

16. **A block of mass m is pulled along a horizontal surface by applying a force at an angle θ with the horizontal. If the block travels with a uniform velocity and has a displacement d and the coefficient of friction is μ, then the work done by the applied force is**

(a) $\dfrac{\mu mgd}{\cos\theta+\mu\sin\theta}$ (b) $\dfrac{\mu mgd\cos\theta}{\cos\theta+\mu\sin\theta}$

(c) $\dfrac{\mu mgd\sin\theta}{\cos\theta+\mu\sin\theta}$ (d) $\dfrac{\mu mgd\cos\theta}{\cos\theta-\mu\sin\theta}$

17. **Pressure versus temperature graph of an ideal gas is as shown in figure. Density of the gas at point A is ρ_0. Density at point B will be**

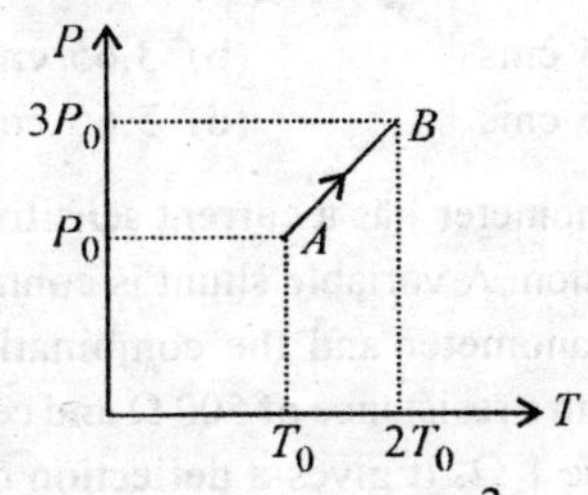

(a) $\dfrac{3}{4}\rho_0$ (b) $\dfrac{3}{2}\rho_0$

(c) $\dfrac{4}{3}\rho_0$ (d) $2\rho_0$

18. **The latent heat of vaporisation of a substance is always**

(a) greater than its latent heat of fusion
(b) greater than its latent heat of sublimation
(c) equal to its latent heat of sublimation
(d) less than its latent heat of fusion

19. **A reversible engine converts one-sixth of the heat input into work. When the temperature of the sink is reduced by 62°C, the efficiency of the engine is doubled. The temperatures of the source and sink are**

(a) 99°C, 37°C (b) 80°C, 37°C
(c) 95°C, 37°C (d) 90°C, 37°C

20. **Graph of specific heat at constant volume for a monoatomic gas is**

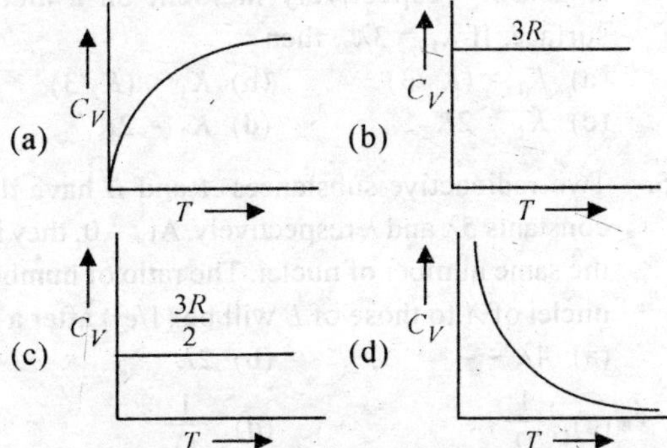

21. **In figure, a particle having mass $m = 5$ g and charge $q' = 2 \times 10^{-9}$ C starts from rest at point a and moves in a straight line to point b. What is its speed v at point b?**

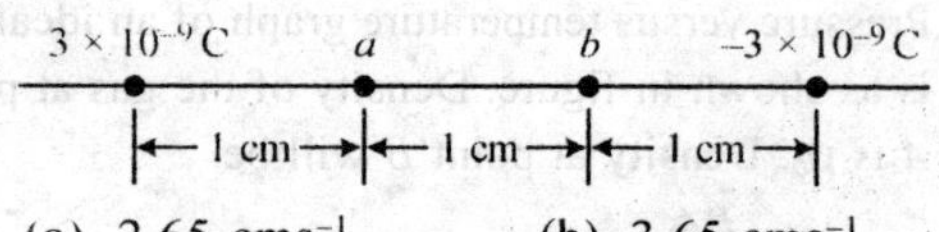

(a) 2.65 cms^{-1} (b) 3.65 cms^{-1}
(c) 4.65 cms^{-1} (d) 5.65 cms^{-1}

22. A galvanometer has a current sensitivity of 1 mA per division. A variable shunt is connected across the galvanometer and the combination is put in series with a resistance of 500 Ω and cell of internal resistance 1 Ω. It gives a deflection of 5 division for shunt of 5 ohm and 20 division for shunt of 25 ohm. The emf of cell is
(a) 47.1 V (b) 57.1 V
(c) 67.1 V (d) 77.1 V

23. A circular coil with a cross-sectional area of 4 cm^2 has 10 turns. It is placed at the center of a long solenoid that has 15 turns/cm and a cross-sectional area of 10 cm^2, as shown in the figure. The axis of the coil conicides with the axis of the solenoid. What is their mutual inductance ?

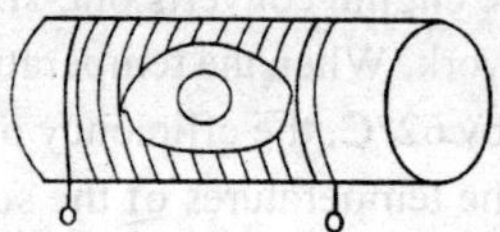

(a) 7.54 μH (b) 8.54 μH
(c) 9.54 μH (d) 10.54 μH

24. If K_1 and K_2 are maximum kinetic energies of photoelectrons emitted when lights of wavelengths λ_1 and λ_2 respectively incident on a metallic surface. If $\lambda_1 = 3\lambda_2$, then
(a) $K_1 > (K_2/3)$ (b) $K_1 < (K_2/3)$
(c) $K_1 = 2K_2$ (d) $K_2 = 2K_1$

25. Two radioactive substances *A* and *B* have decay constants 5λ and λ respectively. At $t = 0$, they have the same number of nuclei. The ratio of number of nuclei of *A* to those of *B* will be $(1/e^2)$ after a time
(a) 4λ (b) 2λ
(c) $\frac{1}{2\lambda}$ (d) $\frac{1}{4\lambda}$

26. The intensity of gamma radiation from a given source is *I*. On passing through 36 mm of lead, it is reduced to *I*/8. The thickness of lead which will reduce the intensity to *I*/2 will be
(a) 18 mm (b) 12 mm
(c) 6 mm (d) 9 mm

27. An electric charge 10^{-3} μC is placed at the origin (0, 0) of (*x*-*y*) co-ordinate system. Two points *A* and *B* are situated at $(\sqrt{2}, \sqrt{2})$ and (2,0) respectively. The potential difference between the points *A* and *B* will be
(a) 4.5 volt (b) 9 volt
(c) zero (d) 2 volt

28. If the energy, $E = G^p h^q c^r$, where *G* is the universal gravitational constant, *h* is the Planck's constant and *c* is the velocity of light, then the values of *p*, *q* and *r* are, respectively
(a) – 1/2, 1/2 and 5/2 (b) 1/2, – 1/2 and – 5/2
(c) – 1/2, 1/2 and 3/2 (d) 1/2, – 1/2 and – 3/2

29. Four holes of radius *R* are cut from a thin square plate of side 4*R* and mass *M*. The moment of inertia of the remaining portion about *z*-axis is

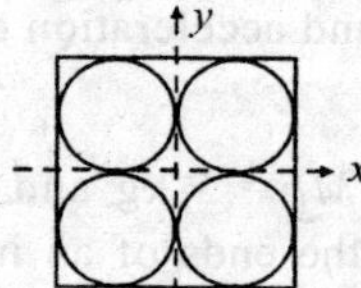

(a) $\frac{\pi}{12}MR^2$ (b) $\left(\frac{4}{3} - \frac{\pi}{4}\right)MR^2$
(c) $\left(\frac{4}{3} - \frac{\pi}{6}\right)MR^2$ (d) $\left(\frac{8}{3} - \frac{10\pi}{16}\right)MR^2$

30. A liquid is kept in a cylindrical vessel which is being rotated about a vertical axis through the centre of the circular base. If the radius of the vessel is *r* and angular velocity of rotation is ω, then the difference in the heights of the liquid at the centre of the vessel and the edge is
(a) $\frac{r\omega}{2g}$ (b) $\frac{r^2\omega^2}{2g}$
(c) $\sqrt{2gr\omega}$ (d) $\frac{\omega^2}{2gr^2}$

31. A block of mass 10 kg is moving in *x*-direction with a constant speed of 10 m/s. It is subjected to a retarding force $F = 0.1x$ joule/metre during its travel from $x = 20$ m to $x = 30$ m. Its final K.E. will be
(a) 475 J (b) 450 J
(c) 275 J (d) 250 J

32. A capillary tube of radius r is immersed in water and water rises in it to a height h. The mass of water in the capillary tube is 5 g. Another capillary tube of radius $2\,r$ is immersed in water. The mass of water that will rise in this tube is

(a) 2.5 g (b) 5.0 g
(c) 10 g (d) 20 g

33. Which of the following pairs does not have same dimensions ?

(a) impulse and momentum
(b) moment of inertia and moment of force
(c) angular momentum and Planck's constant
(d) work and torque.

34. The wavelength of Lymen series for first number is

(a) $\frac{4\times1.097\times10^7}{3}$ m (b) $\frac{3}{4\times1.097\times10^7}$ m
(c) $\frac{4}{3\times1.097\times10^7}$ m (d) $\frac{3}{4}\times1.097\times10^7$ m

35. In the circuit shown, current flowing through 25 V cell is

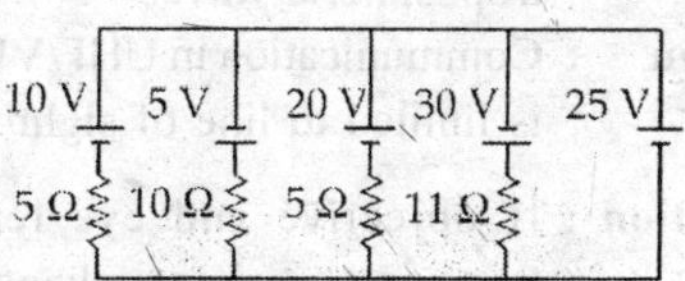

(a) 7.2 A (b) 10 A
(c) 12 A (d) 14.2 A

36. Five sinusoidal waves have the same frequency 500 Hz but their amplitudes are in the ratio $2:\frac{1}{2}:\frac{1}{2}:1:1$ and their phase angles $0, \frac{\pi}{6}, \frac{\pi}{3}, \frac{\pi}{2}$ and π respectively. The phase angle of resultant wave obtained by the superposition of these five waves is

(a) 30° (b) 45°
(c) 60° (d) 90°

37. The second overtone of an open pipe has the same frequency as the first overtone of a closed pipe 2 m long. The length of the open pipe is

(a) 8 m (b) 4 m
(c) 2 m (d) 1 m

38. Let T_1 and T_2 be the time periods of springs A and B when mass M is suspended from one end of each spring. If both springs are taken in series and the same mass M is suspended from the series combination, the time period is T, then

(a) $T_1 + T_2 + T_3$ (b) $\frac{1}{T}=\frac{1}{T_1}+\frac{1}{T_2}$
(c) $T^2 = T_1^2 + T_2^2$ (d) $\frac{1}{T^2}=\frac{1}{T_1^2}+\frac{1}{T^2}$

39. Alternating current cannot be measured by D.C. ammeter because

(a) A.C. cannot pass through D.C. ammeter
(b) A.C. changes direction
(c) average value of current for complete cycle is zero
(d) D.C. ammeter will get damaged

40. The core of any transformer is laminated so as to

(a) reduce the energy loss due to eddy currents
(b) make it light weight
(c) make it robust & strong
(d) increase the secondary voltage

Directions : In the following questions (41-60), a statement of assertion (A) is followed by a statement of reason (R). Mark the correct choice as :

(a) If both assertion and reason are true and reason is the correct explanation of assertion
(b) If both assertion and reason are true but reason is not the correct explanation of assertion
(c) If assertion is true but reason is false
(d) If both assertion and reason are false.

41. Assertion : Two balls of different masses are thrown vertically upward with same speed. They will pass through their point of projection in the downward direction with the same speed.

Reason : The maximum height and downward velocity attained at the point of projection are independent of the mass of the ball.

42. Assertion : In javelin throw, the athlete throws the projectile at an angle slightly more than 45°.

Reason : The maximum range does not depend upon angle of projection.

43. **Assertion** : The apparent weight of a body in an elevator moving with some downward acceleration is less than the actual weight of a body.

Reason : The part of the weight is spent in producing downward acceleration, when body is in elevator.

44. **Assertion** : An electric field is preferred in comparison to magnetic field for detecting the electron beam in a television picture tube.

Reason : Electric field requires low voltage.

45. **Assertion** : A horse has to pull a cart harder during the first few steps of his motion.

Reason : The first few steps are always difficult.

46. **Assertion** : The magnetic poles of earth do not coincide with the geographic poles.

Reason : The discrepancy between the orientation of a compass and true north-south direction is known as magnetic declination.

47. **Assertion** : Electromagnetic waves are transverse in nature

Reason : The electric and magnetic fields of an e.m. wave are perpendicular to each other and also perpendicular to the direction of wave propogation.

48. **Assertion** : A wheel moving down a perfectly frictionless inclined plane will undergo slipping (not rolling motion)

Reason : For perfect rolling motion, work done against friction is zero.

49. **Assertion** : A hollow shaft is found to be stronger than a solid shaft made of same material.

Reason : The torque required to produce a given twist in hollow cylinder is greater than that required to twist a solid cylinder of same size and material.

50. **Assertion** : Water kept in an open vessel will quickly evaporate on the surface of the moon.

Reason : The temperature at the surface of the moon is much higher than boiling point of water.

51. **Assertion** : A pure semiconductor has negative temperature coefficient of resistance.

Reason : On raising the temperature, more charge carriers are released, conductance increases and resistance decreases.

52. **Assertion** : At a fixed temperature, silicon will have a minimum conductivity when it has a smaller acceptor doping.

Reason : The conductivity of an intrinisic semiconductor is slightly higher than that of a lightly doped *p*-type

53. **Assertion** : Communication in UHF/VHF regions can be established by space wave or tropospheric wave.

Reason : Communication in UHF/VHF regions is limited to line of sight distance.

54. **Assertion** : If objective and eye lenses of a microscope are interchanged then it can work as telescope.

Reason : The objective lens of telescope has small focal length.

55. **Assertion** : If a proton and an α-particle enter a uniform magnetic field perpendicularly with the same speed, the time period of revolution of α-particle is double that of proton.

Reason : In a magnetic field, the period of revolution of a charged particle is directly proportional to the mass of the particle and is inversely proportional to charge of particle.

56. **Assertion** : If momentum of a body increases by 50%, its kinetic energy will increase by 125%.

Reason : Kinetic energy is proportional to square of velocity.

57. **Assertion :** The difference in the value of acceleration due to gravity at pole and equator is proportional to square of angular velocity of earth.

Reason : The value of acceleration due to gravity is minimum at the equator and maximum at the pole.

58. **Assertion :** It is advantageous to transmit electric power at high voltage.

Reason : High voltage implies high current.

59. **Assertion :** X-ray astronomy is possible only from satellites orbiting the earth.

Reason : Efficiency of X-rays telescope is large as compared to any other telescope.

60. **Assertion :** The de Broglie equation has significance for any microscopic or sub -microscopic particles.

Reason : The de Broglie wavelengs inversely proportional to the mass of the object if velocity is constant.

CHEMISTRY

61. Butter is an example of which type of colloid?
(a) Solid in liquid (b) Liquid in solid
(c) Liquid in liquid (d) Gas in liquid.

62. What are constituents of 'Mischmetal'?
(a) La, Fe (b) La, Ce
(c) Fe, Ce (d) Ce, Cu

63. For a 1st order reaction if concentration is doubled then rate of reaction becomes
(a) doubles (b) half
(c) four times (d) remains same.

64. In tetragonal crystal system, which of following is not true?
(a) All axial lengths and all axial angles are equal.
(b) All three axial lengths are equal.
(c) All three axial angles are equal.
(d) Two axial angles are equal but the third is different.

65. Which of the following is correct?
(a) Ionic radius is proportional to atomic number.
(b) Ionic radius is inversely proportional to atomic mass.
(c) Ionic radius is inversely proportional to effective nuclear charge.
(d) All are correct.

66. The strained tetracyclic alkane is isomerize thermally to the cyclic alkene. The reaction involves
(a) free radical (b) carbocation
(c) carbanion (d) carbene.

67. [Structure: 3-methoxyphenyl-substituted alkene with terminal =CH–H] $\xrightarrow[HgSO_4]{H_2SO_4,\ H_2O}$ P

The product P is
(a) [Structure with OH and OCH_3]
(b) [Structure with OH, H and OCH_3]
(c) [Structure with OH, H and OCH_3]
(d) none of these.

68. For a reaction X ⟶ Y, the graph of the product concentration (x) versus time (t) came out to be a straight line passing through the origin. Hence the graph of $\frac{-d[X]}{dt}$ and time would be
(a) straight line with a negative slope and an intercept on y-axis
(b) straight line with a positive slope and an intercept on y-axis
(c) a straight line parallel to x-axis
(d) a hyperbola.

69. A factory produces 40 kg of calcium in two hours by electrolysis. How much aluminium can be produced by same current in 2 hours if current efficiency is 50%?
(a) 22 kg (b) 18 kg
(c) 9 kg (d) 27 kg.

70. Equal weight of CO and CH_4 are mixed together in an empty container at 300 K. The fraction of total pressure exerted by CH_4 is

(a) $\frac{16}{17}$ (b) $\frac{7}{11}$

(c) $\frac{8}{9}$ (d) $\frac{5}{16}$

71. Match list I with list II and select the correct answer using the codes given below the lists.

	List I Metal ion		List II Magnetic moment(BM)
A.	Cr^{3+}	1.	$\sqrt{35}$
B.	Fe^{2+}	2.	$\sqrt{30}$
C.	Ni^{2+}	3.	$\sqrt{24}$
D.	Mn^{2+}	4.	$\sqrt{15}$
		5.	$\sqrt{8}$

Codes

(a) A-1, B-3, C-5, D-4
(b) A-2, B-3, C-5, D-1
(c) A-4, B-3, C-5, D-1
(d) A-4, B-5, C-3, D-1

72. Which of the following reactions does not yield an amine?

(a) $R - X + NH_3 \longrightarrow$

(b) $R - CH{=}NOH + [H] \xrightarrow{Na/C_2H_5OH}$

(c) $R - CN + H_2O \xrightarrow{H^+}$

(d) $R - CONH_2 \xrightarrow{LiAlH_4}$

73. The chemical name for melamine is

(a) 1,3,5-Triamino-2,4,6-triazine
(b) 2,4,6-Triamino-1,3,5-triazine
(c) 2-Amino-1,3,5-triazine
(d) 2,4-Diamino-1,3,5-triazine.

74. Bromine is added to cold dilute aqueous solution of NaOH. The mixture is boiled. Which of the following statements is not true?

(a) During the reaction bromine is present in four different oxidation states.
(b) The greatest difference between the various oxidation states of bromine is 5.
(c) On acidification of the final mixture bromine is formed.
(d) Disproportionation of bromine occurs during the reaction.

75. A complex $PtCl_4.5NH_3$ shows a molar conductance of 402 ohm^{-1} cm^2 mol^{-1} in water and precipitates three moles of AgCl with $AgNO_3$ solution. The formula of the complex is

(a) $[Pt(NH_3)_6]Cl_4$ (b) $[Pt(NH_3)_4Cl_2]Cl_2$
(c) $[Pt(NH_3)_5Cl]Cl_3$ (d) $[Pt(NH_3)_3Cl_3]Cl$.

76.

Electrolyte	KCl	KNO_3	HCl	NaOAc	NaCl
Λ^{∞} (S cm^2 mol^{-1})	149.9	145.0	426.2	91.0	126.5

Calculate Λ^{∞}_{HOAC} using appropriate molar conductances of the electrolytes listed above at infinite dilution in H_2O at 25°C.

(a) 517.2 (b) 552.7
(c) 390.7 (d) 217.5

77. In the ground state of Cu^+, the number of shells occupied, subshells occupied, filled orbitals and unpaired electrons respectively are

(a) 4, 8, 15, 0 (b) 3, 6, 15, 1
(c) 3, 6, 14, 0 (d) 4, 7, 14, 2

78. Which of the following conditions is not correct for resonating structures?

(a) The contributing structures must have the same number of unpaired electrons.
(b) The contributing structures should have similar energies.
(c) The contributing structures should be so written that unlike charges reside on atoms that are far apart.
(d) The positive charge should be present on the electropositive element and the negative charge on the electronegative element.

79. CaO and NaCl have the same crystal structure and approximately the same ionic radii. If U is the lattice energy of NaCl, the approximate lattice energy of CaO is

(a) $U/2$ (b) U
(c) $2U$ (d) $4U$

80. The phosphate of a metal has the formula $MHPO_4$. The formula of its chloride would be

(a) MCl (b) MCl_2
(c) MCl_3 (d) M_2Cl_3

81. Two flasks X and Y have capacity 1L and 2L respectively and each of them contains 1 mole of a gas. The temperatures of the flasks are so adjusted that average speed of molecules in X is twice as those in Y. The pressure in flask X would be

(a) same as that in Y (b) half of that in Y
(c) twice of that in Y (d) 8 times of that in Y.

82. Match List I with List II and select the correct answer using the codes given below the lists:

	List I		List II
A.	$\left(\frac{\delta G}{\delta P}\right)_T$	1.	μ_{JT}
B.	$\left(\frac{\delta G}{\delta T}\right)_P$	2.	T
C.	$\left(\frac{\delta H}{\delta S}\right)_P$	3.	$-S$
D.	$\left(\frac{\delta T}{\delta P}\right)_H$	4.	P
		5.	V

	A	B	C	D
(a)	5	1	2	4
(b)	5	3	2	4
(c)	3	5	2	1
(d)	5	3	2	1

83. What is the pH of 0.01 M glycine solution? For glycine $K_{a_1} = 4.5 \times 10^{-3}$ and $K_{a_2} = 1.7 \times 10^{-10}$ at 298 K.

(a) 3.0 (b) 10.0
(c) 7.06 (d) 8.2

84. Which of the following sequence contains atomic number of only representative elements?

(a) 55,12,48,53 (b) 13,33,54,80
(c) 3,33,53,87 (d) 22,33,55,66.

85. 100 cm³ of a given sample of H_2O_2 gives 1000 cm³ of O_2 at S.T.P. The given sample is

(a) 10% H_2O_2 (b) 90% H_2O_2
(c) 10 volume H_2O_2 (d) 100 volume H_2O_2

86. Beryllium and aluminium exhibit many properties which are similar. But the two elements differ in

(a) maximum covalency in compounds
(b) exhibiting amphoteric nature in their oxides
(c) forming covalent halides
(d) forming polymeric hydrides

87. Cyclohexene on ozonolysis followed by reaction with zinc dust and water gives compound E. Compound E on further treatment with aqueous KOH yields compound F. Compound F is

(a) —CHO (b) —CHO
(c) —COOH (d) CO_2H / CO_2H

88. Ethyl ester $\xrightarrow[\text{excess}]{CH_3MgBr}$ P. The product P will be

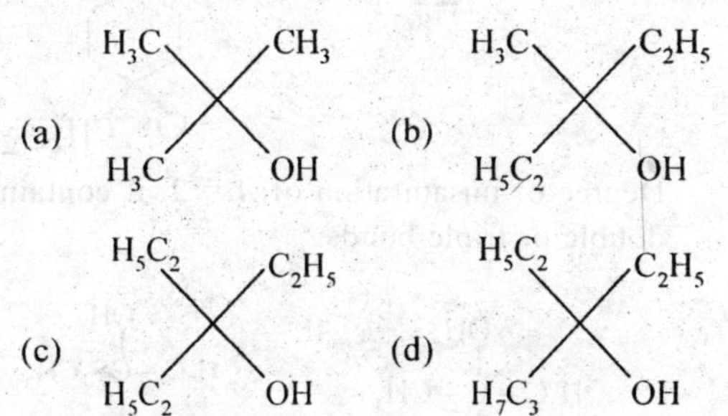

89. The compound which on reaction with aqueous nitrous acid at low temperature produces an oily nitrosoamine is

(a) methyl amine (b) ethyl amine
(c) diethyl amine (d) triethyl amine

90. Compound A (molecular formula C_3H_8O) is treated with acidified potassium dichromate to form a product B (molecular formula C_3H_6O). B forms a shining silver mirror on warming with ammoniacal silver nitrate. B when treated with an aqueous solution of $H_2NCONHNH_2$. HCl and sodium acetate gives a product C. Identify the structure of C.

(a) $CH_3CH_2CH = NNHCONH_2$
(b) $CH_3-\underset{CH_3}{\underset{|}{C}}=NNHCONH_2$
(c) $CH_3-\underset{CH_3}{\underset{|}{C}}=NCONHNH_2$
(d) $CH_3CH_2CH=NCONHNH_2$

91. Assume that you are travelling at a speed of 90 km/h in a small car with a mass of 1050 kg. If the uncertainty in the velocity of the car is 1% ($\Delta v = 0.9$ km/h), what is the uncertainty (in meters) in the position of the car ?

(a) $\Delta x \geq 1\times10^{-35}$ m (b) $\Delta x \geq 2\times10^{-37}$ m
(c) $\Delta x \geq 2\times10^{-36}$ m (d) $\Delta x \geq 4\times10^{-38}$ m

92. When 25 g of Na_2SO_4 is dissolved in 10^3 kg of solution, its concentration will be
(a) 2.5 ppm (b) 25 ppm
(c) 250 ppm (d) 100 ppm

93. $A\ (C_{10}H_{18}O) \xrightarrow{HCl} H_3C-C(Cl)-CH_3$ (attached to a cyclohexane ring bearing Cl and CH_3 at the 4-position)

Degree of unsaturation of A = 2, it contains no double or triple bonds.

(a) $H_3C-C(OH)-CH_3$ on a bicyclic ring (b) $H_3C-C(OH)-CH_3$ on a bicyclic ring
(c) $H_3C-CH-CH_2OH$ on a bicyclic ring (d) none of these.

94. The shape and hybridisation of some xenon oxyfluorides are given. Choose the wrong set.
(a) $XeOF_2$-T-Shape-sp^3d
(b) $XeOF_4$ - Square pyramidal-sp^3d^2
(c) XeO_2F_2 -Distorted trigonal bipyramidal-sp^3d
(d) XeO_3F_2 - Octahedral - sp^3d

95. The standard half-cell reduction potential for $Ag^+|Ag$ is 0.7991 V at 25°C. Given the experimental value $K_{sp} = 1.56\times10^{-10}$ for AgCl, calculate the standard half-cell reduction potential for the Ag|AgCl electrode.
(a) 0.2192 V (b) – 0.2192 V
(c) –1.2192 V (d) 1.2192 V.

96. Which of the following acids will not evolve H_2 gas on reaction with alkali metals?
(a) hydrazoic acid (b) perxenic acid
(c) boric acid (d) none of these

97. The major product of the following reaction is

$Cl-CH_2-\overset{H}{C}-\overset{14}{C}H_2$ (epoxide, O bridging) $\xrightarrow{\overset{\oplus}{Na}\overset{-}{O}C_2H_5,\ \Delta}$ products

(a) $CH_2\overset{14}{C}HCH_2-O-C_2H_5$ (epoxide) (b) $CH_2\overset{14}{C}HCH_2OC_2H_5$ (epoxide)
(c) $CH_2(Cl)-CH(\overset{\oplus}{Na}\overset{-}{O})-\overset{14}{C}H_2-O-C_2H_5$
(d) $CH_2(Cl)-CH(OC_2H_5)-\overset{14}{C}H_2ONa$

98. Stomach acid, a dilute solution of HCl in water, can be neutralized by reaction with sodium hydrogen carbonate,
$NaHCO_{3\,(aq)} + HCl_{(aq)} \rightarrow NaCl_{(aq)} + H_2O_{(l)} + CO_{2\,(g)}$
How many milliliters of 0.125 M $NaHCO_3$ solution are needed to neutralize 18.0 mL of 0.100 M HCl?
(a) 14.4 mL (b) 12.0 mL
(c) 14.0 mL (d) 13.2 mL

99. For the electrochemical cell, $M \mid M^+ \parallel X^- \mid X$, $E°(M^+|M) = 0.44$ V and $E°(X|X^-) = 0.33$ V. From this data one can deduce that
(a) $M + X \rightarrow M^+ + X^-$ is the spontaneous reaction
(b) $M^+ + X^- \rightarrow M + X$ is the spontaneous reaction
(c) $E_{cell} = 0.77$ V (d) $E_{cell} = -0.77$ V

100. Which is optically inactive?
(a) $(a)(b)C=C=C=C=C(a)(b)$
(b) $(a)(b)C=C=C=C(a)(b)$
(c) $(a)(b)C=C=C(a)(b)$ (d) cyclohexane ring bearing a, b and $-N(d)(e)$

Directions : In the following questions (101-120), a statement of assertion (A) is followed by a statement of reason (R). Mark the correct choice as :

(a) If both assertion and reason are true and reason is the correct explanation of assertion

(b) If both assertion and reason are true but reason is not the correct explanation of assertion

(c) **If assertion is true but reason is false**

(d) **If both assertion and reason are false.**

101. Assertion : Magnesium is extracted by the electrolysis of fused mixture of $MgCl_2$, NaCl and $CaCl_2$.

Reason : Calcium chloride acts as a reducing agent.

102. Assertion : The equilibrium constant is fixed and a characteristic for any given chemical reaction at a specified temperature.

Reason : The composition of the final equilibrium mixture at a particular temperature depends upon the starting amount of reactants.

103. Assertion : PCl_5 is covalent in gaseous and liquid states but ionic in solid state.

Reason : PCl_5 in solid state consists of tetrahedral PCl_4^+ cation and octahedral PCl_6^- anion.

104. Assertion : Zinc displaces copper from copper sulphate solution.

Reason : The E^o of zinc is – 0.76 V and that of copper is + 0.34 V.

105. Assertion : $CH_3-\underset{\displaystyle COOC_2H_5}{\underset{|}{C}}=CH-COOH$ is 3-carbethoxy- 2-butenoic acid.

Reason : Principal functional group gets lowest number followed by double bond or triple bond.

106. Assertion : Helium has the highest value of ionisation energy among all the elements known.

Reason : Helium has the highest value of electron affinity among all the elements known.

107. Assertion : The nuclear isomers are the atoms with the same atomic number and same mass number, but with different radioactive properties.

Reason : The nucleus in the excited state will evidently have a different half-life as compared to that in the ground state.

108. Assertion : Conductivity of silicon increases by doping it with group-15 elements.

Reason : Doping means introduction of small amount of impurities like P, As or Bi into the pure crystal.

109. Assertion : The overall order of the reaction is the sum of the exponents of all the reactants in the rate expression.

Reason : There are many higher order reactions.

110. Assertion : Transition metals are poor reducing agents.

Reason : Transition metals form numerous alloys with other metals.

111. Assertion : Aldol condensation can be catalysed both by acids and bases.

Reason : β-Hydroxy aldehydes or ketones readily undergo acid catalysed dehydration.

112. Assertion : The position of an element in periodic table after emission of one α- and two β- particles remains unchanged.

Reason : Emission of one α- and two β-particles give isotope of the element which acquires same position in periodic table.

113. Assertion : S.I. unit of atomic mass and molecular mass is kilograms.

Reason : Atomic mass is equal to the mass of 6.023×10^{24} atoms.

114. Assertion : Bond energy and bond dissociation energy have identical value for diatomic molecules.

Reason : Greater the bond dissociation energy, less reactive is the bond.

115. Assertion : The degree of complex formation in actinides decreases in the order $M^{4+} > MO_2^{2+} > M^{3+} > MO_2^+$.

Reason : Actinides form complexes with π-bonding ligands such as alkyl phosphines and thioethers.

116. Assertion : Benzene on heating with conc. H_2SO_4 gives benzenesulphonic acid which when heated with superheated steam under pressure gives benzene.

Reason : Sulphonation is a reversible process.

117. Assertion : The molality of the solution does not change with change in temperature.

Reason : The molality is expressed in units of moles per 1000 g of solvent.

118. Assertion : Due to Frenkel defect, density of the crystalline solid decreases.

Reason : In Frenkel defect, cation or anion leaves the crystal.

119. Assertion : $\left[(en)_2Co\begin{smallmatrix}NH\\ \\OH\end{smallmatrix}Co(en)_2\right]^{3+}$ is named as tetrakis (ethylenediammine)μ-hydroxo-μ-imido dicobalt (III) ion.

Reason : In naming polynuclear complexes *i.e.*, containing two or more metal atoms joined by bridging ligands, the word μ is added with hyphen before the name of such ligands.

120. Assertion : 2,3-Dimethylbut-2-ene is more stable than but-2-ene.

Reason : Six hyperconjugation structures can be written for 2, 3-dimethylbut-2-ene while but-2-ene has twelve.

BIOLOGY

121. Vitamin B_6 is also called
(a) thiamine (b) pantothenic acid
(c) pyridoxine (d) retinol.

122. Protista differs from monera in having
(a) cell wall (b) autotrophic nutrition
(c) flagella (d) nuclear membrane

123. What does 'T' stands for in DPT vaccine?
(a) tuberculosis (b) typhoid
(c) trachoma (d) tetanus

124. Why are vascular bundles closed in monocots?
(a) xylem and phloem are present
(b) xylem and phloem occur in separate bundles
(c) vascular cambium is present between xylem and phloem
(d) vascular cambium is not present.

125. Who invented electron microscope?
(a) Janssen (b) Edison
(c) Knoll & Ruska (d) Landsteiner

126. What do A, B, C, and D represent in the following figure?

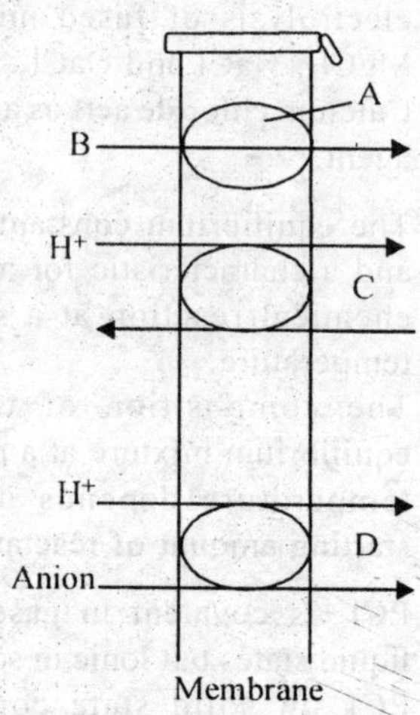

(a) A : carrier protein, B: symport, C: uniport, D : antiport
(b) A : carrier protein, B : uniport, C: antiport, D : symport
(c) A : carrier protein, B : antiport, C: symport, D : uniport
(d) A : carrier protein, B : uniport, C: symport, D : antiport

127. Gametophyte and sporophyte are independent of each other in which of the following groups?
(a) pteridophytes (b) angiosperms
(c) gymnosperms (d) bryophytes

128. Which of the following is correct?
(a) paneth cells secrete pepsinogen
(b) parietal cells secrete hydrochloric acid
(c) argentaffin cells secrete mucus
(d) chief cells secrete gastrin

129. Which of the following has highest diversity in India?
(a) mango (b) dolphin
(c) tiger (d) orchids

130. Which of the following is correct about the given figure?

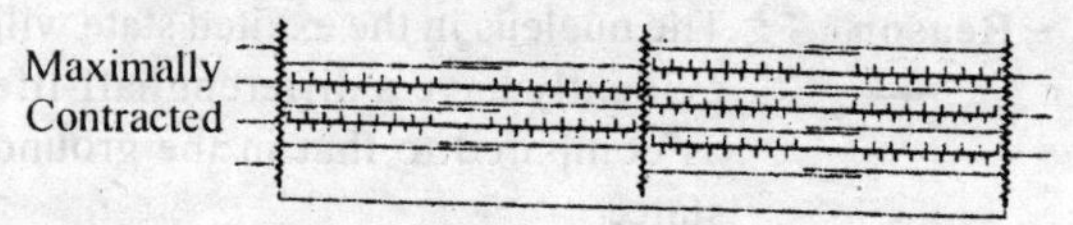

Two sarcomeres

(a) the length of the thick and thin myofilaments has changed.

(b) length of both anisotropic and isotropic band has changed.
(c) the myosin cross-bridges move on the surface of actin and the thin and thick myofilaments slide past each other.
(d) length of the sarcomere remains same.

131. Which of the following disorders are caused due to recessive autosomal mutations?
(a) Turner's syndrome and sickle cell anaemia
(b) Edward's syndrome and Down's syndrome
(c) cystic fibrosis and phenylketonuria
(d) Alzheimer's disease and Huntington's chorea.

132. What is correct about the movement of substance across the membrane in facilitated diffusion?
(a) it is an active transport
(b) it doesn't cause transport of molecules from low concentration to high concentration
(c) it is insensitive to inhibitors
(d) it is a very specific transport

133. Which one is correct?
(a) *Salmonella typhi* and *Haemophilus influenzae* cause pneumonia
(b) Widal test is done for malaria
(c) *Entamoeba histolytica* causes amoebiasis
(d) *Wuchereria* causes enterobiasis.

134. What is the Greek word for ecology?
(a) ethology (b) oekologie
(c) synecology (d) hexicology

135. Which of the following is correct regarding genetic code?
(a) UUU is the initiation codon which also codes for phenylalanine.
(b) there are 64 triplet codons and only 20 amino acids.
(c) three random nitrogen bases specify the placement of one amino acid.
(d) UAA is the nonsense codon which also codes for methionine.

136. The given figure shows L.S of the seed of maize. What do A, B, C and D represent?

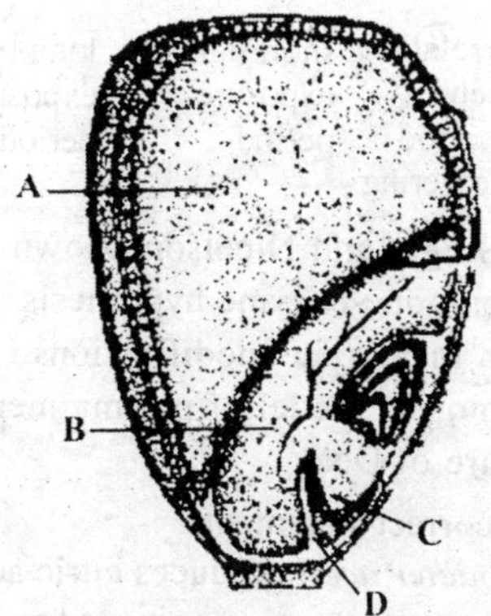

(a) A : endosperm B : scutellum
C : plumule D : coleoptile
(b) A : scutellum B : pericarp
C : radicle D : coleoptile
(c) A : endosperm B : scutellum
C : radicle D : coleorrhiza
(d) A : scutellum B : pericarp
C : plumule D : coleorrhiza

137. Refer the given figures on photoperiodism and select the correct option.

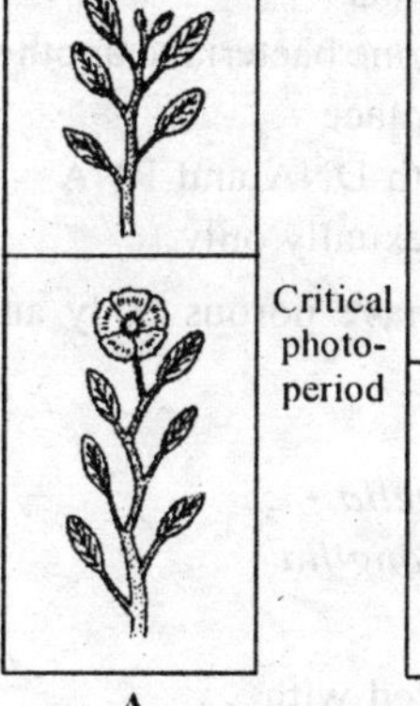

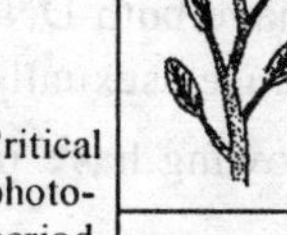

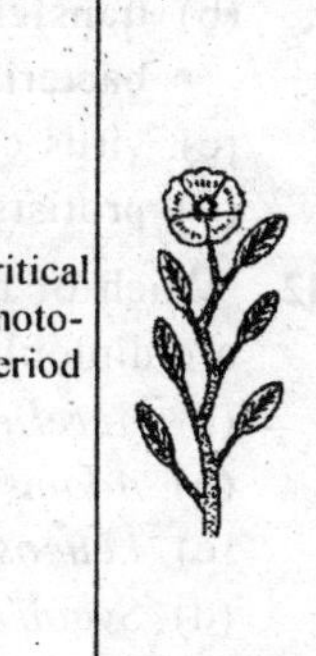

	A	B	C
(a)	no correlation between light period and flowering	long light-exposure period	short light-exposure period
(b)	long light-exposure period	no correlation between light period and flowering	short light-exposure period
(c)	short light-exposure period	long light-exposure period	no correlation between light period and flowering

(d) no correlation between light period and flowering | short light-exposure period | long light-exposure period

138. What are Singer and Nicolson known for?
(a) one-gene-one-enzyme hypothesis
(b) plasma membrane modifications
(c) fluid-mosaic model of plasma membrane
(d) structure of DNA

139. Select the correct statement.
(a) *Acetobacter aceti* produces citric acid
(b) *Saccharomyces cerevisiae* is used as clot buster
(c) *Penicillium notatum* restrict the growth of *Staphylococci*
(d) methanogens are found in aerobic conditions

140. Which of the following diseases is also called Christmas disease?
(a) sickle-cell anaemia
(b) haemoglobinuria
(c) myocardial infarction
(d) haemophilia - B

141. Which of the following is correct?
(a) all fungi are filamentous
(b) transfer of DNA from one bacteria to another bacteria cannot take place
(c) virus cannot have both DNA and RNA
(d) protists reproduce asexually only.

142. Which of the following have porous body and are diploblastic?
(a) *Aurelia* and *Obelia*
(b) *Adamsia* and *Euplectella*
(c) *Leucosolenia* and *Spongilla*
(d) *Sycon* and *Hydra*

143. CD-4 receptor is associated with
(a) AIDS (b) cancer
(c) malaria (d) pneumonia

144. Which one is correct regarding electrocardiograph (ECG)?
(a) P-wave represents the electrical excitation of the ventricle
(b) QRS complex represents repolarisation of the ventricles
(c) T-wave represents repolarisation of the atria
(d) by counting the number of QRS complexes one can determine the pulse rate.

145. Animals take phosphorus from
(a) water (b) plants
(c) rock (d) soil

146. What is the effect of GnRH produced by hypothalamus?
(a) stimulates the synthesis and secretion of androgens
(b) stimulates secretion of milk in mammary glands
(c) stimulates foetal ejection reflex
(d) stimulates synthesis of carbohydrates from non-carbohydrates in liver.

147. Chemosensitive area of respiratory centre in medulla is affected by
(a) less CO_2 and H^+ ions
(b) less O_2 and H^+ ions
(c) excess CO_2 and H^+ ions
(d) excess O_2 and H^+ ions.

148. What do A, B, C and D represent?

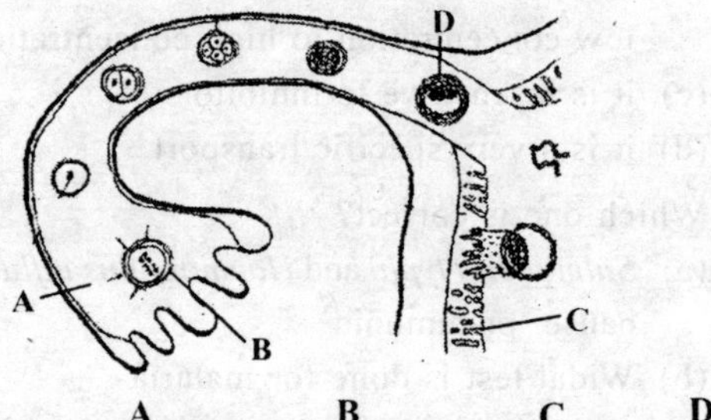

	A	B	C	D
(a)	infundibulum	fertilization	myometrium	morula
(b)	infundibulum	fertilization	endometrium	blastocyst
(c)	isthmus	fertilization	myometrium	blastocyst
(d)	isthmus	fertilization	endometrium	morula

149. Microvilli of intestinal epithelium are similar in function with
(a) typhlosole in earthworm
(b) hepatic caecae in cockroach
(c) intestinal caecum in earthworm
(d) Malpighian tubules in cockroach.

150. The type of epithelial cells which line the inner surface of Fallopian tubes, bronchioles and bronchi are known as
(a) squamous epithelium
(b) ciliated epithelium
(c) columnar epithelium
(d) cubical epithelium.

151. Cyclic photophosphorylation involves
(a) PS I (b) PS II
(c) PS I and PS II (d) P_{680}

152. Which animal has the longest gestation period?
(a) shark (b) walrus
(c) elephant (d) dog

153. What is a plasmid?
(a) bacterial, linear, dsDNA
(b) extrachromosomal linear RNA
(c) extrachromosomal circular dsDNA
(d) autonomously replicating circular RNA.

154. The concept of chemical evolution is based on
(a) interaction of water, air and clay under intense heat
(b) effect of solar radiation on chemicals
(c) possible origin of life by combination of chemicals under suitable environmental conditions
(d) crystallization of chemicals.

155. Which of the following is a correct match between crop, variety and resistance to diseases?

	Crop	Variety	Resistance to diseases
(a)	wheat	himgiri	white rust
(b)	*Brassica*	Pusa sadabahar	black rot
(c)	cowpea	Pusa komal	bacterial blight
(d)	chilli	Pusa swarnim	chilly mosaic virus

156. Recombinant DNA technology involves several steps in which initial step is of isolation of the DNA. Which enzymes are used in the process for the break down of fungal cell, plant cell and bacterial cell respectively?
(a) lysozyme, lipases, trypsin
(b) chitinase, cellulase, lysozyme
(c) chitinase, cellulase, trypsin
(d) trypsin, lipases, cellulase

157. The taxon which includes related species is
(a) class (b) order
(c) family (d) genus

158. Match the following columns and select the correct option

Column I	Column II
(A) *Panthera tigris*	(i) Mango
(B) *Mangifera indica*	(ii) Common Indian frog
(C) *Musca domestica*	(iii) Cockroach
(D) *Periplaneta americana*	(iv) Tiger
(E) *Rana tigerina*	(v) House fly

(a) A - (ii), B - (v), C - (i), D - (iii), E - (iv)
(b) A - (iv), B - (i), C - (v), D - (iii), E - (ii)
(c) A - (ii), B - (v), C - (iii), D - (i), E - (iv)
(d) A - (iv), B - (i), C - (v), D - (ii), E - (iii)

159. Which of the following is correct regarding HIV, hepatitis B, gonorrhoea, trichomoniasis?
(a) trichomoniasis is a STD whereas other are not
(b) gonorrhoea is a viral disease whereas others are bacterial
(c) HIV is a pathogen whereas others are diseases
(d) Hepatitis B is eradicated completely whereas others are not.

160. The first stable product of Calvin cycle is
(a) 3-phosphoglycerate
(b) 1, 3 biphosphoglycerate
(c) glyceraldehyde - 3 phosphate
(d) ribulose - 5- phosphate

Directions : In the following questions (161-180), a statement of assertion (A) is followed by a statement of reason (R). Mark the correct choice as :
(a) If both assertion and reason are true and reason is the correct explanation of assertion
(b) If both assertion and reason are true but reason is not the correct explanation of assertion
(c) If assertion is true but reason is false
(d) If both assertion and reason are false.

161. Assertion : Adrenaline is called an emergency hormone.
Reason : It acts on the cells of skeletal, cardiac, smooth muscles, blood vessels and fat cells.

162. Assertion : Cork prevents the loss of water by evaporation.
Reason : Cork cells contain tannins.

163. Assertion : In cockroach respiratory gases directly comes in contact with the various organs of the body.

Reason : Cockroaches do not have respiratory pigment.

164. Assertion : Interferons are antiviral proteins.
Reason : Interferons are secreted by virus infected cells.

165. Assertion : While on going down the loop of Henle, the filtrate becomes hypotonic.
Reason : The descending limb of loop of Henle is impermeable to both water and electrolytes.

166. Assertion : Shrinkage of the protoplast of a cell occurs under the influence of hypertonic solution.
Reason : Hypertonic solution causes plasmolysis.

167. Assertion : Inbreeding produces pureline.
Reason : It causes homozygosity.

168. Assertion : Parturition is induced by neural signal in maternal pituitary.
Reason : At the end of gestation period, the maternal pituitary release prolactin which causes uterine contractions.

169. Assertion : *Commelina* shows cleistogamy.
Reason : This reduces chances of inbreeding.

170. Assertion : *Antirrhinum* is a good example to understand incomplete dominance.
Reason : Heterozygotes show characteristics of both the alleles.

171. Assertion : Presence of large amounts of nutrients in water body causes excessive growth of planktonic algae.
Reason : It is due to biomagnification.

172. Assertion : Bile is essential for the digestion of lipids.
Reason : Bile juice contains enzymes bilirubin and biliverdin.

173. Assertion : Emphysema is a chronic disorder in which alveolar walls are damaged.
Reason : Emphysema is closely related to cigarette smoking.

174. Assertion : DNA fingerprinting involves identifying differences in specific regions in DNA sequence.
Reason : DNA fingerprinting is the basis of paternity testing.

175. Assertion : All pathogens are parasites but all parasites are not pathogens.
Reason : Majority of the parasites confer benefits to the host.

176. Assertion : Due to pollution atmospheric concentration of CO_2 is increasing which will be harmful for C_4 plants whereas productive for C_3 plants.
Reason : C_4 plants have greater efficiency for CO_2 as CO_2 is fixed by PEP oxygenase.

177. Assertion : Insulin is antagonistic to glucagon.
Reason : It is an anabolic hormone.

178. Assertion : Auditory ossicles are small bones present in the cavity of inner ear.
Reason : Auditory ossicles maintain the balance of air pressure between two sides of ear drum.

179. Assertion : Pharyngeal nephridia play a role in the conservation of water in the earthworm.
Reason : They help the earthworm in keeping the skin moist for cutaneous respiration.

180. Assertion : Pantothenic acid deficiency is probably the most common vitamin deficiency.
Reason : Macrocytic anaemia is a characteristic feature of pantothenic acid deficiency.

GENERAL KNOWLEDGE

181. Which country has three capitals?
(a) S. Africa (b) Switzerland
(c) Netherland (c) Australia

182. Which is the largest desert in the world?
(a) Atacama (b) Thar
(c) Sahara (d) Kalahri

183. Which is the largest lake in the world?
(a) Caspian sea (b) Wular
(c) Lake superior (d) Baikal

184. Which country has won 'Fifa World Cup' maximum times?
(a) Germany (b) Brazil
(c) France (d) Italy

185. 'World population day' is on
(a) 8th March (b) 21st March
(c) 11th July (d) 3rd October

186. Who invented the stethescope?
(a) Reni Laennec (b) Hopkins
(c) Louis Pasteur (d) Hausen

187. Which country has largest number of coal reserves?
(a) USA (b) Russia
(c) China (d) India

188. What term is given to the relationship between culture and food?
(a) astronomy (b) agronomy
(c) gastronomy (d) geology

189. One-rupee note bears the signature of the
(a) Governor of Reserve Bank of India
(b) Finance ministry
(c) Secretary, Ministry of Finance
(d) President of India

190. Which one of the following classical dance forms originated in Andhra Pradesh?
(a) bharatnatyam (b) kathakali
(c) kuchipudi (d) odissi

191. On adding salt to water, the boiling point and freezing point of water will
(a) increase
(b) increase and decrease respectively
(c) decrease
(d) decrease and increase respectively.

192. Chocolates can be bad for health because of a high content of
(a) cobalt (b) nickel
(c) zinc (d) lead

193. The novel Coolie is written by
(a) R. K. Narayan (b) Prem Chand
(c) Jainendra Kumar (d) Mulk Raj Anand

194. Beirut is the capital of
(a) Syria (b) Jordan
(c) Lebanon (d) Libya

195. The first month of Saka year is
(a) vaisakh (b) chaitra
(c) jyeshtha (d) paush

196. Chameli Devi Award is given to an outstanding woman who is a
(a) vocalist (b) lawyer
(c) journalist (d) scientist

197. "Olive Branch" is a sign of
(a) war (b) peace
(c) defeat (d) conquest

198. 800 in Roman number is written as
(a) DDCC (b) DDDC
(c) DCCC (d) DCCD.

199. Santosh Trophy is associated with
(a) hockey (b) cricket
(c) badminton (d) football

200. Which river carries maximum quantity of water in the world?
(a) Nile (b) Amazon
(c) Thames (d) Mississippi

SOLUTIONS

PHYSICS

1. **(b)**

2. **(c)** : In a photon-particle collision (such as photon-electron), the total energy and total momentum are conserved. However, the number of photons may not be conserved in a collision. The photon may be absorbed or a new photon may be created.

3. **(a)** :

Truth Table of this gate

A	B	Y'	Y
0	0	1	0
1	0	0	1
0	1	0	1
1	1	0	1

$Y' = \overline{A+B} = \overline{A} \cdot \overline{B}$

and $Y = \overline{Y'} = \overline{\overline{A} \cdot \overline{B}} = \overline{\overline{A+B}} = A + B$

This is the boolean expression for the OR gate.

4. **(c)** : The power of lens

$P = \frac{1}{f} = \frac{1}{v} - \frac{1}{u} = \left[\frac{1}{25} - \frac{1}{\text{N.P.}}\right]$ where N.P. = Near point of vision

$$P = \left[\frac{1}{25} - \frac{1}{100}\right]$$

$$P = \frac{4-1}{100} = \frac{3}{100\text{ cm}} = \frac{3}{1\text{ m}} = 3\text{ D}$$

5. **(b)** : The kinetic energy of the projectiles is maximum at the point of release.

The ratio of K.E. of projectiles

$$\frac{\frac{1}{2}mu_1^2}{\frac{1}{2}mu_2^2} = \frac{4}{1}$$

$$\frac{u_1^2}{u_2^2} = \frac{4}{1} \quad \text{.... (i)}$$

The ratio of maximum heights of projectiles

$$\frac{H_1}{H_2} = \frac{4}{1}$$

$$\frac{\frac{u_1^2 \sin^2\theta_1}{2g}}{\frac{u_2^2 \sin^2\theta_2}{2g}} = \frac{4}{1}$$

$$\frac{u_1^2}{u_2^2} \cdot \frac{\sin^2\theta_1}{\sin^2\theta_2} = \frac{4}{1}$$

$$\frac{4}{1} \cdot \frac{\sin^2\theta_1}{\sin^2\theta_2} = \frac{4}{1} \quad \text{(from equation (i))}$$

$\sin^2\theta_1 = \sin^2\theta_2$

$\theta_1 = \theta_2$

Now, ratio of ranges of projectiles

$$\frac{R_1}{R_2} = \frac{u_1^2 \sin 2\theta_1}{u_2^2 \sin 2\theta_2}$$

$$\frac{R_1}{R_2} = \frac{u_1^2 \sin 2\theta_1}{u_2^2 \sin 2\theta_1} \quad (\because \theta_1 = \theta_2)$$

$$\frac{R_1}{R_2} = \frac{u_1^2}{u_2^2}, \quad \frac{R_1}{R_2} = \frac{4}{1}$$

6. **(d)**

7. **(c)** : Relative magnetic permeability of diamagnetic substances is always less than unity.

i.e. $\mu_r < 1$

$\mu_r = (1 + \chi_m)$ as $\mu_r < 1$, χ_m is negative.

Hence, susceptibility of diamagnetic substances has a small negative value.

8. **(b)**

9. **(c)** : Fundamental frequency of a vibrating string is expressed as

$$f = \frac{1}{2L}\sqrt{\frac{T}{\mu}} = \frac{1}{LD}\sqrt{\frac{T}{\pi\rho}}$$

where, D = diameter of string

ρ = density of the material of string

As length L and radius are doubled, the new frequency

$$f' = \frac{1}{(2L)(2D)}\sqrt{\frac{T}{\pi\rho}} = \frac{1}{4}f$$

10. (c) : Since the bubbles coalesce in vacuum and there is no change in temperature, hence its surface energy does not change. This means that the surface area remains unchanged. Hence

$4\pi a^2 + 4\pi b^2 = 4\pi R^2$ or $R = \sqrt{a^2 + b^2}$

11. (a) : Capacitors C_1 and C_2 are in parallel, their equivalent capacitance is in series with capacitor C_3. Hence, the equivalent capacitance of the given circuit is

$$C_{eq} = \frac{(C_1 + C_2)C_3}{C_1 + C_2 + C_3}$$

Charge on capacitor C_3 is

$$Q = V C_{eq} = \frac{V(C_1 + C_2)C_3}{C_1 + C_2 + C_3}$$

Voltage across C_3 is

$$= \frac{Q}{C_3} = \frac{V(C_1 + C_2)}{C_1 + C_2 + C_3}$$

12. (c) : For Brackett series, $n_1 = 4$, $n_2 = 5, 6, 7$ ....

$$\frac{1}{\lambda} = R\left(\frac{1}{n_1^2} - \frac{1}{n_2^2}\right)$$

where $R = 1.09678 \times 10^7$ m^{-1}, called Rydberg's constant.

$$\frac{1}{\lambda} = R\left(\frac{1}{4^2} - \frac{1}{n_2^2}\right)$$

For maximum wavelength, $n_2 = 5$

$$\frac{1}{\lambda_{max}} = 1.09687 \times 10^7 \left(\frac{1}{4^2} - \frac{1}{5^2}\right)$$

$\lambda_{max} = 40519$ Å

13. (a) : $r = \frac{n^2}{Z} \times 0.529$

For He$^+$, $n = 2$, $Z = 1$

$$r = \frac{4}{2} \times 0.529 = 1.058 \text{ Å}$$

14. (c) : $x = 3t^2 - 6t$; So (velocity)$_x = \frac{dx}{dt} = 6t - 6$;

$y = t^2 - 2t$

So, (velocity)$_y = \frac{dy}{dt} = 2t - 2$

At time $t = 1$,

$$= \frac{dx}{dt} = 6 \times 1 - 6 = 0 \text{ and } \frac{dy}{dt} = 2 \times 1 - 2 = 0.$$

15. (c) : Since $M_2 > M_1$, therefore M_2 moves downwards and M_1 moves upwards with an acceleration a as shown in the figure.

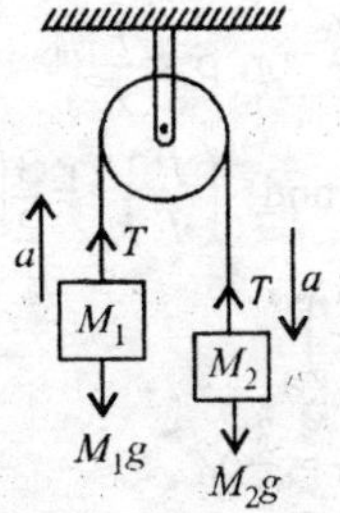

Free body diagram of M_1

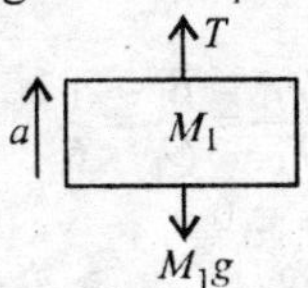

The equation of motion for M_1 is

$T - M_1g = M_1a$ ......(i)

Free body diagram of M_2

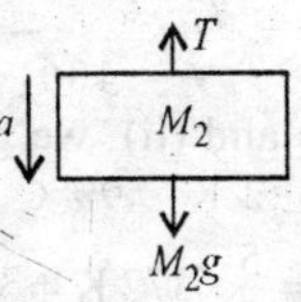

The equation of motion for M_2 is

$M_2g - T = M_2a$ ......(ii)

Adding (i) and (ii), we get

$$a = \frac{(M_2 - M_1)g}{M_2 + M_1} = \frac{(10-5)g}{(10+5)} = \frac{g}{3}$$

16. (b) : Because the block moves with a uniform velocity, the resultant force is zero. Resolving F into horizontal component $F\cos\theta$ and vertical component $F\sin\theta$, we get

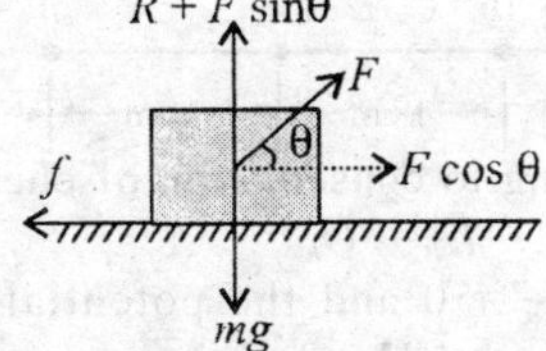

$R + F\sin\theta = mg$ or $R = mg - F\sin\theta$

Also $f = \mu R = \mu(mg - F\sin\theta)$

But $F\cos\theta = f$

or $F\cos\theta = \mu(mg - F\sin\theta)$

or $F(\cos\theta + \mu\sin\theta) = \mu mg$

$$\therefore \quad F = \frac{\mu mg}{\cos\theta + \mu\sin\theta}$$

Work $W = Fs\cos\theta$

$$\therefore \quad W = \frac{\mu mgd\cos\theta}{\cos\theta + \mu\sin\theta}$$

$(\because s = d)$

17. **(b)** : $\rho = \frac{PM}{RT}$ or $\rho \propto \frac{P}{T}$

$\left(\frac{P}{T}\right)_A = \frac{P_0}{T_0}$ and $\left(\frac{P}{T}\right)_B = \frac{3}{2}\left(\frac{P_0}{T_0}\right)$

$\left(\frac{P}{T}\right)_B = \frac{3}{2}\left(\frac{P}{T}\right)_A$

$\therefore\ \rho_B = \frac{3}{2}\rho_A = \frac{3}{2}\rho_0$

18. **(a)**

19. **(a)** : $\eta_1 = 1 - \frac{T_L}{T_H} = \frac{W}{Q_1} = \frac{1}{6}$

or $5T_H - 6T_L = 0$ ...(i)

$\eta_2 = 1 - \frac{T_L - 62}{T_H} = 2\eta_1 = \frac{1}{3}$ (Given)

$\Rightarrow 1 - \frac{1}{3} = \frac{T_L - 62}{T_H}$

or $2T_H - 3T_L = -186$ ...(ii)

Solving (i) and (ii), we get

$\therefore\ T_H = 372\text{ K} = 99°\text{C}$

$T_L = \frac{5}{6}T_H = \frac{5}{6} \times 372\text{ K} = 310\text{ K} = 37°\text{C}$

20. **(c)** :According to first law of thermodynamics

$\Delta Q = \Delta U + P\Delta V$

If ΔQ is absorbed at constant volume, $\Delta V = 0$

$C_V = \left(\frac{\Delta Q}{\Delta T}\right)_V = \left(\frac{\Delta U}{\Delta T}\right)_V = \frac{\Delta U}{\Delta T}$

for an ideal monoatomic gas

$\frac{\Delta U}{\Delta T} = \frac{3}{2}R;\ C_V = \frac{3}{2}R$

21. **(c)** :

3×10^{-9} C, a, b, -3×10^{-9} C; ←1 cm→←1 cm→←1 cm→

According to conservation of energy, we get

$K_a + U_a = K_b + U_b$

Here, $K_a = 0$ and the potential energies are $U_a = q'V_a$ and $U_b = q'V_b$.

$\therefore\ 0 + q'V_a = \frac{1}{2}mv^2 + q'V_b$.

or $v = \sqrt{\frac{2q'(V_a - V_b)}{m}}$

$V_a = (9.0 \times 10^9\ \text{Nm}^2\text{C}^{-2})$

$\left(\frac{3\times10^{-9}\text{ C}}{0.01\text{ m}} + \frac{-3\times10^{-9}\text{ C}}{0.02\text{ m}}\right) = 1350\text{ V}$

$V_b = (9.0 \times 10^9\ \text{Nm}^2\text{C}^{-2})$

$\left(\frac{3\times10^{-9}\text{ C}}{0.02\text{ m}} + \frac{-3\times10^{-9}\text{ C}}{0.01\text{ m}}\right) = -1350\text{ V}.$

$\therefore\ v = \sqrt{\frac{2(2\times10^{-9}\text{ C})(2700\text{ V})}{5\times10^{-3}\text{ kg}}} = 4.65\times10^{-2}\text{ m s}^{-1}$

$= 4.65\text{ cm s}^{-1}$

22. **(a)** :

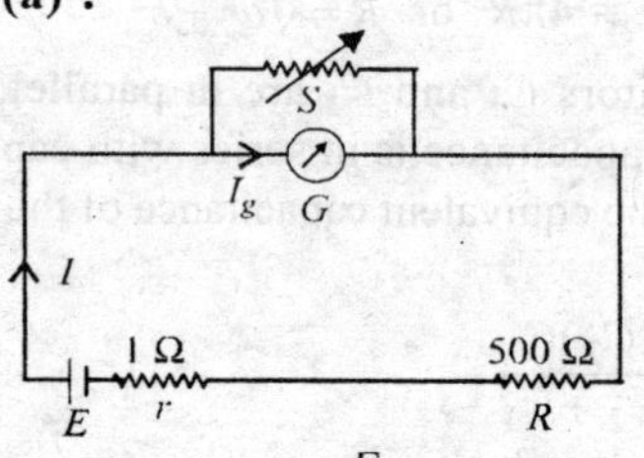

Here, $I = \frac{E}{R + r + \frac{GS}{G+S}}$ and $I_g = \frac{IS}{G+S}$

$I_g = \frac{E}{(R+r) + \frac{GS}{(G+S)}} \times \frac{S}{(G+S)}$

$\therefore\ I_g = \frac{ES}{(R+r)(G+S) + GS}$

For $S = 5$ ohm, $I_g = 5 \times 10^{-3}$ A

and for $S = 25$ ohm,

$I_g = 20 \times 10^{-3}$ A

Hence, $5\times10^{-3} = \frac{E\times5}{501(G+5)+5G}$ ...(i)

and $20\times10^{-3} = \frac{E\times25}{501(G+25)+25G}$ ...(ii)

Dividing and solving,

$G = 88.2\ \Omega$

From (i), we get

$E = 10^{-3}\ [501\ (88.2 + 5) + 5 \times 88.2]$

$= 47.1$ volt

23. **(a)** : Let us refer to the coil as circuit 1 and the solenoid as circuit 2. The field in the central region of the solenoid is uniform, so the flux through the coil is

$\Phi_{12} = B_2A_1 = (\mu_0 n_2 I_2)A_1$

where $n_2 = N_2/l = 1500$ turns/m. The mutual inductance is

$M = \frac{N_1\Phi_{12}}{I_2} = \mu_0 n_2 N_1 A_1$

$= (4\pi \times 10^{-7}\text{T}\cdot\text{m/A})\,(1500\text{ m}^{-1})\,(10)\,(4 \times 10^{-4}\text{ m}^2)$

$= 7.54 \times 10^{-6}$ H

24. **(b)** : $K_1 = \frac{hc}{\lambda_1} - \phi_0$ ....(i)

and $K_2 = \frac{hc}{\lambda_2} - \phi_0$ or $\frac{hc}{\lambda_2} = (K_2 + \phi_0)$ .... (ii)

$\therefore \quad K_1 - K_2 = hc\left[\frac{1}{\lambda_1} - \frac{1}{\lambda_2}\right]$

$= hc\left[\frac{1}{3\lambda_2} - \frac{1}{\lambda_2}\right] = \frac{2hc}{3\lambda_2}$

$= -\frac{2}{3}(K_2 + \phi_0)$ From (ii)

or $K_1 = K_2 - \frac{2}{3}K_2 - \frac{2}{3}\phi_0 = \frac{K_2}{3} - \frac{2}{3}\phi_0$

or $K_1 < \frac{K_2}{3}$

25. **(c)** : At $t = 0$, $N = N_0$ for both the substances A and B

$\therefore \quad N_A = N_0 e^{-\lambda_A t}$ and $N_B = N_o e^{-\lambda_B t}$

$\frac{N_A}{N_B} = \frac{e^{-\lambda_A t}}{e^{-\lambda_B t}} = e^{(\lambda_B - \lambda_A)t} = e^{(\lambda - 5\lambda)t}$

$= e^{-4\lambda t} = \left(\frac{1}{e}\right)^{4\lambda t}$

As $\frac{N_A}{N_B} = \left(\frac{1}{e}\right)^2$ [According to question]

$\therefore \quad 4\lambda t = 2$

or $t = \frac{2}{4\lambda} = \frac{1}{2\lambda}$

26. **(b)** : $\because \; I = I_0 e^{-kx} \Rightarrow \frac{I}{I_0} = e^{-kx}$

$\therefore \quad \ln\left(\frac{I}{I_0}\right) = -kx$

In first case

$\ln\left(\frac{1}{8}\right) = -k \times 36$

$\ln(2^{-3}) = -k \times 36$

or $3\ln 2 = k \times 36$ ....(i)

In second case, $\ln\left(\frac{1}{2}\right) = -k \times x$

or $\ln(2^{-1}) = -kx$

or $\ln 2 = kx$ .... (ii)

From (i) and (ii)

$3 \times (kx) = k \times 36$

or $x = 12$ mm.

27. **(c)** : $\vec{r}_1 = \sqrt{2}\hat{i} + \sqrt{2}\hat{j}$

$|\vec{r}_1| = r_1 = \sqrt{(\sqrt{2})^2 + (\sqrt{2})^2} = 2$

$\vec{r}_2 = 2\hat{i} + 0\hat{j}$

or $|\vec{r}_2| = r_2 = 2$

Y, A, r_1, $(\sqrt{2}, \sqrt{2})$, B, X, (0, 0), (2, 0), r_2

Potential at point A is

$V_A = \frac{1q}{4\pi\varepsilon_0 r_1}$

$= \frac{1}{4\pi\varepsilon_0}\frac{10^{-3} \times 10^{-6}}{2}$

Potential at point B is

$V_B = \frac{1}{4\pi\varepsilon_0}\frac{q}{r_2} = \frac{1}{4\pi\varepsilon_0}\frac{10^{-3} \times 10^{-6}}{2}$

$\therefore \quad V_A - V_B = 0.$

28. **(a)** : $E = G^p h^q c^r$ ...(i)

$[M^1L^2T^{-2}] = [M^{-1}L^3T^{-2}]^p [ML^2T^{-1}]^q [LT^{-1}]^r$

$= M^{-p+q} L^{3p+2q+r} T^{-2p-q-r}$

Applying principle of homogeneity of dimensions, we get

$-p + q = 1$ ...(ii)

$3p + 2q + r = 2$ ...(iii)

$-2p - q - r = -2$ ...(iv)

Add (iii) and (iv), $p + q = 0$ ...(v)

Add (ii) and (v), we get $q = \frac{1}{2}$

From (ii), we get $p = q - 1 = \frac{1}{2} - 1 = -\frac{1}{2}$.

Put in (iii), we get $-\frac{3}{2} + 1 + r = 2, \quad r = 5/2$

29. **(d)** : If M is mass of the square plate before cutting the holes, then mass of portion of each hole,

$m = \frac{M}{16R^2} \times \pi R^2 = \frac{M\pi}{16}$

$\therefore$ Moment of inertia of remaining portion about Z axis

$I = I_{square} - 4\; I_{hole}$

$= \frac{M}{12}(16R^2 + 16R^2) - 4\left[\frac{mR^2}{2} + m(\sqrt{2}R)^2\right]$

$= \frac{M}{12} \times 32R^2 - 10mR^2$

$= \frac{8}{3}MR^2 - \frac{10}{16}MR^2\pi$

$I = \left(\frac{8}{3} - \frac{10\pi}{16}\right)MR^2.$

30. **(b)** : From Bernoulli's theorem,

$P_A + \frac{1}{2}dv_A^2 + dgh_A = P_B + \frac{1}{2}dv_B^2 + dgh_B$

Here, $h_A = h_B$

$\therefore P_A + \frac{1}{2}dv_A^2 = P_B + \frac{1}{2}dv_B^2$

$P_A - P_B = \frac{1}{2}d[v_B^2 - v_A^2]$

Now, $v_A = 0$, $v_B = r\omega$

and $P_A - P_B = hdg$

$\therefore \quad hdg = \frac{1}{2}dr^2\omega^2$ or $h = \frac{r^2\omega^2}{2g}$

31. **(a)** : Initial K.E., $E_1 = \frac{1}{2}mv^2$

$= \frac{1}{2} \times 10 \times (10)^2 = 500$ J

At $x = 20$ m, retarding force,

$F_1 = 0.1 \times 20 = 2$ N

At $x = 30$ m, retarding force,

$F_2 = 0.1 \times 30 = 3$ N.

Average Retarding Force $F = \frac{F_1 + F_2}{2} = \frac{2+3}{2} = 2.5$

Work done by retarding force = loss in K.E.

$= F \times s = 2.5\ (30 - 20) = 25$ J

Final K.E. = E_1 – loss in K.E. = 500 – 25 = 475 J

32. **(c)** : $h = \frac{2S\cos\theta}{r\rho g}$

Mass of water in the first tube,

$m = \pi r^2 h\rho = \pi r^2 \times \left(\frac{2S\cos\theta}{r\rho g}\right) \times \rho$

$= \frac{2\pi r S\cos\theta}{g}$

$\therefore \quad m \propto r$. Hence, $\frac{m'}{m} = \frac{2r}{r} = 2$

or $m' = 2m = 2 \times 5\ g = 10\ g$.

33. **(b)** : Impulse = $F \times t$

$= \frac{m(v_2 - v_1)}{t} \times t = m(v_2 - v_1)$

= change in momentum

$\therefore$ [Impulse] = [Momentum]

Angular momentum, L = mvr

Planck's constant, $[h]$ = [energy] × [time]

$\Rightarrow \quad [F \times r \times \text{time}) = \frac{m(v_2 - v_1)}{t} \times r \times t$

$\Rightarrow m(v_2 - v_1) \times r$ = (change of momentum) × r

$\therefore \quad [h] = [L]$.

Work, $W = \vec{F}.\vec{d}$: Torque, $\tau = \vec{r} \times \vec{F}$

$\therefore \quad [W] = [\tau]$

Moment of inertia, $I = mr^2$ = mass × (distance)^2

Moment of force, $\tau = \vec{r} \times \vec{F}$ = distance × force

$= \text{distance} \times \frac{\text{change of momentum}}{\text{time}}$

$\therefore \quad [I] \neq [\tau]$.

Therefore, moment of inertia and moment of force have different dimensions.

34. **(a)**

35. **(c)** :

Applying *KVL* in loop *ABCDA*, *ABFEA*, *ABGHA* and *ABJIA*, we get

$30 - i_1 \times 11 = -25$ ...(i)

$20 + i_2 \times 5 = 25$ ...(ii)

$5 - i_3 \times 10 = -25$ ....(iii)

$10 + i_4 \times 5 = 25$ ...(iv)

Solving equations (i), (ii), (iii) and (iv) we get $i_1 = 5$ A, $i_2 = 1$ A, $i_3 = 3$ A and $i_4 = 3$ A.

Hence, current flowing through 25 V cell is 12 A.

36. **(b)** :

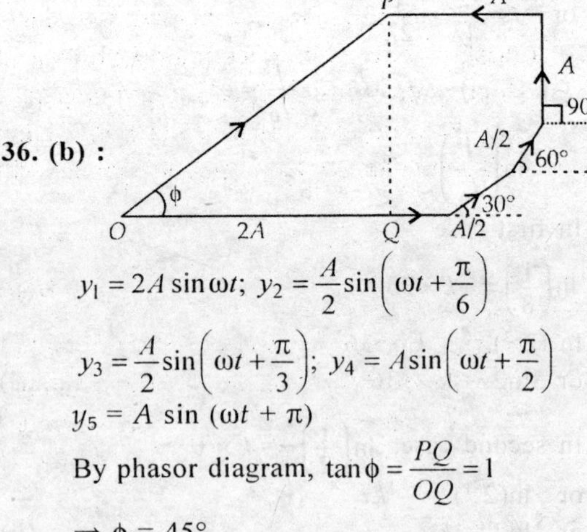

$y_1 = 2A\sin\omega t$; $y_2 = \frac{A}{2}\sin\left(\omega t + \frac{\pi}{6}\right)$

$y_3 = \frac{A}{2}\sin\left(\omega t + \frac{\pi}{3}\right)$; $y_4 = A\sin\left(\omega t + \frac{\pi}{2}\right)$

$y_5 = A\sin(\omega t + \pi)$

By phasor diagram, $\tan\phi = \frac{PQ}{OQ} = 1$

$\Rightarrow \phi = 45°$

37. **(b)** : Let L be the length of the open pipe. The fundamental frequency of the open pipe is given by

$\upsilon = \frac{v}{2L}$, v = velocity of sound in air

The second overtone of the open pipe has a

frequency $3\upsilon_O = \frac{3v}{2L_O}$ Hz

The length of the closed pipe $L_C = 2$ m.

The fundamental frequency of the closed pipe is given by $\upsilon = \frac{v}{4L}$

The first overtone of the closed pipe has a frequency

$$3\upsilon_C = \frac{3v}{4L_C} = \frac{3v}{4\times 2} = \frac{3v}{8} \text{ Hz}$$

Now $3\upsilon_O = 3\upsilon_C$ or $\frac{3v}{2L_O} = \frac{3v}{8}$

or $2L_O = 8$ or $L_O = 4$ m

38. **(c) :** $T_1 = 2\pi\sqrt{\frac{M}{k_1}}$ or $k_1 = \frac{4\pi^2 M}{T_1^2}$

and $k_2 = \frac{4\pi^2 M}{T_2^2}$

In series combination, $k_{eff} = \frac{k_1 k_2}{k_1 + k_2} = \frac{4\pi^2 M}{T_1^2 + T_2^2}$

$\therefore\ T = 2\pi\sqrt{\frac{M}{k_{eff}}} = \sqrt{T_1^2 + T_2^2}$.

39. **(c) :** Average value of A.C. for complete cycle is zero. Hence A.C. can not be measured by D.C. ammeter.

40. **(a) :** The energy loss due to eddy currents is reduced by using laminated core in a transformer.

41. **(a) :** $h = ut - (1/2)gt^2$ and $v^2 = u^2 - 2gh$
The above equations are independent of mass

42. **(d) :** If a body is projected from a place above the surface of earth, then for the maximum range, the angle of projection should be less than 45°.

43. **(b) :** The apparent weight of a body in an elevator moving with downward acceleration a is given by $W = m(g - a)$

44. **(d) :** If electric field is used for detecting the electron beam, then very high voltage will have to be applied or very long tube will have to be taken.

45. **(c) :** In the first few steps, work has to be done against limiting friction and afterwards, work is to be done against dynamic friction, which is smaller than the limiting friction.

46. **(a)**

47. **(a)**

48. **(b) :** Rolling occurs only on account of friction which is a tangential force capable of providing torque when the inclined plane is perfectly smooth, it will simply slip under the effect of its own weight. Once the perfect rolling begins, force of friction becomes zero. Hence, the work done against friction is zero.

49. **(a)**

50. **(a)** Water would evaporate quickly because there is no atmosphere on moon, due to which surface temperature of moon is much higher than earth (maximum surface temperature of moon is 123°C).

51. **(a)**

52. **(c) :** As conductivity of an intrinsic semiconductor is less than that of a lightly doped p-type

53. **(b) :** As UHF/VHF waves are not reflected by ionosphere being of higher frequency.

54. **(d) :** We cannot interchange the objective and eye lenses of a microscope to make a telescope. The reason is that the focal length of lenses in microscope are very small, of the order of mm or a few cm and the difference $(f_O - f_e)$ is very small, while the telescope objective have a very large focal length as compared to eye lens of microscope.

55. **(a) :** The period of a charged particle in a magnetic field is given by $T = \frac{2\pi m}{qB}$, *i.e.*, $T \propto \frac{m}{q}$

We know that, $m_p = m$, $m_\alpha = 4m$, $q_p = e$, $q_\alpha = 2e$

$\therefore\ \frac{T_p}{T_\alpha} = \frac{1}{2}$ or $T_\alpha = 2T_p$

56. **(a) :** As, $p_2 = p_1 + 50\%$ of $p_1 = (3/2)\,p_1$

$\therefore\ v_2 = (3/2)\,v_1$

As, kinetic energy, $K \propto v^2$

$\therefore\ K_2 = \frac{9}{4} K_1$

Increase in K.E. $= \frac{(K_2 - K_1)\times 100}{K_1} = 125\%$.

57. **(b) :** Acceleration due to gravity,
$g' = g - R_e\omega^2 \cos^2\lambda$
At equator, $\lambda = 0°$, $\therefore \cos 0° = 1$
$\therefore\ g_e = g - R_e\,\omega^2$
At poles, $\lambda = 90°$, $\therefore \cos 90° = 0$ $\therefore\ g_p = g$
Thus, $g_p - g_e = g - g + R_e\omega^2 = R_e\omega^2$
Also, the value of g is maximum at poles and minimum at equator.

58. **(c)** : As $P = Vi$, hence for the transmission of same power, high voltage implies less current. Therefore heat energy loses ($H = i^2 Rt / 4.2$) are minimized if power is transmitted at high voltage.

59. **(c)** : The earth's atmosphere is transparent to visible light and radio waves, but absorbs X-rays. Therefore X-rays telescope cannot be used on earth surface.

60. **(a)**

CHEMISTRY

61. **(c)**

62. **(b)** : The constituents of Mischmetal is approximately 50% cerium and 25% lanthanum with small amounts of neodymium and praseodymium.

63. **(a)** : For a first order reaction, rate = $k[A]$, when concentration of A is doubled, the rate becomes double.

64. **(c)** : In tetragonal system, $a = b \neq c$, $\alpha = \beta = \gamma = 90°$

65. **(c)** : (c) is correct answer because $r_{ionic} \propto \frac{1}{Z_{eff}}$

66. **(a)** :

$\xrightarrow{\Delta}$ Free radical

67. **(c)** :

$\xrightarrow{H^+}$ ... $\xrightarrow{-H^+}$ (P)

68. **(c)** : If product concentration is x.

For a zero order reaction $\frac{x}{t} = k$

Thus graph would be a straight line passing through origin. So the given information is for zero order reaction. For a zero order reaction, rate of the reaction is constant. Thus, plot of rate *vs* time, *i.e.*, $-\frac{d[X]}{dt}$ *vs* time will be a straight line parallel to x-axis.

69. **(c)** : $\frac{W_{Ca}}{E_{Ca}} = \frac{W_{Al}}{E_{Al}} \Rightarrow \frac{40}{20} = \frac{W_{Al}}{9} \Rightarrow W_{Al} = 18 \text{ kg}$

As current efficiency is 50% so, $W_{Al} = 9$ kg

70. **(b)** : Let the weight of CO = weight of $CH_4 = a$ g

Moles of CO $= \frac{a}{28}$

Moles of $CH_4 = \frac{a}{16}$

Total moles $= \frac{a}{28} + \frac{a}{16}$

$$x_{CH_4} = \frac{\frac{a}{16}}{\frac{a}{28} + \frac{a}{16}} = \frac{a}{16} \times \frac{28 \times 16}{44a} = \frac{14}{22} = \frac{7}{11}$$

$\therefore$ Fraction of pressure exerted by $CH_4 = 7/11$.

71. **(c)** : For $Cr^{3+} = 3d^3$, $\mu = \sqrt{3(3+2)} = \sqrt{15}$ B.M.

For $Fe^{2+} = 3d^6$, $\mu = \sqrt{4(4+2)} = \sqrt{24}$ B.M.

For $Ni^{2+} = 3d^8$, $\mu = \sqrt{2(2+2)} = \sqrt{8}$ B.M.

For $Mn^{2+} = 3d^5$, $\mu = \sqrt{5(5+2)} = \sqrt{35}$ B.M.

72. **(c)** : Cyanides, on hydrolysis, give acids

$$RCN + 2H_2O \xrightarrow{H^+} RCOOH + NH_3$$

while all other reactions give amines.

73. **(b)** :

2,4,6-triamino-1,3,5-triazine

74. **(b)** :

$$2NaOH_{(dilute)} + Br_2 \xrightarrow{cold} NaBrO + NaBr + H_2O$$

$$\underset{\text{Sodium hypobromide}}{3NaBrO} \xrightarrow{300\text{ K}} 3NaBrO$$

On acidification, the final mixture gives bromine.

$5NaBrO + NaBrO_3 + 6HCl \longrightarrow 6NaCl + 3Br_2 + 3H_2O$

Thus, during the reaction, bromine is present in four different oxidation states *i.e.*, zero in Br_2, +1 in NaBrO, −1 in NaBr and +5 in $NaBrO_3$. The greatest difference between various oxidation states of bromine is 6 and not 5. On acidification of the final mixture, Br_2 is formed and disproportionation of Br_2 occurs during the reaction giving BrO^-, Br^- and BrO_3^- ions.

75. **(c) :** The complex $PtCl_4.5NH_3$ is designated as $[Pt(NH_3)_5Cl]Cl_3$ which ionizes to $[Pt(NH_3)_5Cl]^{3+} + 3Cl^-$ ions. Thus total ions produced are four but three moles of AgCl are produced from $3Cl^-$ ions with $AgNO_3$.

76. **(c) :** $\wedge^{\infty}_{HOAC} = \wedge^{\infty}_{NaOAC} + \wedge^{\infty}_{HCl} - \wedge^{\infty}_{NaCl}$

$= 91.0 + 426.2 - 126.5$ S cm^2 mol^{-1}

$= 390.7$ S cm^2 mol^{-1}

77. **(c) :** $Cu^+ = 1s^2\,2s^2\,2p^6 3s^2 3p^6 3d^{10}$.
Shells occupied =3, sub-shells occupied = 6, filled orbitals = 14. Unpaired $e^- = 0$.

78. **(c) :** There is no restriction that resonating structures should have +ve and −ve charges on atoms that are far apart.

79. **(d) :** Lattice energy $= -\frac{q_1 q_2}{r^2}$

where q_1 and q_2 are charges on ions and r is the distance between them. Since interionic distances in CaO and NaCl are similar, (larger cation has smaller anion and vice versa) therefore, r is almost the same. Therefore, lattice energy depends only on charge. Since the magnitude of charge on Na^+ and Cl^- ions is unity and that on Ca^{2+} and O^{2-} ions is 2 each, therefore, the lattice energy of CaO is four times the lattice energy of NaCl, *i.e.*,4*U*.

80. **(b) :** Since the phosphate of a metal is $MHPO_4$, therefore, metal M must be divalent, *i.e.*, M^{2+}. As a result, the formula of its chloride is MCl_2.

81. **(d) :** $P = \frac{1}{3}\frac{mnu^2}{V}$

$$\frac{P_X}{P_Y} = \frac{n_X u_X V_Y}{n_Y u_Y V_x} = \frac{(N_0/1000)}{(N_0/2000)} \times 2 \times \frac{2}{1} = 8$$

82. **(d) :** From thermodynamics, $dG = VdP - SdT$

At constant T, $dT = 0$ so that $\left(\frac{\delta G}{\delta P}\right)_T = V$

At constant P, $dP = 0$ so that $\left(\frac{\delta G}{\delta T}\right)_P = -S$

Also $\mu_{JT} = \left(\frac{\delta T}{\delta P}\right)_H$

83. **(c) :** Glycine $H_3N^+CH_2COO^-$ is more acidic than basic. Instead of K_b value, the second given K_a value is corresponding to the K_b value $(\because K_a \times K_b = 10^{-14})$. Hence, overall ionization constant,

$K = K_{a_1} \times K_{a_2} = 4.5 \times 10^{-3} \times 1.7 \times 10^{-10}$

$= 7.65 \times 10^{-13}$

$H^+ = \sqrt{KC} = \sqrt{7.65 \times 10^{-13} \times 0.01}$

$= \sqrt{0.765 \times 10^{-14}} = 0.87 \times 10^{-7}$ M

pH = − log (0.87 × 10^{-7}) = 7.06

84. **(c) :** Sequence (c) contains only representative elements.

85. **(c) :** $2H_2O_2 \longrightarrow 2H_2O + O_2$
100 mL 1000 mL

or 1 mL of H_2O_2 will give 10 mL of O_2 at STP

Thus its volume strength is 10 volume.

86. **(a) :** Be exhibits maximum covalency of four whereas Al shows maximum covalency of six.

87. **(a) :**

Cyclohexene $\xrightarrow[2.\ Zn,\ H_2O]{1.\ O_3}$ OHC–(CH$_2$)$_3$–α–CHO (*E*) $\xrightarrow[\text{aldol condensation}]{OH^-}$ [cyclic intermediate with H–C=O and CHO] ≡ 2-hydroxycyclopentane-carbaldehyde (OH, CHO) $\xrightarrow{\Delta}$ cyclopentene–CHO (*F*)

88. **(a) :**

$CH_3C(=O)OC_2H_5 + CH_3MgBr \longrightarrow$ $(:O^-)C(OC_2H_5)(H_3C)(CH_3)$

$$\longrightarrow CH_3-\overset{O}{\overset{\|}{C}}-CH_3 + C_2H_5O^- \xrightarrow{CH_3MgX} (CH_3)_2C(XMgO)CH_3 \xrightarrow{HOH/H^+} (CH_3)_2C(HO)CH_3 \; (P)$$

89. (c) : Secondary (2°) amines (aliphatic as well as aromatic) react with nitrous acid (HNO_2) to form N-nitrosoamines.

$$\underset{(2^\circ \text{ amine})}{(C_2H_5)_2NH} + \underset{(\text{nitrous acid})}{HONO} \longrightarrow \underset{(\text{N-nitrosodiethylamine})}{(C_2H_5)_2N-N{=}O} + H_2O$$

90. (a) :

$$\underset{A}{C_3H_8O} \xrightarrow{K_2Cr_2O_7/H^+} \underset{B}{C_3H_6O} \xrightarrow{\text{amm. }AgNO_3} \text{Silver mirror}$$

$$\underset{B}{C_3H_6O} \xrightarrow{H_2NCONHNH_2\cdot HCl} C$$

Reaction of B indicates that B is an aldehyde thus B should be C_2H_5CHO or CH_3CH_2CHO and therefore C should be $CH_3CH_2CH=NNHCONH_2$.

$$\underset{[A]}{CH_3CH_2CH_2OH} \xrightarrow{[O]} \underset{[B]}{CH_3CH_2CHO} \xrightarrow{\text{Silver mirror test}} CH_3CH_2COOH + 2Ag\downarrow$$

$$CH_3CH_2CHO + \underset{\text{semicarbazide}}{H_2NNHCONH_2} \longrightarrow \underset{\text{semicarbazone } [C]}{CH_3CH_2CH=NNHCONH_2}$$

91. (b) : $\Delta x \geq \dfrac{h}{(4\pi)(m\Delta v)}$

$$\Delta x \geq \frac{6.626\times10^{-34}}{(4\times3.14\times1050)(0.9)\left(\dfrac{1}{3600}\right)\left(\dfrac{1000}{1}\right)}$$

$\Delta x \geq 2\times10^{-37}$ m

The uncertainty in the position of the car is far smaller than the uncertainty in the position of an electron in a hydrogen atom (3×10^{-10} m) and far too small a value to have any measurable consequences.

92. (b) : When a solute is present in very minute amounts (trace quantities), the concentration is expressed in ppm.

$$\text{ppm of } A = \frac{\text{mass of component } A}{\text{total mass of solution}} \times 10^6$$

$$= \frac{0.025}{10^3} \times 10^6 = 25 \text{ ppm}.$$

93. (a) : Degree of unsaturation of $C_{10}H_{18}O = 2$, but it contains no double or triple bond. Hence there are two rings – one six membered as indicated by product and the other three membered which is cleaved by HCl due to strain. Hence A has following structure.

$$H_3C-\underset{|}{\overset{OH}{\overset{|}{C}}}-CH_3 \text{ (attached to bicyclic ring: cyclohexane fused with cyclopropane)}$$

94. (d) : The structure of XeO_3F_2 - $O{=}Xe(F)(F)({=}O)_2$

No. of lone pair of Xe = 0 and no. of bond pair = 5

Hybridisation of Xe = sp^3d

Hence, shape of XeO_3F_2 should be trigonal bipyramidal and not octahedral.

95. (a) : For the desired reaction,

$$AgCl + 1e^- \rightarrow Ag + Cl^-, \quad E^\circ = \frac{-\Delta_r G^\circ}{(1)F}$$

The needed $\Delta_r G^\circ$ can be obtained by adding the values of $\Delta_r G^\circ$ for the reactions

$Ag^+ + 1e^- \rightarrow Ag$; $\Delta G^\circ = -nFE^\circ$

$AgCl \rightarrow Ag^+ + Cl^-$; $\Delta G^\circ = -RT \ln K_{sp}$, giving

$$\Delta_r G^\circ = -(1 \text{ mol})(9.648\times10^4 \text{ J mol}^{-1} \text{ V}^{-1})(0.7991 \text{ V})$$

$$-(8.314 \text{ JK}^{-1}\text{mol}^{-1})(298 \text{ K})\ln(1.56\times10^{-10})$$

$$= -77.10 \text{ kJ} + 55.95 \text{ kJ} = -21.15 \text{ kJ}$$

The potential is $E^\circ = \dfrac{-(-21.15)}{(1)(96.485)} = +0.2192$ V.

96. (d) : None of these acids evolve H_2 gas with alkali metals.

97. (b) : $Cl-CH_2-\overset{H}{\overset{|}{C}}-\overset{14}{C}H_2$ (epoxide, O bridging) $+ \overset{\ominus}{O}C_2H_5 \longrightarrow$

$Cl-CH_2-\overset{H}{\overset{|}{C}}(\overset{\ominus}{O})-\overset{14}{C}H_2-OC_2H_5 \longrightarrow H_2C-CH-\overset{14}{C}H_2-O-C_2H_5$ (epoxide, O bridging H_2C and CH)

98. (a) : Given, $M_{HCl} = 0.1$ M, $V_{HCl} = 18.0$ mL

$M_{NaHCO_3} = 0.125$ M, $V_{NaHCO_3} = ?$

On applying, $M_{HCl} \times V_{HCl} = M_{NaHCO_3} \times V_{NaHCO_3}$
$\Rightarrow 0.1 \times 18 = 0.125 \times V_{NaHCO_3}$
$\Rightarrow M_{NaHCO_3} = 14.4$ mL
Thus, 14.4 mL of the 1.25 M $NaHCO_3$ solution is needed to neutralise 18.0 mL of the 0.100 M HCl solution.

99. (b) : $M^+ + X^- \rightarrow M + X$ is spontaneous because for the cell represented by $M|M^+ \| X^-|X$, the value of $E°$ is positive *i.e.* (0.44 – 0.33) V = 0.11 V.

100. (b) : Allenes with even number of cumulative double bonds are optically active if both sides are disymmetric.

$$\begin{matrix} a \\ b \end{matrix}\!\!>\!C=C=C\!<\!\!\begin{matrix} a \\ b \end{matrix}$$

(horizontal plane) (vertical plane)

(no plane of symmetry)

101. (c) : NaCl and $CaCl_2$ are added to provide conductivity to the electrolyte and also to lower the fusion temperature of anhydrous $MgCl_2$.

102. (b) : The equilibrium constant is always fixed and is characteristic of a reaction at specified temperature. However final composition of a reaction mixture at equilibrium at constant temperature depends on the initial concentration of reactants and products.

103. (a) : PCl_5 is trigonal bipyramidal containing sp^3d hybridized P atom in liquid and gaseous states whereas in solid state it consists of tetrahedral PCl_4^+ cation and octahedral PCl_6^- anion.

104. (a)

105. (a) : $\overset{4}{C}H_3-\underset{\underset{COOC_2H_5}{|}}{\overset{3}{C}}=\overset{2}{C}H-\overset{1}{C}OOH$

Here since —COOH is the principal functional group, it gets the lowest number than the secondary functional group (3-carbethoxy). So it is 3-carbethoxy-2-butenoic acid.

106. (c) : He contains fully filled $1s^2$ orbital which has more penetrating effect and is very close to the nucleus and hence has higher value of ionisation energy.

107. (a) : The nuclear isomerism in the nuclei of same mass number and same atomic number arises due to different radioactive properties. The reason for nuclear isomerism is the different energy states of two isomeric nuclei. One may be in the ground state and other in an excited state. The nucleus in the excited state will have different half-life.

108. (b) : When a silicon crystal is doped with a group-15 elements, such as P, As, Sb or Bi the structure of the crystal lattice is left unchanged but an occasional atom with five valence electrons occupies a site that would normally be occupied by a silicon atom. The foreign atom uses four of its electrons in covalent bonding but the remaining fifth electron becomes delocalised and is thus free to contribute to electrical conduction.

109. (c) : Reactions of higher order are rare because chances for larger number of molecules to come simultaneously for collision are less.

110. (b) : In actual practice transition metals react with acid very slowly and act as poor reducing agents. This is due to the protection of metal as a result of formation of thin oxide protective film. Further, their poor tendency as reducing agent is due to high ionisation energy, high heat of vapourization and low heat of hydration.

111. (b) : Both carbanions (formed in presence of base) and enol form (formed in presence of an acid) act as nucleophiles and hence add on the carbonyl group of aldehydes and ketones to give aldols.

112. (a) : The loss of one α-particle will reduce the mass number by four and atomic number by two. Subsequent two β-emissions will increase the atomic number by two without affecting the mass number. Hence, the new element will be only an isotope of the parent nucleide and hence its position in the periodic table remains unchanged.

113. (d) : Atomic mass and molecular mass are the ratios and have no units.

$$\text{Mol. mass} = \frac{\text{Wt. of one molecule of the substance}}{\frac{1}{12} \times \text{wt. of one atom of C}-12}$$

114. (b) : Bond dissociation energy is the energy required to break a particular bond in one mole of a gaseous molecule. Bond energy is the average values of dissociation energies of the same type of bond present in the molecule. Bond energy of C–H bond in methane is 99.2 kcal/mol. Thus for polyatomic molecules, average bond energy is taken as the dissociation bond energy.

115. (b) : The higher the charge on the metal ion, smaller is the ionic size and more is the complex forming ability. Thus, the degree of complex formation decreases in the order

$M^{4+} > MO_2^{2+} > M^{3+} > MO_2^{+}$

The higher tendency of complex formation of MO_2^{2+} as compared to M^{3+} is due to high concentration of charge on metal atom M in MO_2^{2+}.

116. (a) : Sulphonation of benzene is an electrophilic substitution reaction in which SO_3 acts as the electrophile.

$$C_6H_6 + HOSO_3H \xrightleftharpoons{80^\circ C} C_6H_5SO_3H + H_2O$$

117. (a) : Molality does not depend upon volume thus it does not depend on temperature.

118. (d) : In a Frenkel defect an ion leaves its position in the lattice and occupies normally vacant interstitial position.

119. (a) : $\left[(en)_2Co\begin{smallmatrix}NH\\ \\ OH\end{smallmatrix}Co(en)_2\right]^{3+}$ is named as tetrakis (ethylenediammine)-μ-hydroxo-μ-imido dicobalt (III) ion. For more than one bridging group the word μ is repeated before each bridging group.

120. (c) : Greater the number of hyperconjugating structures, greater is the stability of the compound.

BIOLOGY

121. (c) : Vitamin B_6, also called pyridoxine is widely distributed in cereal grains, yeast, liver, milk, etc. It is a constituent of a coenzyme (pyridoxal phosphate) involved in amino acid metabolism. Deficiency causes retarded growth, dermatitis, convulsions, and other symptoms.

122. (d) : All single-celled eukaryotes are placed under protista. Phylogenetically the kingdom protista acts as a connecting link between the prokaryotic kingdom— Monera and the complex multicellular kingdoms— Fungi, Plantae and Animalia. Being eukaryotes, the protistan cell body contains a well defined nucleus and other membrane-bound organelles. It is surrounded by plasmalemma (cell membrane). Cilia and flagella occur in a number of forms. Nucleus has typical structure—porous nuclear envelope, chromatin, nucleolus and nucleoplasm. Monerans lack nuclear membrane.

123. (d) : DPT vaccine is a combined vaccine against diphtheria, whooping cough (pertussis), and tetanus now replaced by the DTaP/IPV/Hib and DTaP/IPV vaccines.

124. (d) : The vascular system consists of complex tissues, the phloem and the xylem. The xylem and phloem together constitute vascular bundles. In dicotyledonous stems, cambium is present between phloem and xylem. Such vascular bundles because of the presence of cambium possess the ability to form secondary xylem and phloem tissues, and hence are called open vascular bundles. In the monocotyledons, the vascular bundles have no cambium present in them. Hence, since they do not form secondary tissues they are referred to as closed.

125. (c)

126. (a)

127. (a) : Bryophytes are nonvascular terrestrial plants of moist habitats in which a multicellular diploid sporophyte lives as a parasite on an independent multicellular haploid gametophyte that develops multicellular jacketed sex organs. Whereas, in pteridophytes, the main plant body is a sporophyte which is differentiated into true root, stem and leaves and gametophyte is small or inconspicuous, it is usually independent.

128. (b) : Parietal cells are present in the epithelium of the gastric glands. They are large and are most numerous on the side walls of the glands. They are also called oxyntic cells as they stain strongly with eosin. They secrete hydrochloric acid and Castle intrinsic factor.

129. (a) : A single species might show high diversity at the genetic level over its distributional range. India has more than 50,000 genetically different strains of rice, and 1,000 varieties of mango.

130. (c)

131. (c) : Gene related human disorders are determined by mutations in single gene. They are transmitted to the offspring as per Mendelian principles. The pattern of inheritance of such Mendelian disorders can be traced in a family by the pedigree analysis. Cystic fibrosis is an abnormal recessive disorder of infants, children and young adults that is due to an abnormal recessive autosomal allele present on chromosome 7. In 70% of cases, it is due to deletion of three bases. The disease gets its name from the fibrous cysts that appear in the pancreas. It produces a defective glycoprotein. The defective glycoprotein causes formation of thick mucus in skin, lungs, pancreas, liver and other secretory organs. There is maldigestion of food with high fat content in stool. Liver may undergo cirrhosis.

Phenylketonuria is an inborn, autosomal, recessive metabolic disorder in which the homozygous recessive individual lacks the enzyme phenylalanine hydroxylase needed to change phenylalanine to tyrosine in liver. It results in hyperphenylalaninemia which is characterised by accumulation and excretion of phenylalanine, phenylpyruvic acid and related compounds. Lack of the enzyme is due to the abnormal autosomal recessive gene on chromosome 12.

132. **(d) :** In facilitated diffusion special proteins help move substances across membranes along the concentration gradient without expenditure of ATP energy. Facilitated diffusion is very specific, it allows cell to select substances for uptake. It is sensitive to inhibitors which react with protein side chains.

133. **(c) :** *Entamoeba histolytica* is a protozoan parasite in the large intestine of human which causes amoebiasis (amoebic dysentery).

Streptococcus pneumoniae and *Haemophilus influenzae* are responsible for the disease pneumonia in humans which infects the alveoli (air filled sacs) of the lungs. *Plasmodium*, a tiny protozoan is responsible for malaria. Typhoid fever could be confirmed by Widal test.

Wuchereria (*W. bancrofti* and *W. malayi*), the filarial worms cause a slowly developing chronic inflammation of the organs in which they live for many years, usually the lymphatic vessels of the lower limbs and the disease is called elephantiasis or filariasis.

134. **(b) :** The term ecology was coined by combining two Greek words, *oikos* (meaning 'house' or 'dwelling place') and *logos* (meaning 'the study of') to denote such relationships between the organisms and their environment. Thus, literally, ecology is the study of organisms 'at home'.

135. **(b) :** There are 64-triplet codons which code for 20 amino acids. This is due to the degeneracy of code as some amino acids are influenced by more than one codon. Only tryptophan and methionine are specified by single codons. All other amino acids are specified by two (*e.g.*, phenylalanine—UUU, UUC) to six (*e.g.*, arginine—CGU, CGC, CGA, CGG, AGA, AGG) codons.

136. **(c)**

137. **(a)**

138. **(c) :** The most recent model of plasma membrane is fluid-mosaic model which was proposed by Singer and Nicolson in 1972. According to this model, the membrane does not have a uniform disposition of lipids and proteins but is instead a mosaic of the two. Further, the membrane is not solid but is quasifluid.

139. **(c) :** *Penicillium notatum* restrict the growth of *Staphylococci*. *Acetobacter aceti* produces acetic acid. *Saccharomyces cerevisiae* is used for commercial production of ethanol. *Streptococcus* produces streptokinase which is modified by genetic engineering to be used as a 'clot buster' for removing clots from the blood vessels of patients who have undergone myocardial infarction leading to heart attack. Bacteria which produce methane are collectively called methanogens, and one such common bacterium is *Methanobacterium*. These bacteria are commonly found in the anaerobic sludge during sewage treatment.

140. **(d) :** Haemophilia B is due to def
IX (Christmas factor). T
prolong

14

142.

143. (
s

syndrome (a death warrant) is a serious disease (also called slim disease) caused by a retrovirus HIV (human immunodeficiency virus). It is a set of symptoms and infections resulting from the damage to the human immune system by the virus, that depletes primarily the number of T-lymphocytes (CD-4 T cells or helper T-cells) and renders the patient susceptible to opportunistic infections *i.e.*, infection caused by non-pathogens.

144. (d) : The P-wave represents the electrical excitation (or depolarisation) of the atria, which leads to the contraction of both the atria. The QRS complex represents the depolarisation of the ventricles, which initiates the ventricular contraction. The T-wave represents the return of the ventricles from excited to normal state (repolarisation). So, by counting the number of QRS complexes that occur in a given time period, one can determine the heart beat rate of an individual.

145. (b) : Phosphorus is a major constituent of biological membranes, nucleic acids and cellular energy transfer systems. Many animals also need large quantities of this element to make shells, bones and teeth. The natural reservoir of phosphorus is rock, which contains phosphorus in the form of phosphates. When rocks are weathered, minute amounts of these phosphates dissolve in soil solution and are absorbed by the roots of the plants. Herbivores and other animals obtain this element from plants.

146. (a) : Gonadotropin releasing hormone (GnRH), stimulates the anterior lobe of the pituitary gland to secrete two gonadotropic hormones, follicle stimulating hormone (FSH) and luteinising hormone (LH). In male LH activates the Leydig's (interstitial) cells of the testis to secrete androgens.

147. (c) : Human beings have a significant ability to maintain and moderate the respiratory rhythm to suit the demands of the body tissues. A specialised centre present in the medulla region of the brain called respiratory rhythm centre is primarily responsible for this regulation. A chemosensitive area is situated adjacent to the rhythm centre which is highly sensitive to CO_2 and hydrogen ions. Increase in these substances can activate this centre, which in turn can signal the rhythm centre to make necessary adjustments in the respiratory process by which these substances can be eliminated.

148. (b)

149. (a) : Microvilli increases absorptive surface area. Typhlosolar region in earthworm is the middle region of the intestine in which the mid-dorsal wall of the intestine is thrown into a longitudinal fold which is known as typhlosole. The typhlosole increases the absorptive surface of the intestine.

150. (b) : In ciliated epithelium, the cells bear numerous delicate hair like outgrowths, the cilia, arising from basal granules. This epithelium lines most of the respiratory tract and Fallopian tubes (oviducts). It is also present in tympanic cavity of middle ear and auditory tube (Eustachian tube).

151. (a) : Cyclic photophosphorylation is a process of photophosphorylation in which an electron expelled by the excited photocentre is returned to it after passing through a series of electron carriers. Cyclic photophosphorylation is performed by photosystem I only. The electron is circulated within the photosystem and the phosphorylation occurs due to cyclic flow of electron. The excited electron does not pass on to $NADP^+$ but is cycled back to the PS I complex through the electron transport chain. The cyclic flow hence, results only in the synthesis of ATP, but not of $NADPH + H^+$.

152. (c) : Elephant has the longest gestation period among the given animals. The gestation period of an elephant is 624-641 days.

153. (c) : Plasmid is a structure in bacterial cells consisting of DNA that can exist and replicate independently of the chromosome. These are extrachromosomal circular dsDNA which provide genetic instructions for certain cell activities (*e.g.* resistance to antibiotic drugs). They can be transferred from cell to cell in a bacterial colony. Plasmids are widely used as vectors to produce recombinant DNA for gene cloning.

154. (c) : Concept of chemical evolution refers to origin of life from non living matter. First inorganic compounds and then organic compounds were formed in accordance with ever changing environmental conditions.

155. (c)

Crop	Variety	Resistance to diseases
Wheat	Himgiri	Leaf and stripe rust, hill bunt
Brassica	Pusa swarnim	White rust
Cowpea	Pusa komal	Bacterial blight
Chilli	Pusa sadabahar	Chilly mosaic virus

156. (b) : Processes of recombinant DNA technology involves isolation of DNA of a desired DNA fragment. In order to cut the DNA with restriction enzymes, it needs to be in pure form, free from other macro molecules. The DNA is enclosed within the membranes, we have to break the cell open to release DNA along with other macromolecules such as RNA, proteins, polysaccharides and also lipids. This can be achieved by treating the bacterial cells/plant or animal tissue with enzymes such as lysozyme (bacteria), cellulase (plant cells), chitinase (fungus). The RNA can be removed by treatment with ribonuclease whereas proteins can be removed by treatment with protease.

157. (d) : Genus comprises a group of related species which has more characters in common in comparison to species of other genera. In the other words, genera are aggregates of closely related species. For example, potato and brinjal are two different species but both belong to the genus *Solanum*.

158. (b) : *Panthera tigris* - Tiger
Mangifera indica - Mango
Musca domestica - Housefly
Periplaneta americana - Cockroach
Rana tigerina - Common Indian frog

159. (c)

160. (a) : Calvin pathway occurs in all photosynthetic plants which is CO_2 fixation cycle. Carbon dioxide combines with ribulose-1, 5-biphosphate to produce a transient intermediate compound. The intermediate compound splits up immediately in the presence of water to form the two molecules of 3-phosphoglycerate or PGA. It is the first stable product of photosynthesis.

161. (b) : Adrenaline (epinephrine) is a hormone produced by the medulla of the adrenal glands, that increases heart activity, improves the power and prolongs the action of muscles, and increases the rate and depth of breathing to prepare the body for 'fright, fight, or flight.It is secreted at the time of emergency. Hence it is also called emergency hormone.

162. (b) : Cork consists of dead and compactly arranged rectangular cells that possess suberised cell walls. The cork cells contain tannins. Hence, they appear brown or dark brown in colour. The cork cells of some plants are filled with air. Cork prevents the loss of water by evaporation. It also protects the interior against entry of harmful micro-organisms, mechanical injury and extremes of temperature. Cork is light, compressible, nonreactive and sufficiently resistant to fire. It is used as stopper for bottles, shock absorption and insulation.

163. (a) : The blood of cockroach, also called as haemolymph is a mobile connective tissue composed of corpuscles and a colourless fluid, the plasma. It does not contain any respiratory pigment and therefore plays no role in respiration.

The respiratory system consists of a network of trachea, that open through 10 pairs of small holes called spiracles present on the lateral side of the body. Thin branching tubes carry oxygen from the air to all the parts. The opening of the spiracles is regulated by the sphincters. Exchange of gases take place at the tracheoles by diffusion.

164. (a) : Virus infected cells secrete proteins known as interferons which protect non infected cells from further viral infection.

165. (d) : The descending limb of loop of Henle is permeable to water but almost impermeable to electrolytes. This concentrates the filtrate as it moves down.

166. (a) : Shrinkage of the protoplast of a cell under the influence of a hypertonic solution is called plasmolysis. Hypertonic solution causes exosmosis or withdrawal of water from cytoplasm and then the central vacuole of cell. The size of cytoplasm as well as central vacuole and hence protoplast becomes reduced. The pressure on the wall is simultaneously reduced and the elastic wall contracts causing a reduction in cell size.

167. **(a) :** Inbreeding refers to the mating of closely related individuals within the same breed for 4-6 generations. Superior males and superior females of the same breed are identified and mated in pairs. The progeny obtained from such matings are evaluated and superior males and females among them are identified for further mating. Inbreeding increases homozygosity. Thus inbreeding is necessary if we want to evolve a pureline in any animal.

168. **(d) :** The process of delivery of the foetus (childbirth) is called parturition. Parturition is induced by a complex neuroendocrine mechanism. The signals for parturition originate from the fully developed foetus and the placenta which induce mild uterine contractions called foetal ejection reflex. This triggers release of oxytocin from the maternal pituitary. Oxytocin acts on the uterine muscle and causes stronger uterine contractions, which in turn stimulates further secretion of oxytocin. The stimulatory reflex between the uterine contraction and oxytocin secretion continues resulting in stronger and stronger contractions. This leads to expulsion of the baby out of the uterus through the birth canal.

169. **(c)**

170. **(c) :** Incomplete dominance is the phenomenon where none of the two contrasting alleles or factors is dominant. The expression of the character in a hybrid or F_1 individual is intermediate or a fine mixture of the expression of the two factors. The inheritance of flower colour in *Antirrhinum* is a good example to understand incomplete dominance. There are two types of flower colour in pure state, red and white. When the two types of plants are crossed, the hybrid or plants of F_1 generation have pink flowers. The pink colour apparently appears due to mixing of red and white colours (incomplete dominance).

171. **(c) :** Presence of large amounts of nutrients in water causes excessive growth of planktonic (free-floating) algae, called an algal bloom which imparts a distinct colour to the water bodies. Algal blooms cause deterioration of the water quality and fish mortality. Biomagnification refers to increase in concentration of the toxicant at successive trophic levels.

172. **(d) :** Bile (gall) is a bitter-tasting greenish-yellow alkaline fluid produced by the liver, stored in the gall bladder, and secreted into the duodenum of vertebrates. It assists the digestion and absorption of fats by the action of bile salts, which chemically reduce fatty substances and decrease the surface tension of fat droplets so that they are broken down and emulsified. Bile may also stimulate gut muscle contraction (peristalsis). Bile also contains the bile pigments, bilirubin and biliverdin, which are produced by the breakdown of the blood pigment haemoglobin.

173. **(a) :** The word "emphysema" means "inflation" or "full of air". Emphysema is an inflation or abnormal distension of the bronchioles or alveolar sacs of the lungs. It causes irreversible distension and loss of elasticity of alveoli. As a result, the alveolar sacs remain filled with air even after expiration. The exhalation becomes more difficult. The lungs remain inflated. Many of the septa between the alveoli are destroyed and much of the elastic tissue of the lungs is replaced by connective tissue. Major causes are cigarette smoking and the inhalation of other smoke or toxic substances over a period of time.

174. **(b) :** DNA fingerprinting involves identifying differences in some specific regions in DNA sequence called as repetitive DNA, because in these sequences, a small stretch of DNA is repeated many times. These sequences normally do not code for any proteins, but they form a large portion of human genome. These sequence show high degree of polymorphism and form the basis of DNA fingerprinting. As the polymorphisms are inheritable from parents to children, DNA fingerprinting is the basis of paternity testing in case of disputes.

175. **(c) :** Parasitism is a relationship between two living organisms of different species in which one organism called parasite obtains its food directly from another living organism called host.
Majority of the parasites harm the host; they may reduce the survival, growth and reproduction of the host and reduce its population density.
Pathogens are disease-causing microorganisms which get benefit by causing harm to host

organism. Pathogens such as viruses, bacteria, fungi, protozoans, helminths, insects etc., reproduce or multiply inside the host organism and therefore, they get the opportunity to complete the life cycle and spread their population.

176. (c) : CO_2 concentration of the atmosphere is 0.036% or 360 ppm (360 $\mu l \cdot l^{-1}$). It is a limiting factor for C_3 as the available CO_2 concentration is lower than the optimum for photosynthesis. Increase in its concentration upto 0.05% increases the rate of photosynthesis in most C_3 plants. When CO_2 concentration is reduced, there comes a point at which illuminated plant parts stop absorbing carbon dioxide from their environment. It is known as CO_2 compensation point or threshold value. At this value CO_2 fixed in photosynthesis is equal to CO_2 evolved in respiration and photorespiration. The value is 25–100 ppm in C_3 plants and 0–10 ppm in C_4 plants. The reason for low compensation value for C_4 plants is the greater efficiency of CO_2 fixation through PEP-carboxylase.

177. (a) : Glucagon stimulates the liver to convert stored glycogen into glucose. Glucagon is also called an "anti-insulin" hormone. Insulin is antagonistic to glucagon. Insulin converts glucose into glycogen in the liver and muscles.
It promotes protein synthesis in tissue from amino acids.Insulin reduces catabolism of proteins. It is an anabolic hormone. It increase the synthesis of fat in the adipose tissue from fatty acids.
Insulin reduces the breakdown and oxidation of fat.

178. (d) : Auditory ossicles are three small bones present in the middle ear. These three ear ossicles are malleus, the incus and the stapes. These three bones are in the sequence of malleus, incus and stapes and are attached to each other. Their function is to increase the intensity of sound waves. The cavity of middle ear communicates with that of pharynx through the air filled tube called Eustachian tube. The Eustachian tube maintains the balance in the air pressure between two sides of the ear drum and thus allows it to vibrate freely when sound waves impinge on it.

179. (c) : Pharyngeal nephridia occur in three pairs of bunches in the 4th, 5th and 6th segments lying on each side of the alimentary canal. The ducts of the nephridia of the sixth segment open into the buccal cavity while the ducts from the nephridia bunches of the fourth and fifth segments open into the pharynx. These ducts carry excretory products from the pharyngeal nephridia into the gut. Enteronephric condition is an adaptation for the conservation of water which is absorbed by the inner lining of the alimentary canal.
Ectonephric nephridia discharge their contents directly to the outside which help the earthworm in keeping the skin moist for cutaneous respiration only. Integumentary nephridia are ectonephric nephridia while, pharyngeal and septal nephridia are enteronephric.

180. (d) : Pantothenic acid, formerly known as chick anti-dermatitis factor or filtrate factor is widely distributed in nature. It is a surprise to biochemists that despite the involvement of pantothenic acid (as coenzyme A) in a great number of metabolic reactions, its deficiency manifestations have not been reported in humans, presumably because of the wide occurrence of this vitamin in almost all foods and because small amount can be synthesized in the body. Folic acid deficiency is probably the most common vitamin deficiency.
The macrocytic anaemia (abnormally large RBC) associated with megaloblastic changes in bone narrow is a characteristic feature of folate deficiency.

GENERAL KNOWLEDGE

181. (a)	**182.** (c)	**183.** (a)	**184.** (b)	**185.** (c)
186. (a)	**187.** (a)	**188.** (c)	**189.** (c)	**190.** (c)
191. (b)	**192.** (d)	**193.** (d)	**194.** (c)	**195.** (b)
196. (c)	**197.** (b)	**198.** (c)	**199.** (d)	**200.** (b)

☺☺☺

Chapterwise Index - '11

Physics • Chemistry • Biology

Use the index for topicwise analysis of AIIMS paper and refer to these questions when you are practising MCQs chapterwise.

PHYSICS

Chapter's Name	Question No.	Total
Units and Dimensions	1	1
Motion in One Dimension		
Motion in Two Dimensions		
Laws of Motion and Friction	31	1
Work, Power and Energy	44	1
Centre of Mass and Rotational Motion	3, 6	2
Gravitation	43	1
Properties of Matter	4, 5, 40	3
Oscillations	7, 8, 9	3
Waves	30, 32, 41	3
Heat and Thermodynamics	10, 34, 35, 45, 46	5
Electrostatics	11, 48	2
Current Electricity		
Thermal and chemical effects of current		
Magnetic Effects of Current	12, 20, 36, 37, 58	5
Magnetism	24, 25, 60	3
Electromagnetic Induction and Alternating Current	2, 13, 27, 28	4
Electromagnetic Waves		
Ray Optics	21, 22, 42, 51, 52, 59	6
Wave Optics	14, 15	2
Modern Physics	18, 19, 23, 26, 33, 38, 39, 47, 53, 54, 56, 57	12
Solids and Semiconductor Devices	24, 49, 50	3
Universe		
Principles of Communication	16, 17, 55	3

CHEMISTRY

Chapter's Name	Question No.	Total
Basic Concepts	61, 74	2
Atomic Structure	76, 79	2
Periodic Properties		
Chemical Bonding	71	1
Nuclear Chemistry	84	1
Gaseous and Liquid States	80	1
Solid State	83, 104	2
Mole Concept & Solutions	113	1
Colloids, Surface Chemistry & Catalysis	75	1
Equilibrium	77, 78, 82	3
Kinetics	87, 111	2
Energetics	72, 81, 85, 86, 110	5
Electrochemistry	107	1
Redox Reactions	73, 112	2
Metallurgy		
Hydrogen and its Compounds	66, 67, 108	3
s-Block Elements	70	1
p-Block Elements	62, 63, 65, 68, 101, 102, 103, 106, 109	9
d- and *f*-Block Elements	105	1
Complex Compounds	64, 69	2
Purification and Analysis of Organic Compound		
General Organic Chemistry	88, 89, 97, 98, 99, 117	6
Aliphatic Hydrocarbons	100	1
Aromatic Hydrocarbons	96, 116	2
Halogen Derivatives	114	1
Alcohols, Phenols and Ethers	93, 115, 120	3
Aldehydes and Ketones		
Carboxylic acids & their derivatives	95	1
Organic Compounds Containing Nitrogen	94	1
Biochemistry	90, 91, 118, 119	4
Chemistry in Action	92	1
Environmental Chemistry		

BIOLOGY		
Chapter's Name	**Question No.**	**Total**
General Biology	158	1
Biological Classification	123	1
Kingdom Monera		
Kingdom Fungi		
Plant Kingdom	145, 167	2
Cell and its Structural Components	128, 133	2
Cell Reproduction	143	1
Cell Respiration	135	1
Enzymes	161	1
Biomolecules		
Mendelian Genetics	171	1
Hereditary Material		
Anatomy of Flowering Plants	130	1
Morphology of Flowering Plants	129	1
Physiology of Flowering Plants	131, 132, 134, 137, 162, 163, 164	7
Embryology of Flowering Plants		
Growth and Development in Flowering Plants	126, 136, 165, 168	4
Angiosperm Families		
Ecology and Pollution	124, 125, 127, 148, 166, 169, 170	7
Applied Botany	139, 146, 173	3

Chapter's Name	Question No.	Total
Animal Kingdom	150, 154, 175	3
Genes and Chromosomes	144	1
Gene regulation and Applied Genetics	121, 122, 142	3
Human Genetics & Genetic Disorder		
Animal Tissue		
Musculo-Skeletal System	138, 149, 160	3
Digestive System and Nutrition	140, 174	2
Respiration		
Circulatory System and Immunity	155, 159, 176, 177	4
Excretion and Osmoregulation	156	1
Reproduction and Embryonic Development	152, 157, 172, 179	4
Nervous System and Sense Organs	151, 178	2
Endocrine System		
Common Human Disease	147, 180	2
Growth and Regeneration		
Evolution	153	1
Drug Addiction		
Applied Zoology		
Wild Life and Conservation	141	1
Human Population & Growth		

SOLVED PAPER
AIIMS - 2011★

Time : 3½ Hours Max. Marks : 200

PHYSICS

1. What is the dimensions of magnetic field B in terms of C (= coulomb), M, L, T?
(a) $[M^1L^1T^{-2}C]$ (b) $[M^1L^0T^{-1}C^{-1}]$
(c) $[M^1L^0T^{-2}C]$ (d) $[M^1L^0T^{-1}C]$

2. What is the mechanical equivalent of spring constant k in LC oscillating circuit?
(a) $\frac{1}{L}$ (b) $\frac{1}{C}$
(c) $\frac{L}{C}$ (d) $\frac{1}{LC}$

3. What is the moment of inertia for a solid sphere w.r.t. a tangent touching to its surface?
(a) $\frac{2}{5}MR^2$ (b) $\frac{7}{5}MR^2$
(c) $\frac{2}{3}MR^2$ (d) $\frac{5}{3}MR^2$

4. Water is flowing with velocity 4 m s^{-1} in a cylinder of diameter 8 cm, it is connected to a pipe with it end tip of diameter 2 cm, calculate the velocity of water at this free end.
(a) 4 m s^{-1} (b) 8 m s^{-1}
(c) 32 m s^{-1} (d) 64 m s^{-1}

5. A cylindrical wire is twisted with an angle θ, what is torsion produced in it?
(a) $\frac{C}{\theta}$ (b) $C\theta$
(c) $\frac{C}{\theta^2}$ (d) $C\theta^{3/2}$

6. Given, $\vec{\omega} = 2\hat{k}$ and $\vec{r} = 2\hat{i} + 2\hat{j}$. Find the linear velocity.
(a) $4\hat{i} + 4\hat{j}$ (b) $4\hat{i} + 4\hat{k}$
(c) $-4\hat{i} + 4\hat{j}$ (d) $-4\hat{i} - 4\hat{j}$

7. If maximum speed of a particle in SHM is given by V_m, what is its average speed?
(a) $\frac{\pi}{2}V_m$ (b) $\frac{2}{\pi}V_m$
(c) $\frac{\pi}{4}V_m$ (d) $\frac{V_m}{\sqrt{2}}$

8. Which of the following equation does not represent a SHM?
(a) $\cos\omega t + \sin\omega t$ (b) $\sin\omega t - \cos\omega t$
(c) $1 - \sin 2\omega t$ (d) $\sin\omega t + \cos(\omega t + \alpha)$

9. In simple harmonic motion, loss of kinetic energy is proportional to
(a) e^x (b) x^3
(c) $\log x$ (d) x^2

10. Emissive and absorptive power of a material at 2000 K is 8 and 10 respectively, calculate the emissivity of IBB (Ideal black body)
(a) 0.2 (b) 0.4
(c) 0.6 (d) 0.8

11. Energy stored in between the plates of parallel plate capacitor of area A, separated by distance d is
(a) $\frac{1}{2}\varepsilon_0 E^2 Ad$ (b) $\frac{1}{2}\varepsilon_0 E^2 \frac{A}{d}$
(c) $\frac{1}{2}\varepsilon_0 \frac{d}{E^2 A}$ (d) $\frac{1}{2}\frac{Ad}{\varepsilon_0 E^2}$

12. Magnetic energy per unit volume is represented by
(a) $\frac{B^2}{2\mu_0}$ (b) $\frac{B^2}{2\mu_0^2}$
(c) $\frac{2B^2}{\mu_0}$ (d) $\frac{B^2}{\mu_0}$

13. Mutual inductance M between two concentric coils of radii 1 m and 2 m is
(a) $\frac{\mu_0\pi}{2}$ (b) $\frac{\mu_0\pi}{4}$

★ *Based on memory*, Contributed by : **Allen Career Institute**, Kota (Rajasthan)

(c) $\frac{\mu_0 \pi}{8}$ (d) $\frac{\mu_0 \pi}{10}$

14. In an interference, the intensity of two interfering waves are I and $4I$ respectively. They produce intensity at two points A and B with phase angle of $\pi/2$ and π respectively. Then difference in between them is

(a) I (b) $2I$
(c) $4I$ (d) $5I$

15. In a single slit diffraction with $\lambda = 500$ nm and a lens of diameter 0.1 mm then width of central maxima, obtain on screen at a distance of 1 m will be

(a) 5 mm (b) 1 mm
(c) 10 mm (d) 2.5 mm

16. Voltage of modulating wave of 5 V with 10 MHz frequency was superimposed on carrier wave of frequency 20 MHz and voltage 20 V then the modulation index is

(a) 0.25 (b) 1.25
(c) 2.43 (d) 64.0

17. The area covered by a transmitting antenna of height 50 m is

(a) 320π km^2 (b) 1440 km^2
(c) 640π km^2 (d) 120π km^2

18. If we assume kinetic energy of a proton is equal to energy of the photon, the ratio of de Broglie wavelength of proton to photon is proportional to

(a) E (b) $E^{-1/2}$
(c) $E^{1/2}$ (d) $E^{3/2}$

19. The ratio of the masses of the elements having their nuclear radii 2 fermi and 1 fermi is

(a) 8 (b) 2
(c) 3 (d) 4

20. A proton travels few distance in an electric field, then it enters a crossed magnetic field of 1 T and radius 0.2 m, find the velocity of proton.

(a) 0.2×10^8 m s^{-1} (b) 0.2×10^7 m s^{-1}
(c) 0.2×10^6 m s^{-1} (d) 2×10^7 m s^{-1}

21. Two lens of focal lengths –20 cm and +10 cm are put in combination, find the power of the combination.

(a) – 1 D (b) – 2 D
(c) + 5 D (d) + 2 D

22. A far sighted person has his near point 50 cm, find the power of lens he should use to see at 25 cm, clearly.

(a) + 1 D (b) + 2 D
(c) – 2 D (d) – 1 D

23. For a nuclear reactor to run in critical condition the reproduction factor k should be

(a) = 1 (b) > 1
(c) < 1 (d) >>> 1

24. Which of the following substances magnetic susceptibility χ_m is negative?

(a) Diamagnetic (b) Paramagnetic
(c) Ferromagnetic (d) All of these

25. When orientation of dipoles parallel and antiparallel to magnetic field is distributed unequally, then the material is

(a) paramagnetic (b) ferromagnetic
(c) ferrimagnetic (d) antiferromagnetic

26. S^{32} absorbs energy and decays into which element after two α-emissions?

(a) Carbon (b) Aluminium
(c) Oxygen (d) Magnesium

27. Lenz law is consistent with conservation of

(a) energy (b) mass
(c) charge (d) momentum

28. In series LCR circuit, the phase difference between applied voltage and current is

(a) positive when $X_L > X_C$
(b) positive when $X_C > X_L$
(c) 90° (d) 0°

29. Direction of electric field in P-N junction diode is

(a) from P-side to N-side
(b) from N-side to P-side
(c) randomly oriented
(d) electric field does not exist

30. What is your observation when two sources are emitting sound with frequency 499 Hz and 501 Hz?

(a) Frequency of 500 Hz is heard with change in intensity take place twice.
(b) Frequency of 500 Hz is heard with change in intensity take place once.
(c) Frequenc y of 2 Hz is heard with change in intensity take place once.
(d) Frequency of 2 Hz is heard with change in intensity take place twice.

31. A 0.2 kg object at rest is subjected to a force $(0.3\hat{i} - 0.4\hat{j})$ N. What is the velocity after 6 s?
(a) $(9\hat{i} - 12\hat{j})$ (b) $(8\hat{i} - 16\hat{j})$
(c) $(12\hat{i} - 9\hat{j})$ (d) $(16\hat{i} - 8\hat{j})$

32. If man were standing unsymmetrically between parallel cliffs, claps his hands and starts hearing a series of echoes at intervals of 1 s. If speed of sound in air is 340 m s^{-1}, the distance between two cliffs would be
(a) 340 m (b) 510 m
(c) 170 m (d) 680 m

33. Half life of a radioactive material is 5 years, then the percentage of it remained after 25 years will be
(a) 3.125% (b) 6.25%
(c) 1.25% (d) 25%

34. For an adiabatic process
(a) $\Delta S = 0$ (b) $\Delta U = 0$
(c) $Q = 0$ (d) $W = 0$

35. For cyclic process which of the following quantity is zero?
(a) ΔV (b) ΔU
(c) W (d) ΔQ

36. Magnetic field at *a* distance a from long current carrying wire is proportional to
(a) $\frac{1}{a}$ (b) $\frac{1}{a^2}$
(c) $\frac{1}{\sqrt{a}}$ (d) $\frac{1}{a^{3/2}}$

37. When a positively charged particle enters into a uniform magnetic field with uniform velocity, its trajectory can be
(i) a straight line (ii) a circle
(iii) a helix
(a) (i) only (b) (i) or (ii)
(c) (i) or (iii)
(d) any one of (i), (ii) and (iii)

38. Among the following which is used to control the rate of reaction in nuclear fission reactions?
(a) Water (b) Heavy water
(c) Cadmium (d) Graphite

39. The series corresponding to minimum wavelength transition in H-atom
(a) Balmer series (b) Lyman series
(c) Paschen series (d) Brackett series

40. Pressure head in Bernoulli's equation is
(a) $\frac{P\rho}{g}$ (b) $\frac{P}{\rho g}$
(c) ρg (d) $P\rho g$

Directions : In the following questions (41-60), a statement of assertion (A) is followed by a statement of reason (R). Mark the correct choice as :
(a) If both assertion and reason are true and reason is the correct explanation of assertion.
(b) If both assertion and reason are true but reason is not the correct explanation of assertion.
(c) If assertion is true but reason is false.
(d) If both assertion and reason are false.

41. **Assertion** : Transverse sound wave does not occurs in gases.
Reason : Gases cannot sustain shearing strain.

42. **Assertion** : When white light fall on the compact disc, multicolours are seen after reflection.
Reason : CD disc behaves like a prism.

43. **Assertion** : Total energy is conserved in moving a satellite to higher orbit.
Reason : Sum of change in PE and KE is same in magnitude and opposite in nature.

44. **Assertion** : KE is conserved at every instant of (elastic) collision.
Reason : No deformation of matter occurs in elastic collision.

45. **Assertion** : C_P is always greater than C_V in gases.
Reason : Work done at constant pressure is more than at constant volume.

46. **Assertion** : During rapid pumping of air in tyres, air inside the tyre is hotter than atmospheric air.
Reason : Adiabatic process occurs at very high rate.

47. **Assertion** : For nuclear reactor, it is desirable to have $k = 1$.
Reason : Sustained chain reaction occur at this critical condition.

48. Assertion : Gauss's law can't be used to calculate electric field near an electric dipole.

Reason : Electric dipole don't have symmetrical charge distribution.

49. Assertion : Photodiode and photovoltaic cell are based on the same principle.

Reason : Both use same method of operations to work.

50. Assertion : Transistor can be used as a switch.

Reason : Both linear and non-linear voltage bias dependance occurs in it.

51. Assertion : When a white light is passed through a lens, violet light is more refracted than red light.

Reason : Focal length for red light is greater than violet.

52. Assertion : Microscope magnifies the image.

Reason : Angular magnification for image is more than object in microscope.

53. Assertion : Mass defect in nuclear reactions is less than 1%

Reason : In nuclear reaction, change in *BE/N* is generally less than 1%.

54. Assertion : It is very easy to detect neutrino in nature.

Reason : It has high affinity to interact with matter.

55. Assertion : In the transmission of long distance radio signals, short wave band is used.

Reason : In shorter wavelength, attenuation is very less.

56. Assertion : There is a physical significance of matter waves.

Reason : Both interference and diffraction occurs in it.

57. Assertion : It is desirable to slow down fast moving neutrons to sustain controlled chain reactions.

Reason : Slow moving neutrons efficiently collides with U^{235}.

58. Assertion : Magnetic field lines are continuous and closed.

Reason : Magnetic monopole does not exist.

59. Assertion : Magnification of a convex mirror is always positive, but that of a concave mirror may be both positive or negative.

Reason : It depends on the sign convention chosen.

60. Assertion : Magnetic force between two short magnets, when they are co-axial follows inverse square law of distance.

Reason : The magnetic forces between two poles do not follow inverse square law of distance.

CHEMISTRY

61. The compound which does not exist as hydrate form
(a) ferrous sulphate (b) copper sulphate
(c) magnesium sulphate
(d) sodium chloride

62. Iodine oxidises sodium borohydride to give
(a) B_2H_6 (b) sodium hydride
(c) HI (d) I_3^-

63. The wrong statement about fullerene is
(a) it has 5-membered carbon ring
(b) it has 6-membered carbon ring
(c) it has sp^2 hybridization
(d) it has 5-membered rings more than 6-membered rings

64. The wavelength of light absorbed is highest in
(a) $[Co(NH_3)_5Cl]^{2+}$ (b) $[Co(NH_3)_5H_2O]^{3+}$
(c) $[Co(NH_3)_6]^{3+}$ (d) $[Co(en)_3]^{3+}$

65. PCl_3 on hydrolysis gives fumes of
(a) $H_3PO_3 + HCl$ (b) $H_3PO_4 + HCl$
(c) H_3PO_2 and H_3PO_3 (d) $H_3PO_2 + HCl$

66. In solid ice, oxygen atom is surrounded
(a) tetrahedrally by 4 hydrogen atoms
(b) octahedrally by 2 oxygen and 4 hydrogen atoms
(c) tetrahedrally by 2 hydrogen and 2 oxygen atoms
(d) octahedrally by 6 hydrogen atoms

67. Predict the product of reaction of I_2 with H_2O_2 in basic medium.

(a) I^- (b) I_2O_3
(c) IO_3^- (d) I_3^-

68. First compound of Xe synthesized was
(a) $[XeF]^+ [XePtF_5]^-$ (b) $[XeO_2]$
(c) $Xe[PtF_6]$ (d) $O_2[XeF_6]$

69. Which of the following is diamagnetic ?
(a) $[Cu(NH_3)_4]^{2+}$ (b) $[NiCl_4]^{2-}$
(c) $[PtCl_4]^{2-}$ (d) $[Cu(H_2O)_4]^{2+}$

70. Which of the following is not hygroscopic?
(a) $CsCl$ (b) $MgCl_2$
(c) $CaCl_2$ (d) $LiCl$

71. Decreasing order of bond angle is
(a) $BeCl_2 > NO_2 > SO_2$ (b) $BeCl_2 > SO_2 > NO_2$
(c) $SO_2 > BeCl_2 > NO_2$ (d) $SO_2 > NO_2 > BeCl_2$

72. The enthalpy of formation of $CO_{(g)}$, $CO_{2(g)}$, $N_2O_{(g)}$ and $N_2O_{4(g)}$ is –110, –393, +811 and 10 kJ/mol respectively. For the reaction, $N_2O_{4(g)} + 3CO_{(g)} \rightarrow N_2O_{(g)} + 3CO_{2(g)}$. ΔH_r (kJ/mol) is
(a) –212 (b) +212
(c) +48 (d) – 48

73. When $KMnO_4$ reacts with KBr in alkaline medium gives bromate ion. Then oxidation state of Mn changes from +7 to
(a) +6 (b) +4
(c) +3 (d) +2

74. How much amount of $CuSO_4{\cdot}5H_2O$ is required for liberation of 2.54 g of I_2 when titrated with KI?
(a) 2.5 g (b) 4.99 g
(c) 2.4 g (d) 1.2 g

75. Which of the following is incorrect for physisorption?
(a) Reversible
(b) Increases with increase in temperature.
(c) Low heat of adsorption.
(d) Increases with increase in surface area.

76. Smallest wavelength occurs for
(a) Lyman series (b) Balmer series
(c) Paschen series (d) Brackett series

77. K_{sp} of $CaSO_4{\cdot}5H_2O$ is 9×10^{-6}, find the volume for 1 g of $CaSO_4$ (M.wt. = 136).
(a) 2.45 litre (b) 5.1 litre
(c) 4.52 litre (d) 3.2 litre

78. Which of the following is not a characteristic of equilibrium?
(a) Rate is equal in both directions.
(b) Measurable quantities are constant at equilibrium.
(c) Equilibrium occurs in reversible condition.
(d) Equilibrium occurs only in open vessel at constant temperature.

79. Which of the following is wrong for Bohr model?
(a) It establishes stability of atom.
(b) It is inconsistent with Heisenberg uncertainty principle.
(c) It explains the concept of spectral lines for hydrogen like species.
(d) Electrons behave as particle and wave.

80. In the van der Waals equation, 'a' signifies
(a) intermolecular attraction
(b) intramolecular attraction
(c) attraction between molecules and wall of container
(d) volume of molecules

81. For adiabatic process, which is correct?
(a) $\Delta T = 0$ (b) $\Delta S = 0$
(c) $q = 0$ (d) $q_p = 0$

82. 25 mL, 0.2 M $Ca(OH)_2$ is neutralised by 10 mL of 1 M HCl. Then pH of resulting solution is
(a) 1.37 (b) 9
(c) 12 (d) 7

83. Schottky defect is
(a) vacancy of ions
(b) delocalization of ions
(c) interstitial vacancy of ions
(d) vacancy of only cations

84. Which material is used as a neutron moderator?
(a) Graphite (b) Cadmium
(c) Boron (d) Uranium

85. Which of the following is not a thermodynamic function?
(a) Internal energy (b) Work done
(c) Enthalpy (d) Entropy

86. Which of the following is intensive property?
(a) Enthalpy (b) Entropy
(c) Specific heat (d) Volume

87. For a first order gas phase reaction–

$$A_{(g)} \rightarrow 2B_{(g)} + C_{(g)}$$

P_0 be initial pressure of A and P_t the total pressure at time 't'. Integrated rate equation is

(a) $\frac{2.303}{t}\log\left(\frac{P_0}{P_0 - P_t}\right)$

(b) $\frac{2.303}{t}\log\left(\frac{2P_0}{3P_0 - P_t}\right)$

(c) $\frac{2.303}{t}\log\left(\frac{P_0}{2P_0 - P_t}\right)$

(d) $\frac{2.303}{t}\log\left(\frac{2P_0}{2P_0 - P_t}\right)$

88. Decreasing order of nucleophilicity is

(a) $OH^- > NH_2^- > CH_3O^- > RNH_2$

(b) $NH_2^- > OH^- > CH_3O^- > RNH_2$

(c) $NH_2^- > CH_3O^- > OH^- > RNH_2$

(d) $CH_3O^- > NH_2^- > OH^- > RNH_2$

89. Find the number of stereoisomers of 1,2-dihydroxy cyclopentane.

(a) 1 (b) 2
(c) 3 (d) 4

90. Find the hydrolysis product when a phosphodiester bond of nucleotide breaks.

(a) 3-OH-deoxyribose-5-PO_4^{3-}
(b) 5-OH-deoxyribose-3-PO_4^{3-}
(c) 2-OH-deoxyribose-2-PO_4^{3-}
(d) 4-OH-deoxyribose-2-PO_4^{3-}

91. Find the hydrolysis product of maltose.

(a) α-D-glucose + α-D-glucose
(b) α-D-glucose + α-D-fructose
(c) α-D-glucose + α-D-galactose
(d) α-D-fructose + α-D-galactose

92. Isoprene is

(a) 3-methyl-1,2-butadiene
(b) 2-methyl-1,3-butadiene
(c) 3-chloro-1,2-butadiene
(d) 2-chloro-1,3-butadiene

93. Find the product for

$CH_3CH_2–O–CH_2–CH_2–O–CH_2–C_6H_5 + HI$ (excess)

(a) $HO–CH_2CH_2OH, C_6H_5CH_2–I, CH_3CH_2–I$
(b) $C_6H_5CH_2–OH, CH_3CH_2–I, I–CH_2CH_2–OH$
(c) $I–CH_2CH_2–I, C_6H_5CH_2–I, CH_3CH_2–OH$
(d) $HO–CH_2CH_2–OH, C_6H_5CH_2–I, CH_3CH_2–OH$

94. Best method to form aromatic iodide is

(a) $ArN_2^+ + HI \longrightarrow$ (b) $RNH_2 + I_2 \longrightarrow$
(c) $ArN_2^+ + KI \longrightarrow$ (d) $ArN_2^+ + PI_3 \longrightarrow$

95. Maximum decarboxylation occurs in

(a) CH_3COOH (b) C_6H_5COOH
(c) $C_6H_5CH_2COOH$ (d) CH_3COCH_2COOH

96. The correct increasing order of reactivity for the following molecules towards electrophilic aromatic substitution is

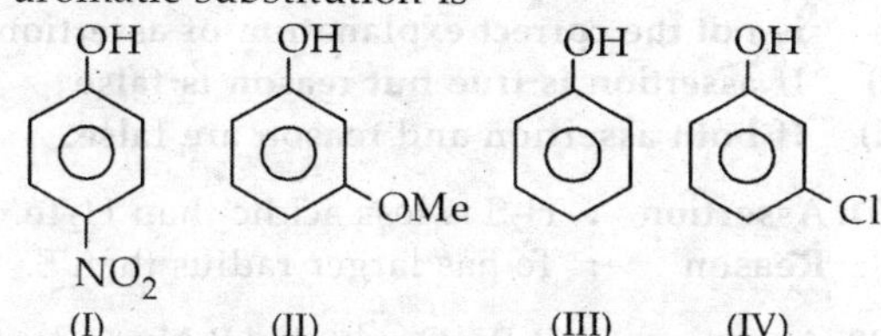

(a) I < IV < II < III (b) I < IV < III < II
(c) I < III < II < IV (d) I < III < IV < II

97.

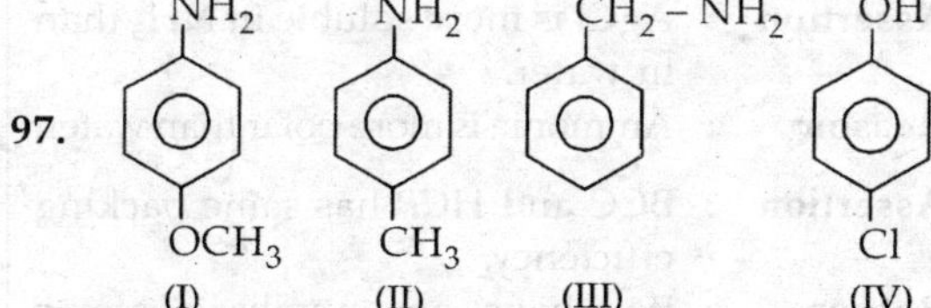

The correct decreasing order of pK_b is

(a) I > II > III > IV (b) III > IV > II > I
(c) II > III > IV > I (d) IV > II > I > III

98. The correct decreasing order of pK_a is

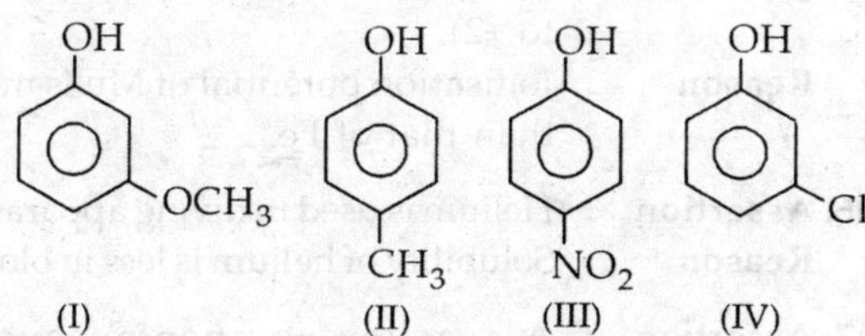

(a) II > IV > I > III (b) IV > II > III > I
(c) III > II > IV > I (d) IV > I > II > III

99. S_N2 reaction readily occurs in

(a) $CH_3CH_2 – O – CH_3$

(b) $CH_3 – C(CH_3)_2 – O – CH_3$

(c) $CH_2{=}CH - CH_2 - O - CH_3$
(d) $Ph - CH_2 - O - CH_2 - CH_3$

100. The number of σ- and π-bonds present in pent-4-ene-1-yne is
(a) 10, 3 (b) 4, 9
(c) 3, 10 (d) 9, 4

Directions : In the following questions (101-120), a statement of assertion (A) is followed by a statement of reason (R). Mark the correct choice as :
(a) If both assertion and reason are true and reason is the correct explanation of assertion
(b) If both assertion and reason are true but reason is not the correct explanation of assertion
(c) If assertion is true but reason is false
(d) If both assertion and reason are false.

101. Assertion : H_2S is less acidic than H_2Te.
Reason : Te has larger radius than S.

102. Assertion : $R_3P{=}O$ exists but $R_3N{=}O$ does not exist.
Reason : P is more electronegative than N.

103. Assertion : AgCl is more soluble in NH_3 than in water.
Reason : Ammonia is more polar than water.

104. Assertion : BCC and HCP has same packing efficiency.
Reason : Both have same number of atoms per unit cell and same arrangement.

105. Assertion : Reduction potential of Mn (+3 to +2) is more positive than Fe (+3 to +2).
Reason : Ionisation potential of Mn is more than that of Fe.

106. Assertion : Helium is used in diving apparatus.
Reason : Solubility of helium is less in blood.

107. Assertion : A reaction is spontaneous if E_{cell} = +ve.
Reason : For E_{cell} = +ve, ΔG is always –ve.

108. Assertion : Sulphur is oxidised by H_2O_2 in presence of Fe (III).
Reason : Fe (III) oxidises sulphur to sulphate.

109. Assertion : Chlorine undergoes disproportionation reaction in alkaline medium.
Reason : Cl_2 is an oxidising agent.

110. Assertion : Entropy is always constant for a closed system.
Reason : Closed system is always reversible.

111. Assertion : Two different reactions can never have same rate of reaction.
Reason : Rate of reaction always depends only on frequency of collision and Arrhenius factor.

112. Assertion : The formal oxidation no. of sulphur in $Na_2S_4O_6$ is 2.5.
Reason : Two S-atoms are not directly linked with O-atoms.

113. Assertion : A non volatile solute is mixed in a solution then elevation in boiling point and depression in freezing point both are 2 K.
Reason : Elevation in boiling point and depression in freezing point both depend on melting point of non-volatile solute.

114. Assertion : Rate of reaction of alkyl halide in Williamson's synthesis reaction is 1°RX > 2°RX > 3°RX.
Reason : It is a type of bimolecular substitution reaction (S_N2).

115. Assertion : Dehydration of alcohols always takes place in basic medium.
Reason : OH^- is a better leaving group.

116. Assertion : Toluene in presence of UV rays forms benzaldehyde.
Reason : Dichlorotoluene is formed as an intermediate.

117. Assertion : $CH_3-C(CH_3)_2-CH_2-Br + NaOH \longrightarrow CH_3-C(CH_3)(OH)-CH_2-CH_3$
Reason : It follows with formation of more stable carbocation.

118. Assertion : β- pleated sheet structure of protein shows maximum extension.

Reason : Intermolecular hydrogen bonding is present in them.

119. Assertion : Fructose is a reducing sugar.
Reason : It has a ketonic group.

120. Assertion : *p*-Nitrophenol gives more electrophilic substituted compound than *m*-methoxyphenol.
Reason : Methoxy group shows only negative *I*-effect.

BIOLOGY

121. What is the source of *Eco* R I?
(a) *Escherichia coli* R I
(b) *Escherichia coli* R I 13
(c) *Escherichia coli* R Y 13
(d) *Escherichia coli* R X 13

122. First clinical gene therapy was given in 1992 to a 4 years old girl for
(a) adenine deficiency
(b) growth deficiency
(c) adenosine deaminase deficiency
(d) adenosine deficiency

123. Bacteria, fungi, lower plants survive in adverse conditions by
(a) diapause (b) suspended growth
(c) migration
(d) formation of thick walled spores

124. What are labelled phases A, B and C in given sigmoidal growth curve?

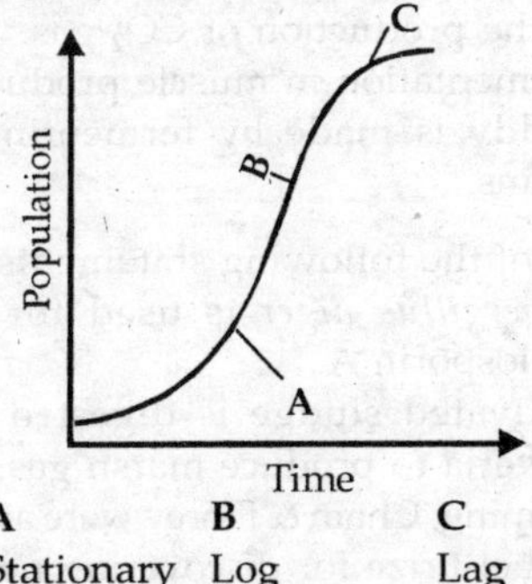

	A	B	C
(a)	Stationary	Log	Lag
(b)	Lag	Stationary	Log
(c)	Log	Lag	Stationary
(d)	Lag	Log	Stationary

125. Monarch butterfly escapes from predators by
(a) foul smell (b) bitter taste
(c) colour combination
(d) rough skin

126. What is the characteristic of tapetum ?
(a) It does not store food
(b) It is multi-nucleated
(c) It is multi-layered structure
(d) It nourishes the megaspore

127. In vehicles, catalytic converters are used
(a) to increase mileage of vehicles
(b) to convert CO_2 into carbonates
(c) to increase the efficiency of lead mixed petrol
(d) to convert CO to CO_2.

128. Cell theory was proposed by
(a) a botanist
(b) a zoologist
(c) a botanist and a zoologist
(d) a psychologist

129. Identify the given figures A, B, C, D and E.

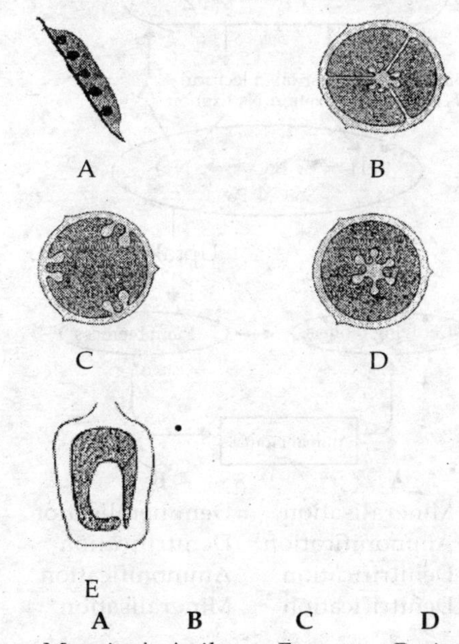

	A	B	C	D	E
(a)	Marginal	Axile	Free central	Parietal	Basal
(b)	Marginal	Parietal	Free central	Axile	Basal
(c)	Marginal	Axile	Parietal	Free central	Basal
(d)	Marginal	Axile	Parietal	Basal	Free central

130. Given figure shows

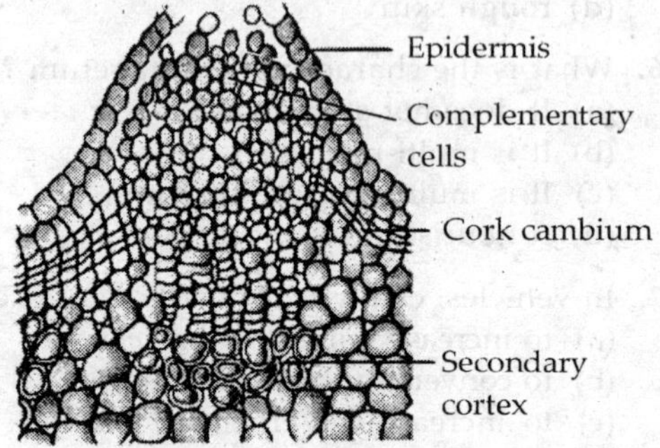

(a) structure of lenticel
(b) hydathode showing gaseous vapour exchange
(c) fungus reproducing by spore formation
(d) algae reproducing by spore formation.

131. In the given diagram A and B represent

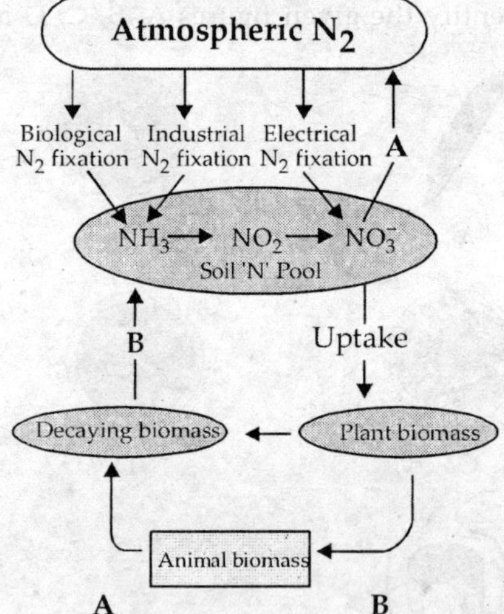

	A	B
(a)	Mineralisation	Demineralisation
(b)	Ammonification	Denitrification
(c)	Denitrification	Ammonification
(d)	Denitrification	Mineralisation

132. In active transport, carrier proteins are used, which use energy in the form of ATP, to
(a) transport molecules against concentration gradient of cell wall.
(b) transport molecules along concentration gradient of cell membrane.
(c) transport molecules against concentration gradient of cell membrane.
(d) transport molecules along concentration gradient of cell wall.

133. In a 50 gm living tissue, what would be the amount of water?
(a) 15 - 25 gm (b) 25 - 30 gm
(c) 35 - 45 gm (d) 70 - 90 gm

134. PS-II occurs only in
(a) stroma (b) granal thylakoids
(c) stromal lamella (d) matrix

135. After glycolysis, fate of glucose in mitochondrial matrix is
(a) oxidation (b) reduction
(c) oxidative decarboxylation
(d) hydrolysis

136. Cleistogamy is leading over anthesis because
(a) pollination agent is not required
(b) it assures heterozygosity
(c) it favours insect pollination
(d) it allows xenogamy.

137. Which of the following statements is correct?
(a) Photorespiration is useful process.
(b) C_4 plants are more efficient than C_3 plants.
(c) C_3 plants are more efficient than C_4 plants.
(d) Photorespiration is absent in C_3 plants but present in C_4 plants.

138. Which of the following statements is incorrect regarding fermentation ?
(a) *Propionibacterium* is used to ferment the cheese.
(b) The puffed-up appearance of dough is due to the production of CO_2 gas.
(c) Fermentation in muscle produces ethanol.
(d) Toddy is made by fermenting sap from palms.

139. Which of the following statements is correct ?
(a) *Aspergillus niger* is used for producing cyclosporin A.
(b) Activated sludge is digested by aerobic bacteria to produce marsh gas.
(c) Fleming, Chain & Florey were awarded with Nobel Prize for discovering penicillin.
(d) BOD is amount of oxygen produced by bacteria on decomposition.

140. Which of the following elements is present in very less quantity in the body ?
(a) K (b) Ca
(c) Mg (d) Cu

141. Which of the following is best method of germplasm conservation ?
(a) herbarium (b) botanical garden
(c) seed bank (d) zoological park

142. Which one of the following options is a correct match of phenomenon and its explanation ?
(a) Reverse Transcription PCR – Many copies of a DNA sequence.
(b) Central dogma – RNA → DNA → Protein → RNA.
(c) RNA silencing – Use of ds-RNA to stop the expression of ss-RNA.
(d) Transcription – Process of formation of RNA & proteins.

143. Which of the following is not a characteristic of meiosis?
(a) It involves two stages of DNA replication one before meiosis-I and another before meiosis-II
(b) It involves recombination and crossing over
(c) Sister chromatids separate during anaphase-II
(d) Nuclear membrane disappears during prophase.

144. Which of the following is correct ?
(a) Henking discovered the small Y-chromosome
(b) *Drosophila* also shows XX-XY sex determination like human
(c) Birds have ZZ-ZW sex determination, where females are ZZ & males are ZW
(d) Grasshoppers show XX-XY sex determination.

145. Which statement is correct regarding mosses ?
(a) They have dominant and independent sporophyte.
(b) Their antherozoids require water for fertilization.
(c) Their archegonia produce many eggs.
(d) Their antherozoids are multiflagellated.

146. Which of the following statements is correct ?
(a) Catalytic converter can separate particulate matter of diameter less than 2.5 micrometers.
(b) Histones are acidic in nature that forms core for DNA packaging.
(c) *Lactobacillus* is not present in dough used in idli formation.
(d) Template with polarity 5′ → 3′ has continuous DNA replication.

147. Which of the following statements is correct ?
1. Common cold – Droplet Infection.
2. Typhoid – Contaminated food & water.
3. AIDS – Shaking hands.
4. Ringworm – Using infected towels.
(a) 1 and 2 (b) 3 and 4
(c) 1 and 3 (d) 1,2 and 4

148. Which of the following statements is correct ?
(a) Lion and leopard show convergent evolution.
(b) Cryptic camouflage is seen in *Biston betularia*.
(c) Natural selection is responsible for extinction of dinosaurs.
(d) *Homo habilis* and *Homo erectus* are closely related.

149. Tendon and ligament are example of
(a) dense regular connective tissue
(b) dense irregular connective tissue
(c) loose connective tissue
(d) specialised connective tissue

150. Kingdom Animalia is characterised by
(a) direct dependence on autotrophs
(b) indirect dependence on autotrophs
(c) absence of chlorophyll
(d) absence of cell wall.

151. If medulla oblongata is destroyed then which of the following functions will be effected ?
(a) No thermoregulation
(b) No vision
(c) No memory
(d) No response when pricked with needle

152. Which of the following statements is correct?
(a) Monkey, apes and humans exhibit estrous cycle.
(b) Urine is pale yellow and slightly alkaline.
(c) Lots of enzymes are present in bile juice.
(d) Ovulation in humans is spontaneous.

153. Which of the following evidences does not favour the Lamarckian concept of inheritance of acquired characters?
(a) absence of limbs in snakes
(b) melanization in peppered moth
(c) presence of webbed toes in aquatic birds
(d) lack of pigment in cave-dwelling animals

154. Which of the following is a correct match?
(a) Frog – External ears
(b) Earthworm – Muscular gizzard, typhlosole.
(c) Human – Fat globule, 10 pairs of cranial nerves.
(d) Cockroach – Chilopoda

155. Which of the following is an incorrect statement?
(a) Blood group 'O' person have A and B antigens on RBCs.
(b) Eosinophils resist infections and are associated with allergic infection.
(c) RBC's contain carbonic anhydrase.
(d) T wave of normal ECG represent of depolarization of ventricle.

156. Which one of the following is correct regarding the excretion ?
(a) Large amount of water from renal filtrate is reabsorbed in DCT and a less amount is reabsorbed by PCT
(b) The descending limb of loop of Henle is completely impermeable to salts.
(c) Malpighian corpuscle is found in medulla region of kidney.
(d) The colour of urine is pale yellow and is slightly alkaline in nature.

157. In assisted reproductive technology where gametes have been fertilized *in vitro*, which of the following is practicable for embryo transplantation in Fallopian tube?
(a) only embryo up to 8 blastomeres if zygote is not transplanted.
(b) only zygote is transplanted not embryo
(c) either embryo or zygote with 8 blastomere phase transplanted.
(d) morulla with 8-24 celled stage is transplanted in Fallopian tube.

158. Which of the following features can be said to be a true defining feature of living beings without any exception ?
(a) they can digest their food.
(b) all of them can reproduce.
(c) they can regenerate.
(d) they can respond to external stimuli

159. The opening between the right atrium and the right ventricle is guarded by the valve named
(a) bicuspid valve (b) tricuspid valve
(c) mitral valve (d) semilunar valve

160. Skeletal muscles appear striated due to presence of two characteristic proteins in alternating dark and light bands. Which of the following is a correct match of the protein with its light refractive property and colour?

	Protein	Colour	Property
(a)	Myosin	Light	Anisotropic
(b)	Actin	Dark	Anisotropic
(c)	Myosin	Dark	Isotropic
(d)	Actin	Light	Isotropic

Directions : In the following questions (161-180), a statement of assertion (A) is followed by a statement of reason (R). Mark the correct choice as :
(a) If both assertion and reason are true and reason is the correct explanation of assertion
(b) If both assertion and reason are true but reason is not the correct explanation of assertion
(c) If assertion is true but reason is false
(d) If both assertion and reason are false.

161. Assertion : Enzymes lower down the activation energy of the reactant molecule to make its transition into product easier.
Reason : Enzymes are highly substrate specific catalysts.

162. Assertion : Water that enters into a plant cell through diffusion makes it turgid.
Reason : Entry of water into the cell through diffusion develops wall pressure inside the cell.

163. Assertion : Movement of materials inside phloem is bidirectional *i.e.* it can be both upwards or downwards.
Reason : Movement of molecules inside xylem is unidirectional *i.e.* always upwards.

164. Assertion : Protons or hydrogen ions produced by photolysis of water accumulate in the lumen of thylakoids.
Reason : Photolysis of water takes place in inner membrane of thylakoid.

165. Assertion : Plant growth as a whole is indefinite.
Reason : Plants retain the capacity of continuous growth throughout their life.

166. Assertion : Amount of organic biodegradable compounds present in water is measured by the BOD of that water.

Reason : During biodegradation of biodegradable organic compounds, oxygen is released by bacteria.

167. Assertion : In angiosperms, transport of food and water is more efficient than gymnosperms and pteridophytes.

Reason : In angiosperms longitudinally arranged sieve elements and vessels with perforated end walls are present.

168. Assertion : In some species of asteraceae and poaceae seeds are formed without fertilization.

Reason : Formation of fruit without fertilization is called parthenocarpy.

169. Assertion : Algal blooms are formed in nutrient-less water.

Reason : Algal blooms in water turn it unfit for human consumption, but cause enormous growth of fish.

170. Assertion : A mangrove tree growing in marshy place has pneumatophores.

Reason : Pneumatophores help in better anchorage to marshy soil.

171. Assertion : A geneticist crossed two plants, he got 50% tall and 50% dwarf progenies.

Reason : It follows Mendelian law as one of the parent plant might be heterozygous.

172. Assertion : Now-a-days amniocentesis is banned.

Reason : Amniocentesis gives the information of any abnormality in the foetus and many other complications regarding pregnancy can be detected.

173. Assertion : A gene from *Bacillus thuringiensis* is incorporated in plant genome to increase their yield.

Reason : *Bacillus thuringiensis* has Bt toxin producing gene, which kills the larva of insects.

174. Assertion : Glycerides are important nutrients for body.

Reason : Glycerides are hydrolysed into glycerol and fatty acids which are further absorbed in intestine by the formation of chylomicron.

175. Assertion : Blood in cockroach is colourless haemolymph with no respiratory pigment.

Reason : Respiration in cockroach occurs through diffusion in haemolymph.

176. Assertion : Blood group 'O' have anti-A & anti-B antibodies.

Reason : It does not have any antigens.

177. Assertion : S.A. node induces excitatory impulses in heart.

Reason : S.A. node is self excitatory.

178. Assertion : Organ of Corti rests on tectorial membrane.

Reason : It helps to maintain equilibrium of body.

179. Assertion : Corpus luteum is produced by Graafian follicle after ovulation.

Reason : It secretes estrogen which is necessary to maintain pregnancy.

180. Assertion : Sporozoites of malarial parasite enter in the human body due to biting of freshly born female *Anopheles* mosquito, whose mother was a carrier of malarial parasite.

Reason : Male and female gametocytes of malarial parasites are formed in the human intestine.

GENERAL KNOWLEDGE

181. Which river derives its name from Sanskrit word "Lavanavari"?

(a) Luni (b) Kosi
(c) Sabarmati (d) Kaveri

182. Which river's name means "containing reed"?

(a) Gangad (b) Betwa
(c) Narmada (d) Luni

183. First Indian woman grandmaster in chess is

(a) Saheli Dhar
(b) Bhagyashree Thipse

(c) Vijaylakshmi Pandit
(d) Amrit Kaur

184. Two letters printed on first postal stamp of India are
(a) Jai hind (b) Jai kisan
(c) Jai bharat (d) Vande matram

185. Which of the following is called 'Floating sanctuary of India'?
(a) Keibul Lamjao (b) Manas
(c) Kaziranga (d) Bharatpur

186. "India wins freedom" this book was written by
(a) Jawahar Lal Nehru (b) Maulana Azad
(c) Sardar Patel (d) Rajendra Prasad

187. Which fruit is often called "love apple" ?
(a) Pineapple (b) Orange
(c) Tomato (d) Papaya

188. Which country was first to adopt family planning programme?
(a) India (b) China
(c) USA (d) Indonesia

189. After whom the atomic energy programme is commissioned in India?
(a) S.N. Bose (b) C.V. Raman
(c) H.G. Khurana (d) H.J. Bhabha

190. After the death of which prime minister did Guljarilal Nanda joined as acting PM for second time?
(a) Indira Gandhi
(b) Jawahar Lal Nehru
(c) Lal Bahadur Shastri
(d) Charan Singh

191. Whom did Jawahar Lal Nehru called father of Indian revolution?
(a) Bal Gangadhar Tilak
(b) Vipin Chandra Pal
(c) Dhondo Keshave Karve
(d) Maulana Abdul Kalam Azad

192. Among these, who had been the last governor general of India?
(a) Dr. Radhakrishnan
(b) R. Gopalachari
(c) Sardar Patel
(d) Dr. Bhim Rao Ambedkar

193. With which of the following religions, "Karamappa" is related?
(a) Jainism (b) Buddhism
(c) Hinduism (d) Christinism

194. Which of the following authors is not born in India?
(a) Rudyard Kipling (b) Ruskin Bond
(c) Gorge Orwell (d) V.S. Naipal

195. Which of the following actress won the best actress award 3 times consecutively?
(a) Rekha (b) Jaya Bachchan
(c) Smita Patil (d) Shabana Azmi

196. Which woman won the Sahitya Kala Academy award first time?
(a) Amrita Pritam (b) Sarojini Naidu
(c) Kamla Mehta (d) Geeta Das

197. To which gharana " Kishori Amonkar '" belongs to ?
(a) Kirana (b) Jaipur-Attrivi
(c) Lucknow (d) Gwalior

198. Who is the author of the book "Siddhant Shiromani"?
(a) Bhaskaracharya - II
(b) Bhaskaracharya - I
(c) Aryabhatt (d) Ramanujan

199. Which of the following has introduced transcendental meditation?
(a) Rajneesh Osho
(b) Swami Chinmiyanand
(c) Vivekanand
(d) Maharishi Mahesh Yogi

200. Which of the following animal's body secretion is oily red, commonly known as "Sweat blood"?
(a) Rhinoceros (b) Hippopotamus
(c) Cow (d) Tiger

SOLUTIONS

PHYSICS

1. **(b)** : $B = \frac{F}{qv} = \frac{[MLT^{-2}]}{[AT][LT^{-1}]} = [ML^0T^{-2}A^{-1}]$

But $[A] = [C\ T^{-1}]$

$\therefore\ [B] = [ML^0T^{-1}C^{-1}]$

2. **(b)** : The mechanical equivalent of spring constant in LC oscillating circuit is, $k = \frac{1}{C}$.

3. **(b)** :

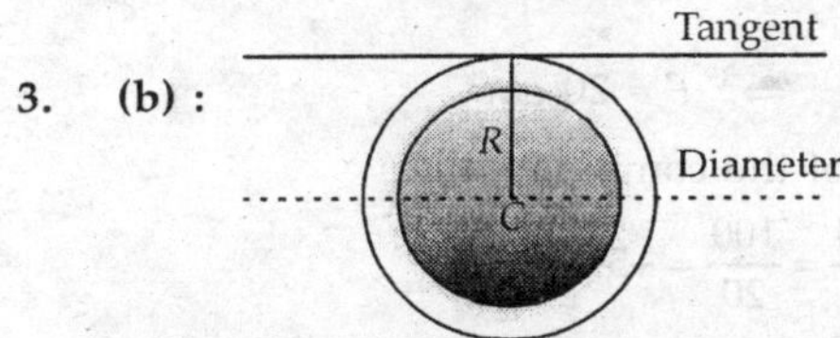

The moment of inertia for a solid sphere along its diameter is

$I_{diameter} = \frac{2}{5}MR^2$

Moment of inertia about a tangent touching to its surface,

$I_{tangent} = I_{diameter} + MR^2$

(using theorem of parallel axes)

$= \frac{2}{5}MR^2 + MR^2 = \frac{7}{5}MR^2$

4. **(d)** : Here, $v_1 = 4$ m s^{-1}, $A_1 = \pi r_1^2 = 16\pi \times 10^{-4}$ m^2

$A_2 = \pi r_2^2 = \pi \times 10^{-4}$ m^2

Using, $A_1v_1 = A_2v_2$

$\therefore v_2 = \frac{A_1v_1}{A_2} = \frac{16\pi \times 10^{-4} \times 4}{\pi \times 10^{-4}} = 64\,\text{m s}^{-1}$

Velocity of water at free end, $v_2 = 64$ m s^{-1}

5. **(b)** : The torsion produced in wire is directly proportional to the twist

i.e, $\tau \propto \theta$

or $\tau = C\theta$, where C is restoring couple per unit twist.

6. **(c)** : Here, $\omega = 2\hat{k}$

$\vec{r} = 2\hat{i} + 2\hat{j}$

Linear velocity, $\vec{v} = \vec{\omega} \times \vec{r}$

$= 2\hat{k} \times (2\hat{i} + 2\hat{j})$

$= -4\hat{i} + 4\hat{j}$

7. **(b)** : The average velocity in simple harmonic motion is given by

$$V_{av} = \frac{2}{\pi}V_m$$

8. **(c)** : (a) $(\cos\omega t + \sin\omega t)$ is a periodic function. It can also be written as

$= \frac{\sqrt{2}}{\sqrt{2}}\sin\omega t + \frac{\sqrt{2}}{\sqrt{2}}\cos\omega t$

$= \sqrt{2}\left(\cos\frac{\pi}{4}\sin\omega t + \sin\frac{\pi}{4}\cos\omega t\right)$

$= \sqrt{2}\sin\left(\omega t + \frac{\pi}{4}\right) = \sqrt{2}\sin\left(\omega t + \frac{\pi}{4} + 2\pi\right)$

$= \sqrt{2}\sin\left[\omega\left(t + \frac{2\pi}{\omega}\right) + \frac{\pi}{4}\right]$

This represent a simple harmonic function with period $\frac{2\pi}{\omega}$ and phase $\frac{\pi}{4}$.

(b) $\sin\omega t - \cos\omega t$ is a periodic function. It can be written as

$= \sqrt{2}\left[\sin\omega t\cos\frac{\pi}{4} - \cos\omega t\sin\frac{\pi}{4}\right]$

$= \sqrt{2}\sin\left(\omega t - \frac{\pi}{4}\right) = \sqrt{2}\sin\left[\omega\left(t + \frac{2\pi}{\omega}\right) - \frac{\pi}{4}\right]$

This represent a simple harmonic function with period $\frac{2\pi}{\omega}$.

(c) $F(t) = 1 - \sin 2\omega t$

This is a non periodic function.

(d) $F(t) = \sin\omega t + \cos(\omega t + \alpha)$

also represent a simple harmonic function.

9. **(d)** : In simple harmonic motion, loss of kinetic energy is proportional to the square of amplitude of oscillation.

i.e., loss of kinetic energy $\propto x^2$

10. **(d)** : The ratio of emissive power to absorptive power is the same for all surfaces at the same temperature and is equal to the emissivity for a perfectly black body at that temperature.

i.e, $\frac{e}{a} = \varepsilon$

Here, $e = 8$, $a = 10$

$\therefore\ \varepsilon = \frac{e}{a} = \frac{8}{10} = 0.8$

11. **(a) :** Energy stored in capacitor of capacitance C with voltage V is, $U=\frac{1}{2}CV^2$

but $C=\frac{\varepsilon_0 A}{d}, V=Ed$

where A is the area of capacitor plate and d is the distance of separation and E is the electric field.

$\therefore \quad U=\frac{1}{2}\frac{\varepsilon_0 A}{d}E^2d^2=\frac{1}{2}\varepsilon_0 E^2 Ad$

12. **(a)**

13. **(b) :** Here, r_1 = 1 m, r_2 = 2 m

Mutual inductance, $M=\frac{\mu_0\pi r_1^2}{2r_2}$

$=\frac{\mu_0\pi\times 1}{2\times 2}=\frac{\mu_0\pi}{4}$

14. **(c) :** Resultant intensity,

$I=I_1+I_2+2\sqrt{I_1I_2}\cos\phi$

Here, $I_1=I, I_2=4I, \phi_1=\frac{\pi}{2}$ and $\phi_2=\pi$

At A intensity,

$I_A=I+4I+2\sqrt{4I^2}\cos\frac{\pi}{2}=5I$

At B intensity,

$I_B=I+4I+2\sqrt{4I^2}\cos\pi=5I-4I=I$

Therefore, difference between intensities is $I_A-I_B=5I-I=4I$

15. **(c)**

16. **(a) :** Given, A_m = 5 V, A_c = 20 V

$\therefore$ Modulation index, $\mu=\frac{A_m}{A_c}=\frac{5}{20}=0.25$

17. **(c) :** Here, h = 50 m

Area covered = $\pi d^2=\pi\times 2hR \quad (\because d^2=2hR)$

where $R=6.4\times 10^6$ m (radius of earth)

$\therefore$ area covered $=\pi\times 2hR=\pi\times 2\times 50\times 6.4\times 10^6$

$=640\pi\times 10^6\ \text{m}^2=640\pi\ \text{km}^2$

18. **(c) :** For photon, $\lambda_P=\frac{hc}{E}$

Here, E is energy of photon.

For proton, $\lambda_p=\frac{h}{\sqrt{2mK}}$

Here, m and K be mass and kinetic energy of proton respectively.

$\therefore \quad \frac{\lambda_p}{\lambda_P}=\frac{E}{c}\sqrt{2mK}\propto E^{1/2} \quad (\because E=K \text{ Given})$

19. **(a) :** Here R_1 = 2 fm, R_2 = 1 fm

The radius of nucleus is, $R\propto A^{1/3}$

$\therefore \quad \frac{A_1}{A_2}=\left(\frac{R_1}{R_2}\right)^3=\left(\frac{2}{1}\right)^2=8$

20. **(a) :** Given, B = 1 T, r = 0.2 m

$r=\frac{mv}{qB}$

i.e, $v=\frac{0.2\times 1.6\times 10^{-19}\times 1}{1.6\times 10^{-27}}=0.2\times 10^8\ \text{m s}^{-1}$

21. **(c) :** Here f_1 = – 20 cm, f_2 = + 10 cm

Focal length of combination is,

$\frac{1}{F}=\frac{1}{f_1}+\frac{1}{f_2}=\frac{1}{-20}+\frac{1}{10}$

$\frac{1}{F}=\frac{1}{20} \Rightarrow F=20$ cm

Power of the combination,

$P=\frac{100}{F}=\frac{100}{20}=+5\,\text{D}$

22. **(b) :** Here u = – 25 cm, v = –50 cm

We have $\frac{1}{f}=\frac{1}{-u}+\frac{1}{v}$

i.e, $\frac{1}{f}=\frac{1}{25}-\frac{1}{50}$ or f = 50 cm

Power of lens he should use,

$P=\frac{100}{f}=\frac{100}{50}=+2\,\text{D}$

23. **(a) :** At k = 1, the chain reaction will be steady or sustained and the size of the fissionable material used is said to be the critical size.

24. **(a) :** Susceptibility χ_m is small and negative for diamagnetic substances.

25. **(c) :** The orientation of dipoles parallel and antiparallel to magnetic field is distributed unequally in ferrimagnetic materials.

26. **(d) :** The α-emission of S^{32} is as follows :

${}_{16}S^{32}\rightarrow {}_{14}Si^{28}+{}_2He^4$

${}_{14}Si^{28}\rightarrow {}_{12}Mg^{24}+{}_2He^4$

So after the emission of two α-particle ${}_{12}Mg^{24}$ is formed.

27. **(a) :** Lenz's law is accordance with the principle of conservation of energy.

28. **(a) :** In series LCR circuit, the phase angle ϕ is given by

$$\tan\phi = \frac{X_L - X_C}{R}$$

When $X_L > X_C$, $\tan\phi$ is positive. Therefore the phase difference is positive.

29. **(b)** : The direction of electric field is from *N*-side to *P*-side in *PN* junction diode.

30. **(a)** : Here, $\upsilon_1 = 499$ Hz, $\upsilon_2 = 501$ Hz

$$\text{Frequency heard} = \frac{\upsilon_1 + \upsilon_2}{2} = \frac{499 + 501}{2} = 500 \text{ Hz}$$

Since the difference in intensity is 2, change in intensity take place twice.

31. **(a)** : Here, $m = 0.2$ kg, $u = 0$

$\vec{F} = (0.3\hat{i} - 0.4\hat{j})$

$\vec{v} = ?, t = 6$ s

$$\vec{a} = \frac{\vec{F}}{m} = \frac{(0.3\hat{i} - 0.4\hat{j})}{0.2} = \left(\frac{3}{2}\hat{i} - 2\hat{j}\right)$$

From $\vec{v} = \vec{u} + \vec{a}t$

$$\vec{v} = 0 + \left(\frac{3}{2}\hat{i} - 2\hat{j}\right) \times 6 = 9\hat{i} - 12\hat{j}$$

32. **(b)** : Let x be distance of person from one cliff and y be distance of person from 2nd cliff. Let $y > x$.

$\therefore \quad x + x = v \times t_1 = 340 \times 1 = 340$

$x = 170$ m

$y + y = v \times t_2 = 340 \times 2 = 680$

$y = 340$ m.

Distance between two cliffs

$= x + y = 170 + 340 = 510$ m

33. **(a)** : Here, $t = 25$ years, $T_{1/2} = 5$ years

$$\text{Number of half lives, } n = \frac{t}{T_{1/2}} = \frac{25}{5} = 5$$

Percentage of radio active material remained after 25 years is $= \left(\frac{1}{2}\right)^n \times 100$

$$= \left(\frac{1}{2}\right)^5 \times 100 = 3.125\%$$

34. **(a)** : For an adiabatic process, change in entropy of the system is zero,

i.e, $\Delta S = 0$

35. **(b)** : As internal energy is a state variable and final state coincides with the initial state in cyclic process, $\therefore \Delta U = 0$

36. **(a)** : The expression for magnetic field is case of a long current carrying wire is $B = \frac{\mu_0 I}{2\pi a}$

i.e, $B \propto \frac{1}{a}$

37. **(d)**

38. **(c)** : In nuclear reactor, to control the chain reaction from becoming violent, rods of boron or cadmium called control rods are inserted in the holes of reactor core.

39. **(b)** : Lyman series is obtained when an electron jumps to the first orbit ($n_1 = 1$) from any outer orbit ($n_2 = 2, 3, 4...$)

$$\frac{1}{\lambda} = RZ\left[\frac{1}{n_1^2} - \frac{1}{n_2^2}\right]$$

For H, $Z = 1$ and R is the Rydberg's constant $R = 1.097 \times 10^7 \text{ m}^{-1}$. In this series, the shortest wavelength or the limit of this series (For $n_1 = 1$ and $n_2 = \infty$) is nearly = 911Å

40. **(b)** : Bernoulli's equation is

$$P + \rho gh + \frac{1}{2}\rho v^2 = \text{ a constant,}$$

or $$\frac{P}{\rho g} + h + \frac{1}{2}\frac{v^2}{g} = \text{constant,}$$

Here, $\frac{P}{\rho g}$ is called pressure head.

41. **(b)** : In gases, sound waves are always longitudinal because, gases cannot sustain shearing strain.

42. **(a)** : The CD acts like a prism because the narrow grooves are so close to each other that you cannot see the separation. But, white light fall on the CD will be separated by multicolours by grooves.

43. **(c)** : Total energy is given by

$$E = -\frac{GMm}{2R}$$

where R is the radius of orbit.

44. **(d)** : Kinetic energy is not conserved at every instant of elastic collision because there will be friction and deformation losses of energy.

45. **(a)** : When we heat the gas at constant volume, the heat is supplied to raise the temperature of gas only. When we heat the gas at constant pressure, the volume of the gas apart from temperature of the gas rises. When the gas

expands, it does some external work for increasing the volume. So in this case, the heat is supplied.

(a) to raise the temperature of the gas.

(b) to do the mechanical work for expansion.

As a result more amount of heat is required to increase the temperature of the gas through the same amount when the pressure is kept constant. Hence C_P is always greater than the value of C_V.

46. (a)

47. **(a) :** Multiplication factor (k) is a measure of the growth rate of neutrons in the reactor. For $k = 1$; the operation of the reaction is said to be critical condition at which sustained chain reaction occurs. If k becomes greater than the reaction rate and reactor power increases exponentially.

48. **(a) :** Gauss's law is applicable for any closed surface. Gauss's law is most useful in situation where the charge distribution has spherical or cylindrical symmetry or is distributed uniformly over the plane. Whereas electric dipole is a system of two equal and opposite point charges separated by a very small and finite distance.

49. (a)

50. **(b) :** The transistor can be used as a switch, amplifier and oscillator.

51. **(a) :** When white light is passed through a lens, violet light is more refracted than red light because wavelength of violet is less than red light and therefore focal length for red light is greater than violet.

52. **(a) :** Microscope is an optical instrument which forms a magnified image of a small nearby object and thus, increases the visual angle subtended by the image at the eye so that the object is seen to be bigger and distinct. Therefore angular magnification for image is more than object.

53. (a)

54. (d)

55. **(a) :** The sky waves are the radio waves used for very long distance radio communication at medium and high frequencies (*i.e.*, shortwave band). In shorter wavelength, attenuation is very less.

56. (a)

57. **(c) :** The average energy of a neutron produced in fission of U^{235} is 2 MeV. These neutrons unless slowed down will escape from the reactor without interacting with uranium nuclei, unless a large amount of fissionable material is used for sustaining the chain reaction. What we needs to do is to slow down the fast neutrons by elastic scattering with light nuclei. Chadwick's experiment showed that in an elastic collision with hydrogen neutron almost come to rest.

58. (a)

59. **(b) :** The sign of magnification depend on the sign convention chosen. According to the new Cartesian sign conventions, magnification for a convex mirror is positive because image formed by a convex mirror is always virtual and erect. A concave mirror can form virtual or erect images and also real, inverted images. In the latter case, its magnification becomes negative. The reason though correct does not explain the assertion properly.

60. **(d) :** It does not follow inverse square law of distance. The assertion is false. The reason is also false.

CHEMISTRY

61. **(d) :** Ferrous sulphate $\rightarrow FeSO_4{\cdot}7H_2O$

Copper sulphate $\rightarrow CuSO_4{\cdot}5H_2O$

Magnesium sulphate $\rightarrow MgSO_4{\cdot}7H_2O$

Sodium chloride $\rightarrow NaCl$

62. **(a) :** The oxidation of sodium borohydride with iodine in diglyme gives diborane.

$$2NaBH_4 + I_2 \xrightarrow{\text{Diglyme}} B_2H_6 + 2NaI + H_2$$

63. **(d) :** Fullerene consists of 12 five-membered rings and 20 six-membered rings. So it has five membered rings less than six membered rings.

64. **(a) :** As in complex $[Co(NH_3)_5Cl]^{2+}$ unpaired electrons are present, so it requires less energy for excitation. Thus, the wavelength of light absorbed will be highest (*i.e.*, $E \propto 1/\lambda$).

65. **(a) :** Phosphorus trichloride reacts violently with water forming phosphorous acid.

$$PCl_3 + 3HOH \longrightarrow H_3PO_3 + 3HCl$$

66. **(a) :** X-ray studies have shown that in ice, four hydrogen atoms tetrahedrally surround each oxygen atoms.

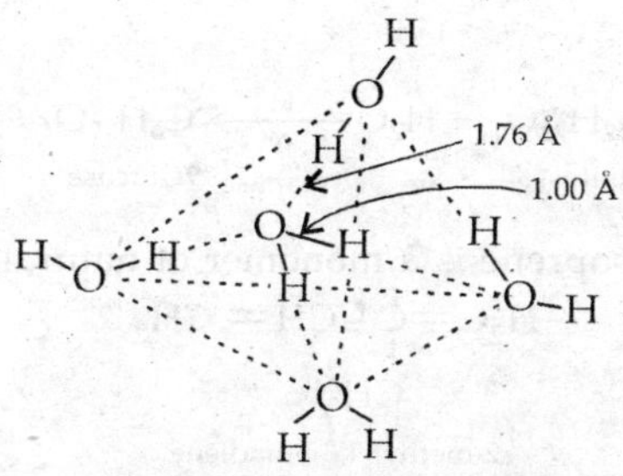

Tetrahedral arrangement of water

67. **(a) :** $I_{2(s)} + H_2O_{2(aq)} + 2OH^-_{(aq)} \longrightarrow 2I^-_{(aq)} + 2H_2O_{(l)} + O_{2(g)}$

68. **(c) :** $XePtF_6$ was first real compound of any of the noble gases.

69. **(c) :** $[Cu(NH_3)_4]^{2+}$

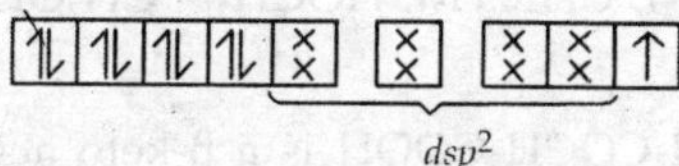

No. of unpaired electrons = 1

So, $[Cu(NH_3)_4]^{2+}$ is paramagnetic.

$[NiCl_4]^{2-}$: [⇅|⇅|⇅|↑|↑] [×] [×|×|×] (sp^3)

No. of unpaired electrons = 2

So, $[NiCl_4]^{2-}$ is paramagnetic.

$[PtCl_4]^{2-}$: [⇅|⇅|⇅|⇅|×] [×] [×|×|] (dsp^2)

No. of unpaired electrons = 0

So, $[PtCl_4]^{2-}$ is diamagnetic.

$[Cu(H_2O)_4]^{2+}$: [⇅|⇅|⇅|⇅|↑] [×] [×|×|×] (sp^3)

No. of unpaired electrons = 1

So, $[Cu(H_2O)_4]^{2+}$ is paramagnetic.

70. **(a) :** CsCl is not hygroscopic in nature while $MgCl_2$, $CaCl_2$ and LiCl are hygroscopic in nature.

71. **(a) :** Compound : $BeCl_2 > NO_2 > SO_2$

Angle : 180° > 132° > 119.5°

72. **(d) :** $N_2O_{4(g)} + 3CO_{(g)} \longrightarrow N_2O_{(g)} + 3CO_{2(g)}$

$\Delta H_{reaction} = \Sigma_{\text{Heat of formation of products}} - \Sigma_{\text{Heat of formation of reactants}}$

$\Delta H_{reaction} = [\Delta H_f N_2O + 3 \times \Delta H_f CO_2] - [\Delta H_f N_2O_4 + 3 \times \Delta H_f CO]$

$\Delta H_r = [+811 + 3(-393)] - [10 + 3(-110)]$

$= [811 - 1179] - [-320] = -368 + 320$

$= -48$ kJ/mol

73. **(b) :** $2\overset{+7}{Mn}O_4^- + Br^- + H_2O \longrightarrow 2\overset{+4}{Mn}O_2 + BrO_3^- + 2OH^-$

74. **(b) :** $2CuSO_4 \cdot 5H_2O + 4KI \longrightarrow Cu_2I_2 + 2K_2SO_4 + I_2 + 10H_2O$

254 g

Molecular weight of $2CuSO_4 \cdot 5H_2O$

$[2(63.5 + 32 + 64) + 10(18)]$ g = 499 g

254 g of I_2 is liberated by 499 g $CuSO_4 \cdot 5H_2O$

2.54 g of I_2 will be liberated by x g $CuSO_4 \cdot 5H_2O$

$x = \frac{499}{254} \times 2.54 = 4.99$ g

75. **(b) :** Since, the adsorption process is exothermic, the physical adsorption occurs readily at low temperature and decreases with increase in temperature (Le-Chatelier's principle).

76. **(a) :** Series → Lyman, Balmer, Paschen, Brackett, Pfund

$\xrightarrow{\text{Increasing wavelength}}$

77. **(a) :** $CaSO_{4\,(s)} \rightleftharpoons Ca^{2+}_{(aq)} + SO_4^{2-}{}_{(aq)}$

$S \quad S$

$K_{sp} = S^2 = 9 \times 10^{-6}$

$S = 3 \times 10^{-3}$ mol L^{-1}

Solubility in g litre^{-1} = molecular mass × S

$= 136 \times 3 \times 10^{-3} = 408 \times 10^{-3}$ g L^{-1}

408×10^{-3} g of $CaSO_4$ present in 1 litre

1 g of $CaSO_4$ present is $\frac{1}{408 \times 10^{-3}} = 2.45$ litre.

78. **(d) :** Equilibrium state can only be achieved if a reversible reaction is carried out in a closed space.

79. **(d) :** (a) It successfully explained the stability of atoms.

(b) It is not in agreement with Heisenberg's uncertainty principle.

(c) It does not explain the spectra of multi-electron atoms.

(d) It does not explain de Broglie concept of the dual character of matter.

80. **(a) :** In van der Waal's equation, a signifies the intermolecular force of attraction.

81. **(c) :** For adiabatic process, no exchange of heat takes place between the system and surroundings. *i.e.* $q = 0$.

82. **(d) :** Number of millimoles of base (*i.e.*, $Ca(OH)_2$) $= N_1V_1 = 2 \times M_1 \times V_1 = 2 \times 0.2 \times 25 = 10$

Number of millimoles of acid (*i.e.*, HCl) = N_2V_2
= 10 × 1 = 10

As, no. of millimoles of acid = no. of millimoles of base

∴ Acid is completely neutralised by base forming a neutral solution.

∴ pH of the resulting solution = 7.

83. **(a) :** In Schottky defect, some of the lattice points are unoccupied (vacancies or holes). The number of missing cations and anions is the same, thus crystal remains neutral.

84. **(a) :** Neutron moderators slow down the speed of neutrons by collisions. They do not absorb neutrons. *e.g.* water and graphite.

85. **(b) :** Thermodynamic functions are : Internal energy, enthalpy, entropy, pressure, volume, temperature, free energy, number of moles.

86. **(c) :** Intensive property : Specific heat
Extensive property : Enthalpy, entropy, volume.

87. **(b) :**

$$\begin{array}{llll} & A_{(g)} \longrightarrow & 2B_{(g)} + & C_{(g)} \\ \text{Initial :} & P_0 & 0 & 0 \\ & P_0 - P & 2P & P \end{array}$$

Total pressure at time $(t) = P_0 - P + 2P + P = P_t$

$\Rightarrow \quad P_t = P_0 + 2P$

$$P_t - P_0 = 2P \Rightarrow P = \frac{P_t - P_0}{2}$$

$$k = \frac{2.303}{t}\log\left[\frac{P_0}{P_0 - P}\right] = \frac{2.303}{t}\log\left[\frac{P_0}{P_0 - \left(\frac{P_t - P_0}{2}\right)}\right]$$

$$= \frac{2.303}{t}\log\left(\frac{2P_0}{2P_0 - P_t + P_0}\right) = \frac{2.303}{t}\log\left(\frac{2P_0}{3P_0 - P_t}\right)$$

88. **(c) :** If the nucleophilic atoms are in the same row of the periodic table, nucleophilicity is approximately in order of basicity. So, the order is $NH_2^- > CH_3O^- > OH^- > RNH_2$.

89. **(c) :** Symmetrical molecule

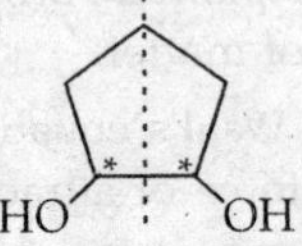

Number of chiral carbon atoms = 2 (even)

$$\text{Number of stereoisomers} = 2^{n-1} + 2^{\frac{n}{2}-1}$$

$$= 2^{2-1} + 2^{\frac{2}{2}-1} = 2^1 - 2^0 = 2 + 1 = 3$$

90. **(a)**

91. **(a) :** $\underset{\text{Maltose}}{C_{12}H_{22}O_{11}} + H_2O \xrightarrow[\text{maltase}]{H^+ \text{ or}} \underset{\text{Glucose}}{C_6H_{12}O_6} + \underset{\text{Glucose}}{C_6H_{12}O_6}$

92. **(b) :** Isoprene is a monomer of natural rubber.

$$H_2C{=}\underset{\underset{CH_3}{|}}{C}{-}CH{=}CH_2$$

2-methyl-1,3-butadiene

93. **(a) :** Presence of excess of HI favours S_N1 mechanism.
So, formation of products is controlled by the stability of the carbocation resulting in the cleavage of C – O bond in protonated ether.
Thus the product for given equation are $C_6H_5CH_2I$, CH_3CH_2I, $HOCH_2 - CH_2OH$.

94. **(c)**

95. **(d) :** CH_3COCH_2COOH is a β-keto acid. Thus decarboxylation is maximum in a carboxylic acid containing an electron withdrawing group such as >CO or – COOH at the β-carbon atom with respect to the – COOH group.

96. **(b) :** Greater is the electron density on aromatic ring, greater is the reactivity towards electrophilic aromatic substitution.

97. **(d) :** Substituent with strong +*R* effect, +*I* effect and weaker –*I* effect increases the basicity. Hence pK_b decreases. Also, alkylamines are stronger bases than arylamines. So, the order is (d).

98. **(a) :** Weaker acids have higher pK_a. – OCH_3 at *meta*-position exerts only –*I* effect, hence increases the acidity.
–*I* effect order : – NO_2 > – OCH_3 > – Cl.
– CH_3 has +*I* effect.
So order is (a).

99. **(a)**

100. **(a) :** Pent-4-ene-1-yne

$$\overset{1}{CH} \equiv \overset{2}{C} - \overset{3}{CH_2} - \overset{4}{CH} = \overset{5}{CH_2}$$

No. of σ-bonds – 4 (C – C) + 6 (C – H) = 10

No. of π-bonds – 1 (C=C) + 2 (C≡C) = 3

101. **(b) :** As the size of the atom *M* in H_2M increases, the strength of the H – *M* bond decreases.

102. **(c) :** The electronegativity of N (3.0) is much higher than P (2.1).

103. (c) : Solubility of AgCl (at 25°C) in H_2O
= 0.0020 g AgCl per litre of H_2O
Solubility of AgCl in NH_3 (at 25°C)
= 14.00 g AgCl dissolved per kg of NH_3
Ammonia is less polar than water, as oxygen is more electronegative than nitrogen.

104. (d) : BCC has 68% and HCP has 74% packing efficiency.
BCC - 2 atoms per unit cell, HCP - 4 atoms per unit cell
In BCC, particles are present at corners and one particle is present at the centre within the body of the unit cell. In HCP, the packing gives a hexagonal pattern.

105. (c) : Mn^{2+} = [Ar] $3d^5$, Mn^{3+} = [Ar] $3d^4$
Fe^{2+} = [Ar] $3d^6$, Fe^{3+} = [Ar] $3d^5$
Thus, Mn^{2+} has more stable configuration than Mn^{3+} while Fe^{3+} has more stable configuration than Fe^{2+}. Hence, reduction potential for Mn^{3+}/Mn^{2+} couple is more positive than Fe^{3+}/Fe^{2+}.

106. (a) : A mixture of 2% O_2 and 98% He is used in diving apparatus which gives the same partial pressure of O_2 as in normal air at 1 atm. Due to high partial pressure and greater solubility, N_2 gets dissolved in blood and form bubbles (bends or decompression sickness). Hence, N_2 is replaced by helium which is much less soluble in biological fluids.

107. (a) : For a redox reaction to be spontaneous, the EMF of the cell must be positive.
As, $-\Delta G = nFE_{cell}$
Therefore, for E_{cell} = +ve, ΔG is always negative.

108. (a) : H_2O_2 oxidises sulphur to sulphate in presence of Fe^{3+} ions.

109. (b) : $Cl_2 + 2NaOH \text{ (dil.)} \xrightarrow{\text{cold}} NaCl + NaOCl + H_2O$

$3Cl_2 + 6NaOH \text{ (conc.)} \xrightarrow{\text{heat}} 5NaCl + NaClO_3 + 3H_2O$

Chlorine undergoes the simultaneous oxidation-reduction. Chlorine is simultaneously reduced to chloride ion (Cl^-) and is oxidised to either ClO^- or ClO_3^- ion. Halogens (*e.g.* Cl) have a strong tendency to accept electrons, so they act as strong oxidising agents.

110. (d) : For a closed system, the entropy can increase, decrease or remain constant.
Closed system can be reversible or irreversible.

111. (d) : Two different reactions can have same rate of reaction. Rate of reaction depends upon many factors like nature and concentration of reactants, temperature, catalyst, energy factors, orientation factor, etc.

112. (a) : $\overset{+}{Na}\overset{-}{O} - \overset{O}{\underset{O}{\overset{\|+5}{S}}} - \overset{0}{S} - \overset{0}{S} - \overset{O}{\underset{O}{\overset{\|+5}{S}}} - \overset{-}{O}\overset{+}{Na}$

Formal oxidation number of sulphur

$$= \frac{2 \times 5 + 2 \times 0}{4} = 2.5$$

113. (d) : Elevation in boiling point $(\Delta T_b) = K_b \times m$
Depression in freezing point $(\Delta T_f) = K_f \times m$.
Elevation in boiling point and depression in freezing point are colligative properties *i.e.*, they depend only on the number of particles of the solute. Value of K_b and K_f are different, so ΔT_b and ΔT_f are also different.

114. (a) : Williamson's synthesis occurs by S_N2 mechanism and primary alkyl halides are most reactive in S_N2 reactions.

115. (d) : Dehydration of alcohols can be carried out either with protonic acids such as conc. H_2SO_4, H_3PO_4 or catalysts such as anhydrous zinc chloride or alumina.

116. (d) : Oxidation of toluene using CrO_3 in acetic anhydride or CrO_2Cl_2 in CCl_4 or CS_2 and then hydrolysis gives benzaldehyde. No such intermediate is formed.

117. (a) : $CH_3 - \underset{CH_3}{\overset{CH_3}{\overset{|}{\underset{|}{C}}}} - CH_2 - Br + NaOH \xrightarrow{S_N1}$
1° alkyl halide

$CH_3 - \underset{CH_3}{\overset{CH_3}{\overset{|}{\underset{|}{C}}}} - \overset{\oplus}{C}H_2 \longrightarrow CH_3 - \underset{\oplus}{\overset{CH_3}{\overset{|}{C}}} - CH_2 - CH_3$
alkyl migration — 3° alkyl carbocation

$\downarrow OH^-$

$CH_3 - \underset{OH}{\overset{CH_3}{\overset{|}{\underset{|}{C}}}} - CH_2 - CH_3$
2-methylbutanol-2

Neopentyl bromide being primary alkyl halide does not undergo S_N2 reaction but proceeds via S_N1 path because of steric hindrance caused by the bulky nature of tertiary butyl group.

118. (b) : In β-pleated sheet structure, the polypeptide chains are held together by intermolecular H-bonds. Extension and contraction of β-pleated sheet structure of protein depends on the size of *R*.

119. (b) : All those carbohydrates which contain aldehydic or ketonic group in the hemiacetal or hemiketal form and reduce Tollen's or Fehling's solutions are reducing sugars. All monosaccharides are reducing sugars (whether aldoses or ketoses).

Fructose is a monosaccharide with keto group.

120. (d) : In *p*-nitrophenol, $-NO_2$ group has $-I$ effect, as a result of which electron density decreases on the benzene ring, hence reactivity towards electrophilic substitution decreases. Methoxy group shows both $+R$ (due to lone pair of electrons on O) and $-I$ effect (due to greater electronegativity of O).

$-OCH_3$ at *meta*-position shows only $-I$ effect but lesser than $-I$ effect of $-NO_2$ group.

BIOLOGY

121. (c) : *Eco* R I is type II restriction endonuclease enzyme extracted from *Eco* R Y 13 bacteria. It can recognize and cleave 5′-GAATTC-3' palindromic sequence and is widely used in biotechnology experiments.

122. (c) : Gene therapy is a procedure of introducing copies of a healthy gene to replace defective gene responsible for disease development. The first clinical gene transfer took place on 22nd May 1992 for correction of adenosine deaminase (ADA) enzyme deficiency.

123. (d) : Bacteria, fungi and lower plants survive in adverse conditions through formation of thick walled spores. Algae form resting spore or akinetes which are thick walled spores and store food material. In fungi, thick walled perennating spores called chlamydospores are formed. Bacteria form endospores which is probably the most resistant living thing known. They may remain alive in boiling water for more than 2 hours.

124. (d) : When a graph is plotted taking into consideration time on one hand and growth rate on the other hand, a 'S' shaped curve is obtained. It is called "grand period of growth". This total growth period is divided into three stages.

(1) Initial lag phase

(2) Middle log phase

(3) Final stationary phase.

125. (b) : Monarch butterfly escapes from predators because of its bitter taste. Viceroy butterfly (*Basilarchia archippus*) mimics monarch butterfly to escape from predators.

126. (b) : Tapetum is the innermost one cell thick layer of microsporangium wall. The cells of this layer are radially enlarged and store food. The cells are multinucleated and provide nourishment to developing microspores or pollen grains.

127. (d) : Catalytic converters have platinum-palladium and rhodium metals as catalyst. It converts more harmful carbon monoxide and unburnt hydrocarbons into less harmful carbon dioxide and water.

128. (c) : Cell theory was proposed by a German botanist M.J. Schleiden and another German, a zoologist T.S. Schwann in 1839.

129. (c) : These are different arrangements of ovule attachment to inner surface of ovary wall. (A) represents marginal, (B) represents axile, (C) represents parietal, (D) represents free central, (E) represents basal placentation.

130. (a) : The figure shows structure of lenticel which facilitates gaseous exchange and transpiration These are aerating pores in the bark of woody trees. These are surrounded by loosely arranged thin walled complementary cells enclosing intercellular spaces for gaseous exchange

131. (c) : In given diagram (A) represents denitrification and (B) represents ammonification. Denitrification is conversion of nitrates into nitrogen gas by some microorganisms *e.g., Pseudomonas denitrificans, Thiobacillus denitrificans, Micrococcus denitrificans.* Ammonification is conversion of dead remains of living organisms into ammonia with the help of microorganisms like *Bacillus ramosus, B. vulgaris, B. mesentericus* etc.

132. (c) : In active transport, carrier proteins which are located at membrane, use energy in the form of ATP to transport molecules against concentration gradient of cell membrane. Transportation rate reaches maximum when all carrier proteins are being used or are saturated. These proteins are very specific to certain substances and are sensitive to inhibitors.

133. (c) : Water is the most abundant chemical compound in living organism. In a cell, water occupies 70–90% of the cellular mass. So, in 50 gm of living tissue 35–45 gm of water would be present.

134. (b) : Photosystem II mostly occurs in the appressed regions of granal thylakoids.

135. (a) : After glycolysis, pyruvate forms acetyl Co-A which undergoes oxidation to form CO_2 and H_2O through Krebs' cycle in mitochondrial matrix.

136. (a) : Cleistogamous flowers do not open at all. In such flowers, the anthers and stigma lie close to each other. Anthers when dehisce in the flower buds, pollen grains come in contact with the stigma to effect pollination Thus, cleistogamous flowers are autogamous as there is no chance of cross-pollination. So, no pollination agent is required in these flowers.

137. (b) : C_4 plants are more efficient than C_3 plants because they have little photorespiration while in C_3 plants more than half of photosynthetic carbon get lost in photorespiration. C_4 plants are more efficient in picking up CO_2, even in low CO_2 concentration because of high affinity of CO_2 with PEP (phosphoenol pyruvic acid).

138. (c) : Fermentation in muscle produces lactic acid. In our bodies certain muscle cells, called fast twitch muscles, have less capability for storing and using oxygen than other muscles. When we run, these muscles run short of oxygen, the fast twitch muscles begin using lactic acid fermentation. This allows the muscle to continue to function by producing ATP by glycolysis.

139. (c) : *Aspergillus niger* is used for commercial and industrial production of certain chemicals like citric acid. Activated sludge is digested by anaerobic bacteria to produce marsh gas. BOD is amount of oxygen required by bacteria for decomposition.

140. (d) : Trace elements or microelements (*e.g.* iron, iodine, zinc, manganese, cobalt, copper, molybdenum, etc.) are required in very small amounts to our body.

141 (c) : Endangered plants may be preserved in part through seed bank or germplasm bank. The term seed bank sometimes refers to a cryogenic laboratory facility in which the seeds of certain species can be preserved for up to a century or more without losing their fertility. It can also be used to refer to a special type of arboretum where seeds are harvested and the crop is rotated. For plants that cannot be preserved in seed banks, the only other option for preserving germplasm is *in vitro* storage, where cuttings of plants are kept under strict conditions in glass tubes and vessels.

142. (a) Reverse Transcription Polymerase Chain Reaction (RT-PCR) is a variant of Polymerase Chain Reaction (PCR), a laboratory technique commonly used in molecular biology to generate many copies of a DNA sequence, a process termed "amplification". In RT-PCR, however, an RNA strand is first reverse transcribed into its DNA complement (complementary DNA, or *c*DNA) using the enzyme reverse transcriptase, and the resulting *c*DNA is amplified using traditional PCR or Real-Time PCR. Reverse transcription PCR (RT-PCR)is not to be confused with Real-Time Polymerase Chain Reaction (Q-PCR/qRT-PCR),RNA silencing (also called as post-transcriptional gene silencing PTGS) refers to a family of gene silencing effects by which the expression of one or more genes is down regulated or entirely suppressed by the introduction of an antisense (single stranded) RNA molecule. Transcription is the process of creating a complementary RNA copy of a sequence of DNA.

143. (a) : Chromosome replication occurs once but meiosis has two M-phases each with its own karyokinesis and cytokinesis. As a result chromosome number is halved. The transition period between M-phase I (meiosis I) and M-phase II (meiosis II) is short and without DNA replication. It is called interkinesis.

144. (b) : Hermann Henking discovered the X chromosome while studying insects in the early 1890s. The sex chromosomes in birds are opposite of that in humans. Human males are heterogametic (XY), females are homogametic (XX), in birds males are homogametic (ZZ) and females are heterogametic (ZW). The "W" is the sex determining chromosome just as the Y in humans. A bird with a W is always a female. In grasshoppers, there is no Y chromosome, so a grasshopper with one X chromosome (symbolized as XO) is normally a male, while a grasshopper with two X chromosomes (XX) is normally a female.

145. (b) : In mosses the sporophytes (*i.e.* the diploid body) are short-lived and dependent on the gametophyte. In the presence of water, sperms from the antheridia swim to the archegonia and fertilization occurs, leading to the production of a diploid sporophyte. The sperm of mosses is biflagellate, *i.e.* they have two flagella that aid in propulsion. Since the sperms must swim to the archegonium, fertilization cannot occur without water.

146. (a) : According to Central Pollution Control Board (CPCB), particulate size 2.5 micrometers or less in diameter (PM 2.5) are responsible for causing the greatest harm to human health. These fine particulates can be inhaled deep into the lungs and can cause breathing and respiratory symptoms, such as irritation, inflammations and damage to the lungs and premature deaths.

147. (d) : Common cold can take place from one person to other as it is a communicable in nature. A healthy person can get infected by being in close vicinity of infected person when he/she sneezes, coughs, as the droplets generated by sneeze and cough contain infecting agents. Typhoid occurs by the intake of contaminated water & food. While ringworm is one of the skin disease which can transfer from one person to other by the use of infected towel & handkerchief. AIDS (Acquired Immuno deficiency) does not occur or transfer by shaking hands.

148. (b) : The peppered moth (*Biston betularia*) is a temperate species of night-flying moth. Peppered moth evolution is often used by educators as an example of natural selection. Peppered moths are cryptically camouflaged against their backgrounds when they rest on the tree trunk.

149. (a) : Fibres and fibroblasts are compactly packed in the dense connective tissues. Orientation of fibres show a regular or irregular pattern and are called dense regular and dense irregular tissues. In the dense regular connective tissues, the collagen fibres are present in rows between many parallel bundles of fibres. Tendons, which attach skeletal muscles to bones and ligaments which attach one bone to another are examples of this tissue.

150. (d) : The main criteria for classification used by Whittaker includes cell structure, thallus organization, mode of nutrition, reproduction and phylogenetic relationships. So, the absence of cell wall is one of the main characteristics of animal kingdom.

151. (d) : Medulla oblongata is part of the vertebrate brain stem, derived from the hindbrain, that is continuous with the spinal cord. Its function is to regulate the reflex responses controlling respiration, heart beat, blood pressure, and other involuntary processes. It gives rise to many of the cranial nerves.

152. (d) : Great apes, humans goes through a menstrual cycle while monkey goes through estrous cycle. Urine is light yellow colored watery fluid which is slightly acidic. Bile juice does not contain any digestive enzymes.

153. (b) : Industrial melanism is an adaptation where the moths living in the industrial areas developed melanin pigments to match their body to the soot-covered surroundings. The phenomenon provides an excellent example of operation of selection in natural conditions.

Industrial melanism, therefore, presents an excellent example of natural selection (proposed by Darwin), but it is not the example of acquired characters proposed by Lamarck.

In caves, due to absence of light, the body of the animal lacks pigmentation. *e.g. Proteus anguinus*. In pythons and related snakes rudimentary pelvic girdle and traces of hind limb are present. They form small clawed projections externally, but internally there are vestiges of an ilium, femur, tibia and a claw. In aquatic birds and flying frog, the feet are webbed which sustain it in the prolonged leaps to which it is adapted.

154. (b) : Frogs do not have external ears. Instead, they have an eardrum of sorts, called a tympanum, which is just behind each eye. Typhlosole are internal folds of the intestine or intestinal inner wall. Typhlosole occurs in bivalve mollusks, lampreys and some annelids and echinoderms. The gizzard, also referred to as the ventriculus, gastric mill, and gigerium, is an organ found in the digestive tract of some animals, including birds, reptiles, earthworms and some fish. This specialized organ constructed of thick, muscular walls is used for grinding up food; often rocks are instrumental in this process. In certain insects and mollusks, the gizzard features chitinous plates or teeth. Humans have 12 pairs of cranial nerves. Cockroach belongs to class insecta of phylum arthropoda.

155. (d) : The T wave represents the repolarization (or recovery) of the ventricles. The end of the T-wave marks the end of systole. The P-wave represents the electrical excitation (or depolarisation) of the atria, which leads to the contraction of both the atria. The QRS complex represents the depolarisation of the ventricles, which initiates the ventricular contraction.

156. (b) : In descending limb of loop of Henle, the water is reabsorbed from filtrate flowing in it due to increasing osmolarity of interstitial fluid. Sodium and other solutes are not reabsorbed here. The filtrate becomes hypertonic to blood plasma. All nephrons have their renal Malphigian corpuscles in the cortex. Cortical nephrons have their loop of Henle in the renal medulla near its junction with the renal cortex, while the loop of Henle of juxtamedullary nephrons is located deep in the renal medulla; they are called juxtamedullary because their renal corpuscle is located near the medulla (but still in the cortex).

157. (a) : In *in vitro* fertilization (IVF-fertilization outside the body in almost similar conditions as that in the body) followed by embryo transfer (ET), ova from the wife/donor (female) and sperms from the husband/donor (male) are collected and are induced to form zygote under simulated conditions in the laboratory. The zygote or early embryos (with upto 8 blastomeres) could then be transferred into the Fallopian tube (ZIFT-Zygote Intra Fallopian Transfer) and embryos with more than 8 blastomeres, into the uterus (IUT-Intra Uterine Transfer), to complete its further development.

158. (d) : The most obvious and technically complicated feature of all living organisms is their ability to sense their surroundings or environment and respond to these environmental stimuli which could be physical, chemical or biological. All organisms, from the prokaryotes to the most complex eukaryotes can sense and respond to environmental cues *eg*. Photoperiod affects reproduction in seasonal breeders, both plants and animals. Consciousness therefore, becomes the defining property of living organisms. There are many organisms which do not reproduce *e.g.* mule. Thus, reproduction cannot be an all-inclusive defining characteristic of living organisms. However no non-living object is capable of reproducing or replicating by itself.

159. (b) : The opening between the right atrium and right ventricle is guarded by a valve formed of three muscular flaps or cusps, the tricuspid valve.

160. (d) : Each actin (thin) filament is a polymerised protein made up of two 'F' (fibrous) actin strands helically wound to each other. Each 'F' actin is a polymer of monomeric 'G' (globular) actins. It is light in colour & shows isotropic property.

161. (b) : Enzymes are highly substrate specific *i.e.* they catalyze the reaction of a particular substrate only. They facilitate occurrence of a reaction and transition of reactant into product. A chemical reaction $S \rightarrow P$ (where S is the substrate and P the product or products) will take place when a certain number of S molecules at any given instant possess enough energy to attain an activated condition called the 'transition state'. The enzyme combines transiently with the substrate to produce a transient state having a lower energy of activation than that of substrate alone. This results in acceleration of the reaction. Once the products are formed, the enzyme (or catalyst) is free or regenerated to combine with another molecule of the substrate and repeat the process.

162. (c) : Cell's turgidity is due to turgor pressure. Turgor pressure is the pressure which develops in the confined part of an osmotic system due to osmotic entry of water into it. It is also called hydrostatic pressure or pressure potential. The force exerted by the cell wall over the protoplast is called wall pressure. Normally wall pressure is equal and opposite to turgor pressure except when the cell becomes flaccid.

163. (b) : Long distance bulk movement of substances that occurs through conducting or vascular tissues of plants is called translocation. There are two vascular tissues, xylem and phloem. Xylem translocation is mainly from roots to aerial parts. It passes water with mineral salts, some organic nitrogen and hormones *i.e.* unidirectional. Phloem translocates organic substances and inorganic solutes first from leaves to all other parts of the plant and storage organs. Storage organs re-export organic nutrients to those parts which require the same as newly formed leaves and fruits *i.e.* it is bidirectional.

164. (b) : The first step in photosynthesis is the light-driven oxidation (splitting or photolysis) of water. It provides the electrons for the photosynthetic electron transport chains as well as protons for the establishment of a proton gradient. It occurs on the lumenal side of the thylakoid membrane. During photolysis, water is oxidised to oxygen, protons and electrons. Protons accumulate in the lumen.

165. (a) : Unlike animals, plants do not stop growing after reaching maturity. They continue to grow and bear new roots, leaves, branches, flowers, etc. While roots, stems and their branches have indefinite growth, other organs like leaves, flowers and fruits show limited or definite growth. They appear and fall off periodically and sometimes repeatedly. In lower plants, growth is diffused as every cell can divide and enlarge. Higher plants possess specific areas which take part in the formation of new cells. These areas are called meristems. Meristems are of three types– apical, intercalary and lateral. Cells of the meristematic region have the capacity to divide and self perpetuate. They produce cells which lose the capacity to divide and enter G_0 phase for undergoing differentiation to form particular tissues and organs. The meristem which is consumed in the formation of an organ is called determinate meristem. The meristem which continues its activity throughout life of the plant is called indeterminate meristem. It is the reason behind indefinite growth of plants.

166. (c) : Organic biodegradable (*i.e.* they can be degraded by decomposers) pollutants in water are measured by BOD. BOD(biological oxygen demand) is the oxygen demanded or required by bacteria and other decomposers to oxidise pollutants.

167. (a) : Vessels are much elongated tubes which are closed at either end and are formed by the union of several short, wide and thickened cells called vessel elements. The end walls of vessel elements are transverse or oblique. They are often completely dissolved. The condition is called simple perforation plate. In a few cases the end walls remain intact and possess several pores in reticulate, scalariform or forminate forms. Such an end wall is called multiple perforation plate. Sieve tubes are elongated tubular conducting channels of phloem formed of several cells called sieve tube elements or members or sieve tube cells. Sieve tube members are placed end to end. The end walls are generally bulged out. They may be transverse or oblique. They have many small pores or sieve pits. Due to the presence of sieve pits the end walls are commonly called sieve plates. In some cases the end walls of sieve elements possess more than one porous area. Such an end wall is called compound sieve plate. Gymnosperms & pteridophytes lack these two vascular structures *i.e.* vessels and sieve elements. In angiosperms presence of vessels & sieve elements in addition to all other vascular tissues make their food & water transport more efficient.

168. (b) : Formation of seeds without fertilization is called apomixis. It leads to clonal reproduction in which all offsprings are by and large genetically identical to the parent. The egg contains a full complement of genes and does not need to fuse with a sperm to produce a zygote. Apomixis provides for the perpetuation of traits favourable to individual survival but eliminates the longer-term evolutionary advantage of biparental inheritance. In asteraceae, various genera and individual species of the order asterales are known to reproduce by apomixis (the setting of seeds without fertilization), either completely or in addition to normal sexual means. In poaceae about 35 genera produce seeds without fertilization. On the other hand, parthenocarpy is development of fruits without fertilization. The fruit resembles a normally produced fruit but is seedless, *e.g.* pineapple, banana, cucumber, grape, orange, grapefruit etc.

169. **(d)** : Algal blooms are a result of eutrophication. Eutrophication involves change in biological productivity and nutrient content of a water body. Eutrophication literally means 'well nourished or enriched'. Eutrophication become excessive, when abnormally high amount of nutrients from sewage, fertilizers, animal wastage and detergent, enter streams and lakes causing excessive growth or blooms of microorganisms. They are harmful for both humans and aquatic organisms. Eutrophication results in higher BOD and reduced dissolved oxygen in water body. It causes death of fish and other aquatic animals.

170. **(c)** : Mangroves which form shallow littoral forests near sea shores areas are halophytes. Mangrove grow in physiologically dry environment (water is available in plenty but in the form of strong salt solution). These plants develop shallow rootings due to water logged environment where oxygen scarcity prevails. To ensure proper aeration in root system, plants produce respiratory roots or pneumatophores which are negatively geotropic peg-like projections above ground with numerous pores or lenticels for gaseous exchange.

171. **(a)** : It can be explained as follows

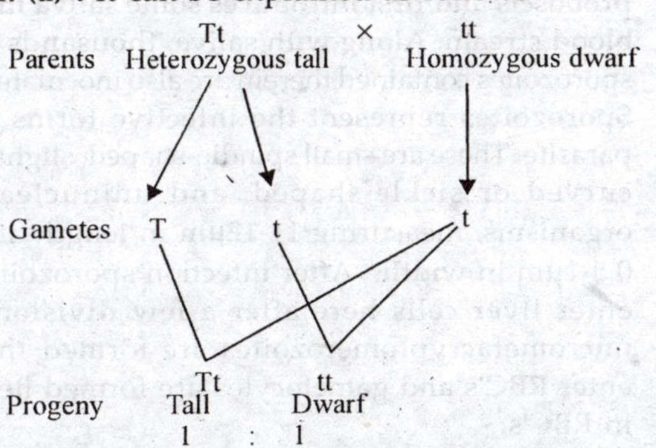

or 50% tall, 50% dwarf progeny.

172. **(b)** : Amniocentesis is a foetal sex determination and disorder test based on the chromosomal pattern in the amniotic fluid surrounding the developing embryo. The amniotic fluid contains cells from foetus skin and respiratory tract. These cells are cultured and are used to determine chromosomal abnormalities (Down's syndrome, Klinefelter's syndrome, etc.) and metabolic disorders (phenylketonuria, sickle cell anaemia, etc.) of the foetus. But now-a-days instead of positive uses of amniocentesis it is being used for female foeticide. Sex of the foetus is determined using amniocentesis and then if it turns out to been a female one, foetus is aborted. That is why amniocentesis has been banned in India.

173. **(a)** : *Bacillus thuringiensis* is a bacterium found in soil worldwide. Several strains can infect and kill insects. Due to this property, through genetic engineering, gene coding for insecticide is incorporated into plant genome. Plant having this gene are insect resistant thus high yielding *e.g.* Bt cotton is usually resistant to bollworm disease of cotton. It is the first genetically modified crop of India. This produces its own insecticide, as it contain a gene from soil bacterium *Bacillus thuringiensis*.

174. **(c)** : Glycerides, mainly triglycerides are a principle form of fats present in our food. During digestion, fats are digested to form monoglycerides and free fatty acids. They first become dissolved in the central lipid portions of bile micelles which are soluble in chyme. In this form, the monoglycerides and free fatty acids are carried to the surfaces of the microvilli of the intestinal cell brush border and then penetrate into the interior of the epithelial cells, which is possible because the lipids are also soluble in the epithelial cell membrane. This leaves the bile micelles still in the chyme, where they function again and to help absorb still more monoglycerides and fatty acids.
After entering the epithelial cell, the fatty acids and monoglycerides are taken up by the cell's smooth endoplasmic reticulum; here they are mainly used to form new triglycerides that are subsequently released in the form of chylomicrons through the base of the epithelial cell, to flow upward through the thoracic lymph duct and empty into the circulating blood. Thus, chylomicrons help in transport of glycerides through blood circulation to various body parts.

175 **(c)** : The colourless blood or haemolymph of cockroach has a clear plasma and numerous white corpuscles called haemocytes. Being devoid of any respiratory pigment, it does not serve for gaseous exchange. Its plasma contains

about 70% water. Rest of it is composed of amino acids, uric acid, proteins, sugars, fats, and salts of sodium, potassium, calcium and magnesium. Transportation of these materials between different parts of body is the main function of haemolymph. In all terrestrial insects, like cockroach, every tissue of body is in direct contact with atmospheric air for gaseous exchange. A complicated system of numerous shiny, transparent and branched air tubes or tracheae is found for this purpose in the haemocoel cavity. Atmospheric air enters into and escapes out from this system through ten pairs of slit-like apertures called stigmata or spiracles, located on lateral sides of body.

176. (b) : ABO blood groups are determined by the gene *I* (isoagglutinin). There are three alleles, I^A, I^B and I^O of this gene. Proteins produced by the I^A and I^B alleles are called A antigen and B antigen. People with blood group A have the A antigen on the surface of their RBCs, and antibodies against antigen B in their plasma. Persons with blood group B have B antigen on their RBCs, and antibodies against A antigen in their plasma. Individuals with AB blood group have both antigen A and antigen B on their RBCs, and no antibodies for either of the antigens in their plasma. Type O individuals are without A and B antigens on their RBCs, but have antibodies for both these antigens in their plasma.

177. (b) : Sinu-auricular node or S-A node is located in the wall of the right auricle below the opening of the superior vena cava. The S-A node has unique property of self excitation, which enables it to act the "pacemaker" of the heart. It spontaneously initiates a wave of contraction which spreads over both the auricles more or less simultaneously along the muscle fibres that fan out from the pacemaker.

178. (d) : The organ of Corti lies on the basilar membrane. It contains a series of electromechanically sensitive cells *i.e.* hair cells. They are the receptive end organs that generate nerve impulses in response to sound vibrations. Thus, organ of Corti is actually the organ that perceives sound. Minute hairs project upward from hair cell and they are embedded in the tectorial membrane. Equilibrium of body is maintained with the help of semicircular canals, utricle and saccule of internal ear.

179. (b) : After ovulation, the empty Graafian follicle contains a blood clot which is called corpus haemorrhagic. Its granulosa cells continue to proliferate, develop yellow carotene pigment or lutein and get converted into lutein cells. This converts the ruptured follicle into yellow body called corpus luteum. It becomes a temporary endocrine gland secreting progesterone with small quantity of estrogen. in absence of fertilization, after few days, corpus luteum ultimately stops activity, loses yellow colour, begins to degenerate, then it is called corpus albicans. If fertilization occurs and foetus is implanted in the endometrium, the trophoblast cells of the developing placenta secrete a hormone human chorionic gonadotrophin (hCG). This hormone, like LH, maintains the corpus luteum and the secretion of progesterone and estradiol by it. These two hormones check the breakdown of the endometrium of the uterus. Thus corpus luteum helps to maintain pregnancy.

180. (b) : A healthy person acquires infection when a female *Anopheles* mosquito, containing infective stages of parasite (sporozoites) in its salivary glands, bites him for sucking his blood. The mosquito punctures the host's skin by its proboscis and first introduces some saliva into blood stream. Along with saliva, thousands of sporozoites contained therein are also inoculated. Sporozoites represent the infective forms of parasite. These are small spindle-shaped, slightly curved or sickle-shaped, and uninucleate organisms, measuring 11-12μm in length and 0.5-1μm in width. After infection sporozoites enter liver cells here after a few divisions, micrometacryptomerozoites are formed that enter RBC's and gametocytes are formed here in RBC's.

GENERAL KNOWLEDGE

181. (a)	**182.** (b)	**183.** (c)	**184.** (a)	**185.** (a)
186. (b)	**187.** (c)	**188.** (a)	**189.** (d)	**190.** (c)
191. (a)	**192.** (b)	**193.** (b)	**194.** (d)	**195.** (d)
196. (a)	**197.** (b)	**198.** (a)	**199.** (d)	**200.** (b)

☺☺☺

Chapterwise Index - '12

Physics • Chemistry • Biology

Use the index for topicwise analysis of AIIMS paper and refer to these questions when you are practising MCQs chapterwise.

PHYSICS

Chapter's Name	Question No.	Total
Units and Dimensions	11	1
Motion in One Dimension		
Motion in Two Dimensions		
Laws of Motion and Friction	45	1
Work, Power and Energy	47	1
Centre of Mass and Rotational Motion	24, 30	2
Gravitation	19, 27	2
Properties of Matter	22, 43, 60	3
Oscillations	16, 33	2
Waves	3	1
Heat and Thermodynamics	28, 32, 34, 35, 36, 41, 51	7
Electrostatics	13, 23, 26, 53, 57	5
Current Electricity	29	1
Thermal and chemical effects of current	31	1
Magnetic Effects of Current	10, 12, 18, 44, 46, 54	6
Magnetism	52	1
Electromagnetic Induction and Alternating Current	2, 9, 14, 39	4
Electromagnetic Waves	37, 56	2
Ray Optics	4, 42, 49	3
Wave Optics	5, 25	2
Modern Physics	6, 8, 15, 17, 20, 21, 40, 48, 50, 55, 58, 59	12
Solids and Semiconductor Devices	1, 7, 38	3
Universe		
Principles of Communication		

CHEMISTRY

Chapter's Name	Question No.	Total
Basic Concepts		
Atomic Structure	61, 70, 105, 113	4
Periodic Properties	88	1
Chemical Bonding	89, 107, 108	3
Nuclear Chemistry		
Gaseous and Liquid States	67, 120	2
Solid State	66, 74, 82	3
Mole Concept & Solutions	118	1
Colloids, Surface Chemistry & Catalysis	83	1
Equilibrium	64, 75, 80, 91	4
Kinetics	72, 81, 101	3
Energetics	68	1
Electrochemistry	79	1
Redox Reactions	111, 114	2
Metallurgy		
Hydrogen and its Compounds		
s-Block Elements	98	1
p-Block Elements	63, 69, 73, 87, 93, 94, 103, 104, 110	9
d- and *f*-Block Elements	71, 84, 85, 112, 115	5
Complex Compounds	116, 117	2
Purification and Analysis of Organic Compound		
General Organic Chemistry	78, 86, 90, 92, 106	5
Aliphatic Hydrocarbons	102, 119	2
Aromatic Hydrocarbons		
Halogen Derivatives	100	1
Alcohols, Phenols and Ethers	96, 109	2
Aldehydes and Ketones		
Carboxylic acids & their derivatives	65, 77	2
Organic Compounds Containing Nitrogen	62, 97, 99	3
Biochemistry		
Chemistry in Action	95	1
Environmental Chemistry	76	1

BIOLOGY		
Chapter's Name	**Question No.**	**Total**
General Biology		
Biological Classification	171	1
Kingdom Monera		
Kingdom Fungi	125	1
Plant Kingdom		
Cell and its Structural Components	129, 132	2
Cell Reproduction	142, 151, 152	3
Cell Respiration	134	1
Enzymes		
Biomolecules	160	1
Mendelian Genetics		
Hereditary Material		
Anatomy of Flowering Plants		
Morphology of Flowering Plants	122, 131, 145, 157	4
Physiology of Flowering Plants	126, 137, 141, 147, 168	5
Embryology of Flowering Plants		
Growth and Development in Flowering Plants		
Angiosperm Families		
Ecology and Pollution	124, 130, 140, 158, 172	5
Applied Botany	153, 154, 155	3

Chapter's Name	Question No.	Total
Animal Kingdom	121, 128, 149, 163, 165	5
Genes and Chromosomes	135	1
Gene regulation and Applied Genetics		
Human Genetics & Genetic Disorder	167, 169	2
Animal Tissue		
Musculo-Skeletal System	138	1
Digestive System and Nutrition	150, 177, 178	3
Respiration	146, 176	2
Circulatory System and Immunity	144, 156	2
Excretion and Osmoregulation	170	1
Reproduction and Embryonic Development	123, 127	2
Nervous System and Sense Organs	133, 139, 164, 179	4
Endocrine System	143. 166, 175, 180	4
Common Human Disease	173, 174	2
Growth and Regeneration		
Evolution	148	1
Drug Addiction		
Applied Zoology	136, 159, 162	3
Wild Life and Conservation	161	1
Human Population & Growth		

SOLVED PAPER

AIIMS - 2012★

Time : 3½ Hours

Max. Marks : 200

PHYSICS

1. Which of the following current must be zero in an unbiased *PN* junction diode?
(a) Current due to majority charge carriers (both electrons and holes).
(b) Current due to minority charge carriers (both electrons and holes).
(c) Current due to majority and minority charge carriers.
(d) Current due to majority and minority charge carriers (only holes).

2. In an *AC* circuit, voltage $V = V_0 \sin \omega t$ and inductor *L* is connected across the circuit. Then the instantaneous power will be
(a) $\frac{V_0^2}{2\omega L} \sin \omega t$ (b) $\frac{-V_0^2}{2\omega L} \sin \omega t$
(c) $\frac{-V_0^2}{2\omega L} \sin 2\omega t$ (d) $\frac{V_0^2}{\omega L} \sin 2\omega t$

3. Two sinusoidal waves of intensity *I* having same frequency and same amplitude interferes constructively at a point. The resultant intensity at a point will be
(a) *I* (b) 2*I* (c) 4*I* (d) 8*I*

4. In a convex lens of focal length *F*, the minimum distance between an object and its real image must be
(a) 3*F* (b) 4*F* (c) $\frac{3}{2}F$ (d) 2*F*

5. In Young's double slit experiment, fringe order is represented by *m*, then fringe width is
(a) Independent of *m*.
(b) Directly proportional to *m*.
(c) Directly proportional to (2*m* + 1).
(d) Inversely proportional to (2*m* + 1).

6. Half life of a radio-active element is 8 years, how much amount will be present after 32 years?
(a) $\frac{1}{4}$ (b) $\frac{1}{8}$ (c) $\frac{1}{16}$ (d) $\frac{1}{32}$

7. In the given circuit, the voltage across the load is maintained at 12 V. The current in the zener diode varies from 0-50 mA. What is the maximum wattage of the diode?

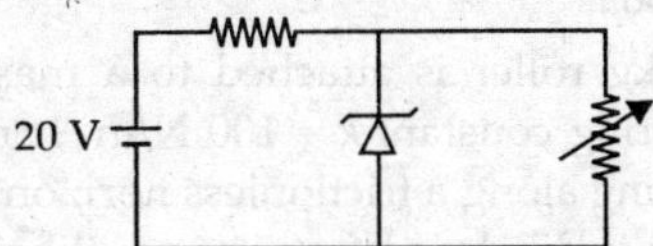

(a) 12 W (b) 6 W (c) 0.6 W (d) 1.2 W

8. A photon is incident having frequency 1×10^{14} sec^{-1}. Threshold frequency of metal is 5×10^{13} sec^{-1}. Find the kinetic energy of the ejected electron.
(a) 3.3×10^{-21} J (b) 6.6×10^{-21} J
(c) 3.3×10^{-20} J (d) 6.6×10^{-20} J

9. In a given series *LCR* circuit $R = 4\ \Omega$, $X_L = 5\ \Omega$ and $X_C = 8\ \Omega$, the current
(a) Leads the voltage by $\tan^{-1}(3/4)$.
(b) Leads the voltage by $\tan^{-1}(5/8)$.
(c) Lags the voltage by $\tan^{-1}(3/4)$.
(d) Lags the voltage by $\tan^{-1}(5/8)$.

10. A wire of mass 100 g, length 1 m and current 5 A is balanced in mid air by a magnetic field *B*, then find the value of *B*.
(a) 0.2 T (b) 0.1 T (c) 0.5 T (d) 0.6 T

11. Dimensional formula of ΔQ, heat supplied to the system is given by
(a) $[M^1L^2T^{-2}]$ (b) $[M^1L^1T^{-2}]$
(c) $[M^1L^2T^{-1}]$ (d) $[ML^1T^{-1}]$

12. A toroid with mean radius r_0, diameter 2*a* have *N* turns carrying current *I*. What is the magnetic field *B* inside the toroid?
(a) $\frac{NI}{2\pi r_0}$ (b) $\frac{NI}{2\pi(r_0 + a)}$
(c) $\frac{NI}{\pi(r_0 + a)}$ (d) zero

13. Identify incorrect for electric charge *q*
(a) quantised (b) conserved
(c) additive (d) non-transferable.

★ *Based on memory. Courtesy : Allen Career Institute, Kota (Rajasthan)*

14. Which of the following parameter in the series *LCR* circuit is analogous to driving force *F*(*t*) in mechanics?

(a) $\frac{V_0}{L}$ (b) inductance *L*
(c) capacitance *C* (d) voltage V_0

15. The minimum magnetic dipole moment of electron in hydrogen atom is

(a) $\frac{eh}{2\pi m}$ (b) $\frac{eh}{4\pi m}$
(c) $\frac{eh}{\pi m}$ (d) 0

16. A 4 kg roller is attached to a massless spring of spring constant k = 100 N/m. It rolls without slipping along a frictionless horizontal road. The roller is displaced from its equilibrium position by 10 cm and then released. Its maximum speed will be

(a) 0.5 m s^{-1} (b) 0.6 m s^{-1}
(c) 0.4 m s^{-1} (d) 0.8 m s^{-1}

17. Total energy of the electron in hydrogen atom above 0 eV leads to

(a) continuation of energy states.
(b) large number of discrete ionised states.
(c) balmar series. (d) paschen series.

18. Two wires carrying

(a) Parallel current repel each other.
(b) Antiparallel current attract each other.
(c) Antiparallel current repel each other.
(d) Equal magnitudes of antiparallel current attract each other.

19. A particle is thrown vertically upwards with velocity 11.2 km s^{-1} from the surface of earth. Calculate its velocity at height 3 *R*. Where *R* is the radius of earth.

(a) ≈ 9.25 km s^{-1} (b) ≈ 5.6 km s^{-1}
(c) ≈ 11.2 km s^{-1} (d) ≈ 4.3 km s^{-1}

20. Gamma decay takes place

(a) Prior to alpha decay.
(b) Prior to beta decay.
(c) Prior to positron decay.
(d) Due to de-excitment of nuclear levels.

21. Calculate the kinetic energy of the electron having wavelength 1 nm.

(a) 2.1 eV (b) 3.1 eV
(c) 1.5 eV (d) 4.2 eV

22. A spherical body of diameter *D* is falling in viscous medium. Its terminal velocity is proportional to

(a) $V_t \propto D^{1/2}$ (b) $V_t \propto D^{3/2}$
(c) $V_t \propto D^2$ (d) $V_t \propto D^{5/2}$

23. Electric field outside a long wire carrying charge *q* is proportional to

(a) $\frac{1}{r}$ (b) $\frac{1}{r^2}$
(c) $\frac{1}{r^{3/5}}$ (d) $\frac{1}{r^{3/2}}$

24. If 2 kg mass is rotating on a circular path of radius 0.8 m with angular velocity of 44 rad/sec. If radius of the path becomes 1 m, then what will be the value of angular velocity?

(a) 28.16 rad/sec (b) 19.28 rad/sec
(c) 8.12 rad/sec (d) 35.26 rad/sec

25. A light ray is incident on a glass slab, it is partially reflected and partially transmitted. Then the reflected ray is

(a) completely polarised and highly intense.
(b) partially polarised and poorly intense.
(c) partially polarised and highly intense.
(d) completely polarised and poorly intense.

26. An electron projected with velocity $\vec{v} = v_0\,\hat{i}$ in the electric field $\vec{E} = E_0\,\hat{j}$. Trace the path followed by the electron E_0.

(a) Parabola (b) Circle
(c) Straight line in + *y* direction.
(d) Straight line in – *y* direction.

27. Find out the correct relation for the dependance of change in acceleration due to gravity on the angle at the latitude, due to rotation of earth

(a) $dg \propto \cos\phi$ (b) $dg \propto \cos^2\phi$
(c) $dg \propto \cos^{3/2}\phi$ (d) $dg \propto \frac{1}{\cos\phi}$

28. Two conductors having same width and length, thickness d_1 and d_2, thermal conductivity K_1 and k_2 are placed one above the another. Find the equivalent thermal conductivity.

(a) $\frac{(d_1+d_2)(K_1d_2+K_2d_1)}{2(K_1+K_2)}$

(b) $\frac{(d_1-d_2)(K_1d_2+K_2d_1)}{2(K_1+K_2)}$

(c) $\frac{K_1d_1+K_2d_2}{d_1+d_2}$ (d) $\frac{K_1+K_2}{d_1+d_2}$

29. Calculate I for the given circuit diagram.

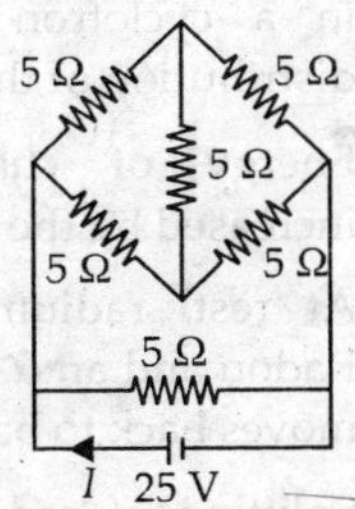

(a) 10 A (b) 5 A (c) 2.5 A (d) 20 A

30. A solid cylinder, a circular disc, a solid sphere and a hollow cylinder of the same radius are placed on an inclined plane. Which of the following will have maximum acceleration at the bottom of the plane?
(a) Circular disc. (b) Solid cylinder.
(c) Solid sphere. (d) Hollow cylinder.

31. Calculate the heat emitted by a bulb of 100 W in 1 min.
(a) 100 J (b) 1000 J
(c) 600 J (d) 6000 J

32. Degree of freedom for polyatomic gas
(a) ≥ 4 (b) ≥ 5 (c) ≥ 6 (d) ≥ 7

33. A particle moving about its equilibrium position with equation $y = -ax - bt$. Interpret the condition
(a) It will always perform the SHM.
(b) It can never perform the SHM.
(c) It can perform SHM only when $t \geq \frac{bx}{a}$
(d) It can perform SHM only when $t \leq \frac{bx}{a}$.

34. Conversion of water to steam is accompanied by which process?
(a) Adiabatic. (b) Isothermal.
(c) Isochoric. (d) Cyclic.

35. An ideal gas is taken through the cycle $A \to B \to C \to A$, as shown in figure. If the net heat supplied to the gas in the cycle is 5 J the work done by the gas in the process $A \to B$ is

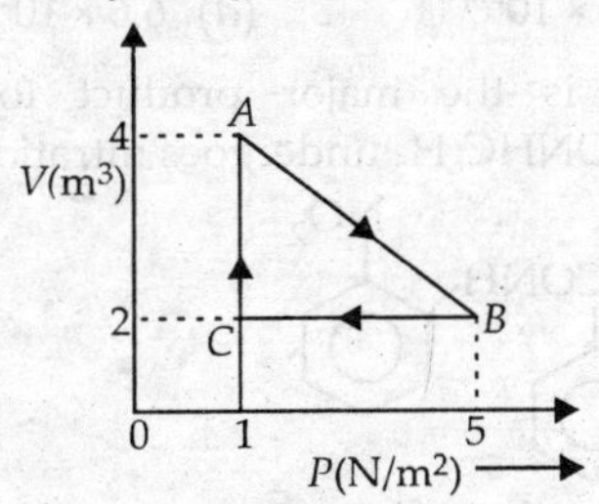

(a) 2 J (b) 3 J (c) 4 J (d) 5 J

36. What is the slope for an isothermal process?
(a) $\frac{P}{V}$ (b) $-\frac{P}{V}$ (c) Zero (d) ∞

37. The frequency order for X-rays (A), γ-rays (B), UV rays (C) is
(a) $B > A > C$ (b) $A > B > C$
(c) $C > B > A$ (d) $A > C > B$

38. For a common-emitter transistor, input current is 5 μA, β = 100 circuit is operated at load resistance of 10 kΩ, then voltage across collector emitter will be
(a) 5 V (b) 10 V (c) 12.5 V (d) 7.5 V

39. Find the voltage drop across a capacitor connected with a resistance and a battery of 60 V in series after a long time.
(a) 0 V (b) 60 V (c) 30 V (d) 38 V

40. The nucleus ${}^{m}_{n}X$ emits one α particle and 2β-particles. The resulting nucleus is
(a) ${}^{m-4}_{n-2}Y$ (b) ${}^{m-6}_{n-4}Z$
(c) ${}^{m-6}_{n}Z$ (d) ${}^{m-4}_{n}X$

Directions : In the following questions (41-60), a statement of assertion (A) is followed by a statement of reason (R). Mark the correct choice as :

(a) If both assertion and reason are true and reason is the correct explanation of assertion.
(b) If both assertion and reason are true but reason is not the correct explanation of assertion.
(c) If assertion is true but reason is false.
(d) If both assertion and reason are false.

41. **Assertion :** Maximum air flow due to convection does not occur at the north pole but it occurs at 30° N.

Reason : There is maximum temperature difference between equator and 30° N

42. **Assertion :** A thick lens shows more chromatic aberration.

Reason : Thick lens behave as many thin lenses.

43. **Assertion :** Surface energy of an oil drop is same whether placed on glass or water surface.

Reason : Surface energy is dependent only on the properties of oil.

44. Assertion : Magnetic force is always perpendicular to the magnetic field.

Reason : Electric force is along the direction of electric field.

45. Assertion : Animate object can accelerate in the absence of external force.

Reason : Newton's second law is not applicable on animate object.

46. Assertion : A planar circular loop of area A and carrying current I is equivalent to magnetic dipole of dipole moment $M = IA$.

Reason : At large distances, magnetic field of circular loop and magnetic dipole is same.

47. Assertion : In elastic collision, kinetic energy is conserved.

Reason : Energy is always conserved.

48. Assertion : Bohr's atomic model cannot be used to explain multiple electron species.

Reason : It does not take inter-electronic interactions in account.

49. Assertion : The focal length of objective lens in telescope is much more than that of eye piece.

Reason : Telescope has high resolving power due to large focal length.

50. Assertion : Total energy of electron in an hydrogen atom is negative.

Reason : It is bounded to the nucleus.

51. Assertion : Vibrational energy of diatomic molecule corresponding to each degree of freedom is k_BT.

Reason : For every molecule, vibrational degree of freedom is 2.

52. Assertion : A superconductor is a perfect diamagnetic substance.

Reason : A superconductor is a perfect conductor.

53. Assertion : An electrostatic field line never form closed loop.

Reason : Electrostatic field is a conservative field.

54. Assertion : A charged particle can be accelerated in a cyclotron by the alternate distribution of the field.

Reason : Energy of charged particle is increased by the field applied.

55. Assertion : At rest, radium is decayed into Radon and an α-particle. They both moves back to back of each other.

Reason : Splitting of radioactive particle is based on conservation of linear momentum.

56. Assertion : In electromagnetic waves electric field and magnetic field lines are perpendicular to each other.

Reason : Electric field and magnetic field are self sustaining.

57. Assertion : Gauss's law shows diversion when inverse square law is not obeyed.

Reason : Gauss's law is a consequence of conservation of charges.

58. Assertion : More energy is released in fusion than fission.

Reason : More number of nucleons take part in fission.

59. Assertion : γ-radiation emission occurs after α and β decay.

Reason : Energy levels occur in nucleus.

60. Assertion : Turbulence is always dissipative.

Reason : High reynold number promotes turbulence.

CHEMISTRY

61. Threshold frequency of a metal is 5×10^{13} s^{-1} upon which 1×10^{14} s^{-1} frequency light is focused. Then the maximum kinetic energy of emitted electron is

(a) 3.3×10^{-21} (b) 3.3×10^{-20}
(c) 6.6×10^{-21} (d) 6.6×10^{-20}

62. Which is the major product formed when $C_6H_5CONHC_6H_5$ undergoes nitration?

(a) 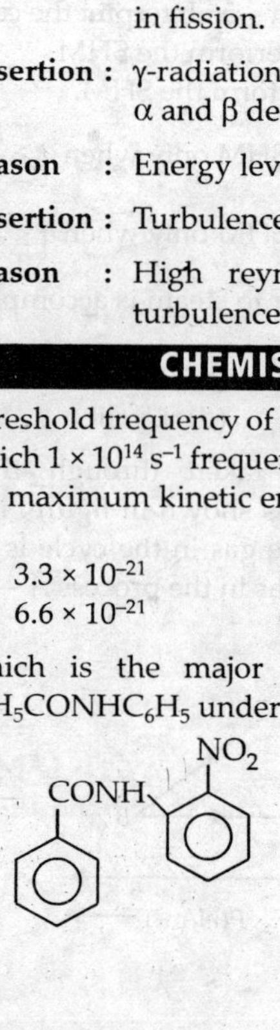 [structure: C_6H_5–CONH–C_6H_4 with NO_2 ortho]

(b) [Structure: benzene ring with CONH– linked to a benzene ring bearing NO_2]

(c) [Structure: benzene ring with CO–NH– linked to benzene ring, O_2N ortho on first ring]

(d) [Structure: benzene ring with CO–NH– linked to benzene ring, NO_2 para on first ring]

63. How many P = O bond present in $(HPO_3)_3$?
(a) 0 (b) 3 (c) 6 (d) 9

64. At equilibrium which is correct?
(a) $\Delta G = 0$ (b) $\Delta S = 0$
(c) $\Delta H = 0$ (d) $\Delta G° = 0$

65. If phthalic acid is treated with NH_3 and then it is first heated weakly then strongly, the final product formed is

(a) [Structure: benzene with two ortho $CONH_2$ groups] (b) [Structure: benzene with $CONH_2$ and –CO–NH– as shown]

(c) [Structure: benzene with COOH and $CONH_2$ ortho] (d) [Structure: phthalimide, benzene fused with C(=O)–NH–C(=O)]

66. In *bcc* structure contribution of corner and central atom is
(a) $\frac{1}{8}, 1$ (b) $\frac{1}{4}, \frac{1}{8}$ (c) $\frac{1}{8}, \frac{1}{2}$ (d) $1, \frac{1}{2}$

67. Arrange the following gases in order of their critical temperature.
NH_3, H_2O, CO_2, O_2
(a) $NH_3 > H_2O > CO_2 > O_2$
(b) $O_2 > CO_2 > H_2O > NH_3$
(c) $H_2O > NH_3 > CO_2 > O_2$
(d) $CO_2 > O_2 > H_2O > NH_3$

68. Bond dissociation energy of CH_4 is 360 kJ/mol and C_2H_6 is 620 kJ/mol. Then bond dissociation energy of C — C bond is
(a) 170 kJ/mol (b) 50 kJ/mol
(c) 80 kJ/mol (d) 220 kJ/mol

69. For silicon which is not correct?
(a) It is a type of silicate.
(b) It is thermally unstable.
(c) It is hydrophilic.
(d) Repeating unit is R_2SiO.

70. In Bohr's orbit, $\frac{nh}{2\pi}$ indicates
(a) Momentum (b) Kinetic energy
(c) Potential energy (d) Angular momentum

71. Which is not stable under ambient condition?
(a) TiO_2, Ti^{+4} (b) VO, V^{+4}
(c) VO_2, V^{+5} (d) Cu_2O, Cu^{+2}

72. For a reaction, $r = k(CH_3COCH_3)^{3/2}$ then unit of rate of reaction and rate constant respectively is
(a) mol L^{-1} s^{-1}, $mol^{-1/2}$ $L^{1/2}$ s^{-1}
(b) mol^{-1} L^{-1} s^{-1}, $mol^{-1/2}$ $L^{-1/2}$ s^{-1}
(c) mol L^{-1} s^{-1}, $mol^{+1/2}$ $L^{1/2}$ s^{-1}
(d) mol L s, $mol^{+1/2}$ $L^{1/2}$ s

73. Which of the following is the correct statement for PH_3?
(a) It is less poisonous than NH_3.
(b) It is less basic than NH_3.
(c) Electronegativity of $PH_3 > NH_3$.
(d) It does not show reducing properties.

74. If Si is doped with B,
(a) *n*-type semiconductor is formed
(b) *p*-type semiconductor is formed
(c) insulator is formed
(d) polymer is formed.

75. Which has the highest pH?
(a) CH_3COOK (b) Na_2CO_3
(c) NH_4Cl (d) $NaNO_3$

76. Living in the atmosphere of CO is dangerous, because it
(a) combines with O_2 present inside to form CO_2
(b) reduces organic matter of tissues
(c) combines with haemoglobin and makes it incapable to absorb oxygen
(d) dries up the blood.

77. In a set of reactions, acetic acid yielded a product *S*.

$$CH_3COOH \xrightarrow{SOCl_2} P \xrightarrow[\text{Anhy. AlCl}_3]{\text{Benzene}} Q \xrightarrow{HCN} R \xrightarrow{HOH} S$$

The structure of *S* would be

(a) [Structure: C_6H_5–C(OH)(CH_3)–COOH]

(b) $C_6H_5-CH_2-C(OH)(COOH)-CH_3$

(c) $C_6H_5-CH_2-C(OH)(CN)-CH_3$

(d) $C_6H_5-C(CN)(OH)-CH_3$

78. Which of the following is a chiral compound?
(a) Hexane (b) *n*-Butane
(c) Methane
(d) 2,3,4-Trimethylhexane.

79. For $Zn^{2+} | Zn$, $E° = -0.76$ V then EMF of the cell Zn/Zn^{2+} (1M) | $2H^+$ (1M) | H_2 (1 atm) will be
(a) -0.76 V (b) 0.76 V
(c) 0.38 V (d) -0.38 V

80. $\frac{K_p}{K_c}$ for following reaction will be
$$CO_{(g)} + \frac{1}{2}O_{2(g)} \rightarrow CO_{2(g)}$$
(a) RT (b) $\frac{1}{RT}$ (c) $\frac{1}{\sqrt{RT}}$ (d) $\frac{RT}{2}$

81. If $t_{1/2}$ *vs* $\frac{1}{a^2}$ is a straight line graph then determine the order of reaction.
(a) Zero order (b) First order
(c) Second order (d) Third order

82. CsCl has *bcc* arrangement. Its unit cell edge length is 400 pm. Its inter-ionic distance is
(a) 400 pm (b) 800 pm
(c) $\sqrt{3} \times 100$ pm (d) $\frac{\sqrt{3}}{2} \times 400$ pm

83. A colloidal solution is kept in dark and is illuminated by a beam of light then brightness appears at the right angle of direction of light. This effect is called
(a) Tyndall effect (b) Brownian effect
(c) Hardy-Schulze effect
(d) None of these

84. MnO_3 in an acidic medium dissociates into
(a) MnO_2 and MnO_4^- (b) MnO and MnO_4^-
(c) MnO_2 and MnO (d) MnO_2 and MnO_3

85. Magnetic moment of Cr^{2+} is nearest to
(a) Fe^{2+} (b) Mn^{2+} (c) Co^{2+} (d) Ni^{2+}

86. Which of the following compounds are optically active?

(1) H on top, H at bottom; upper carbon: F (left), I (right); lower carbon: F (left), I (right)
(2) H on top, H at bottom; upper carbon: I (left), F (right); lower carbon: F (left), I (right)
(3) H on top, H at bottom; upper carbon: F (left), I (right); lower carbon: I (left), F (right)
(4) H on top, H at bottom; upper carbon: I (left), F (right); lower carbon: I (left), F (right)

(a) 1 and 2 (b) 2 and 3
(c) 3 and 4 (d) 1 and 4

87. Which will not form precipitation after addition of $(NH_4)_2CO_3$ in presence of NH_4Cl?
(a) Mg (b) Ba (c) Sn (d) Sr

88. Difference in atomic radius is maximum for
(a) Rb-Cs (b) K-Rb
(c) Na-K (d) Li-Na

89. The dipole moment is minimum in
(a) NH_3 (b) NF_3 (c) SO_2 (d) BF_3

90. Number of isomers of C_5H_6
(a) 2 (b) 3 (c) 4 (d) 5

91. At 60° and 1 atm, N_2O_4 is 50% dissociated into NO_2 then K_p is
(a) 1.33 atm (b) 2 atm
(c) 2.67 atm (d) 3 atm

92. pK_a increases in benzoic acid when substituent "*x*" is bonded at *para*-position, then "*x*" is
(a) –COOH (b) $-NO_2$
(c) –CN (d) $-OCH_3$

93. $S_2O_8^{2-}$ have
(a) S–S bond (b) S–O bridge
(c) O–O bridge
(d) All S–O bond lengths are same.

94. N–N bond length is minimum in
(a) N_2O (b) N_2O_3
(c) N_2O_4 (d) N_2O_5

95. Which is correct example of condensation polymer?
(a) Nylon, Buna–S (b) Teflon, Buna–N
(c) Nylon 6,6, Dacron (d) Neoprene, Buna–S

96. But-1-ene $\xrightarrow[H_3O^+]{(CH_3COO)_2Hg}$?

The product in the above reaction is

(a) $CH_3CH_2CH_2CH_2OH$

(b) $CH_3CH_2\underset{\underset{OH}{|}}{CH}-CH_3$

(c) $CH_2=CH-\underset{\underset{OH}{|}}{CH}-CH_3$

(d) $CH_3-CH=\underset{\underset{OH}{|}}{C}-CH_3$

97. Nitrobenzene ($PhNO_2$) $\xrightarrow{Zn + NH_4Cl}$ P

P will be

(a) $C_6H_5NH_2$ (b) C_6H_5NHOH

(c) $C_6H_5-N=O$ (d) C_6H_6

98. Which is correct order of solubility in water?

(a) $Ba(OH)_2 < Mg(OH)_2$

(b) $BaCO_3 > CaCO_3$

(c) $CaSO_4 < MgSO_4$

(d) $Ca(OH)_2 \simeq Mg(OH)_2$

99. $PhCH_2Cl \xrightarrow{aq.\ NaCN} ? \xrightarrow{\text{Catalytic hydrogenation}} (U)$

The final product (U) is :

(a) $C_6H_5CH_2CH_2NH_2$

(b) $C_6H_5CH_2CONH_2$

(c) $C_6H_5CH_2NH_2$

(d) $C_6H_5CH_2NHCH_3$

100. An aromatic compound $C_7H_6Cl_2$ (A), gives AgCl on boiling with alcoholic $AgNO_2$ solution and yields C_7H_7OCl on treatment with sodium hydroxide. (A) on oxidation gives monochlorobenzoic acid. The compound (A) is:

(a) benzene ring with CH_2Cl and Cl (para)

(b) benzene ring with CH_2Cl, –Cl, –Cl and Cl

(c) benzene ring with CH_3, Cl and Cl

(d) benzene ring with $CHCl_2$

Directions : In the following questions (101-120), a statement of assertion (A) is followed by a statement of reason (R). Mark the correct choice as :

(a) If both assertion and reason are true and reason is the correct explanation of assertion

(b) If both assertion and reason are true but reason is not the correct explanation of assertion

(c) If assertion is true but reason is false

(d) If both assertion and reason are false.

101. Assertion : Rate of reaction doubles when concentration of reactant is doubled if it is a first order reaction.

Reason : Rate constant also doubles.

102. Assertion : Sodium acetate on Kolbe's electrolysis gives methane.

Reason : Methyl free radical is formed at cathode.

103. Assertion : H_3PO_2 has strong reducing property but H_3PO_4 does not.

Reason : P–OH bond present in H_3PO_4.

104. Assertion : Diamond and graphite do not have the same crystal structure.

Reason : Diamond is crystalline while graphite is amorphous.

105. Assertion : Bohr model fails in case of multi-electron species.

Reason : It does not mention electron-electron interactions.

106. Assertion : 1, 2-dichloroethane is optically active.

Reason : Meso compound is optically active.

107. Assertion : ClF_3 has T-shape structure.

Reason : It has two lone pairs arranged at 180° angle.

108. Assertion : O_2 is paramagnetic.

Reason : It has one unpaired electron.

109. Assertion : Phenol is more reactive than benzene towards electrophilic substitution reaction.

Reason : In the case of phenol, the intermediate carbocation is more resonance stabilised.

110. Assertion : H_2Se is less acidic than H_2S.

Reason : S is less electronegative than Se.

111. Assertion : Fluorine is a stronger oxidizing agent than iodine.

Reason : Fluorine has greater electronegativity than iodine.

112. Assertion : Ce^{4+} is used as an oxidising agent in volumetric analysis.

Reason : Ce^{4+} has the tendency of attaining + 3 oxidation state.

113. Assertion : The spectrum of He^+ is expected to be similar to that of hydrogen.

Reason : He^+ is also one electron system.

114. Assertion : Cl_2 gas bleaches the articles permanently.

Reason : Cl_2 is a strong reducing agent.

115. Assertion : $La(OH)_3$ is more basic than $Lu(OH)_3$.

Reason : Size of Lu^{3+} increases and shows more covalent character.

116. Assertion : F^- ion is a weak ligand and forms outer orbital complex.

Reason : F^- ion cannot force the electrons of d_{z^2} and $d_{x^2-y^2}$ orbitals of the inner shell to occupy d_{xy}, d_{yz} and d_{zx} orbitals of the same shell.

117. Assertion : $[Fe(H_2O)_5NO]SO_4$ is paramagnetic.

Reason : The Fe in $[Fe(H_2O)_5NO]SO_4$ has three unpaired electrons.

118. Assertion : The solubility of a gas in a liquid increases with increase of pressure.

Reason : The solubility of a gas in a liquid is directly proportional to the pressure of the gas.

119. Assertion : $HC\equiv C^-$ is more stable than $H_2C=CH^-$.

Reason : $HC\equiv C^-$ has more *s*-character than $H_2C=CH^-$.

120. Assertion : In a pressure cooker, the water is brought to boil. The cooker is then removed from the stove. Now on removing the lid of pressure cooker, the water starts boiling again.

Reason : The impurities in water bring down its boiling point.

BIOLOGY

121. Which of the following is correct regarding respiration in adult frog?
(a) In water- Skin, gills
(b) On land - Skin, buccal cavity
(c) In water- Skin, buccal cavity
(d) On land- Skin, lungs, gills.

122. Which of the following is correctly matched?
(a) *Monstera*- Fibrous root
(b) *Dahlia*- Fasciculated root
(c) *Azadirachta* - Adventitious root
(d) Basil- Prop roots

123. The 'cells of Rauber' are
(a) secretory cells of endometrium in uterus
(b) inner cell mass of blastocoel
(c) outer cells of trophoblast in contact with uterine wall
(d) cells of trophoblast, in contact with inner cell mass of blastocyst.

124.

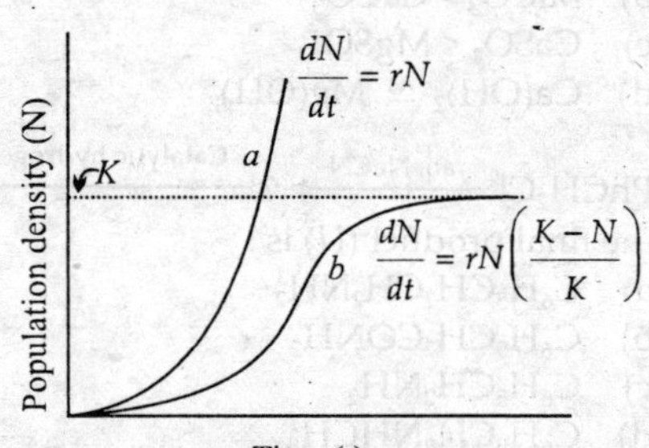

Which is correctly labelled with respect to the given diagram?
(a) B : Logistic curve
(b) C : Carrying capacity
(c) C : Exponential curve
(d) A : Carrying capacity

125. Deuteromycetes are known as fungi imperfecti because
(a) their zygote undergoes meroblastic and holoblastic cleavage
(b) only asexual stages are known
(c) they have aseptate mycelium
(d) they are autotrophic.

126. Abscisic acid is known as the stress hormone because it
(a) breaks seed dormancy
(b) induces flowering
(c) promotes leaf fall
(d) promotes closure of stomata.

127. Choose the correct statement.
(a) hPL plays a major role in parturition.
(b) Foetus shows movements first time in the 7th month of pregnancy.
(c) Signal for parturition comes from fully developed foetus and placenta.
(d) Embryo's heart is formed by the 2nd month of pregnancy.

128. One of the world's most poisonous fish toxins is released by
(a) clown fish (b) sword fish
(c) eel fish (d) puffer fish.

129. Na^+/K^+ pump is associated with
(a) passive transport (b) active transport
(c) osmosis (d) imbibition.

130. Which one has the largest species variety in India?
(a) Wheat (b) Maize
(c) Rice (d) Potato.

131. Photorespiration shows formation of
(a) sugar but not ATP
(b) ATP but not sugar
(c) both ATP and sugar
(d) neither ATP nor sugar.

132. The microscope usually used for seeing living cells or tissues is
(a) compound microscope
(b) electron micrscope
(c) phase contrast microscope
(d) light microscope.

133.

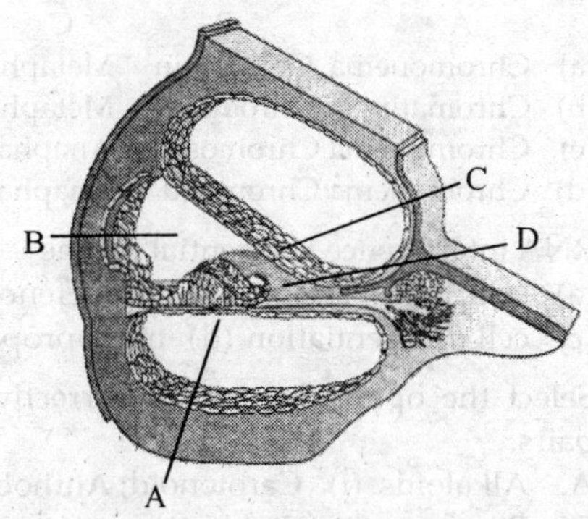

Which of the following is correctly labelled?
(a) A : Reissner's membrane
(b) B : Scala vestibuli
(c) C : Basilar membrane
(d) D : Tectorial membrane.

134. In aerobic respiration, total number of ATP molecules formed from 1 glucose molecule is
(a) 28 (b) 32
(c) 36 (d) 30.

135. Which of the following cartoon characters does not share its name with that of a gene?
(a) Tintin (b) Popeye
(c) Asterix (d) Obelix

136. Apiculture is associated with which of the following groups of plants?
(a) Grapes, maize, potato
(b) Sugarcane, paddy, banana
(c) Guava, sunflower, strawberry
(d) Pineapple, sugarcane, strawberry.

137.

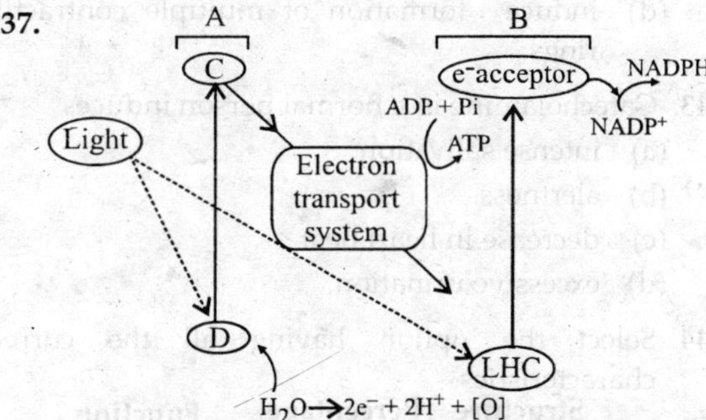

Which of the following is correctly labelled for the given figure?
(a) A : PS II ; B : PS I ; C : e^- acceptor; D: LHC
(b) A : LHC; B : e^- acceptor; C : PS I; D : PS II
(c) A : PS I ; B : PS II ; C : e^- acceptor; D : LHC
(d) A : e^-acceptor; B : LHC; C : PS II; D : PS I

138. During muscular contraction, which of the following events occur?
(i) H-zone disappears
(ii) A band widens
(iii) I band reduces in width
(iv) Width of A band is unaffected
(v) M line and Z line come closer.
(a) (i), (iii), (iv) and (v)
(b) (i), (ii) and (v)
(c) (ii), (iv) and (v)
(d) (i), (ii) and (iii).

139. The release of chemical messenger from synaptic vesicles is under the influence of these ion(s).
(a) Cl^- (b) Fe^{++} and S^{++}
(c) Ca^{++} (d) Mg^{++} and Sr^{++}

140. Cattle ranches are known to causes acute green house effect. This is due to
(a) mechanized milking practices
(b) methanogenic bacteria in rumen
(c) decomposition of left over fodder
(d) decomposition of organic remains in faeces.

141. Kranz anatomy is usually associated with
(a) C_3 plants
(b) C_4 plants
(c) CAM plants
(d) C_3-C_4 intermediate plants.

142. Microtubule depolymerizing drug such as colchicine is expected to
(a) inhibit spindle formation during mitosis
(b) inhibit cytokinesis
(c) allow mitosis beyond metaphase
(d) induce formation of multiple contractile rings.

143. Catecholamine in a normal person induces
(a) intense salivation
(b) alertness
(c) decrease in heart beat
(d) excessive urination.

144. Select the option having all the correct characteristics.

	Structure	Percentage	Function
(a)		0.3 – 0.5	Phagocytic
(b)		0.5 – 1.0	Secrete histamine and serotonin
(c)		30 – 40	Defence against parasites
(d)		30 – 40	Allergic reactions

145. Plants with inferior ovary usually bear
(a) pseudocarps (b) berries
(c) aggregate fruits (d) seedless fruits.

146. Oxygen binding to haemoglobin in blood is
(a) directly proportional to the concentration of CO_2 in the medium
(b) inversely proportional to the concentration of CO_2 in the medium
(c) directly proportional to the concentration of CO in the medium
(d) independent of the concentration of CO in the medium.

147. Leghaemoglobin is produced in response to
(a) respiration (b) photosynthesis
(c) fatty acid synthesis (d) N_2 fixation.

148. The extinct human ancestor, who ate only fruits and hunted with stone weapons was
(a) *Ramapithecus* (b) *Australopithecus*
(c) *Dryopithecus* (d) *Homo erectus.*

149. What is common between earthworm and *Periplaneta*?
(a) Both have red coloured blood
(b) Both possess anal styles
(c) Both have malpighian tubules
(d) Both have segmented body.

150. In a normal adult, ascending order of concentration of following molecules is
(a) K > Na > Fe > Cu (b) Na > K > Cu > Fe
(c) Fe > Na > K > Cu (d) Na > Fe > K > Cu

151. Which of the following statements is incorrect about G_0 phase?
(a) Mitosis occurs after G_0 phase.
(b) Biocatalysts can be used to exit G_0 phase.
(c) Cell volume keeps on increasing during this phase.
(d) Cell metabolism occurs continuously in G_0 phase.

152. Beads on string like structures of *A* are seen in *B*, which further condense to form chromosomes in *C* stage of cell division.

	A	B	C
(a)	Chromonema	Chromatin	Metaphase
(b)	Chromatin	Chromatid	Metaphase
(c)	Chromonema	Chromosome	Anaphase
(d)	Chromonema	Chromatid	Anaphase.

153. RNA interference is essential for the
(a) cell proliferation (b) cell defence
(c) cell differentiation (d) micropropagation.

154. Select the option having all correctly matched pairs.
A. Alkaloids (i) Carotenoid; Anthocyanin
B. Pigments (ii) Vinblastin; curcumin
C. Drugs (iii) Morphine; Codeine
(a) A-i; B-ii; C-iii (b) A-ii; B-iii; C-i
(c) A-iii; B-i; C-ii (d) A-i; B-iii; C-ii.

155. Dust, oolong and brick are varieties of
(a) coffee (b) pepper
(c) tea (d) lavang.

156. Ventricular diastole occurs due to a/an
(a) organ system (b) cell organelle
(c) tissue (d) organ.

157.

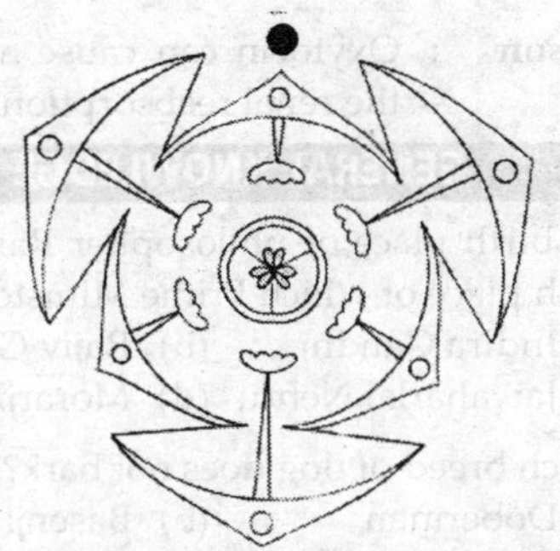

Plants having the above given floral diagram are
(a) leguminous
(b) dicots
(c) medicinal and perennial
(d) having pinnately compound leaves.

158. Select the correct statement.
(a) Particulate matter of size 10 μm can create severe damage to the lungs.
(b) Particulate matter of size greater than 2.5 μm can get trapped in lungs and cause problems.
(c) Particulate matter of size less than 2.5 μm penetrate deep into lungs.
(d) None of the above.

159. Pebrine in silkworms is caused by
(a) *Dugesia* (b) *Monocystis*
(c) *Nosema* (d) *Plasmodium.*

160. Which of the following is a homopolysaccharide?
(a) Heparin (b) Inulin
(c) Pectin (d) Hyaluronic acid.

Direction : In the following questions (161-180), a statement of assertion (A) is followed by a statement of reason (R). Mark the correct choice as :
(a) If both assertion and reason are true and reason is the correct explanation of assertion
(b) If both assertion and reason are true but reason is not the correct explanation of assertion
(c) If assertion is true but reason is false
(d) If both assertion and reason are false.

161. **Assertion :** There are 34 biodiversity hotspots in the world.
Reason : High level of species richness is a criteria for selection of a biodiversity hotspot.

162. **Assertion :** Inbreeding increases homozygosity, thus exposes harmful recessive genes, which are eliminated by selection.
Reason : Continued inbreeding reduces fertility and productivity.

163. **Assertion :** Some marine animals find it difficult to live in fresh water and *vice versa.*
Reason : Some animals can tolerate a narrow salinity range, while others can tolerate a wide salinity range.

164. **Assertion :** Mylein sheath insulates the nerve fibre and prevents its depolarisation.
Reason : Nerve impulses are conducted more rapidly in non - myelinated nerve fibres than in myelinated ones.

165. **Assertion :** Frog can change its colour, according to its surroundings.
Reason : It is a way of mimicry to capture preys.

166. **Assertion :** Less iodine intake causes goitre.
Reason : Less iodine in body decreases thyroxine secretion.

167. **Assertion :** Hb^s Hb^s denotes the homozygous condition for sickle-cell anaemia.
Reason : It occurs due to substitution of glutamic acid by valine at the 6th position of β-chain of Hb.

168. **Assertion :** Excess Mn in soil, can adversely decrease Mg, Fe and Cu concentrations in the soil.
Reason : Mn increases rate of photosynthesis, thereby increasing absorption of Mg, Fe and Ca from soil.

169. **Assertion :** A middle aged woman is reported to have small breasts and undersized uterus.
Reason : Her genotypic analysis shows XO condition of allosomes.

170. Assertion : In proximal convoluted tubule glomerular filtrate becomes hypertonic to blood plasma.

Reason : HCO_3^- is absorbed only in the proximal convoluted tubule.

171. Assertion : Complexity of classification increases from kingdom to species.

Reason : Common characters increase from kingdom to species.

172. Assertion : In a terrestrial ecosystem, detritus food chain is the major conduit for energy flow.

Reason : Solar energy is the direct source for energy supply in a detritus food chain.

173. Assertion : Filarial worm is transmitted to humans by *Culex* mosquito.

Reason : *Culex* prefers to breed in fresh water.

174. Assertion : AIDS is caused by the HIV, a retro-virus.

Reason : Retroviruses have RNA genome.

175. Assertion : A male is found to be lacking facial hair and pubic hair.

Reason : It is a case of hyposecretion of testosterone from Leydig's cells of testes.

176. Assertion : Extra oxygen consumption in human body is known as oxygen debt.

Reason : The extra oxygen is required by the body to oxidise the accumulated lactic acid produced during strenuous exercise.

177. Assertion : Emulsification is necessary for the digestion of fats.

Reason : After fats are emulsified, the action of enzyme amylase gets significantly increased.

178. Assertion : In jaundice, the skin and mucous membranes assume a yellowish hue.

Reason : Yellow pigment bilirubin imparts pale yellow colour to blood plasma.

179. Assertion : No taste sensation is evoked when drop of distilled water is put on human tongue.

Reason : Man does not possess taste buds for tasting water.

180. Assertion : Oxytocin is also known as Anti-diuretic hormone (ADH).

Reason : Oxytocin can cause an increase in the renal reabsorption of water.

GENERAL KNOWLEDGE

181. The birth place of philosopher Ramanuja is the death place of which Prime Minister?
(a) Indira Gandhi (b) Rajiv Gandhi
(c) Jawaharlal Nehru (d) Morarji Desai.

182. Which breed of dog does not bark?
(a) Doberman (b) Basenji
(c) German Shepherd
(d) Dalmatian.

183. Which author of Indian origin was born in the Caribbean Nation of Trinidad and Tobago?
(a) Salman Rushdie (b) V.S. Naipaul
(c) Shashi Tharoor (d) Nirad C. Chaudhuri.

184. Tezpur in north-east is famous for
(a) hottest chilli in the world
(b) sweetest apple
(c) largest producer of gold
(d) largest producer of coal

185. Belt and Jacket, Catch-hold and loose styles are the basic types of which sport?
(a) Boxing (b) Wrestling
(c) Kho-Kho (d) Kabaddi.

186. Kashmiri stag is also known as
(a) Hangul (b) Nilgai
(c) Sambhar (d) Chital.

187. Who was the first Indian Prime Minister to lose an election?
(a) Lal Bahadur Shastri
(b) V.P. Singh
(c) Morarji Desai (d) Indira Gandhi.

188. The city of Mysore has derived its name from the sanskrit word, for which of these?
(a) Beautiful town (b) Buffalo town
(c) Great town (d) Golden town.

189. Which of the following persons founded Indian National Orchestra?

(a) Zubin Mehta (b) Shankar Mahadevan
(c) A.R. Rehman (d) Ravi Shankar.

190. Which is the second highest civilian award in India?
(a) Bharat Ratna (b) Padma Vibhushan
(c) Padma Bhushan (d) Padma Shri.

191. Surface of which gemstone is called orient?
(a) Emerald (b) Emethyst
(c) Pearl (d) Diamond.

192. Which of the following states is the highest producer of soyabean in India?
(a) Uttar Pradesh (b) Andhra Pradesh
(c) Rajasthan (d) Madhya Pradesh.

193. Who captained India in woman cricket world cup 2000?
(a) Anju Jain (b) Neetu David
(c) Shantha Rangaswami
(d) Poornima Rao.

194. Which Union Territory has its name of the basis of a temple in the village Manimajra?
(a) Chandigarh (b) Lakshdweep
(c) Pondicherry (d) Daman and Diu.

195. In tricolour flag of India, saffron colour is a symbol of
(a) unity (b) sacrifice
(c) peace (d) prosperity.

196. Which of the following languages is not based on Devanagari script?
(a) Hindi (b) Sanskrit
(c) Nepali (d) Urdu.

197. Which one of the following is a military alliance?
(a) ASEAN (b) SAARC
(c) NATO (d) NAFTA.

198. 'Fanning and Dust', these terms are associated with
(a) tea (b) coffee
(c) soup (d) cold drink.

199. Which one of the following footballers is awarded Arjuna Award 2011?
(a) Sunil Chhetri (b) Baichung Bhutia
(c) Bruno Coutinho (d) I.M. Vijayan.

200. 'Cix's Bazar' is situated in
(a) Pakistan (b) Sri Lanka
(c) Bangladesh (d) Indonesia.

SOLUTIONS

PHYSICS

1. **(b)** : In an unbiased *PN* junction diode current flow due to minority charge carriers (electron in the *P*-region and holes in the *N*-region).

2. **(c)** : If $\frac{dI}{dt}$ is the rate of change of current through inductor *L* of any instant, then induced emf in the inductor of the same instant is

$$= \left(-\frac{L\,dI}{dt}\right)$$

To maintain the flow of current in the circuit applied voltage must be equal and opposite to the induced voltage.

$$\therefore \quad V = -\left(-L\frac{dI}{dt}\right)$$

Given, $V = V_0 \sin\omega t$ ...(i)

$$\therefore \quad V_0 \sin\omega t = \frac{L\,dI}{dt}$$

$$\frac{dI}{dt} = \frac{V_0}{L}\sin\omega t$$

$$\text{or } I = \frac{-V_0}{L}\frac{\cos\omega t}{\omega} \qquad \text{...(ii)}$$

Instantaneous power,

$$\because \quad P = VI$$

$$= (V_0 \sin\omega t)\left(-\frac{V_0\cos\omega t}{L\omega}\right) \quad \text{(Using (i) \& (ii))}$$

$$= \frac{-V_0^2 \sin 2\omega t}{2L\,\omega}$$

3. **(c)** : The resultant intensity is given by

$$I_R = I_1 + I_2 + 2\sqrt{I_1 I_2}\,\cos\phi$$

For constructive interference, $\cos\phi = 1$

$$\therefore \quad I_R = I_1 + I_2 + 2\sqrt{I_1 I_2}$$

or $I_R = 4I$ (Given $I_1 = I_2 = I$)

4. **(b)** : Let *L* is the distance between a real object and its real image formed by a convex lens, then as

$$L = (|u| + |v|)$$

$$= (\sqrt{u} - \sqrt{v})^2 + 2\sqrt{uv} \qquad \text{...(i)}$$

L will be minimum, when

$$(\sqrt{u} - \sqrt{v})^2 = 0$$

i.e., $u = v$

Putting, $u = -u$ and $v = +u$ in lens formula,

$$\frac{1}{v} - \frac{1}{u} = \frac{1}{F}$$

$$\frac{1}{u} - \frac{1}{-u} = \frac{1}{F}$$

$$u = 2F$$

$$\therefore \quad (L)_{min} = 2\sqrt{2F \times 2F} = 4F \qquad \text{(Using (i))}$$

5. **(a)** : The fringe width is given by

$$\beta = \frac{\lambda D}{d}$$

Here *D* is the separation between screen and slits and *d* is the separation between slits.

6. **(c)** : Here, $T_{1/2} = 8$ years

$t = 32$ years

$$\text{Using, } N = N_0\left(\frac{1}{2}\right)^{\frac{t}{T_{1/2}}}$$

$$\left(\frac{N}{N_0}\right) = \left(\frac{1}{2}\right)^{\frac{32}{8}}$$

$$= \left(\frac{1}{2}\right)^4$$

$$\left(\frac{N}{N_0}\right) = \frac{1}{16}$$

7. **(c)** : In the circuit, the zener diode is used as power regular therefore,

$$P = VI$$

$$= 12 \times 0.05 = 0.6 \text{ W.}$$

8. **(c)** : The relation between kinetic energy, threshold frequency and frequency of photon is given as

$$\frac{1}{2}mv^2 = (h\upsilon - h\upsilon_0)$$

$$= h\,(1 \times 10^{14} - 5 \times 10^{13})$$

$$k = h\,(5 \times 10^{13})$$

$$= 6.67 \times 10^{-34} \times 5 \times 10^{13}$$

$$= 3.3 \times 10^{-20} \text{ J.}$$

9. **(a)** : The phase angle

$$\theta = \tan^{-1}\left(\frac{X_C - X_L}{R}\right)$$

$= \tan^{-1}\left(\frac{8-5}{4}\right)$

$\theta = \tan^{-1}\left(\frac{3}{4}\right)$

Therefore, the current leads the voltage by $\tan^{-1}\left(\frac{3}{4}\right)$.

10. **(a) :** Here, $m = 100$ g $= 10^{-1}$ kg, $l = 1$ m, $I = 5$ A
For a wire balanced midway air by a magnetic field is
$mg = IlB$.

or $B = \frac{mg}{Il}$

$= \frac{10^{-1} \times 10}{5 \times 1}$

$B = 0.2$ T.

11. **(a) :** Heat supplied to a system is in the form of energy.
∴ Dimensional formula is = $[M L^2 T^{-2}]$.

12. **(d) :** The magnetic field at any point inside the toroid is zero.

13. **(d)**

14. **(a)**

15. **(b) :** Magnetic dipole moment of electron in an atom is given as

$M = \frac{n\,eh}{4\pi m} = n\mu_B$

where, n = number of orbit
μ_B = Bohr Magneton
For minimum dipole moment, $n = 1$

∴ $M = \frac{eh}{4\pi m}$

16. **(a)**

17. **(a) :** Total energy of an electron in hydrogen atom above 0 eV leads to continuation of energy states.

18. **(c) :** Two parallel current carrying wires in the same direction attract each other whereas two parallel current carrying wires in the opposite direction repel each other.

19. **(b) :** Let a particle of mass m is thrown vertically upwards with velocity v. Let its velocity be v' at a height $3R$ from the surface of the earth.
According to the conservation of energy,

$$\frac{1}{2}mv^2 - \frac{GMm}{R} = \frac{1}{2}mv'^2 - \frac{GMm}{(R+3R)}$$

$$v^2 - \frac{2GM}{R} = v'^2 - \frac{2GM}{4R}$$

$$v^2 - v'^2 = \frac{-2GM}{4R} + \frac{2GM}{R} = \frac{6}{4}\frac{GM}{R}$$

$$v'^2 = v^2 - \frac{6}{4}\frac{GM}{R}$$

$$v'^2 = \sqrt{(11.2)^2 - \frac{3}{2}gR} \quad \left(\because g = \frac{GM}{R^2}\right)$$

$$= \sqrt{(11.2)^2 - \frac{3}{2} \times \frac{9.8 \times 6400}{1000}}$$

$$= \sqrt{(11.2)^2 - (94.08)}$$

$= 5.6$ km s^{-1}

20. **(d) :** The Gamma decay due to instability of nucleus is excess energy of nucleus.

21. **(c) :** de broglie wavelength,

$\lambda = \frac{h}{\sqrt{2mk}}$

or $k = \frac{h^2}{2m\lambda^2}$

$= \frac{(6.67 \times 10^{-34})^2}{2 \times 9.1 \times 10^{-31} \times (1 \times 10^{-9})^2} = 1.5$ eV.

22. **(c) :** Terminal velocity
$V_t \propto D^2$.

23. **(a) :** Electric field due to a long charged wire is given as

$E = \frac{\lambda}{2\pi \epsilon_0 r}$

where, λ = linear charge density.
r = distance from the wire.

∴ $E \propto \frac{1}{r}$

24. **(a) :** Mass $(m) = 2$ kg; initial radius of the path $(r_1) = 0.8$ m; initial angular velocity $(\omega_1) = 44$ rad/sec and final radius of the path $(r_2) = 1$ m.
Moment of inertia, $I_1 = mr_1^2 = 2 \times (0.8)^2$ $= 1.28$ kg m^2 and $I_2 = mr_2^2 = 2 \times (1)^2 = 2$ kg m^2
Therefore from the law of conservation of angular momentum $I_1\omega_1 = I_2\omega_2$

or $\omega_2 = \frac{I_1 \times \omega_1}{I_2} = \frac{1.28 \times 44}{2}$

$\omega_2 = 28.16$ rad/sec

25. (b)

26. (a) : Since, $\vec{v} = v_0 \hat{i}$

$$\vec{E} = E_0 \hat{j}$$

The electron is moving in x-direction perpendicular to the electric field which is in y-direction.

Thus, the path of electron moving perpendicular to field will be a parabola.

27. (b) : Effective acceleration due to gravity due to rotation earth is given as

$$g' = g - R\omega^2\cos^2\phi$$

$\therefore$ Change in acceleration, $dg = R\omega^2\cos^2\phi$

$\therefore$ $dg \propto \cos^2\phi$

28. (c) : Let t be the width and L be the length of each conductor.

Effective thermal resistance, $R_p = \dfrac{R_1R_2}{R_1+R_2}$

$\because$ $R = \dfrac{L}{KA}$

where k = thermal conductivity

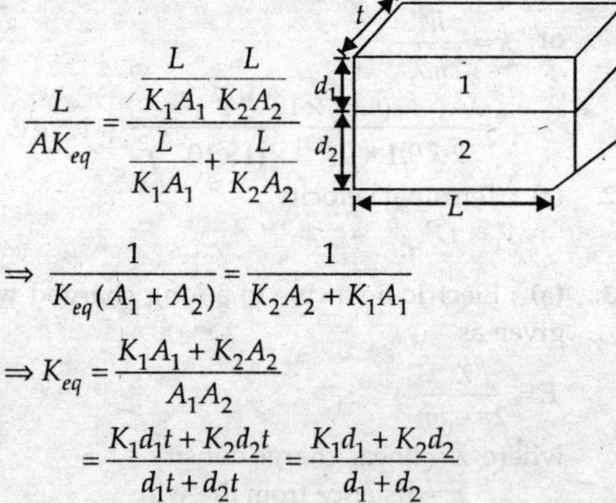

$$\frac{L}{AK_{eq}} = \frac{\frac{L}{K_1A_1}\frac{L}{K_2A_2}}{\frac{L}{K_1A_1}+\frac{L}{K_2A_2}}$$

$$\Rightarrow \frac{1}{K_{eq}(A_1+A_2)} = \frac{1}{K_2A_2+K_1A_1}$$

$$\Rightarrow K_{eq} = \frac{K_1A_1+K_2A_2}{A_1A_2}$$

$$= \frac{K_1d_1t+K_2d_2t}{d_1t+d_2t} = \frac{K_1d_1+K_2d_2}{d_1+d_2}$$

29. (a) : It is a balanced Wheatstone bridge. Hence no current flows through resistance of arm BD and the resistance of arm BD is ineffective.

$$\therefore \frac{R_{AB}}{R_{BC}} = \frac{R_{AD}}{R_{DC}}$$

$$\Rightarrow \frac{5\,\Omega}{5\,\Omega} = \frac{5\,\Omega}{5\,\Omega}$$

Resistance of arm $ABC = 5\,\Omega + 5\,\Omega = 10\,\Omega$

Resistance of arm $ADC = 5\,\Omega + 5\,\Omega = 10\,\Omega$

The effective resistance between A and C is

$$\frac{1}{R_{AC}} = \frac{1}{10} + \frac{1}{10} \text{ or } R_{AC} = 5\,\Omega$$

Now the equivalent circuit becomes

$\therefore$ The equivalent resistance of the circuit

$$\frac{1}{R} = \frac{1}{5} + \frac{1}{5} \text{ or } R = 2.5\,\Omega$$

Current in the circuit,

$$I = \frac{V}{R} = \frac{25}{2.5} = 10\text{ A}$$

30. (c) : Let the inclination of the inclined plane be θ. Acceleration of a rolling body is given as

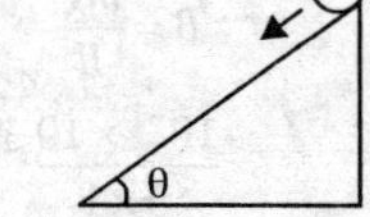

$$a = \frac{g\sin\theta}{(1+K^2/R^2)}$$

Here, K is radius of gyration.

For circular disc

$$I = \frac{1}{2}MR^2 \therefore \frac{K^2}{R^2} = \frac{1}{2}$$

$$\therefore a = \frac{2}{3}g\sin\theta \quad \text{...(i)}$$

For solid cylinder

$$I = \frac{1}{2}MR^2 \therefore \frac{K^2}{R^2} = \frac{1}{2}$$

$$\therefore a = \frac{2}{3}g\sin\theta \quad \text{...(ii)}$$

For solid sphere

$$I = \frac{2}{5}MR^2 \therefore \frac{K^2}{R^2} = \frac{2}{5}$$

$$\therefore a = \frac{5}{7}g\sin\theta \quad \text{...(iii)}$$

For hollow cylinder

$$I = MR^2 \therefore \frac{K^2}{R^2} = 1$$

$$\therefore a = \frac{1}{2}g\sin\theta \quad \text{...(iv)}$$

Hence, from (i), (ii), (iii) and (iv) we conclude that the solid sphere will reach the bottom with maximum acceleration.

31. (d) : Here, $P = 100$ W, $t = 10$ min $= 60$ s

Heat developed in time t

$$H = P \times t = (100\text{ W})(60\text{ s}) = 6000\text{ J}$$

32. (c) : A polyatomic gas has 3 translational. 3 rotational degrees of freedom and a certain number (f) of vibrational modes. Hence, the degree of freedom for polyatomic gas is ≥ 6.

33. (b)

34. (b)

35. (b) :

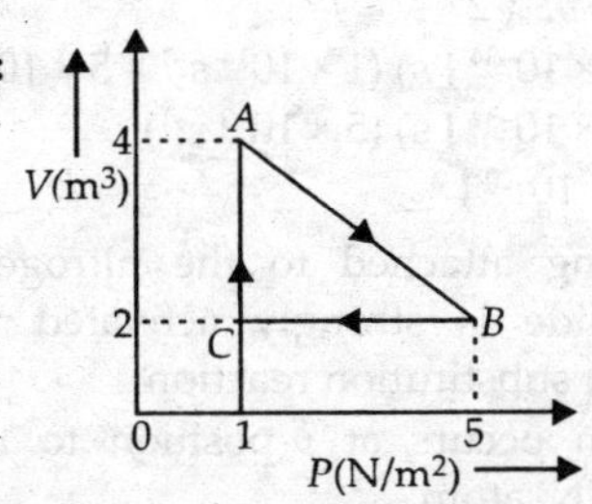

Process $B \to C$ occurs at constant volume

Hence, $W_{BC} = 0$

Process $C \to A$ occurs at constant process.

Hence the work done in the process is

$W_{CA} = P\Delta V = (1)(V_A - V_C) = (1)(4-2) = 2\text{ J}$

For a cyclic process, $\Delta U = 0$

According to the first law of thermodynamics

$$\Delta Q = \Delta W + \Delta U$$
$$\Delta Q = \Delta W$$
$$= W_{AB} + W_{BC} + W_{CA}$$
$$5 = W_{AB} + 0 + 2 \text{ or } W_{AB} = 3\text{ J}$$

36. (b) : For an isothermal process, the slope is $-\dfrac{P}{V}$.

37. (a) : The frequency order for given electromagnetic waves is as follows.

$\upsilon_{\gamma\text{-rays}} > \upsilon_{\text{X-Rays}} > \upsilon_{\text{UV}}$

$B > A > C$

38. (a) : Here, $I_B = 5\ \mu\text{A} = 5 \times 10^{-6}\text{ A}$

$\beta = 100$

$R_L = 10\text{ k}\Omega = 10 \times 10^3\ \Omega$

As $\beta = \dfrac{I_C}{I_B}$

or $I_C = (100)(5 \times 10^{-6}\text{ A}) = 5 \times 10^{-4}\text{ A}$

The voltage across collector emitter is

$V_{CE} = R_L I_C = (10 \times 10^3\ \Omega)(5 \times 10^{-4}\text{ A}) = 5\text{ V}$

39. (b) : After a long time the capacitor has become fully charged, the entire battery voltage 60 V appears across the capacitor.

40. (d) : Emission of α-particle decreases the mass number and the atomic number by 4 and 2 respectively. Emission of β-particle increases the atomic number by 1 while the mass number remains unchanged.

After the emission of the one α-particle and two β-particles

Decreases in mass number = 4 – 0 = 4

Decreases in atomic number = 2 – 2 = 0

$\therefore$ The resulting the nucleus is ${}^{m-4}_{n}X$.

i.e. the isotope of the given nucleus.

41. (a) : Maximum air flow due to convection does not occur at the north pole but it occurs at 30° N pole because there is a maximum temperature difference between equator and 30°N at poles.

42. (c) : Lenses have different refractive index for different wavelengths of light. The refractive index decreases with increasing wavelength. So red light will bend least and violet the most. This will result is slight dispersion which will be seen as chromatic aberration.

43. (d) : If a material is in contact with another material, the surface energy depends on the interaction of molecules of the materials. If the molecules of the materials attract each other, surface energy is reduced and when they repel each other, the surface energy is increased. Thus the surface energy depends on both the materials, so both the assertion and reason are false.

44. (b)

45. (a) : Animate object do not obey Newton's second law, so it can accelerate in the absence of external force.

46. (a) : Magnetic field due to a circular loop carrying current I is given as

$$B = \frac{\mu_0}{4\pi}\frac{2\pi I r^2}{(r^2 + x^2)^{3/2}}$$

where, r = radius of loop

x = distance from centre of loop

For large distances, $(x >> r)$,

$$\therefore\ B = \frac{\mu_0}{4\pi}\frac{2IA}{x^3} = \frac{\mu_0}{4\pi}\frac{2M}{x^3}$$

where $M = IA$ = magnetic dipole moment of current loop which is equal to the magnetic field due to magnetic dipole.

Thus, the current loop can be considered as a magnetic dipole.

47. (b)

48. (b)

49. (b) : In telescope to have a large magnifying power, focal length of objective lens is kept large. To increase the magnifying power and resolving power, aperture of the objective lens is made large.

50. **(a) :** We know that $E = -\frac{13.6}{n^2}$ eV

It shows that total energy of electron in a stationary orbit in a hydrogen atom is negative, which means the electron is bound to the nuclear and is not free to leave it.

51. **(c) :** According to law of equipartition of energy, in thermal equilibrium, at temperature T, each degree of freedom of translational, rotational and vibrational motion contributes an average energy equal to $\frac{1}{2}k_BT$. The vibrational motion has two types of energy associated with the vibrations along the length of the molecule-kinetic energy and potential energy. Thus, it contributes two degrees of freedom. Thus vibrational energy

$= 2 \times \frac{1}{2}k_BT = k_BT.$

52. **(b) :** Superconductor is both a perfect diamagnetic substance as well as a perfect conductor.

53. **(b) :** Electrostatic field is a conservative field which means work done by an electrostatic field in moving a charge from one point to another depends only on the initial and the final positions and is independent at the path taken to go from one point to the another.

54. **(a) :** Cyclotron is used to accelerate charged particles to high energies. It uses both electric and magnetic fields together to increase the energy of the charged particle.

55. **(a)**

56. **(b) :** Electromagnetic waves are those waves in which there are sinusoidal variation of electric and magnetic field vectors at right angles to each other as well as at right angles to the direction of wave propagation. They are self-sustaining oscillations of electric and magnetic fields in free space or vacuum.

57. **(b) :** Gauss's theorem is based on inverse square dependence of electric field on distance.

58. **(b)**

59. **(a)**

60. **(b)**

CHEMISTRY

61. **(b) :** Following the conservation of energy principle,

Kinetic energy $\left(\frac{1}{2}m_e v^2\right) = h(\upsilon - \upsilon_0)$

$= (6.626 \times 10^{-34}\text{ J s})(1 \times 10^{14}\text{ s}^{-1} - 5 \times 10^{13}\text{ s}^{-1})$

$= (6.626 \times 10^{-34}\text{ J s})(5 \times 10^{13}\text{ s}^{-1})$

$= 3.313 \times 10^{-20}$ J

62. **(b) :** The ring attached to the nitrogen atom in benzanilide is strongly activated towards electrophilic substitution reaction.

$\therefore$ Nitration occurs at *p*-position to the ring attached to 'N' atom.

C_6H_5–CO–NH–C_6H_5 $\xrightarrow[H_2SO_4]{HNO_3}$ C_6H_5–CO–NH–C_6H_4–NO_2

63. **(b) :**

(cyclic structure: three P atoms linked by O bridges; each P bears =O and –OH)

$(HPO_3)_3$

64. **(a)**

65. **(d)**

$C_6H_4(COOH)_2$ (Phthalic acid) $\xrightarrow{NH_3}$ $C_6H_4(COONH_4)_2$ $\xrightarrow{\text{Weakly heated}}$ $C_6H_4(CONH_2)_2$ $\xrightarrow[573\text{ K}]{\Delta\text{ strongly,}}$ $C_6H_4(CO)_2NH$

66. **(a) :** *bcc* has eight atoms at corners and each is shared by 8 unit cells so that the contribution of each atom at corner is $\frac{1}{8}$.

67. **(c) :** Greater are the intermolecular forces of attraction, higher is the critical temperature.

68. **(c) :** Dissociation energy of methane = 360 kJ mol^{-1}

$\therefore$ Bond energy of C — H bond $= \frac{360}{4} = 90$ kJ

Bond energy of ethane,

1(C — C) + 6 (C — H) = 620 kJ/mol

(C — C) + 6 × 90 = 620

(C — C) + 540 = 620

C — C = 620 – 540

C — C = 80 kJ mol^{-1}.

Bond dissociation of C — C bond = 80 kJ mol^{-1}.

69. **(c) :** Silicon is hydrophobic.

70. **(d) :** $mvr = \frac{nh}{2\pi}$

71. **(d) :** Copper (I) compounds are unstable in aqueous solution and undergo disproportionation.

$2Cu^+ \rightarrow Cu^{2+} + Cu$

The greater stability of $Cu^{2+}_{(aq.)}$ than $Cu^+_{(aq.)}$ is due to much more *–ve* $\Delta_{hyd}H$ of $Cu^{2+}_{(aq.)}$ than $Cu^+_{(aq.)}$, which more than compensates for the second ionisation enthalpy of Cu.

72. **(a) :** Rate $= \frac{\text{concentration}}{\text{time}} = \frac{\text{mol L}^{-1}}{\text{s}}$

$= \text{mol L}^{-1}\text{ s}^{-1}$

The units of rate constant for the reaction of the order = $(\text{mol L}^{-1})^{1-n}\text{ s}^{-1}$

here, $n = \frac{3}{2}$

$\therefore$ Unit of rate constant $= (\text{mol L}^{-1})^{1-3/2}\text{ s}^{-1}$

$= (\text{mol L}^{-1})^{-1/2}\text{ s}^{-1}$

$= \text{mol}^{-1/2}\text{ L}^{1/2}\text{ s}^{-1}$

73. **(b) :** Nitrogen is more electronegative and smaller in size than phosphorus. Therefore, the lone pair is concentrated on a small region and has maximum electron density. So, NH_3 is more basic than PH_3.

74. **(b) :** Silicon belongs to group 14, it is doped with a group 13 element like B which contains only three valence electrons. The place where the fourth valence e^- is missing is called electron hole. Under the electric field, e^- holes moves toward the negatively charged plate, which implies that e^- holes are positively charged, thus it is a *p*-type semiconductor.

75. **(b) :** NH_4Cl solution is acidic, its pH < 7. $NaNO_3$ solution is neutral, its pH = 7. CH_3COOK and Na_2CO_3 solutions are basic their pH > 7. But Na_2CO_3 solution is more basic, its pH > pH of CH_3COOK solution.

76. **(c) :** Carbon monoxide combines with haemoglobin of blood to form a complex called carboxy-haemoglobin. Formation of this complex makes the haemoglobin incapable of oxygen transport. Due to which there will be oxygen deficiency in the blood.

77. **(a) :**

$CH_3COOH \xrightarrow{SOCl_2} CH_3COCl$ (*P*) $\xrightarrow[\text{Anhyd. AlCl}_3]{\text{Benzene}}$ $C_6H_5COCH_3$ (*Q*) $\xrightarrow{HCN}$ $C_6H_5C(OH)(CH_3)CN$ (*R*) $\xrightarrow{HOH}$ $C_6H_5C(OH)(CH_3)COOH$ (*S*)

78. **(d) :** Chiral compound contains one or more 'chiral' carbon atom(s). Chiral carbon atoms are usually bonded to four different atoms or group of atoms.

$CH_3 - CH_2 - CH_2 - CH_2 - CH_2 - CH_3$ (Hexane) (Achiral)

$CH_3 - CH_2 - CH_2 - CH_3$ (*n*-Butane) (Achiral)

CH_4 (Methane) (Achiral)

$CH_3 - CH(CH_3) - C^*H(CH_3) - C^*H(CH_3) - CH_2 - CH_3$

(Chiral)

(2, 3, 4-Trimethylhexane.)

79. **(b) :** $E^\circ_{cell} = E^\circ_{right} - E^\circ_{left}$

$E^\circ_{cell} = 0 - (0 - 0.76) = 0.76$ V

80. **(c)** : $\Delta_{n_g} = n_p - n_r = 1 - \frac{3}{2}$

$\Delta_{n_g} = \frac{-1}{2}$. Hence $K_p = K_c(RT)^{-1/2}$

$\frac{K_p}{K_c} = \frac{1}{(RT)^{1/2}} = \frac{1}{\sqrt{RT}}$

81. **(d)** : For a nth order reaction,

$t_{1/2} \propto \frac{1}{[a]^{n-1}}$

where n = order of reaction

$t_{1/2} \propto \frac{1}{[a]^{3-1}}$ $[\because n = 3]$

$t_{1/2} \propto \frac{1}{[a]^2}$

82. **(c)** : In the body-centred cubic unit cell,

$a\sqrt{3} = 4r$

$r = \frac{a\sqrt{3}}{4} = \frac{400\sqrt{3}}{4} = 100\sqrt{3}$ pm

83. **(a)**

84. **(a)** : In acidic solution, manganese (VI) becomes unstable and undergo disproportionation to form manganese (VII) and manganese (IV)

$5\overset{VI}{Mn}O_3 + 2H^+ \longrightarrow 3\overset{IV}{Mn}O_2 + 2\overset{VII}{Mn}O_4^- + H_2O$

85. **(a)** : $Cr^{2+} = 3d^4$, No. of unpaired electrons $(n) = 4$

Magnetic moment $= \sqrt{n(n+2)}$ BM

$= \sqrt{4(4+2)} = \sqrt{24} = 4.89$ BM

$Fe^{2+} = 3d^6$, No. of unpaired electrons $(n) = 4$

Magnetic moment $= \sqrt{4(4+2)}$ BM

$= \sqrt{24} = 4.89$ BM

$Mn^{2+} = 3d^5$, No. of unpaired electrons $(n) = 5$

Magnetic moment $= \sqrt{5(5+2)}$ BM

$= \sqrt{35} = 5.91$ BM

$Co^{2+} = 3d^7$, No. of unpaired electrons $(n) = 3$

Magnetic moment $= \sqrt{3(3+2)}$ BM

$= \sqrt{15} = 3.87$ BM

$Ni^{2+} = 3d^8$, No. of unpaired electrons $(n) = 2$

Magnetic moment $= \sqrt{2(2+2)}$ BM

$= \sqrt{8} = 2.82$ BM

86. **(b)** : (1) and (4) compounds are *meso*-compounds, they possesses a plane of symmetry and is consequently optically inactive and superimposes on its mirror image (*i.e.*, they are identical).

87. **(c)**

88. **(c)** : The difference in atomic radius is maximum between Na and K.

89. **(d)** : BF_3 has zero dipole moment.

90. **(b)** : Isomers of C_5H_6 :

; CH_3 ; $CH=CH_2$

91. **(b)**: $N_2O_4 \rightleftharpoons 2NO_2$

	N_2O_4	$2NO_2$
Initially	1	0
At equilibrium	$1-\alpha$	2α

N_2O_4 is 50% dissociated, so $\alpha = \frac{1}{2}$

$$K_p = \frac{p^2_{NO_2}}{p_{N_2O_4}} = \frac{\left(2\times\frac{1}{2}\right)^2}{\left(1-\frac{1}{2}\right)} = 2 \text{ atm}$$

92. **(d)** : Larger the value of pK_a, smaller will be its acidity. Out of the four groups, –COOH, $-NO_2$ and –CN are e^- withdrawing which makes benzoic acid more acidic whereas $-OCH_3$ is e^- donating which reduces the acidity (makes H^+ less easily available). pK_a value increases if $-OCH_3$ is present at *para*-position of benzoic acid.

93. **(c)** : The structure of peroxodisulfate anion is:

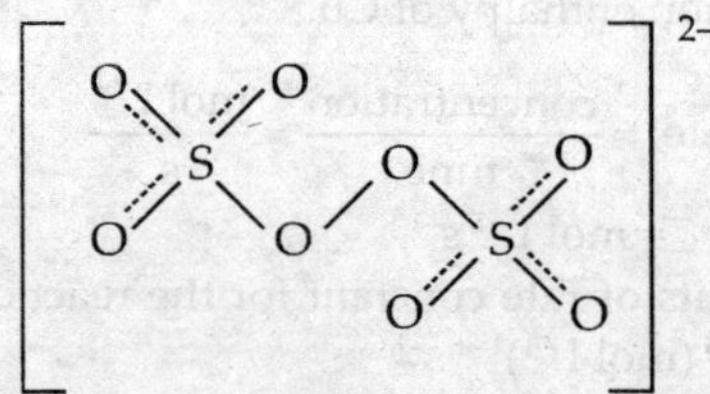

It has a O–O bridge.

94. **(a)** : N—N bond length is minimum in N_2O.

Compound	Structure
N_2O	N —113 pm— N —119 pm— O Linear
N_2O_3	O, 121 pm, 130°, N, 186 pm, 105°, 114 pm, N, O, 117°, O Planar

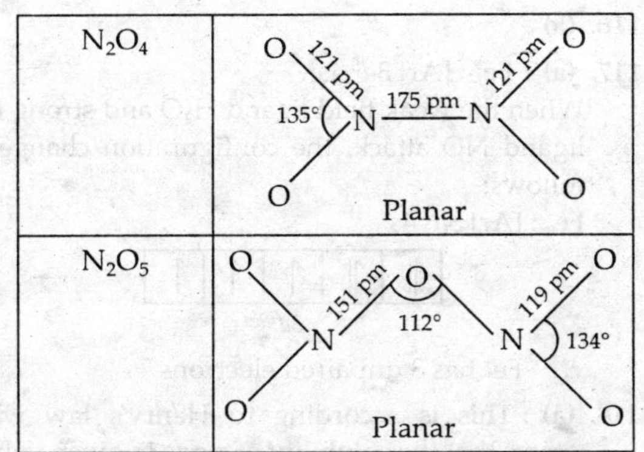

95. (c) : Nylon 6, 6 and dacron are the examples of condensation polymers.
Condensation polymers are formed by condensation of two or more bifunctional monomers with the elimination of simple molecules like H_2O, NH_3, alcohol, etc.
Dacron is formed from ethylene glycol and terephthalic acid with the removal of H_2O.
Nylon 6, 6 is formed from hexamethylenediamine and adipic acid with the removal of H_2O.

$[n\ HOCH_2CH_2OH]$ + n [HOOC–C_6H_4–COOH]
Ethylene glycol — Terephthalic acid

$\downarrow$

$-[OCH_2CH_2-O-C(=O)-C_6H_4-C(=O)]-_n + n\,H_2O$
Dacron

$n\,H_2N-(CH_2)_6-NH_2$ +
Hexamethylenediamine

$n\,HO-C(=O)-(CH_2)_4-C(=O)-OH$
Adipic acid

$\downarrow$

$-[N(H)-(CH_2)_6-N(H)-C(=O)-(CH_2)_4-C(=O)]-_n$
Nylon – 6, 6

96. (b) :

$CH_3CH_2CH=CH_2 \xrightarrow[H_3O^+]{Hg(OAc)_2} H_3C-CH_2-CH(OH)-CH_3$
But-1-ene — Butan-2-ol

97. (b) : Nitrobenzene ($C_6H_5NO_2$) + 4 [H] $\xrightarrow{Zn/NH_4Cl}$ Phenyl hydroxylamine (C_6H_5NHOH)

In neutral medium, nitrobenzene reduces to phenyl hydroxylamine.

98. (c) : $MgSO_4$ is readily soluble in water. The solubility of the sulphates of alkaline earth metals decrease with increase in size of the central metal ion. The greater hydration enthalpies of Mg^{2+} ions overcome the lattice enthalpy factor and therefore $MgSO_4$ is more soluble in water.

99. (a) : $PhCH_2Cl \xrightarrow{aq.\ NaCN} PhCH_2CN \xrightarrow[\text{Cat. hydrogenation}]{H_2,\ Pd} PhCH_2CH_2NH_2$ (U)

100. (a) : p-$ClC_6H_4CH_2Cl$ (A) $\xrightarrow[AgNO_2]{\Delta}$ p-$ClC_6H_4CH_2NO_2$ + AgCl

p-$ClC_6H_4CH_2Cl$ (A) $\xrightarrow{NaOH(aq.)}$ p-$ClC_6H_4CH_2OH$

p-$ClC_6H_4CH_2Cl$ (A) $\xrightarrow[KMnO_4/[H^+]]{[O]}$ p-ClC_6H_4COOH
Monochlorobenzoic acid

101. (c) : For first order reaction,
Rate$_1 = k[A_1]$
According to question,
$[A_2] = [2A_1]$
$\therefore$ Rate$_2 = k[2A_1]$
$\Rightarrow$ Rate$_2$ = 2 Rate$_1$
For a given reaction, rate constant is constant and independent of the concentration of reactant.

102. (d) : Sodium acetate on Kolbe's electrolysis gives ethane. It is formed at anode.

103. (b) : (H_3PO_2): P(=O)(H)(H)(OH) — (H_3PO_4): P(=O)(OH)(OH)(OH)

Oxoacids of phosphorus which contain P – H bond act as reducing agents and reduce metal salts to free metals. Thus, H_3PO_2 act as reducing agent while H_3PO_4 does not.

104. (c) : In diamond, C-atoms are sp^3 hybridized while in graphite, they are sp^2 hybridized.

105. (b) : Bohr model does not explain the spectra of multi-electron atoms.

106. (d) : $\overset{1}{C}H_2(Cl)-\overset{2}{C}H_2(Cl)$

Since it has no chiral carbon, it is optically inactive. Meso compounds are optically inactive.

107. (c) : ClF_3 (T-shape)

The lone pairs are at equatorial position (120° angle).

108. (c) : Oxygen has two unpaired electrons. So it is paramagnetic.

109. (b) : –OH group shows $+M$ effect and is an activating group, moreover the arenium ion of phenolic substitution is more stable.

110. (c) : S is more electronegative than Se.

111. (b) : Fluorine has higher standard electrode potential (reduction potential) than iodine.

112. (a) : The element which can reduce itself acts as an oxidising agent.

113. (a) : All species like He^+, Li^{2+}, Be^{3+} having one electron are expected to have similar spectrum as that of hydrogen.

114. (c) : Cl_2 is an oxidising agent. It bleaches the articles permanently by oxidation in presence of moisture.

115. (a) : Due to lanthanide contraction, the size of Lu^{3+} is increased and therefore $Lu(OH)_3$ shows more covalent character (Large cation, more is covalent character - Fajan's rule). Thus $La(OH)_3$ is more ionic and thus more basic.

116. (a)

117. (a) : Fe^+ : [Ar] $3d^6\,4s^1$

When the weak field ligand H_2O and strong field ligand NO attack, the configuration changes as follows:

Fe^+ : [Ar] $3d^7\,4s^0$

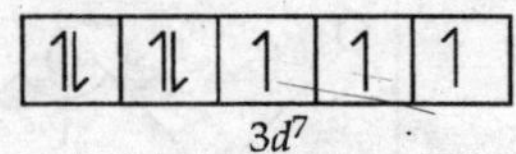

∴ Fe^+ has 3 unpaired electrons.

118. (a) : This is according to Henry's law which states that the solubility of a gas in given volume of a liquid at a particular temperature is directly proportional to the pressure of gas above the liquid. $m \propto p$, $m = kp$ where k = Henry's constant.

119. (a) : $HC\equiv C^-$ has 50% *s*-character and $H_2C=CH^-$ has 33% *s*-character. Stability of carbanions increases with an increase in the *s*-character at the carbanion. So $HC\equiv C^-$ is more stable than $H_2C=CH^-$.

120. (c) : In pressure cooker, water boils above 100°C. When the lid of cooker is opened, pressure is lowered so that boiling point decreases and water boils again.

BIOLOGY

121. (b) : In frog three types of respiration occurs to suit its amphibious mode of life. These are cutaneous, buccopharyngeal and pulmonary respiration. Cutaneous respiration occurs through the thin, moist, highly vascular and naked skin. It takes place in water as well as on land. Buccopharyngeal respiration occurs on land *via* thin, vascular, moist lining of buccopharyngeal cavity. Pulmonary respiration takes place when the frog is outside the water. It occurs by lungs of adult frog.

122. (b) : Fasciculated root is a type of adventitious root. In this case, roots are swollen which occur in clusters from lower nodes of stems, e.g., *Asparagus, Dahlia*, etc.

123. (d) : The blastomeres in the blastocyst are arranged into an outer layer called trophoblast and an inner group of cells attached to trophoblast called the inner cell mass. Inner cell mass looks like a small knob at one pole which gives rise to the embryo and is called the embryonal knob. The trophoblast does not take part in the formation of the embryo proper. It remains external to the embryo and gives rise to the extraembryonic membranes, namely, chorion and amnion, for the protection and nourishment of the embryo. The trophoblast cells in contact with the embryonal knob are known as cells of Rauber.

124. **(d) :** The given figure shows population growth curve, in which A is carrying capacity, B is exponential growth curve and C is logistic growth curve.

125. **(b) :** Deuteromycetes are commonly known as imperfect fungi because only the asexual or vegetative stages of these fungi are known. The deuteromycetes reproduce only by asexual spores known as conidia. The mycelium is septate and branched. Some members are saprophytes or parasites while a large number of them are decomposers of litter and help in mineral cycling. Some examples are *Alternaria, Colletotrichum* and *Trichoderma.*

126. **(d) :** Abscisic acid acts as a general plant growth inhibitor and an inhibitor of plant metabolism. ABA inhibits seed germination. ABA stimulates the closure of stomata in the epidermis and increases the tolerance of plants to various kinds of stresses. Therefore, it is also called the stress hormone.

127. **(c) :** Parturition is induced from the fully developed foetus and the placenta. Parturition involves foetal ejection reflex which are mild contractions of the placenta. This reflex triggers release of oxytocin from the maternal pituitary which acts on the uterine muscles and causes stronger uterine contractions and that further stimulates secretion of oxytocin. This stimulatory reflex between uterine muscle contraction and oxytocin secretion continues resulting in stronger contractions and eventually leading into expulsion of the baby out of the uterus.

128. **(d)**

129. **(b) :** Sodium-potassium pump (Na^+–K^+) is a membrane transport protein that exchanges sodium ions (Na^+) for potassium ions (K^+). It transports 3 Na^+ outwards for $2K^+$ into the cell, thus maintaining the differential concentrations of each ion across the plasma membrane. The process requires energy in the form of ATP, being a form of active transport.

130. **(c)**

131. **(d) :** Photorespiration is the light dependent process of oxygenation of ribulose biphosphate (RuBP) and release of carbon dioxide by the photosynthetic organs of a plant. Normally photosynthetic organs do the reverse in the light, i.e., uptake of CO_2 and release of O_2. At high temperature, RuBP carboxylase functions as oxygenase and instead of fixing carbon dioxide (C_3 cycle), oxidises ribulose 1, 5-biphosphate to produce a 3-carbon phosphoglyceric acid and a 2-carbon phosphoglycolate.

Photorespiration does not produce energy or reducing power. Rather, it consumes energy. Further, it undoes the work of photosynthesis. There is 25% loss of fixed CO_2. Therefore, photorespiration is a highly wasteful process. This happens only in case of C3 plants. C4 plants have overcome the problem of photorespiration.

132. **(c) :** Phase contrast microscope was developed by Zernicke (1935, Nobel Prize 1953) to observe living cells and the events occurring in them (e.g., Spindle formation, movement of chromosomes, endocytosis, exocytosis). It is similar to optical microscope except that it has an annular diaphragm in the condenser and a transparent phase plate at the back focal plane of objective. The microscope converts differences in refractive indices into differences in brightness.

133. **(d) :** A - Basilar membrane
B - Scala media
C - Reissner's membrane
D - Tectorial membrane

134. **(c) :** The net gain from complete oxidation of a glucose molecule in aerobic respiration is 36 ATP molecules. 10 molecules of $NADH_2$ (2 from Glycolysis + 8 from Krebs' cycle) yield $= 10 \times 3 = 30$ ATP, 2 molecules of $FADH_2$ yield $= 2 \times 2 = 4$ ATP and glycolysis also yields 2 ATP. Therefore, total release of ATP per hexose will be $= 30 + 4 + 2 = 36$ ATP.

135. **(a)**

136. **(c)**

137. **(c) :** A - Photosystem I (PS I)
B - Photosystem II (PS II)
C - e– acceptor
D - LHC(Light Harvesting Complex).

138. **(a) :** Muscle contraction is brought about by sliding of the actin filaments over myosin filaments. When a muscle fibril contracts, its A band remains constant and I band shortens. H zone also disappears as the actin filaments of both sides in each sarcomere may overlap each other at M line.

139. (c) : When an impulse arrives at the synaptic knob of the axon, it depolarizes the presynaptic membrane and increases its permeability to calcium ions (Ca^{2+}). Ca^{2+} ions from the synaptic cleft pass into the synaptic knob via voltage-gated channels. Sudden rise in the cytosolic concentration of Ca^{2+}, causes the release of a chemical, called neurotransmitter substance, from small synaptic vesicles present there into the synaptic cleft by exocytosis through the presynaptic membrane.

140. (b) : Cattle ranching refers to practice of raising grazing livestock such as cattle or sheep for meat and wool, etc. The area of landscape meant primarily for cattle ranching is called a ranch. The practice has lead to accelerated deforestation and contributed to increased methane gas concentration in atmosphere. Whatever cattle eat; is subjected to the action of methanogens (bacteria) harbouring the stomach (rumen) of cattle. The action of these bacteria on food material produces methane gas which is released through cattle fart into the earth's atmosphere where it absorbs heat just like carbon dioxide, contributing to global warming.

141. (b) : The C_4 plants are adapted to dry tropical regions and have greater productivity of biomass. They have special type of leaf anatomy known as Kranz anatomy. In this type of anatomy the bundle sheath cells form several layers around the vascular bundles; they are characterized by having a large number of chloroplasts, thick walls impervious to gaseous exchange and no intercellular spaces.

142. (a) : Colchicine is an alkaloid derived from the autumn crocus, *Colchicum autumnale*. It inhibits spindle formation in cells during mitosis so that chromosomes cannot separate during anaphase, thus inducing multiple sets of chromosomes. It does not affect cytokinesis.

143. (b) : The adrenal medulla secretes two hormones called adrenaline or epinephrine and noradrenaline or norepinephrine. These are commonly called as catecholamines. These are rapidly secreted in response to stress of any kind and during emergency situations and are called emergency hormones or hormones of fight or flight. These hormones increase alertness, pupillary dilation, piloerection (raising of hairs), sweating, etc. Both the hormones increase the heart beat, the strength of heart contraction and the rate of respiration. Catecholamines also stimulate the breakdown of glycogen, lipids and proteins.

144. (b) : The structure in option (b) is of a basophil. Basophils are granular WBCs and are the least (0.5– 1 per cent) of the total WBCs. They secrete histamine, serotonin, heparin, etc. and are involved in inflammatory reactions.

145. (a)

146. (b) : Bohr's effect is the phenomenon whereby the affinity of the respiratory pigment i.e., haemoglobin in the blood for oxygen is reduced when the level of carbon dioxide is increased. An increase in carbon dioxide concentration makes the blood more acidic which results in decrease in the efficiency of the uptake of oxygen by haemoglobin molecules. This facilitates gaseous exchange, because more oxygen is released in the tissues where the amount of carbon dioxide is rising due to metabolic activity. In its reverse, more oxygen is taken up at the lungs where the amount of carbon dioxide is low.

147. (d) : Bacteria like *Rhizobium* and *Frankia* live free as aerobes in the soil but are unable to fix nitrogen. They develop the ability to fix nitrogen only as a symbiont when they become anaerobic. They are unable to fix nitrogen by themselves. Roots of a legume secrete chemical attractants. Bacteria collect over the root hairs and form an infection thread enclosing the bacteria. Infection thread grows alongwith multiplication of bacteria. Bacteria stop dividing and form irregular polyhedral structures called bacteroids. In an infected cell bacteriods occur in groups surrounded by host membrane. The host cell develops a pinkish pigment called leghaemoglobin (Lb). It is oxygen scavenger and is related to blood pigment haemoglobin. It protects nitrogen fixing enzyme nitrogenase from oxygen.

148. (b)

149. (d) : Segmentation occurs in three highly organized phyla-annelida (earthworm), arthropoda (*Periplaneta*) and chordates. The body is often divided both externally and internally into a number of segments (metameres) *e.g.*, annelids. Segmentation is mostly external in arthropods and mainly internal in man and other chordates.

150. (a)

151. (a) : G_0 phase is the stage of inactivation of cell cycle due to non-availability of mitogens and energy rich compounds. The cells in this phase remain metabolically active and usually grow in size assuming particular shape (cell differentiation). Cell enters G_0 phase from a cell cycle checkpoint in the G_1 phase. G_1 phase checkpoint (restriction point) takes the key decision whether the cell should divide, delay division or enter resting stage. Cells then remain in G_0 phase until there is a reason for them to divide. Several biocatalysts can help a cell in G_0 phase to proceed through cell division when required.

152. (a) : The "beads-on-a-string" structure is seen in electron microscope of isolated metaphase chromosomes. The chromonema form the gene bearing portions of the chromosome. Basically chromonema is made up of nucleosome chains. Nucleosome chain gives a beads on string appearance under electron microscope. Nucleosome is the fundamental packaging unit in eukaryotic chromosomes.

153. (b) : RNAi is a regulatory mechanism for an estimated 30% of all protein-coding genes(in mammals). It helps to protect cells against certain viruses by targeting viral RNA for destruction. It helps to silence potentially disruptive transposons in the genome by destroying RNA copies arising from transposon replication. RNAi is a precise and efficient tool for knockout of specific genes when studying gene function in experimental organisms. It also has potential for new forms of targeted gene therapy.

154. (c) : Alkaloids - Morphine, Codeine
Pigments- Carotenoids, Anthocyanin
Drugs- Vinblastin, Curcumin.

155. (c) : Four main types of commercial tea are generally recognized in the trade. These are black tea (China, India, Sri Lanka), green tea (China, Japan and Taiwan), oolong tea (Taiwan) and brick tea (China). Dust or fannings are left over small part of tea leaves, which are also widely used.

156. (c) : The cardiac cycle consists of one heart beat or one cycle of contraction and relaxation of the cardiac muscle. The contraction phase is called the systole while the relaxation phase is called the diastole.

157. (c) : The given floral diagram is of liliaceae family. This family is a characteristic representative of monocot plants. Most plants of this family are good ornamentals, source of medicine, vegetables and colchicine.

158. (c) : Particulate matter mainly includes dust, soot particles, volatile hydrocarbons, some sulphate and metallic residues emitted into the air by sources such as factories, power plants, vehicles, etc. PM is usually divided into different classes based on size ranging from total suspended matter (TSP) to PM-10 (particles with diameter of 10 μ or less) to PM-2.5 (particles with diameter of 2.5 μ or less). Smallest particles pose highest human health risk. Larger particles (≤ 10 μ) can easily be expelled from lungs through mucus but finer particles (≤ 2.5 μ) penetrate deep in lungs and can cause severe lung damage including lung cancer.

159. (c) : Pebrine or pepper disease is caused by protozoan *Nosema bombycis*. The parasite infects eggs and is therefore, transmitted to next generation. It kills caterpillars.

160. (b) : Homopolysaccharides or homoglycans are those complex carbohydrates which are formed by polymerization of only one type of monosaccharide monomers. For example, starch, glycogen, inulin, cellulose, chitin, etc.

Agar, pectin, hyaluronic acid, heparin, etc., are heteropolysaccharides.

161. (b) : Hot spots are areas with high density of biodiversity or megadiversity which are also the most threatened ones. Ecologically hot spots are determined by four factors.

(i) Number of species/species diversity.
(ii) Degree of endemism
(iii) Degree of threat to habitat due to its degradation and fragmentation.
(iv) Degree of exploitation.

Myers (1988) initially identified 12 hot spots. Today the number of hotspots identified by ecologists is 34 covering an area less than 2% of land surface with about 20% of human population living there.

162. (b) : When the offsprings are produced by self fertilization or breeding between closely related parents it is called inbreeding. Inbreeding results in increase in homozygosity. The most revealing impact of inbreeding is the loss of vigour and physiological efficiency of the organisms characterized by reduction in size. A number of lethal and defective characters appear in the population which has undergone inbreeding (selfing). This loss of fitness in the progenies or decline in character expression with decreased heterozygosity arising from self mating is known as inbreeding depression or inbreeding decline. Continued inbreeding reduces fertility and even productivity. But the inbreeding progeny with lethal and harmful recessive genes being homozygous express these traits which otherwise remain hidden in heterozygous individuals. Natural selection works upon these individuals and eliminate them. Gradually, such genes get eliminated from the population.

163. (a) : For aquatic organism salt concentration (measured as salinity in parts per thousand) is a major factor for their survival. Salinity of different aquatic habitats varies greatly. It is less than 5 per thousand parts, in inland waters, 30–35 per thousand parts in the sea and more than 100 per thousand parts in some hypersaline lagoons. Many fresh water animals cannot live for long in sea water and vice versa because of the osmotic problems they would face due to the change in relative tonicity of the surrounding water with cytoplasm. It may result into endosmosis or exosmosis according to the conditions. The tolerance of organisms to the salinity range varies. Some organisms are tolerant of a wide range of salinities and are called euryhaline e.g. salmon, while some can tolerate only a narrow range of salinity i.e., stenohaline e.g., shark.

164. (c) : In non-myelinated nerve fibres, the ionic changes are repeated over the membrane all along the length of the fibre. So, the action potential flows all along the membrane over the entire length of the fibre. But in myelinated fibres, the ionic changes and the consequent depolarisation can take place only at the nodes of Ranvier free from myelin sheath, because the myelin sheath between the nodes insulates the fibre and prevents its depolarisation. So, the action potential in effect jumps from one node to the next.This is called saltatory conduction of nerve impulses. Because of this, nerve impulses do not have to run all along the myelinated nerve fibre. This is why nerve impulses are conducted far more rapidly in myelinated fibres than in the non - myelinated ones.

165. (c) : Frogs are able to change the colour of their skins to match with that of the surroundings. It makes them hard to be noticed by enemies. This is a type of protective colouration known as camouflage not mimicry. Changes in colour are possible by dispersion or concentration of special amoeboid pigment cells in their skin.

166. (a) : Simple goitre or endemic goitre is the enlargement of thyroid gland accompanied with cretinism or myxoedema. It occurs in case of hyposecretion of thyroxine. To compensate for lower secretion of thyroxine from cells, thyroid gland enlarges to accommodate more secretory cells. It is caused due to dietary deficiency of iodine. To form normal quantities of thyroxine about 1 mg/week of ingested iodine is required in the form of iodides.

167. (b) : Sickle cell anaemia is an autosomal hereditary disorder in which the erythrocytes become sickle shaped. The disorder or disease is caused by the formation of an abnormal haemoglobin called haemoglobin–s denoted as Hbs. Thus, the genotype of an individual homozygous for sickle cell anaemia is written as HbsHbs.

168. (d) : Manganese (Mn) is a micronutrient. Excess of it in soil can cause manganese toxicity characterized by brown spots surrounded by chlorotic veins. It occurs due to (i) reduction in uptake of iron and magnesium (ii) inhibition of binding of magnesium to specific enzymes (iii) inhibition of calcium translocation into shoot apex. Therefore excess of manganese (Mn) causes deficiency of iron (Fe), magnesium (Mg) and calcium (Ca).

Hence the toxicity symptoms of Mn are actually combined deficiency symptoms of Fe, Mg and Ca.

169. (a) : Females having 45 chromosomes (2A + X0) are affected with Turner's syndrome. Individuals having Turner's syndrome have female sexual differentiation but ovaries are rudimentary. Other associated phenotypes of this condition are short stature, webbed-neck, broad chest, lack of secondary sexual characteristics and sterility. Thus, any imbalance in the copies of the sex chromosomes may disrupt the genetic information necessary for normal sexual development.

170. (d) : In proximal convoluted tubule (PCT) about 65% of the glomerular filtrate is reabsorbed normally. Here most of the solutes are reabsorbed making the filtrate isotonic to blood plasma. HCO–3 is not absorbed in PCT.

171. (b) : Classification involves hierarchy of steps, in which each step represents a rank or category, called taxonomic category or taxon. All taxa together constitute a taxonomic hierarchy as follows:

Species → Genus → Family → Order → Class → Phylum or division → Kingdom.

Most common characters among individual members are found in taxon species. Common characters decrease from species to kingdom and members of a kingdom have least number of common characters. Similarly, complexity of classification decreases from species to kingdom.

172. (c) : There are two types of food chains: grazing food chain and detritus food chain. Detritus food chains are those which start from the dead bodies of animals or fallen leaves etc. In terrestrial ecosystems, detritus food chain is the major conduit of energy flow, while in aquatic ecosystems, grazing food chain is the major conduit of energy flow. As the detritus food chains depend upon the dead organic matter hence, these are not directly dependent upon solar energy.

173. (c) : *Wuchereria* (*W.bancrofti* & *W.malayi*), the filarial worms cause a slowly developing chronic inflammation of the organs in which they live for many years, usually the lymphatic vessels of the lower limbs, and the disease is called filariasis. The pathogen spread from one human being to another through mosquitoes like Culex and to a less extent by *Anopheles* and *Aedes*. The parasite resides in lymph vessels, connective tissues and mesentery. It is manifestated by lymphoedema accompanied by thickening of subcutaneous tissues and skin so that there is permanent swelling mostly of feet, legs, thighs, scrotal sacs, breast etc. In Culex and other mosquitoes females are blood sucking while males suck juices of flowers and fruits. Female Culex carries filarial worm from one person to another. It prefers to breed in dirty water near human habitation.

174. (b) : Retrovirus is an RNA-containing virus that converts its RNA into DNA by means of the enzyme reverse transcriptase. This enables it to become integrated into its host's DNA. Some retroviruses can cause cancer in animals they contain oncogenes (cancer-causing genes), which are activated when the virus enters its host cell and starts to replicate. The special properties of retroviruses make them useful as vectors for inserting genetic material into eukaryotic cells. The best-known retrovirus is HIV, responsible for AIDS in humans.

175. (a) : Leydig's cells or interstitial cells of testes are large, polygonal cells that lie in the connective tissue present between the seminiferous tubules. They secrete androgens, the male sex hormones e.g., testosterone into the blood. Androgens control male sexual characteristics including facial and pubic hairs.

176. (a) : During strenuous exercise, the muscle does not get sufficient oxygen to meet its energy needs immediately. So, it contracts anaerobically and accumulates lactic acid. During recovery, the oxygen consumption of the muscle far exceeds than that in the resting state. The extra oxygen consumed during recovery is called oxygen debt of the muscle.

177. (c) : Being insoluble in water, fats and oils form large immiscible droplets in aqueous media but the enzymes which hydrolyse fats and oils (called lipases) are insoluble in fats and soluble in water. Therefore, lipases can act only on the water adjoining surfaces of fat droplets. Evidently, the larger the surface area of fat droplets, the greater is the action of the lipase on them. We know that the smaller the size of a droplet, the larger is its surface area relative to its mass. Thus lipases can digest fat in significant amounts only when large fat droplets are broken into tiny droplets to form a fine emulsion. This is the reason why emulsification is so necessary for the digestion of fats. Enzyme amylase, on the other hand, is a starch - hydrolysing enzyme which has no role in fat digestion.

178. **(b)** : Bilirubin is a yellow pigment which arises from the catabolism of red pigment haemoglobin of old and worn out RBCs. The pale yellow colour of blood plasma is largely due to the presence of bilirubin. It has to be excreted into the bile and from there it is excreted out of the body along with the faecal matter. If, all of the bilirubin can not be excreted from the body then the skin and mucous membranes assume a yellowish hue, giving rise to the condition called jaundice.

179. **(a)** : No taste sensation is evoked when distilled water is put on human tongue because man does not possess taste buds for tasting water. The taste buds present on the tongue send nerve impulses to the brain which actually preceives the taste sensation. Some mammals such as rhesus monkeys, pigs, cats and dogs possess some taste buds which send nerve impulses to the brain when distilled water is applied on them. It seems, therefore, that water may stimulate these taste buds to evoke taste sensation in these animals.

180. **(d)** : It is not oxytocin, but the hormone vasopressin (also known as antidiuretic hormone, ADH) because it reduces the volume of urine by increasing the reabsorption of water from the urine in the distal convoluted tubules, collecting tubules and collecting ducts in the kidney. It does so by rendering the walls of those tubules permeable to water. Failure of secretion of vasopressin leads to a reduced renal reabsorption of water and a consequent elimination of a large volume of very dilute (hypotonic) urine.

Oxytocin is another hormone released by the posterior lobe of pituitary gland. Oxytocin contracts the mammary glands, smooth muscles of uterus. Uterine contractions, stimulated by oxytocin at the end of pregnancy, help in the child-birth or parturition, hence also called birth hormone. The oxytocin - induced contractions of the mammary gland muscles help in the flow of stored milk from the mammary glands, hence also called milk ejection hormone.

GENERAL KNOWLEDGE

181. (b)	182. (b)	183. (b)	184. (a)	185. (b)
186. (a)	187. (d)	188. (b)	189. (d)	190. (b)
191. (c)	192. (d)	193. (a)	194. (a)	195. (b)
196. (d)	197. (c)	198. (a)	199. (a)	200. (c)

Chapterwise Index - '13

Physics • Chemistry • Biology

Use the index for topicwise analysis of AIIMS paper and refer to these questions when you are practising MCQs chapterwise.

PHYSICS

Chapter's Name	Question No.	Total
Units and Dimensions	8	1
Motion in One Dimension		0
Motion in Two Dimensions	30, 36	2
Laws of Motion and Friction	4	1
Work, Power and Energy	57	1
Centre of Mass and Rotational Motion	18, 46, 56	3
Gravitation	11, 40	2
Properties of Matter		0
Oscillations	29, 58	2
Waves		0
Heat and Thermodynamics	13, 14, 15, 16, 17, 21, 35, 37, 39, 45	10
Electrostatics	7, 25, 43, 44, 48	5
Current Electricity	33, 53, 54	3
Thermal and chemical effects of current		0
Magnetic Effects of Current		0
Magnetism	9, 47, 59	3
Electromagnetic Induction and Alternating Current	12, 22, 32	3
Electromagnetic Waves	31, 52	2
Ray Optics	42, 50, 55, 60	4
Wave Optics	23, 27	2
Modern Physics	2, 3, 6, 24, 28, 38, 49, 51	8
Solids and Semiconductor Devices	10. 26, 34	3
Universe		0
Principles of Communication	1, 5, 19, 20, 42	5

CHEMISTRY

Chapter's Name	Question No.	Total
Basic Concepts		0
Atomic Structure	92, 117	2
Periodic Properties	64	1
Chemical Bonding	66, 67	2
Nuclear Chemistry		0
Gaseous and Liquid States	113	1
Solid State	90, 111	2
Mole Concept & Solutions	88, 89	2
Colloids, Surface Chemistry & Catalysis	91, 96	2
Equilibrium	94, 105	2
Kinetics	61, 98, 115	3
Energetics	95, 112, 114, 116	4
Electrochemistry	93	1
Redox Reactions	68, 74, 118	3
Metallurgy	99, 119	2
Hydrogen and its Compounds	97	1
s-Block Elements	71	1
p-Block Elements	69, 101, 102, 120	4
d- and *f*-Block Elements	62, 63, 65, 70, 73	5
Complex Compounds	72, 103, 104	3
Purification and Analysis of Organic Compound		0
General Organic Chemistry		0
Aliphatic Hydrocarbons	85	1
Aromatic Hydrocarbons		0
Halogen Derivatives		0
Alcohols, Phenols and Ethers	76, 80, 81, 87, 109	5
Aldehydes and Ketones	78, 79, 107	3
Carboxylic acids & their derivatives	82, 106, 108	3
Organic Compounds Containing Nitrogen	83, 84, 86	3
Biochemistry	77, 110	2
Chemistry in Action	100	1
Environmental Chemistry	75	1

BIOLOGY		
Chapter's Name	**Question No.**	**Total**
General Biology		0
Biological Classification	150, 152	2
Kingdom Monera		0
Kingdom Fungi		0
Plant Kingdom	142	1
Cell and its Structural Components	154, 157, 170	3
Cell Reproduction	133, 172	2
Cell Respiration		
Biomolecules	132, 178, 179	3
Principles of Inheritance and Variation	144, 175	2
Molecular Basis of Inheritance		0
Plant Anatomy	153, 168	2
Plant Morphology	147	1
Plant Physiology	139, 159, 162, 176	4
Sexual Reproduction in Flowering Plants	131, 134, 135, 136	4
Ecology and Environment	123, 124, 158, 160, 169, 171	6
Animal Kingdom	121, 126, 161	3
Animal Tissue		0
Musculo-Skeletal System	149	1
Digestive System and Nutrition	143, 163, 177, 180	4
Respiratory System	155	1
Circulatory System	125, 151, 156, 164	4
Excretion and Osmoregulation	145	1
Nervous System and Sense Organs	148, 174	2
Endocrinc System	140	1
Reproduction and Embryonic Development	127, 128, 165, 173	4
Human Health and Diseases	130	1
Evolution	129	1
Biotechnology	122, 137, 138	3
Applied Biology	141, 146, 166, 167	4

SOLVED PAPER
AIIMS - 2013★

Time : 3½ Hours

Max. Marks : 200

PHYSICS

1. For satellite communication which wave is used?
(a) Space wave (b) Sky wave
(c) Ground wave (d) Microwave

2. In nuclear fission, which of the following quantity is conserved?
(a) Energy
(b) Mass
(c) Momentum
(d) Both energy and mass.

3. When a slow neutron is captured by a $^{235}_{92}U$ nucleus, a fission energy releasing 200 MeV. If power of nuclear reactor is 100 W then rate of nuclear fission is
(a) $3.6 \times 10^6\ s^{-1}$ (b) $3.1 \times 10^{12}\ s^{-1}$
(c) $1.8 \times 10^4\ s^{-1}$ (d) $4.1 \times 10^6\ s^{-1}$

4. A ball of mass m is tied up with string and rotated along a horizontal circle of radius r. At an instant, its velocity is v, and tension in string is T, the force required for circular motion is
(a) $T-\frac{mv^2}{r}$ (b) $T+\frac{mv^2}{r}$
(c) $\frac{mv^2}{r}$ (d) zero

5. If modulation index is 1/2 and power of carrier wave is 2 W. Then what will be the total power in modulated wave?
(a) 0.5 W (b) 1 W
(c) 0.25 W (d) 2.25 W

6. If velocity of a particle is three times of that of electron and ratio of de Broglie wavelength of particle to that of electron is 1.814×10^{-4}. The particle will be
(a) Neutron (b) Deutron
(c) Alpha (d) Tritium

7. A dipole of dipole moment 'p' is placed in non-uniform electric field along x-axis. Electric field is increasing at the rate of $1\ V\ m^{-1}$ then the force on dipole is
(a) 0 (b) $2p$
(c) $p/2$ (d) p

8. Dimensional formula of angular momentum is
(a) ML^2T^{-1} (b) $M^2L^2T^{-2}$
(c) ML^2T^{-3} (d) MLT^{-1}

9. Relation between magnetic moment and angular velocity is
(a) $M \propto \omega$ (b) $M \propto \omega^2$
(c) $M \propto \sqrt{\omega}$ (d) None of these

10. In an intrinsic semiconductor band gap is 1.2 eV then ratio of number of charge carriers at 600 K and 300 K is
(a) 10^4 (b) 10^7 (c) 10^5 (d) 10^3

11. Gravitational potential of the body of mass m at a height h from surface of earth of radius R is (Take g = acceleration due to gravity at earth's surface)
(a) $-g(R + h)$ (b) $-g(R - h)$
(c) $g(R + h)$ (d) $g(R - h)$

12. Which of the following is the best method to reduce eddy currents?
(a) Laminating core (b) Using thick wires
(c) Reducing hysteresis loss
(d) None of these

13. In a cyclic process, work done by the system is
(a) zero
(b) more than the heat given to the system
(c) equal to heat given to the system
(d) independent of heat given to system

14. In a cylinder their are 60 g Ne and 64 g O_2. If pressure of mixture of gases in cylinder is 30 bar then in this cylinder partial pressure of O_2 is (in bar)
(a) 30 (b) 20 (c) 15 (d) 12

★ *Based on memory.* Courtesy : ***Allen Career Institute**, Kota (Rajasthan)*

15. A gas mixture contain one mole O_2 gas and one mole He gas. Find the ratio of specific heat at constant pressure to that at constant volume of the gaseous mixture.
(a) 2 (b) 1.5
(c) 2.5 (d) 4

16. One mole of oxygen of volume 1 litre at 4 atm pressure to attains 1 atm pressure by result of isothermal expansion. Find work done by the gas.
(a) $\approx$ 155 J (b) $\approx$ 206 J
(c) $\approx$ 355 J (d) $\approx$ 552 J

17. Graph of specific heat at constant volume for a monoatomic gas is

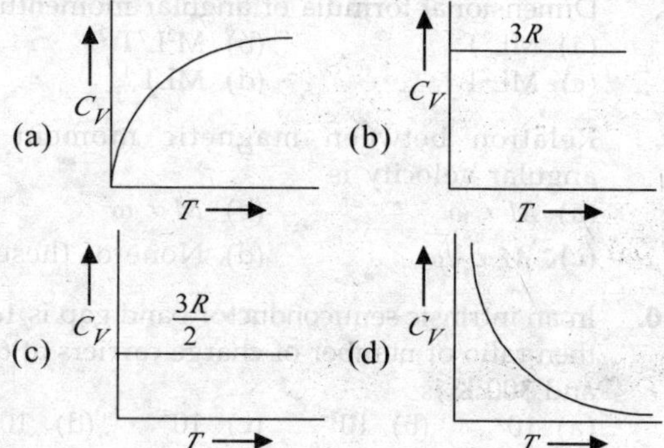

18. Given that force $(5\hat{i}+7\hat{j}-3\hat{k})$ N acts on a particle at position $(\hat{i}+\hat{j}-\hat{k})$ m. Find torque of this force on the particle about origin.
(a) $4\hat{i}-2\hat{j}+2\hat{k}$ (b) $2\hat{i}-3\hat{j}+4\hat{k}$
(c) $5\hat{i}-2\hat{j}+3\hat{k}$ (d) $6\hat{i}-4\hat{j}+4\hat{k}$

19. Astronomical wavelength increase due to doppler effect known as
(a) Red shift (b) Voilet shift
(c) UV (d) IR shift

20. Long distance communication between two point on earth is achieved by
(a) Space wave communication
(b) Sky wave communication
(c) Satellite wave communication
(d) Line of sight transmission

21. Which of the following is not a state function?
(a) Work-done in adiabatic process.
(b) Work done in isothermal process.
(c) Heat at constant pressure.
(d) Heat at constant volume.

22. In an oscillating system, a restoring force is a must. In an L-C circuit, restoring force is provide by
(a) capacitor (b) inductance
(c) resistance (d) both (a) and (b)

23. Polaroid glass is used in sun glasses because
(a) it reduces the light intensity to half on account of polarisation
(b) it is fashionable
(c) it has good colour
(d) it is cheaper

24. Which of the following statement is incorrect?
(a) Neutron is less stable than proton
(b) Neutron can cause fission in nuclear reactors but proton can not.
(c) A free proton can emit beta particle.
(d) A bound proton can emit beta particle.

25. Electric field at a distance r from infinitely long conducting sheet is proportional to
(a) r^{-1} (b) r^{-2}
(c) $r^{-3/2}$ (d) independent of r

26. Given that the mobility of electrons in Ge is 0.4 m^2 V^{-1} s^{-1} and electronic charge is 1.6×10^{-19}C. The number of donor atom (per m^3) semiconductor of conductivity 500 mho/m is
(a) 8×10^{21} (b) 8×10^{15}
(c) 5×10^{21} (d) 8×10^{16}

27. In a Young's double slit experiment the spacing between the slits is 0.3 mm and the screen is kept at a distance of 1.5 m. The second bright fringe is found 6 mm from the central fringe. The wavelength of the light used in the experiment is
(a) 625 nm (b) 600 nm
(c) 550 nm (d) 500 nm

28. In beta plus decay
(a) antineutrino is produced with electron
(b) neutrino is produced with positron
(c) neutron is produced with electron
(d) none of these

29. A simple pendulum performs simple harmonic motion about $x = 0$ with an amplitude 'a' and time period 'T'. The speed of the pendulum at $x = a/2$ will be
(a) $\frac{\pi a}{T}$ (b) $\frac{3\pi^2 a}{T}$

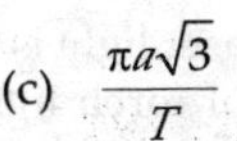

(c) $\frac{\pi a\sqrt{3}}{T}$ (d) $\frac{\pi a\sqrt{3}}{2T}$

30. A particle is projected from the ground with an initial speed of 'v' at angle θ with horizontal. The average velocity of the particle between its point of projection and height point of trajectory is

(a) $\frac{v}{2}\sqrt{1+2\cos^2\theta}$ (b) $\frac{v}{2}\sqrt{1+\cos^2\theta}$

(c) $\frac{v}{2}\sqrt{1+3\cos^2\theta}$ (d) $v\cos\theta$

31. The frequency of a light wave in a material is 2×10^{14} Hz and wavelength is 5000 Å. The refractive index of material will be

(a) 1.50 (b) 3.00 (c) 1.33 (d) 1.40

32. Two solenoids of equal number of turns having their length and the radii in the same ratio 1 : 2. The ratio of their self-inductance will be

(a) 1 : 2 (b) 2 : 1 (c) 1 : 1 (d) 1 : 4

33. A circuit consisting of five resistors each of resistance R, forming a Wheatstone bridge. What is the equivalent resistance of the circuit?

(a) $2R$ (b) R
(c) $2R/3$ (d) $R/2$

34. The circuit as shown in figure, the equivalent gate is

(a) NOR gate (b) OR gate
(c) AND gate (d) NAND gate

35. An engine has an efficiency of 1/6. When the temperature of sink is reduced by 62°C, its efficiency is doubled. The temperature of source will be

(a) 37° C (b) 62° C
(c) 99° C (d) 124° C

36. If a vector $2\hat{i}+3\hat{j}+8\hat{k}$ is perpendicular to the vector $4\hat{i}-4\hat{j}+\alpha\hat{k}$, then value of α is

(a) –1 (b) $\frac{1}{2}$ (c) $-\frac{1}{2}$ (d) 1

37. 1 g of steam is sent into 1 g of ice. At thermal equilibrium, the resultant temperature of mixture is

(a) 270°C (b) 230°C
(c) 100°C (d) 120°C

38. Ratio of longest wavelengths corresponding to Lyman and Balmer series in hydrogen spectrum is

(a) $\frac{7}{29}$ (b) $\frac{9}{31}$ (c) $\frac{5}{27}$ (d) $\frac{3}{23}$

39. The molar specific heats of an ideal gas at constant pressure and volume are denoted by C_P and C_V respectively. If $\gamma = \frac{C_P}{C_V}$ and R is the universal gas constant, then C_V is equal to

(a) $\frac{(\gamma-1)}{R}$ (b) γR

(c) $\frac{1+\gamma}{1-\gamma}$ (d) $\frac{R}{(\gamma-1)}$

40. A body of mass m is taken from the earth's surface to the height equal to twice the radius(R) of the earth. The change in potential energy of body will be

(a) $3mgR$ (b) $\frac{1}{3}mgR$

(c) $2mgR$ (d) $\frac{2}{3}mgR$

Directions : In the following questions (41-60), a statement of assertion (A) is followed by a statement of reason (R). Mark the correct choice as :

(a) If both assertion and reason are true and reason is the correct explanation of assertion.

(b) If both assertion and reason are true but reason is not the correct explanation of assertion.

(c) If assertion is true but reason is false.

(d) If both assertion and reason are false.

41. Assertion : In a communication system based on amplitude modulation the modulation index is kept < 1.

Reason : It ensures minimum distortion of signal.

42. Assertion : If optical density of a substance is more than that of water then the mass density of substance can be less than water.

Reason : Optical density and mass density are not related.

43. **Assertion** : On going away from a point charge or a small electric dipole, electric field decreases at the same rate in both the cases.

Reason : Electric field is inversely proportional to square of distance from the charge or on electric dipole.

44. **Assertion** : If a conductor is given charge then no excess inner charge appears.

Reason : Electric field inside conductor is zero.

45. **Assertion** : Water kept in an open vessel will quickly evaporate on the surface of the moon.

Reason : The temperature at the surface of the moon is much higher than the boiling point of water.

46. **Assertion** : Moment of inertia is always constant.

Reason : Angular moment is conserved that is why moment of inertia is constant.

47. **Assertion** : Magnetic lines forms closed loops in nature.

Reason : Mono-magnetic pole does not exist in nature.

48. **Assertion** : Gaussian surface is considered carefully.

Reason : The point where electric field to be calculated should be with in the surface.

49. **Assertion** : $^{60}_{27}Co$ is a source of gamma radiation.

Reason : Gamma emission is due to nuclear decay.

50. **Assertion** : When light ray is incident at polarising angle on glass, refracted light is partially polarised.

Reason : The intensity of light decreases in polarisation.

51. **Assertion** : A laser beam of 0.2 W power can drill holes through a metal sheet, whereas a 1000 W torch-light cannot.

Reason : The frequency of laser light is much higher than that of torch light.

52. **Assertion** : Electromagnetic radiations exert pressure.

Reason : Electromagnetic-waves carry both momentum and energy.

53. **Assertion** : Electric appliances with metallic body. *e.g.,* heaters, presses etc., have three pin connections, whereas an electric bulb has a two pin connection.

Reason : Three pin connections reduce heating of connecting cables.

54. **Assertion** : Total current entering a circuit is equal to leaving the circuit by Kirchhoff's law.

Reason : It is based on conservation of energy.

55. **Assertion** : The sun rises some time before the actual sun-rise.

Reason : Because of the refraction through the different layers of atmosphere.

56. **Assertion** : Centre of mass of a system does not move under the action of internal forces.

Reason : Internal forces are non conservative forces.

57. **Assertion** : Total energy is negative for a bound system.

Reason : Potential energy of a bound system is negative and more than kinetic energy.

58. **Assertion** : A undamped spring-mass system is simplest free vibration system.

Reason : It has three degrees of freedom.

59. **Assertion** : Magnetic field is useful in producing parallel beam of charged particle.

Reason : Magnetic field inhibits the motion of charged particle moving across it.

60. **Assertion** : Resolving power of a telescope depends only on wavelength.

Reason : This is proportional to square of wavelength.

CHEMISTRY

61. The plot of a concentration of the reactant versus time for a reaction is a straight line with a negative slope. The reaction follows a
(a) first order rate equation
(b) zero order rate equation
(c) second order reaction
(d) third order rate equation

62. Which of the following element has lowest melting point?
(a) Cr (b) Fe
(c) Ni (d) Cu

63. Maximum number of unpaired electrons are present in
(a) Gd^{3+} (b) Yb^{2+}
(c) Tb^{2+} (d) Pm^{3+}

64. The first ionisation enthalpy of Na, Mg and Si are 496, 737, 776 kJ/mol respectively. What will be the first ionisation enthalpy potential of Al in kJ/mol?
(a) > 766 kJ/mol
(b) > 496 and < 737 kJ
(c) > 737 and < 766 kJ/mol
(d) > 496 kJ/mol

65. When calomel is treated with ammonium hydroxide, a black substance is formed. The black substance is
(a) Hg + HgO (b) $HgO.HgCl_2$
(c) $H_2N - Hg - Cl + Hg$
(d) $Hg(NH_2)_2 + HgO$

66. Total number of antibonding electrons present in O_2 will be
(a) 6 (b) 8
(c) 4 (d) 2

67. In BF_3, the B – F bond length is 1.30 Å, when BF_3 is allowed to be treated with Me_3N, it forms an adduct, $Me_3N \rightarrow BF_3$, the bond length of B – F in the adduct is
(a) greater than 1.30 Å
(b) smaller than 1.30 Å
(c) equal to 1.30 Å
(d) none of these.

68. Oxidation state of iron in haemoglobin is
(a) 0 (b) +2
(c) –2 (d) +3

69. Which of the following statement is not true for hydrolysis of XeF_6?
(a) $XeOF_4$ is formed. (b) XeO_2F_2 is formed.
(c) It is a redox reaction.
(d) XeO_3 is formed.

70. Which of the following is most basic?
(a) $Al(OH)_3$ (b) $Cr(OH)_3$
(c) $La(OH)_3$ (d) $Fe(OH)_3$

71. Bleaching powder does not contain
(a) $CaCl_2$ (b) $Ca(OH)_2$
(c) $Ca(OCl)_2$ (d) $Ca(ClO_3)_2$

72. Which of the following metal ion forms unstable complex with CN^-?
(a) Ag(I) (b) Zn(II)
(c) Cu(II) (d) Cr(II)

73. Which of the following ion does not exist?
(a) $[CuI_4]^{2-}$ (b) VO_4^{3-}
(c) WO_4^{2-} (d) CrO_4^{2-}

74. $K_2Cr_2O_7$ in acidic medium converts into
(a) Cr^{2+} (b) Cr^{3+}
(c) Cr^{4+} (d) Cr^{5+}

75. Which of the following is not a green house gas?
(a) Hydrogen (b) Carbon dioxide
(c) Methane
(d) Nitrous oxide or N_2O

76. Phenol (OH on benzene ring) $\xrightarrow{\text{dil. } HNO_3}$ *A* (Major product)

A is

(a) OH, NO_2 (ortho-nitrophenol) (b) OH, NO_2 (para-nitrophenol)

(c) OH, NO_2, NO_2 (2,4-dinitrophenol) (d) OH, NO_2 (meta-nitrophenol)

77. Which of the following is a non-reducing sugar?
(a) Sucrose (b) Maltose
(c) Lactose (d) Mannose

78. Arrange the following compounds in increasing order of reactivity towards nucleophilic addition reaction.

(I) $C_6H_5COCH_3$ (II) $CH_3CO-C_2H_5$
(III) C_6H_5CHO (IV) $Cl-CH_2-CHO$
(a) IV > III > II > I (b) IV > II > III > I
(c) I > II > III > IV (c) III > IV > II > I

79. Toluene ($C_6H_5CH_3$) $\xrightarrow[\text{(ii) } Ac_2O/H_3O^{\oplus}]{\text{(i) } CrO_3}$ *A*; Product *A* is

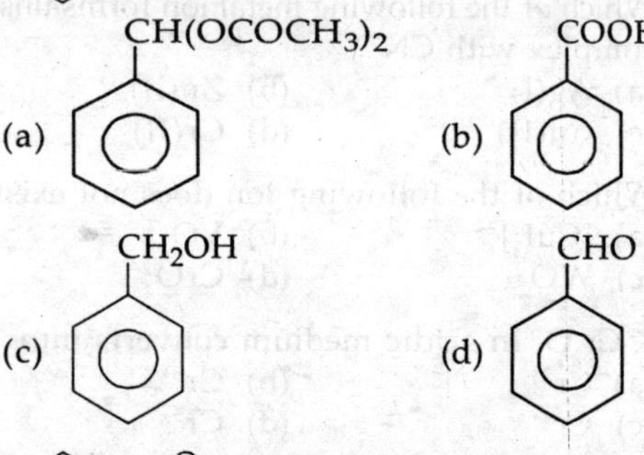

(a) $C_6H_5CH(OCOCH_3)_2$ (b) C_6H_5COOH
(c) $C_6H_5CH_2OH$ (d) C_6H_5CHO

80. 1,3-Benzodioxole $\xrightarrow[\Delta]{\text{HI (excess)}}$

(a) 2-hydroxybenzyl alcohol (OH, CH_2OH on benzene) + CH_2I_2
(b) 2-iodobenzyl iodide (I, CH_2-I on benzene) + HCHO
(c) 2-(iodomethyl)phenol (OH, CH_2-I on benzene) + $I-CH_2-OH$
(d) 2-iodobenzyl alcohol (I, CH_2OH on benzene) + $I_2 + CH_3OH$

81. Which of the following reaction will not produce ethylene glycol?

(a) CH_2-CH_2 (epoxide, O bridging) $\xrightarrow[\text{heat}]{H_3O^+}$

(b) $ClCH_2CH_2Cl \xrightarrow[\text{heat}]{OH^-}$

(c) $HO-CH_2-CH_2-OCH_3 \xrightarrow[\text{heat}]{OH^-}$

(d) $CH_2=CH_2 \xrightarrow[KMnO_4]{\text{alkaline}}$

82. Salicylic acid can be easily prepared by reaction between

(a) phenol and CO_2
(b) benzoic acid and H_2O_2
(c) benzene diazonium chloride and CO_2
(d) phenol and formic acid.

83. Reaction of aniline with HNO_2 followed by treatment of dilute acid gives

(a) C_6H_5NHOH (b) C_6H_5OH
(c) $C_6H_5NHNH_2$ (d) C_6H_6

84. Which of the following will give carbylamine test?

(a) CH_3NH_2 (b) CH_3NHCH_3
(c) $CH_3N(CH_3)CH_3$ (d) CH_3CONH_2

85. When *trans*-2-butene is reacted with Br_2 then product formed is

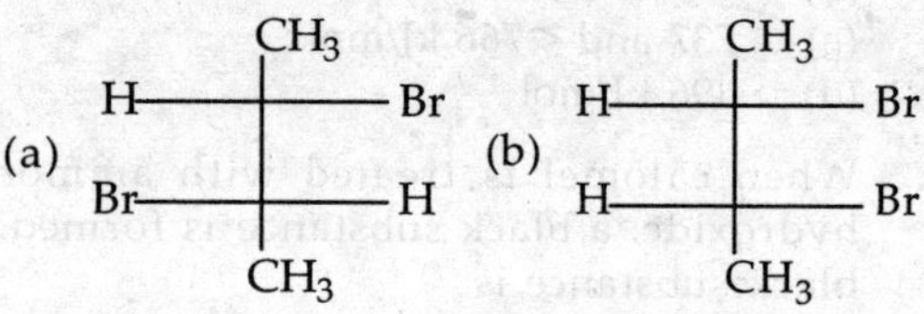

(a) Fischer projection: top CH_3; H—Br; Br—H; bottom CH_3 (b) Fischer projection: top CH_3; H—Br; H—Br; bottom CH_3

(c) Meso compounds (d) both (b) and (c)

86. Which of the following does not give nitroalkane?

(a) $CH_3-N(CH_3)-CH_3 \xrightarrow{KMnO_4}$

(b) $C_2H_5I \xrightarrow{\text{alc. } AgNO_2}$

(c) $CH_3-CH_3 \xrightarrow{\text{Fuming } HNO_3}$

(d) Both (a) and (b)

87. A compound containing two –OH groups attached with one carbon atom is unstable but which one of the following is stable?

(a) $CH_3CH(OH)_2$ (b) $CH_3-C(OH)_3$

(c) $Cl_3CH(OH)_2$ (d) None of these.

88. Which of the following is true for an ideal solution?

(a) $\Delta H_{(mix)} = 0$ (b) $\Delta S_{(mix)} = 0$
(c) $\Delta G_{(mix)} = 0$ (d) None of these

89. Boiling point of benzene is 353.23 K. When 1.8 g of non-volatile solute is dissolved in 90 g of benzene. Then boiling point is raised to 354.11 K. Given K_b (benzene) = 2.53 kg mol^{-1}. The molecular mass of non-volatile substance is

(a) 58 g mol^{-1} (b) 120 g mol^{-1}
(c) 116 g mol^{-1} (d) 60 g mol^{-1}.

90. In a solid, atom M occupies *ccp* lattice and 1/3rd of tetrahedral voids are occupied by atom N. Find the formula of solid formed by M and N.

(a) M_3N_2 (b) M_2N_3
(c) M_4N_3 (d) M_3N_4

91. Hair cream is

(a) gel (b) emulsion
(c) solid sol (d) sol.

92. A particle is moving 3 times faster than the speed of electron. If the ratio of wavelength of particle and electron is 1.8×10^{-4}, then particle is

(a) Neutron (b) α-particle
(c) Deuteron (d) Tritium

93. Electrode potential of hydrogen electrode is 18 mV, then $[H^+]$ is

(a) 0.2 (b) 1
(c) 2 (d) 5

94. What will be the solubility product of AX_3?

(a) $27S^4$ (b) $4S^3$
(c) $36S^4$ (d) $9S^3$

95. Which thermodynamic parameter is not a state function?

(a) q at constant pressure
(b) q at constant volume
(c) W at adiabatic
(d) W at isothermal

96. According to Hardy schulze law, the flocculating power of an ion increases with

(a) decreases in size
(b) increase in size
(c) decrease in charge
(d) increase in charge.

97. Strength of H_2O_2 is 15.18 g L^{-1}, then it is equal to

(a) 1 volume (b) 10 volume
(c) 5 volume (d) 7 volume

98. Energy of activation of forward reaction for an endothermic process is 50 kJ. If enthalpy change for forward reaction is 20 kJ then enthalpy change for backward reaction will be

(a) 30 kJ (b) 20 kJ
(c) 70 kJ (d) 50 kJ

99. What is the role of aniline or cresol when added in a froth floatation process?

(a) Stabilizer (b) Depressant
(c) Wetting agent (d) All of these.

100. Non-stick cookwares generally have a coating of a polymer, whose monomer is

(a) $CH_2=CH_2$ (b) $CH_2=CHCN$
(c) $CH_2=CHCl$ (d) $CF_2=CF_2$

Directions : In the following questions (101-120), a statement of assertion (A) is followed by a statement of reason (R). Mark the correct choice as :

(a) If both assertion and reason are true and reason is the correct explanation of assertion.
(b) If both assertion and reason are true but reason is not the correct explanation of assertion.
(c) If assertion is true but reason is false.
(d) If both assertion and reason are false.

101. Assertion : Bond dissociation energy is $F_2 > Cl_2$.
Reason : Cl_2 has more electronic repulsion than F_2.

102. Assertion : Bond lengths of P$-$Cl bonds in gaseous PCl_5 and solid PCl_5 are not equal.
Reason : Because in solid state two PCl_5 molecules are associated.

103. Assertion : EDTA forms complex with divalent metals of 3*d*-series in the ratio of 1:1
Reason : EDTA has 4 $-$COOH groups.

104. Assertion : In a mixture of Cd(II) and Cu(II), Cd^{2+} gets precipitated in presence of KCN by H_2S.
Reason : The stability constant of $[Cu(CN)_4]^{3-}$ is greater than $[Cd(CN)_4]^{2-}$.

105. Assertion : Aq. solution of $CoCl_2$ is pink in colour. It turns blue in presence of conc. HCl.

Reason : It is due to the formation of $[CoCl_4]^{2-}$.

106. Assertion : Acetamide on reaction with KOH and bromine gives acetic acid.

Reason : Bromine catalyses hydrolysis of acetamide.

107. Assertion : Mixture of benzaldehyde and acetaldehyde in hot alkaline medium gives cinnamaldehyde.

Reason : Benzaldehyde is strong electrophile than acetaldehyde.

108. Assertion : *cis*-3-chloroprop-2-enoic acid is less stable than its *trans*-form.

Reason : Dipole moment of *cis*-form is greater than *trans*-form.

109. Assertion : Aryl sulphonic acid gives phenol on reacting with NaOH at high temperature.

Reason : This reaction is electrophilic substitution reaction.

110. Assertion : All enzymes are made up of proteins and all proteins have three dimensional structures.

Reason : Secondary structures of protein are sequence of amino acids.

111. Assertion : The presence of a large number of Schottky defects in NaCl lowers its density.

Reason : In NaCl, there are approximately 10^6 Schottky pairs per cm^3 at room temperature.

112. Assertion : For an isolated system, q is zero.

Reason : In an isolated system, change in U and V is zero.

113. Assertion : At critical point the densities of substance in gaseous and liquid states are same.

Reason : Critical temperature is the temperature at which the real gas exhibit ideal behaviour for considerable range of pressure.

114. Assertion : Entropy of system increases for a spontaneous reaction.

Reason : Enthalpy of reaction always decreases for spontaneous reaction.

115. Assertion : Catalyst changes Gibbs free energy of system.

Reason : Catalyst changes pre-exponential factor of a chemical reaction.

116. Assertion : A process is called adiabatic if the system does not exchange heat with the surroundings.

Reason : It does not not involve increase or decrease in temperature of the system.

117. Assertion : Number of radial and angular nodes for $3p$-orbital are 1, 1 respectively.

Reason : Number of radial and angular nodes depends only on principal quantum number.

118. Assertion : Cu is stronger reducing agent than H_2.

Reason : $E°$ of Cu^{2+}/Cu is negative.

119. Assertion : Magnesium is extracted by the electrolysis of fused mixture of $MgCl_2$, NaCl and $CaCl_2$.

Reason : Calcium chloride acts as a reducing agent.

120. Assertion : Phosphoric acid has no reducing properties.

Reason : Phosphoric acid does not contain P—H bonds.

BIOLOGY

121. Stinging capsules (nematocysts) are found in
(a) wasp and honeybee
(b) scorpion and cobra
(c) sea pen and sea fan
(d) cactus and Venus flytrap.

122. Which of the following is a cloning vector?
(a) DNA of *Salmonella typhimurium*
(b) *Ti* plasmid
(c) Amp^r and Tet^r loci
(d) *Ori* minus pBR322

123. India is one of the twelve megadiversity countries with ____ of genetic resources of the world.
(a) 12.1% (b) 18.1% (c) 38.1% (d) 8.1%

124. Which of the following is not an invasive species?
(a) *Parthenium hysterophorus*
(b) *Nelumbo* (lotus)
(c) *Lantana camara* (d) *Eichhornia crassipes*

125. Intercalated discs are characteristic of muscles found in
(a) heart (b) thigh
(c) urinary bladder (d) stomach.

126. In which of the following sets of organisms, does the external fertilization occur?
(a) Echinodermata and mosses
(b) Hemichordata and ferns
(c) Amphibians and algae
(d) Reptiles and gymnosperms

127. Starting from the maximum, arrange the following male reproductive accessory organs in the correct order, based on the amount of secretion poured into urethra.
(i) Prostrate gland
(ii) Seminal vesicle
(iii) Bulbourethral gland
(a) (i) > (ii) > (iii) (b) (iii) > (ii) > (i)
(c) (ii) > (iii) > (i) (d) (ii) > (i) > (iii)

128. Which of the following contraceptive devices make uterus unsuitable for implantation?
(a) Progestasert (b) CuT
(c) Lippe's loop (d) Multiload

129. In Miller's experiment, he used a mixture of CH_4, NH_3, H_2 and water vapour in a closed flask to mimic early earth conditions. What was the temperature at which this flask was kept?
(a) 800°C (b) 1200°C (c) 200°C (d) 400°C

130. Sexual stage (gametocytes) of *Plasmodium* occurs in
(a) Salivary glands of mosquito
(b) Human RBC
(c) Intestine of mosquito
(d) Human liver

131. Occurrence of triploid (3n) primary endosperm nucleus is a characteristic feature of
(a) Algae (b) Gymnosperms
(c) Angiosperms (d) Bryophytes.

132. From the following groups, select the one which has only secondary metabolites?
(a) Arbrin, cellulose, arginine, tyrosine
(b) Glycine, gums, serine, diterpenes
(c) Carotenoids, phenylalanine, curcumin, rubber
(d) Conclavin-A, morphine, codeine, vinblastin

133. In a diploid cell, at which stage of cell cycle, the amount of DNA is doubled?
(a) G_1 and G_2 phase (b) G_0 phase
(c) S, G_2 and M phase (d) S phase

134. Sporopollenin is a constituent of pollen exine. It can be degraded by the action of
(a) enzymes (b) high temperature
(c) strong acids
(d) cannot be degraded.

135. The pollen grains of rice and wheat lose their viability in ___ minutes of their release.
(a) 30 (b) 10 (c) 60 (d) 90

136. After double fertilization, a mature ovule has
(a) 1 diploid and 1 haploid cell
(b) 1 diploid and 1 triploid cell
(c) 2 haploid and 1 triploid cell
(d) 1 haploid and 1 triploid cell.

137. Genetically modified (GM) crops can be produced by
(a) recombinant DNA technology
(b) somatic hybridization
(c) cross breeding (d) micropropagation.

138. Which of the following is a palindromic sequence?
(a) 5′ - CGTATG - 3′ (b) 5′ - CGAATG - 3′
3′ - GCATAC - 5′ 3′ - CGAATG - 5′
(c) 5′ - GAATTC - 3′ (d) 5′ - GACTAC - 3′
3′ - CTTAAG - 5′ 3′ - TACGAC - 5′

139. C_4 plants have better productivity because
(a) C_4 plants absorb more light
(b) C_4 plants absorb more CO_2
(c) C_4 plants does not carry photorespiration
(d) C_4 plants have more amount of RuBisCO.

140. Match the source gland with its respective hormone and function and select the correct option.

	Source gland	Hormone	Function
(a)	Anterior pitutary	Oxytocin	Contraction of uterine muscles
(b)	Anterior pitutary	Vasopressin	Induces reabsorption of water in nephron
(c)	Thymus	Thymosin	Proliferation of T-lymphocytes
(d)	α-cells of islets of Langerhans	Glucagon	Uptake of glucose into the cell.

141. Which of the following microbes is correctly paired with its function?

(a) *Aspergillus niger* – Production of lactic acid
(b) *Trichoderma polysporum* – Lowers blood cholesterol
(c) *Saccharomyces cerevisiae* – Production of citric acid
(d) Methanogenic bacteria – Gobar gas formation

142. Match Column - I with Column - II and select the correct option from the codes given below.

	Column - I		Column - II
A.	Chlorophyta	(i)	*Equisetum*
B.	Lycopsida	(ii)	*Chara*
C.	Phaeophyta	(iii)	*Selaginella*
D.	Sphenopsida	(iv)	*Ectocarpus*

(a) A - (ii), B - (iii), C - (iv), D - (i)
(b) A - (iv), B - (i), C - (ii), D - (iii)
(c) A - (ii), B - (iii), C - (i), D - (iv)
(d) A - (iv), B - (i), C - (iii), D - (ii)

143. Which of the following gastric secretions is correctly matched with its source?

(a) Pepsin – Chief cells
(b) Chymotrypsin – Parietal cells
(c) HCl – Goblet cells
(d) Mucus – Oxyntic cells

144. Which of the following is true for a recessive disease in family A and B?

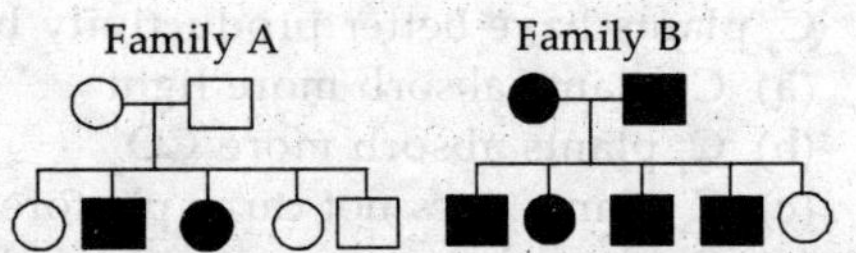

(a) In family A, both the parents are homozygous recessive.
(b) In family B, both the parents are homozygous dominant.
(c) In family B, both the parents are heterozygous recessive.
(d) In family A, both the parents are heterozygous recessive.

145. Which of the following is true for excretion in humans?

(a) Glucose and amino acids are reabsorbed in PCT by simple diffusion.
(b) DCT is impermeable to water.
(c) On an average, 25-30 gm of urea is excreted out per day.
(d) Maximum reabsorption occurs in the loop of Henle.

146. Which of the following is not true for inbreeding?

(a) It causes inbreeding depression after a few generations.
(b) It always increases the productivity.
(c) It is used to produce a pure line.
(d) It leads to homozygosity.

147. Which of the following is the correct floral formula for the floral diagram given below?

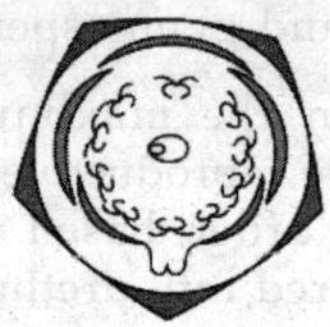

(a) Br $\oplus$ ⚥ Epi $K_{5 \text{ or } (5)} \widehat{C_5 A}_{(\infty)} \underline{G}_{(2\ \infty)}$
(b) $\oplus$ ⚥ $K_{(5)} \widehat{C_5 A}_{(5)} \underline{G}_{(2)}$
(c) % ⚥ $K_{(5)} C_{1+2+(2)} A_{(9)+1} \underline{G}_1$
(d) $\oplus$ ⚥ $\widehat{P_{3+3 \text{ or } (3+3)} A}_{3+3} \underline{G}_{(3)}$

148. Which of the following is true for the function of labelled parts in the diagram below?

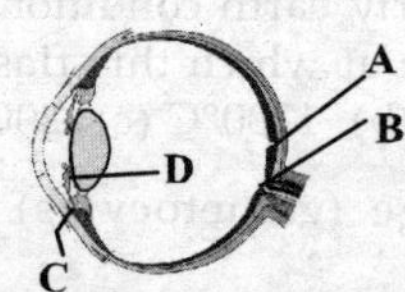

(a) **A** - Blind spot – Image is formed here
(b) **B** - Fovea – No visual activity is present
(c) **C** - Cornea – Helps to hold lens in place
(d) **D** - Iris – Visible coloured portion of eye

149. Which of the following is true for the labelled parts in the figure below?

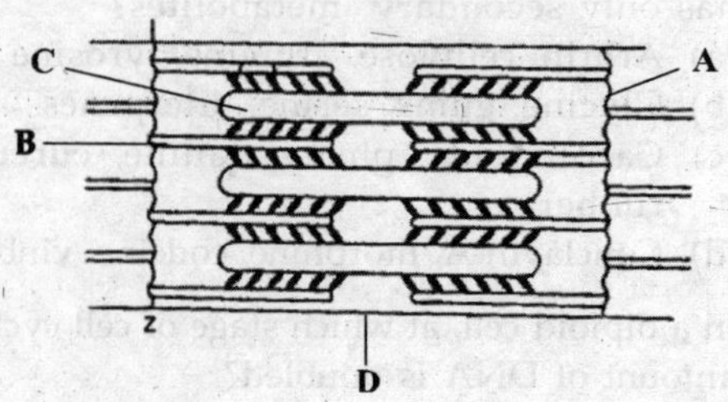

(a) **A** - Z-line – located at centre of I - band
(b) **B** - Thin filament – occurs in A-band only
(c) **C** - Thick filament – confined to I-band
(d) **D** - H-zone – located at centre of M-line

150. Which of the following is correctly matched without exception in regard to plant classification?
(a) Family – Poaceae - ae
(b) Division – Pteridophyta - phyta
(c) Class – Bryopsida - sida
(d) Genus – *Solanum* - um

151. What is the oxidation state of iron in haemoglobin?
(a) Fe^- (b) Fe^{2+}
(c) Fe^{3+} (d) Fe^{4+}

152. In the given table, some organisms are classified into categories. However, there is one exception. Select the option with correctly mentioned exceptional organism.

	Organisms	Category	Exception
(a)	*Penicillium, Aspergillus, Mucor*	Fungi	Mucor
(b)	Cacti, Venus flytrap	Plants	Cacti
(c)	*Ascaris, Neresis, Wuchereria*	Aschelminthes	*Neresis*
(d)	Scorpion, Prawn, *Anopheles*	Arthropoda	Prawn

153. Select the correct pair amongst the following.
(a) Spring wood – light colour, high density
(b) Spring wood – dark colour, low density
(c) Autumn wood – light colour, high density
(d) Autumn wood – dark colour, high density.

154. Which of the following organelles contain DNA?
(i) Mitochondria (ii) Chloroplasts (iii) Golgi bodies (iv) Ribosomes
(a) (i) and (ii)
(b) (ii) and (iii)
(c) (i) only
(d) (iv) only.

155. Carbon dioxide (CO_2) diffuses into blood from tissue site and passes to alveolar site in the form of
(a) bicarbonate; 70%
(b) bicarbonate; 20 – 25%
(c) carbaminohaemoglobin; 60 – 70%
(d) carbaminohaemoglobin; 7%.

156. Select the option having all the correct characteristics.

	Structure	Percentage of WBCs	Function
(a)	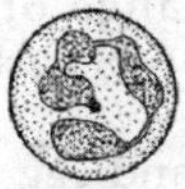	0.3 – 0.5	Phagocytic
(b)	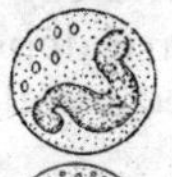	0.5 – 1.0	Secrete histamine and serotonin
(c)	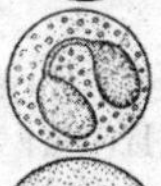	30 – 40	Defence against parasites
(d)	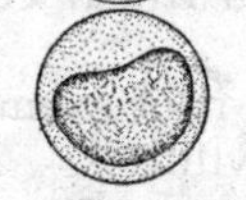	30 – 40	Allergic reactions

157. Chromatin is made up of:
(a) DNA and protein
(b) DNA and histone
(c) DNA, RNA, protein
(d) RNA, histone and oil bodies.

158. A large quantity of urban sewage is drained to nearby village river. Which among the given conditions would happen after mixing of sewage into the river?
(i) Biochemical oxygen demand (BOD) of receiving water body increases.
(ii) Dissolved oxygen of receiving water body decreases.
(iii) It will not cause mortality among fishes and other aquatic creatures.
(iv) It will lead to nutrient enrichment of receiving water body.
(a) (i), (ii) and (iii) (b) (i), (ii) and (iv)
(c) (ii) and (iii) (d) (iii) and (iv).

159. Which of the following plant growth regulators (PGRs) promotes root initiation, flowering and induced parthenocarpy?
(a) Gibberellin (b) Auxin
(c) Cytokinin (d) Ethylene.

160. Which of the following is a secondary pollutant?
(a) Carbon dioxide
(b) Nitrogen oxides
(c) Peroxyacyl nitrates
(d) All of these.

Directions : In the following questions (161-180), a statement of assertion (A) is followed by a statement of reason (R). Mark the correct choice as :

(a) If both assertion and reason are true and reason is the correct explanation of assertion.

(b) If both assertion and reason are true but reason is not the correct explanation of assertion.

(c) If assertion is true but reason is false.

(d) If both assertion and reason are false.

161. Assertion : A mutual exchange of sperms occurs between two earthworms during mating.

Reason : Mature sperms and egg cells and nutritive fluid are deposited in cocoons produced by gland cells of clitellum.

162. Assertion : On plotting the length of the root against time, a linear curve is obtained.

Reason : An elongating root exemplifies arithmetic growth.

163. Assertion : Small intestine is the principal organ for absorption of nutrients.

Reason : Absorption of water, simple sugars and alcohol etc. takes place in small intestine.

164. Assertion : On touching radial artery in our wrist, we feel pulse waves.

Reason : The heart beats originate from the sinoatrial node (SA node) on the right atrium.

165. Assertion : In a regular medical examination of a small population, a 35 years old lady was found to have higher levels of oestrogens, progesterone in her blood.

Reason : The lady is 12 weeks pregnant.

166. Assertion : While working on *Staphylococci*, Alexander Fleming observed that *Penicillium notatum* inhibits the growth of the bacteria.

Reason : This inhibiting chemical was commercially extracted and its full potential was established by Alexander Fleming.

167. Assertion : *Saccharomyces cerevisiae* produces acetic acid.

Reason : *Trichoderma polysporum* produces blood cholestrol lowering agent.

168. Assertion : Protostele is the simplest stele.

Reason : Protostele is the most advanced type of stele.

169. Assertion : Rice field is an ecosystem for plants and animals.

Reason : Gut of human/animals is an ecosystem for flora and fauna.

170. Assertion : Mitochondria and chloroplasts have their own genome.

Reason : Endoplasmic reticulum and Golgi body are the cell organelles which have their own DNA.

171. Assertion : Now-a-days, the biodiversity is declining with an accelerated rate.

Reason : Exotic species are considered to be a major cause of extinction of species.

172. Assertion : Meiosis II is similar to mitosis.

Reason : Meiosis I cannot occur in haploid cells.

173. Assertion : Periodic abstinence is a natural method where couples abstain from coitus

Reason : Coitus from day 5–10 should be avoided because this is the time of ovulation.

174. Assertion : Corpus callosum connects the two cerebral hemispheres.

Reason : Association areas are responsible for complex functions like intersensory association of memory and communication.

175. Assertion : Only a boy child could be born with a substitution of glutamic acid by valine on 6th codon of beta-chain of haemoglobin.

Reason : The gene for the above mutation is found on Y-chromosome.

176. Assertion : The efficiency of C_4 plant is more than those of C_3 plant.

Reason : C_4 plants are more efficient in picking CO_2.

177. Assertion : Cattles feed on leaves of maize to get nutrition for growth and development.

Reason : A number of symbiotic bacteria are present in rumen of cattle.

178. Assertion : All proteinecous enzymes have a three-dimensional structure.

Reason : The secondary structure of protein is according to amino acid present inside the polypeptides.

179. Assertion : Glutamine contains amide group.

Reason : Isoelectric point of glutamine is 7.

180. Assertion : Duodenum is the main organ of small intestine.

Reason : In duodenum, digestion and absorption mainly occurs.

GENERAL KNOWLEDGE

181. From whom does the Indian government take advice on legal issues?
(a) Chief Justice of Court apex
(b) Solicitor General
(c) Chairman of Planning Commission
(d) Attorney General

182. The Vice President of India is the Chairman of
(a) Lok Sabha (b) Rajya Sabha
(c) Vidhan Sabha
(d) Legislative Assembly

183. Which of the following players won Miami Men's Double tennis – 2012 title?
(a) Daniel Nestor and Radek Stepanek
(b) Radek Stepanek and Leander Paes
(c) Daniel Nestor and Max Mirnyi
(d) Rohan Bopanna and Mahesh Bhupathi

184. Which ancient Indian sage authored 'Yog Sutra'?
(a) Patanjali (b) Kapil Muni
(c) Saatchi dananda (d) Gautam

185. Which Indian Mathematician first time in the world used zero as a number and showed its mathematical operation?
(a) Aryabhatt (b) Ramanuja
(c) Bhaskaracharya (d) Brahmagupta

186. Which Indian freedom fighter was popularly called "Mahamana"?
(a) Bal Gangadhar Tilak
(b) Madan Mohan Malviya
(c) Jawahar lal Nehru
(d) Mahatma Gandhi

187. The book "Big Egos, Small Men" is written by
(a) Mani Shankar Aiyr
(b) Kapil Sibal
(c) Ram Jethmalani (d) Soli Sorabjee

188. Which is the largest buddhist monastery in India?
(a) Rumtek Monastery, Sikkim
(b) Tawang Monastery, Arunachal Pradesh
(c) Thiksey Monastery, Jammu and Kashmir
(d) Ghoom Monastery, West Bengal

189. 'Van Mahotsav' Day is observed on
(a) 1st December (b) 1st July
(c) 23rd February (d) 14th March

190. The famous Kashi Vishwanath temple at Varanasi is dedicated to which Hindu god?
(a) Lord Shiva (b) Lord Vishnu
(c) Lord Brahma (d) Lord Krishna

191. Which Indian State celebrated its 77th foundation day on 1st April, 2013?
(a) Guajrat (b) Odisha
(c) Rajasthan (d) Tamil Nadu

192. According to Mahabharat who constructed the unparalled palace of the Pandavas?
(a) Vishwakarma (b) Krishna
(c) Indra (d) Maya Danava

193. Where was first share market of India established?
(a) Mumbai (b) Kolkata
(c) Delhi (d) Chennai

194. Garampani Sanctuary is located at
(a) Diphu, Assam (b) Junagarh, Gujrat
(c) Kohima, Nagaland
(d) Gangtok, Sikkim

195. Maximum sugarcane production occurs in which country?
(a) India (b) China
(c) Brazil (d) Indonesia

196. Which of the following is not a green house gas?
(a) Carbon dioxide (CO_2)
(b) Nitrous oxide (N_2O)
(c) Methane (CH_4)
(d) Hydrogen (H_2)

197. Which first woman singer got the Bharat Ratna award and is also known as nightingale of carnatic music?

(a) M.S. Subbulaxmi (b) Shubha Mudgal
(c) N. Rajam (d) Vasundhara Devi

198. For seeing objects on the surface of water from submarine, the instrument used is
(a) kaleidoscope (b) periscope
(c) telescope (d) spectroscope

199. Under the tenure of which Prime Minister did Indo-Pak war (1965) take place which ended with Tashkent Treaty?
(a) Lal Bahadur Shastri
(b) Jawaharlal Nehru
(c) Gulzarilal Nanda (d) Morarji Desai

200. A famous writer who travelled to India with Mahmood Ghazni and wrote a book "Tareekh-al-Hind"
(a) Abdul Hai Lakhnawi
(b) Al - Biruni
(c) Riyad-us-Saliheen
(d) Ibn Kathir

SOLUTIONS

PHYSICS

1. **(a) :** A space wave travels in a straight line from transmitting antenna to the receiving antenna. Space waves are used for line of sight communication as well as satellite communication.

2. **(d) :** In nuclear fission or fusion both energy and mass are conserved.

3. **(b) :** Number of fission per second

$$= \frac{\text{total power}}{\text{energy/fission}}.$$

Here, total power = 100 W

energy/fission = 200 MeV = $200 \times 10^6 \times 1.6 \times 10^{-19}$ J
$= 3.2 \times 10^{-11}$ J.

$$\therefore \quad \text{fission rate} = \frac{100}{3.2 \times 10^{-11}} = 3.1 \times 10^{12}\ \text{s}^{-1}$$

4. **(c) :** From figure,

$$\therefore \quad T \sin\theta = \frac{mv^2}{r}$$

θ, $T\cos\theta$, r, O, $T\sin\theta$, mg

5. **(d)**

6. **(a) :** de brogile wavelength, $\lambda = \frac{h}{p}$

or $\lambda = \frac{h}{mv}$

$$\therefore \quad \frac{\lambda_p}{\lambda_e} = \frac{m_e v_e}{m_p v_p}$$

$$\Rightarrow \quad m_p = \frac{m_e v_e}{v_p} \times \frac{\lambda_e}{\lambda_p}$$

Here, $m_e = 9.1 \times 10^{-31}$ kg, $v_p = 3v_e$

and $\frac{\lambda_p}{\lambda_e} = 1.814 \times 10^{-4}$

$$\therefore \quad m_p = \frac{9.1 \times 10^{-31}}{1.814 \times 10^{-4} \times 3} = 1.672 \times 10^{-27}\ \text{kg}$$

Thus, the particle is neutron.

7. **(d)**

8. **(a) :** Angular momentum = moment of inertia × angular velocity

$= [ML^2] \times [T^{-1}] = [ML^2T^{-1}]$.

9. **(a) :** Magnetic moment,

$$M = IA = I(\pi r^2) = \frac{q}{T} \times \pi r^2 \qquad (\because q = It).$$

As $\omega = \frac{2\pi}{T}$

$$\therefore \quad M = \frac{q\omega r^2}{2}$$

or $M \propto \omega$

10. **(c)**

11. **(b) :** If a point mass m is placed at a height h from surface of earth, the potential energy is

$$U_h = -\frac{GMm}{(R+h)} = \frac{-gR^2m}{R\left(1+\frac{h}{R}\right)} = \frac{-gR^2m}{R}\left(1+\frac{h}{R}\right)^{-1}$$

$$\left(\because g = \frac{GM}{R^2}\right)$$

$$U_h = \frac{-gR^2m(R-h)}{R^2}$$

$= -gm(R-h)$

$$\therefore \quad V = \frac{U_h}{m} = \frac{-gm(R-h)}{m} = -g(R-h)$$

12. **(a) :** To reduce the eddy currents in the metal armature of motors the wire is wrapped around a number of thin metal sheets called lamination.

13. **(c)**

14. **(d)**

15. **(b) :** For mixture of gases,

$$C_V = \frac{\frac{3}{2}R + \frac{5}{2}R}{1+1} = 2R$$

$$C_P = 2R + R = 3R$$

$$\therefore \quad \frac{C_P}{C_V} = \frac{3}{2}\frac{R}{R} = 1.5$$

16. **(d)**

17. **(c)** :According to first law of thermodynamics

$\Delta Q = \Delta U + P\Delta V$

If ΔQ is absorbed at constant volume, $\Delta V = 0$

$$C_V = \left(\frac{\Delta Q}{\Delta T}\right)_V = \left(\frac{\Delta U}{\Delta T}\right)_V = \frac{\Delta U}{\Delta T}$$

for an ideal monoatomic gas

$$\frac{\Delta U}{\Delta T} = \frac{3}{2}R;\ C_V = \frac{3}{2}R$$

18. **(a)** : Torque, $\vec{\tau} = \vec{r} \times \vec{F}$

$$= (\hat{i}+\hat{j}-\hat{k}) \times (5\hat{i}+7\hat{j}-3\hat{k})$$

$$= \hat{i}(-3+7) - \hat{j}(-3+5) + \hat{k}(7-5)$$

$$\vec{\tau} = 4\hat{i} - 2\hat{j} + 2\hat{k}$$

19. **(a)** : In physics (namely astrophysics), redshift happens when light or other electromagnetic radiation from an object moving away from the observer is increased in wavelength or shifted to the red end of the spectrum.

20. **(b)** : Sky waves are of practical importance of large distance communication.

21. **(d)**

22. **(b)** : Restoring force is produced by inductor as it acts as a source of energy.

23. **(a)** : Polaroid glass is used in sun glasses because it reduces the light intensity to half on account of polarisation.

24. **(c)** : A free neutron is unstable $(n \rightarrow p + \bar{e} + \bar{\nu})$. But a simlar free proton decay is not possible, since a proton is (slightly) lighter than a neutron.

25. **(d)** : From Gauss's law, E is independent of r.

26. **(a)** : Using, $\sigma = n_e q \mu_e$

Here, $\sigma = 500$ mho/m

$e = 1.6 \times 10^{-19}$ C

$\mu_e = 0.4\ \text{m}^2\ \text{V}^{-1}\ \text{s}^{-1}$

$$\therefore \quad n_e = \frac{500}{1.6 \times 10^{-19} \times 0.4}$$

$$= 7.8 \times 10^{21} \simeq 8 \times 10^{21}\ \text{m}^{-3}$$

27. **(b)** **28.** **(b)**

29. **(c)** : As simple pendulum performs simple harmonic motion.

$\therefore$ velocity, $v = \omega\sqrt{a^2 - x^2}$

At, $x = \frac{a}{2}$

$$v = \frac{2\pi}{T}\sqrt{a^2 - \left(\frac{a}{2}\right)^2} = \frac{2\pi}{T}\frac{\sqrt{3a^2}}{2} = \frac{\pi a\sqrt{3}}{T}$$

30. **(c)** : From figure,

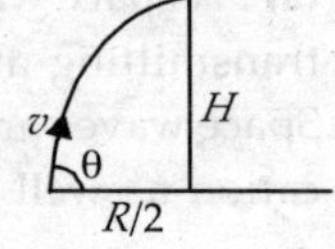

average velocity,

$$v_{av} = \frac{\sqrt{H^2 + R^2/4}}{T/2} \quad ...(i)$$

Here, $H = \frac{u^2 \sin^2\theta}{2g}$

$$R = \frac{u^2 \sin 2\theta}{g} \text{ and } T = \frac{2u\sin\theta}{g}$$

Putting these value in (i), we get

$$v_{av} = \frac{v}{2}\sqrt{1 + 3\cos^2\theta}$$

31. **(b)** : Using, $\mu = \frac{c}{v}$

Here, $c = 3 \times 10^8\ \text{m s}^{-1}$

$v = \upsilon\lambda = 2 \times 10^{14}\ \text{Hz} \times 5000 \times 10^{-10}\ \text{m}$

$= 1 \times 10^8\ \text{m s}^{-1}$

$$\therefore \quad \mu = \frac{3 \times 10^8\ \text{m s}^{-1}}{1 \times 10^8\ \text{m s}^{-1}} = 3$$

32. **(a)** : For solenoids, self inductance is given by,

$$L = \frac{\mu_0 N^2 A}{l}$$

$$\therefore \quad \frac{L_1}{L_2} = \frac{\left(\frac{\pi r_1^2}{l_1}\right)}{\left(\frac{\pi r_2^2}{l_2}\right)} = \frac{\left(\frac{r_1^2}{l_1}\right)}{\left(\frac{r_2^2}{l_1}\right)}$$

$$\text{or} \quad \frac{L_1}{L_2} = \frac{1}{2} \quad \left(\because \frac{r_1^2}{l_1} \Big/ \frac{r_2^2}{l_2} = 1/2\right)$$

33. **(b)** :

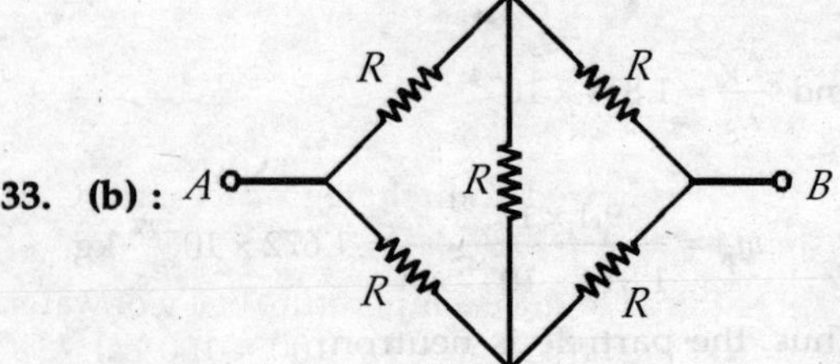

Equivalent circuit,

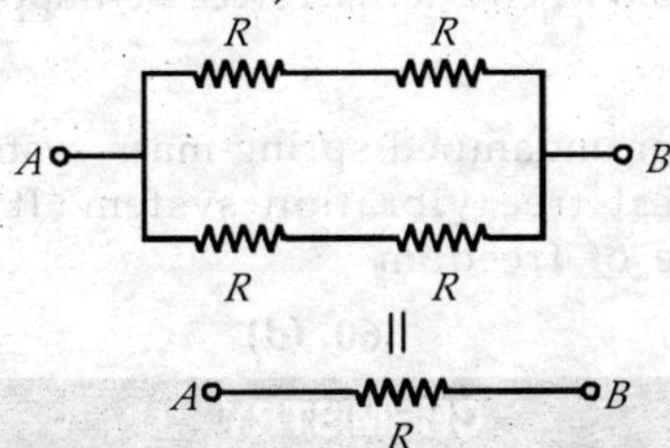

34. **(a) :** From circuit diagram,

A, B → $\overline{A+B}$ → $\overline{A+B}$ → $\overline{A+B}$

Output, $Y = \overline{A+B}$

Thus, circuit behave like NOR gate.

35. **(c) :** Using, $\eta = 1 - \frac{T_2}{T_1}$

or $\frac{T_2}{T_1} = 1 - \eta$

According to first case

$$\frac{T_2}{T_1} = 1 - \frac{1}{6} = \frac{5}{6} \quad \text{...(i)}$$

According to second case

$$\frac{T_2 - 62}{T_1} = 1 - 2 \times \frac{1}{6} = \frac{2}{3} \quad \text{...(ii)}$$

$$\frac{T_2}{T_1} - \frac{62}{T_1} = \frac{2}{3}$$

From equations (i) and (ii), we get

$$\frac{5}{6} - \frac{62}{T_1} = \frac{2}{3} \Rightarrow \frac{5}{6} - \frac{2}{3} = \frac{62}{T_1}$$

$$\Rightarrow \quad \frac{1}{6} = \frac{62}{T_1}$$

$T_1 = 372$ K or $T_1 = 372 - 273$

$T_1 = 99°$C

36. **(b) :** For perpendicular vectors.

$\vec{A} \cdot \vec{B} = 0$

$$\therefore \quad (2\hat{i} + 3\hat{j} + 8\hat{k}) \cdot (4\hat{i} - 4\hat{j} + \alpha\hat{k}) = 0$$

$8 - 12 + 8\alpha = 0$

$-4 + 8\alpha = 0$

$\alpha = \frac{1}{2}$.

37. **(c) :** Heat required to melt 1 g of ice at 0°C to water at 0°C = 1 × 80 cal.

Heat required to raise temperature of 1 g of water from 0°C to 100°C = 1 × 1 × 100 = 100 cal.

Total heat required for maximum temperature of 100°C = 80 + 100 = 180 cal.

As one gram of steam gives 540 cal of heat when it is converted to water at 100°C, therefore, temperature of the mixture = 100°C.

38. **(c) :** The transition equation for Lyman series is given by

$$\frac{1}{\lambda} = R\left(\frac{1}{1^2} - \frac{1}{n^2}\right)$$

for largest wavelength, n = 2.

$$\therefore \quad \frac{1}{\lambda_{max}} = R\left(\frac{1}{1^2} - \frac{1}{2^2}\right)$$

The transition equation for Balmer series is given by

$$\frac{1}{\lambda} = R\left(\frac{1}{2^2} - \frac{1}{n^2}\right)$$

for largest wavelength, n = 3

$$\therefore \quad \frac{1}{\lambda_{max}} = R\left(\frac{1}{2^2} - \frac{1}{3^2}\right)$$

Therefore, $$\frac{\lambda_{L_{max}}}{\lambda_{B_{max}}} = \frac{\left(\frac{1}{2^2} - \frac{1}{3^2}\right)}{\left(\frac{1}{1^2} - \frac{1}{2^2}\right)} = \frac{\frac{5}{36}}{\frac{3}{4}} = \frac{5}{27}$$

39. **(d) :** Using,

$$C_P - C_V = R$$

$$\Rightarrow \quad C_V\left(\frac{C_P}{C_V} - 1\right) = R$$

$$(\gamma - 1) = \frac{R}{C_V} \quad \left[\because \quad \frac{C_P}{C_V} = \gamma\right]$$

or $$C_V = \frac{R}{(\gamma - 1)}$$

40. **(d)**

41. **(a) :** The modulation index in practice, is kept ≤ 1 to avoid distortion.

42. **(a) :** Optical density and mass density are not related to each other mass density is mass per unit volume. It is not possible that mass density of an optically denser medium may be less than that of an optically rarer medium (optical density is the ratio of the speed of light in two media). *e.g.*, turpentine and water. Mass density of turpentine is less than that of water but its optical density is higher.

43. (d)

44. (b) : When a conductor is charged the excess charge can reside only on the surface. The electric field inside conductor is zero.

45. (c) : Since the escape velocity on the surface of the moon is much less than that on earth, so the water molecules get evaporated faster.

46. (d) : The moment of inertia is not a fixed quantity but depends on the orientation and position of the axis of rotation with respect to the body as a whole.

47. (c) : The magnetic field lines form closed loops unlike electrostatic field lines which originate from the charge and end at charge. Mono-magnetic pole does not exist in nature.

48. (a)

49. (c) : The emission of γ rays by a $^{60}_{27}Co$ nucleus is subsequent to beta decay.

50. (d) : Light reflected (in the rarer medium) is completely polarised. The intensity of light does not change in polarisation.

51. (c) : A laser is a highly monochromatic and near-perfect parallel beam of light, due to which the beam can be focussed by a converging lens to a very small spot. As the intensity of the beam is too high, it can drill holes through a metal sheet even if the power is 0.2 W. But even a torch-light of 1000 W power cannot drill holes in such a metal sheet, because the light is less intense and the beam is not parallel.

52. (b) : Electromagnetic wave transport energy, momentum and information. Electromagnetic waves exert radiation pressure on surface.

53. (c)

54. (a) : The sum of all the currents directed towards a point in circuit is equal to the sum of all the currents directed away from that point. It is based on conservation of electrical energy.

55. (a) : This is because refraction through the different layers of atmosphere.

56. (d) : Centre of mass of a body is a point that moves when external forces are applied on the body as though all the mass concentrated at that point and when external forces were applied there.

57. (a)

58. (c) : An undamped spring-mass system is the simplest free vibration system. It has one degree of freedom

59. (a) **60. (d)**

CHEMISTRY

61. (b) : A straight line plot of $[A]$ *vs* t with negative slope is for a reaction of zero-order.

62. (d) : Cu has lowest melting point because it has lowest enthalpy of atomisation (*i.e.*, heat required to break the metal lattice to get free atoms) among the elements.

	Ni	> Fe	> Cr	> Cu
Enthalpy of atomisation : (in kJ mol^{-1})	430	416	397	339

63. (a) :

		No. of unpaired electrons
Gd^{3+} : $[Xe]4f^7$	1 1 1 1 1 1 1	7
Yb^{2+} : $[Xe]4f^{14}$	1l 1l 1l 1l 1l 1l 1l	0
Tb^{2+} : $[Xe]4f^9$	1l 1l 1 1 1 1 1	5
Pm^{3+} : $[Xe]4f^4$	1 1 1 1	4

64. (c) : Na, Mg, Al and Si are in period 3 and as we move across the period, the atomic size decreases and hence ionisation enthalpy increases. So, the order is Na < Mg < Al < Si Hence, *IE* of Al is greater than that of Mg (737 kJ/mol) and lower than that of Si (776 kJ/mol).

65. (c) :

$$\underset{\text{Calomel}}{Hg_2Cl_2} + 2NH_4OH \longrightarrow \underbrace{Hg\begin{matrix}NH_2\\Cl\end{matrix} + Hg}_{\text{Black}} + NH_4Cl + 2H_2O$$

66. (a) : O_2 $(\sigma1s)^2(\sigma^*1s)^2(\sigma2s)^2(\sigma^*2s)^2(\sigma2p_z)^2(\pi2p_x^2 = \pi2p_y^2)$ $(\pi^*2p_x^{\,1} = \pi^*2p_y^1)$

Thus, there are total 6 electrons in antibonding orbitals.

67. (a) : In BF_3, there is back bonding in between fluorine and boron due to presence of *p*-orbital in boron.

F, F>B—F, back bonding imparts double bond characteristics.

As BF_3 forms adduct the back bonding is no longer present and thus double bond characteristic disappears. Hence, bond becomes a bit longer than earlier (1.30 Å).

68. **(b) :** Oxidation state of iron in haemoglobin is +2.

69. **(c) :** Hydrolysis of XeF_6 is not a redox reaction. XeF_6 reacts violently with water, but slow hydrolysis by atmospheric moisture gives highly explosive solid, XeO_3.

$XeF_{6(s)} + 3H_2O_{(l)} \longrightarrow XeO_{3(s)} + 6HF_{(aq)}$

Partial hydrolysis of XeF_6 yields $XeOF_4$ and XeO_2F_2.

$XeF_6 + H_2O \longrightarrow XeOF_4 + 2HF$

$XeF_6 + 2H_2O \longrightarrow XeO_2F_2 + 4HF$

70. **(c) :** $La(OH)_3$ is the most basic as it has the largest atomic size. $Al(OH)_3$ is amphoteric in nature.

71. **(d) :** Bleaching powder is a mixture of calcium hypochlorite, $Ca(OCl)_2$ and the basic chloride $CaCl_2$, H_2O with some slaked lime, $Ca(OH)_2$.

72. **(a) :** Except Ag(I), all ions form stable complexes with CN^-.

73. **(a) :** $[CuI_4]^{2-}$ does not exist because I^- being a stronger reducing agent reduces Cu^{2+} to Cu^+.

$2CuI_2 \longrightarrow 2CuI + I_2$

74. **(b) :** $Cr_2O^{2-}_7 + 14H^+ + 6e^- \longrightarrow 2Cr^{3+} + 7H_2O$

75. **(a) :** Carbon dioxide, methane, water vapour, nitrous oxide, CFCs and ozone are green house gases.

76. **(a) :** Phenol $\xrightarrow[298\ K]{dil.HNO_3}$ o-Nitrophenol (40%, major) + p-Nitrophenol (13%, minor)

o-Nitrophenol (40%, major)

p-Nitrophenol (13%, minor)

77. **(a) :** All the monosaccharides (aldoses and ketoses) and disaccharides except sucrose reduce Fehling's solution or Tollens' reagent and hence are reducing sugars.

78. **(a) :** Two electron releasing alkyl groups in ketones make the carbon less electron deficient in comparison to aldehydes. Therefore ketones are less reactive than aldehydes towards nucleophilic addition reactions.

Aromatic aldehydes and ketones are less reactive than corresponding aliphatic aldehydes and ketones due to +*R* effect of benzene ring.

Aromatic aldehydes are more reactive than alkyl aryl ketones which in turn are more reactive than diaryl ketones.

Since –Cl is more electronegative than carbon, it increases the reactivity.

So, the order is

$\underset{(IV)}{Cl-CH_2-CHO} > \underset{(III)}{C_6H_5CHO} > \underset{(II)}{CH_3COC_2H_5} > \underset{(I)}{C_6H_5COCH_3}$

79. **(d) :**

$C_6H_5CH_3 \xrightarrow[(CH_3CO)_2O]{CrO_3,\ [O]} C_6H_5CH(OCOCH_3)_2 \xrightarrow[Hydrolysis]{OH^-/H_2O} C_6H_5CHO + 2CH_3COOH$

80. **(b) :**

1,3-Benzodioxole $\xrightarrow[\Delta]{HI\ (excess)}$ o-iodobenzyl iodide ($C_6H_4(I)CH_2-I$) + HCHO

Ethers are readily cleaved by action of HI to form alcohol and alkyl halide.

$R-O-R + HX \longrightarrow RX + R-OH$

If excess of halogen acid is used, then alcohol formed reacts further with halogen acid to produce alkyl halide.

81. **(c) :**

82. **(a) :**

$C_6H_5OH \xrightarrow{NaOH} C_6H_5O^-Na^+ \xrightarrow[125°C,\ 6\ atm]{CO_2} o\text{-}HOC_6H_4COONa \xrightarrow{dil.\ HCl} o\text{-}HOC_6H_4COOH$

Salicylic acid

83. **(b) :** $NaNO_2 + HCl \longrightarrow NaCl + HNO_2$

$$C_6H_5NH_2 + NaNO_2 + 2HCl \xrightarrow{0-5°C} C_6H_5N_2^+Cl^- + 2H_2O + 2NaCl$$

$$C_6H_5N_2^+Cl^- \xrightarrow[\Delta]{H_2O, H^+} C_6H_5OH$$

Phenol

84. **(a) :** Only primary amines will give carbylamine test.

$$CH_3NH_2 + CHCl_3 + 3KOH \longrightarrow \underset{\text{(offensive smell)}}{CH_3N \equiv C} + 3KCl + 3H_2O$$

85. **(d) :** With *trans*-but-2-ene, the product of Br_2 addition is optically inactive due to the formation of symmetric meso-compounds.

$$\underset{\textit{Trans}\text{-but-2-ene}}{H-C(CH_3)=C(H)-CH_3} + Br_2 \longrightarrow \text{(Meso)}$$

(Fischer projections: CH_3 top; H–C–Br; H–C–Br; CH_3 bottom and CH_3 top; Br–C–H; Br–C–H; CH_3 bottom)

86. **(a) :** Tertiary amines are not oxidised by $KMnO_4$.

87. **(c) :** Chloral hydrate is stable due to hydrogen bonding.

($Cl_2C(H)-C(H)(OH)_2$ structure with intramolecular H-bonds O–H···Cl)

88. **(a) :** For an ideal solution, $\Delta H_{mix} = 0$ and $\Delta V_{mix} = 0$.

89. **(a) :** $T_b° = 353.23$ K, $W_B = 1.8$ g,
$W_A = 90$ g, $T_b = 354.11$ K,
$K_b = 2.53$ kg mol^{-1}
$\Delta T_b = T_b - T_b° = 354.11 - 353.23 = 0.88$ K

$$M_B = \frac{W_B \times K_b \times 1000}{\Delta T_b \times W_A} = \frac{1.8 \times 2.53 \times 1000}{0.88 \times 90}$$

$= 57.5 \approx 58$ g mol^{-1}

90. **(a) :** Suppose number of M atoms = n
Then number of tetrahedral sites = $2n$
Number of N atoms $= \frac{1}{3}(2n)$
Ratio $M : N = n : \frac{2}{3}n = 3:2$,
i.e., formula is M_3N_2

91. **(b) :** Hair cream is an emulsion in which both dispersed phase and dispersion medium are liquids.

92. **(a) :** Given : $\frac{\lambda_{particle}}{\lambda_{electron}} = 1.8 \times 10^{-4}$

and $\frac{v_{particle}}{v_{electron}} = 3$

According to de-Broglie equation,

$$\lambda = \frac{h}{mv}$$

$$\frac{\lambda_{particle}}{\lambda_{electron}} = \frac{h}{m_{particle} \times v_{particle}} \times \frac{m_{electron} \times v_{electron}}{h}$$

$$= \frac{m_{electron}}{m_{particle}} \times \frac{v_{electron}}{v_{particle}}$$

$$\Rightarrow 1.8 \times 10^{-4} = \frac{9.1 \times 10^{-31} \text{ kg}}{m_{particle}} \times \frac{1}{3}$$

$$m_{particle} = \frac{9.1 \times 10^{-31}}{1.8 \times 10^{-4} \times 3}$$

$= 1.6852 \times 10^{-27}$ kg

Actual mass of neutron is 1.67493×10^{-27} kg.
Hence, the particle is neutron.

93. **(c) :** Given : $E_{H^+/H_2} = 18 \times 10^{-3}$ V, $[H^+] = ?$

Applying Nernst equation,

$$E_{H^+/H_2} = E°_{H^+/H_2} - \frac{0.0591}{1} \log \frac{1}{[H^+]}$$

18×10^{-3} V $= 0 + 0.0591 \log [H^+]$
18×10^{-3} V $= 0.0591 \log [H^+]$
$\log [H^+] = 0.3046$
$\therefore$ $[H^+]$ = antilog (0.3046) = 2.02 = 2.0

94. **(a) :** $AX_3 \rightleftharpoons \underset{S}{A^{3+}} + \underset{3S}{3X^-}$
$K_{sp} = [A^{3+}][X^-]^3$
$= (S)\cdot(3S)^3 = 27S^4$

95. **(d) :** H and U are state functions but W and q are not state functions.
From the equation, $\Delta H = \Delta U + \Delta PV$
At constant pressure, $\Delta H = \Delta U + P\Delta V$
At constant volume, $\Delta H = \Delta U + V\Delta P$
At constant pressure, $\Delta P = 0$, $\Delta H = q_p$
so, it is a state function.

At constant volume, $\Delta V = 0$, $\Delta U = q_v$, so, it is a state function.
Work done in any adiabatic process is state function.
$\Delta U = q - W \quad (\because q = 0)$
$\Delta U = -W$
Work done in isothermal process is not a state function.
$W = -q \quad (\because \Delta T = 0, q \neq 0)$

96. **(d) :** Greater the valency of the flocculating ion, greater is its flocculating power.

97. **(c) :** Volume strength $= \dfrac{5.6 \times \text{Strength in g L}^{-1}}{\text{Eq. wt. of } H_2O_2}$

$= \dfrac{5.6 \times 15.18}{12} = 5$ volumes

98. **(a) :**

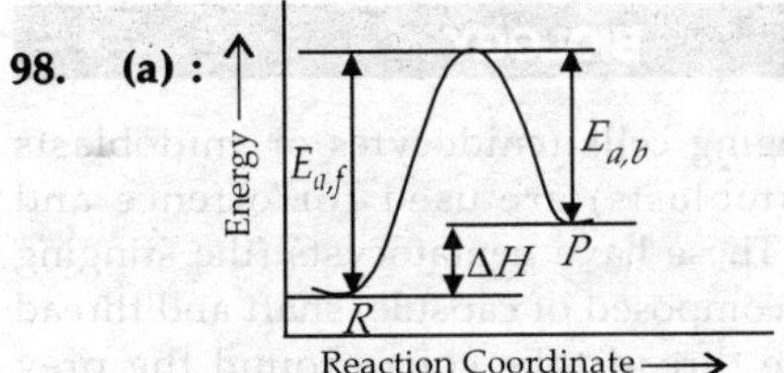

For endothermic reaction,
$E_{a,b} = E_{a,f} - \Delta H°$
$= 50 \text{ kJ} - 20 \text{ kJ} = 30 \text{ kJ}$

99. **(a)**

100. **(d) :** $nCF_2{=}CF_2 \longrightarrow {-}\!\!\left[CF_2 - CF_2\right]\!\!{-}_n$ (Teflon)
Teflon is used for non-sticking cookwares.

101. **(d) :** Bond dissociation energy is $F_2 < Cl_2$ because of relatively large electron-electron repulsion among the lone pairs in F_2 molecule where they are much closer to each other than in Cl_2.

102. **(a) :** As in solid state, PCl_5 exists as an ionic solid $[PCl_4]^+[PCl_6]^-$ in which the cation, $[PCl_4]^+$ is tetrahedral and the anion, $[PCl_6]^-$ is octahedral. PCl_5 in gaseous state has trigonal bipyramidal structure in which three equatorial bonds are equivalent, while the two axial bonds are longer than equatorial bonds due to more bond pair repulsion.

103. **(b) :** EDTA is a hexadentate ligand. It forms complex with central metal in the ratio 1 : 1 in which it binds through two nitrogen atoms and four oxygen atoms.

104. **(a) :** $Cd^{2+} + 2CN^- \longrightarrow Cd(CN)_2\downarrow$
$Cd(CN)_2\downarrow + 2CN^- \longrightarrow [Cd(CN)_4]^{2-}$
$[Cd(CN)_4]^{2-}$ is colourless compound and not too stable. When hydrogen sulphide gas is added, cadmium sulphide is precipitated.
$[Cd(CN)_4]^{2-} + H_2S \longrightarrow CdS\downarrow + 2H^+ + 4CN^-$
But in case of Cu^{2+},
$Cu^{2+} + 2CN^- \longrightarrow Cu(CN)_2\downarrow$
$2Cu(CN)_2\downarrow \xrightarrow[\text{decomposes}]{\text{Quickly}} 2CuCN\downarrow + (CN)_2\uparrow$
$CuCN\downarrow + 3CN^- \longrightarrow [Cu(CN)_4]^{3-}$
This complex is so stable (*i.e.*, $[Cu^+]$ is too low) that H_2S cannot precipitate Cu(I) sulphide (Cu_2S).

105. **(a) :**
$$\underset{\text{Pink}}{[Co(H_2O)_6]^{2+}} + 4Cl^- \rightleftharpoons \underset{\text{Blue}}{[CoCl_4]^{2-}} + 6H_2O$$
According to Le Chatelier's principle, on adding conc. HCl, the equilibrium shifts in forward direction giving blue colour. And when this blue colour is diluted, equilibrium shifts in backward direction leading to pink colour.

106. **(d) :**
$$\underset{\text{Acetamide}}{CH_3-\overset{\overset{O}{||}}{C}-NH_2} + Br_2 + 4KOH \longrightarrow \underset{\text{Methanamine}}{CH_3NH_2} + K_2CO_3 + 2KBr + 2H_2O$$

107. **(a) :** This is a Claisen-Schmidt reaction.
$$C_6H_5-\overset{\overset{O}{||}}{C}-H + CH_2CHO \xrightarrow{\text{hot alkali}}$$
Benzaldehyde (Electrophile as it does not contain α-hydrogen) Acetaldehyde (Nucleophile as it contains α-hydrogen)
$$C_6H_5-\overset{OH}{\overset{|}{C}H}-\overset{H}{\overset{|}{C}H}-CHO$$
Aldol (unstable)
$$\xrightarrow[-H_2O]{\Delta,\ H^+} C_6H_5CH{=}CHCHO$$
Cinnamaldehyde

108. **(b) :** Assertion is true because usually, for acrylic systems *trans*-isomers are more stable than *cis*-isomers. This is due to increased unfavourable steric interaction of the substituents in *cis*-isomer. Reason is also true because generally the dipole moment of *trans*-form is zero (or less) depending whether the substituents on both sides of double bond are same or not while *cis*-forms are polar in nature with certain value of dipole moment.

109. (c) :

$$C_6H_5SO_3H \xrightarrow[H_2O]{NaOH} C_6H_5SO_3^-Na^+ \xrightarrow[350°C]{NaOH} C_6H_5O^-Na^+ \xrightarrow{H_3O^+} C_6H_5OH$$

This is nucleophilic aromatic substitution reaction and occurs *via* the addition-elimination mechanism with SO_3^{2-} as the leaving group.

110. (d) : All enzymes are made up of proteins and all proteins do not have 3-dimensional structures as proteins are classified into primary, secondary, tertiary and quaternary structures and only tertiary has 3-dimensional structure. The sequence in which the amino acids are arranged in a protein is called primary structure of protein.

111. (b) : When an atom or an ion is missing from its normal lattice site, a lattice vacancy or defect is created, which is called Schottky defect. Due to missing density of crystal will be lowered.

112. (b) : For an isolated system,
$W = q = 0$
$\Delta U = q + W$
Hence, $\Delta U = 0$
$W = P\Delta V$
as $W = 0$ so, $\Delta V = 0$

113. (c) : Temperature at which the real gas exhibit ideal behaviour for considerable range of pressure is known as Boyle's temperature.

$T_b = \frac{a}{bR}$ a, and b are van der Waal's constant.

Critical temperature is the temperature above which the gas cannot be liquefied, how so ever high pressure may be applied : $T_c = \frac{8a}{27Rb}$.

114. (a) : ΔS is +ve and ΔH is –ve for a spontaneous reaction at all temperatures.

115. (d) : Catalyst have no effects on Gibb's free energy of system and pre-exponential factor of a chemical reaction.

116. (c) : It may involve increase or decrease in temperature of the system. Systems in which such process occur, are thermally insulated from the surroundings.

117. (c) : For $3p$-orbital, number of radial nodes $= n - l - 1 = 3 - 1 - 1 = 3 - 2 = 1$

Number of angular nodes $= l = 1$

Number of radial and angular nodes depend on both n and l.

118. (d) : $E°$ of Cu^{2+}/Cu is + 0.34 V and positive $E°$ means that the redox couple is a weaker reducing agent than the H^+/H_2 couple.

119. (c) : NaCl and $CaCl_2$ are added to provide conductivity to the electrolyte and also to lower the fusion temperature of anhydrous $MgCl_2$.

120. (a) : Phosphoric acid is a tribasic acid, *i.e,*. 3 hydroxyl groups are present.

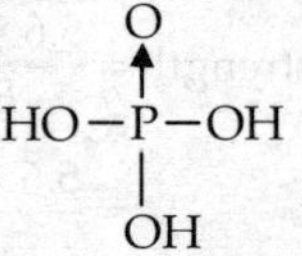

BIOLOGY

121. (c) : Stinging cells (cnidocytes or cnidoblasts or nematoblasts) are used for offence and defence. These have nematocysts (the stinging organs), composed of capsule, shaft and thread tube. The thread tube coils around the prey or attaches to it or injects a toxin, called hypnotoxin which paralyzes the victim. They are found in cnidarians- sea pen (*Pennatula*), sea fan (*Gorgonia*), etc.

122. (b) : The DNA used as a carrier for transferring a fragment of foreign DNA into a suitable host is called vehicle DNA or cloning vector or gene carrier. The *Ti* plasmid (tumour inducing plasmid) is present in *Agrobacterium tumefaciens*, a Gram negative soil bacterium that infects a wide range of plants and causes tumorous growth specially at the root /stem junction (crown gall). The *Ti* plasmid comprises the gene responsible for the tumorous growth, gets incorporated into the genome of infected plant cells. This property is of interest for genetic engineering as *Ti* plasmid can be used as DNA vector by replacing the tumour inducing genes with the gene of interest and a marker gene to enable selection of transformed cells. The *Ti* plasmid, is widely used in plant genetic engineering as a vector, novel plant genes being spliced into the plasmid sequence by gene manipulation and thus carried into the host plant cells. This provides the opportunity to develop new and better species.

123. (d) : The total number of species estimated is about 1.74 million. Out of these, the number of known species in India is 1,42,000 or roughly 8.1% of the total though India has only 2.4% land area. India with about 45000 species of plants and twice as many species of animals is one of the 12 megadiversity countries of the world.

124. (b) : Non-native or alien species are often introduced inadvertently for their economic and other uses. They often become invasive and drive away the local species. These species are considered to be second major cause of extinction of species (the first being habitat destruction). *Lantana camara* has replaced many species in forests of Central India. *Parthenium hystero-phorus* has pushed out several herbs and shrubs from open places in the plains. Water hyacinth (*Eichhornia crassipes*) was introduced in Indian waters to reduce pollution. It clogged water bodies including wetlands at many places resulting in death of several aquatic plants and animals. *Nelumbo* (lotus) is not an invasive species.

125. (a) : Cardiac muscle fibres are found in the wall of heart. They have dark intercalated discs at intervals. These are specialized regions of cell membranes of two adjacent fibres. They permit the wave of muscle contraction to be transmitted from one cardiac fibre to another.

126. (c) : When fertilization occurs outside the body of the organism, this type of gametic fusion is called external fertilization or external syngamy. The external medium such as water is required for this type of fertilization. Thus, in most aquatic organisms such as a majority of algae, fishes and amphibians, external fertilization occurs.

127. (d) : Seminal vesicles produce an alkaline secretion which forms 60% of the volume of semen. The secretion of the seminal vesicles contains fructose, prostaglandins, citrate, inositol, and clotting proteins. Prostate gland produces a milky and slightly alkaline secretion which forms 25% of the volume of semen. It possesses calcium, phosphate, bicarbonate, enzymes prefibrolysin, clotting enzymes, and prostaglandins. Bulbourethral glands or Cowper's glands also secrete an alkaline fluid which neutralizes acids from urine in the urethera. Their secretion contributes the least to semen but is very important.

128. (a) : All the options are examples of intra-uterine contraceptive devices (IUCDs). These are plastic or metal objects which are inserted by doctors in the uterus through vagina. Lippe's loop is non-medicated IUCD. CuT and Multiload are copper releasing IUCDs, which suppress motility and fertilizing capacity of sperms. Progestasert is a hormone releasing IUCD which makes the uterus unsuitable for implantation and cervix hostile to the sperms.

129. (a)

130. (b) : Inside the red blood cells, oval-shaped merozoites stop proceeding with erythrocytic cycle to increase in size and become rounded gametocytes. Male gametocytes or microgametocytes are smaller and contain a large diffused nucleus. Female gametocytes (or mega gametocytes) are larger with a small compact peripheral nucleus. These do not divide but remain as intracellular parasites within their host's blood corpuscles, until they either die or are ingested by the vectors. They give rise to gametes in insects.

131. (c) : Endosperm is the food laden tissue which is meant for nourishing the embryo in seed plants. In gymnosperms, it represents the female gametophyte and thus is haploid(n). In angiosperms, the endosperm is a special tissue which is formed as a result of fusion of a male gamete with diploid secondary nucleus of the central cell (vegetative fertilization or triple fusion). The fusion product is primary endosperm cell having a triploid (3n) endosperm nucleus.

132. (d) : Secondary metabolites are derivatives of primary metabolites which have no direct function in growth and development of plants. These compounds are accessory rather than central to the functioning, *e.g.*, arbrin, cellulose, gums, diterpenes, carotenoids, curcumin, rubber etc. Arginine, tyrosine, glycine, serine and phenylalanine are amino acids, which are primary metabolites.

133. (d) : S-phase is known as synthetic phase. In this stage replication of DNA takes place on the template of the existing DNA and thus the amount of DNA per cell doubles. If the initial amount of DNA is denoted as 2C, then it increases to 4C.

134. (d) : The outer layer of pollen grain is called exine. It is thick and smooth and culticularised. The cutin is called sporopollenin. It is not degraded by any enzyme. It is not affected by high temperature, strong acid or strong alkali. Thus, it is resistant to chemical and biological decomposition. Because of sporopollenin, pollen grains are well preserved as microfossils.

135. (a) : Pollen viability is the period for which pollen grains retain the ability to germinate. Pollen viability is little in flowers which are pollinated in bud condition. It is 30 minutes in rice and wheat. It depends upon environmental conditions of temperature and humidity.

136. (b) : Double fertilization is the fusion of two male gametes brought about by a pollen tube fusing to two different cells of the same female gametophyte in order to produce two different structures. It is found only in angiosperms. In angiosperms, the pollen tube bursts open in one of the two synergids to release the two male gametes. One male gamete fuses with the egg or oosphere to form a diploid zygote or oospore. It is called generative fertilization. The second male gamete descends down and fuses with the diploid secondary nucleus of the central cell to form a triploid primary endosperm cell. It is known as vegetative fertilization. Thus, after double fertilization, a mature angiospermous ovule contains one diploid cell (zygote) and one triploid cell (endosperm). The haploid cells of the ovule such as antipodals and synergids degenerate after fertilization.

137. (a) : Transgenic plants or genetically modified (GM) crops are those plants in which a foreign gene has been introduced and integrated into the host DNA *via* recombinant DNA technology. The transfer or introduction of a foreign gene results in the production of desirable traits like disease resistance, insect resistance, herbicide resistance, etc.

138. (c) : The palindromes in DNA are base pair sequences that are the same when read forward (left to right) or backward (right to left) from a central axis of symmetry. The following sequence reads the same on the two strands in 5′ → 3′ direction. This is also true when we read in the 3′ → 5′ direction.

$$\begin{array}{l} \longleftarrow \\ 5' - GAATTC - 3' \\ 3' - CTTAAG - 5' \\ \longrightarrow \end{array}$$

Palindromic sequence

Restriction endonuclease enzymes recognize palindromic sequences in DNA and cut them.

139. (c) : Presence of photorespiration is considered as a wasteful and energy consuming process in crop plants which ultimately leads to reduction in final yield of crops. It is estimated that during C_3 photosynthesis, upto 50% of the CO_2 fixed may have to pass through photorespiratory process, thereby resulting in considerable decrease in photosynthetic productivity. In C_3 plants, there is little loss of photosynthetic activity on account of photorespiration which is absent in C_4 plants and hence they have better productivity.

140. (c) : Oxytocin is released by posterior pituitary. Vasopressin decreases the amount of urine by increasing reabsorption of water from DCT and collecting tubules. It also stimulates the contraction of walls of blood vessels, thereby raising the blood pressure. Glucagon stimulates liver to convert stored glycogen into glucose and thus raises the blood sugar level. Thymus releases thymosin which aids in proliferation of T-lymphocytes.

141. (d) : *Aspergillus niger* carries out fermentation to form citric acid. Fungus *Trichoderma polysporum* produces cyclosporin through fermentative activity. Cyclosporin-A has antifungal, anti-inflammatory and immuno-suppressive properties. *Saccharomyces cerevisiae* (baker's yeast/brewer's yeast) is used in production of bread/alcohol. Methanogenic bacteria carry out microbial decomposition of organic matter and aids in gobar gas production.

142. (a)

143. (a) : Parietal cells (or oxyntic cells) secrete hydrochloric acid (HCl) and Castle's intrinsic factor. Chief cells (or peptic cells) secrete gastric digestive enzymes as proenzymes — pepsinogen and prorennin. HCl helps in converting pepsinogen to pepsin. Goblet cells secrete mucus which helps to neutralise acid in stomach and protects stomach wall against HCl action.

144. (d) : In family A, if both the parents are

homozygous recessive, then both should be diseased and should have 100% diseased progeny. In family B, if both parents are homozygous dominant, they would not have got the recessive disease in first place. In family B, if both are heterozygous recessive, then also they would not have got the disease, neither 80% of progeny would be diseased.

145. **(c) :** Glucose and amino acids are reabsorbed in PCT by secondary active transport. Water, sodium and chloride ions are reabsorbed in DCT. It is permeable to water. Maximum reabsorption takes place within the PCT. Humans are ureotelic and excrete out 25-30 gm of urea per day.

146. **(b):** Inbreeding leads to increase in homozygosity. This, in recessive alleles, may cause expression of harmful effects. Also, inbreeding depression may lead to loss of fitness in progenies, thus decreasing productivity in some cases.

147. **(c) :** The given floral diagram is of family Fabaceae. Flower – zygomorphic, bisexual. Sepals - five, fused. Petals - five, polypetalous, papillionaceous corolla. Androecium - ten, diadelphous. Gynoecium - ovary superior, monocarpellary, unilocular, marginal placentation, with many ovules.

148. **(d) :** A - Fovea centralis : Sharpest vision occurs here.

B - Blindspot : No image is formed here.

C - Ciliary body: It helps to hold the lens in position.

D - Iris : Visible coloured portion of eye.

149. **(a) :** A - Z line : located at centre of I-band.

B - Thin filament : occurs in both I-band and A-band.

C - Thick filament : occurs in A-band.

D - H-zone - present at the centre of A-band.

150. **(a) :** All plant families end with –ae suffix. However, it differs for division, class and genus.

151. **(b) :** RBCs contain haemoglobin. It has four polypeptide chains and four haem groups attached to it or 4 atoms of iron in ferrous form (Fe^{2+}), thus it can react with 4 molecules of oxygen to form oxyhaemoglobin.

152. **(c) :** *Nereis* is classified under Phylum Annelida. It is a unisexual annelid and its reproductive phase is called *Heteronereis*. It is usually called clam worm or sand worm or rag worm which is found on the sea shore in the tubular burrows. Except the peristomium (first segment) and last anal segment, each segment bears laterally one pair of fleshy projections, the parapodia, used in swimming.

153. **(d) :** The yearly growth of secondary xylem is distinct in the area which experiences two seasons, one favourable (spring or rainy season) and the other unfavourable (autumn, winter and dry summer). The wood formed in a single year consists of two types of wood, spring wood and autumn wood. The spring or early wood is much wider than the autumn or late wood. It is lighter in colour and of lower density. Spring wood consists of larger and wider xylem elements. The autumn or late wood is dark coloured and of higher density. It contains compactly arranged smaller and narrower elements which have comparatively thicker walls. In autumn wood, tracheids and fibres are more abundant than those found in the spring wood.

154. **(a) :** Both mitochondria and chloroplast are semi-autonomous organelles as they possess their own DNA, RNA and 70S ribosomes to have sufficient functional independence from cellular machinery. Chloroplasts DNA is bigger than mitochondrial DNA. However, genetic information contained in these DNAs is limited. DNA is naked (without histone proteins) in both.

155. **(a) :** Blood is the medium of transport of O_2 and CO_2. Nearly 20-25% of CO_2 is transported by RBCs as carbaminohaemoglobin whereas 70% of it is carried as bicarbonate through plasma. About 7% of CO_2 is carried in dissolved state through plasma. The largest fraction of CO_2 is converted to bicarbonate ions (HCO^-_3) and transported in plasma. When CO_2 diffuses into the RBCs, it combines with H_2O, forming carbonic acid (H_2CO_3). H_2CO_3 is unstable and quickly dissociates into hydrogen ions and bicarbonate ions.

156. **(b) :** Options (a), (b), (c) and (d) show neutrophil, basophil, eosinophil and monocyte respectively. Neutrophils are the most abundant cells (60-65%) of the total WBCs and basophils are the least (0.5 - 1%) among them. Neutrophils and monocytes (6 - 8%) are phagocytic cells. Which destroy foreign organisms entering the body. Basophils secrete histamine, serotonin, heparin, etc. and are involved in inflammatory reactions. Eosinophils (2 - 3%) resist infections and are also associated with allergic reactions.

157. (c) : Nucleus contains nucleoli and chromatin network. Chromatin contains DNA and some basic proteins called histones, some non-histone proteins and also RNA.

158. (b) : When sewage, having biodegradable organic matter is released in water body, micro-organisms involved in biodegradation of organic matter in the receiving water body consume a lot of oxygen to decompose the sewage and as a result there would be a sharp decline in dissolved oxygen downstream from the point of sewage discharge, and biological oxygen demand (BOD) would increase. Presence of large amount of nutrients in water causes excessive growth of planktonic (free-floating) algae, called algal bloom. Algal bloom causes deterioration of water quality and fish mortality.

159. (b): Auxins promote root initiation at a concentration which otherwise is inhibitory for growth of intact root. Auxins are often employed for inducing flowering in litchi and pineapple. Application of auxins to unpollinated pistils make them develop into seedless fruits or parthenocarps.

160.(c): Secondary air pollutants are photochemically produced from primary pollutants and are thus called photochemical oxidants. Ozone, peroxyacyl nitrates, aldehydes and phenols are produced due to photochemical reactions between nitrogen oxides and unsaturated hydrocarbons.

161. (b): The earthworms are bisexual or hermaphrodite or monoecious and protandrous. The self-fertilization is not possible in the earthworm because of the relative position of openings of male and female reproductive organs, hence cross fertilization takes place.

During mating, two worms attach themselves with their ventral surfaces and become opposed to each other in opposite direction to exchange packets of sperms called spermatophores. Mature sperm and egg cells and nutritive fluid are deposited in cocoons, produced by the gland cells of clitellum. The ova (eggs) are fertilized by the sperm cells within the cocoon which then slips off the worm and is deposited in or on the soil. The cocoon holds the worm embryos. After about 3 weeks, each cocoon produces two to twenty baby worms with an average of four.

162. (a): In arithmetic growth, following mitotic cell division, only one daughter cell continues to divide while the other differentiates and matures. The simplest expression of arithmetic growth is exemplified by a root elongating at a constant rate. On plotting the length of the organ against time, a linear curve is obtained.

163. (c): Absorption of substances takes place in different parts of the alimentary canal, like mouth, stomach, small intestine and large intestine. However, maximum absorption occurs in the small intestine. Hence, small intestine is the principal organ for absorption of nutrients. The digestion is completed here and the final products of digestion such as glucose, fructose, fatty acids, glycerol and amino acids are absorbed through the mucosa into the blood stream and lymph. Absorption of water, single sugars and alcohol, etc. takes place in stomach. In larger intestine, absorption of water, some minerals and drugs takes place.

164. (b): Pulse is the rhythmic contraction and relaxation in the aorta and its main arteries. It is a regular jerk of an artery. The pulse rate is exactly the same as the heart rate because an artery pulses every time the heart beats. Pulse is usually taken on the radial artery in the wrist but it can be taken on any artery that flows near enough to the surface of the body to be felt. The heart beat originates from the sinoatrial node (SA Node) - pacemaker, which lies in the wall of the right atrium near the opening of the superior vena cava. The SA node is a mass of neuromuscular tissue. Another mass of neuromuscular tissue, the atrioventricular node (AV node) is situated in the wall of the right atrium. The AV node picks up the wave of contraction propagated by SA node. A mass of specialized fibres, the bundle of His, originates from the AV node. The bundle of His divides into two branches, one going to each ventricle. Within the myocardium of the ventricles, the branches of bundle of His divides into a network of fine fibres called the Purkinje fibres. The bundle of His and the Purkinje fibres convey impulse of contraction from the AV node to the myocardium of the ventricles.

165. (a): One of the hormones released by the placenta is human chorionic gonadotropin (hCG). This hormone is secreted by the trophoblast cells even before they become the chorion, and is the hormone assayed in the pregnancy test. Because its action is almost identical to that of luteinizing hormone (LH), hCG maintains the mother's corpus luteum. The corpus luteum, in turn, continues to secrete oestrogens and progesterone, thereby preventing menstruation and further ovulations. At around 10th week, the secretion of human chorionic gonadotropin (hCG) by placenta declines, and the corpus luteum regresses as a result. However, menstruation does not occur because placenta itself secretes oestrogens and progesterone. In fact, the amounts of these two hormones secreted by the placenta far exceed the amounts that are ever secreted by the ovaries. The high levels of oestrogens and progesterone in the blood during pregnancy continue to inhibit the release of FSH and LH, thereby preventing ovulation. They also help maintain the uterus and eventually prepare it for labor and delivery, and they stimulate the development of the mammary glands in the preparation for lactation after delivery.

166. (c): Alexander Fleming while working on *Staphylococci* bacteria, once observed a mould growing in one of his unwashed culture plates around which *Staphylococci* could not grow. He found out that it was due to a chemical produced by the mould and he named it Penicillin after the mould *Penicillium notatum*. However, its full potential as an effective antibiotic was established much later by Ernest Chain and Howard Florey.

167. (d): Yeast (*Saccharomyces cerevisiae*) is used for commercial production of ethanol. A bioactive molecule, cyclosporin A which is used as an immunosuppressive agent in organ-transplant patients, is produced by the fungus *Trichoderma polysporum*.

168. (c): Protostele is the simplest and considered to be the most primitive type of stele. It consists of a solid core of xylem surrounded by the cylinder of phloem, enclosing no pith. All other types of steles have evolved from it in the course of evolutionary specialization. Protosteles may be found in *Selaginella, Lycopodium, Gleichenia* and *Lygodium* among present day forms.

169. (b): The human digestive system carries about trillions of microorganisms colonising the gut making an amazing ecosystem that live together in harmony. In this context human intestine is said to be rich in flora and fauna. The microorganisms perform a host of useful functions, such as fermenting unused energy substrates, training the immune system, preventing growth of harmful, pathogenic bacteria, regulating the development of the gut, producing vitamins for the host (such as biotin and vitamin K), and producing hormones to direct the host to store fats.
Fish culture is sometimes done in combination with a rice crop, so that fish are grown in the water in the paddy field. Thus, a rice field is an example of ecosystem inhabiting both plants and animals.

170. (c) : *Refer answer 154.*

171. (b): The world is facing accelerated rates of species extinctions, largely due to human interference. There are four major causes – (i) habitat loss and fragmentation, (ii) over-exploitation, (iii) alien species invasions and (iv) co-extinctions.
Non-native of alien species are often introduced inadvertently for their economic and other uses. They often become invasive and drive away the local species. The exotic species are considered to be second major cause of extinction of species (the first being habitat destruction).

172. (b): Meiosis consists of two divisions, meiosis I and meiosis II. The first division of meiosis is called heterotypic or reduction division. During this division the number of chromosomes is reduced to half. The two chromatids of a chromosome become genetically different due to crossing over. These chromatids are separated in the second division of meiosis. The second meiotic division is known as homotypic or equational division, because the chromosome number remains the same as produced after the end of the first division. Though meiosis II is similar to mitosis, meiosis II is not mitosis because (i) it always occurs in haploid cells, (ii) it is not preceded by DNA replication, (iii) the two chromatids of a chromosome are often dissimilar, (iv) the daughter cells formed after meiosis II are neither similar to each other nor similar to the parent cell.

173. (c): Periodic abstinence is a natural method of birth control in which the couples avoid or abstain from coitus (copulation or intercourse) from day 10 to 17 of the menstrual cycle because ovulation can occur during this period. The chances of fertilization are very high during this period, therefore, it is called the fertile period.

174. (b): The cerebrum is the largest and most complex of all the parts of the human brain. It consists of left and right hemispheres connected by a large bundle of myelinated fibres, the corpus callosum. Association areas interpret the input, store the input and initiate a response in light of similar past experience. Thus, the association areas are involved in memory, learning and reasoning.

175. (d): Sickle cell anaemia is an autosomal recessive hereditary disorder in which the erythrocytes become sickle-shaped under oxygen deficiency as during strenuous exercise and at high altitudes. The disorder or disease is caused by the formation of an abnormal haemoglobin called haemoglobin-S. As found out by Ingram (1958), haemoglobin-S differs from normal haemoglobin-A in only one amino acid – 6th amino acid of β-chain, glutamic acid, is replaced by valine due to substitution (transversion) of T by A in the second position of the triplet codon (CTC) which is changed to CAC in the β-haemoglobin gene situated on chromosome 11.

176. (a) : The efficiency of C_4 plants is more than those of C_3 plants because (i) C_4 plants are more efficient in picking up CO_2 even when it is found in low concentration because of the high affinity of PEP, (ii) concentric arrangement of mesophyll cells produces a smaller area in relation to volume for better utilization of available water and reduce the intensity of solar radiations, (iii) they can tolerate excess salts because of the presence of organic acids, (iv) normal oxygen concentration is not inhibitory for the growth in contrast to C_3 plants, (v) they are adapted to high temperature and intense radiation of tropics.

177. (a) : The cattles, buffaloes, goats, sheep, deer and camels are herbivorous animals that feed on plant leaves, twigs, etc. Their stomach consists of 4 chambers: rumen (paunch), reticulum (honeycomb), omasum (psalterium) and abomasum (rennet). In the rumen, food undergoes mechanical and chemical breakdown. Mechanical breakdown results from thorough churning brought about by muscular contractions and aided by cornified surface of villi. Chemical breakdown is caused by symbiotic micro-organisms bacteria such as *Ruminococcus* and ciliate such as *Entodinium caudatum.* These micoorganisms live as symbionts in the rumen and reticulum of the stomach of the ruminants (*e.g.*, cows and buffaloes) and in the large intestine of other herbivorous mammals (*e.g.*, horses and donkeys) and release enzymes, cellulases, which act on cellulose and simplify it to short-chain fatty acids. Cellulose is not digested in human being.

178. (b) : The secondary structure of proteins is the development of new stearic relationships of amino acids present in the linear sequence inside the polypeptides. Some of the new relationship are of regular nature and give periodicity to the structure. There are three types of secondary structures – α-helix, β-pleated and collagen helix. They are held in a particular structure due hydrogen bonds between oxygen of carboxylic group (–CO group) of one amino acid residue and >NH group of another amino acid.

The protein enzymes have active sites which are capable of attracting and holding particular substrate molecules by is specific charge, size and shape so as to allow the chemical change. An active site consists of a few amino acids and their side groups which are brought together in a particular fashion due to secondary and tertiary folding of a protein molecule and its association with the cofactor, if any. Tertiary structure is bending and folding of various types to form spheres, rods or fibres. It further brings new stearic relationships of amino acids specially those which are far apart in the linear sequence. Tertiary structure is stabilized by several types of bonds— hydrogen bonds, ionic bonds, van der Waal's interactions, covalent bonds, hydrophobic bonds. Tertiary structure gives the protein a three dimensional conformation.

179. (c) : Glutamine is one of the 20 amino acids. Its side chain is an amide formed by replacing the side chain hydroxyl of glutamic acid with an amine functional group, making it the amide of glutamic acid. In human blood, glutamine is the most abundant free amino acid. The isoelectric point is the pH at which a particular molecule or surface carries no net electrical charge. The isoelectric point (pI) of glutamine is 5.65.

180. (d) : Principal organ for digestion and absorption for nutrients is small intestine. Small intestine is distinguishable into three regions, a 'U' shaped duodenum, a long coiled middle portion jejunum and a highly coiled ileum. Mainly iron, calcium and amino acids are absorbed in duodenum; fatty acids, glycerol, monosaccharides and vitamins are absorbed in jejunum, and absorption of vitamin B_{12}, bile salts and water occur in ileum.

GENERAL KNOWLEDGE

181. (d)	**182. (b)**	**183. (b)**	**184. (b)**	**185. (d)**
186. (b)	**187. (c)**	**188. (b)**	**189. (b)**	**190. (a)**
191. (b)	**192. (d)**	**193. (a)**	**194. (a)**	**195. (c)**
196. (d)	**197. (a)**	**198. (b)**	**199. (a)**	**200. (b)**

Chapterwise Index - '14

Physics • Chemistry • Biology

Use the index for topicwise analysis of AIIMS paper and refer to these questions when you are practising MCQs chapterwise.

PHYSICS

Chapter's Name	Question No.	Total
Units and Dimensions	1	1
Motion in One Dimension	37, 54	2
Motion in Two Dimensions	4, 25	2
Laws of Motion and Friction	2, 46	2
Work, Power and Energy	3, 27, 45	3
Centre of Mass and Rotational Motion	26, 28, 35, 44	4
Gravitation	5, 29	2
Properties of Matter	11, 55	2
Oscillations	14, 30, 38, 56	4
Waves	6, 31, 58	3
Heat and Thermodynamics	12, 13, 39, 57	4
Electrostatics	22, 23, 51, 53	4
Current Electricity	7, 52	2
Thermal and chemical effects of current		
Magnetic Effects of Current	8, 24, 40	3
Magnetism		
Electromagnetic Induction and Alternating Current	9, 20, 21	3
Electromagnetic Waves	43	1
Ray Optics	10, 19, 32, 60	4
Wave Optics	34	1
Modern Physics	16, 17, 18, 36, 42, 48, 59	7
Solids and Semiconductor Devices	15, 33, 49	3
Universe		
Principles of Communication	41, 47, 50	3

CHEMISTRY

Chapter's Name	Question No.	Total
Basic Concepts	86	1
Atomic Structure	84	1
Periodic Properties	70	1
Chemical Bonding	85, 87, 103	3
Nuclear Chemistry		
Gaseous and Liquid States		
Solid State	63, 105	2
Mole Concept & Solutions	93, 113	2
Colloids, Surface Chemistry & Catalysis	74, 95, 107	3
Equilibrium	81, 108	2
Kinetics	82, 83	2
Energetics	77	1
Electrochemistry	94, 115	2
Redox Reactions	88	1
Metallurgy	72	1
Hydrogen and its Compounds	89, 116	2
s-Block Elements	90	1
p-Block Elements	65, 68, 69, 71, 73, 76, 109, 120	8
d- and ***f***-Block Elements	66, 78, 79, 101, 102, 106	6
Complex Compounds	67, 117	2
Purification and Analysis of Organic Compound	91, 92, 118	3
General Organic Chemistry		
Aliphatic Hydrocarbons	111, 114	2
Aromatic Hydrocarbons	98	1
Halogen Derivatives	110	1
Alcohols, Phenols and Ethers	99	1
Aldehydes and Ketones	75, 100	2
Carboxylic acids & their derivatives	112	1
Organic Compounds Containing Nitrogen	97	1
Biochemistry	64, 104	2
Chemistry in Action	61, 62, 96, 119	4
Environmental Chemistry	80	1

BIOLOGY

Chapter's Name	Question No.	Total
General Biology		
Biological Classification		
Kingdom Monera		
Kingdom Fungi	175	1
Plant Kingdom	125, 167	2
Cell and its Structural Components		
Cell Reproduction	121	1
Cell Respiration	168	1
Biomolecules	133, 149	2
Principles of Inheritance and Variation	123, 161	2
Molecular Basis of Inheritance	171	1
Plant Anatomy		
Plant Morphology	127	1
Plant Physiology	126, 130, 177, 178	4
Sexual Reproduction in Flowering Plants	137	1
Ecology and Environment	122, 129, 135, 148, 150, 172, 174	7
Animal Kingdom	136, 143	2
Animal Tissue		
Musculo-Skeletal System	144, 176	2
Digestive System and Nutrition	154, 162	2
Respiratory System		
Circulatory System	145, 153, 166, 169, 179	5
Excretion and Osmoregulation	146	1
Nervous System and Sense Organs	152, 163	2
Endocrine System	141, 159, 180	3
Reproduction and Embryonic Development	124, 134	2
Human Health and Diseases	140, 155, 160, 164, 165, 170	6
Evolution	142	1
Biotechnology	132, 151, 156, 158, 173	5
Applied Biology	128, 131, 138, 139, 147, 157	6

SOLVED PAPER
AIIMS - 2014★

Time : 3½ Hours | Max. Marks : 200

PHYSICS

1. If the units of length, mass and force are chosen as fundamental units, the dimensions of time would be
(a) $[M^{1/2}L^{-1/2}F^{1/2}]$ (b) $[M^{1/2}L^{1/2}F^{1/2}]$
(c) $[M^{1/2}L^{1/2}F^{-1/2}]$ (d) $[M^{1/2}L^{-1/2}F^{-1/2}]$

2. A block of mass 2 kg is placed on the floor. The coefficient of static friction is 0.4. If a force of 2.8 N is applied on the block parallel to the floor, the force of friction between the block and the floor is (g = 10 m s^{-2})
(a) 2.8 N (b) 2 N (c) 8 N (d) Zero

3. A heavy truck moving with a velocity of 60 km h^{-1} collides with a light drum at rest. If the collision be elastic, then the velocity of the drum immediately after collision will be
(a) zero (b) 60 km h^{-1}
(c) 120 km h^{-1} (d) uncertain

4. A cyclist is moving in a circular track of radius 80 m with a velocity of 36 km h^{-1}. He has to lean from the vertical approximately through an angle (Take g = 10 m s^{-2})
(a) $\tan^{-1}(4)$ (b) $\tan^{-1}(1/8)$
(c) $\tan^{-1}(1/4)$ (d) $\tan^{-1}(2)$

5. A satellite is in an orbit around the earth. If its kinetic energy is doubled, then
(a) it will maintain its path
(b) it will fall on the earth
(c) it will rotate with a great speed
(d) it will escape out of earth's gravitational field.

6. Two waves represented by $y = a\sin(\omega t - kx)$ and $y = a\cos(\omega t - kx)$ are superposed. The resultant wave will have an amplitude
(a) a (b) $\sqrt{2}a$ (c) $2a$ (d) zero

7. 2, 4 and 6 S are the conductances of three conductors. When they are joined in parallel, their equivalent conductance will be
(a) 12 S (b) (1/12) S
(c) (12/11) S (d) 11/12 S

8. Two parallel long wires A and B carry currents i_1 and $i_2 (< i_1)$. When i_1 and i_2 are in the same direction, the magnetic field at a point mid way between the wires is 10 μT. If i_2 is reverse the field becomes 30 μT. The ratio i_1/i_2 is
(a) 1 (b) 2 (c) 3 (d) 4

9. Two conducting circular loops of radii R_1 and R_2 are placed in the same plane with their centres coinciding. If $R_1 > R_2$, the mutual inductance M between them will be directly proportional to
(a) $\frac{R_1}{R_2}$ (b) $\frac{R_2}{R_1}$ (c) $\frac{R_1^2}{R_2}$ (d) $\frac{R_2^2}{R_1}$

10. The length of deviation for a glass prism is equal to its refracting angle. The refractive index of glass is 1.5. Then the angle of prism is
(a) $2\cos^{-1}(3/4)$ (b) $\sin^{-1}(3/4)$
(c) $2\sin^{-1}(3/2)$ (d) $\cos^{-1}(3/2)$

11. A steel wire with cross-section 3 cm^2 has elastic limit 2.4×10^8 N m^{-2}. The maximum upward acceleration that can be given to a 1200 kg elevator supported by this cable wire if the stress is not to exceed one-third of the elastic limit is (Take g = 10 m s^{-2})
(a) 12 m s^{-2} (b) 10 m s^{-2}
(c) 8 m s^{-2} (d) 7 m s^{-2}

12. 70 calories of heat are required to raise the temperature of 2 moles of an ideal gas at constant pressure from 30°C to 35°C.

★ Based on memory.

The amount of heat required to raise the temperature of the same sample of the gas through the same range at constant volume is (Gas constant = 1.99 cal/K-mole)
(a) 30 cal (b) 50 cal
(c) 70 cal (d) 90 cal

13. 3 mole of hydrogen is mixed with 1 mole of neon. The molar specific heat at constant pressure is
(a) $\frac{9R}{4}$ (b) $\frac{9R}{2}$ (c) $\frac{13R}{4}$ (d) $\frac{13R}{2}$

14. A bottle weighing 220 g and of area of cross-section 50 cm^2, and height 4 cm oscillates on the surface of water in vertical position. Its frequency of oscillation is
(a) 1.5 Hz (b) 2.5 Hz
(c) 3.5 Hz (d) 4.5 Hz

15. Which logic gate is represented by the following combination of logic gates in figure?
(a) OR
(b) NAND
(c) AND
(d) NOR

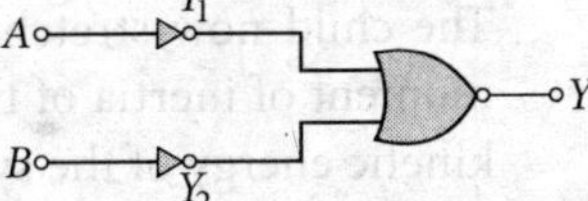

16. If the wavelength of 1st line of Balmer series of hydrogen is 6561 Å, the wavelength of the 2nd line of series will be
(a) 9780 Å (b) 4860 Å
(c) 8857 Å (d) 4429 Å

17. n-alpha particles per second are emitted from N atoms of a radioactive element. The half-life of the radioactive element is
(a) $\frac{n}{N}$ s (b) $\frac{N}{n}$ s
(c) $\frac{0.693\,N}{n}$ s (d) $\frac{0.693\,n}{N}$ s

18. The light of wavelength 4000 Å falls on a photosensitive substance whose work function is 2 eV. Its stopping potential is
(a) 1.1 V (b) 1.8 V
(c) 1.26 V (d) 0.8 V

19. Resolving power of reflecting microscope increases with
(a) decrease in wavelength of incident light
(b) increase in wavelength of incident light
(c) increase in diameter of objective lens
(d) none of these

20. The most suitable metal for making electro-magnets and transformer cores is
(a) steel (b) iron
(c) copper (d) aluminium

21. An inductive circuit contains a resistance of 10 Ω and an inductance of 2 H. If an AC voltage of 120 V and frequency 60 Hz is applied to this circuit, the current would be nearly
(a) 0.72 A (b) 0.16 A
(c) 0.48 A (d) 0.80 A

22. The diameter of the plate of a parallel plate condenser is 6 cm. If its capacity is equal to that of a sphere of diameter 200 cm, the separation between the plates of the condenser is
(a) 4.5×10^{-4} m (b) 2.25×10^{-4} m
(c) 6.75×10^{-4} m (d) 9×10^{-4} m

23. In a uniform electric field a charge of 3 C experiences a force of 3000 N. The potential difference between two points 1 cm apart along the electric line of force will be
(a) 10 V (b) 30 V (c) 300 V (d) 100 V

24. A long straight wire carries 10 A d.c. current an electron travels perpendicular to the plane of this wire at a distance 0.1 m with velocity 5.0×10^6 m s^{-1}. Force acting on the electron due to current in wire is
(a) zero N (b) 0.6×10^{-17} N
(c) 2.4×10^{-17} N (d) 2.2×10^{-17} N

25. An arrow is projected into air. Its time of flight is 5 s and range 200 m. What is the maximum height reached by it? (Take $g = 10$ m s^{-2})
(a) 31.25 m (b) 24.5 m
(c) 18.25 m (d) 46.75 m

26. A particle moves in a circular path with decreasing speed. Choose the correct statement.
(a) Angular momentum remains constant
(b) Acceleration $\vec{a}$ is towards the centre
(c) Particle moves in a spiral path with decreasing radius
(d) The direction of angular momentum remains constant

27. A body of mass 2 kg is thrown up vertically with kinetic energy of 490 J. The height at which the kinetic energy of the body becomes half of its original value is
(a) 50 m (b) 12.25 m
(c) 25 m (d) 10 m

28. Two homogeneous spheres A and B of masses m and $2m$ having radii $2a$ and a respectively are placed in touch. The distance of centre of mass from first sphere is
(a) a (b) $2a$
(c) $3a$ (d) none of these

29. What will be the effect on the weight of a body placed on the surface of earth, if earth suddenly stops rotating?
(a) No effect
(b) Weight will increase
(c) Weight will decrease
(d) Weight will become zero

30. The time period of a particle undergoing SHM is 16 s. It starts motion from the mean position. After 2 s, its velocity is 0.4 m s^{-1}. The amplitude is
(a) 1.44 m (b) 0.72 m
(c) 2.88 m (d) 0.36 m

31. A 5.5 metre length of string has a mass of 0.035 kg. If the tension in the string is 77 N, the velocity of the wave on the string is
(a) 210 m s^{-1} (b) 40 m s^{-1}
(c) 110 m s^{-1} (d) 55 m s^{-1}

32. The near point of distinct vision is at 1 m for an elderly person. What power of lens is to be used to bring the near point to the minimum distance of distinct vision (25 cm)?
(a) 2.5 D (b) 3 D
(c) 3.5 D (d) 4 D

33. Which of the given statements about transistor is not true?
(a) Emitter is heavily doped.
(b) Base is thin.
(c) Base is lightly doped.
(d) Collector region is smaller comparative to emitter in size.

34. In a Young's double slit experiment the intensity of light when slit is at distance λ from central is I. What will be the intensity at the distance of slit is $\frac{\lambda}{6}$?
(a) $\frac{I}{6}$ (b) $\frac{I}{12}$ (c) $\frac{3}{4}I$ (d) $\frac{I}{8}$

35. A child is standing with folded hands at the centre of a platform rotating about its central axis. The kinetic energy of the system is K. The child now stretches his arms so that the moment of inertia of the system doubled. The kinetic energy of the system now is
(a) $2K$ (b) $\frac{K}{2}$ (c) $\frac{K}{4}$ (d) $4K$

36. A triply ionized beryllium (Be^{3+}) has the same orbital radius as the ground state of hydrogen. Then the quantum state n of Be^{3+} is
(a) $n = 1$ (b) $n = 2$ (c) $n = 3$ (d) $n = 4$

37. A particle is moving eastwards with a velocity of 5 m/s. In 10 s, the velocity changes to 5 m/s northwards. The average acceleration in this time is
(a) zero
(b) $\frac{1}{\sqrt{2}}$ m s^{-2} towards north-west
(c) $\frac{1}{\sqrt{2}}$ m s^{-2} towards north-east
(d) $\frac{1}{\sqrt{2}}$ m s^{-2} towards north

38. A spring of spring constant 5×10^3 N m^{-1} is stretched initially by 5 cm from the unstretched position. The work required to stretch it further by another 5 cm is
(a) 6.25 N m (b) 1250 N m
(c) 18.75 N m (d) 25.00 N m

39. According to kinetic theory of gases, molecules of a gas behave like
(a) inelastic spheres
(b) perfectly elastic rigid spheres
(c) perfectly elastic non-rigid spheres
(d) inelastic non-rigid spheres

40. A particle of charge q and mass m starts moving from the origin under the action of an electric field $\vec{E} = E_0 \hat{i}$ and $\vec{B} = B_0 \hat{i}$ with a velocity $\vec{v} = v_0 \hat{j}$. The speed of the particle will become $\frac{\sqrt{5}}{2} v_0$ after a time
(a) $\frac{mv_0}{qE_0}$ (b) $\frac{mv_0}{2qE_0}$
(c) $\frac{\sqrt{3}mv_0}{2qE_0}$ (d) $\frac{\sqrt{5}mv_0}{2qE_0}$

Directions: In the following questions (41-60), a statement of assertion is followed by a statement of reason. Mark the correct choice as :
(a) If both assertion and reason are true and reason is the correct explanation of assertion.
(b) If both assertion and reason are true but reason is not the correct explanation of assertion.
(c) If assertion is true but reason is false.
(d) If both assertion and reason are false.

41. **Assertion :** Sky wave signals are used for long distance radio communication. These signals are in general, less stable than ground wave signals.
Reason : The state of ionosphere varies from hour to hour, day to day and season to season.

42. **Assertion :** The ratio for time taken for light emission from an atom to that for release of nuclear energy in fission is 1 : 100.
Reason : Time taken for the light emission from an atom is of the order of 10^{-8} s.

43. **Assertion :** Static crashes are heard on radio, when lightning flash occurs in the sky.
Reason : Electromagnetic waves having frequency of radio wave range interfere with radio waves.

44. **Assertion :** The velocity of a body at the bottom of an inclined plane of given height is more when it slides down the plane compared to when it is rolling down the same plane.
Reason : In rolling down, a body acquires both kinetic energy of translation and rotation.

45. **Assertion :** A quick collision between two bodies is more violent than a slow collision, even when the initial and the final velocities are identical.
Reason : The rate of change of momentum is greater in the first case.

46. **Assertion :** A body subject to three concurrent forces may be in equilibrium.
Reason : For equilibrium, the sum of all the concurrent forces acting at a point should be zero.

47. **Assertion :** Long distance transmission of a.c. is carried out at extremely high voltages.
Reason : Because when the distance is large, voltage has to be large.

48. **Assertion :** An electron microscope is based on de Broglie hypothesis.
Reason : A beam of electrons behaves as a wave which can be converged by electric and magnetic lenses.

49. Assertion : The resistance of a junction of a spoiled transistor is low when forward biased or reverse biased.

Reason : The resistance of a junction of a transistor in working order is high always.

50. Assertion : Short wave communication over long distance is not possible via ground waves.

Reason : The ground waves can bend round the corners of the objects on earth.

51. Assertion : A charged particle free to move in an electric field always moves along an electric field line.

Reason : The electric field lines diverge from a negative charge and converge at a positive charge.

52. Assertion : Current is passed through a metallic wire so that it becomes red hot. When cold water is poured on half of its portion, the rest of the half portion becomes more hot.

Reason : Resistance decreases due to decrease in temperature.

53. Assertion : If an electron and proton possessing same kinetic energy enter an electric field in a perpendicular direction, the path of the electron is more curved than that of the proton.

Reason : Electron forms a larger curve due to its small mass.

54. Assertion : The relative velocity between any two bodies moving in opposite direction is equal to sum of the velocities of two bodies.

Reason : Sometimes relative velocity between two bodies is equal to difference in velocities of the two bodies.

55. Assertion : When height of a tube is less than liquid rise in the capillary tube, the liquid does not overflow.

Reason : Product of radius of meniscus and height of liquid in the capillary tube always remain constant.

56. Assertion : The periodic time of a hard spring is less as compared to that of a soft spring.

Reason : The periodic time depends upon the spring constant, which is large for hard spring.

57. Assertion : It is not possible for a system, unaided by an external agency to transfer heat from a body at lower temperature to another body at a higher temperature.

Reason : It is not possible to violate the second law of thermodynamics.

58. Assertion : To hear distinct beats, difference in frequencies of two sources should be less than 10.

Reason : More the number of beats per sec more difficult to hear them.

59. Assertion : γ-radiation emission occurs after α and β decay.

Reason : Energy levels occur in nucleus.

60. Assertion : The edges of the images of white object formed by a concave mirror on the screen appear white.

Reason : Concave mirror does not suffer from chromatic aberration.

CHEMISTRY

61. Which is a bactericidal antibiotic?
(a) Penicillin (b) Erythromycin
(c) Tetracycline (d) Chloramphenicol

62. Monomers of nylon 2-nylon 6 are
(a) glycine and amino caproic acid
(b) glycine and caproic acid
(c) hexamethylene diamine and adipic acid
(d) alanine and amino caproic acid.

63. *A* forms *hcp* lattice and *B* are occupying 1/3rd of tetrahedral voids, then the formula of compound is
(a) AB (b) A_3B_2 (c) A_2B_3 (d) AB_4

64. Maltose is made of the units
(a) α-*D* glucose and β-*D* glucose
(b) α-*D* glucose and β-*D* fructose
(c) α-*D* glucose and α-*D* glucose
(d) α-*D* glucose and β-*D* galactose.

65. Rhombic sulphur dissolves best in
(a) CS_2 (b) H_2O (c) ethanol (d) ether.

66. $KMnO_4$ in alkaline medium changes to
(a) Mn^{3+} (b) MnO_2
(c) MnO_4^{2-} (d) $Mn(OH)_4^-$

67. Least coordination number is shown by
(a) $Co_2(CO)_8$ (b) $Mn_2(CO)_{10}$
(c) $[Fe(en)_2NH_3]$ (d) $[Cr(OH)_3(NH_3)_3]$

68. Enrichment of U^{235} is done by
(a) IF_7 (b) ClF_3 (c) IF_5 (d) ClF_5

69. Which halogen forms only one oxoacid (HO*X*)?
(a) F (b) Cl (c) Br (d) I

70. Which is correct regarding size of atom?
(a) N < O (b) B < Ne
(c) V > Ti (d) Na > K

71. Which is correct regarding acidity?
(a) $H_2S < H_2Se$ (b) $H_2S > H_2Se$
(c) $H_2Se > H_2Te$ (d) None of these.

72. Slag formed in blast furnace, removes the impurity of
(a) SiO_2 (b) CaO (c) CO_2 (d) FeO

73. When CO_2 is passed through solution of sodium aluminate precipitate of which compound is formed?
(a) $Al(OH)_3$ (b) Al_2O_3
(c) Na_2CO_3 (d) No ppt.

74. Purification of colloids is done by
(a) dialysis (b) peptisation
(c) electrophoresis (d) coagulation.

75. Which does not give Cannizzaro reaction?
(a) HCHO (b) $C_6H_5\underset{\underset{O}{\|}}{C}—CHO$
(c) Ph—CHO (d) $Ph—CH_2—CHO$

76. Which of the following is not sp^2 hybridised?
(a) Graphite (b) Graphene
(c) Fullerene (d) Dry ice

77. A diatomic gas at pressure *P*, compressed adiabatically to half of its volume, what is the final pressure?
(a) $(2)^{1.4}P$ (b) $P/(2)^{1.4}$
(c) $(2)^{5/3}P$ (d) $P/(2)^{5/3}$

78. Choose the correctly paired gaseous cation and its magnetic (spin only) moment (in B.M.)
(a) Ti^{2+}, 3.87 B.M. (b) Cr^{2+}, 4.90 B.M.
(c) Co^{3+}, 3.87 B.M. (d) Mn^{2+}, 4.90 B.M.

79. In presence of acidic medium, $KMnO_4$ converts H_2S into
(a) Mn only (b) MnS only
(c) MnS + S (d) S only.

80. Which of the following has highest concentration of PAN?
(a) Smoke
(b) Ozone
(c) Photochemical smog
(d) Reducing smog

81. The equilibrium constant for the reaction,
$$\frac{1}{2}H_{2(g)} + \frac{1}{2}I_{2(g)} \rightleftharpoons HI_{(g)} \text{ is } K_c.$$
Equilibrium constant for the reaction,
$2HI_{(g)} \rightleftharpoons H_{2(g)} + I_{2(g)}$ will be
(a) $1/K_c$ (b) $1/(K_c)^2$ (c) $2/K_c$ (d) $2/(K_c)^2$

82. 75% of a zero order reaction complete in 4 h 87.5% of the same reaction completes in
(a) 6 h (b) 12 h (c) 8 h (d) 2 h

83. For the reaction $A_{(g)} \longrightarrow B_{(g)} + C_{(g)}$, the rate constant is given as (P_i is initial pressure and P_t is pressure at time *t*)

(a) $k=\frac{2.303}{t}\log\frac{P_i}{P_t}$

(b) $k=\frac{2.303}{t}\log\frac{P_i}{(2P_i-P_t)}$

(c) $k=\frac{2.303}{t}\log\frac{2P_i-P_t}{P_i}$

(d) $k=\frac{2.303}{t}\log\frac{P_i-P_t}{2P_i}$

84. Which of the following pairs represent isotones?
(a) ${}^{77}_{33}As$, ${}^{78}_{34}Se$ (b) ${}^{195}_{78}Pt$, ${}^{190}_{76}Os$
(c) ${}^{108}_{47}Ag$, ${}^{112}_{48}Cd$ (d) ${}^{178}_{72}Hf$, ${}^{137}_{56}Ba$

85. In O_3 molecule, the formal charge on the central O-atom is
(a) 0 (b) –1 (c) –2 (d) +1

86. The number of atoms in 52 g of He is
(a) 78.299×10^{24} atoms
(b) 7.820×10^{-24} atoms
(c) 7.829×10^{24} atoms
(d) 78.234×10^{25} atoms

87. Which of the following represents the correct bond order?
(a) $O_2^+ < O_2^- > O_2^{2-}$ (b) $O_2^- > O_2^{2-} > O_2^+$
(c) $O_2^{2-} > O_2^+ > O_2^-$ (d) $O_2^+ > O_2^- > O_2^{2-}$

88. What is the oxidation number of Br in $KBrO_4$?
(a) +6 (b) +7 (c) +5 (d) +8

89. Which of the following reactions increases the production of dihydrogen from synthesis gas?
(a) $CH_{4(g)} + H_2O_{(g)} \xrightarrow[Ni]{1270\text{ K}} CO_{(g)} + H_{2(g)}$
(b) $C_{(s)} + H_2O_{(g)} \xrightarrow{1270\text{ K}} CO_{(g)} + H_{2(g)}$
(c) $CO_{(g)} + H_2O_{(g)} \xrightarrow[\text{Catalyst}]{673\text{ K}} CO_{2(g)} + H_{2(g)}$
(d) $C_2H_6 + 2H_2O \xrightarrow[Ni]{1270\text{ K}} 2CO + 5H_2$

90. Which of the following statements is incorrect?
(a) Li^+ has minimum degree of hydration.
(b) The oxidation state of K in KO_2 is +1.
(c) Na is used to make a Na/Pb alloy.
(d) $MgSO_4$ is readily soluble in water.

91. The purity of an organic compound is determined by
(a) chromatography (b) crystallisation
(c) melting or boiling point
(d) both (a) and (c).

92. The IUPAC name of the given compound is $(CH_3)_3CCH_2C(CH_3)_3$
(a) 2, 3, 4, 4-tetramethylpentane
(b) 1, 2, 2, 4-tetramethylpentene
(c) 2, 2, 4, 4-tetramethylpentane
(d) 3, 3-dimethylpentane.

93. The value of Henry's constant K_H is
(a) greater for gases with higher solubility
(b) greater for gases with lower solubility
(c) constant for all gases
(d) not related to the solubility of gases.

94. Which cell will measure standard electrode potential of copper electrode?
(a) $Pt_{(s)} | H_{2(g,\ 0.1\text{ bar})} | H^+_{(aq.,\ 1\text{ M})} || Cu^{2+}_{(aq.,\ 1\text{ M})} | Cu_{(s)}$
(b) $Pt_{(s)} | H_{2(g,\ 1\text{ bar})} | H^+_{(aq.,\ 1\text{ M})} || Cu^{2+}_{(aq.,\ 2\text{ M})} | Cu_{(s)}$
(c) $Pt_{(s)} | H_{2(g,\ 1\text{ bar})} | H^+_{(aq.,\ 1\text{ M})} || Cu^{2+}_{(aq.,\ 1\text{ M})} | Cu_{(s)}$
(d) $Pt_{(s)} | H_{2(g,\ 1\text{ bar})} | H^+_{(aq.,\ 0.1\text{ M})} || Cu^{2+}_{(aq.,\ 1\text{ M})} | Cu_{(s)}$

95. Which one of the following is an example for homogeneous catalysis?
(a) Manufacture of ammonia by Haber's process.
(b) Manufacture of sulphuric acid by contact process.
(c) Hydrogenation of oil.
(d) Hydrolysis of sucrose in presence of dilute hydrochloric acid.

96. Which one of the following is not employed as antihistamine?
(a) Dimetane (b) Chloramphenicol
(c) Seldane (d) Both (a) and (b)

97. Which one of the following forms propanenitrile as the major product?
(a) Propyl bromide + alcoholic KCN
(b) Ethyl bromide + alcoholic KCN
(c) Ethyl bromide + alcoholic AgCN
(d) Propyl bromide + alcoholic AgCN

98. What is '*A*' in the following reaction?

$$C_6H_5-CH_2-CH=CH_2 + HCl \longrightarrow A$$

(a) $CH_2-CH=CH_2$ attached to benzene ring with Cl on the ring (ortho)

(b) $C_6H_5-CH_2-CH_2-CH_2-Cl$

(c) $C_6H_5-CH_2-CH(Cl)-CH_3$

(d) $C_6H_5-CH(Cl)-CH_2-CH_3$

99. During the dehydration of alcohols to alkenes by heating with conc. H_2SO_4, the initiating step is
(a) elimination of water
(b) protonation of an alcohol molecule
(c) formation of an ester
(d) formation of carbocation.

100. In Clemmensen reduction, carbonyl compound is treated with
(a) zinc amalgam + HCl
(b) sodium amalgam + HCl
(c) zinc amalgam + HNO_3
(d) sodium amalgam + HNO_3.

Directions : In the following questions (101-120), a statement of assertion is followed by a statement of reason. Mark the correct choice as :
(a) If both assertion and reason are true and reason is the correct explanation of assertion.
(b) If both assertion and reason are true but reason is not the correct explanation of assertion.
(c) If assertion is true but reason is false.
(d) If both assertion and reason are false.

101. **Assertion :** Co(IV) is known but Ni(IV) is not.
Reason : Ni(IV) has d^4 electronic configuration.

102. **Assertion :** The correct order of oxidising power is : $VO_2^+ < Cr_2O_7^{2-} < MnO_4^-$
Reason : The oxidation state of Mn is +7.

103. **Assertion :** O_2 has higher bond length than O_3.
Reason : O_3 is paramagnetic.

104. **Assertion :** Insulin is water soluble.
Reason : Insulin is a globular protein.

105. **Assertion :** Monoclinic sulphur is an example of monoclinic crystal system.
Reason : For a monoclinic system, $a \neq b \neq c$ and $\alpha = \gamma = 90°, \beta \neq 90°$.

106. **Assertion :** Chemistry of actinoids is more complicated than lanthanoids.
Reason : Actinoid elements are radioactive.

107. **Assertion :** Coagulation power of Al^{3+} is more than Na^+.
Reason : Greater the valency of the flocculating ion added, greater is its power to cause precipitation (Hardy-Schulze rule).

108. **Assertion :** Mixture of CH_3COOH and CH_3COONH_4 is an example of acidic buffer.
Reason : Acidic buffer contains equimolar mixture of weak acid and its salt with weak base.

109. Assertion : Al becomes passive in conc. HNO_3.

Reason : Conc. HNO_3 has no action on aluminium metal.

110. Assertion : Chloroform is stored in dark coloured bottles.

Reason : Chronic chloroform exposure may cause damage to liver and kidneys.

111. Assertion : Saturated hydrocarbons are chemically less reactive.

Reason : All isomeric paraffins have same parent name.

112. Assertion : $(CH_3)_3CCOOH$ does not give HVZ reaction.

Reason : $(CH_3)_3CCOOH$ does not have α-hydrogen atom.

113. Assertion : An ideal solution obeys Raoult's law.

Reason : In an ideal solution, solute-solute as well as solvent-solvent interactions are similar to solute-solvent interactions.

114. Assertion : All the hydrogen atoms in $CH_2=C=CH_2$ lie in one plane.

Reason : All the carbon atoms in its are sp^2 hybridized.

115. Assertion : Conductivity of all electrolytes decreases on dilution.

Reason : On dilution number of ions per unit volume decreases.

116. Assertion : Permanent hardness of water is removed by treatment with washing soda.

Reason : Washing soda reacts with soluble calcium and magnesium chlorides and sulphates in hard water to form insoluble carbonates.

117. Assertion : Linkage isomerism arises in coordination compounds containing ambidentate ligand.

Reason : Ambidentate ligand has two different donor atoms.

118. Assertion : *Ortho* and *para*-nitrophenol can be separated by steam distillation.

Reason : *Para*-nitrophenol is steam volatile due to intramolecular hydrogen bonding.

119. Assertion : Natural rubber is a polymer of isoprene.

Reason : Isoprene is a pentene.

120. Assertion : H_3PO_3 is dibasic acid.

Reason : Two hydrogen atoms are directly attached to the P.

BIOLOGY

121. Which is the longest phase of the cell cycle?
(a) M-phase (b) Interphase
(c) Leptotene (d) S-phase

122. The total number of biodiversity hotspots in the world are
(a) 72 (b) 34 (c) 52 (d) 24.

123. Which of the following occurs due to monosomy of sex chromosome?
(a) Down's syndrome (b) Turner's syndrome
(c) Haemophilia (d) Sickle cell anaemia

124. During menstrual cycle, levels of LH and estrogen are highest around
(a) 14th day (b) 21st day
(c) 7th day (d) 28th day.

125. Which of the given genera is homosporous?
(a) *Cycas* (b) *Pinus*
(c) *Selaginella* (d) *Lycopodium*

126. Which of the following are a group of micronutrients for plants?
(a) Fe, Mn, Cu, Mo, Zn
(b) Fe, Mn, Cu, O, C
(c) Cu, B, Cl, Fe, Ca
(d) Ca, Mg, Fe

127. Match Column - I with Column - II and choose the correct option from below.

Column - I	Column - II
A. Marginal placentation	(i) Sunflower
B. Axile placentation	(ii) Mustard
C. Parietal placentation	(iii) Lemon
D. Basal placentation	(iv) Pea

(a) A - (iv), B - (iii), C - (ii), D - (i)
(b) A - (iv), B - (iii), C - (i), D - (ii)
(c) A - (iv), B - (i), C - (ii), D - (iii)
(d) A - (iii), B - (iv), C - (ii), D - (i)

128. Somaclones are prepared by
(a) callus culture
(b) sexual reproduction
(c) micropropagation
(d) somatic hybridisation.

129. Plants do not get benefit from
(a) N_2 in air (b) O_2 in air
(c) CO_2 in air (d) O_3 in air.

130. Vernalisation is subjected to plants growing in
(a) tropical areas
(b) sub tropical areas
(c) temperate areas
(d) hot areas/arctic region.

131. The phenomenon that operates in the formation of root or shoot in a callus culture is
(a) differentiation (b) re-differentiation
(c) de-differentiation (d) re-juvenation.

132. Which of the following genes do not occur naturally in living organisms?
(a) *Bt* genes
(b) RNA*i* genes
(c) Cry genes
(d) Endogeneous cytoplasmic defense genes

133. DNA and RNA comprise of
(a) sugar, phosphate, base
(b) sugar, phosphate
(c) base, phosphate
(d) sugar, base.

134. Choose the correct pair.
(a) Coconut, cucurbits - dioecious
(b) Honeybee, Rotifers - parthenogenesis
(c) *Ornithorhyncus*, Whale - viviparity
(d) Frog, Peacock - external fertilisation

135. Which of the following associations shows mutualism?
(a) Fig and wasp
(b) Barnacles on whale
(c) Roundworms in human intestine
(d) Orchids on mango tree

136. Select the incorrect statement.
(a) *Periplaneta* has compound eyes.
(b) Earthworm shows segmentation.
(c) *Ascaris* shows sexual dimorphism.
(d) Liver fluke has a complete alimentary canal.

137. How many haploid nuclei are present in a mature pollen grain?
(a) One (b) Two (c) Three (d) Four

138. In cloning of cattle a fertilized egg is taken out of the mother's womb and
(a) in the eight cell stage, cells are separated and cultured untill small embryos are formed which are implanted into the womb of other cows
(b) in the eight cell stage the individual cells are separated under electrical field for further development in culture media
(c) from this upto eight identical twins can be produced
(d) the egg is divided into 4 pairs of cells which are implanted into the womb of other cows.

139. Select the correct pair of microorganism and the product obtained from it.
(a) *Monascus purpureus* - produces large holes in Swiss cheese.
(b) *Saccharomyces cerevisiae* - used for making wine and beer after distillation.
(c) *Streptococcus* - produces streptokinase which is used to remove clots.
(d) *Aspergillus niger* - produces citric acid and butyric acid.

140. Choose the correctly matched pair from the following.
(a) Gonorrhoea, hepatitis B - sexually transmitted diseases
(b) AIDS, gonorrhoea - viral infection
(c) Diphtheria, ringworm - fungal infection
(d) Diphtheria, tuberculosis - protozoan infection

141. Select the correct statement about hormones and their actions.
(a) Parathyroid hormone increases K^+ absorption of the body.
(b) Insulin and glucagon helps to maintain blood sugar levels.
(c) Old aged people have weak immunity due to increased activity of thymus.
(d) Osteoporosis in women occurs due to increased levels of oestrogens.

142. Select the correct sequence for *Homo erectus*.
(a) Erectus → homo → primata → chordata → animalia
(b) Homo → erectus → primata → animalia → chordata
(c) Homo → erectus → primata → chordata → animalia
(d) Erectus → homo → animalia → primata → chordata

143. Refer the given figure of digestive system of earthworm and identify the part labelled X.

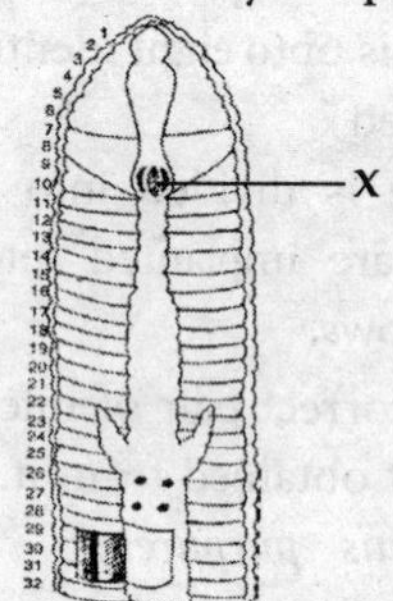

(a) Intestinal caecae (b) Typhlosole
(c) Gizzard (d) Pharynx.

144. Select the correct option regarding A, B and C.

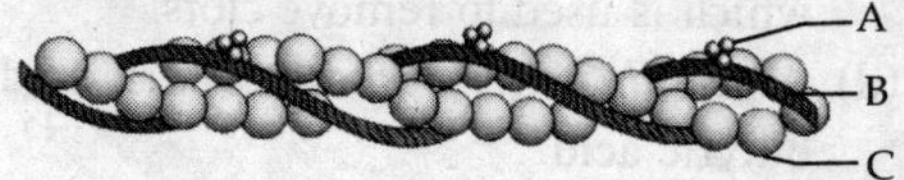

(a) A-Tropomyosin-runs close to F-actin throughout its length
(b) B-Troponin-complex protein distributed at regular interval of tropomyosin
(c) C-F actin - polymer of monomeric G-actin helically bound to each other
(d) None of these

145. Identify the given figure and select the correct option.

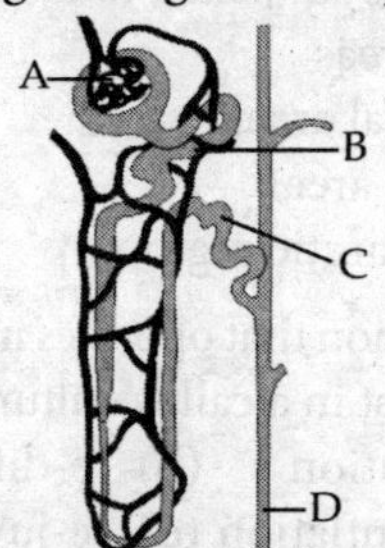

(a) Neutrophil - phagocytic cell which destroy foreign organisms entering the body.
(b) Eosinophil - their number increases during allergic infection.
(c) Lymphocyte - small sized non-motile and non-phagocytic.
(d) Monocyte - motile and phagocytic in nature.

146. Refer the given figure of nephron.

A
B
C
D

Identify A, B, C and D and select the correct option regarding them
(a) A-Glomerulus - a tuft of capillaries formed by afferent arteriole.
(b) B-PCT-reabsorption of HCO_3^- and selective secretion of H^+ and K^+ occurs here.
(c) C-DCT-almost all glucose, amino acids, water, Na^+, K^+ and uric acid are absorbed here.
(d) D-collecting duct-extends from the cortex of the kidney to the inner parts of medulla. Large amount of water is secreted in this region.

147. Which antibiotic has bactericidal effect?
(a) Erythromycin (b) Penicillin
(c) Streptomycin (d) Chloramphenicol

148. Which of the following statements is not true?
(a) The biodiversity decreases with increasing latitude.
(b) The biodiversity decreases with increasing altitude.
(c) The fishes show greatest biodiversity among vertebrates.
(d) The biodiversity of bryophytes is greater than that of angiosperms.

149. Which of the following options consist of non-essential amino acids only?
(a) Valine, leucine, glycine, alanine
(b) Glycine, serine, proline, glutamic acid
(c) Proline, aspartic acid, glutamic acid, methionine
(d) Cysteine, tyrosine, alanine, isoleucine

150. Photochemical smog formed in congested metropolitan cities mainly consists of
(a) ozone, peroxyacyl nitrate and NO_x
(b) smoke, peroxyacyl nitrate and SO_2
(c) hydrocarbons, SO_2 and CO_2
(d) hydrocarbons, ozone and SO_x.

151. How are transformants selected from non-transformants?
(a) Presence of more than one recognition site in the vector DNA.
(b) Presence of alien DNA into the vector DNA results into insertional inactivation of selectable marker.
(c) Antibiotic resistance gene gets inactivated due to insertion of alien DNA.
(d) Both (b) and (c).

152. Given is the diagrammatic representation of the sectional view of cochlea. Select the correct option regarding it.

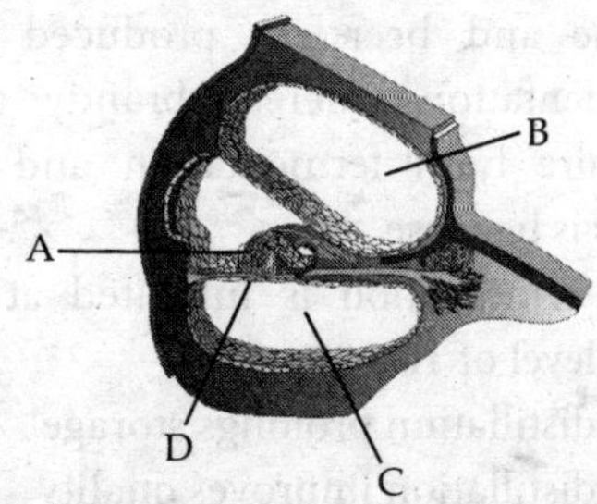

(a) A - Organ of corti-responsible for maintenance of balance of the body and posture.
(b) B - Scala vestibuli-filled with perilymph that ends at the oval window.
(c) C - Scala tympani - terminates at the round window which opens to the middle ear.
(d) D - Basilar membrane - nerve impulses are generated against it.

153. In a standard ECG which one of the following alphabets is the correct representation of the respective activity of the human heart?
(a) S - start of systole (b) T - end of diastole
(c) P - depolarisation of the atria
(d) R - repolarisation of ventricles

154. Which one of the following vitamins is anti-haemorrhagic?
(a) Vitamin B_{12} (b) Vitamin B_5
(c) Vitamin C (d) Vitamin K

155. Which of the following is not a character of cancerous cells in our body?
(a) Contact inhibition
(b) Neoplasia
(c) Metastasis
(d) Inability for differentiation

156. What is true about Bt toxin?
(a) Bt protein exists as active toxin in the *Bacillus*.
(b) The activated toxin enters the ovaries of the pest to sterilise it and thus prevent its multiplication.
(c) The concerned *Bacillus* has antitoxins.
(d) The inactive protoxin gets converted into active form in the insect gut.

157. Wine and beer are produced directly by fermentation whereas brandy and whisky require both fermentation and distillation. This is because
(a) fermentation is inhibited at an alcohol level of 10-18%
(b) distillation prolongs storage
(c) distillation improves quality
(d) distillation purifies the beverage.

158. Which of the following is not a characteristic of pBR322 vector?
(a) It is the first artificial cloning vector constructed in 1977 by Boliver and Rodriguez.
(b) It is the most widely used, versatile and easily manipulated vector.
(c) It has two antibiotic resistance genes, tet^R and amp^R.
(d) It does not have restriction site for *Sal I.*

159. Which of the following pairs of hormones can easily pass through the cell membrane and binds to a receptor inside it (mostly in the nucleus)?
(a) Insulin, glucagon
(b) Thyroxine, insulin
(c) Somatostatin, oxytocin
(d) Cortisol, testosterone

160. Which one of the following immune system components does not correctly match with its respective role?
(a) Interferons - secreted by virus-infected cells and protect non-infected cells from further viral infection
(b) B-lymphocytes-produces antibodies in response to pathogens into blood to fight with them
(c) Macrophages-mucus secreting cells that trap microbes entering in the body
(d) IgA-present in colostrum in early days of lactation and protect infant from diseases

Directions: In the following questions (161-180), a statement of assertion is followed by a statement of reason. Mark the correct choice as :
(a) If both assertion and reason are true and reason is the correct explanation of assertion.
(b) If both assertion and reason are true but reason is not the correct explanation of assertion.
(c) If assertion is true but reason is false.
(d) If both assertion and reason are false.

161. Assertion : In a pedigree analysis, ⟨5⟩ represents five unaffected offsprings.
Reason : In a pedigree analysis, the offsprings are numbered with arabic numerals (1, 2, 3.....) and a generation is numbered with roman numerals (I, II, III...).

162. Assertion : HCl converts pepsinogen into active enzyme pepsin.
Reason : Pepsin converts protein into proteoses and peptones.

163. Assertion : The optic nerves leave the eye at the point called blind spot.
Reason : Only cone are densely packed at the blind spot, hence is the name.

164. Assertion : Smoking causes oxygen deficiency in the body.
Reason : Carbon monoxide when inhaled while smoking, combines with haemoglobin to form chemically stable compound.

165. Assertion : The immune responses of old persons become weak.
Reason : Thymus is degenerated in old individuals resulting in a decreased production of thymosin.

166. Assertion : The enlarged Q and R waves indicate myocardial infarction.
Reason : The QRS complex represents ventricular repolarisation.

167. Assertion : The leaves in gymosperms are well-adapted to withstand extremes of temperature, humidity and wind.

Reason : Unlike bryophytes and pteridophytes, in gymnosperms the male and female gametophytes do not have an independent free-living existence.

168. Assertion : Glucose is the favoured respiratory substrate.

Reason : When glucose is used as respiratory substrate and is completely oxidized, the RQ is 1.

169. Assertion : Human heart is myogenic.

Reason : The contraction is initiated by a specialized patch of modified heart muscles without requiring stimulation from nerve cells.

170. Assertion : AIDS and hepatitis B are sexually transmitted diseases.

Reason : There is no permanent cure for both of them.

171. Assertion : One codon may code for more than one amino acid.

Reason : A codon is degenerate and ambiguous.

172. Assertion : Interspecific competition is the only potent force in organic evolution.

Reason : Unexceptionally two closely related species competing for the same resources cannot co-exist indefinitely.

173. Assertion : GM crops can affect human health by causing allergic reactions.

Reason : Transgenes in commercial crops can endanger native species *e.g.*, the *Bt* toxin gene expressed in pollen might endanger pollinators like honeybees.

174. Assertion : Secondary air pollutants are formed by interaction among the primary pollutants and are more toxic.

Reason : DDT is a secondary air pollutant.

175. Assertion : In basidiomycetes, basidiospores are produced endogenously in the basidium.

Reason : In ascomycetes, ascospores are produced exogenously in ascus.

176. Assertion : In a pivot joint, rounded or pointed bone fits into a shallow depression in another bone.

Reason : Pivot joints are present between the metacarpals and phalanges of the fingers.

177. Assertion : Deficiency symptoms of N, K and Mg are first visible in the senescent leaves.

Reason : Biomolecules containing these elements are broken down in the older leaves, making these elements available for mobilising to younger leaves.

178. Assertion : Photorespiration interferes with the successful functioning of Calvin cycle.

Reason : Photorespiration oxidises ribulose-1,5 biphosphate which is an acceptor of CO_2 in Calvin cycle.

179. Assertion : Pulmonary circulation consists of flow of deoxygenated blood from right ventricle to the lungs and flow of oxygenated blood from lungs to the left atrium.

Reason : Systemic circulation consists of flow of oxygenated blood from the left ventricle to all parts of the body and deoxygenated blood from different parts to right atrium.

180. Assertion : Adrenocorticotropic-Releasing Hormones (ARH) excite the anterior lobe of pituitary gland to produce adrenocorticotropic hormone (ACTH).

Reason : ACTH stimulates the adrenal cortex to secrete its glucocorticoid and mineralocorticoid hormones.

GENERAL KNOWLEDGE

181. The Dandi March by Gandhiji began on
(a) 12th March, 1930 (b) 1st March, 1930
(c) 26th January, 1930 (d) 10th May, 1930

182. Who was the first Home Minister of India after independence?
(a) Dr. V.V. Giri (b) Dr. Zakir Hussain
(c) Morarji Desai
(d) Sardar Vallabhbhai Patel

183. Which of the following is an outcome of the rotation of the earth?
(a) Eclipse (b) Gravitational force
(c) Coriolis force (d) Tidal force

184. Aluminium oxide is a/an
(a) Basic oxide (b) Amphoteric oxide
(c) Neutral oxide (d) Acidic oxide

185. The Forward Bloc was founded by
(a) Bhagat Singh
(b) Jai Prakash Narayan
(c) Subhas Chandra Bose
(d) Ram Manohar Lohia

186. World Environment Day is celebrated on
(a) June 5 (b) October 5
(c) July 7 (d) March 7

187. Who wrote 'Indica'?
(a) Vishakhadatta (b) Chanakya
(c) Ashoka (d) Megasthenes

188. Kalachakra ceremony is associated with
(a) Jainism (b) Buddhism
(c) Sikhism (d) Din-e-ilahi

189. Which of the following states does not have an Upper House (Vidhan Parishad)?
(a) Andhra Pradesh (b) Bihar
(c) Uttar Pradesh (d) Odisha

190. Who wrote 'Natya Shastra'?
(a) Bharata Muni (b) Ravi Shankar
(c) Kalidasa (d) Manmohan Ghosh

191. In which year did the adult suffrage change from 21 to 18 in India?
(a) 1978 (b) 2000
(c) 1989 (d) 1984

192. Who was the first woman Prime Minister in the world?
(a) Indira Gandhi
(b) Gold Meir
(c) Margaret Thatcher
(d) Sirimavo Bandaranaike

193. Who presides over the joint session of Lok Sabha and Rajya Sabha?
(a) President (b) Vice President
(c) Speaker (d) Chief Justice

194. Which of the following authorities, has the right to issue 'aadhar card' to the residents of India?
(a) Intelligence Bureau
(b) Planning Commission
(c) State Government
(d) Election Commission

195. In which city Ashoka Pillar is believed to have originated?
(a) Varanasi (b) Sanchi
(c) Sarnath (d) Vaishali

196. Who has won Nobel Prize award twice?
(a) Marie Curie (b) Neil Bohr
(c) Ernest Rutherford (d) Albert Einstein

197. Where will the next to next summer olympics take place?
(a) Rio de Janeiro (b) Tokyo
(c) Ryeongchang (d) Beijing

198. Ramesh Agrawal won green Nobel Prize award for blocking a major Indian company, India Steel & Power Ltd., from opening a second coal mine in which of the following states?
(a) Jharkhand (b) Odisha
(c) Chhattisgarh (d) Bihar

199. Who won the Dada Saheb Phalke award for contribution to Indian Cinema in the year 2014?
(a) Asha Bhosle (b) Pran
(c) Gulzar (d) Jagjit Singh

200. In which country is 'Pali' language taught?
(a) Myanmar (b) Malaysia
(c) Vietnam (d) China

SOLUTIONS

PHYSICS

1. **(c) :** As $F = [MLT^{-2}]$ or $[T^2] = \frac{[ML]}{[F]}$

or $[T] = [M^{1/2}L^{1/2}F^{-1/2}]$

2. **(a) :** As $f_{ms} = \mu_s mg = 0.4 \times 2 \times 10 = 8$ N.
The applied force of 2.8 N is less than f_{ms} (= 8 N) and as such the block does not move. When the block is at rest,
frictional force = applied force = 2.8 N

3. **(c) :** In an elastic collision of a very heavy body with a very light body at rest, the speed of lighter body becomes twice the speed of the heavier body, *i.e.*, $v_2 = 2u_1 = 120$ km h^{-1}.

4. **(b) :** Here, $r = 80$ m, $v = 36$ km h^{-1} = $36 \times (5/18)$ m s^{-1} = 10 m s^{-1}

$$\therefore \quad \tan\theta = \frac{v^2}{rg} = \frac{(10)^2}{80 \times 10} = \frac{1}{8}$$

or $\theta = \tan^{-1}\left(\frac{1}{8}\right)$

5. **(d) :** Kinetic energy, $K = \frac{1}{2}mv_0^2$

or $v_0 = \sqrt{\frac{2K}{m}}$

When kinetic energy is doubled, then

$$v_0' = \sqrt{\frac{2 \times 2K}{m}} = \sqrt{2}\sqrt{\frac{2K}{m}} = \sqrt{2}v_0$$

But $\sqrt{2}v_0 = v_e$ (escape velocity)
Hence satellite will escape out of earth's gravitational field.

6. **(b) :** Given,

$y = a\sin(\omega t - kx)$ and $y = a\cos(\omega t - kx)$

Here, the phase difference between the two waves is $\frac{\pi}{2}$.

So, the resultant amplitude,

$$A = \sqrt{a_1^2 + a_2^2 + 2a_1a_2\cos\phi}$$

Here $a_1 = a$, $a_2 = a$, $\phi = \frac{\pi}{2}$

$$\therefore \quad A = \sqrt{a^2 + a^2 + 2a^2\cos\frac{\pi}{2}}$$

or $A = \sqrt{a^2 + a^2 + 0} \Rightarrow A = \sqrt{2}a$

7. **(a) :** Here, $R_1 = 1/2\ \Omega$, $R_2 = 1/4\ \Omega$; $R_3 = 1/6\ \Omega$

In parallel; $\frac{1}{R_p} = \frac{1}{R_1} + \frac{1}{R_2} + \frac{1}{R_3} = 2 + 4 + 6 = 12$

or equivalent conductance, $G = \frac{1}{R_p} = 12\ S$

8. **(b) :** $\frac{\mu_0}{4\pi}\frac{2i_1}{r} - \frac{\mu_0}{4\pi}\frac{2i_2}{r} = 10\ \mu T$

$\frac{\mu_0}{4\pi}\frac{2i_1}{r} + \frac{\mu_0}{4\pi}\frac{2i_2}{r} = 30\ \mu T$

On solving $i_1 = 20$ A and $i_2 = 10$ A. $\therefore$ $i_1/i_2 = 2$

9. **(d) :** Magnetic field at the centre of primary coil $B = \mu_0 i_1/2R_1$. Considering it to be uniform, magnetic flux passing through secondary coil is

$$\phi_2 = BA = \frac{\mu_0 i_1}{2R_1}(\pi R_2^2)$$

Now, $M = \frac{\phi_2}{i_1} = \frac{\mu_0 \pi R_2^2}{2R_1}$ $\therefore$ $M \propto \frac{R_2^2}{R_1}$.

10. **(a) :** Here, $\delta_m = A$, $\mu = 1.5$

$$\therefore \ \mu = \frac{\sin\frac{(A+\delta_m)}{2}}{\sin\frac{A}{2}} = \frac{\sin\frac{(A+A)}{2}}{\sin\frac{A}{2}}$$

$$= \frac{2\sin\left(\frac{A}{2}\right)\cos\left(\frac{A}{2}\right)}{\sin\left(\frac{A}{2}\right)}$$

$$\frac{3}{2}=2\cos\frac{A}{2} \qquad \left(\because \mu=1.5=\frac{3}{2}\right)$$

$$\cos\frac{A}{2}=\frac{3}{4}$$

$$\frac{A}{2}=\cos^{-1}\left(\frac{3}{4}\right) \text{ or } A=2\cos^{-1}\left(\frac{3}{4}\right)$$

11. **(b) :** Maximum tension an elevator can tolerate is

$$T=\frac{1}{3}\text{stress}\times\text{area of cross-section}$$

$$=\frac{1}{3}\times(2.4\times10^{8})\times(3\times10^{-4}) = 2.4\times10^{4}\text{ N}$$

If a is the maximum upward acceleration of elevator then $T = m(g + a)$

or $2.4\times10^4 = 1200(10 + a)$

On solving, $a = 10$ m s^{-2}.

12. **(b) :** As $dQ = C_P m\Delta T$

$\therefore \quad 70 = C_P \times 2(35 - 30)$

$\therefore \quad C_P = 7$ cal/mole/°C

$C_V = C_P - R$

$= 7 - 1.99 = 5.01$ cal mol^{-1} °C^{-1}

$\therefore \quad dQ' = C_V m\Delta T$

$= 5.01 \times 2 \times (35 - 30) = 50.1$ cal

13. **(c) :** For mixture, $C_V=\dfrac{n_1C_{V_1}+n_2C_{V_2}}{n_1+n_2}$

$$=\frac{3\times\frac{5}{2}R+1\times\frac{3}{2}R}{3+1}=\frac{9R}{4}$$

$$C_P=C_V+R=\frac{9R}{4}+R=\frac{13R}{4}$$

14. **(b) :** Let h be the depth of bottle in water then

$A h\rho g = mg$ or $h=\dfrac{m}{A\rho}=\dfrac{200}{50\times1}=4$ cm.

Now time period,

$$T=2\pi\sqrt{\frac{h}{g}} \text{ or } \upsilon=\frac{1}{T}=\frac{1}{2\pi}\sqrt{\frac{g}{h}}$$

$$=\frac{7}{2\times22}\sqrt{\frac{980}{4}}=2.5\text{ Hz}$$

15. **(c) :**

A	B	Y_1	Y_2	$Y=\overline{Y_1+Y_2}$
0	0	1	1	0
0	1	1	0	0
1	0	0	1	0
1	1	0	0	1

According to truth table,

$Y = A{\cdot}B$, the given combination of logic gates represents AND gate.

16. **(b) :** For the first line of Balmer series,

$$\frac{1}{\lambda_1}=R\left(\frac{1}{2^2}-\frac{1}{3^2}\right)=\frac{5R}{36}$$

For the second line of Balmer series.

$$\frac{1}{\lambda_2}=R\left(\frac{1}{2^2}-\frac{1}{4^2}\right)=\frac{3R}{16}$$

$$\therefore \frac{\lambda_2}{\lambda_1}=\frac{5R/36}{3R/16}=\frac{20}{27};$$

$$\text{or } \lambda_2=\frac{20}{27}(6561\text{ Å}) = 4860\text{ Å}$$

17. **(c) :** As $R = \lambda N$, $n = \lambda N$, or $\lambda = (n/N)$

$$T_{1/2}=\frac{0.693}{\lambda}=\frac{0.693\,N}{n}\text{s}$$

18. **(a) :** As $K_{\max}=\dfrac{hc}{\lambda}-\phi_0$

$= 3.1\text{ eV} - 2\text{ eV} = 1.1\text{ eV}$

$V_0 = 1.1$ V

19. **(a) :** RP of a reflecting microscope $=\dfrac{2\mu\sin\theta}{\lambda}$

20. **(b) :** Iron is most suitable for electromagnets and transformers, because of low energy losses.

21. **(b) :** Here, $R = 10\ \Omega$, $L = 2$ H,

$V = 120$ V, $\upsilon = 60$ Hz

$$X_L=\omega L=2\pi\upsilon L=2\times\frac{22}{7}\times60\times2 = 754.3\ \Omega$$

$$Z=\sqrt{R^2+X_L^2}=\sqrt{10^2+(754.3)^2}=754.35\ \Omega$$

$$I_V=\frac{V}{Z}=\frac{120}{754.3}\text{A}=0.16\text{ A}$$

22. **(b)**: As $\frac{\varepsilon_0 A}{d} = 4\pi\varepsilon_0 R$

$$d = \frac{A}{4\pi R} = \frac{\pi(6/2)^2}{4\pi(100)} = 2.25\times10^{-2}\text{ cm}$$

$= 2.25 \times 10^{-4}$ m

23. **(a)**: As $E = \frac{F}{q} = \frac{3000\text{ N}}{3\text{C}} = 1000\text{ N C}^{-1}$

$dr = 1$ cm $= 10^{-2}$ m

$dV = E(dr) = 1000 \times 10^{-2} = 10$ V

24. **(a)**: Force on the electron $\vec{F} = -e(\vec{v}\times\vec{B})$. As electron is travelling in a plane perpendicular to the plane of wire, so angle θ between $\vec{v}$ and $\vec{B}$ is either 0° or 180° and sin 0° or sin 180° = 0.

25. **(a)**: Given, $5 = \frac{2u\sin\theta}{g}$ or $\frac{u\sin\theta}{g} = \frac{5}{2}$

Maximum height $= \frac{u^2\sin^2\theta}{2g} = \frac{g}{2}\times\left(\frac{u^2\sin^2\theta}{g^2}\right)$

$$= \frac{g}{2}\times\left(\frac{5}{2}\right)^2 = \frac{10}{2}\times\frac{25}{4} = 31.25\text{ m}$$

26. **(d)**: Angular momentum is an axial vector, so its direction is along the axis, perpendicular to the plane of motion which is not changing because of change of speed. Therefore, the direction of angular momentum remains the same and its magnitude may vary.

27. **(b)**: Potential energy at the required height

$$= \frac{490}{2} = 245\text{ J}$$

Again, $245 = 2 \times 10 \times h$

or $h = \frac{245}{20}\text{ m} = 12.25\text{ m}$

28. **(b)**

29. **(b)**: The value of g at latitude λ is

$g' = g - R\omega^2\cos^2\lambda$.

If earth stops rotating, $\omega = 0$; $g' = g$.

It means the weight of body will increase.

30. **(a)**: Velocity, $v = r\omega\cos\omega t$

$$0.4 = r\times\frac{2\pi}{16}\cos\frac{2\pi}{16}\times2 = r\times\frac{2\pi}{16}\times\frac{1}{\sqrt{2}}$$

or $r = \frac{0.4\times16\times\sqrt{2}}{2\pi} = \frac{3.2\sqrt{2}}{\pi} = 1.44\text{ m}$

31. **(c)**: Here, $m = \frac{0.035}{5.5}, T = 77\text{ N}$

∴ Velocity on the string is

$$v = \sqrt{T/m} = \sqrt{\frac{77}{0.035/5.5}} = \sqrt{\frac{77\times5.5}{0.035}} = 110\text{ m s}^{-1}$$

32. **(b)**: Here, $u = -25$ cm $v = -1$ m $= -100$ cm

$$\therefore \frac{1}{f} = \frac{1}{v} - \frac{1}{u} = \frac{1}{-100} + \frac{1}{25} = \frac{3}{100}$$

or $f = \frac{100}{3}\text{ cm} = \frac{1}{3}\text{ m}$

Therefore, required power,

$$P = \frac{1}{f(\text{m})} = \frac{1}{1/3}$$

$P = 3$ D

33. **(d)**

34. **(c)**: As, $\phi = \frac{2\pi}{\lambda}\Delta x \Rightarrow \phi = \frac{2\pi}{\lambda}\lambda$

$\phi = 2\pi$

$\therefore I = I_1 + I_2 + 2\sqrt{I_1I_2}\cos\phi$

$= I' + I' + 2I'\cos2\pi$

$I = 2I' + 2I' = 4I'$

When $\Delta x = \frac{\lambda}{6}$, then

$$\phi = \frac{2\pi}{\lambda}\times\frac{\lambda}{6} = \frac{2\pi}{6}$$

$$\therefore\quad I_1 = I' + I' + 2\sqrt{I'I'}\cos\frac{2\pi}{6}$$

$I_1 = 2I' + 2I'(1/2)$

$I_1 = 3I'$

$$\therefore\quad \frac{I_1}{I} = \frac{3I'}{4I'} = \frac{3}{4}$$

or $I_1 = \frac{3}{4}I$

35. (b) : According to the principle of conservation of angular momentum, $I\omega$ = constant
As I is doubled, ω becomes half

Now K.E. of rotation, $K = \frac{1}{2}I\omega^2$

Since I is doubled and ω is halved, K.E. will become half *i.e.* $\frac{K}{2}$.

36. (b) : Radius of nth orbit in hydrogen like atoms is

$$r_n = \frac{a_0 n^2}{Z}$$

where a_0 is the Bohr's radius
For hydrogen atom, $Z = 1$

$\therefore\ r_1 = a_0 \quad (\because n = 1 \text{ for ground state})$

For Be^{3+}, $Z = 4$

$$\therefore\ r_n = \frac{a_0 n^2}{4}$$

According to given problem

$$r_1 = r_n$$

$$a_0 = \frac{n^2 a_0}{4}$$

$$n = 2$$

37. (b) : Velocity in eastward direction $= 5\hat{i}$
velocity in northward direction $= 5\hat{j}$

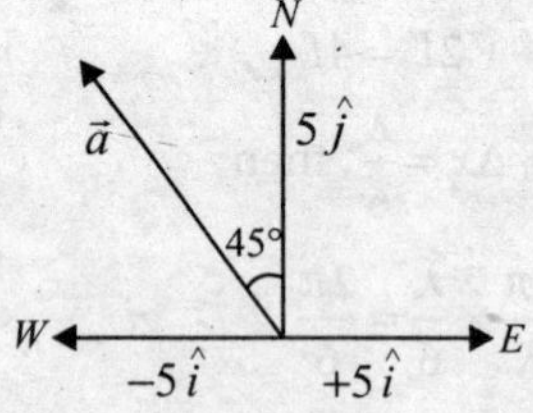

$\therefore$ Acceleration $\vec{a} = \frac{5\hat{j} - 5\hat{i}}{10}$

or $\vec{a} = \frac{1}{2}\hat{j} - \frac{1}{2}\hat{i}$ or $|\vec{a}| = \sqrt{\left(\frac{1}{2}\right)^2 + \left(-\frac{1}{2}\right)^2}$

or $|\vec{a}| = \frac{1}{\sqrt{2}}$ m s^{-2} towards north-west.

38. (c) : $U_1 = \frac{1}{2}kx_1^2 = \frac{1}{2} \times (5\times 10^3) \times (5\times 10^{-2})^2$
$= 6.25$ N m

$U_2 = \frac{1}{2}kx_2^2 = \frac{1}{2} \times 5\times 10^3 \times (5+5)^2 \times 10^{-4}$
$= 25$ N m

$\therefore$ Work done $= U_2 - U_1 = 25.0 - 6.25$
$= 18.75$ N m

39. (b) : According to kinetic theory of gases, gas molecules behave as a perfectly elastic rigid spheres.

40. (b) : Here, $\vec{E}$ and $\vec{B}$ are acting along x-axis and $\vec{v}$ is along y-axis *i.e.* perpendicular to both $\vec{E}$ and $\vec{B}$. Therefore, the path of charged particle is a helix with increasing speed. Speed of particle at time t is

$$v = \sqrt{v_x^2 + v_y^2} \quad \text{...(i)}$$

Here, $v_y = v_0; v_x = \frac{qE_0}{m}t$ and $v = \frac{\sqrt{5}}{2}v_0$

Putting values in (i), we get

$$t = \frac{mv_0}{2qE_0}$$

41. (b) : Since ionospheric properties change with time, the sky wave signals are in general less stable than ground wave signals.

42. (a) : Time taken for the light emission from an atom $\approx 10^{-8}$ s.
Time taken for release of energy in fission $\approx 10^{-6}$

Required ratio $= \frac{10^{-8}}{10^{-6}} = \frac{1}{100} = 1:100$

43. (a)

44. (b) : When a body slides, its entire PE is converted into KE of translation. But when it rolls down, some part of its PE is converted into its KE of rotation, thereby reducing its KE of translation and hence its linear velocity.

45. (a) : As $\Delta p = m\Delta v$, $\Delta p \propto \Delta v$, and $F = \frac{\Delta p}{\Delta t}$ the rate of change of momentum is greater in a quicker collision between two bodies. The quicker collision between two bodies is more violent due to greater force.

46. (a) : A body subjected to three concurrent forces is in equilibrium if their resultant is zero.

47. (b) : Reason is false. When voltage is extremely high, current is extremely weak. Therefore, energy loss in long distance transmission of a.c. becomes negligible.

48. (a) : Both the assertion and reason are true and latter explains the former correctly.

49. (c) : The reason is not true. The junction of a transistor in working order has low resistance, when forward biased and it has high resistance, when reverse biased. The assertion, however is true.

50. (a) : Assertion and Reason both are correct and Reason is the correct explanation of assertion.

51. (d) : Only a charged particle initially at rest moves along the electric field line. In case, the charged particle is in motion and its initial velocity is at an angle with the electric field line, the particle may follow a parabolic path.

52. (a) : The resistance of that half portion of the metallic wire (heated red hot) on which cold water is poured decreases due to fall in its temperature. This results in a decrease in the resistance of the entire wire. As a result, the current in the wire increases and the other half portion becomes hotter than before.

53. (d) : As

$$qE = \frac{mv^2}{r}, r = \frac{mv^2}{qE} = \frac{2K}{qE} \text{(where } K = \frac{1}{2}mv^2\text{)}$$

i.e., $r \propto \frac{1}{q}$.

Since electron and proton have equal charge, r is the same for both of them.

Here, r depends on K(which is given to be the same for both the particles) and as such not on their masses.

54. (b) : When two bodies are moving in opposite directions, relative velocity between them is equal to sum of the velocity of bodies. But if the bodies are moving in same direction their relative velocity is equal to difference in velocity of the bodies.

55. (a) : As

$$hR = \frac{2S}{\rho g} = \text{a finite constant.}$$

Hence when the tube is of insufficient length, radius of curvature of the liquid meniscus increases, so as to maintain the product hR a finite constant, *i.e.*, as h decreases, R increases and the liquid meniscus becomes more and more flat, but the liquid does not overflow.

56. (b) : The time period of a oscillating spring is given by,

$T = 2\pi\sqrt{\frac{m}{k}}$ *i.e.* $T \propto \frac{1}{\sqrt{k}}$. Since the spring constant is large for hard spring, therefore hard spring has a less periodic time as compared to soft spring.

57. (a) : Second law of thermodynamics can be explained with the help of example of refrigerator, as we know that in refrigerator, the working substance extracts heat from colder body and rejects a large amount of heat to a hotter body with the help of an external agency *i.e.*, the electric supply of the refrigerator. No refrigerator can ever work without external supply of electric energy to it.

58. (a) : According to the property of persistence of hearing, the impression of a sound heard persists on our mind for $\frac{1}{10}$ sec. Therefore, number of beats per sec should be less than 10. Hence difference in frequencies of two sources must be less than 10. [beats per sec = $\upsilon_2 - \upsilon_1$]

59. (a)

60. (a) : The rays of all colours incident on a concave mirror at the same angle are reflected at the same angle. As there is no chromatic aberration, the reflected image is white.

CHEMISTRY

61. (a) : Penicillin is a bactericidal whereas erythromycin, tetracycline and chloramphenicol are bacteriostatic antibiotics.

62. (a) : Nylon 2-nylon 6 is an alternating polyamide copolymer of glycine ($H_2N—CH_2—COOH$) and amino caproic acid [$H_2N(CH_2)_5COOH$].

63. (b) : Let no. of atoms of A used in close packing $= n$

Number of tetrahedral voids = $2n$

Number of atoms of $B = \frac{1}{3} \times 2n = \frac{2}{3}n$

$A : B = n : \frac{2}{3}n = 3 : 2$

Formula of the compound = A_3B_2

64. (c) : The disaccharide maltose (malt sugar) is formed by the condensation of two molecules of α-*D*-glycopyranose in which C_1 of one glucose unit is connected to C_4 of the other glucose unit.

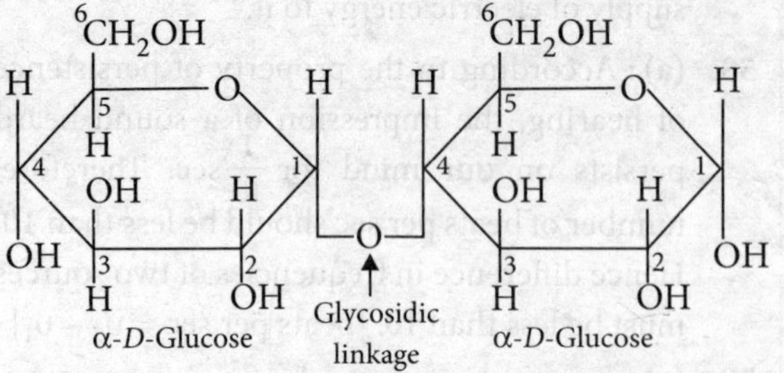

Structure of α-*D*-maltose

65. (a) : Rhombic sulphur is insoluble in water but readily soluble in carbon disulphide, CS_2. It dissolves to some extent in benzene, alcohol and ether also.

66. (b) : In alkaline solution, $KMnO_4$ is first reduced to manganate and then to insoluble manganese dioxide.

$$2KMnO_4 + H_2O \xrightarrow{\text{alkaline}} 2MnO_2 + 2KOH + 3[O]$$

67. (a) :

Complex	Coordination no.
$Co_2(CO)_8$	4
$Mn_2(CO)_{10}$	5
$[Fe(en)_2NH_3]$	5
$[Cr(OH)_3(NH_3)_3]$	6

68. (b) : ClF_3 and BrF_3 are used for the production of UF_6 in the enrichment of U^{235}.

$$U_{(s)} + 3ClF_{3(l)} \longrightarrow UF_{6(g)} + 3ClF_{(g)}$$

69. (a) : Due to high electronegativity and small size, fluorine forms only one oxoacid, HOF known as fluoric(I) acid or hypofluorous acid.

70. (b) : The atomic radii of noble gases are by far the largest in their respective periods. This is due to the reason that noble gases have only van der Waals radii.

71. (a) : Due to decrease in bond ($H—E$, where E = O, S, Se, Te) dissociation enthalpy down the group, acidic character increases.

Hence, the order is :

$H_2O < H_2S < H_2Se < H_2Te$

72. (a) : In the blast furnace, SiO_2 is removed as calcium silicate.

$$\underset{\text{Flux}}{CaO} + \underset{\substack{\text{Gangue} \\ \text{(Impurity)}}}{SiO_2} \longrightarrow \underset{\text{(Slag)}}{CaSiO_3}$$

73. (a) : In Hall's process, for purifying the bauxite ore, the solution containing sodium meta aluminate is warmed to 50-60°C and carbon dioxide is circulated through it, $Al(OH)_3$ separates out as precipitate.

$$2NaAlO_2 + CO_2 + 3H_2O \longrightarrow 2Al(OH)_3 + Na_2CO_3$$

74. (a) : Colloidal solutions are prepared by peptisation method, whereas coagulation and electrophoresis are the properties of colloidal solution.

75. **(d) :** Aldehydes having no α – H atoms undergo Cannizzaro reaction. Hence all the given compounds (except $PhCH_2CHO$ has α–H atom) will undergo Cannizzaro reaction.

76. **(d) :** Solid CO_2 is dry ice in which carbon atom undergoes *sp*-hybridisation.

77. **(a) :** For adiabatic conditions, PV^γ = Constant

$$P_1V_1^\gamma = P_2V_2^\gamma\ ;\ V_2 = \frac{1}{2}V_1$$

$$P_2 = P_1\left(\frac{V_1}{V_2}\right)^\gamma \quad \text{[For diatomic gas, } \gamma = 1.4]$$

$$P_2 = P_1\left(\frac{V_1 \times 2}{V_1}\right)^{1.4}$$

$$P_2 = P_1\,(2)^{1.4} = (2)^{1.4}\,P$$

78. **(b) :** Using expression, $\mu = \sqrt{n(n+2)}$ B.M. (where, n = no. of unpaired electrons)

Ion	Outer configuration	n	μ
$_{22}Ti^{2+}$	$3d^2$	2	2.84
$_{24}Cr^{2+}$	$3d^4$	4	4.90
$_{27}Co^{3+}$	$3d^6$	4	4.90
$_{25}Mn^{2+}$	$3d^5$	5	5.92

79. **(d) :** Acidified $KMnO_4$ oxidises H_2S to S only.

$$2KMnO_4 + 3H_2SO_4 + 5H_2S \longrightarrow K_2SO_4 + 2MnSO_4 + 5S + 8H_2O$$

80. **(c) :** The main component of photochemical smog is peroxyacetyl nitrate, (PAN). The other components are ozone, nitric oxide, acrolein and formaldehyde.

81. **(b) :** The given reaction is,

$$\frac{1}{2}H_{2(g)} + \frac{1}{2}I_{2(g)} \rightleftharpoons HI_{(g)} \quad \text{... (i)}$$

$$\text{Hence, } K_c = \frac{[HI]}{[H_2]^{1/2}[I_2]^{1/2}} \quad \text{... (ii)}$$

Now, reverse the eqn. (i) and multiply by 2, we get

$$2HI \rightleftharpoons H_{2(g)} + I_{2(g)}$$

$$\text{Hence, } K_c' = \frac{[H_2][I_2]}{[HI]^2} \quad \text{...(iii)}$$

Equating equations (ii) and (iii), we get

$$K_c' = \frac{1}{(K_c)^2}$$

82. **(a) :** Using the relation,

$$t_{87.5\%} = \frac{3}{2}t_{75\%}$$

$$t_{87.5\%} = \frac{3}{2} \times \frac{4}{1} = 6\text{ h}$$

83. **(b) :** For the reaction, $A_{(g)} \longrightarrow B_{(g)} + C_{(g)}$

$t = 0$: P_i, 0, 0

t: $(P_i - x)$, x, x

Given: P_i is initial pressure at time, $t = 0$ and P_t is pressure at time 't'.

$$P_t = (P_i - x) + x + x = P_i + x$$

$$x = P_t - P_i$$

Here, $P_A = P_i - x \Rightarrow P_i - (P_t - P_i)$

$$P_A = 2P_i - P_t$$

$$k = \frac{2.303}{t}\log\frac{P_i}{P_A}$$

$$k = \frac{2.303}{t}\log\frac{P_i}{(2P_i - P_t)}$$

84. **(a) :** Isotones have the same number of neutrons.

As = 77 – 33 = 44 ; Se = 78 – 34 = 44

85. **(d) :** Lewis gave the structure of O_3 molecule as

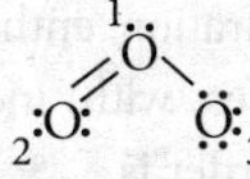

Using the relation,

Formal charge = [Total no. of valence electrons in the free atom] – [Total no. of non-bonding (lone pair) electrons] – $\frac{1}{2}$ [Total no. of bonding (shared) electrons]

The formal charge on central O –atom *i.e.*, no. 1

$$= 6 - 2 - \frac{1}{2}(6) = +1$$

86. **(c) :** Number of atoms $= \dfrac{N_A \times \text{mass}}{\text{At. mass}}$

$$= \frac{6.023 \times 10^{23} \times 52}{4} = 7.829 \times 10^{24}\text{ atoms}$$

87. (d):

Ion	Total no. of electrons	MO configuration	B.O.
O_2^+	15	$KK\,\sigma 2s^2\ \sigma^*2s^2\ \sigma 2p_z^2$ $\pi 2p_x^2 = \pi 2p_y^2\ \pi^*2p_x^1$ $= \pi^*2p_y^0$	2.5
O_2^-	17	$KK\,\sigma 2s^2\ \sigma^*2s^2\ \sigma 2p_z^2$ $\pi 2p_x^2 = \pi 2p_y^2\ \pi^*2p_x^2$ $= \pi^*2p_y^1$	1.5
O_2^{2-}	18	$KK\,\sigma 2s^2\ \sigma^*2s^2\ \sigma 2p_z^2$ $\pi 2p_x^2 = \pi 2p_y^2\ \pi^*2p_x^2$ $= \pi^*2p_y^2$	1.0

Hence, the correct B.O. is $O_2^+ > O_2^- > O_2^{2-}$.

88. (b): Let the oxidation no. of Br be x.

In $KBrO_4$, $+1 + x + 4(-2) = 0$, $-7 + x = 0$,

$x = +7$

89. (c): The production of dihydrogen can be increased by reacting carbon monoxide of syngas mixtures with steam in the presence of iron chromate as catalyst.

$$CO_{(g)} + H_2O_{(g)} \xrightarrow[\text{Catalyst}]{673\text{ K}} CO_{2(g)} + H_{2(g)}$$

This is called water-gas shift reaction.

90. (a): The hydration enthalpies of alkali metal ions decreases with increase in ionic sizes Hence, the order is

$Li^+ > Na^+ > K^+ > Rb^+ > Cs^+$.

Therefore, Li^+ has maximum degree of hydration.

91. (d): Most of the pure compounds have sharp melting and boiling points. Chromatographic and spectroscopic techniques are the new methods of checking the purity.

92. (c): $\overset{5}{C}H_3-\overset{4}{C}(CH_3)_2-\overset{3}{C}H_2-\overset{2}{C}(CH_3)_2-\overset{1}{C}H_3$

2, 2, 4, 4- Tetramethylpentane

93. (b): $p = K_H x$

Higher the value of K_H at a given pressure, lower is the solubility of the gas in the liquid.

94. (c): To calculate the standard electrode potential of the given cell it is coupled with the standard hydrogen electrode in which pressure of hydrogen gas is one bar and the conc. of H^+ ion in the solution is one molar and also the concentrations of the oxidised and the reduced forms of the species in the right hand half-cell are unity.

95. (d): $\underset{\text{Sucrose}}{C_{12}H_{22}O_{11(aq)}} + H_2O_{(l)} \xrightarrow{HCl_{(aq)}} \underset{\text{Glucose}}{C_6H_{12}O_{6(aq)}} + \underset{\text{Fructose}}{C_6H_{12}O_{6(aq)}}$

96. (b): Chloramphenicol is a bacteriostatic antibiotic drug.

97. (b): $\underset{\text{Ethyl bromide}}{C_2H_5Br} + KCN_{(alco.)} \xrightarrow{\Delta} \underset{\substack{\text{Propanenitrile}\\ \text{(Major product)}}}{C_2H_5CN} + KBr$

98. (c): According to Markovnikov's rule,

$C_6H_5-CH_2-CH=CH_2 + HCl \longrightarrow \underset{(A)}{C_6H_5-CH_2-CH(Cl)-CH_3}$

99. (b): The mechanism of dehydration of alcohol involves the following steps-

1. Formation of protonated alcohol
2. Formation of carbocation
3. Formation of ethene by elimination of a proton.

100. (a): In Clemmensen reduction, the carbonyl group of aldehydes and ketones is reduced to $>CH_2$ group on treatment with zinc amalgam and concentrated hydrochloric acid.

$$>C=O \xrightarrow[\text{HCl}]{\text{Zn-Hg}} >CH_2 + H_2O$$

101. (d): Both Co and Ni have (IV) oxidation state. Ni (IV) has $3d^6$ electronic configuration.

Metals	Outer electronic configuration	Oxi. states
Co	$3d^7 4s^2$	+2, +3, +4
Ni	$3d^8 4s^2$	+2, +3, +4

102. (b): The oxidation states of the given compounds are

$VO_2^+ : x + 2(-2) = +1$

$\Rightarrow x = +5$

$Cr_2O_7^{2-} : 2x + 7(-2) = -2$

$\Rightarrow 2x = +12$

$\Rightarrow x = +6$

$MnO_4^- : x + 4(-2) = -1$

$x = -1 + 8 = +7$

The correct order of oxidising power is

$VO_2^+ < Cr_2O_7^{2-} < MnO_4^-$

due to the increasing stability of the lower species to which they are reduced.

103. (d): The resonance forms do not show any unshared electrons. Hence, O_2 molecule does not show any paramagnetic properties.

Str.	O=O 121 pm	O=O–O ≡ O···O···O (128 pm, 128 pm)
B.O.	2.0	1.5

The bond length decreases as bond order increases. Hence, bond length of O_3 is higher than O_2.

104. (b): Insulin is a globular protein. This protein has three-dimensional folded structure. These are stabilised by internal hydrogen bonding. Hence, they are water soluble.

105. (a)

106. (b): Chemistry of actinoids is more complicated due to the possibility of large number of oxidation states.

107. (a)

108. (d): CH_3COOH/CH_3COONH_4 is not an example of acidic buffer. Acidic buffer contains equimolar mixture of weak acid and its salt with strong base. *e.g.* CH_3COOH/CH_3COONa.

109. (c) : Al metal is rendered passive when treated with conc. HNO_3 because concentrated HNO_3 is oxidising agent and produces a protective layer of oxide on the surface.

110. (b): Chloroform is slowly oxidised by air in the presence of light to an extremely poisonous gas 'phosgene'. Therefore, it is stored in dark bottles, completely filled so that air is kept out.

111. (b): Less reactivity of saturated hydrocarbons are due to presence of single bonds between carbon atoms.

112. (a)

113. (a)

114. (d): The two H-atoms on first carbon and the two H-atoms on the third carbon atom lie in perpendicular planes. The central carbon atom is *sp*-hybridized while terminal carbon atoms are sp^2-hybridized.

115. (a)

116. (a) : $MCl_2 + Na_2CO_3 \rightarrow MCO_3\downarrow + 2NaCl$

$MSO_4 + Na_2CO_3 \rightarrow MCO_3\downarrow + Na_2SO_4$

(where, M = Mg, Ca)

117. (a)

118. (c) : *o*-Nitrophenol is steam volatile due to intramolecular hydrogen bonding while *p*-nitrophenol is less volatile due to intermolecular hydrogen bonding.

119. (c) : Isoprene is 2-methyl-1, 3-butadiene.

$CH_2{=}C(CH_3){-}CH{=}CH_2$

120. (c) : Structure of H_3PO_3 is

$H{-}P(=O)(OH){-}OH$

Due to the presence of two hydroxyl protons it is dibasic acid.

BIOLOGY

121. (b) : Cell cycle is divided into 2 phases. (i) Interphase (a period of preparation for cell division), (ii) M phase (the actual period of cell division). The interphase cell is metabolically quite active. Interphase is the long non-dividing phase further divided into G_1, S and G_2. It occupies 75 to 95% of entire cell division time.

122. (b) : Biodiversity hotspots are the areas of high endemism and high levels of species richness. Initially 25 biodiversity hotspots were identified, but subsequently nine more have been added to list bringing the total number of biodiversity hotspots in the world to 34.

123. (b) : Turner's syndrome is caused due to the absence of one of the X chromosomes *i.e.*, 45 chromosomes total with sex chromosomes as XO. Such females are sterile as ovaries are rudimentary. Besides this, other features include lack of other secondary sexual characters, etc.

124. (a) : The secretion of gonadotropins (LH and FSH) increases gradually during the follicular phase and stimulates follicular development as well as secretion of estrogens by the growing follicles. Both LH and FSH attain a peak level in the middle of the cycle (about 14th day). Rapid secretion of LH leading to its maximum level during mid-cycle called LH surge induces rupture of Graafian follicle and thereby the release of ovum (ovulation). Concentration of estrogen in blood is also high around 14th day and reaches its peak.

125. (d) : In pteridophytes, majority of plants are homosporous (producing similar kind of spores) *e.g.*, *Lycopodium*. However, plants of genera like *Selaginella* and *Salvinia* are heterosporous (producing macro and micro spores). *Pinus* and *Cycas*, which are gymnosperms, are also heterosporous.

126. (a) : Micronutrients or trace elements are needed in very small amounts (less than 10 mmole kg^{-1} of dry matter). These are 8 in number and include iron, manganese, copper, molybdenum, zinc, boron, chlorine and nickel.

127. (a) :

Pea	–	Marginal placentation
Lemon	–	Axile placentation
Mustard	–	Parietal placentation
Sunflower	–	Basal placentation

128. (c) : Somaclones are genetically identical plants developed from any part of a plant by tissue culture/micropropagation. This type of micropropagation is also called somaclonal propagation.

129. (d) : Ozone is a harmful secondary air pollutant. Ozone, being a strong oxidant destroys chlorenchyma, produces necrosis, hardens rubber, damages textiles, corrodes the surface of marble statues and heritage buildings.

130. (c) : Vernalisation refers specially to the promotion of flowering by exposure to a period of low temperature. Many temperate plants have vernalisation requirement and must experience a period of low temperature in winter, to initiate or accelerate flowering process, or in many fruit tree species, to induce dormancy and then break dormancy prior to flowering.

131. (a) : The cells derived from root apical and shoot apical meristems and cambium differentiate and mature to perform special functions. This act leading to maturation is termed as differentiation. During differentiation, cells undergo few to major structural changes both in their cell walls and protoplasm.

132. (d) : Bt genes, RNA*i* genes and *Cry* genes occur naturally in living organisms. Bt toxic gene of bacterium *Bacillus thuringiensis* has been cloned from bacteria, and expressed in plants, to provide resistance to insects without the need of insecticides. The choice of genes depends upon the crop and the targeted pest as most Bt toxins are insect group specific. The toxin is coded by a gene named *Cry*. RNA*i* takes place in all eukaryotic organisms as a method of cellular defense. This method involves silencing of a specific *m*RNA due to a complementary dsRNA molecule that binds to and prevents translation of the *m*RNA (silencing).

133. (a) : DNA and RNA are nucleic acids which are found in living systems. DNA is a long polymer of deoxyribonucleotides and RNA is a long polymer of ribonucleotides. A nucleotide has 3 components – a nitrogenous base, a pentose sugar and a phosphate group.

134. (b) : Coconut and cucurbits are monoecious plants. *Ornithorhynchus* is an egg-laying mammal. Whale is a viviparous mammal. Frog shows external fertilisation. It takes place in water. Peacock shows internal fertilisation.

135. (a) : Mutualism is an interaction between two organisms of different species in which both the partners are benefitted, with none of the two capable of living separately. In many species of fig trees there is a relationship with the pollinator species of wasp. The female wasp uses the fruit not only as an oviposition site but uses the developing seeds within the fruit for nourishing its larvae. The wasp pollinates the fig inflorescence, while searching for suitable egg-laying sites. The fig returns this favour of pollination by offering the wasp some of its developing seeds, as food for the developing wasp larvae.

136. (d) : Liver fluke has an incomplete alimentary canal.

137. (b)

138. (a)

139. (c) : Statins produced by the yeast *Monascus purpureus* are used as blood-cholestrol lowering agents. *Saccharomyces cerevisiae* is used for making bread and ethanol. *Aspergillus niger* (a fungus) produces citric acid.

140. (a) : AIDS is caused by HIV virus. Gonorrhoea is caused by bacteria *Neisseria gonorrhoeae*. Diphtheria is caused by bacteria *Corynebacterium diphtheria*. Ringworm disease is caused by fungus *Trichophyton*, *Epidermophyton* and *Microsporum*. Tuberculosis is caused by a bacterium called *Mycobacterium tuberculosis*.

141. (b) : Parathyroid hormone (PTH) stimulates the reabsorption of Ca^{2+} by renal tubules and increases Ca^{2+} absorption from digested food. It means PTH increases the blood Ca^{2+} level. Old aged persons have weak immunity because thymus is degenerated in old individuals resulting in a decreased production of thymosin. Oestoporosis in women occurs due to decreased level of estrogen.

142. (a) : Taxonomical hierarchy shows arrangement in ascending order.

Species → Genus → Family → Order → Division → Kingdom

143. (c)

144. (c) : A – Troponin

B – Tropomyosin

C – F-actin

Two filaments of protein tropomyosin run close to F-actins throughout its length. A complex protein troponin is distributed at regular intervals on the tropomyosin. In the resting state, a subunit of troponin masks the active binding sites for myosin on the actin filaments.

145. (a) : Neutrophil is a phagocytic cell which destroys foreign organisms entering the body. It has many lobed nucleus, fine granules in cytoplasm and it takes acidic as well as basic stains.

146. (a)

147. (b) : Penicillin has bactericidal effect *i.e.*, they kill bacteria.

148. (d) : The biodiversity of bryophytes is less than that of angiosperms. Bryophytes are plants that can live in soil but are dependent on water for sexual reproduction.

Angiosperms are much advanced plant species which consist of male sex organ (stamen) and female sex organ (pistil) borne in a flower.

149. (b) : Non-essential amino acids are those amino acids which can be synthesized by human body from raw materials. Glycine, serine, proline, glutamic acid all are non-essential amino acids.

150. (a) : Photochemical smog is a grey or yellowish brown opaque smog having oxidizing environment but little smokes. It is formed at high temperature over cities and towns due to still air, emission of NO_2 oxides and hydrocarbons from automobile exhausts. Nitrogen dioxide splits into nitric oxide and nascent oxygen. Nascent oxygen combines with molecular oxygen to form ozone. Ozone reacts with hydrocarbons to form aldehydes and ketones. Nitrogen oxides, oxygen and ketones combine to form peroxy-acyl-nitrates (PAN).

151. (d)

152. (c)

153. (c) : A normal electrogram (ECG) is composed of a P wave, a QRS wave (complex) and a T wave. The P-wave represents the electrical excitation or depolarisation of the atria. The QRS complex represents the depolarisation of the ventricles which initiates the ventricular contraction. The contraction starts shortly after Q and marks the beginning of the systole. The T-wave represents the repolarisation of ventricles. The end of the T-wave marks the end of systole.

154. (d) : Anti-haemorrhagic vitamins are those substances which promote haemostasis or stop beeding. Vitamin K is one of them.

155. (a) : Normal cells show the property of contact inhibition, by virtue of which contact with other cells inhibits their uncontrolled growth. Cancer cells appears to have lost this property.

156. (d) : Some strains of *Bacillus thuringiensis* produce proteins that kill certain insects like lepidopterans and coleopterans, etc. *Bacillus thuringiensis* forms some protein crystals. These crystals contain a toxic insecticidal protein. Bt toxin proteins exist as inactive protoxins, but once an insect ingests the inactive toxin it is converted to active form of toxin due to the alkaline pH of the alimentary canal that solublizes the crystals.

157. (d) : Beverages like beer, wine are fermented but not distilled. They have relatively low alcohol content typically less than 100%. Hard liquor like brandy and whisky are produced by both fermentation and distillation. Distillation process purifies them and removes diluting components like water and increases the alcohol content.

158. (d) : pBR322 has a restriction site for *Sal* I.

159. (d) : Cortisol and testosterone are steroidal in nature. Steroid hormones are lipid soluble and easily pass through cell membrane of a target cell into the cytoplasm. In the cytoplasm they bind to specific intracellular receptors (proteins) to form a hormone receptor complex that enters the nucleus.

160. (c) : Macrophages are cells produced by differentiation of monocytes in tissues. They are present throughout the body with large numbers in the lymph nodes, bone marrow and spleen. These are specialized phagocytic cells that attack foreign substances.

161. (b)

162. (b) : Pepsin is a digestive enzyme that is released in stomach as proenzyme-pepsinogen. HCl which is secreted by gastric glands of stomach converts proenzyme pepsinogen into the active enzyme pepsin. Pepsin converts proteins into proteoses and peptones.

163. (c) : The nerve fibres from all parts of the retina converge to leave through a point called blindspot. It is the place in the visual field that corresponds to the lack of light detecting photo receptor cells on the optic disc of the retina.

164. (a)

165. (a)

166. (c) : The enlarged Q and R waves indicate a myocardial infarction (heart attack). QRS complex begins as small downward deflection (Q) and continues as large upright (R) and triangular wave ending as downward wave (S) at its base. It represents ventricular depolarisation (ventricular contraction).

167. (b) : The leaves in gymnosperms are well-adapted to withstand extremes of temperature, humidity and wind. In conifers, the needle-like leaves reduce the surface area. Their thick cuticle and sunken stomata also help to reduce water loss. Unlike bryophytes and pteridophytes, in gymnosperms the male and the female gametophytes do not have an independent free-living existence. They remain within the sporangia retained on the sporophytes.

168. (a) : The ratio of the volume of CO_2 evolved to the volume of O_2 consumed in respiration is called the respiratory quotient (RQ) or respiratory ratio.

$$RQ = \frac{\text{Volume of } CO_2 \text{ evolved}}{\text{Volume of } O_2 \text{ consumed}}$$

The respiratory quotient depends upon the type of respiratory substrate used during respiration. When carbohydrates are used as substrate and are completely oxidised, the RQ will be 1, because equal amounts of CO_2 and O_2 are evolved and consumed.

$$C_6H_{12}O_6 + 6O_2 \rightarrow 6CO_2 + 6H_2O + \text{Energy}$$

$$RQ = \frac{6CO_2}{6O_2} = 1.0$$

169. (a) : The mammalian heart is myogenic. It means the heart beat originates from a specialised muscles (nodal tissue). It is regulated by the nerves.

170. (b) : Diseases or infections which are transmitted through sexual intercourse are called sexually transmitted diseases (STDs). AIDS and hepatitis-B are sexually transmitted diseases. Hepatitis-B and AIDS can also be transmitted by sharing of injection needles, surgical instruments with infected persons, transfusion of blood, etc. There is no permanent cure for AIDS and hepatitis-B.

171. (d) : The relationship between the sequence of amino acids in a polypeptide and nucleotide sequence of DNA or *m*RNA is called genetic code. The genetic code is triplet. One codon codes for only one amino acid, hence it is unambiguous and specific. Some amino acids are coded by more than one codon, hence the code is degenerate.

172. (d) : Darwin was convinced that interspecific competition is a potent force in organic evolution. It is generally believed that competition occurs when closely related species compete for the same resources that are limiting, but it is not entirely true. Totally unrelated species could also compete for the same resource. Gause's 'Competitive Exclusion Principle' states that two closely related species competing for the same resources cannot co-exist indefinitely and the competitively inferior one will be eliminated eventually. This may be true if resources are limiting, but not otherwise.

173. (b) : The transgenic food may cause toxicity or produce allergies. The enzyme produced by the antibiotic resistance can cause allergies, because it is a foreign protein. The introduction of transgenic plants into agriculture is creating some issues. One of them is the potential risk of transgene in commercial crops endangering native or nontarget species. For example the gene for Bt toxin expressed in pollen might endanger pollinators like honeybees.

174. (c) : Secondary air pollutants are produced photo-chemically from primary pollutants. Smog, photochemical smog, ozone and PAN all are secondary air pollutants. DDT is a primary soil pollutant.

175. (d) : In ascomycetes ascospores are produced internally in each ascus (sporangial sac). In Basidiomycetes, basidiospores are produced exogenously at tips of fine outgrowths called sterigmata.

176. (c) : The joints between the atlas and axis and between the radius and ulna just below the elbow are the examples of pivot joints.

177. (a) : The parts of the plants that show the deficiency symptoms also depend on the mobility of the element in the plant. For elements that are actively mobilised within the plants and exported to young developing tissues, the deficiency symptoms tend to appear first in the older tissues. For example, the deficiency symptoms of nitrogen, potassium and magnesium are visible first in the senescent leaves. In the older leaves, biomolecules containing these elements are broken down, making these elements available for mobilising to younger leaves.

178. (a) **179. (b)** **180. (b)**

GENERAL KNOWLEDGE

181. (a)	**182. (d)**	**183. (c)**	**184. (b)**	**185. (c)**
186. (a)	**187. (d)**	**188. (b)**	**189. (d)**	**190. (a)**
191. (c)	**192. (d)**	**193. (c)**	**194. (b)**	**195. (c)**
196. (a)	**197. (b)**	**198. (c)**	**199. (c)**	**200. (a)**